Optum

Desk Reference

Coders' Desk Reference for HCPCS Level II

Answers to your toughest HCPCS Level II coding questions

AF864873

2023

optumcoding.com

Publisher's Notice

Coders' Desk Reference for HCPCS was conceived to be an authoritative source of information about coding and reimbursement issues. Every effort has been made to verify accuracy, and information is believed reliable at the time of publication. Absolute accuracy cannot be guaranteed, however. This publication is made available with the understanding that the publisher is not engaged in rendering legal or other services requiring a professional license. Please address questions regarding this product to the Optum customer service department at 1.800.464.3649, option 1 or email us at customerservice@optum.com.

Our Commitment to Accuracy

Optum is committed to producing accurate and reliable materials.

To report corrections, please email customerassistance@optum.com. You can also reach customer service by calling 1.800.464.3649, option 1.

Copyright

Made in the USA.
ISBN 978-1-62254-793-7

Acknowledgments

Denise Smith, RN, BSN, *Senior Product Manager*
Stacy Perry, *Manager, Desktop Publishing*
LaJuana Green, RHIA, CCS, *Subject Matter Expert*
Elizabeth Leibold, RHIT, *Subject Matter Expert*
Tracy Betzler, *Senior Desktop Publishing Specialist*
Hope M. Dunn, *Senior Desktop Publishing Specialist*
Katie Russell, *Desktop Publishing Specialist*
Kimberli Turner, *Editor*

Subject Matter Experts

LaJuana Green, RHIA, CCS

Ms. Green is a Registered Health Information Administrator with over 35 years of experience in multiple areas of information management. She has proven expertise in the analysis of medical record documentation, assignment of ICD-10-CM and PCS codes, DRG validation, and CPT code assignment in ambulatory surgery units and the hospital outpatient setting. Her experience includes serving as a director of a health information management department, clinical technical editing, new technology research and writing, medical record management, utilization review activities, quality assurance, tumor registry, medical library services, and chargemaster maintenance. Ms. Green is an active member of the American Health Information Management Association (AHIMA).

Elizabeth Leibold, RHIT

Ms. Leibold has more than 30 years of experience in the health care profession. She has served in a variety of roles, ranging from patient registration to billing and collections, and has an extensive background in physician and hospital outpatient coding and compliance. She has worked for large health care systems and health information management services companies, and has wide-ranging experience in facility and professional component coding, along with CPT expertise in interventional procedures, infusion services, emergency department, observation, and ambulatory surgery coding. Her areas of expertise include chart-to-claim coding audits and providing staff education to tenured and new coding staff. She is an active member of the American Health Information Management Association (AHIMA) and Tennessee Health Information Management Association (THIMA).

Contents

Introduction **1**
Format 1
Using HCPCS Codes 1
Using HCPCS Modifiers 1
Glossary and Reimbursement Terms 1
HCPCS Lay Descriptions 1

Using HCPCS Codes **3**
Keeping Current in Coding 3
The HCPCS Book Format 3

Using HCPCS Modifiers **7**
Ambulance Modifiers 7
HCPCS Level II Modifiers 7

Durable Medical Equipment, Prosthetics, Orthotics, and Supplies (DMEPOS) **21**
The DMEPOS Industry 21
Special Federal and Third-Party Payer Definitions 21
Documentation Standards 23
DMEPOS Resources 27

Other Selected Topics for Medicare **29**

Glossary and Reimbursement Terms **31**

HCPCS Lay Descriptions **51**

Introduction

Coding is a complicated business. It is not enough to have current copies of the International Classification of Diseases, 10th Revision, Clinical Modification (ICD-10-CM), *Current Procedural Terminology*, Fourth Edition (CPT®), and Healthcare Common Procedure Coding System (HCPCS Level II) books. Medical coders also need dictionaries and specialty texts if they are to accurately translate physicians' operative reports or patient charts into reimbursement codes.

That's why Optum has developed the *Coders' Desk Reference* series—to provide a one-stop resource with answers to a wide variety of coding questions. Optum polled the medical reimbursement community and our technical staff to determine the issues causing bottlenecks in a coder's workload.

Experienced coders are frustrated by limited definitions accompanying many HCPCS Level II codes. Beginning coders need guidelines on reporting HCPCS Level II codes as well as basic information about medical and reimbursement issues. Everyone requires up-to-date information about the anticipated changes to this coding systems.

Coders' Desk Reference for HCPCS answers the questions of both experienced and novice medical coders concerning medical supplies and equipment, as well as select services provided on an outpatient basis. It is a compendium of answers to a wide variety of coding questions and an introduction to new systems in coding structures. In order to code accurately, coders must first have an understanding of the coding systems involved.

Format

Since the first release of *Coders' Desk Reference for HCPCS*, coders' corrections, suggestions, and tips have been incorporated into every printing, making this book as informative and useful as possible. Changes reflecting the dynamic world of coding are ongoing, and Optum encourages input for inclusion in future editions of the book. Information in this product has been updated to reflect 2023 HCPCS codes.

Coders' Desk Reference for HCPCS is divided into convenient sections for easy use, with each section organized alphanumerically. Simply access the section by thumbing through the convenient tabbing system to find the specific item of interest.

Using HCPCS Codes

For the new coder, and even for the veteran, this chapter provides an overview of the HCPCS book—what it is and how best to use this coding system for identifying procedures.

Using HCPCS Modifiers

Modifiers augment HCPCS codes to the satisfaction of private and government payers. Optum coding experts interpret HCPCS modifiers and identify their advantage in reimbursement.

Glossary and Reimbursement Terms

To get reimbursed in a timely manner, it is important to have a clear understanding of the terminology used by medical providers, major insurers, and the federal government. This section includes up-to-date terminology that will help coders have a better understanding of the complex reimbursement climate.

HCPCS Lay Descriptions

The lay descriptions contained in the *Coders' Desk Reference for HCPCS Level II* are written by Optum technical staff to provide a common or generally accepted method of accomplishing the service indicated by the HCPCS codes description. In cases where more than one procedure or method is reported by a single code, one example of those methods or procedures may be given in the lay description. No lay description in this product is intended to give an absolute, required method of performing the service described in the HCPCS code. Reflecting the full spectrum of variations in technology and of professional techniques would be impossible in a book this size. Each HCPCS code is followed by a detailed description of the supply, service, or procedure that code represents.

Coders' Desk Reference for HCPCS was developed to help providers comply with the emerging standards by which Durable Medical Equipment, Prosthetics, Orthotics, and Supplies (DMEPOS), medications, provider services, temporary Medicare codes, and other disparate items and services are coded, reported, and paid. Remember that *Coders' Desk Reference for HCPCS* is a post-treatment medical reference and, as such, it is inappropriate to use this manual to select medical treatment.

The dental (D) codes are not included in the official HCPCS Level II code set. The American Dental Association (ADA) holds the copyright on those codes and instructed CMS to remove them. As a result, Optum has removed them from this product; however, Optum has additional resources available for customers requiring the dental codes. Please visit www.optumcoding.com or call 1.800.464.3649.

Using HCPCS Codes

HCPCS is an acronym (pronounced "hick-picks") for the Healthcare Common Procedure Coding System. This coding system presents national codes used to report supplies and equipment, as well as select services provided on an outpatient basis. HCPCS codes are published by CMS and updated quarterly. These codes can be obtained through the federal government and through publishers such as Optum, which produce a complete annual edition of the HCPCS Level II codes.

HCPCS Level II codes may be reported throughout the United States in all Medicare regions. They consist of one alpha character (A through V) followed by four digits. For example:

C1824 Generator, cardiac contractility modulation (implantable)

J0172 Injection, aducanumab-avwa, 2 mg

HCPCS Level II codes describe:

- DME equipment, devices, accessories, supplies, and repairs; prosthetics; orthotics; medical and surgical supplies
- Medications
- Provider services
- Temporary Medicare codes (most commonly found in the G codes)
- Other disparate items and services, such as ambulance services
- Temporary national codes (non-Medicare) (S codes)

The majority of services and procedures performed are reported with CPT codes. However, because the CPT coding system does not describe specific drugs, durable medical equipment (DME), prosthetics, orthotics, supplies, and certain other services, the HCPCS Level II coding system must be used.

CPT and HCPCS Level II codes are designated code sets for use in electronic HIPAA complaint transactions. CPT codes are widely accepted by third-party payers with minimal problems. HIPAA covered entities are by law required to accept HCPCS Level II codes. However, providers may encounter problems with some HCPCS Level II codes. For example, Medicare does not accept HCPCS Level II codes that begin with an S and many third-party payers do not accept codes that begin with a G.

Payers who accept HCPCS Level II codes require the code that most accurately describes the item provided. For example, a Medicare patient is given a physician's order for a gastrostomy tube. Durable medical equipment Medicare administrative contractors (DME MAC) instructs providers to report HCPCS code B4087 *Gastrostomy/jejunostomy tube, standard, any material, any type, each*. If this patient had been a non-Medicare beneficiary covered by a plan that did not accept HCPCS Level II codes, the CPT code 99070 *Supplies and materials (except spectacles), provided by the physician or other qualified health care professional over and above those usually included with the office visit or other services rendered (list drugs, trays, supplies, or materials provided)*, would be reported with a description of the gastrostomy tube.

Keeping Current in Coding

The various coding systems change quarterly. To correctly report and be reimbursed for DMEPOS services and items, providers and suppliers must keep up-to-date with respect to these changes. Additionally, to maintain compliance in reporting services and items furnished to patients—especially Medicare and state Medicaid patients—providers and suppliers are required to report the most current codes and be knowledgeable about appropriate code reporting.

Some of the changes these coding systems undergo include:

- Code and modifier additions
- Code and modifier deletions
- Revisions of code and modifier descriptions
- Changes in grammar
- Parenthetical and instructional note changes
- Guideline changes
- Index entry changes

Providers and suppliers can choose from a variety of coding resources and educational seminars to keep up-to-date on quarterly changes. Providers and suppliers of DMEPOS should attend, at a minimum, an annual Medicare update for correct coding and billing procedures. This will help ensure compliance with federal standards.

The HCPCS Book Format

The HCPCS book is self-referencing. Its introductory material provides information about its rules, format, and guidelines. The introduction to the HCPCS book should be carefully studied at least once by medical coders and reviewed annually for changes. Classes and correspondence courses teach medical coding and several introductory coding books convey the

HCPCS book fundamentals. Additionally, the Centers for Medicare and Medicaid Services (CMS) and private consultants sponsor coding seminars to discuss changes and methods to implement these changes into regular coding practice.

Below is a glossary of the HCPCS book terminology. Consult these listings, along with the HCPCS book, as needed to solve coding problems.

The alphabetic sections of the HCPCS book are:

- A Codes
  - Transportation Services Including Ambulance
  - Medical and Surgical Supplies
- B Codes
  - Enteral and Parenteral Therapy
- C Codes
  - Outpatient PPS
- E Codes
  - Durable Medical Equipment
- G Codes
  - Procedures/Professional Services (Temporary)
- H Codes
  - Alcohol and Drug Abuse Treatment Services
- J Codes
  - J Codes Drugs
  - J Codes Chemotherapy Drugs
- K Codes
  - Temporary Codes
- L Codes
  - Orthotic Procedures and Devices
  - Prosthetic Procedures
- M Codes
  - Medical Services
  - Quality Measures
- P Codes
  - Pathology and Laboratory Services
- Q Codes
  - Q Codes (Temporary)
- R Codes
  - Diagnostic Radiology Services
- S Codes
  - Temporary National Codes (Non-Medicare)
- T Codes
  - National T Codes Established for State Medicaid Agencies
- U Codes
  - Coronavirus Services
- V Codes
  - Vision Services
  - Hearing Services

Index

Because HCPCS is organized by code number rather than by service or supply name, the index enables the coder to locate any code without looking through individual ranges of codes. Just look up the medical or surgical supply, service, orthotic, or prosthetic in question to find the appropriate code(s). This index also refers to many of the brand names by which these items are known.

Table of Drugs and Biologicals

The table lists HCPCS codes from any available section under brand and generic names with the dose amount, route of administration, and code numbers. The brand names of drugs and biologicals listed are examples only and may not include all products available for that type. While every effort is made to make the table comprehensive, it is not all-inclusive.

Symbols, Icons, and Appendix 5

Symbols alert users to changes or other attributes of a code. The symbols appear in the left margin, just in front of the code number, as shown here:

● A closed circle designates a new code.

▲ A closed triangle indicates a code description has been changed or altered.

❍ An open circle designates a code that has been reinstated or recycled by CMS.

In Optum's *HCPCS Level II* book, additional icons are provided to assist with reimbursement issues. These icons appear to the right of the code descriptor, as shown here:

☑ A blue box with a check mark indicates a quantity alert – the quantity indicated in the code descriptor may not coincide with quantities available in the marketplace.

♀ Female Only icons – Identifies procedures that some payers may consider female only.

♂ Male Only icons – Identifies procedures that some payers may consider male only.

[A] An "A" in an orange box indicates an age edit – this code is intended for use with a specific age group.

[M] An "M" in an orange box indicates procedures that should, in general, only be used for maternity patients between 12 and 55 years of age.

♿ A wheelchair identifies when to consult the CMS DMEPOS for payment of the durable medical item. Additionally, required modifiers for new, used, and rented equipment are provided next to this icon.

⊘ A circle with a strike through indicates items and services excluded from SNF consolidated billing that may be reported directly to the Medicare contractor by the provider or supplier.

A2–Z3 ASC Payment Indicators – a green box with an alphanumeric code to indicate how the ASC payment rate was derived and/or how the procedure, item, or service is treated under the ASC payment system. For more information, consult Optum's *Revenue Cycle Pro*.

A-Y OPPS Status Indicators – a purple box with an alphanumeric code to indicate how HCPCS codes are paid or not paid under the OPPS.

Color Coverage Bars

In Optum's *HCPCS Level II* book, color bars are added over the code to indicate the Coverage Indicator as provided by CMS. The colors indicate the following:

- Green – Special Coverage Instructions: Special coverage instructions apply and can typically be found in the Medicare Internet Only Manuals (IOMs)
- Yellow – Carrier Discretion: Contact the carrier for specific coverage information.
- Pink – Not Covered: These codes are not covered or are invalid for Medicare.

These symbols and icons may have a bearing on assignment of codes for a practice. In addition, codes that are deleted effective January 1st of the current year, or that were deleted during the previous year, will appear in the book with a strikethrough. Consult Appendix 5 for a summary of the additions, deletions, and revisions made to the current HCPCS edition.

Using HCPCS Modifiers

The HCPCS Level II codes are alphanumeric codes developed by CMS as a complementary coding system to the AMA's CPT codes. HCPCS Level II codes describe procedures, services, and supplies not found in the CPT® manual.

Similar to the CPT coding system, HCPCS Level II codes contain modifiers that serve to further define services and items without changing the basic meaning of the HCPCS Level II code with which they are reported.

It is important to note that HCPCS Level II modifiers may be reported in conjunction with both CPT and HCPCS Level II codes. In some cases, documentation may be required to accompany the claim to support the need for a particular modifier's use, especially in cases when the presence of a modifier causes suspension of the claim for manual review and pricing.

Ambulance Modifiers

For ambulance services modifiers, there are single alpha characters with distinct definitions that are paired together to form a two-character modifier. The first character indicates the origination of the patient (e.g., private residence, physician office, etc.) and the second character indicates the destination of the patient (e.g., hospital, skilled nursing facility, etc.). When reporting ambulance services, the name of the hospital or facility should be included on the claim. If reporting the scene of an accident or acute event (character S) as the origin of the patient, a written description of the actual location of the scene or event must be included with the claim.

Ambulance modifiers must be reported as two characters. For example, an ambulance transport from an accident scene to an acute care hospital would have modifier SH appended to the ambulance HCPCS code.

In addition, institutional-based providers must report one of the following modifiers with every HCPCS code to describe whether the service was provided under arrangement or directly:

QM Ambulance service provided under arrangement by a provider of services

QN Ambulance service furnished directly by a provider of services

Ambulance Modifier Listing

D Diagnostic or therapeutic site other than "P" or "H" when reported as origin codes

E Residential, domiciliary, custodial facility (other than 1819 facility)

G Hospital-based ESRD facility

H Hospital

I Site of transfer (for example, airport or helicopter pad) between modes of ambulance transport

J Freestanding ESRD facility

N Skilled nursing facility

P Physician's office

R Residence

S Scene of accident or acute event

X Intermediate stop at physician's office on way to hospital (destination code only). Note: Modifier X can only be reported as a designation code in the second position of a modifier

HCPCS Level II Modifiers

Alphabetical Listing

A1 Dressing for one wound

A2 Dressing for two wounds

A3 Dressing for three wounds

A4 Dressing for four wounds

A5 Dressing for five wounds

A6 Dressing for six wounds

A7 Dressing for seven wounds

A8 Dressing for eight wounds

A9 Dressing for nine or more wounds

AA Anesthesia performed personally by anesthesiologist

- CPT codes approved for reporting with modifier AA are 00100–01999.
- If an anesthetist assists the physician in the care of a single patient, the service is considered personally performed by the physician. The anesthesiologist should report this service with modifier AA and the appropriate CPT code from series 00100–01999.
- Modifier AA affects Medicare payment.

AB Audiology service furnished personally by an audiologist without a physician/NPP order for nonacute hearing assessment unrelated to disequilibrium, or hearing aids, or examinations for the purpose of prescribing, fitting, or changing hearing aids; service may be performed once every 12 months, per beneficiary

AD Medical supervision by a physician; more than four concurrent anesthesia procedures
- Modifier AD affects Medicare payment as a distinct fee schedule amount exists.

AE Registered dietitian

AF Specialty physician

AG Primary physician

AH Clinical psychologist

AI Principal physician of record

AJ Clinical social worker
- Medicare limits allowable to 75 percent of the physician fee schedule.

AK Nonparticipating physician

AM Physician, team member service
- The physician member of a team is required to perform one out of every three visits made by a team member.
- Modifier AM should be appended to indicate a team member visit was performed by the physician.
- Team member visits will be denied if only one person rendering services is billing for team services, as this is inappropriate billing practice.
- Modifier AM has no effect on payment.

AO Alternate payment method declined by provider of service

AP Determination of refractive state was not performed in the course of diagnostic ophthalmological examination
- Modifier AP has no effect on payment.

AQ Physician providing a service in an unlisted health professional shortage area (HPSA)

AR Physician provider services in a physician scarcity area

AS Physician assistant, nurse practitioner, or clinical nurse specialist services for assistant at surgery

AT Acute treatment (This modifier should be used when reporting services 98940, 98941, 98942)
- Modifier AT has no effect on payment for Medicare and many third-party carrier claims.

AU Item furnished in conjunction with a urological, ostomy, or tracheostomy supply

AV Item furnished in conjunction with a prosthetic device, prosthetic, or orthotic

AW Item furnished in conjunction with a surgical dressing

AX Item furnished in conjunction with dialysis services

AY Item or service furnished to an ESRD patient that is not for the treatment of ESRD

AZ Physician providing a service in a dental health professional shortage area for the purpose of an electronic health record incentive payment

BA Item furnished in conjunction with parenteral enteral nutrition (PEN) services

BL Special acquisition of blood and blood products

BO Orally administered nutrition, not by feeding tube

BP The beneficiary has been informed of the purchase and rental options and has elected to purchase the item

BR The beneficiary has been informed of the purchase and rental options and has elected to rent the item

BU The beneficiary has been informed of the purchase and rental options and after 30 days has not informed the supplier of his/her decision

CA Procedure payable only in the inpatient setting when performed emergently on an outpatient who expires prior to admission

CB Service ordered by a renal dialysis facility (RDF) physician as part of the ESRD beneficiary's dialysis benefit, is not part of the composite rate, and is separately reimbursable

CC Procedure code change (Use CC when the procedure code submitted was changed either for administrative reasons or because an incorrect code was filed)
- Modifier CC is used by the carrier when the procedure code submitted had to be changed for administrative reasons or because an incorrect code was submitted.
- Payment rule: Payment determination will be based on the new code used by the contractor carrier/fiscal intermediary.
- Modifier CC has no effect on payment.

CD AMCC test has been ordered by an ESRD facility or MCP physician that is part of the composite rate and is not separately billable

CE AMCC test has been ordered by an ESRD facility or MCP physician that is separately reimbursable based on medical necessity

CF AMCC test has been ordered by an ESRD facility or MCP physician that is not part of the composite rate and is separately billable

CG Policy criteria applied

CH 0 percent impaired, limited or restricted

CI At least 1 percent but less than 20 percent impaired, limited or restricted

CJ At least 20 percent but less than 40 percent impaired, limited or restricted

CK At least 40 percent but less than 60 percent impaired, limited or restricted

CL At least 60 percent but less than 80 percent impaired, limited or restricted

CM At least 80 percent but less than 100 percent impaired, limited or restricted

CN 100 percent impaired, limited or restricted

- These modifiers are to be appended to the functional limitation HCPCS codes reported by therapists.

CO Outpatient occupational therapy services furnished in whole or in part by an occupational therapy assistant

CQ Outpatient physical therapy services furnished in whole or in part by a physical therapist assistant

CR Catastrophe/disaster related

CS Cost-sharing waived for specified COVID-19 testing-related services that result in an order for, or administration of, a COVID-19 test and/or used for cost-sharing waived preventive services furnished via telehealth in Rural Health Clinics and Federally Qualified Health Centers during the COVID-19 public health emergency

CT Computed tomography services furnished using equipment that does not meet each of the attributes of the national electrical manufacturers association (NEMA) XR-29-2013 standard

DA Oral health assessment by a licensed health professional other than a dentist

E1 Upper left, eyelid

E2 Lower left, eyelid

E3 Upper right, eyelid

E4 Lower right, eyelid

EA Erythropoetic stimulating agent (ESA) administered to treat anemia due to anticancer chemotherapy

EB Erythropoetic stimulating agent (ESA) administered to treat anemia due to anticancer radiotherapy

EC Erythropoetic stimulating agent (ESA) administered to treat anemia not due to anticancer radiotherapy or anticancer chemotherapy

- Report modifiers EA, EB, and EC when ESA is administered to a patient who is not ESRD or who is not on maintenance dialysis. Report these modifiers with HCPCS Level II codes J0881 and J0885 only.

ED Hematocrit level has exceeded 39% (or hemoglobin level has exceeded 13.0 g/dl) for three or more consecutive billing cycles immediately prior to and including the current cycle

EE Hematocrit level has not exceeded 39% (or hemoglobin level has not exceeded 13.0 g/dl) for three or more consecutive billing cycles immediately prior to and including the current cycle

- Report modifier ED or EE on claims for EPO for ESRD patients receiving dialysis in renal dialysis facilities. Claims reporting no modifier or both modifiers will be returned to the provider for correction.

EJ Subsequent claims for a defined course of therapy (e.g., EPO, sodium hyaluronate, infliximab)

EM Emergency reserve supply (for ESRD benefit only)

EP Service provided as part of Medicaid Early Periodic Screening Diagnosis and Treatment (EPSDT) program

ER Items and services furnished by a provider-based, off-campus emergency department

ET Emergency services

- This modifier should be applied to report dental procedures performed in emergency situations.

EX Expatriate beneficiary

EY No physician or other licensed health care provider order for this item or service

FA Left hand, thumb

F1 Left hand, second digit

F2 Left hand, third digit

F3 Left hand, fourth digit

F4 Left hand, fifth digit

F5 Right hand, thumb

F6 Right hand, second digit

F7 Right hand, third digit

F8 Right hand, fourth digit

F9 Right hand, fifth digit

FB Item provided without cost to provider, supplier or practitioner, or full credit received for replaced device (examples, but not limited to, covered under warranty, replaced due to defect, free samples)

- Modifier FB is appended to indicate a device used in a procedure was provided without cost.
- Report modifier FB with the procedure.

FC Partial credit received for replaced device

- Report modifier FC when a credit greater than or equal to 50 percent and less than 100 percent has been given for a replaced device.
- Report modifier FC with the procedure.

FP Service provided as part of family planning program

FQ The service was furnished using audio-only communication technology

FR The supervising practitioner was present through two-way, audio/video communication technology

FS Split (or shared) evaluation and management visit

FT Unrelated evaluation and management (E/M) visit during a postoperative period, or on the same day as a procedure or another E/M visit. (Report when an E/M visit is furnished within the global period but is unrelated, or when one or more additional E/M visits furnished on the same day are unrelated)

FX X-ray taken using film

FY X-ray taken using computed radiography technology/cassette-based imaging

G0 Telehealth services for diagnosis, evaluation, or treatment of symptoms of an acute stroke

G1 Most recent URR reading of less than 60

G2 Most recent URR reading of 60 to 64.9

G3 Most recent URR reading of 65 to 69.9

G4 Most recent URR reading of 70 to 74.9

G5 Most recent URR reading of 75 or greater

G6 ESRD patient for whom less than six dialysis sessions have been provided in a month

- URR is the urea reduction ratio, a calculation that demonstrates the effectiveness of renal dialysis.
- ESRD facilities must append modifiers to reflect the most recent urea reduction ratio (URR), along with CPT code 90999 *Unlisted dialysis procedure inpatient or outpatient*, on all claims filed to Medicare for hemodialysis. Consequently, it will be necessary for ESRD facilities to also report a HCPCS code with the dialysis revenue code (0820, 0821, and 0829). ESRD facilities (both hospital-based and free-standing) should report CPT code 90999 and one of the G modifiers as appropriate, on all claims filed for hemodialysis services. This information will provide data to CMS regarding the adequacy of hemodialysis for quality improvement initiatives. ESRD facilities must monitor hemodialysis adequacy monthly for all facility patients. Home hemodialysis patients may be monitored less frequently, but not less often than quarterly.

G7 Pregnancy resulted from rape or incest, or pregnancy certified by physician as life threatening

- This modifier is appended to the CPT procedure code for abortion services and indicates that the pregnancy resulted from rape or incest, or that the physician considers the pregnancy to be life threatening to the mother.
- Reporting this modifier on a claim communicates to the contractor that the physician certifies that the abortion meets Medicare's coverage policy. Medicare will cover an abortion when:
  - the pregnancy is the result of an act of rape or incest
  - the woman suffers from a physical disorder, physical injury, or physical illness, including a life-endangering physical condition caused by or arising from the pregnancy itself, that would, as certified by a physician, place the woman in danger of death unless an abortion is performed
- Claims submitted with modifier G7 for abortion services may be subject to postpayment review by the contractor.
- Third-party payers, other than Medicare, may not accept this modifier. Individual payers should be queried for claim submission requirements.

G8 Monitored anesthesia care (MAC) for deep complex, complicated, or markedly invasive surgical procedure

G9 Monitored anesthesia care for patient who has a history of severe cardiopulmonary condition

GA Waiver of liability statement issued as required by payer policy, individual case

- This modifier indicates that the provider or supplier has a required signed advance beneficiary notice (ABN) retained in the patient's chart.
- The purpose of the waiver of liability is to ensure that the provider will be paid for the services performed, and to protect the beneficiary from receiving unnecessary services. Providers who acquire a waiver of liability for a covered service should append modifier GA directly following a procedure code to indicate that a beneficiary has signed a waiver of liability form. The provider should keep the form on file. No other statement regarding the waiver of liability is required when modifier GA is reported. Modifier GA at the end of a procedure code is sufficient evidence that the beneficiary has signed an advance notice. If the beneficiary subsequently requests a review of the denial, Medicare will request the provider or supplier to forward a copy of the notice for their files.
- An advanced notice may be applied to an extended course of treatment provided the notice identifies each service for which Medicare is likely to deny payment. A separate notice is required, however, if additional services for which Medicare is likely to deny payment are furnished later in the course of treatment.
- Medicare will deny payment for services reported with modifier GA. The beneficiary can appeal the denial.

GB Claim being resubmitted for payment because it is no longer covered under a global payment demonstration

GC This service has been performed in part by a resident under the direction of a teaching physician

- When a teaching physician's services are billed using this modifier, the teaching physician is certifying that he or she was present during the key portion of the service and was immediately available during the other portions of the service.
- When an anesthesiologist appends modifier QK for two to four medically directed procedures, he or she would not also append modifier GC to the anesthesia code. Only modifier QK is appended.
- When there is a one-on-one situation with a resident and a teaching anesthesiologist (teaching setting), the anesthesiologist would append modifier GC only.
- Modifiers QK and GC are never appended together.
- Modifier GC has no effect on payment.

GE This service has been performed by a resident without the presence of a teaching physician under the primary care exemption

- This modifier identifies services being billed under the primary care exception to the guideline for governing presence during the key portion of a service by the teaching physician.
- Modifier GE has no effect on payment.

GF Nonphysician (e.g., nurse practitioner (NP), certified registered nurse anesthetist (CRNA), certified registered nurse (CRN), clinical nurse specialist (CNS), physician assistant (PA)) services in a critical access hospital

GG Performance and payment of a screening mammogram and diagnostic mammogram on the same patient, same day

- Report modifier GG when the radiologist who interprets a screening mammography orders and interprets additional films based on the results of the screening mammogram while the beneficiary is still at the facility for the screening exam. When this occurs, Medicare will pay for both the screening and diagnostic mammograms.

GH Diagnostic mammogram converted from screening mammogram on same day

- Report modifier GH when the radiologist's interpretation results in additional films and no additional payment is requested. When this modifier is reported, Medicare pays only for the diagnostic mammogram.
- The radiologist is considered the ordering physician in this situation and must furnish his or her national provider identifier (NPI) for Medicare claims. Diagnostic mammography claims submitted to Medicare without the ordering physician's NPI will be denied and returned as unprocessable.

GJ "Opt out" physician or practitioner emergency or urgent service

- Append for claims submitted to Medicare for services rendered by an opt out provider who has not signed a private contract with the Medicare patient requiring emergent or urgent medical care.
- The provider may not charge the Medicare beneficiary more than what a nonparticipating provider would be permitted to charge and must submit the claim to Medicare on the beneficiary's behalf.
- If modifier GJ is not reported on the claim for emergency or urgent care rendered to a Medicare beneficiary by the opt out provider, the claim will be denied and returned as unprocessable.

GK Reasonable and necessary item/service associated with a GA or GZ modifier

GL Medically unnecessary upgrade provided instead of nonupgraded item. No charge. No advance beneficiary notice (ABN).

GM Multiple patients on one ambulance trip

GN Services delivered under an outpatient speech-language pathology plan of care

GO Services delivered under an outpatient occupational therapy plan of care

GP Services delivered under an outpatient physical therapy plan of care

GQ Via asynchronous telecommunications system

GR This service was performed in whole or in part by a resident in a department of veteran's affairs medical center or clinic, supervised in accordance with VA policy

GS Dosage of erythropoietin stimulating agent has been reduced and maintained in response to hematocrit or hemoglobin level

GT Via interactive audio and video telecommunication systems

GU Waiver of liability statement issued as required by payer policy, routine notice

GV Attending physician not employed or paid under arrangement by the patient's hospice provider

GW Service not related to hospice patient's terminal condition

GX Notice of liability issued, voluntary under payer policy

- Append when the provider has a signed voluntary advance beneficiary notice (ABN) in the patient's chart.
- Append if the provider wants a patient's statement of liability for services that are excluded by statute.

- Services with modifier GX will be denied.

GY Item or service statutorily excluded, does not meet the definition of any Medicare benefit or, for non-Medicare insurers, is not a contract benefit

GZ Item or service expected to be denied as not reasonable and necessary

H9 Court-ordered

HA Child/adolescent program

HB Adult program, non-geriatric

HC Adult program, geriatric

HD Pregnant/parenting women's program

HE Mental health program

HF Substance abuse program

HG Opioid addiction treatment program

HH Integrated mental health/substance abuse program

HI Integrated mental health and intellectual disability/developmental disabilities program

HJ Employee assistance program

HK Specialized mental health programs for high-risk populations

HL Intern

HM Less than bachelor's degree level

HN Bachelor's degree level

HO Master's degree level

HP Doctoral level

HQ Group setting

HR Family/couple with client present

HS Family/couple without client present

HT Multi-disciplinary team

HU Funded by child welfare agency

HV Funded state addictions agency

HW Funded by state mental health agency

HX Funded by county/local agency

HY Funded by juvenile justice agency

HZ Funded by criminal justice agency

J1 Competitive acquisition program (CAP) no-pay submission for a prescription number

J2 Competitive acquisition program (CAP), restocking of emergency drugs after emergency administration

J3 Competitive acquisition program (CAP), drug not available through CAP as written, reimbursed under average sales price methodology

J4 DMEPOS item subject to DMEPOS competitive bidding program that is furnished by a hospital upon discharge

J5 Off-the-shelf orthotic subject to DMEPOS competitive bidding program that is furnished as part of a physical therapist or occupational therapist professional service

JA Administered intravenously

JB Administered subcutaneously

- Report modifier JA or JB to indicate the route of administration when erythropoiesis-stimulating agents (ESA), such as epoetin alfa and darbepoetin alfa, are reported. When both methods of administration are used, such as in a renal dialysis facility, report separate lines to identify the number of administrations provided using each method.

JC Skin substitute used as a graft

JD Skin substitute not used as a graft

JE Administered via dialysate

JG Drug or biological acquired with 340B drug pricing program discount, reported for informational purposes

JW Drug amount discarded/not administered to any patient

JZ Zero drug amount discarded/not administered to any patient

K0 Lower extremity prosthesis functional level-0: does not have the ability or potential to ambulate or transfer safely with or without assistance and a prosthesis does not enhance their quality of life or mobility

K1 Lower extremity prosthesis functional level-1: has the ability or potential to use a prosthesis for transfers or ambulation on level surfaces at fixed cadence. Typical of the limited and unlimited household ambulator

K2 Lower extremity prosthesis functional level-2: has the ability or potential for ambulation with the ability to traverse low level environmental barriers such as curbs, stairs or uneven surfaces. Typical of the limited community ambulator

K3 Lower extremity prosthesis functional level-3: has the ability or potential for ambulation with variable cadence. Typical of the community ambulator who has the ability to traverse most environmental barriers and may have vocational, therapeutic, or exercise activity that demands prosthetic utilization beyond simple locomotion

K4 Lower extremity prosthesis functional level-4: has the ability or potential for prosthetic ambulation that exceeds the basic ambulation skills, exhibiting high impact, stress, or energy levels, typical of the prosthetic demands of the child, active adult, or athlete

KA Add-on option/accessory for wheelchair

KB Beneficiary requested upgrade for ABN, more than four modifiers identified on claim

KC Replacement of special power wheelchair interface

KD Drug or biological infused through DME

KE Bid under round one of the DMEPOS competitive bidding program for use with noncompetitive bid base equipment

KF Item designated by FDA as Class III device

KG DMEPOS item subject to DMEPOS competitive bidding program number 1

KH DMEPOS item, initial claim, purchase or first month rental
- DMEPOS is the acronym for durable medical equipment, prosthetics, orthotics, and supplies
- Report with modifier RR for rented DME.

KI DMEPOS item, second or third month rental
- Report with modifier RR for rented DME.

KJ DMEPOS item, parenteral enteral nutrition (PEN) pump or capped rental, months four to 15

KK DMEPOS item subject to DMEPOS competitive bidding program number 2

KL DMEPOS item delivered via mail

KM Replacement of facial prosthesis including new impression/moulage

KN Replacement of facial prosthesis using previous master model

KO Single drug unit dose formulation

KP First drug of a multiple drug unit dose formulation

KQ Second or subsequent drug of a multiple drug unit formulation

KR Rental item–billing for partial month

KS Glucose monitor supply for diabetic beneficiary not treated with insulin

KT Beneficiary resides in a competitive bidding area and travels outside that competitive bidding area and receives a competitive bid item

KU DMEPOS item subject to DMEPOS competitive bidding program number 3

KV DMEPOS item subject to DMEPOS competitive bidding program that is furnished as part of a professional service

KW DMEPOS item subject to DMEPOS competitive bidding program number 4

KX Requirements specified in the medical policy have been met

KY DMEPOS item subject to DMEPOS competitive bidding program number 5

KZ New coverage not implemented by managed care

LC Left circumflex coronary artery

LD Left anterior descending coronary artery

LL Lease/rental (Use the LL modifier when DME equipment rental is to be applied against the purchase price)

LM Left main coronary artery
- Report modifiers LC, LD, LM, RC, and RI to indicate which coronary artery was involved in the percutaneous coronary intervention (PCI). PCI codes are in the range of 92920–92944.

LR Laboratory round trip

LS FDA-monitored intraocular lens implant

LT Left side (used to identify procedures performed on the left side of the body)
- This modifier indicates the side of the body on which a procedure is performed. It does not indicate a bilateral procedure.
- Modifiers LT and RT have no effect on payment; however, failure to append when appropriate could result in delay or denial (or partial denial) of the claim.

LU Fractionated payment of CAR-T therapy

M2 Medicare secondary payer (MSP)

MA Ordering professional is not required to consult a clinical decision support mechanism due to service being rendered to a patient with a suspected or confirmed emergency medical condition

MB Ordering professional is not required to consult a clinical decision support mechanism due to the significant hardship exception of insufficient internet access

MC Ordering professional is not required to consult a clinical decision support mechanism due to the significant hardship exception of electronic health record or clinical decision support mechanism vendor issues

MD Ordering professional is not required to consult a clinical decision support mechanism due to the significant hardship exception of extreme and uncontrollable circumstances

ME The order for this service adheres to appropriate use criteria in the clinical decision support mechanism consulted by the ordering professional

MF The order for this service does not adhere to the appropriate use criteria in the clinical decision support mechanism consulted by the ordering professional

MG The order for this service does not have applicable appropriate use criteria in the qualified clinical decision support mechanism consulted by the ordering professional

MH Unknown if ordering professional consulted a clinical decision support mechanism for this service, related information was not provided to the furnishing professional or provider

MS Six-month maintenance and servicing fee for reasonable and necessary parts and labor which are not covered under any manufacturer or supplier warranty

N1 Group 1 oxygen coverage criteria met

N2 Group 2 oxygen coverage criteria met

N3 Group 3 oxygen coverage criteria met

NB Nebulizer system, any type, FDA-cleared for use with specific drug

NR New when rented (use the NR modifier when DME which was new at the time of rental is subsequently purchased)

NU New equipment

P1 Anesthesia physical status—Normal, healthy patient

P2 Anesthesia physical status—Patient with mild, systemic disease

P3 Anesthesia physical status—Patient with severe, systemic disease

P4 Anesthesia physical status—Patient with severe, systemic disease that is a constant threat to life

P5 Anesthesia physical status—Moribund patient who is not expected to survive without the operation

P6 Anesthesia physical status—Declared brain-dead patient whose organs are being removed for donor purposes

PA Surgical or other invasive procedure on wrong body part

- Medicare will not pay for surgery performed on the wrong patient or wrong body part, or an incorrect procedure performed on a patient. All payments for these mistakenly performed procedures and any related services will be denied.
- For outpatient services, one of the three modifiers (PA, PB, or PC) should be appended to line items related to the surgical error.

PB Surgical or other invasive procedure on wrong patient

- Medicare will not pay for surgery performed on the wrong patient or wrong body part, or an incorrect procedure performed on a patient. All payments for these mistakenly performed procedures and any related services will be denied.
- For outpatient services, one of the three modifiers (PA, PB, or PC) should be appended to line items related to the surgical error.

PC Wrong surgery or other invasive procedure on patient

- Medicare will not pay for surgery performed on the wrong patient or wrong body part, or an incorrect procedure performed on a patient. All payments for these mistakenly performed procedures and any related services will be denied.
- For outpatient services, one of the three modifiers (PA, PB, or PC) should be appended to line items related to the surgical error.

PD Diagnostic or related nondiagnostic item or service provided in a wholly owned or operated entity to a patient who is admitted as an inpatient within 3 days

- Modifier PD must be appended to physician preadmission diagnostic and admission-related nondiagnostic services, reported with HCPCS/CPT codes, that are subject to the three-day inpatient payment window policy. When modifier PD is present, Medicare pays only the professional component for CPT/HCPCS codes with a technical component (TC)/professional component (PC) split that are provided in the three-day (one-day in the case of non-IPPS hospitals) payment window, or the facility rate for codes without a TC/PC split.

PI Positron Emission Tomography (PET) or PET/Computed Tomography (CT) to inform the initial treatment strategy of tumors that are biopsy proven or strongly suspected of being cancerous based on other diagnostic testing

PL Progressive addition lenses

PM Post-mortem

PN Nonexcepted service provided at an off-campus, outpatient, provider-based department of a hospital

PO Excepted service provided at an off-campus, outpatient, provider-based department of a hospital

- Modifier PO is to be reported only by facilities on institutional/facility claims. Physician and professional claims should report new place of service (POS) code set 19 for Off Campus-Outpatient Hospital and revised POS code 22 for On Campus-Outpatient Hospital.

PS Positron Emission Tomography (PET) or PET/Computed Tomography (CT) to inform the subsequent treatment strategy of cancerous tumors when the beneficiary's treating physician determines that the PET study is needed to inform subsequent antitumor strategy

PT Colorectal cancer screening test; converted to diagnostic test or other procedure

- Append HCPCS Level II modifier PT to the diagnostic procedure code reported instead of the colorectal cancer screening. When reported with modifier PT, the deductible will be waived for all surgical services on the same date as the planned screening colonoscopy, planned flexible sigmoidoscopy, or barium enema.

Q0 Investigational clinical service provided in a clinical research study that is in an approved clinical research study

Q1 Routine clinical service provided in a clinical research study that is in an approved clinical research study

Q2 Demonstration procedure/service

Q3 Live kidney donor surgery and related services

- Append to identify postoperative live kidney donor services that are reimbursed at 100 percent of the Medicare fee schedule amount.

Q4 Service for ordering/referring physician qualifies as a service exemption

- Append when the ordering or referring provider has a financial relationship with the entity performing the service, and for which the service qualifies as one of the service-related exemptions.

Q5 Service furnished under a reciprocal billing arrangement by a substitute physician or by a substitute physical therapist furnishing outpatient physical therapy services in a health professional shortage area, a medically underserved area, or a rural area

- Modifier Q5 is to be applied to the end of a procedure code to indicate that the service was provided by a substitute physician. The regular physician should keep a record on file of each service provided by the substitute physician, associated with the substitute physician's UPIN, and make this record available to Medicare upon request.
- This modifier has no effect on payment.

Q6 Service furnished under a fee-for-time compensation arrangement by a substitute physician or by a substitute physical therapist furnishing outpatient physical therapy services in a health professional shortage area, a medically underserved area, or a rural area

- Locum tenens physicians generally have no practice of their own; they usually move from area to area as needed. The patient's regular physician may submit a claim and receive Medicare Part B payment for a covered and medically necessary visit of a locum tenens physician who is not an employee of the regular physician and whose services for patients of the regular physician are not restricted to the regular physician's office. The locum tenens physician should not provide the visit services to Medicare patients for a continuous period of longer than 60 days.
- This modifier has no effect on payment.

Q7, Q8, and Q9—Foot care

- Documentation of the systemic conditions and class findings must be in the patient's record. The record must be maintained in the physician's office and available for medical review by the carrier. Documentation should indicate the course of treatment and length of treatment for infectious conditions. Documentation should include the affected toe, including the clinical evidence of mycosis, the manner in which and to what extent the nail was debrided, and the antifungal agent used in the office note/progress note.
- A description of the qualifying symptoms should be documented.
- Ambulatory patients must exhibit a marked limitation in ambulation, pain, or secondary infection resulting from the thickening and dystrophy.
- Non-ambulatory patients must suffer from pain or secondary infection resulting from the thickening and dystrophy of the infected nail plate.
- Routine foot care is excluded from Medicare coverage.
- General diagnosis such as ASHD, circulatory problems, vascular disease, and venous insufficiency are not sufficient to permit payment for routine foot care.

Q7 One Class A finding

- Class A findings: Nontraumatic amputation of foot or integral skeletal portions thereof.
- This modifier was established to allow the provider to report class findings without having to write a narrative description on the claim form or submit additional documentation with the claim. This modifier should be appended to foot care procedures (e.g., 11720, 11721) to indicate the severity of the patient's systemic condition and justify the medical necessity of a procedure that is usually denied as routine.

Q8 Two Class B findings

- Class B findings:
  - absent posterior tibial pulse
  - absent dorsalis pedis pulse
  - advance trophic changes such as (three required):
    - hair growth (decrease or absence)
    - nail changes (thickening)
    - pigmentary changes (discoloration)
    - skin texture (thin, shiny)
    - skin color (rubor or redness)
- This modifier was established to allow the provider to report class findings without having to write a narrative description on the claim form or submit additional documentation with the claim. This modifier should be appended to foot care procedures (e.g., 11720, 11721) to indicate the severity of the patient's systemic condition and to justify the medical necessity of a procedure that is usually denied as routine.

Q9 One Class B and two Class C findings
- Class C findings:
  - claudication
  - temperature changes (e.g., cold feet)
  - edema
  - paresthesia
  - burning
- This modifier was established to allow the provider to report class findings without having to write a narrative description on the claim form or submit additional documentation with the claim. This modifier should be appended to foot care procedures (e.g., 11720, 11721) to indicate the severity of the patient's systemic condition and to justify the medical necessity of a procedure that is usually denied as routine.

QA Prescribed amounts of stationary oxygen for daytime use while at rest and nighttime use differ and the average of the two amounts is less than 1 liter per minute (LPM)

QB Prescribed amounts of stationary oxygen for daytime use while at rest and nighttime use differ and the average of the two amounts exceeds 4 liters per minute (LPM) and portable oxygen is prescribed

QC Single channel monitoring

QD Recording and storage in solid state memory by a digital recorder
- This modifier has no effect on payment.

QE Prescribed amount of stationary oxygen while at rest is less than 1 liter per minute (LPM)

QF Prescribed amount of stationary oxygen while at rest exceeds 4 liters per minute (LPM) and portable oxygen is prescribed

QG Prescribed amount of stationary oxygen while at rest is greater than 4 liters per minute (LPM)

QH Oxygen conserving device is being used with an oxygen delivery system

QJ Services/items provided to a prisoner or patient in state or local custody, however the state or local government, as applicable, meets the requirements in 42 CFR 411.4 (B)

QK Medical direction of two, three, or four concurrent anesthesia procedures involving qualified individuals

QL Patient pronounced dead after ambulance called

QM Ambulance service provided under arrangement by a provider of services
- Modifiers QM and QN should be appended when a patient has an inpatient status at one hospital and is transferred to another hospital or facility for tests or treatment and then is returned to the first hospital.
- This modifier is valid for Medicare; however, the service would be denied under Medicare Part B since it is considered a Medicare Part A expense.

QN Ambulance service furnished directly by a provider of services
- Modifiers QM and QN should be appended when a patient has an inpatient status at one hospital and is transferred to another hospital or facility for tests or treatment, and then is returned to the first hospital.
- This modifier is valid for Medicare; however, the service would be denied under Medicare Part B since it is considered a Medicare Part A expense.

QP Documentation is on file showing that the laboratory test(s) was ordered individually or ordered as a CPT-recognized panel other than automated profile codes 80002-80019, G0058, G0059, and G0060
- Sufficient documentation would be the requisition form showing that the physician had individually ordered tests either by code or the corresponding code definition.
- The individual tests that constitute an organ or disease related CPT panel do not need to be ordered individually in order for the laboratory to append modifier QP. The laboratory may bill using the CPT code for organ or disease oriented panel with modifier QP when the physician orders the components of the panel.
- CMS does not require laboratories to append this modifier, but some contractors (fiscal intermediary or carrier) strongly advise its use.

QQ Ordering professional consulted a qualified clinical decision support mechanism for this service and the related data was provided to the furnishing professional

QR Prescribed amounts of stationary oxygen for daytime use while at rest and nighttime use differ and the average of the two amounts is greater than 4 liters per minute (LPM)

QS Monitored anesthesia care services
- Monitored anesthesia care (MAC) services will be closely watched to ensure medical necessity is documented. ICD-10-CM codes should accurately describe the condition requiring MAC anesthesia. CMS collects data for MAC, even though it is paid the same as general anesthesia. The anesthesiologist or CRNA monitors the patient's vital signs, furnishes the preanesthesia exam, prescribes the necessary anesthesia care, administers medications, and furnishes required postoperative anesthesia care.

QT Recording and storage on tape by an analog tape recorder
- This modifier has no effect on payment.

QW CLIA waived test

QX CRNA service: with medical direction by a physician
- Payment rule: Limits payment to 55 percent of the amount that would have been allowed if personally performed by a physician or nonsupervised CRNA.

QY Medical direction of one certified registered nurse anesthetist (CRNA) by an anesthesiologist

QZ CRNA service: without medical direction by a physician
- Payment rule: No effect on payment. Payment would be equal to the amount that would have been allowed if personally performed by a physician.

RA Replacement of a DME, orthotic or prosthetic item

RB Replacement of a part of a DME, orthotic or prosthetic item furnished as part of a repair

RC Right coronary artery

RD Drug provided to beneficiary, but not administered "incident-to"

RE Furnished in full compliance with FDA-mandated risk evaluation and mitigation strategy (REMS)

RI Ramus intermedius coronary artery
- Report modifiers LC, LD, LM, RC, and RI to indicate which coronary artery was involved in the percutaneous coronary intervention (PCI). PCI codes are in the range of 92920–92944.

RR Rental (use the "RR" modifier when DME is to be rented)
- Append in conjunction with the appropriate "rental" modifiers KH, KI, and KJ.
- Modifier RR is placed directly after the HCPCS Level II code for the DME followed by the appropriate rental modifier as above.

RT Right side (Used to identify procedures performed on the right side of the body)
- There are many procedure codes that require a physician to indicate the side of the body on which a procedure was performed by appending modifiers RT and LT.
- When billing for a separately identifiable/unrelated surgical procedure performed during the postoperative period of another surgical procedure, procedure code modifiers RT (right) and LT (left) must be indicated on the claim as appropriate. In addition, modifier 79 (unrelated procedure or service by the same physician during the postoperative period) must be submitted on the subsequent claim.
- This modifier indicates the side of the body on which a procedure is performed. It does not indicate a bilateral procedure.
- Modifiers LT and RT have no effect on payment; however, failure to append when appropriate could result in delay or denial (or partial denial) of the claim.

SA Nurse practitioner rendering service in collaboration with a physician

SB Nurse midwife

SC Medically necessary service or supply

SD Services provided by registered nurse with specialized, highly technical home infusion training

SE State and/or federally-funded programs/services

SF Second opinion ordered by a professional review organization (PRO) per section 9401, p.l. 99-272 (100% reimbursement—no Medicare deductible or coinsurance)
- Append when the second opinion is ordered or requested by QIO.
- For Medicare beneficiaries, when this modifier is reported the service is eligible for 100 percent reimbursement. The usual deductible and/or coinsurance amounts are not applied.

SG Ambulatory surgery center (ASC) facility service
- This modifier is no longer required on Medicare claims. Physician and nonphysician practitioner fees must be billed on a separate claim form from the ASC facility fees.

SH Second concurrently administered infusion therapy

SJ Third or more concurrently administered infusion therapy

SK Member of high risk population (use only with codes for immunization)

SL State supplied vaccine

SM Second surgical opinion

SN Third surgical opinion

SQ Item ordered by home health

SS Home infusion services provided in the infusion suite of the IV therapy provider

ST Related to trauma or injury

SU Procedure performed in physician's office (to denote use of facility and equipment)

SV Pharmaceuticals delivered to patient's home but not utilized

SW Services provided by a certified diabetic educator

SY Persons who are in close contact with member of high-risk population (use only with codes for immunization)

TA Left foot, great toe

T1 Left foot, second digit

T2 Left foot, third digit

T3 Left foot, fourth digit

T4 Left foot, fifth digit

T5 Right foot, great toe

T6 Right foot, second digit

T7 Right foot, third digit

T8 Right foot, fourth digit

T9 Right foot, fifth digit

TB Drug or biological acquired with 340B drug pricing program discount, reported for informational purposes for select entities

TC Technical component;
Under certain circumstances, a charge may be made for the technical component alone. Under these circumstances, the technical component charge is identified by adding modifier TC to the usual procedure number. Technical component charges are institutional charges and not billed separately by physicians. However, portable x-ray suppliers only bill for technical component and should utilize modifier TC. The charge data from portable x-ray suppliers will then be used to build customary and prevailing profiles.

- There are stand-alone procedure codes that describe technical component only codes (e.g., staff and equipment costs) of diagnostic tests. They also identify procedures that are covered only as diagnostic tests and, therefore, do not have a related professional component. The use of modifier TC on these codes is not appropriate, nor is it correct coding. Technical component services only are institutional and should not be billed separately by the physicians. However, portable x-ray suppliers only bill for the technical component and should append modifier TC.

TD RN

TE LPN/LVN

TF Intermediate level of care

TG Complex/high tech level of care

TH Obstetrical treatment/services, prenatal or postpartum

TJ Program group, child and/or adolescent

TK Extra patient or passenger, non-ambulance

TL Early intervention/individualized family service plan (IFSP)

TM Individualized education program (IEP)

TN Rural/outside providers' customary service area

TP Medical transport, unloaded vehicle

TQ Basic life support transport by a volunteer ambulance provider

TR School-based individualized education program (IEP) services provided outside the public school district responsible for the student

TS Follow-up service

TT Individualized service provided to more than one patient in same setting

TU Special payment rate, overtime

TV Special payment rates, holidays/weekends

TW Back-up equipment

U1 Medicaid level of care 1, as defined by each state

U2 Medicaid level of care 2, as defined by each state

U3 Medicaid level of care 3, as defined by each state

U4 Medicaid level of care 4, as defined by each state

U5 Medicaid level of care 5, as defined by each state

U6 Medicaid level of care 6, as defined by each state

U7 Medicaid level of care 7, as defined by each state

U8 Medicaid level of care 8, as defined by each state

U9 Medicaid level of care 9, as defined by each state

UA Medicaid level of care 10, as defined by each state

UB Medicaid level of care 11, as defined by each state

UC Medicaid level of care 12, as defined by each state

UD Medicaid level of care 13, as defined by each state

UE Used durable medical equipment

- Append when the used equipment is purchased by a beneficiary.

UF Services provided in the morning

UG Services provided in the afternoon

UH Services provided in the evening

UJ Services provided at night

UK Services provided on behalf of the client to someone other than the client (collateral relationship)

UN Two patients served

UP Three patients served

UQ Four patients served

UR Five patients served

US Six or more patients served

V1 Demonstration modifier 1

V2 Demonstration modifier 2

V3 Demonstration modifier 3

V4 Demonstration modifier 4

V5 Vascular catheter (alone or with any other vascular access)

V6 Arteriovenous graft (or other vascular access not including a vascular catheter)

V7 Arteriovenous fistula only (in use with two needles)

- ESRD facilities are required to append V5, V6, or V7 for the type of vascular access used for the delivery of hemodialysis at the last hemodialysis session of the month. The modifier must be appended to the latest line-item date of service billing for revenue code 0821.

VM Medicare diabetes prevention program (MDPP) virtual make-up session

VP Aphakic patient

X1 Continuous/broad services: for reporting services by clinicians, who provide the principal care for a patient, with no planned endpoint of the relationship; services in this category represent comprehensive care, dealing with the entire scope of patient problems, either directly or in a care coordination role; reporting clinician service examples include, but are not limited to: primary care, and clinicians providing comprehensive care to patients in addition to specialty care

X2 Continuous/focused services: for reporting services by clinicians whose expertise is needed for the ongoing management of a chronic disease or a condition that needs to be managed and followed with no planned endpoint to the relationship; reporting clinician service examples include but are not limited to: a rheumatologist taking care of the patient's rheumatoid arthritis longitudinally but not providing general primary care services

X3 Episodic/broad services: for reporting services by clinicians who have broad responsibility for the comprehensive needs of the patient that is limited to a defined period and circumstance such as a hospitalization; reporting clinician service examples include but are not limited to the hospitalist's services rendered providing comprehensive and general care to a patient while admitted to the hospital

X4 Episodic/focused services: for reporting services by clinicians who provide focused care on particular types of treatment limited to a defined period and circumstance; the patient has a problem, acute or chronic, that will be treated with surgery, radiation, or some other type of generally time-limited intervention; reporting clinician service examples include but are not limited to, the orthopedic surgeon performing a knee replacement and seeing the patient through the postoperative period

X5 Diagnostic services requested by another clinician: for reporting services by a clinician who furnishes care to the patient only as requested by another clinician or subsequent and related services requested by another clinician; this modifier is reported for patient relationships that may not be adequately captured by the above alternative categories; reporting clinician service examples include but are not limited to, the radiologist's interpretation of an imaging study requested by another clinician

XE Separate encounter, a service that is distinct because it occurred during a separate encounter

XP Separate practitioner, a service that is distinct because it was performed by a different practitioner

XS Separate structure, a service that is distinct because it was performed on a separate organ/structure

XU Unusual non-overlapping service, the use of a service that is distinct because it does not overlap usual components of the main service

Durable Medical Equipment, Prosthetics, Orthotics, and Supplies (DMEPOS)

The DMEPOS Industry

Wheelchairs, artificial limbs, braces, surgical dressings, and medications are all examples of durable medical equipment, prosthetics, orthotics, and supplies, known by the acronyms DME and POS, or simply DMEPOS.

The DMEPOS industry includes manufacturers, pharmaceutical companies, medical equipment and supply companies (suppliers and vendors), and providers. Entities peripheral to the DMEPOS industry, but having direct impact on its operations, include the Food and Drug Administration (FDA), which approves the use of medical devices and pharmaceuticals in the United States, and federal and state health care programs such as Medicare and Medicaid, which provide DMEPOS coverage and/or reimbursement for millions of beneficiaries. Other third-party payers, various preferred provider organizations (PPOs), workers' compensation carriers, and managed care organizations (MCOs) also influence the DMEPOS industry.

Health insurance benefits for DMEPOS, in general, are entangled in a mesh of rules and regulations governing coverage and reimbursement. The Centers for Medicare and Medicaid Services (CMS) is the federal agency that runs the Medicare program and oversees the Medicaid program. CMS has strict criteria that must be met by both suppliers and providers of DMEPOS, as well as numerous rules and regulations covering every aspect of the DMEPOS reimbursement process. These include coding, claims preparation, provider and supplier certifications, options for equipment rental and purchase, and a host of other billing directives. CMS's model of DMEPOS reimbursement, viewed as generally effective even if somewhat cumbersome, has inspired a number of third-party payers to pattern their own reimbursement protocol after it to some degree. While a state Medicaid program has some degree of flexibility, many will follow the Medicare program guidelines.

Special Federal and Third-Party Payer Definitions

For federally funded health care programs, such as Medicare and the Children's Health Insurance Program (CHIP), and for programs that are partially funded by the federal government, such as state Medicaid programs, there are strict definitions of what constitutes DMEPOS. A number of commercial insurance plans also follow this same framework, or a similar one, constructed around the prescription, dispensation, reporting, and reimbursement of DMEPOS.

Defining DME

According to CMS, DME must meet specific criteria to be eligible for coverage. These criteria are shown here in the form of questions. The provider or supplier must be able to answer yes to all of these questions for the equipment or device to be recognized as eligible for reimbursement under the Medicare program:

- **Can the medical equipment withstand repeated use?** Medicare Fact: Many items, though durable in nature, such as braces (orthoses) and prostheses, are not considered DME. These items fall into different categories of DMEPOS classifications. Medical supplies such as incontinent pads, catheters, bandages, stockings, irrigating kits, sheets, and bags are expendable in nature and do not qualify as DME.
- **Is the medical equipment primarily and customarily used for medical purposes?** Medicare Fact: Certain types of medical equipment are considered "presumptively medical," meaning the sole purpose of the equipment is to provide medical benefits to the patient. A variety of devices and equipment fall into this category, including hospital beds, respirators, nebulizers, commodes, traction devices, and oxygen tents. Other types of medical equipment are considered "presumptively nonmedical," meaning that the devices and equipment are not only used for medical benefits, but also for purposes of personal comfort, ambient control, environmental enhancement, or convenience. For example, an air conditioner might yield certain medical benefits to a patient recuperating from a cardiac event. The air conditioner will lower the room temperature, which may in turn assist the patient with fluid retention by minimizing

DMEPOS

fluid loss. However, because the primary and customary use of the air conditioner is not for the purpose of body fluid maintenance, it is not considered DME and payment will not be made for this equipment under the Medicare program.

- **Is the medical equipment not of use to a person without illness or injury or in need of improvement of a malformed body part?** Medicare Fact: An order or CMN on its own will not justify medical necessity even if the physician signs it. There must be documentation in the patient's medical record to substantiate the medical necessity for the item.
- **Is the medical equipment appropriate for home use?** Medicare Fact: For a patient's DME rental or purchase to be eligible for coverage under this criterion, the patient's home must be a personal dwelling or apartment, a relative's home, a home for the aged, or some other type of institution fulfilling the domiciliary needs of the patient. However, it cannot be a skilled nursing facility or a hospital.

An answer of no to any of the preceding questions could render the DME as ineligible for Medicare coverage.

Orthotic and prosthetic devices are not subject to the home use requirement for coverage and payment purposes.

Special exceptions can be made by the Medicare program, some state Medicaid programs, and other third-party payers even when the DME equipment or device does not meet the accepted definition of DME by specifically contradicting two of the criteria: (1) the equipment or devices are not primarily and customarily used for medical purposes, and/or (2) the equipment or devices can be used in the absence of illness, injury, or deformity. A DMEPOS item, described by one or both of these contradicting criteria, may be eligible for Medicare coverage if the therapeutic purpose is clearly distinguished, such as in the use of a heat lamp where the medical need for heat therapy has been established. The fact that the patient's course of treatment is under the supervision of the physician must also be in evidence.

Defining Prostheses

Prosthetic devices, as recognized by CMS and many third-party payers, are those devices that replace all or part of an internal body organ, or replace all or part of the function of a permanently inoperative or malfunctioning internal body organ. This category of devices includes:

- Artificial limbs
- Breast and eye prostheses
- Maxillofacial devices
- Joint implants
- Devices that replace all or part of the ear or nose
- Ostomy and colostomy bags
- Irrigation and flushing equipment directly related to ostomy/colostomy care

An example of a prosthesis is a urinary collection and retention system that replaces the function of the bladder in cases of permanent urinary incontinence. Replacement of a prosthetic device may be covered, but only when the replacement is required because of a change in the beneficiary's physical condition. Adjustments to an artificial limb or other prosthetic device required by wear or by a change in the beneficiary's physical condition may be likewise covered when ordered by a physician.

While parenteral and enteral nutrition (PEN) is covered by the Medicare program in many instances, there is a disparity between information in the Code of Federal Regulations (CFR) and information provided by the durable medical equipment Medicare administrative contractors (DME MAC) in the classification of PEN as a prosthetic. The CFR, in chapter 42, section 414.202, states that PEN and related accouterments are not considered to be prosthetic, while the Durable Medical Equipment Regional Carriers (DMERC) supplier manuals list these items as general prosthetics. The Medicare Internet-Only Manuals (IOMs) likewise details PEN as covered under the prosthetic device benefit. The conditions for coverage are not affected by this classification disparity. PEN is covered for patients who, due to chronic illness or injury, cannot take in sustenance through oral feeding and/or who have a permanently inoperative internal body organ or function and must receive life-sustaining nutrients via parenteral or enteral means.

Defining Orthoses

An orthosis or orthotic device is used for the correction or prevention of skeletal deformities. This includes braces for the neck, shoulder and arm, forearm, wrist and hand, hip, leg, ankle, and foot, as well as spinal or back devices. If there is a change in the beneficiary's physical condition that requires replacements and adjustments, those may also be covered. However, according to CMS, to be classified as an orthotic, the brace must be a rigid or semi-rigid device used for supporting a weak or deformed body member, or for restricting or eliminating motion in a diseased or injured part of the body.

Orthoses can be classified as prefabricated or custom fabricated. A prefabricated orthosis is typically manufactured and sold without specific patient data, or in other words, without the patient's personal measurements and orthotic requirements. These devices and appliances can usually be bent, trimmed, and molded many times (with or without heat) to meet specific patient physical and therapeutic needs. An orthosis that is assembled at the point of service from prefabricated component parts is still considered to be a prefabricated orthosis.

A custom fabricated orthosis is one that has been made by following a specific patient's physical measurements and therapeutic requirements. These devices and appliances require more than bending, trimming, or simple molding to properly fit the specific patient. The creation of custom fabricated orthoses involves a significant amount of detailed work, such as building each orthotic device from component materials of plastic, metal, and fabrics. A molded-to-patient, custom, fabricated orthosis is one in which an impression of the patient's body part is taken and the resultant impression cast is used to construct the orthosis.

Defining Supplies

Within the DMEPOS industry, a supply is an item or accessory needed for the effective use of a DME, prosthetic or orthotic device, or appliance. Such supplies include those drugs and biologicals that must be placed directly into equipment to achieve the therapeutic benefit of the DME or to ensure the proper functioning of the equipment. An example of this is the use of heparin within a home dialysis system. To be eligible for coverage by Medicare, Medicaid, and third-party payers, supplies must be medically necessary and must be prescribed by the treating provider. Supplies eligible for reimbursement by these programs and payers are typically not those bought off the shelf or over the counter at local drug stores and grocery stores, with the exception of recent additions to the list of covered supplies for a patient's home use, such as supplies needed with a glucometer for the monitoring of diabetes mellitus.

Medical supplies are considered to be part of a provider's practice expense, and payment for many supplies by the Medicare program and most state Medicaid programs is included in the practice expense portion of the payment or fee schedule amount reimbursed to the provider for the primary medical or surgical service. The supplies are considered incidental to the primary medical or surgical service. Other third-party payers follow the definition of billable medical and surgical supplies found in the CPT book, which is stated in CPT guidelines as "supplies and materials provided by the physician (e.g., sterile trays/drugs), over and above those usually included with the office visit or other services rendered." Many payers require the use of CPT code 99070 *Supplies and materials (except spectacles), provided by the physician or other qualified health care professional over and above those usually included with the office visit or other services rendered (list drugs, trays, supplies, or materials provided)* or 99072 *Additional supplies, materials, and clinical staff time over and above those usually included in an office visit or other nonfacility service(s), when performed during a Public Health Emergency, as defined by law, due to respiratory-transmitted infectious disease.* Because these CPT codes are general in their descriptions, additional documentation or a special notation in the appropriate field for electronic claims is needed to describe the specific supply being reported.

Health care facilities must follow federal guidelines for each type of facility (hospital inpatient, hospital outpatient, ASC, skilled nursing facility, etc.) when reporting supplies to Medicare for separate payment.

Defining Customized DME

In accordance with a longstanding definition in 42 CFR, Section 414.224, the criteria listed in 42 CFR, Section 414.224(a) state, "To be considered a customized item for payment purposes under paragraph (b) of this section, a covered item (including a wheelchair) must be uniquely constructed or substantially modified for a specific beneficiary according to the description and orders of a physician and be so different from another item used for the same purpose that the two items cannot be grouped together for pricing purposes. (b) Payment is made on a lump sum basis for the purchase of a customized item based on the carrier's individual consideration and judgment of a reasonable payment amount for each customized item. The carrier's individual consideration takes into account written documentation on the costs of the item including at least the cost of labor and materials used in customizing an item."

The Omnibus Budget Reconciliation Act (OBRA) of November 1990 amended the criteria for treatment of wheelchair as a customized item. This alternative definition of customized wheelchairs was never adopted for Medicare payment purposes and should not be confused with the definition of customized items referenced above.

Documentation Standards

Documentation in the medical record must contain information justifying hospitalization, an observation stay, an encounter or visit, or services provided for a patient. It must indicate that services are provided using current medical knowledge and treatment for the condition or injury, and that the services are medically necessary. In addition, the documentation must stand up to the scrutiny of others.

To meet the requirements of medical necessity for all health care services reported to the Medicare program, the patient's medical record must reflect the nature and extent of the diagnosis or injury, with clear documentation of the following patient-specific facts:

- Physical examination findings
- Diagnostic tests/analyses results
- Relation of diagnosis to the DMEPOS item

- Complicating comorbidities
- Physical functional abilities and/or limitations (ability to ambulate or transfer, amount of time needed to be spent in a bed, extent of use of a wheelchair, types/frequencies of activities recommended for outside the home, etc.)
- Duration of the diagnosis (acute, acute but refractory to treatment, chronic)
- Overall expected course/prognosis
- Rehabilitation potentials

In most instances, an evaluation and management (E/M) service is rendered before or during the same session that an order for DMEPOS is given. Requirements for the correct reporting of E/M services are beyond the scope of this publication; however, in addition to the criteria listed above for medical record documentation, an appropriate patient history must be obtained.

In general, the following three criteria (known as key elements of E/M documentation) should appear in the patient's medical record to correctly report an E/M service:

- Patient history
- Physical examination
- Level of medical decision-making

This is a requirement under both the American Medical Association's (AMA) and the Centers of Medicare and Medicaid Services' (CMS) guidelines.

Providers who dispense DMEPOS should take note that during audits of E/M services, a prevalent finding is the lack of review of systems information. This is an integral part of the patient's history. The absence or inadequate documentation of this part of the patient's history will cause an auditor to downgrade the original level of E/M, resulting in an overpayment situation in which the provider will have to refund the reimbursement difference to the payer or the patient.

Providers may receive requests from DMEPOS suppliers for copies of patient medical records that support the medical necessity of the provider's order. This is generally in response to a direct demand made upon the supplier from the Medicare contractor to substantiate the need for DMEPOS items. Providers should respond promptly to any requests made by the DMEPOS supplier for additional information. Suppliers do report certain difficulties in obtaining copies of medical records from provider offices.

General DME Documentation Standards

The following documentation is necessary for DMEPOS items regardless of the payer:

- The provider should sign and date an order for the DMEPOS item
- If the treating provider is also supplying the item, the clinical notes should substantiate the need for the item
- The diagnosis establishing the medical necessity for the item must be documented in the medical record
- If the medical necessity for the item, as determined by the payer, cannot be established due to the nature of the patient's condition, injury, or illness, then the patient must sign a waiver before receiving the item. For Medicare patients, this waiver is called the advance beneficiary notice (ABN). This document must be kept on file in case the Medicare contractor, Medicaid agency, third-party payer, or managed care plan requests proof of the advance notice
- It is recommended that the provider keep a copy of the Certificate of Medical Necessity (CMN) in the patient's medical record. An order or CMN on its own will not justify medical necessity even if the physician signs it
- If a DME Information Form (DIF) is used instead of or in conjunction with the CMN, a copy of the DIF should be kept in the patient's medical record. In some cases, the DIF replaces the CMN for certain DME supplies. The DIF must be signed by the supplier. The DIF contains much of the same information and does not require a narrative description of the equipment, cost, or a physician signature. *See the section below for more information on DIFs*
- Provider records must substantiate the information and answers contained in the CMN

Provider Orders for DMEPOS

Provider orders for DMEPOS usually take the form of clinical record or progress note annotations, or they can take the form of separate, individual orders. These separate orders can be written on:

- Prescription forms
- Internally generated practice DMEPOS order forms
- Forms supplied by the third-party payer for DMEPOS authorization and reimbursement

In any case, a copy of the order may have to accompany the claim to the payer (if a paper claim) or must be retained on file (if an electronic claim).

For DMEPOS items billed to third-party payers, the provider must have documentation that adequately demonstrates the medical necessity of the item. This is true for any medical service. This information must be a permanent part of the patient's medical record, as should the original order for the DMEPOS item.

An order or CMN on its own will not justify medical necessity even if the physician signs it.

In many instances, an entry made directly into the clinical record notes or progress notes can aptly serve as the provider order for the DMEPOS item, especially in situations where the DMEPOS supplier and the health care provider are one and the same. In these cases, the medical record entry must be complete and disclose all of the same information necessary for separate provider order documents.

Face-to-Face Encounter

42 CFR 410.38(g) currently states that "as a requirement for payment, CMS may determine through carrier instructions, or carriers may determine that an item of durable medical equipment requires a written physician order before delivery of the item." For covered items as defined in 42 CFR 410.38(g), a physician must document that the physician, physician assistant (PA), nurse practitioner (NP), or clinical nurse specialist (CNS) had a face-to-face encounter with the beneficiary within six months prior to completing the detailed written order. On claims selected for review if there is no face-to-face encounter, contractors shall deny the claim.

The contractor will ensure that the physician saw the beneficiary (including through the appropriate use of telehealth) and conducted a face-to-face assessment. Face-to-face documentation includes information supporting that the beneficiary was evaluated or treated for a condition that supports the item(s) of DME ordered. If this information is not included, the contractor shall deny the claim. If the physician completed the detailed written order before the face-to-face encounter, the contractor shall deny the claim.

If the DMEPOS item was ordered by a PA, NP, or CNS, the physician must sign or cosign and date the portion of the medical record that indicates that the face-to-face assessment occurred. If this information is not included, the contractor shall deny the claim. (*Medicare Program Integrity Manual*, Pub. 100-08, chap. 05, sec. 5.2.4-5.2.5.2)

Detailed Written Order

Any detailed written order must contain:

- Patient's name; insured's name
- Other patient identifying information (third-party payer ID number, patient's Social Security number, date of birth, patient's address and telephone number)
- DMEPOS item ordered with full description
- DMEPOS options or features that will be billed separately or that may require an upgraded HCPCS Level II code—if these codes are recognized by the payer—for the item
- Expected duration of use of the DMEPOS item; prognosis as it is known at the time of the DMEPOS order
- Patient's diagnosis, including ICD-10-CM code and narrative description
- Start date of DMEPOS order
- Prescribing practitioner's NPI number
- Signature of the ordering practitioner (physician, PA, NP, or CNS)

Medicare requires that the detailed written order be completed after the face-to-face encounter. If the date of the detailed written order is prior to the date of the face-to-face encounter, the claim will be denied. (*Medicare Program Integrity Manual*, Pub. 100-08, chap. 05, sec. 5.2.4-5.2.5.2)

Orders for supplies to be used on a continuing or periodic basis must contain information about the quantities of the supplies needed, frequency of change (for dressings, pads, and so on), and expected duration of use.

If the DMEPOS item is a drug, the order must specify the name of the drug, concentration (if applicable), dosage, frequency of administration, and duration of infusion (if applicable).

Someone other than the physician may complete the detailed description of the item. However, the treating physician must review the detailed description and personally sign and date the order to indicate agreement.

The *Medicare Program Integrity Manual*, Pub. 100-08, chapter 5, section 5.2.2, advises that except as noted below, suppliers may dispense most items of DMEPOS based on a verbal order. This verbal dispensing order must include:

- A description of the item
- The patient's name
- The physician's name
- The start date of the order

Suppliers must maintain written documentation of the verbal order and this documentation must be available to Medicare upon request. For items that are dispensed based on a verbal order, the supplier must obtain a written order that meets the requirements of this section.

Verbal orders are unacceptable for certain DME billable to Medicare. A written order prior to delivery is required for:

- Pressure reducing pads
- Mattress overlays, mattresses, and beds
- Seat lift mechanisms
- TENS units

- Power operated vehicles and power wheelchairs
- Other items as denoted by contractor local or regional coverage decisions

For these items, the supplier must have received a written order that has been both signed and dated by the treating physician before dispensing the item.

If replacement supplies are needed for the use of purchased DMEPOS, the provider must specify on the prescription, or on the CMN, the type of supplies needed and the frequency with which they must be replaced, used, or consumed. "As needed" or "PRN" statements are not acceptable.

A new order is required when:

- There is a change in the order for the accessory, supply, drug, or item
- An item is replaced
- There is a change in the supplier
- The documentation section of a particular medical policy may require a new order on a regular basis (even if there is no change in the order)

For items that require a CMN, and for accessories, supplies, and drugs related to an item requiring a CMN, the CMN may serve as the written order IF the narrative description of the item is detailed enough. This applies to both hard copy and electronic orders and CMNs.

For DMEPOS products that are supplied as refills to the original order, suppliers must not automatically ship the refills, even if authorized by the patient. Suppliers must contact the patient prior to dispensing the refill. This will be done to ensure that the refilled item remains reasonable and necessary, existing supplies are approaching exhaustion, and to confirm any changes or modifications to the order. Contact with the patient or designee regarding refills must take place no sooner than 14 calendar days prior to the delivery or shipping date. The supplier must deliver the refill no sooner than 10 calendar days prior to the end of usage for the current product, regardless of which delivery method is utilized.

Separate Physician and Provider Orders

Suppliers of DMEPOS must conform to the demands of their participating contracts with the various third-party payers. DMEPOS items require an official order signed and dated by the ordering provider. The order must detail the patient's identifying information, including but not limited to a description of the DMEPOS item and the reason the patient requires the DMEPOS prescription. The provider's signature may or may not be a stamp facsimile or other substitute; some payers require an original signature. A faxed copy of the original order is usually sufficient for suppliers to fill the DMEPOS order and submit their claim for the item furnished.

However, in the case of illegible or faded faxed copies of DMEPOS orders, suppliers should insist on the original order being mailed or delivered by courier in prompt fashion. When the payer requires special forms (supplied by the payer) to be completed before the authorization, dispensation, and reimbursement of the DMEPOS item, these forms are generally viewed as a substitution for the provider order. The forms are usually supplied in duplicate or triplicate so the physician or provider has an immediate copy; the copy must become a permanent part of the patient's medical record.

Maintenance of Ordering and Certifying Documentation

The physician who writes the orders, as well as the provider or supplier that furnishes covered ordered items of durable medical equipment, prosthetics, orthotics and supplies (DMEPOS), clinical laboratory, imaging services, or covered ordered or certified home health services, is required to maintain documentation for seven years from the date of service. The parties must provide access to that documentation upon the request of CMS or a Medicare contractor.

The maintained documentation must include written and electronic documents related to written orders, certifications, and requests for payment; the National Provider Identifier (NPI) of the physician who ordered/certified the home health services; and the NPI of the physician or other eligible professional (when permitted) who ordered items of DMEPOS or clinical laboratory or imaging services.

Medicare billing privileges may be revoked if the provider, supplier, physician, or eligible professional (as applicable) fails to maintain this documentation or to furnish this documentation upon request. Documentation cannot be requested for written orders and certifications dated prior to July 6, 2010.

A contractor may request documentation if it has reason to believe that the provider, supplier, physician, or eligible professional is not maintaining the documentation. A request may also be appropriate when:

- The contractor has detected an unusually high number of denied claims, or the Fraud Prevention System has generated an alert with respect to the provider
- The provider has been the subject of a recent Zone Program Integrity Contractor referral
- The provider maintains an elevated surety bond amount

The contractor will prepare and send a request letter to the provider via mail when it believes that a request for documentation is warranted. The provider has 30 calendar days from the date of the contractor's request to respond. If the provider fails to respond within the time limit, the contractor can revoke the provider's Medicare billing privileges and bar reenrollment for one year. (*Medicare Program Integrity Manual,* pub. 100-08, chap. 15, sec. 15.18)

DMEPOS Resources

For additional information on DMEPOS including coding and reimbursement policies and regulations, as well as links to CMS Manuals, Transmittals, DME Medicare Administrative Contractor (MAC) websites, and other information, please visit the Durable Medical Equipment (DME) Center at https://www.cms.gov/Center/Provider-Type/Durable-Medical-Equipment-DME-Center.

For information on the DMEPOS Competitive Bidding Program, visit https://www.cms.gov/medicare/medicare-fee-for-service-payment/dmeposcompetitivebid.

For information on the DMEPOS fee schedule, visit https://www.cms.gov/medicare/medicare-fee-for-service-payment/dmeposfeesched.

Other Selected Topics for Medicare

Below is a list of selected Medicare-related topics and the websites to visit. As policies and fee schedules can change often, please confirm information to ensure claims are reported based on the most current information.

Ambulance Services
https://www.cms.gov/Center/Provider-Type/Ambulances-Services-Center

Appeals:

- Original Medicare (Fee-for-service)
  https://www.cms.gov/Medicare/Appeals-and-Grievances/OrgMedFFSAppeals
- Managed Care
  https://www.cms.gov/medicare/appeals-and-grievances/mmcag

Demonstration Projects
https://www.cms.gov/medicare/demonstration-projects/demoprojectsevalrpts

Electronic Billing and EDI Transactions
https://www.cms.gov/medicare/billing/electronicbillingeditrans

ESRD
https://www.cms.gov/Center/Special-Topic/End-Stage-Renal-Disease-ESRD-Center

Federally Qualified Health Centers (FQHC)
https://www.cms.gov/Center/Provider-Type/Federally-Qualified-Health-Centers-FQHC-Center

Fee Schedules
https://www.cms.gov/medicare/medicare-fee-for-service-payment/feeschedulegeninfo

Fraud and Abuse
https://www.cms.gov/About-CMS/Components/CPI or the Office of Inspector General at https://oig.hhs.gov/fraud/

Glucose Monitor Coverage
https://www.cms.gov/medicare-coverage-database/view/article.aspx?articleId=52464

Home Health
https://www.cms.gov/Medicare/Medicare-Fee-for-Service-Payment/HomeHealthPPS

Home Infusion Therapy
https://www.cms.gov/Medicare/Medicare-Fee-for-Service-Payment/Home-Infusion-Therapy/Overview

Medicare Coverage Topics Medicare Coverage Center
https://www.cms.gov/Center/Special-Topic/Medicare-Coverage-Center

Opioid Treatment Programs (OTP)
https://www.cms.gov/medicare/medicare-fee-for-service-payment/opioid-treatment-program

Pass-Through Payment Status
https://www.cms.gov/Medicare/Medicare-Fee-for-Service-Payment/HospitalOutpatientPPS

Prior Authorization and Pre-Claim Review
https://www.cms.gov/Research-Statistics-Data-and-Systems/Monitoring-Programs/Medicare-FFS-Compliance-Programs/DMEPOS/Prior-Authorization-Process-for-Certain-Durable-Medical-Equipment-Prosthetic-Orthotics-Supplies-Items

Preventive Services
https://www.cms.gov/Medicare/Prevention/PrevntionGenInfo

Prospective Payment Systems
https://www.cms.gov/medicare/medicare-fee-for-service-payment/prospmedicarefeesvcpmtgen

Quality Payment Program (QPP)
https://qpp.cms.gov/

Rural Health Clinics
https://www.cms.gov/Center/Provider-Type/Rural-Health-Clinics-Center

Skilled Nursing Facility (SNF)
https://www.cms.gov/Center/Provider-Type/Skilled-Nursing-Facility-Center

Glossary and Reimbursement Terms

An increasingly complex reimbursement climate means new terminology develops every year. The following glossary includes terms not only used when coding, it includes terms used by major insurers and the federal government.

AAPA. American Academy of Physician Assistants.

AAPC. American Academy of Professional Coders. National organization for coders and billers offering certification (CPC, CPC-H, and CPC-P) based upon physician-, outpatient facility-, or payer-specific guidelines.

AAPCC. Adjusted average per capita cost. Estimated average cost of Medicare benefits for an individual, based upon criteria including age, sex, institutional status, Medicaid, disability, and end-stage renal failure.

AAPPO. American Association of Preferred Provider Organizations.

abduction. Pulling away from a central reference line, such as moving away from the midline of the body.

abduction pillow. Device that immobilizes the hips and legs of hip surgery patients postoperatively.

ABN. Advance beneficiary notice.

abstractor. Person who selects and extracts specific data from the medical record and enters the information into computer files.

accrual. Amount of money set aside to cover a health care benefit plan's expenses based upon estimates using a combination of data, including the claims system and the plan's prior history. In facility accounting, accrual accounting records the expenses as they are incurred and the revenue as it is generated. This contrasts with cash accounting where expenses are recorded only when payment is made or revenues are recorded only when payment is received.

ACLS. Advanced cardiac life support. Certification for health care professionals who have achieved proficiency in providing emergent care of cardiac and respiratory systems and medication management.

ACR. ***1)*** American College of Radiology. ***2)*** Adjusted community rate, calculation of what premium the plan charges to provide Medicare-covered benefits for greater frequency of use by participants.

activities of daily living. Self-care activities often used to determine a patient's level of function such as bathing, dressing, using a toilet, transferring in and out of bed or a chair, continence, eating, and walking.

actuarial assumptions. Characteristics used in calculating the risks and costs of a plan, including age, sex, and occupation of enrollees; location; utilization rates; and service costs.

adduction. Pulling toward a central reference line, such as toward the midline of the body.

adjudication. Processing and review of a submitted claim resulting in payment, partial payment, or denial. In relationship to judicial hearings, it is the process of hearing and settling a case through an objective, judicial procedure.

admission. Formal acceptance of a patient by a health care facility.

ADS. Alternative delivery system. Any health care delivery system other than traditional fee-for-service.

advance beneficiary notice. Written communication with a Medicare beneficiary given before Part B services are rendered, informing the patient that the provider (including independent laboratories, physicians, practitioners, and/or suppliers) believes Medicare will not pay for some or all of the services to be rendered. Form CMS-R-131 (revised 03/2011) may be used for all situations where Medicare payment is expected to be denied.

adverse selection. In health care contracting, the risk of enrolling members who are sicker than assumed and who will utilize expensive services more frequently.

age restriction. In health care contracting, limitation of benefits when a patient reaches a certain age.

age/sex rating. In health care contracting, structuring capitation payments based on members' ages and genders.

aggregate amount. Contracted maximum for which a member is insured for any single event in a health plan.

AHA. American Hospital Association. Health care industry association that represents the concerns of institutional providers. The AHA hosts the National

Uniform Billing Committee (NUBC), which has a formal consultative role under HIPAA. The AHA also publishes *Coding Clinic* for ICD-10 and HCPCS.

AHIMA. American Health Information Management Association. Association of health information management professionals that offers professional and educational services, providing these certifications: RHIA, RHIT, CCS, CCS-P, CCA, CHDA, and CHPS.

Al-Anon, Alateen. Alcoholic support groups.

AMA. American Medical Association. Professional organization for physicians. The AMA is the secretariat of the National Uniform Claim Committee (NUCC), which has a formal consultative role under HIPAA. The AMA also maintains the Current Procedural Terminology (CPT) coding system.

ambulatory surgery. Surgical procedure in which the patient is admitted, treated, and released on the same day.

AMCRA. American Managed Care Review Association.

ANA. American Nursing Association.

AOA. American Osteopathic Association.

AP-DRG. All patient diagnosis-related group. 3M HIS made revisions and adjustments to the DRG system, now referred to as the All Patient DRGs. Early features of AP-DRGs included MDC 24, specifically devoted to HIV, and restructuring of the major diagnostic categories governing newborns.

APA. American Psychiatric Association.

APG. Ambulatory patient group. Reimbursement methodology developed for the Centers for Medicare and Medicaid Services.

apnea. Absence of breathing or breath.

apnea monitor. Device used to monitor breathing during sleep that sounds an alarm if breathing stops for more than the specified amount of time.

appeal. Specific request made to a payer for reconsideration of a denial or adverse coverage or payment decision and potential restriction of benefit reimbursement.

appropriateness of care. Proper setting of medical care that best meets the patient's care or diagnosis, as defined by a health care plan or other legal entity.

APR. Average payment rate. Amount of money CMS could pay an HMO for services provided to Medicare recipients under a risk contract.

ART. Accredited record technician. Former AHIMA certification describing medical records practitioners; now known as a registered health information technician (RHIT).

AS. Associate of Science.

ASN. Associate of Science, Nursing.

ASO. Administrative services only. Contractual agreement between a self-funded plan and an insurance company in which the insurance company assumes no risk and provides administrative services only.

assignment. In medical reimbursement, the arrangement in which the provider submits the claim on behalf of the patient and is reimbursed directly by the patient's plan. By doing so, the provider agrees to accept what the plan pays.

assignment of benefits. Authorization from the patient allowing the third-party payer to pay the provider directly for medical services. Under Medicare, an assignment is an agreement by the hospital or physician to accept Medicare's payment as the full payment and not to bill the patient for any amounts over the allowance amount, except for deductible and/or coinsurance amounts or noncovered services.

at risk. In medical reimbursement, a type of contract between Medicare and a payer or a payer and a provider in which the payer (in the case of Medicare) and the provider (in the case of the payer contracts) gets paid a set amount for care of a patient base. If costs exceed the amount the payer or provider were paid, the patients still receive care during the term of the contract.

attained age. In medical reimbursement, the age of the member as of the last birthday.

auditor. Professional who evaluates a provider's utilization, quality of care, or level of reimbursement.

AWP. ***1)*** Average wholesale price. Pharmaceutical price based on common data that is included in a pharmacy provider contract. ***2)*** Any willing provider. Describing statutes requiring a provider network to accept any provider who meets the network's usual selection criteria.

backlog. In medical reimbursement, the queue of claims that have not been adjudicated.

balance billing. Arrangement prohibited in Medicare regulations and some payer contracts whereby a provider bills the patient for charges not reimbursed by the payer.

basic coverage. Insurance providing coverage for hospital care.

basic health services. Defined set of benefits all federally qualified HMOs must offer enrollees.

BCBS. Blue Cross Blue Shield.

binder. Broad bandage that supports a body part.

board certification. Certification in a particular specialty based on the physician's demonstration of expertise and experience.

boarder. Individual who receives lodging, such as a parent, caregiver, or other family member, who is not a patient but may wish or need to be near the patient.

book of business. Payer's list of clients and contracts.

brace. Orthotic device that supports, in correct position, any moveable body part, and allows for limited movement. Medicare has a strict definition of a brace that includes only rigid or semirigid devices.

BSN. Bachelor of Science, Nursing.

Buck traction. Type of skin traction of the extremities maintained by using an apparatus such as a special splint, applied by dressings to the affected body part. Buck traction may be used on burn patients to hold the arm in a suspended upward position to prevent swelling, reduce skin shrinkage, and allow for greater range of motion with healing.

bundled. ***1)*** Gathering of several types of health insurance policies under a single payer. ***2)*** Inclusive grouping of codes related to a procedure when submitting a claim.

business coalition. Employers who form a cooperative to purchase health care less expensively.

cafeteria plan. Employer's offer of various services of many payers as separate elements in a health care plan.

Cap. ***1)*** Capitation. ***2)*** Contract maximum.

capitation. Contractual agreement whereby the provider is paid a fixed amount for treating enrolled patients regardless of utilization.

carve-out. Medical benefits for a specific type of care considered covered by separate guidelines or not covered by the payer.

case management. Ongoing review of cases by professionals to assure the most appropriate utilization of services

case manager. Medical professional (usually a nurse or social worker) who reviews cases every few days to determine necessity of care and to advise providers on payers' utilization restrictions. Certifies ongoing care.

casting. Material used for encasing a body part to immobilize it for injury repair; usually made from plaster or fiberglass.

casting tape. Material used for molding casts, usually made from fiberglass, but can be composed of plaster strips.

catastrophic case management. Method of reviewing ongoing cases in which the patient sustains catastrophic or extremely costly medical problems.

catchment area. Geographical area from which a health care organization draws its members.

CC. Complication or comorbid condition.

CDC. Centers for Disease Control and Prevention.

census. In medical reimbursement, number and demographics of patients or members.

CERT. Comprehensive error rate testing.

Certificate of Medical Necessity. Form required by Medicare to establish the medical necessity of certain DMEPOS. It is completed by both the physician and the supplier, detailing the medical diagnosis and other information specific to the device ordered.

certification. Approval by a payer's case manager to continue care for a given number of days or visits.

CFR. Code of Federal Regulations.

churning. ***1)*** Performance-based reimbursement system emphasizing provider productivity. ***2)*** When a provider sees a patient more than medically necessary with the intent of generating more revenue.

Civilian Health and Medical Program of the Uniformed Services. Federal program that covered the health benefits for families of all uniformed service employees. The program has been replaced by TRICARE.

CLA. Certified laboratory assistant.

claim. Statement of services rendered requesting payment from an insurance company or a government entity.

claim lag. Time incurred between the date of a claim and its submission for payment.

claim manual. Administrative guidelines used by claims processors to adjudicate claims according to company policy and procedure.

claims manager. Payer's manager who oversees the employee who processes routine claims.

claims reviewer. Payer employee who reviews claims like an auditor, looking at coding, prior authority, contract violations, etc.

CLIA. Clinical Laboratory Improvement Amendments. Requirements set in 1988, CLIA imposes varying levels of federal regulations on clinical procedures. Few laboratories, including those in physician offices, are exempt. Adopted by Medicare and Medicaid, CLIA regulations redefine laboratory testing in regard to laboratory certification and accreditation, proficiency testing, quality assurance, personnel standards, and program administration.

closed claim. Claim for which all apparent benefits have been paid.

closed panel. Arrangement in which a managed care organization contracts providers on an exclusive basis, restricting the providers from seeing patients enrolled in other payers' plans.

closed treatment. Realignment of a fracture or dislocation without surgically opening the skin to reach the site. Treatment methods employed include with or without manipulation and with or without traction.

CMA. Certified medical assistant.

CMN. Certificate of medical necessity.

CMP. Competitive medical plan. Federal designation allowing plans to obtain eligibility to receive a Medicare risk contract without having to qualify as an HMO.

CMS. Centers for Medicare and Medicaid Services. Federal agency that administers the public health programs.

CMS-1500. Universal form used to file professional claims.

COA. Certificate of authority. State license to operate as an HMO.

COB. Coordination of benefits. In health care contracting, method of integrating benefits payable when there is more than one group insurance plan so that the insured's benefits and the payment of insurance benefits from all sources do not exceed 100 percent of the allowed medical expenses.

COBRA. Consolidated Omnibus Reconciliation Act. Federal law that allows and requires past employees to be covered under company health insurance plans for a set premium, allowing individuals to remain insured when their current plan or position has been terminated.

coder. Professional who translates documented, written diagnoses and procedures into numeric and alphanumeric codes.

coding conventions. Each space, typeface, indentation, and punctuation mark determining how ICD-10-CM codes are interpreted. These conventions were developed to help match correct codes to the diagnoses documented.

coinsurance. Percentage of the allowed charges paid by a beneficiary toward the cost of care.

collagen. Protein based substance of strength and flexibility that is the major component of connective tissue, found in cartilage, bone, tendons, and skin.

collar. Device that encircles the neck to immobilize it, provide support, and/or severely limit its mobility.

commercial carriers. For-profit insurance companies issuing health coverage.

common working file. System of local databases containing total beneficiary histories developed by CMS to improve Medicare claims processing. Medicare fiscal intermediaries, and/or carriers, interact with these databases to obtain data on eligibility, utilization, Medicare secondary payer (MSP), and other detailed claims information.

community rating. Methodology of state and federal governments that require qualified HMOs to request the same amount of money for each member in a plan.

comparative performance report. Report that provides an annual comparison of a physician's services and procedures with those of another physician in the same specialty and geographic area.

complex repair. Surgical closure of a wound requiring more than layered closure of the deeper subcutaneous tissue and fascia (i.e., debridement, scar excision, placement of stents or retention sutures, and sometimes site preparation or undermining that creates the defect requiring complex closure).

complication. Condition arising after the beginning of observation and treatment that modifies the course of the patient's illness or the medical care required, or an undesired result or misadventure in medical care.

component code. In the National Correct Coding Initiative (NCCI), the column II code that cannot be charged to Medicare when the column I code is reported.

component coding. Coding a service that represents only a portion of the entire service provided, meant to standardize the reporting of interventional radiology services. Component coding allows a physician, regardless of specialty, to specifically identify and report those aspects of the service he or she provided, whether the procedural component, the radiological component, or both.

comprehensive codes. In the National Correct Coding Initiative (NCCI), the column I code that is reported to Medicare and precludes reporting column II codes.

consultation. Advice or opinion regarding diagnosis and treatment or determination to accept transfer of care of a patient rendered by a medical professional at the request of the primary care provider.

continuity of coverage. In health care contracting, transfer of benefits from one plan to another without a lapse in coverage.

continuous positive airway pressure device. Pressurized device used to maintain the patient's airway for spontaneous or mechanically aided breathing. Often used for patients with mild to moderate sleep apnea.

contractor. Entity who enters into a contractual agreement with CMS to service a component of the Medicare program administration, for example, fiscal intermediaries, carriers, program safeguard coordinators.

conversion. In health care contracting, shifting a member under a group contract to an individual contract in accordance with contract terms and occurring with a change in employer benefits or when the covered person leaves the group.

conversion factor. ***1)*** Dollar value for each relative value unit. When this dollar amount is multiplied by the total relative value units, it yields the reimbursement rate for the service. ***2)*** National multiplier that converts the geographically adjusted relative value units into Medicare fee schedule dollar amounts that applies to all services paid under the MPFS.

coordinated care. In health care contracting, system of health care delivery that influences utilization, quality of care, and cost of services. Managed care integrates financing and management with an employed or contracted organized provider network that delivers services to an enrolled population.

copayment. Cost-sharing arrangement in which a covered person pays a specified portion of allowed charges. In relation to Medicare, the copayment designates the specific dollar amount that the patient must pay and coinsurance designates the percentage of allowed charges.

Correct Coding Initiative. Official list of codes from the Centers for Medicare and Medicaid Services' (CMS) National Correct Coding Policy Manual for Medicare Services that identifies services considered an integral part of a comprehensive code or mutually exclusive of it.

corridor deductible. Fixed out-of-pocket amount the member must pay before benefits are available.

COT. Certified ophthalmic technician.

COTA. Certified occupational therapy assistant.

counseling. Discussion with a patient and/or family concerning one or more of the following areas: diagnostic results, impressions, and/or recommended diagnostic studies; prognosis; risks and benefits of management (treatment) options; instructions for management (treatment) and/or follow-up; importance of compliance with chosen management (treatment) options; risk factor reduction; and patient and family education.

Coverage Issues Manual. Revised and renamed the National Coverage Determination Manual in the CMS manual system, it contained national coverage decisions and specific medical items, services, treatment procedures, or technologies paid for under the Medicare program. This manual has been converted to the Medicare National Coverage Determinations Manual (NCD manual), Pub. 100-03.

covered charges. Charges for medical care and supplies that are medically necessary and met coverage and program guidelines.

covered person. Any person entitled to benefits under the policy, whether a member or dependent.

CPR. Cardiopulmonary resuscitation. Substitutionary action made for both the heart and lungs in sudden death cases by artificial respiration and external cardiac compression.

CPT. Current Procedural Terminology. Definitive procedural coding system developed by the American Medical Association that lists descriptive terms and identifying codes to provide a uniform language that describes medical, surgical, and diagnostic services for nationwide communication among physicians, patients, and third parties, used in outpatient reporting of services.

CPT codes. Codes maintained and copyrighted by the AMA and selected for use under HIPAA for noninstitutional and nondental professional transactions.

CPT modifier. Two-character code used to indicate that a service was altered in some way from the stated CPT or HCPCS Level II description, but not enough to change the basic definition of the service.

credentialing. ***1)*** Reviewing the medical degrees, licensure, malpractice, and any disciplinary record of medical providers for panel and quality assurance purposes and to grant hospital privileges. ***2)*** Coding certification.

CRNA. Certified registered nurse anesthetist. Nurse trained and specializing in the administration of anesthesia. Anesthesia services rendered by a CRNA must be reported with HCPCS Level II modifier QX, QY, or QZ.

crosswalk. Cross-referencing of CPT codes with ICD-10-CM, anesthesia, dental, or HCPCS Level II codes.

CRT. Certified respiratory therapist.

CSO. Clinical service organization. Health care organization developed by academic medical centers to integrate medical school, faculty practice plan, and hospital.

CST. Certified surgical technologist.

CTLSO. Cervical-thoracic-lumbar-sacral orthosis.

custom fitted. Premanufactured orthotics that can be adjusted to fit the patient by bending, trimming, or other minimal efforts.

cutback. Reduction of the amount or type of insurance for a member who attains a specified age or condition (e.g., age 65, retirement).

daily benefit. Specified maximum benefit payable for room and board charges at a hospital.

DAW. Dispense as written. Notation from a physician to a pharmacist requesting that the brand name medication be given in lieu of a generic medication.

DC. ***1)*** Doctor of chiropractic medicine. ***2)*** Discontinue. ***3)*** Direct current.

decubitus ulcer. Progressively eroding skin lesion produced by inflamed necrotic tissue as it sloughs off caused by continual pressure to a localized area, especially over bony areas, where blood circulation is cut off when a patient lies still for too long without changing position.

deductible. Predetermined dollar amount of covered billed charges that the patient must pay toward the cost of care.

diagnosis. Determination or confirmation of a condition, disease, or syndrome and its implications.

diagnostic. Examination or procedure to which the patient is subjected, or which is performed on materials derived from a hospital outpatient, to obtain information to aid in the assessment of a medical condition or the identification of a disease. Among these examinations and tests are diagnostic laboratory services such as hematology and chemistry, diagnostic x-rays, isotope studies, EKGs, pulmonary function studies, thyroid function tests, psychological tests, and other tests given to determine the nature and severity of an ailment or injury.

direct contract model. Plan that contracts directly with individual private practice physicians rather than through an intermediary.

disarticulation. Removal of a limb through a joint.

discharge plan. Treatment plan by the provider for continued patient care after discharge that may include home care, the services of case managers or other health care providers, or transfer to another facility.

discharge status. Disposition of the patient at discharge (e.g., left against medical advice, discharged home, transferred to an acute care hospital, expired).

discharge transfer. Discharge of a patient from one facility to another.

disposition of patient. Description of the patient's status and destination at discharge (e.g., discharged to home) used for data and quality assurance purposes.

DME. Durable medical equipment. Medical equipment that can withstand repeated use, is not disposable, is used to serve a medical purpose, is generally not useful to a person in the absence of a sickness or injury, and is appropriate for use in the home. Examples of durable medical equipment include hospital beds, wheelchairs, and oxygen equipment.

DME MAC. Durable medical equipment Medicare administrative contractor. Entity where claims for specific DMEPOS must be submitted for processing and reimbursement.

DMEPOS. Durable medical equipment, prosthetics, orthotics, and supplies.

DO. Doctor of osteopathy.

DOS. Date of service. In health care contracting, day the encounter or procedure is performed or the day a supply is issued.

DPM. Doctor of podiatric medicine.

drug formulary. List of prescription medications preferred for use by a health plan and dispensed through participating pharmacies to covered persons.

dual option. Offering of an HMO and traditional plan by one carrier.

dual-lead device. Implantable cardiac device (pacemaker or implantable cardioverter-defibrillator [ICD]) in which pacing and sensing components are placed in only two chambers of the heart.

DUR. Drug utilization review. Review to assure prescribed medications are medically necessary and appropriate.

DVM. Doctor of Veterinary Medicine.

dynamic flexion device. Highly specialized orthotic brace that allows for a controlled range of motion of a joint or joints during postoperative or post-traumatic convalescence.

e.g.. For example.

E/M. Evaluation and management services. Assessment, counseling, and other services provided to a patient and reported through CPT codes.

E/M service components. Key components in determining the correct level of E/M codes are history, examination, and medical decision-making.

EAP. Employee assistance program. Services designed to help employees, their family members, and employers find solutions for workplace and personal problems that affect morale, productivity, or financial issues such as workplace stress, family/marital concerns, legal or financial problems, elder care, child care, substance abuse, emotional/stress issues, and other daily living concerns.

ecchymosis. Bruise.

EdD. Doctor of education.

EDI. Electronic data interchange. Transference of claims, certifications, quality assurance reviews, and utilization data via computer in X12 format. May refer to any electronic exchange of formatted data.

EHO. Emerging healthcare organizations. Hospitals and other providers that are emerging or affiliating.

electronic media claim. Automated claims processing method that uses a data storage tool to transfer claims data to the payer. EMC has been replaced by electronic data interchange (EDI).

emergency department. Organized hospital-based facility for the provision of unscheduled episodic services to patients who present for immediate medical attention. The facility must be available 24 hours a day.

emergency outpatient. Patient admitted for diagnosis and treatment of a condition requiring immediate attention but who will not stay at that facility or be transferred to another.

EMT. Emergency medical technician.

EMT-P. Paramedic.

encounter. Direct personal contact between a registered hospital outpatient (in a medical clinic or emergency department, for example) and a physician (or other person authorized by state law and hospital bylaws to order or furnish services) for the diagnosis and treatment of an illness or injury. Visits with more than one health professional that take place during the same session and at a single location within the hospital are considered a single visit.

enrollee. In medical reimbursement, person who subscribes to a specific health plan.

enrollment. Number of lives covered by the plan.

enteral nutrition. Feeding of a nutrient mixture directly into or just proximal to the upper end of the small bowel via a tube or through an existing stoma. Patients are usually able to absorb the nutrients.

EOB. Explanation of benefits. Statement mailed to the member and provider explaining claim adjudication and payment.

EOMB. Explanation of Medicare benefits. Explanation of Medicaid benefits. Explanation of member benefits. Typically sent to the provider and the patient, an explanation of how Medicare, Medicaid, or member benefits were paid, that is, the allowable amount paid, the coinsurance due to the provider or payable by the patient, or the reason why a claim may have been rejected or paid less or more than the original amount charged.

episode of care. One or more health care services received during a period of relatively continuous care by a hospital or health care provider.

EPO. ***1)*** Epoetin alpha. ***2)*** Exclusive provider organization. In health care contracting, an organization similar to an HMO, but the member must remain within the provider network to receive benefits. EPOs are regulated under insurance statutes rather than HMO legislation.

ERISA. Employee Retirement Income Security Act of 1974, Public Law 93-406. Mandates reporting, disclosure of grievance and appeals requirements, fiduciary standards for private group life and health plans, and preempts state benefit mandates and premium tax laws for self-funded group health plans.

ESRD. End stage renal disease. Progression of chronic renal failure to lasting and irreparable kidney damage that requires dialysis or renal transplant for survival.

established patient. ***1)*** Patient who has received professional services in a face-to-face setting within the last three years from the same physician/qualified health care professional or another physician/qualified health care professional of the exact same specialty and subspecialty who belongs to the same group practice. ***2)*** For OPPS hospitals, patient who has been registered as an inpatient or outpatient in a hospital's provider-based clinic or emergency department within the past three years.

exclusions. Services excluded from a plan's coverage by the employer or payer because of risk or cost.

experience rating. In medical reimbursement, designation of a group's previous claims history to help determine premium rates.

explanation of benefits. Statement mailed to the member and provider explaining claim adjudication and payment.

explanation of Medicare benefits. Medicare statement mailed to the member and provider explaining claim adjudication and payment.

extrication collar. Cervical collar with opening at the throat for patients who have a tracheotomy or tracheostomy.

fab fragment. Immunoglobulin molecule fragment that is antigen binding with a light and heavy chain.

facility. Place of patient care, including inpatient and outpatient, acute or long term.

fact-oriented V codes. Codes that do not describe a problem or a service; they simply state a fact. These generally do not serve as an outpatient primary or inpatient principal diagnosis.

FAR. Federal acquisition regulations. Regulations of the federal government's acquisition of services.

FDA. Food and Drug Administration. Federal agency responsible for protecting public health by substantiating the safety, efficacy, and security of human and veterinary drugs, biological products, medical devices, national food supply, cosmetics, and items that give off radiation.

Federal Register. Government publication listing changes in regulations and federally mandated standards, including coding standards such as HCPCS Level II and ICD-10-CM.

federally qualified HMO. HMO that meets CMS guidelines for Medicare reimbursement.

fee for service. Payment model where each service performed is individually paid. Fee-for-service arrangements may be discounted or undiscounted rates.

fee schedule. List of codes and related services with pre-established billing amounts by a provider, or payment amounts by a payer that could be percentages of billed charges, flat rates, or maximum allowable amounts established by third-party payers. Medicare fee schedules apply to clinical laboratory, radiology, and durable medical equipment services.

FEHB. Federal Employee Health Benefits Program. Provides health plans to federal workers.

FEHBAR. Federal Employee Health Benefits Acquisition Regulations. Federal regulations for acquisition of health services used by government agencies and subcontractors.

FFS. Fee for service. ***1)*** Payment for services, usually physician services, on a service-by-service basis rather than an alternative payment system like capitation. Fee-for-service arrangements may be discounted or undiscounted rates. ***2)*** Situation in which the payer pays full charges for medical services.

FO. Finger orthosis.

formulary. List of prescription medications preferred for use by the health plan and dispensed through participating pharmacies to covered persons.

fraternal insurance. Cooperative plan provided to members of an association or fraternal group.

FTE. Full time employee. Accounting equivalent of one full time employee that includes wages, benefits, and other costs.

gatekeeper. Primary care physician in a health care system in which a member's care must be provided by a primary care physician unless the physician refers the member to a specialist or approves the care provided by a specialist.

GHAA. Group Health Association of America. HMO trade organization.

global surgery package. Services included in a surgical procedure that include all of the elements needed to perform the procedure and routine follow-up care.

gm. Gram.

government mandates. Services mandated by state or federal law.

grace period. Set number of days past the due date of a premium payment during which medical coverage may not be canceled and the premium payment may be made, or after employment termination. It varies by health plan contract and state law but is generally 30 to 60 days.

group model. HMO that contracts with a group of providers.

group practice. Group of providers that shares facilities, resources, and staff, and who may represent a single unit in a managed care network.

HCl. Hydrochloric acid.

HCPCS. Healthcare Common Procedure Coding System. ***HCPCS Level I:*** Healthcare Common Procedure Coding System Level I. Numeric coding system used by physicians, facility outpatient departments, and ambulatory surgery centers (ASC) to code ambulatory, laboratory, radiology, and other diagnostic services for Medicare billing. This coding system contains only the American Medical Association's Current Procedural Terminology (CPT) codes. ***HCPCS Level II:*** Healthcare Common Procedure Coding System Level II. National coding system, developed by CMS, that contains alphanumeric codes for physician and nonphysician services not included in the CPT coding system. HCPCS Level II codes cover such things as ambulance services, durable medical equipment, and orthotic and prosthetic devices. ***HCPCS modifiers:*** Two-character alpha or alphanumeric code that identifies circumstances that alter or enhance the description of a service or supply. They are recognized by carriers nationally.

Hct. Hematocrit.

Health Insurance Portability and Accountability Act of 1996. Federal law that allows persons to qualify immediately for comparable health insurance coverage when they change their employment relationships. Title II, subtitle F, of HIPAA gives the Department of Health and Human Services the authority to mandate the use of standards for the electronic exchange of health care data; to specify what medical and administrative code sets should be used within those standards; to require the use of national identification systems for health care patients, providers, payers (or plans), and employers (or sponsors); and to specify the types of measures required to protect the security and privacy of personally identifiable health care information.

heel cup. Plastic or rubber cup that fits into the back portion of the patient's shoe to provide protection, support, and stabilization.

HFO. Hand-finger orthosis.

HHA. Home health agency. Health care provider, licensed under state or local law, that provides skilled nursing and other therapeutic services. HHAs include visiting nurse associations and hospital-based home care programs. To participate in Medicare, an HHA must meet health and safety standards established by the U.S. Department of Health and Human Services (HHS). Home health services usually are provided in the patient's home, although some outpatient services performed in a hospital, SNF or rehabilitation center may be covered under home health if the equipment is required and cannot be used in the patient's home.

HHS. Health and Human Services. Cabinet department that oversees the operating divisions of the federal government responsible for health and welfare. HHS oversees the Centers for Medicare and Medicaid Services, Food and Drug Administration, Public Health Service, and other such entities.

HIAA. Health Insurance Association of America. Trade organization for payers.

hierarchy. Ranking or ordering of information or people.

HIPAA. Health Insurance Portability and Accountability Act of 1996. Federal law that allows persons to qualify immediately for comparable health insurance coverage when they change their employment relationships. Title II, subtitle F, of HIPAA gives the Department of Health and Human Services the authority to mandate the use of standards for the electronic exchange of health care data; to specify what medical and administrative code sets should be used within those standards; to require the use of national identification systems for health care patients, providers, payers (or plans), and employers (or sponsors); and to specify the types of measures required to protect the security and privacy of personally identifiable health care information.

HKAFO. Hip-knee-ankle foot orthosis.

HMO. Health maintenance organization. Medical health insurance coverage that pays claims based on a provider cost, per diem, or charge basis. Hospitals contract with an HMO to provide care at a contractually reduced price. HMO members pay a set monthly amount for coverage and are treated without additional cost, except for a copayment or deductible amount, payable by the patient. Like all managed care organizations, HMOs use a variety of mechanisms to control costs, including utilization management, discounted provider fee schedules, and financial incentives. HMOs use primary care physicians as gatekeepers and tend to emphasize preventive care.

hold harmless. Contractual clause stating that if either party is held liable for malpractice, the other party is absolved.

home health. Palliative and therapeutic care and assistance in the activities of daily life to home bound Medicare and private plan members.

horseshoe. U-shaped device that stabilizes or immobilizes the patella when used with a knee orthosis.

hospice. Organization that furnishes inpatient, outpatient, and home health care for the terminally ill. Hospices emphasize support and counseling services for terminally ill people and their families, pain relief, and symptom management. When the Medicare beneficiary chooses hospice benefits, all other Medicare benefits are discontinued, except physician services and treatment of conditions not related to the terminal illness.

hypopnea. Abnormal respiratory event lasting at least 10 seconds, with at least a 30 percent reduction in thoracoabdominal movement or airflow as compared to a baseline, and with at least a 4 percent oxygen desaturation.

IA. Intra-arterial.

IBNR. Incurred but not reported. Amount of money the payer's plan accrues to forestall unknown medical expenses.

ICD-10. International Classification of Diseases, 10th Revision. Classification of diseases by alphanumeric code, used by the World Health Organization.

ICD-10-CM. International Classification of Diseases, 10th Revision, Clinical Modification. Clinical modification of the alphanumeric classification of diseases used by the World Health Organization, already in use in much of the world, and used for mortality reporting in the United States.

ICF. Intermediate care facility. Health care facility that furnishes services to patients who do not require the degree of care provided by a hospital or skilled nursing facility or a step-down facility for patients who are leaving the hospital but who cannot be discharged to home because of continuing medical needs.

ID card. Wallet card carried by a plan member providing name, member and group numbers, effective dates, deductibles, and other information.

immobilizer. Device used to restrain a part of the body, keeping the body part from moving.

implant. Material or device inserted or placed within the body for therapeutic, reconstructive, or diagnostic purposes.

in plan. Services chosen from a network provider.

incontestable clause. Provision in a policy that prohibits the plan from disputing coverage for certain conditions after a specified period of time.

INF. ***1)*** Inferior. ***2)*** Infusion.

infusion pump. Device that delivers a measured amount of drug or intravenous solution through injection over a period of time.

inpatient hospitalization. Period in which a patient is housed in a single hospital usually without interruption.

insoles. Rubber or plastic orthotics that fit inside the shoes to correct a deformity or help aid in the healing of an injury.

insurance carrier. Insurer or health plan that may underwrite, administer, or sell a range of health benefit programs.

intermediate repair. ***1)*** Surgical closure of a wound requiring closure of one or more of the deeper subcutaneous tissue and non-muscle fascia layers in addition to the skin. ***2)*** Contaminated wounds with single layer closure that need extensive cleaning or foreign body removal.

internal skeletal fixation. Repair involving wires, pins, screws, and/or plates placed through or within the fractured area to stabilize and immobilize the injury.

IOL. Intraocular lens.

IPA. Individual practice association. Organization made up of providers who, along with the rest of a group, contract with payers at a discounted fee-for-service or capitated rate.

IPO. Individual practice organization. Organization made up of providers who, along with the rest of a group, contract with payers at a discounted fee-for-service or capitated rate.

IS. Information services. Administrators of the computer systems used by payers and providers.

IV. ***1)*** Intravenous. ***2)*** Cranial nerve on the brainstem responsible for motor control of the superior oblique muscle (trochlear).

JCAHO. Joint Commission on Accreditation of Healthcare Organizations. Organization that accredits health care organizations. In the future, the JCAHO may play a role in certifying these organizations' compliance with the HIPAA A/S requirements. Previously known as the Joint Commission for the Accreditation of Hospitals.

JD. Doctor of jurisprudence.

KAFO. Knee-ankle-foot orthosis. External apparatus utilized to improve motor control, gait stabilization, and reduce pain. The device is attached to the leg in order to help correct flexible deformities and to halt the progression of fixed deformities.

key components. Three components of history, examination, and medical decision making are considered the keys to selecting the correct level of E/M codes. In most cases, all three components must be addressed in the documentation. However, in established, subsequent, and follow-up categories, only two of the three must be met or exceeded for a given code.

KOH. Potassium hydroxide.

lapse. Terminated policy.

late effect. Abnormality, dysfunction, or other residual condition produced after the acute phase of an illness, injury, or disease is over. There is no time limit on when late effects can appear.

LCD. Local coverage determination. Published decision by a Medicare contractor regarding coverage guidelines for a particular service and is valid only in the contractor's jurisdiction. LCDs replaced local medical review policies for CMS as of 2006.

LCSW. Licensed clinical social worker.

limiting charge. Maximum amount a nonparticipating physician or provider can charge for services rendered to a Medicare patient.

limits. In medical reimbursement, the ceiling for benefits payable under a plan.

line of business. Different health plans offered by a larger insurer or insurance broker as a product line.

lives. Unit of measurement used by plans to determine the number of people covered. Calculated by multiplying the number of members by 2.5.

local coverage determination. Decision of coverage and related usage specific to a Medicare administrative contractor (MAC), fiscal intermediary or carrier, or in a designated geographic area.

long-term care facility. Nursing home or, more specifically, a facility offering extended, nonacute care to a resident patient whose illness does not require acute care.

loss ratio. Ratio between the cost to deliver medical care and the amount of money taken in by the plan.

LPN. Licensed practical nurse.

LSO. Lumbar sacral orthosis.

LVN. ***1)*** Licensed visiting nurse. ***2)*** Licensed vocational nurse.

MA. ***1)*** Master of arts degree. ***2)*** Medical assistant. ***3)*** Mental age.

MAC. Medicare administrative contractor. One of 15 jurisdictional organizations that contract with CMS to adjudicate professional claims under Part A and Part B, responsible for daily claims processing, utilization review, record maintenance, dissemination of information based on CMS regulations, and whether services are covered and payments are appropriate. Four of the jurisdictions also include home health services. There are four separate MAC jurisdictions for DME services.

malingering. Feigning of illness, as the result of intentional deceit or as the result of mental illness.

managed health care. ***1)*** Managing active cases to ensure care is the most appropriate, efficient, and effective. ***2)*** System of health care meant to manage overall cost. ***3)*** Method of health care whereby contracted physicians participate in managing health care costs.

mandated benefits. Services mandated by state or federal law such as child abuse or rape, not necessarily covered by insurers.

maximum allowable charge. Amount set by the insurer as the highest amount that can be charged for a particular medical service or by a pharmacy vendor.

mcCi. Microcurie.

MCE. Medical care evaluation.

mcg. Microgram.

mCi. Millicurie.

MCO. Managed care organization. Generic term for various health benefit plans that provide coverage for health care services in conjunction with management and review of services provided to ensure that services are medically necessary and appropriate.

MD. Medical doctor.

ME. Medical examiner.

MEd. Master of education.

Medicaid. Joint federal and state program that covers medical expenses for people with low incomes and limited resources who meet the criteria. The benefits for recipients vary from state to state.

medical consultation. Advice or an opinion rendered by a physician at the request of the primary care provider.

medical loss ratio. Ratio between the cost to deliver medical care and the amount of money taken in by the plan.

medical necessity. Medically appropriate and necessary to meet basic health needs; consistent with the diagnosis or condition and national medical practice guidelines regarding type, frequency, and duration of treatment; rendered in a cost-effective manner.

Medicare. Federally funded program authorized as part of the Social Security Act that provides for health care services for people age 65 or older, people with disabilities, and people with end-stage renal disease (ESRD).

Medicare administrative contractor. Uniform type of Medicare administrative entity that processes both institutional and professional claims in specified geographic jurisdictions of the country. There are 15 A/B MACs that are scheduled to be combined into a total of 10 A/B MACS, while maintaining four DME MACs, and four home health/hospice MACs.

Medicare fee schedule. Fee schedule based upon physician work, expense, and malpractice designed to slow the rise in cost for services and standardize payment to physicians regardless of specialty or location of service with geographic adjustments.

Medicare Part A. Hospital insurance coverage that includes hospital, nursing home, hospice, home health, and other inpatient care. Claims are submitted to intermediaries for reimbursement.

Medicare Part B. Supplemental medical insurance that includes outpatient hospital care and physician and other qualified professional care. Claims from providers or suppliers other than a hospital are submitted to carriers for reimbursement. Hospital outpatient claims are submitted to their FI/MAC.

Medicare secondary payer. Specified circumstance when other third-party payers have the primary responsibility for payment of services and Medicare is the secondary payer. Medicare is secondary to workers' compensation, automobile, medical no-fault and liability insurance, EGHPs, LGHPs, and certain employer health plans covering aged and disabled beneficiaries. The MSP program prohibits Medicare payment for items or services if payment has been made or can reasonably be expected to be made by another payer, as described above.

Medicare supplement. Private insurance coverage that pays the Medicare deductible and copayments and may also pay the costs of services not covered by Medicare.

Medigap policy. Health insurance or other health benefit plan offered by a private company to those entitled to Medicare benefits. The policy covers charges not payable by Medicare because of deductibles, coinsurance amounts, or other Medicare-imposed limitations.

member. In medical reimbursement, subscriber of a health plan.

member months. In medical reimbursement, total of months each member was covered.

member services. In health care contracting, the payer department that works as a patient advocate to solve problems and may take claims appeals to a final committee after all other processes have been exhausted.

mental health substance abuse. Payer term for services rendered to members for emotional problems or chemical dependency.

mental or nervous. Payer term for services rendered to members for emotional problems or chemical dependency.

mEq. Milliequivalent.

MeSH. Medical staff-hospital organization.

MET. Multiple employer trust. Group of employers that join together to purchase health insurance using a self-funded approach to lower costs by the broadening membership pool to prevent an adverse selection.

MEWA. Multiple employer welfare association. Group of employers that join together to purchase health insurance using a self-funded approach to lower costs by the broadening membership pool to prevent an adverse selection.

mg. Milligram.

MHA. Master of health administration.

minor procedure. Self-limited procedure, usually with an assignment of 0 or 10 follow-up days by payers. A minor procedure may be considered by many payers to be part of the global package for a primary surgical service and cannot be billed separately from the primary procedure.

MIS. Management information system. Hardware and software facilitating claims management.

mixed model. HMO that includes both an open panel and closed panel option.

ml. Milliliter.

MLP. Midlevel practitioners. Professionals such as nurse practitioners, nurse midwives, physical therapists, physician assistants, and others who provide medical care but do so with physician input.

MLT. Medical laboratory technician.

modality. ***1)*** Form of imaging (e.g., x-ray, fluoroscopy, ultrasound, nuclear medicine, duplex Doppler, CT, and MRI). ***2)*** Any physical agent applied to produce therapeutic changes to biologic tissue including, but not limited to, thermal, acoustic, light, mechanical, or electric energy.

modifier. Two characters that can be appended to a HCPCS code as a means of identifying circumstances that alter or enhance the description of a service or supply.

morbidity rate. In health care contracting, an actuarial term describing predicted medical expense rate.

MP. Metacarpal phalangeal.

MPH. Master of public health. Advanced degree.

MSA. Medical savings account.

MSN. Master of science in nursing.

MSW. Master's in social work.

MT. ***1)*** Medical technologist. ***2)*** Medical transcriptionist.

multiple birth. Two or more infants delivered at the same time.

multiple employer group. Group of employers who contract together to subscribe to a plan, broadening the risk pool and saving money. Different from a multiple employer trust.

multiple-lead device. Implantable cardiac device (pacemaker or implantable cardioverter-defibrillator [ICD]) in which pacing and sensing components are placed in at least three chambers of the heart.

NA. Nurse assistant.

NAHMOR. National Association of HMO Regulators.

NAIC. National Association of Insurance Commissioners. Organization of state insurance regulators.

national coverage determination. National policy statement regarding the circumstances under which a service, item, or test is considered reasonable and necessary or otherwise not covered for Medicare purposes.

National Supplier Clearinghouse. Entity that approves providers and medical equipment vendors as "suppliers" under the Medicare program, issuing an identification number to approved applicants.

national supplier identification number. Number with which providers or other health care professionals who disperse DMEPOS submit their claims. This number is obtained through an application to the National Supplier Clearinghouse, a centralized agency for DMEPOS suppliers.

NBICU. Newborn intensive care unit. Special care unit for premature and seriously ill infants.

NCD. National coverage determinations. National policy statements granting, eliminating, or excluding Medicare coverage for a service, item, or test and indicate CMS policy regarding the circumstances under which the service, item, or test is considered reasonable and necessary or otherwise not covered for Medicare purposes.

NCHS. National Center for Health Statistics. Division of the Centers for Disease Control and Prevention that compiles statistical information used to guide actions and policies to improve the public health of U.S. citizens. The NCHS maintains the ICD-10-CM coding system.

NCQA. National Committee for Quality Assurance. Organization that accredits managed care plans, or HMOs. In the future, the NCQA may play a role in certifying these organizations' compliance with the HIPAA A/S requirements.

ND. Doctor of naturopathy.

nebulization device. Device used to vaporize liquid medication for the airborne delivery of the medication to the patient. The medication is absorbed into the body via the respiratory tract. Medications can also be administered with a nebulizer to fragment and mobilize thick, excess mucous in the respiratory tract; these medications are broadly termed mucolytics.

NEC. Not elsewhere classifiable. Condition or diagnosis that is not provided with its own specified code in ICD-10-CM, but included in a more broadly defined code for other specified conditions.

neonatal period. Period of an infant's life from birth to the age of 27 days, 23 hours, and 59 minutes.

network model. Plan that contracts with multiple groups of providers, or networks, to provide care.

new patient. Patient who is receiving face-to-face care from a provider/qualified health care professional or another physician/qualified health care professional of the exact same specialty and subspecialty who belongs to the same group practice for the first time in three years. For OPPS hospitals, a patient who has not been registered as an inpatient or outpatient, including off-campus provider based clinic or emergency department, within the past three years.

NOS. Not otherwise specified. Condition or diagnosis remains ill-defined and is unspecified without the necessary information for selecting a more specific code.

NP. ***1)*** Nurse practitioner. ***2)*** Neuropsychiatry.

NPI. National provider identifier. Standard eight-digit alphanumeric provider identifier implemented under the Health Insurance Portability and Accountability Act of 1996 (HIPAA) requirements. The first seven digits identify the provider and the eighth position is a check digit. Providers are required to report their NPI number for electronic and paper billing.

O_2. Oxygen.

occupational therapy. Training, education, and assistance intended to assist a person who is recovering from a serious illness or injury perform the activities of daily life.

OIG. Office of Inspector General. Agency within the Department of Health and Human Services that is ultimately responsible for investigating instances of fraud and abuse in the Medicare and Medicaid and other government health care programs. OIG work plan Annual plan released by the Office of Inspector General (OIG) that details the areas of focus for fraud and abuse investigations.

open enrollment period. Time period during which subscribers in a health benefit program have the opportunity to re-enroll or select an alternative health plan being offered to them, usually without evidence of insurability or waiting periods.

open panel. Arrangement in which a managed care organization that contracts with providers on an exclusive basis is still seeking providers.

OPL. Other party liability. In coordination of benefits, the decision that the other plan is the primary plan.

orthosis. Derived from a Greek word meaning "to make straight," it is an artificial appliance that supports, aligns, or corrects an anatomical deformity or improves the use of a moveable body part. Unlike a prosthesis, an orthotic device is always functional in nature.

orthotic. Associated with the making and fitting of an orthosis(es).

osteogenesis stimulator. Device used to stimulate the growth of bone by electrical impulses or ultrasound.

ostomy. Artificial (surgical) opening in the body used for drainage or for delivery of medications or nutrients.

OTR. Occupational therapist registered.

OUD. Opioid use disorder.

out of plan. In health care contracting, services of a provider who is not a member of the preferred provider network.

out of service area. In health care contracting, medical care received out of the geographic area that may or may not be covered, depending on the plan.

outpatient. Person who has not been admitted as an inpatient but who is registered on the hospital or CAH records as an outpatient and receives services (rather than supplies alone) directly from the hospital or CAH. (Code of Federal Regulations, section 410.*2)*

outpatient visit. Encounter in a recognized outpatient facility.

overutilization. Services rendered by providers more frequently than usual.

PA. ***1)*** Physician assistant. Medical professional who receives additional training and can assess, treat, and prescribe medications under a physician's review. ***2)*** Posteroanterior. ***3)*** Pulmonary artery. ***4)*** HCPCS Level II modifier used to denote a surgical or other invasive procedure that was performed on the wrong body part.

paneled. In health care contracting, provider contracted with an HMO.

par provider. Provider who is participating in a health plan or Medicare program.

parenteral nutrition. Nutrients provided subcutaneously, intravenously, intramuscularly, or intradermally for patients during the postoperative period and in other conditions, such as shock, coma, and renal failure.

partial disability. Congenital or acquired inability to perform part of one's job.

partial hospitalization. Situation in which the patient only stays part of each day over a long period. Cardiac, rehabilitation, and chronic pain patients, for example, could use this service.

partial payment. Payment to a provider or member with the expectation that other payments will be forthcoming before the claim is closed.

PATOS. Payment (received) at the time of service.

PBM. Prescription benefit managers. HMO staff who monitor amount and use of drugs prescribed.

PCP. Primary care physician. Physician who makes an initial diagnosis and referral and retains control over the patient and utilization of services both in and outside of the plan.

pediatric patient. Patient usually younger than 14 years of age.

peer review. Evaluation of the quality of the total health care provided by medical staff with equivalent training, such as a physician-to-physician or nurse-to-nurse evaluation.

PEPM. Per employee per month.

PEPP. Payment error prevention program. Program to help reduce Medicare PPS inpatient hospital payment errors.

per diem reimbursement. In health care contracting, reimbursement to an institution based on a set rate per day rather than on a charge-by-charge basis.

percutaneous skeletal fixation. Treatment that is neither open nor closed and the injury site is not directly visualized. Fixation devices (pins, screws) are placed through the skin to stabilize the dislocation using x-ray guidance.

pessary. Device placed in the vagina to support and reposition a prolapsing or retropositioned uterus, rectum, or vagina.

PharmD. Doctor of pharmacy.

PhD. Doctor of philosophy.

PHO. Physician-hospital organization.

physician assistant. Medical professional who receives additional training and can assess, treat, and prescribe medications under a physician's review.

PIN. Physician identification number.

plan manager. Payer employee managing all of the contracts and contract negotiations for one or more specific plans.

PMPM. Per member per month.

PMPY. Per member per year.

pneumatic splint. Splint filled with air or gas to provide circumferential protection and support.

pooling. Health payers' practice of combining risk.

POS. Point of service. Health benefit plan allowing the covered person to choose to receive a service from a participating or nonparticipating provider, with different benefit levels associated with the use of participating providers.

posting date. Date a charge is posted to a patient account by the provider, frequently not the same as the actual date of service, but usually within five days of the actual date of service.

PPA. Preferred provider arrangement. Similar to a PPO.

PPO. Preferred provider organization. Program that establishes contracts with providers of medical care. Usually the benefit contract provides significantly better benefits and lower member cost for services received from preferred providers, encouraging covered persons to use these providers, who may be reimbursed on a discounted basis.

PPS. Prospective payment system. Reimbursement methodology that uses predetermined rates for each type of discharge, procedure, service, or item based on a standard type of case. For hospital inpatients, the Medicare PPS system of DRGs was implemented in 1983 to hold down the rising cost of health care. For hospital outpatients, OPPS has been based on ambulatory payment classifications effective August 1, 2000. For skilled nursing facilities, it is based on the RUG-IV system, and for home health it is based on the HHRGs.

precertification. Confirmation that a payer covers a given procedure for a given patient, including admission or continued stay.

preexisting condition. Symptom that causes a person to seek diagnosis, care, or treatment for which medical advice or treatment was recommended or received by a physician within a certain time period before the effective date of medical insurance coverage. The preexisting condition waiting period is the time the beneficiary must wait after buying health insurance before coverage begins for a condition that existed before coverage was obtained.

prehensile. Ability to grasp, seize, or hold.

presenting problem. Disease, condition, illness, injury, symptom, sign, finding, complaint, or other reason for the patient encounter

primary care. Basic or general health care, traditionally provided by family practice, pediatrics, and internal medicine practitioners.

primary diagnosis. Current, most significant reason for the services or procedures provided.

principal diagnosis. Condition established after study to be chiefly responsible for occasioning the admission of the patient to the hospital for care.

principal procedure. Procedure performed for definitive treatment rather than for diagnostic or exploratory purposes, or that was necessary to treat a complication. Usually related to the principal diagnosis.

prodrug. Inactive drug that goes through a metabolic process when given resulting in a chemical conversion that changes the drug into an active pharmacological agent.

professional association plans. Plan provided by a professional association that affords self-employed professionals (e.g., physicians, CPAs, lawyers) less expensive coverage.

program safeguard coordinator. Contractor charged with maintaining the integrity of the Medicare program. Duties include data analysis, audit, review, and monitoring related to beneficiary information (such as COB data), medical review, cost reports, provider education, and fraud detection and prevention.

prosthetic. Device that replaces all or part of an internal body organ or body part, or that replaces part of the function of a permanently inoperable or malfunctioning internal body organ or body part.

provider. All-inclusive, generic term for people or institutions that provide health care. The provider may be a physician, hospital, pharmacy, other facility, or other health care provider.

PSC. Program safeguard coordinators.

PT. Physical therapy.

PTA. Physical therapy assistant.

PTMPY. Per thousand members per year.

QA. Quality assurance. Monitoring and maintenance of established standards of quality for patient care.

QM. Quality management. Monitoring and maintenance of established standards of quality.

RAC. Recovery Audit Contractors.

RBRVS. Resource-based relative value scale. Fee schedule introduced by CMS to reimburse physician Medicare fees based on the amount of time and resources expended in treating patients with adjustments for overhead costs and geographical differences.

reasonable and customary. Fees charged for medical services that are considered normal, common, and in line with the prevailing fees in the provider's geographical area.

referral. Approval from the primary care physician to see a specialist or receive certain services. May be required for coverage purposes before a patient receives care from anyone except the primary physician.

rehabilitation. Restoration of physical and mental functions to allow the usual daily activities of life.

reimbursement. Payment of actual charges or allowable incurred as a result of accident or illness.

reinsurance. Insurance purchased by an HMO, insurance company, or self-funded employer from another insurance company to protect itself against all or part of the losses that may be incurred in the process of honoring the claims of its participating providers, policy holders, or employees and covered dependents.

residual limb. Portion of an arm or leg that remains attached to the body after an amputation.

review committee. Multidisciplinary committee that considers denied cases being appealed, catastrophic cases, or fee-for-service cases.

RHIA. Registered health information administrator. Accreditation for medical record administrators, previously known as a registered records administrator (RRA), through AHIMA.

RHIT. Registered health information technician. Accreditation for medical records practitioners, previously known as accredited records technician (ART), through AHIMA.

rib belt. Device that encircles the abdomen and provides support for injured ribs while they heal.

risk contract. Contract between Medicare and a payer or a payer and a provider in which the payer (in the case of Medicare) and the provider (in the case of the payer contracts) receive a set amount for care of a patient base. If costs exceed the amount the payer or provider was paid, the patients still receive care during the term of the contract.

risk factor reduction. Reduction of risk in the pool of health plan members.

risk manager. Person charged with keeping financial risk low, including malpractice cases.

risk pool. Pool of people who will be in the insured group, their medical and mental histories, other factors such as age, and their predicted health.

RN. Registered nurse.

RPh. Registered pharmacist.

RPT. Registered physical therapist.

RRA. Registered records administrator.

RRT. Registered respiratory therapist.

rush charge. Charge for expeditious test results.

RVS. Relative value study. Guide that shows the relationship between the time, resources, competency, experience, severity, and other factors necessary to perform procedures that is multiplied by a dollar conversion factor to determine a monetary value for the procedure.

RVU. Relative value unit. Value assigned a procedure based on difficulty and time consumed. Used for computing reimbursement under a relative value study.

SACH. Solid ankle, cushion heel.

sanction. Imposition of penalties or exclusion of a provider for fraud or infractions such as an inappropriate use of services, providing procedures that may harm the patient, or applying inferior techniques.

schedule. Listing of amounts payable for specific procedures.

second opinion. Medical opinion obtained from another health care professional, relevant to clinical evaluation, before the performance of a medical service or surgical procedure. Includes patient education regarding treatment alternatives and/or to determine medical necessity.

secondary insurer. In a COB arrangement, the insurer that reimburses for benefits pending after payment by the primary insurer.

self-funded plan. Plan where the risk is assumed by the employer rather than the insurer. The employer generally pays claims directly from a general fund account that may be managed by a third party.

self-insured. Individual or organization that assumes the financial risk of paying for health care.

self-pay patients. Patients who pay for medical care out-of-pocket.

SEO. Shoulder-elbow orthosis.

service date. Date a charge is incurred for a service.

service plan. ***1)*** Plan that has contracts with providers but is not a managed care plan. ***2)*** Another name for Blue Cross/Blue Shield plans.

shadow pricing. Setting rates just below a competitor's rates. Maximizes profits but raises medical costs.

simple repair. Surgical closure of a superficial wound, requiring single layer suturing of the skin (epidermis, dermis, or subcutaneous tissue).

skeletal traction. Applying direct pulling force on the long axis of bones by inserted wires or pins and using weights and pulleys to keep the bone in proper alignment.

skin traction. Application of a pulling force to a limb accomplished by a device fixed to felt dressings or strappings applied to the body surface.

small subscriber group aggregate. Aggregate of professional associations, small business, or other entities formed to be considered a single, large subscriber group.

SNF. Skilled nursing facility. Institution or a distinct part of an institution that is primarily engaged in providing skilled nursing care and related services for residents who require medical or nursing care; or rehabilitation services for the rehabilitation of injured, disabled, or sick persons.

SO. ***1)*** Shoulder orthosis. ***2)*** Sacroiliac orthosis.

SOF. Signature on file.

softgoods or soft goods. DMEPOS industry term for medical devices such as braces, splints, joint supports and protectors, cervical pillows, and other similar orthopaedic-oriented items.

specimen. Tissue cells or sample of fluid taken for analysis, pathologic examination, and diagnosis.

splint. Brace or support for an anatomical structure after surgery or injury.

split inventory technique. Keeping highly-utilized DMEPOS easily accessible to staff, while keeping surplus in a central storage area.

SSA. Social Security Act.

SSN. Social security number.

staff model. HMO that employs its own providers.

standard anesthesia formula. Reimbursement formula that consists of base units plus time units plus modifying units (e.g., physical status and qualifying circumstances) plus other allowed unit/charges that is multiplied by a conversion factor.

stat charge. Charge for expeditious test results.

state insurance commission. State group that approves insurance certificates for each state and regulates the industry based on statutes.

steering. Providing financial incentives to plan members to use the managed care provider panel.

stockinet. Material used to wrap an injured body part before applying a cast; usually of breathable material to wick moisture away from skin.

stop loss. In health care contracting, a form of reinsurance that protects health insurance above a certain limit and minimizes risks for providers.

subrogation. Recovery of monies or benefits from a third party who is liable for the payment.

subsidiary codes. Services that are not included as part of the primary procedure but that are not performed alone and may be identified as each additional, or list-in-addition-to services. Phrases that help identify subsidiary codes include, but are not limited to: each additional, list in addition to, and done at time of other major procedure

subtraction. Process of using an image to remove an overlying structure in another image to better visualize the area underneath the overlying structure.

superbill. Multipurpose sheet used for all patient encounters that typically contains a check-off list of ICD-10-CM diagnosis codes, evaluation and management codes, and procedure and HCPCS Level II codes in the outpatient setting.

supplemental health services. Optional services that a health plan may cover or provide.

support. Article that provides stabilization, but not immobilization, to an injured or disabled body part.

surgical package. Normal, uncomplicated performance of specific surgical services, with the assumption that, on average, all surgical procedures of a given type are similar with respect to skill level, duration, and length of normal follow-up care.

TCC. Transitional care center. Facility used in lieu of an extended care facility or before discharge to an extended care facility.

technical component. Portion of a health care service that identifies the provision of the equipment, supplies, technical personnel, and costs attendant to the performance of the procedure other than the professional services.

TEFRA. Tax Equity and Fiscal Responsibility Act. Protects the rights of full-time employees to remain on the company's health plan to age 69.

terminal device. Addition to an upper limb prosthesis that replaces the function and/or appearance of a missing hand.

tertiary care facility. Hospital providing specialty care to patients referred from other hospitals because of the severity of their injuries or illnesses.

therapeutic. Act meant to alleviate a medical or mental condition.

therapeutic procedure. Treatment of a pathological or traumatic condition through the use of activities performed to treat or heal the cause or to effect change through the application of clinical skills or services that attempt to improve function.

therapeutic services. Services performed for treatment of a specific diagnosis. These services include performance of the procedure, various incidental elements, and normal, related follow-up care.

thermoplastic. Item that can be softened by heat, but hardens upon cooling.

third-party administrator. Firm that performs administrative functions for a self-funded plan but assumes no risk.

third-party payer. Public or private organization that pays for or underwrites coverage for health care expenses for another entity, usually an employer (e.g., Blue Cross Blue Shield, Medicare, Medicaid, commercial insurers).

THKAO. Thoracic-hip-knee-ankle orthosis.

time limit. In health care contracting, a set number of days in which a claim can be filed according to the payer or state insurance commission.

TPA. Third-party administrator. Firm that performs administrative functions for a self-funded plan but assumes no risk.

TPL. Third party liability. Payer liable for the cost of an illness or injury, such as auto or homeowner insurer.

TQM. Total quality management. Concept that quality is an organic part of a plan's service and a provider's care and can be quantified and constantly improved.

traction. Drawing out or holding tension on an area by applying a direct therapeutic pulling force.

transaction standard. Set of rules, conditions, or requirements describing the classification and components or a transaction. Transaction standards define the data elements and code sets that must be used in a transaction.

transcutaneous electrical nerve stimulator. Device that delivers a controlled amount of electricity to an area of the body to stimulate healing and/or to mitigate post-surgical or post-traumatic pain.

transfer. Situation in which the patient is transferred to another acute care hospital for related care.

treatment plan. Plan of care established by the provider outlining specific deficits and planned treatment that may be submitted to the case manager when seeking certification for a plan member.

triage. Medical screening of patients to determine priority of treatment based on severity of illness or injury and resources at hand.

triple option. Offering of an HMO, indemnity plan, and preferred provider organization by one insurance firm.

type A emergency department. Emergency department licensed and advertised to be available to provide emergent care 24 hours a day, seven days a week. Type A emergency departments must meet both the CPT book definition of an emergency department and the EMTALA definition of a dedicated emergency department.

type B emergency department. Emergency department licensed and advertised to provide emergent care less than 24 hours a day, seven days a week. Type B emergency departments must meet the EMTALA definition of a dedicated emergency department.

uCi. Microcurie.

UCR. Usual, customary, and reasonable. Fees charged for medical services that are considered normal, common, and in line with the prevailing fees in a given geographical area.

unbundling. Separately packaging costs or services that might otherwise be billed together including billing separately for health care services that should be combined according to the industry standards or commonly accepted coding practices.

underwriting. Evaluating and determining the financial risk a member or member group has on an insurer.

unlisted procedure. Procedural descriptions used when the overall procedure and outcome of the procedure are not adequately described by an existing procedure code. Such codes are used as a last resort and only when there is not a more appropriate procedure code.

unspecified. Codes for use when documentation is insufficient to assign a more specific code.

upcoding. Practice of billing a code that represents a higher reimbursement than the code for the procedure actually performed.

URAC. Utilization Review Accreditation Commission. Accrediting body of case management.

urgent admission. Admission in which the patient requires immediate attention for treatment of a physical or psychiatric problem.

USP. United States pharmacopoeia.

USPHS. United States Public Health Service.

utilization review. Formal assessment of the medical necessity, efficiency, and/or appropriateness of health care services and treatment plans on a prospective, concurrent, or retrospective basis.

utilization review nurse. Nurse who evaluates cases for appropriateness of care and length of service and can plan discharge and services needed after discharge.

volume. ***1)*** Number of services performed. ***2)*** Number of patients. ***3)*** Number of patients in a DRG during a specific time.

weighting. Assigning more worth to a fee based on the number of times it is charged, weighting the resource-based relative value fees for an area.

withhold. Percentage of payment to providers held by an HMO until the cost of referral or services has been determined. If the provider goes over the amount determined appropriate, the HMO keeps that amount.

workers' compensation. State-governed system designated to administer and regulate the provision and cost of medical treatment and wage losses arising from a worker's job-related injury or disease, regardless of who is at fault. In exchange, the employer is protected from being sued.

wraparound plan. Insurance or health plan coverage for copays and deductibles not covered under a member's base plan.

ZPIC. Zone Program Integrity Contractor. CMS contractor that replaced the existing Program Safeguard Contractors (PSC). Contractors are responsible for ensuring the integrity of all Medicare-related claims under Parts A and B (hospital, skilled nursing, home health, provider, and durable medical equipment claims), Part C (Medicare Advantage health plans), Part D (prescription drug plans), and coordination of Medicare-Medicaid data matches (Medi-Medi).

HCPCS Lay Descriptions

A

A0021

A0021 Ambulance service, outside state per mile, transport (Medicaid only)

This code represents a per mile charge for ambulance transportation outside of the state where the ambulance provider is based and is reported only for Medicaid claims. Consult the local Medicaid office in the state that the provider is located for further definition and usage requirements.

A0080-A0210

A0080 Nonemergency transportation, per mile - vehicle provided by volunteer (individual or organization), with no vested interest

A0090 Nonemergency transportation, per mile - vehicle provided by individual (family member, self, neighbor) with vested interest

A0100 Nonemergency transportation; taxi

A0110 Nonemergency transportation and bus, intra- or interstate carrier

A0120 Nonemergency transportation: mini-bus, mountain area transports, or other transportation systems

A0130 Nonemergency transportation: wheelchair van

A0140 Nonemergency transportation and air travel (private or commercial) intra- or interstate

A0160 Nonemergency transportation: per mile - caseworker or social worker

A0170 Transportation ancillary: parking fees, tolls, other

A0180 Nonemergency transportation: ancillary: lodging-recipient

A0190 Nonemergency transportation: ancillary: meals, recipient

A0200 Nonemergency transportation: ancillary: lodging, escort

A0210 Nonemergency transportation: ancillary: meals, escort

These codes provide for reporting nonemergency transportation and related ancillary services. Different types of vehicles used and/or the areas traveled, as well as additional fees are specified in these codes. This range reports nonemergency transport services such as a vehicle provided by a volunteer or family member; wheelchair van, taxi, bus, or air transport (private or commercial); mountainous area transport, or transportation outside the state. Examples of ancillary services include parking fees and tolls, lodging or meals for the recipient or for the escort, and per mile transportation of a caseworker or social worker.

A0225

A0225 Ambulance service, neonatal transport, base rate, emergency transport, one way

Report this code for the emergency transport of a neonate by ambulance, one way only, at base rate.

A0380

A0380 BLS mileage (per mile)

A basic life support (BLS) ambulance provides transportation plus the equipment and staff needed for basic life support services, such as controlling bleeding, splinting fractures, treating shock, delivering babies, and performing cardio-pulmonary resuscitation (CPR). BLS transport is reported on a per mile basis.

A0382

A0382 BLS routine disposable supplies

Basic life support (BLS) routine disposable supplies include such items as cervical collar, gauze, dressings, and ice packs. Report a unit of one for all routine disposable supplies that are used.

A0384

A0384 BLS specialized service disposable supplies; defibrillation (used by ALS ambulances and BLS ambulances in jurisdictions where defibrillation is permitted in BLS ambulances)

Specialized disposable basic life support (BLS) defibrillation supplies include such items as defibrillator electrodes (AED), pacing pads, combination pads, and gel pads. This code is reported in jurisdictions where defibrillation is permitted in BLS ambulances.

A0390

A0390 ALS mileage (per mile)

Advanced life support (ALS) mileage is paid on a per mile basis based on the patient's condition. Some local governments may require an ALS response for all calls, but Medicare pays only for the level of service provided, and only when the service is medically necessary. This applies to ground and air transports.

A0392

A0392 ALS specialized service disposable supplies; defibrillation (to be used only in jurisdictions where defibrillation cannot be performed in BLS ambulances)

Specialized disposable advanced life support (ALS) defibrillation supplies include such items as defibrillator electrodes (AED), pacing pads, combination pads, and gel pads.

A0394

A0394 ALS specialized service disposable supplies; IV drug therapy

Specialized disposable advanced life support (ALS) IV drug therapy supplies include items such as IV start kits, IV tubing, disposable armboard, catheter, pump sets, micro drip, and Y-site tubing. Report this code once for all IV drug therapy supplies used.

A0396

A0396 ALS specialized service disposable supplies; esophageal intubation

Specialized disposable advanced life support (ALS) esophageal intubation supplies, which are used for airway management, include such items as esophageal obturator, esophageal gastric tube, stylette, inflation syringe, endotracheal tube, laryngoscope blade, cricotracheotomy kits, and disposable bag valve mask.

A0398

A0398 ALS routine disposable supplies

Advanced life support (ALS) routine disposable supplies include such items as EKG electrodes, cervical collar, gauze, and dressings. Report a unit of one for all routine disposable supplies that are used.

A0420

A0420 Ambulance waiting time (ALS or BLS), one-half (1/2) hour increments

This code reports ambulance waiting time for both BLS and ALS services. Time is reported in one-half hour increments. Do not report waiting time of less than one-half hour. Report one unit for each half-hour increment or portion thereof for waiting times of one-half hour or more.

A0422

A0422 Ambulance (ALS or BLS) oxygen and oxygen supplies, life sustaining situation

This code reports the oxygen and oxygen supplies used in a life-sustaining situation during ambulance transportation (ALS or BLS). There are two levels of ambulance service, basic medical care or basic life support (BLS) and advanced emergency medical care or advanced life support (ALS).

A0424

A0424 Extra ambulance attendant, ground (ALS or BLS) or air (fixed or rotary winged); (requires medical review)

This code reports charges for an additional ambulance attendant for both ground (BLS and ALS) and air (fixed wing and rotary transports). The need for an additional ambulance attendant must be substantiated by report.

A0425

A0425 Ground mileage, per statute mile

This code reports ground mileage. Mileage and reimbursement rates are generally defined by and under the jurisdiction of state statutes.

A0426-A0427

A0426 Ambulance service, advanced life support, nonemergency transport, level 1 (ALS 1)

A0427 Ambulance service, advanced life support, emergency transport, level 1 (ALS 1 - emergency)

Advanced life support, non-emergency transport, level 1 (ALS 1) is the transportation by ground ambulance vehicle and the provision of medically necessary supplies and services. Report these codes for advanced life support, emergency ambulance transport, level 1 (ALS 1-emergency), which includes the provision of an ALS assessment or at least one ALS intervention. Advanced life support intervention means a procedure that is in accordance with state and local laws, beyond the scope of authority of an emergency medical technician-basic (EMT-basic).

A0428-A0429

A0428 Ambulance service, basic life support, nonemergency transport, (BLS)

A0429 Ambulance service, basic life support, emergency transport (BLS, emergency)

Basic life support, non-emergency transport (BLS) is transportation by ground ambulance vehicle and the provision of medically necessary supplies and services, including BLS ambulance services as defined by state laws. The ambulance must be staffed by an individual who is qualified in accordance with state and local laws as an emergency medical technician-basic (EMT-basic). These laws may vary from state to state or within a state. For example, only in some jurisdictions is an EMT-basic permitted to operate limited equipment on board the vehicle, assist more qualified personnel in performing assessments and interventions, and establish a peripheral intravenous (IV) line.

A0430-A0431

A0430 Ambulance service, conventional air services, transport, one way (fixed wing)

A0431 Ambulance service, conventional air services, transport, one way (rotary wing)

Fixed wing (FW) ambulance (airplane) conventional air service is the transportation by a fixed wing aircraft that is certified by the Federal Aviation Administration (FAA) as a fixed wing air ambulance along with the provision of medically necessary services and supplies. Rotary wing (RW) ambulance (helicopter) conventional air service is the transportation by helicopter that is certified by the Federal Aviation Administration (FAA) as a rotary wing ambulance, including the provision of medically necessary supplies and services.

A0432

A0432 Paramedic intercept (PI), rural area, transport furnished by a volunteer ambulance company which is prohibited by state law from billing third-party payers

Paramedic intercept (PI) services are advanced life support (ALS) services provided with the ambulance transport by a volunteer ambulance company that is prohibited from doing any third-party billing by state laws. Report this code for PI services provided in a rural area.

A0433

A0433 Advanced life support, level 2 (ALS 2)

Advanced life support, level 2 (ALS 2) is the transportation by ground ambulance vehicle and the provision of medically necessary supplies and services including at least three separate administrations of one or more medications by intravenous push/bolus or by continuous infusion (excluding crystalloid fluids), or ground ambulance transport and the provision of at least one ALS 2 procedure, such as manual defibrillation/cardioversion, endotracheal intubation, central venous line, cardiac pacing, chest decompression, surgical airway, or intraosseous line.

A0434

A0434 Specialty care transport (SCT)

Specialty care transport (SCT) is hospital-to-hospital transportation of a critically injured or ill beneficiary by a ground ambulance vehicle, including the provision of medically necessary supplies and services, at a level of service beyond the scope of the EMT paramedic. SCT is necessary when a beneficiary's condition requires ongoing care that must be furnished by one or more health professionals in an appropriate specialty area (e.g., emergency or critical care nursing, emergency medicine, respiratory care, cardiovascular care, or a paramedic with additional training).

A0435-A0436

A0435 Fixed wing air mileage, per statute mile

A0436 Rotary wing air mileage, per statute mile

Report these codes for each statutory mile a patient is transported in a fixed wing or a rotary wing aircraft.

A0888

A0888 Noncovered ambulance mileage, per mile (e.g., for miles traveled beyond closest appropriate facility)

Mileage for an ambulance trip is covered only to the nearest appropriate facility. However, there are instances when a beneficiary requests to be transported to a facility that is not the closest appropriate facility. In these situations, there is additional mileage that is not covered. Report this code for these additional, noncovered miles. This policy applies to both ground and air ambulance services.

A0998

A0998 Ambulance response and treatment, no transport

Report this code when an ambulance is dispatched and treatment is provided to the patient without the patient being transported to another site.

A0999

A0999 Unlisted ambulance service

This code is reported for any ambulance service that is not described by other HCPCS Level II codes. It should be reported as a last resort and only when there is not a more appropriate procedure code. When reporting an unlisted code, provide a detailed explanation of the services in remarks, billing notes, or as an attachment.

A2001

A2001 InnovaMatrix AC, per sq cm

InnovaMatrix™ AC is a skin substitute created from extracellular matrix (ECM) found in porcine placenta. The material is processed to remove all cells and then dehydrated. This leaves a matrix or scaffold material that the body uses to surround cells, binding it to tissue and replacing ECM. ECM is a necessary component in wound healing. InnovaMatrix™ AC is used to treat nonhealing wounds such as diabetic, venous, and pressure ulcers, as well as second-degree burns and other traumatic wounds. After debriding the wound of necrotic, damaged, or infected tissue, the provider applies InnovaMatrix™ AC to the wound and a small area of surrounding tissue. The dehydrated sheet is fixed into place using the provider's preferred method of fixation and rehydrated with sterile saline. The wound is covered with a nonadherent dressing and covered with a secure secondary dressing. InnovaMatrix™ AC is absorbed and forms a gel, leaving ECM material. It may be reapplied every seven days over the top of the ECM gel.

A2002

A2002 Mirragen Advanced Wound Matrix, per sq cm

Mirragen® Advanced Wound Matrix is a synthetic, resorbable skin substitute made of biocompatible and resorbable borate-based glass fibers and particulates. The material covers the wound, absorbs exudate, and provides a matrix or scaffold material that the body uses for revascularization and soft tissue regeneration. It is used to treat nonhealing wounds such as diabetic, venous, and pressure ulcers, as well as second-degree burns and other traumatic wounds. After debriding the wound of necrotic, damaged, or infected tissue, the provider ensures the wound and/or product is moistened with sterile saline and applies Mirragen® to the wound, filling areas of tunneling or undermining first, and conforming the material to the wound shape. The wound is covered with a secondary dressing that will maintain a moist environment. Mirragen® should reapplied every three to seven days depending on wound location, moisture/leakage, size and depth, and the frequency of other therapies.

A2004

A2004 XCelliStem, 1 mg

XCelliStem® is a proprietary blend of extracellular matrix (ECM) materials, derived from multiple porcine sources, used to provide a matrix or scaffold material that the body uses for revascularization and soft tissue regeneration. The product easily conforms to irregular wound shapes and can be used to treat wounds such as diabetic, venous, and pressure ulcers, as well as second-degree burns, tunneled/undermined wounds, partial and full-thickness wounds, and other surgical/traumatic wounds. Code A2004 represents 1 mg of product.

A2005

A2005 Microlyte Matrix, per sq cm

Microlyte® Matrix is a wound dressing made of bioresorbable polyvinyl alcohol with a polymeric surface coating that contains ionic and metallic silver, which helps prevent or minimize microbial growth. The product absorbs wound fluid and forms a matrix that conforms to the surface of the wound, helping to maintain a moist environment. Microlyte® Matrix can be used to treat wounds such as diabetic, venous, and pressure ulcers, as well as second-degree burns and other traumatic wounds. After debriding the wound of necrotic, damaged, or infected tissue, the provider ensures the wound and/or product is moistened with sterile saline and applies the matrix to the wound. The wound is covered with a secondary dressing that will maintain a moist environment. Microlyte® Matrix should be evaluated weekly for reapplication. Products containing iodophore should not be used with Microlyte® Matrix as they may reduce the effectiveness of the silver.

A2006

A2006 NovoSorb SynPath dermal matrix, per sq cm

NovoSorb® SynPath is a synthetic dermal matrix comprised of a porous network of nontoxic, biodegradable synthetic polymers that acts as a scaffold to support the proliferation of cells involved in cellular repair. After preparing the wound, the matrix is applied directly to the surface of the wound and the provider secures it in place using their choice of fixation. A temporary, nonbiodegradable sealing membrane is applied over the matrix to limit moisture loss and prevent infection. The wound is then covered with a secondary closure. It is intended to treat wounds such as diabetic, venous, and pressure ulcers, as well as second-degree burns and other traumatic wounds.

A2007

A2007 Restrata, per sq cm

Restrata® is synthetic, resorbable fiber matrix that resembles human extracellular matrix (ECM) and acts as a scaffold material the body uses for revascularization and soft tissue regeneration. The matrix is cut to the desired wound shape and applied to the wound bed, rehydrated, and anchored with the provider's preferred fixation method. After application, the wound is covered with a secondary closure. Restrata® should be reapplied approximately every seven days, as necessary. It is intended to treat wounds such as diabetic, venous, and pressure ulcers, as well as second-degree burns and other traumatic wounds.

A2008

A2008 TheraGenesis, per sq cm

TheraGenesis® is a bilayered wound matrix comprised of a biodegradable porcine tendon-derived atelocollagen layer and a silicone film layer. The collagen matrix acts as a scaffold material the body uses for revascularization and soft tissue regeneration. The silicone layer contains a nonadhesive mesh that helps better adhere the matrix and chosen fixation to the wound. It is intended to treat wounds such as diabetic, venous, and pressure ulcers, as well as second-degree burns and other traumatic wounds.

A2009

A2009 Symphony, per sq cm

Symphony™ is a bioengineered skin substitute that is composed of ovine-derived extracellular matrix (ECM) and hyaluronic acid (HA). It consists of three layers with more than 150 ECM proteins that aid in the wound healing process. It is intended for use in acute and chronic wounds.

A2010

A2010 Apis, per sq cm

Apis® is an absorbable, biodegradable skin substitute comprised of gelatin (porcine derived), Manuka honey, and hydroxyapatite. Skin substitutes are used to protect large or nonhealing wounds or burns.

A2011

A2011 Supra SDRM, per sq cm

Supra SDRM® is a synthetic, resorbable skin substitute made of a tripolymer of polylactide, trimethylene carbonate, E-caprolactone, and polyvinyl alcohol. The material has a microporous structure that provides a protective barrier, allowing the wound to heal and enabling growth of blood vessels. It adheres to the wound bed without direct fixation and should be covered with a secondary, nonadherent mesh dressing. Supra SDRM® is indicated for the treatment of nonhealing wounds such as ulcers, partial- and full-thickness wounds, partial-thickness burns, as well as other traumatic and surgical wounds. It may be reapplied every seven days or as needed. It is available in sizes ranging from 1 x 1 cm to 18 x 18 cm.

A2012

A2012 SUPRATHEL, per sq cm

SUPRATHEL® is a synthetic, resorbable skin substitute made of a tripolymer of polylactide, trimethylene carbonate, and E-caprolactone. The material is highly permeable to oxygen and water vapor, providing an environment favorable for wound healing. It is fully malleable at room temperature, more pliable at body temperature, and can be conformed three dimensionally, which allows application over multiple anatomical orientations. SUPRATHEL® is indicated for the treatment of nonhealing wounds such as split-thickness skin graft donor sites, partial- and full-thickness wounds, burns, as well as other traumatic and surgical wounds. It may be reapplied every seven days or as needed. It is available in four sheet sizes: 5 x 5 cm, 9 x 10 cm, 18 x 10 cm, and 18 x 23 cm.

A2013

A2013 Innovamatrix FS, per sq cm

InnovaMatrix FS is a skin substitute created from a biomaterial found in porcine placental tissue. The material is processed to remove all cells and then dehydrated. This leaves a matrix or scaffold material that the body uses to surround cells, binding it to tissue and replacing extracellular matrix (ECM). ECM is a necessary component in wound healing. It is intended for the treatment of nonhealing wounds such as diabetic, venous, and pressure ulcers, partial- and full-thickness wounds, surgical and traumatic wounds, as well as second-degree burns. The product is fully absorbable and does not require removal. It is supplied in a variety of sizes of fenestrated sheets.

A2014

A2014 Omeza Collagen Matrix, per 100 mg

Omeza Collagen Matrix is a wound care matrix derived from hydrolyzed fish collagen infused with cod liver oil. The matrix acts as an anhydrous skin protectant and is naturally incorporated into the wound over time. It is indicated for the treatment of partial- and full-thickness wounds that are surgical or traumatic; burns; venous, vascular, diabetic, or pressure ulcers; and draining wounds. It is supplied in 1.6 g (2 ml) vials and is spread evenly across the wound bed. No more than two vials should be used in one day and no more than four vials should be used in one week. It should not be used in patients with known sensitivity to fish collagen or cod liver oil and should not be used for the treatment of third-degree burns.

A2015

A2015 Phoenix Wound Matrix, per sq cm

Phoenix Wound Matrix is a 3D electrospun synthetic polymer matrix that consists of bioresorbable synthetic polymers that degrade into alpha-hydroxy and fatty acids that aid in the acceleration of wound healing. It is indicated for the treatment of partial to full-thickness acute and chronic burns and other wounds, including venous, vascular, diabetic, or pressure ulcers, surgical and traumatic wounds, and second-degree burns. The sheet can be trimmed to fit the wound size and applied and rinsed with sterile saline, covered with a nonadherent dressing, and a secondary dressing is applied to provide adherence and protect the wound. The matrix can be reapplied every seven to 14 days, as needed. It is supplied in a 16 mm disc, and sheets in sizes ranging from 2.5 cm X 2.5 cm to 10 cm X 20 cm.

A2016-A2018

A2016 PermeaDerm B, per sq cm
A2017 PermeaDerm Glove, each
A2018 PermeaDerm C, per sq cm

PermeaDerm is a biosynthetic temporary skin substitute comprised of a nylon mesh with silicone. The mesh contains slits in the membrane that allows the provider to adjust porosity by stretching it from zero to the amount required by the specific wound. Through the slits, exudate escapes and is captured by a secondary dressing. It is also transparent, allowing providers to inspect the wound without removing the skin substitute. Three forms are currently available: PermeaDerm B, PermeaDerm C, and PermeaDerm Glove. B and Glove are intended for use in the treatment of donor site wounds, partial thickness burns, and meshed autograft coverage. C is intended for use in the treatment of a range of acute and cleanly debrided chronic wounds, including surgical and traumatic wounds, various types of ulcers, second-degree burns, and draining wounds. It is placed on the wound and can be secured with gauze, skin adhesive, steri-strips, etc. It is then covered with a nonadherent dressing, as well as a secondary absorbent dressing. PermeaDerm B is available in 12.7 cm X 25.4 cm, 25.4 cm X 38.1 cm, and 38.1 cm X 76.2 cm sizes. PermeaDerm G is available in 6.35 cm X 12.7 cm and 12.7 cm X 12.7 cm sizes. PermeaDerm Glove is available in extra-small to extra-large sizes, two each per box.

A4100

A4100 Skin substitute, FDA-cleared as a device, not otherwise specified

This code represents skin substitutes that are not specifically identified by other HCPCS Level II codes. Skin substitutes may or may not contain bioactive tissue, cells, or matrices from human or animal sources. The skin substitutes are used to protect large or non-healing wounds or burns. Some products promote cellular growth and wound repair. Most substitutes are used in place of grafts.

A4206-A4209

A4206 Syringe with needle, sterile, 1 cc or less, each

A4207 Syringe with needle, sterile 2 cc, each

A4208 Syringe with needle, sterile 3 cc, each

A4209 Syringe with needle, sterile 5 cc or greater, each

A sterile syringe with a needle is used for injecting or withdrawing liquids into or from any vessel or cavity. Each may vary in size and content capacity.

A4210

A4210 Needle-free injection device, each

This code reports a needle free injection instrument. These could be injectors such as hypodermic jet pressure powered devices for insulin injections.

A4211

A4211 Supplies for self-administered injections

Patients may administer injectable medications, such as insulin or calcitonin, themselves. Supplies for self-administered injections are rarely covered unless an emergency situation exists.

A4212

A4212 Noncoring needle or stylet with or without catheter

Noncoring needles or stylets are most often used to cleanly penetrate rubber self-sealing septums that are part of indwelling ports and pumps. The reservoirs on these surgically implanted devices can be refilled numerous times when noncoring needles are used.

A4213

A4213 Syringe, sterile, 20 cc or greater, each

This code reports supply of a sterile syringe with a capacity of 20 cc or greater. Syringes of this size may be used for injection of medications by intravenous or intra-arterial push. These types of syringes may also be used for wound irrigation.

A4215

A4215 Needle, sterile, any size, each

This code reports any size sterile needle. This code is for a single needle and may be reported multiple times or with multiple units if more than one needle is used.

A4216-A4217

A4216 Sterile water, saline and/or dextrose, diluent/flush, 10 ml

A4217 Sterile water/saline, 500 ml

Report these codes for sterile water, saline, or dextrose for injection or irrigation.

A4218

A4218 Sterile saline or water, metered dose dispenser, 10 ml

A metered dose dispenser of sterile saline or water may be used with a nebulizer or inhaler for dispensing inhalation medications. A metered dose dispenser delivers a precise amount of sterile saline or water for use in the device. This allows proper dilution of the medication.

A4220

A4220 Refill kit for implantable infusion pump

Implantable infusion pumps are typically small, biocompatible, stainless steel units that are surgically placed subcutaneously near the target drug delivery area. A refillable reservoir delivers a constant, prescribed rate of liquid drug to the target site. Drug delivery may be by spring or piston pressure against the reservoir. Routes of administration include intravenous, intra-arterial, intraperitoneal, and intraventricular. The refill kit may contain appropriate noncoring needles, filters, connectors, and other items, but not the drug itself.

A4221

A4221 Supplies for maintenance of noninsulin drug infusion catheter, per week (list drugs separately)

Drug infusion catheters embrace a range of approaches, including peripheral intravenous lines, peripherally inserted central catheters (PICC), and centrally inserted intravenous lines. Maintenance supplies for such drug infusion catheters may include flush solutions, dressings, cannulas, and needles. List any drugs administered separately.

A4222-A4223

A4222 Infusion supplies for external drug infusion pump, per cassette or bag (list drugs separately)

A4223 Infusion supplies not used with external infusion pump, per cassette or bag (list drugs separately)

These codes report infusion supplies for external drug infusion pumps, which may be portable units worn on belts outside of the body or larger stationary units. They also report infusion supplies not used with an external infusion pump, per cassette or bag. Report per cassette or bag, with drugs, such as diluting solutions, tubing, and other administration supplies, such as port caps, listed separately. These codes are not drug specific.

A4224

A4224 Supplies for maintenance of insulin infusion catheter, per week

Insulin infusion catheters embrace a range of approaches, including peripheral intravenous lines, peripherally inserted central catheters (PICC), and centrally inserted intravenous lines. Maintenance supplies for such insulin infusion catheters may include flush solutions, dressings, cannulas, and needles.

A4225

A4225 Supplies for external insulin infusion pump, syringe type cartridge, sterile, each

This code reports infusion supplies pertaining to external insulin pumps. These are portable, battery-operated devices worn by the patient on a belt or sling. The device connects to a drug reservoir and the system is designed to deliver continuous subcutaneous insulin therapy over an extended period of time. The device usually delivers insulin into subcutaneous fat in the abdominal region and the infusion set must be changed out every few days. Cassettes or bags are included, as are diluting solutions, tubing, and other administration supplies, such as port caps. This code is drug specific to insulin.

A4226

A4226 Supplies for maintenance of insulin infusion pump with dosage rate adjustment using therapeutic continuous glucose sensing, per week

This code reports medical supplies for the weekly maintenance of an insulin infusion pump. The pump may consist of a transmitter, receiver, and smartphone application. The continuous glucose monitor (CGM) transmitter sends encrypted data received from the sensor to the patient's receiver for the patient to adjust insulin dose or to a connected insulin pump, which autonomously adjusts the patient's insulin dose or alerts the patient for further action. The smartphone allows the patient to share glucose data with caregivers and physicians wirelessly. The patient inserts the CGM sensor under the skin. The sensor generates a biometric signal, which it passes to the CGM transmitter, smartphone, and/or a medical device. The transmitter measures and converts the biometric signal into glucose data, encrypted on send, decrypted upon receipt, and readable by the patient. The device may be worn under the patient's clothing.

A4230-A4231

A4230 Infusion set for external insulin pump, nonneedle cannula type

A4231 Infusion set for external insulin pump, needle type

These codes report infusion supplies pertaining to external insulin pumps. These are portable, battery-operated devices worn by the patient on a belt or sling. The device connects to a drug reservoir and the system is designed to deliver continuous subcutaneous insulin therapy over an extended period of time. The device usually delivers insulin into subcutaneous fat in the abdominal region and the infusion set must be changed out every few days. Cassettes or bags are included, as are diluting solutions, tubing, and other administration supplies, such as port caps. These codes are drug specific to insulin.

A4232

A4232 Syringe with needle for external insulin pump, sterile, 3 cc

This code is designated for a syringe with needle for external insulin pump, sterile, 3 cc, and describes the insulin reservoir for use with the external insulin infusion pump. The reservoir may be either glass or plastic and includes the needle for drawing up the insulin. This code does not include the insulin for use in the reservoir.

A4233-A4236

A4233 Replacement battery, alkaline (other than J cell), for use with medically necessary home blood glucose monitor owned by patient, each

A4234 Replacement battery, alkaline, J cell, for use with medically necessary home blood glucose monitor owned by patient, each

A4235 Replacement battery, lithium, for use with medically necessary home blood glucose monitor owned by patient, each

A4236 Replacement battery, silver oxide, for use with medically necessary home blood glucose monitor owned by patient, each

Glucometers with associated accessories and supplies are used for patients with all types of diabetes mellitus to monitor blood glucose, and are available in a variety of models. A replacement battery for a medically necessary, patient-owned home blood glucose monitor (glucometer) is reported based on the type of battery required.

A4238-A4239

A4238 Supply allowance for adjunctive, nonimplanted continuous glucose monitor (CGM), includes all supplies and accessories, 1 month supply = 1 unit of service

A4239 Supply allowance for nonadjunctive, nonimplanted continuous glucose monitor (CGM), includes all supplies and accessories, 1 month supply = 1 unit of service

Continuous glucose monitoring (CGM) systems make continuous measurements of glucose levels. Many of these devices take measurements from subcutaneous tissue rather than from blood. Most systems consist of a sensor that is attached to the back of the arm or abdomen. The sensor has a very thin wire that is inserted subcutaneously. The wire measures the glucose level in interstitial fluid that exits between the cells. The sensor is attached to a transmitter that sends the glucose readings to a wireless receiver. The receiver is a small, computerized device that records and stores the glucose readings. CGMs are classified as adjunctive (do not replace standard blood glucose monitors for treatment decisions) or nonadjunctive (can replace standard blood glucose monitors for treatment decisions). These codes report a one-month supply of accessory/supply components for an adjunctive, nonimplanted CGM system (A4238) or a nonadjunctive, nonimplanted CGM system (A4239).

A4244-A4248

A4244 Alcohol or peroxide, per pint

A4245 Alcohol wipes, per box

A4246 Betadine or pHisoHex solution, per pint

A4247 Betadine or iodine swabs/wipes, per box

A4248 Chlorhexidine containing antiseptic, 1 ml

Glucometers and associated accessories and supplies are used for patients with all types of diabetes mellitus to monitor blood glucose levels. Supplies used in monitoring blood glucose levels include a variety of antiseptics and antimicrobials to cleanse the skin prior to piercing the skin to obtain a blood sample to perform the glucose test. Betadine, pHisoHex, and iodine are other types of anti-infective solutions used on the skin and are available in both pints or individually wrapped swabs or wipes. A chlorhexidine containing antiseptic such as Hibiclens may also be used to prevent skin infections. Chlorhexidine has antiseptic activity and an antimicrobial effect against a wide range of microorganisms.

A4250-A4259

A4250 Urine test or reagent strips or tablets (100 tablets or strips)

A4252 Blood ketone test or reagent strip, each

A4253 Blood glucose test or reagent strips for home blood glucose monitor, per 50 strips

A4255 Platforms for home blood glucose monitor, 50 per box

A4256 Normal, low, and high calibrator solution/chips

A4257 Replacement lens shield cartridge for use with laser skin piercing device, each

A4258 Spring-powered device for lancet, each

A4259 Lancets, per box of 100

Glucometers and associated accessories and supplies are used for patients with all types of diabetes mellitus to monitor blood glucose levels, and are available in a variety of models. Accessories and supplies for these devices range from alcohol prep pads to lancets for piercing the skin to obtain the required blood sample to perform the test. Many of these supplies must be used each time the test is performed and are not reusable. Many diabetics require frequent, if not daily, blood glucose monitoring, whether or not the patient is on insulin. For Type I diabetes mellitus patients who require insulin (the patient's body does not manufacture insulin and therefore it must come from an external source, such as injections), blood glucose monitoring is a life-sustaining requirement. The accessories and supplies are medically necessary to properly and accurately perform the blood glucose monitoring. Blood glucose test or reagent strips are used with home glucose monitoring devices and are usually covered for insulin-dependent diabetics whose monitor has been prescribed by the physician. Platforms are used with lancing devices to prevent cross infection and to control depth of penetration of the lancing device. Calibrator solutions or chips are used with a home glucose monitoring device to check the integrity of the glucometer and the test strips. Calibrator solutions or chips are provided in normal, low, and high levels. Lancing devices use lasers or springs. Use of a laser device requires a lens shield cartridge. A lancet is a pointed surgical knife with two edges.

A4261

A4261 Cervical cap for contraceptive use

A cervical cap is a thimble shaped latex device that covers the cervix and is used with a spermicide as a barrier method of contraception.

A4262-A4263

A4262 Temporary, absorbable lacrimal duct implant, each

A4263 Permanent, long-term, nondissolvable lacrimal duct implant, each

Report A4262 for use of a temporary, absorbable tear duct implant. Report A4263 when a permanent, long-term nondissolvable lacrimal duct implant is used.

A4264

A4264 Permanent implantable contraceptive intratubal occlusion device(s) and delivery system

An intratubal occlusion device is a permanent, implantable, contraceptive occlusive device and system used for nonincisional sterilization. This process is performed using a hysteroscopic approach. The system is comprised of a micro-insert implantable stainless steel inner coil with polyester fibers and a super-elastic nitinol outer anchoring coil. The micro-insert, when released, expands to conform and anchor in the fallopian tube.

A4265

A4265 Paraffin, per pound

Paraffin is a waxy, white, tasteless, odorless mixture of solid hydrocarbon made from petroleum. It is often used as the base for an ointment or wound dressing.

A4266

A4266 Diaphragm for contraceptive use

A diaphragm is a rubber or plastic cup that fits over the cervix uteri and is used for contraceptive purposes.

A4267-A4268

A4267 Contraceptive supply, condom, male, each

A4268 Contraceptive supply, condom, female, each

A condom is a thin, flexible sheath used by a man to prevent pregnancy and/or sexually transmitted diseases. A female condom is made for sheathing the internal anatomy of the female.

A4269

A4269 Contraceptive supply, spermicide (e.g., foam, gel), each

Spermicides are contraceptive agents used to kill spermatozoa.

A4270

A4270 Disposable endoscope sheath, each

This code reports the use of a disposable sheath that covers an endoscope, a device consisting of a tube and optical system for viewing the inside of a hollow organ or cavity.

A4280

A4280 Adhesive skin support attachment for use with external breast prosthesis, each

This code reports the adhesive skin support attachment used with a breast prosthesis, a man-made substitute for a missing breast.

A4281-A4286

A4281 Tubing for breast pump, replacement

A4282 Adapter for breast pump, replacement

A4283 Cap for breast pump bottle, replacement

A4284 Breast shield and splash protector for use with breast pump, replacement

A4285 Polycarbonate bottle for use with breast pump, replacement

A4286 Locking ring for breast pump, replacement

A breast pump is a mechanical device used to extract milk from a lactating mother. Pumps may be manual, electronic, or battery-powered. These codes represent replacement parts for the breast pump.

A4290

A4290 Sacral nerve stimulation test lead, each

There are five pairs of spinal or sacral nerves. Report this code for each test lead used in a sacral nerve stimulation examination.

A4300

A4300 Implantable access catheter, (e.g., venous, arterial, epidural subarachnoid, or peritoneal, etc.) external access

A catheter is a tube inserted into the body to evacuate or inject fluids into body cavities.

A4301

A4301 Implantable access total catheter, port/reservoir (e.g., venous, arterial, epidural, subarachnoid, peritoneal, etc.)

This code reports the supply of an integrated vascular port/reservoir and catheter designed for subdermal implantation. The system is designed for patients requiring regular or continuous intravenous or intra-arterial infusion of drugs. The system may be used to deliver any of a variety of medicines, particularly those for oncology therapy. In some instances, the implanted port and catheter delivers drugs to the spinal cord (epidural), the brain (subarachnoid), or to the abdominal (peritoneal) cavity. Implantable infusion pumps are typically small biocompatible stainless steel units that are surgically placed subcutaneously near the site of optimal drug delivery. The port and reservoir can be smaller in diameter than a nickel coin. A refillable reservoir delivers a constant, prescribed rate of liquid drug to the target site. Typically, the reservoir features a rubber diaphragm that can be penetrated by a non-coring needle to refill the drug.

A4305-A4306

A4305 Disposable drug delivery system, flow rate of 50 ml or greater per hour

A4306 Disposable drug delivery system, flow rate of less than 50 ml per hour

These disposable drug delivery systems comprise devices that deliver liquid drugs by the elastic pressure of the reservoir container. The term elastomeric infusion pump may be used. These codes are not drug specific.

A4310-A4316

A4310 Insertion tray without drainage bag and without catheter (accessories only)

A4311 Insertion tray without drainage bag with indwelling catheter, Foley type, two-way latex with coating (Teflon, silicone, silicone elastomer or hydrophilic, etc.)

A4312 Insertion tray without drainage bag with indwelling catheter, Foley type, two-way, all silicone

A4313 Insertion tray without drainage bag with indwelling catheter, Foley type, three-way, for continuous irrigation

A4314 Insertion tray with drainage bag with indwelling catheter, Foley type, two-way latex with coating (Teflon, silicone, silicone elastomer or hydrophilic, etc.)

A4315 Insertion tray with drainage bag with indwelling catheter, Foley type, two-way, all silicone

A4316 Insertion tray with drainage bag with indwelling catheter, Foley type, three-way, for continuous irrigation

Urinary catheters and external urinary collection devices are used to drain or collect urine from a patient who has permanent urinary incontinence or permanent urinary retention. Supplies or accessories are also used with the catheters and are part of the service provided.

A4320-A4322

A4320 Irrigation tray with bulb or piston syringe, any purpose

A4321 Therapeutic agent for urinary catheter irrigation

A4322 Irrigation syringe, bulb or piston, each

These codes are reported for cleaning and irrigation items for incontinence care.

A4326

A4326 Male external catheter with integral collection chamber, any type, each

Male external catheters (condom-type) are used by patients who have permanent urinary incontinence as an alternative to an indwelling catheter. A male external catheter is used over the external genitalia as an incontinence guard. This code reports a male external catheter with integral collection chamber, any type, each.

A4327-A4328

A4327 Female external urinary collection device; meatal cup, each

A4328 Female external urinary collection device; pouch, each

A female external urinary collection device is used to collect urine as it passes to the outside of the body.

A4330

A4330 Perianal fecal collection pouch with adhesive, each

A perianal pouch is applied to the outside of the body with adhesive to manage stool incontinence.

A4331

A4331 Extension drainage tubing, any type, any length, with connector/adaptor, for use with urinary leg bag or urostomy pouch, each

Extension drainage tubing is used with a urostomy pouch or latex urinary leg bag for patients who are ambulatory or are chair or wheelchair bound but not bedridden. Report this code for any type, any length of extension drainage tubing with the connector or adaptor.

A4332-A4334

A4332 Lubricant, individual sterile packet, each

A4333 Urinary catheter anchoring device, adhesive skin attachment, each

A4334 Urinary catheter anchoring device, leg strap, each

Urinary catheters may be held in place by means of an adhesive patch or a strap that goes around the leg. Lubricant is used for the insertion of the catheter into the bladder.

A4335

A4335 Incontinence supply; miscellaneous

Incontinence supplies are leak proof undergarments worn by the patient who cannot retain or control the release of urine, semen, or feces. This code reports miscellaneous incontinence supplies.

A4336

A4336 Incontinence supply, urethral insert, any type, each

Urethral inserts are designed for the female patient to manage and/or treat urinary incontinence. A self-inserted, single use, disposable intra-urethral device results in instant control of severe stress urinary incontinence (SUI).This insert is a small, latex free, narrow silicone tube that is totally encased in a soft, thin, mineral oil-filled sleeve. The sleeve forms a balloon at the internal tip and a soft, oval shaped external retainer at the opposite end. The device is inserted using a disposable applicator.

A4337

A4337 Incontinence supply, rectal insert, any type, each

Fecal incontinence is the uncontrollable discharge of stool from the rectum. Rectal inserts made of soft silicone or foam resembling a suppository is inserted into the rectum, wearable day or night. Some variations are discharged with regular bowel movements, while others are removed by the patient to allow for bowel movement.

A4338-A4346

A4338 Indwelling catheter; Foley type, two-way latex with coating (Teflon, silicone, silicone elastomer, or hydrophilic, etc.), each

A4340 Indwelling catheter; specialty type, (e.g., Coude, mushroom, wing, etc.), each

A4344 Indwelling catheter, Foley type, two-way, all silicone, each

A4346 Indwelling catheter; Foley type, three-way for continuous irrigation, each

Urinary catheterization involves insertion of a drainage tube up the urethra and into the bladder where it is often held in place by an inflated balloon. For these indwelling catheters, a reservoir is typically attached to contain the drained urine, which, for many patients, may be monitored for volume and tested for content. A topical anesthetic may be employed and the catheter is lubricated.

A4349

A4349 Male external catheter, with or without adhesive, disposable, each

Male external catheters (condom-type) are used by patients who have permanent urinary incontinence as an alternative to an indwelling catheter. A male external catheter is used over the external genitalia as an incontinence guard.

A4351-A4353

A4351 Intermittent urinary catheter; straight tip, with or without coating (Teflon, silicone, silicone elastomer, or hydrophilic, etc.), each

A4352 Intermittent urinary catheter; Coude (curved) tip, with or without coating (Teflon, silicone, silicone elastomeric, or hydrophilic, etc.), each

A4353 Intermittent urinary catheter, with insertion supplies

Urinary catheterization involves insertion of a drainage tube up the urethra and into the bladder where it is often held in place by an inflated balloon. For these indwelling catheters, a reservoir is typically attached to contain the drained urine, which, for many patients, may be monitored for volume and tested for content. This code range, however, reports intermittent catheterization, a treatment approach for certain urinary disorders, and patient profiles. The catheter is inserted using antiseptic technique by the patient or a caregiver four times a day, or more often as needed. A topical anesthetic may be employed and the catheter is lubricated. The bladder is completely voided into a container and the catheter withdrawn after each procedure. The catheter may be disinfected and reused or discarded.

A4354

A4354 Insertion tray with drainage bag but without catheter

This code reports the supply of a urinary catheterization insertion tray. This type of sterile tray typically includes a preloaded syringe, absorbent pads, drapery, gloves, and lubricants. A drainage bag or graduated container is included in the code description, but the catheter itself is specifically excluded.

A4355

A4355 Irrigation tubing set for continuous bladder irrigation through a three-way indwelling Foley catheter, each

This code reports the supply of a specific continuous bladder irrigation set. Bladder catheterization is generally called for in patients unable to void urine naturally and following certain surgeries. Continuous irrigation is usually temporary and may be required in certain circumstances involving obstructions. The bladder is a sterile environment and sterile hardware and technique is ordinarily required to catheterize it. A Foley catheter features a balloon tip that is inflated upon entry into the bladder to hold the device in place (indwelling). A three-way catheter features a lumen for urine drainage, one to inflate and deflate the Foley balloon, and one for irrigation fluids and medications.

A4356

A4356 External urethral clamp or compression device (not to be used for catheter clamp), each

This code reports the supply of external urethral clamps, also known as penile clamps, incontinence clamps, or Cunningham clamps. These reusable metal devices fit over the penis. Typically, soft foam that contours to the shape of the penis is compressed, closing off the urethra. Compression on the devices must be relieved every several hours.

A4357

A4357 Bedside drainage bag, day or night, with or without antireflux device, with or without tube, each

Patients with urinary ostomies may use a bedside drainage bag during the day or night. The bedside drainage bag is used for the collection of urinary output from a urinary pouch. It is sometimes necessary, especially at night, for the bag to be connected to the pouch to prevent urinary overflow and excessive weight in the pouch, which could cause urinary leakage and disruption of the pouch seal. The bag is made of a high grade PVC and can hold up to 2,000 cc. The anti-reflux device prevents backflow.

A4358

A4358 Urinary drainage bag, leg or abdomen, vinyl, with or without tube, with straps, each

Leg or abdomen urinary drainage bags are indicated for patients who are ambulatory or are chair or wheelchair bound but not bedridden. The vinyl bag can be used with a suprapubic or Foley catheter for urine collection. It typically holds up to 1,000 cc. The bag is held in place next to the abdomen or around the leg by woven straps. This code describes a drainage bag, with or without tubing.

A4360

A4360 Disposable external urethral clamp or compression device, with pad and/or pouch, each

A disposable, external urethral clamp or compression device is designed for a male patient to manage and/or treat light to moderate urinary incontinence. It works by minimizing urinary incontinence by means of mechanical compression of the urethra, eliminating the leakage of urine and allowing the bladder to fill. If there is leakage that breaks through from the urethra, the moisture is restricted to the disposable pouch or pad.

A4361

A4361 Ostomy faceplate, each

An ostomy faceplate is a solid interface between the patient's skin and the pouch. It is usually made of plastic, rubber, or encased metal. It does not have an adhesive property and there is no pectin-based or karaya material that is an integral part of the faceplate. It can be taken off the skin and reattached repeatedly. It is held on by means of a separate adhesive and/or an elastic belt.

A4362

A4362 Skin barrier; solid, 4 x 4 or equivalent; each

Skin barriers are an interface between the patient's skin and the pouching system. They are used to create an adhesive seal between the skin and the pouch. Barriers can be curved with a built-in convexity creating a more adhesive bond to the patient's skin and better protrusion of the stoma. These codes represent solid ostomy skin barriers that are used independently, usually with a pouch that does not have its own integral skin barrier.

A4363

A4363 Ostomy clamp, any type, replacement only, each

An ostomy clamp is a closure accessory used to prevent spillage from an open-ended (drainable) ostomy pouch. An ostomy clamp is provided with the purchase of an ostomy bag and is not billed separately. This code reports the replacement of the ostomy clamp.

A4364

A4364 Adhesive, liquid or equal, any type, per oz

Adhesive liquids are applied directly to the skin or to a protective barrier, such as a disk or foam pad, providing increased bonding of ostomy devices. These adhesives are in liquid form or are equal to a liquid available in bottles or spray cans. They are rubber based or acrylic based and non-toxic. Proper application of adhesives is a thin, light coat on the desired area. Adhesives can be removed with petroleum-based solvents.

A4366

A4366 Ostomy vent, any type, each

A separate ostomy vent can be added to the ostomy pouch to allow the release of gas. This code must not be used for pouches in which a vent with a filter is incorporated in the pouch by the manufacturer.

A4367

A4367 Ostomy belt, each

An ostomy belt is used to secure and conceal ostomy appliances. They are made of lightweight cotton and Lycra/elastic. Belts are designed to be used with one or two-piece systems for left, right, or center stomas and vary in width depending on the patient's need. Some belts provide a pocket for the appliance that has a Velcro closure that allows for easy emptying.

A4368

A4368 Ostomy filter, any type, each

An ostomy filter prevents the buildup of gas trapped in the pouch by allowing the gas to be effectively expelled through a vent. Filters may be incorporated into a pouch, inserted into a venting ring on the pouch, or attached to the pouch exterior. They may also include deodorizing materials such as charcoal for the vented gas.

A4369-A4373

A4369 Ostomy skin barrier, liquid (spray, brush, etc.), per oz

A4371 Ostomy skin barrier, powder, per oz

A4372 Ostomy skin barrier, solid 4 x 4 or equivalent, standard wear, with built-in convexity, each

A4373 Ostomy skin barrier, with flange (solid, flexible or accordion), with built-in convexity, any size, each

This range of codes reports skin care and conditioning supplies for patients fitting adhesive pouches over an ostomy, a surgically created opening through the skin to divert bowel contents into an external container or pouch. Peristomal skin can become difficult to care for over time due to the irritating nature of fecal material, enzymes, and the repeated application and removal of adhesives. Barriers are an interface between the patient's skin and the pouching system and have a variety of options such as built-in convexity, locking or non-locking flanges, and use with or without faceplates. Barriers offer a level of protection to the skin while providing a surface to adhere the ostomy faceplate.

A4375-A4378

A4375 Ostomy pouch, drainable, with faceplate attached, plastic, each

A4376 Ostomy pouch, drainable, with faceplate attached, rubber, each

A4377 Ostomy pouch, drainable, for use on faceplate, plastic, each

A4378 Ostomy pouch, drainable, for use on faceplate, rubber, each

These codes represent drainable ostomy pouches. Ostomy pouches are used by patients who have had a surgically created opening for diversion of the urine or feces. An ostomy faceplate is a solid interface between the patient's skin and the pouch. It is usually made of plastic, rubber, or encased metal. It can be taken off the skin and reattached repeatedly. It is held on by means of a separate adhesive and/or an elastic belt.

A4379-A4384

A4379 Ostomy pouch, urinary, with faceplate attached, plastic, each

A4380 Ostomy pouch, urinary, with faceplate attached, rubber, each

A4381 Ostomy pouch, urinary, for use on faceplate, plastic, each

A4382 Ostomy pouch, urinary, for use on faceplate, heavy plastic, each

A4383 Ostomy pouch, urinary, for use on faceplate, rubber, each

A4384 Ostomy faceplate equivalent, silicone ring, each

These codes represent urinary ostomy pouches for use on barrier, with flange. Urinary ostomy pouches are used by patients who have had a surgically created opening for diversion of the urine. An ostomy faceplate is a solid interface between the patient's skin and the pouch. It is usually made of plastic, heavy plastic, rubber, or silicone. It can be taken off the skin and reattached repeatedly. It is held on by means of a separate adhesive and/or an elastic belt.

A4385

A4385 Ostomy skin barrier, solid 4 x 4 or equivalent, extended wear, without built-in convexity, each

An ostomy is a surgically created opening through the skin to divert bowel contents into an external container or pouch. Peristomal skin can become difficult to care for over time due to the irritating nature of fecal material, enzymes, and the repeated application and removal of adhesives. Barriers are an interface between the patient's skin and the pouching system and have a variety of options, such as built-in convexity, locking or non-locking flanges, and use with or without faceplates. Barriers offer a level of protection to the skin while providing a surface to adhere the ostomy faceplate.

A4387-A4390

A4387 Ostomy pouch, closed, with barrier attached, with built-in convexity (one piece), each

A4388 Ostomy pouch, drainable, with extended wear barrier attached, (one piece), each

A4389 Ostomy pouch, drainable, with barrier attached, with built-in convexity (one piece), each

A4390 Ostomy pouch, drainable, with extended wear barrier attached, with built-in convexity (one piece), each

An ostomy pouch is a device used for the collection of stomal or urinary output for patients who have undergone procedures causing a temporary or permanent interference with normal excretion. The ostomy pouch with barrier attached is a one-piece system in which a solid barrier serving to create an adhesive seal is part of the ostomy pouch. The barrier may be pectin-based or karaya-based for normal wear, or pectin-based with special additives for extended wear. The pouch may contain an opening at the bottom through which the contents can be drained, or be sealed without an outlet.

A4391-A4393

A4391 Ostomy pouch, urinary, with extended wear barrier attached (one piece), each

A4392 Ostomy pouch, urinary, with standard wear barrier attached, with built-in convexity (one piece), each

A4393 Ostomy pouch, urinary, with extended wear barrier attached, with built-in convexity (one piece), each

Urinary ostomy pouches are for use with patients who have had a surgically created opening for diversion of the urine. The ostomy pouch with barrier attached is a one-piece system in which a solid barrier serving to create an adhesive seal is part of the pouch. The barrier may be pectin-based or karaya-based for normal wear, or pectin-based with special additives for extended wear. The use of convexity is commonly indicated when a pouch seal is unable to fasten properly for an acceptable length of time or when persistent skin irritation occurs even without leakage.

A4394-A4395

A4394 Ostomy deodorant, with or without lubricant, for use in ostomy pouch, per fl oz

A4395 Ostomy deodorant for use in ostomy pouch, solid, per tablet

These codes report deodorants for use with ostomy pouches, devices for collecting stomal or urinary output in patients who have undergone procedures causing a temporary or permanent interference with normal excretion. Deodorants are available in liquid or solid form and eliminate urine and fecal odors.

A4396

A4396 Ostomy belt with peristomal hernia support

This code reports an ostomy belt with peristomal hernia support. Ostomy belts are used to secure and conceal ostomy appliances. They are made of lightweight cotton and Lycra/elastic. Belts are designed to be used with one or two-piece systems for left, right, or center stomas and vary in width depending on the patient's need. Some belts provide a pocket for the appliance that has a Velcro closure that allows for easy emptying. This ostomy belt utilizes a rigid hernia support plate in the pouch pocket of the belt to provide necessary support for a herniated stoma.

A4398-A4400

A4398 Ostomy irrigation supply; bag, each

A4399 Ostomy irrigation supply; cone/catheter, with or without brush

A4400 Ostomy irrigation set

Irrigation sets are used in the cleaning and maintenance of sigmoid colostomies. Full kits include all supplies necessary for proper irrigation of colostomies, such as a water bag regulator, cone, faceplate, and belts. An irrigation bag is used for holding the warm water necessary for flushing out the ostomy. The replacement of an irrigation ostomy bag or cone/catheter, including brush, would be appropriate every three months.

A4402

A4402 Lubricant, per oz

The lubricants used for ostomy supplies are water soluble, greaseless, odorless gels. These gels lubricate ostomy supplies such as catheters to reduce irritation.

A4404

A4404 Ostomy ring, each

This code reports an ostomy ring. An "o" ring is a round rubber ring used as an additional security measure to hold a pouch clip closed.

A4405-A4406

A4405 Ostomy skin barrier, nonpectin-based, paste, per oz

A4406 Ostomy skin barrier, pectin-based, paste, per oz

Pastes are applied directly to the skin to act as a protective sealant beneath ostomy appliances. They may have a synthetic or natural base. Non-pectin based paste (e.g., karaya) is required for skin sensitive to synthetic barriers.

A4407-A4411

A4407 Ostomy skin barrier, with flange (solid, flexible, or accordion), extended wear, with built-in convexity, 4 x 4 in or smaller, each

A4408 Ostomy skin barrier, with flange (solid, flexible or accordion), extended wear, with built-in convexity, larger than 4 x 4 in, each

A4409 Ostomy skin barrier, with flange (solid, flexible or accordion), extended wear, without built-in convexity, 4 x 4 in or smaller, each

A4410 Ostomy skin barrier, with flange (solid, flexible or accordion), extended wear, without built-in convexity, larger than 4 x 4 in, each

A4411 Ostomy skin barrier, solid 4 x 4 or equivalent, extended wear, with built-in convexity, each

An ostomy skin barrier (wafer) with built-in convexity is one in which an outward curve is usually achieved with plastic embedded in the barrier, allowing better protrusion of the stoma and adherence to the skin. Skin barriers are an interface between the patient's skin and the pouching system. They are used to create an adhesive seal between the skin and the pouch.

A4412-A4413

A4412 Ostomy pouch, drainable, high output, for use on a barrier with flange (two-piece system), without filter, each

A4413 Ostomy pouch, drainable, high output, for use on a barrier with flange (two-piece system), with filter, each

These codes report the supply of a high-output, drainable ostomy pouch to be used with a two-piece barrier with flange system. These pouches have been specifically designed for high stomal output. A high-output ostomy pouch must have a capacity of greater than or equal to 0.75 liters, an anti-reflux valve, and a large bore solid spout with cap or plug.

A4414-A4415

A4414 Ostomy skin barrier, with flange (solid, flexible or accordion), without built-in convexity, 4 x 4 in or smaller, each

A4415 Ostomy skin barrier, with flange (solid, flexible or accordion), without built-in convexity, larger than 4 x 4 in, each

These codes represent ostomy skin barriers with a flange, solid, flexible, or accordion type, without built-in convexity, not specified as extended wear. Skin barriers are an interface between the patient's skin and the pouching system. They are used to create an adhesive seal between the skin and the pouch.

A4416-A4420

A4416 Ostomy pouch, closed, with barrier attached, with filter (one piece), each

A4417 Ostomy pouch, closed, with barrier attached, with built-in convexity, with filter (one piece), each

A4418 Ostomy pouch, closed; without barrier attached, with filter (one piece), each

A4419 Ostomy pouch, closed; for use on barrier with nonlocking flange, with filter (two piece), each

A4420 Ostomy pouch, closed; for use on barrier with locking flange (two piece), each

These codes represent ostomy pouches that are for use with patients who have had a surgically created opening for diversion of stool. Ostomy pouches collect the stomal output, in this case feces, and can be drainable or closed. Drainable pouches have an opening at the bottom through which fecal contents can be emptied. Closed pouches have a sealed bottom with no outlet for feces. There are also one-piece and two-piece systems. One-piece systems are supplied "with barrier attached" or "without barrier attached." Two-piece systems have a locking or non-locking flange that is coupled to a skin barrier with flange. Skin barriers are an interface between the patient's skin and the pouching system and have a variety of different options such as built-in convexity, filters, locking or non-locking flanges, and use with or without faceplates.

A4421

A4421 Ostomy supply; miscellaneous

Report this code for miscellaneous ostomy supplies for which a more specific code is not available.

A4422

A4422 Ostomy absorbent material (sheet/pad/crystal packet) for use in ostomy pouch to thicken liquid stomal output, each

Absorbent material such as sheets, pads, or crystals is added to the ostomy pouch to thicken the liquid output from the stoma. These materials draw liquid away from the stoma to minimize irritation, reduce splashing when emptying the pouch, and facilitate in venting of gas. Report this code for absorbent material, any type.

A4423

A4423 Ostomy pouch, closed; for use on barrier with locking flange, with filter (two piece), each

Ostomy pouches collect the stomal output, in this case feces, and can be drainable or closed. Drainable pouches have an opening at the bottom through which fecal contents can be emptied. Closed pouches have a sealed bottom with no outlet for feces. There are also one-piece and two-piece systems. One-piece systems are supplied "with barrier attached" or "without barrier attached." Two-piece systems have a locking or non-locking flange that is coupled to a skin barrier with flange. Skin barriers are an interface between the patient's skin and the pouching system and have a variety of different options, such as built-in convexity, filters, locking or non-locking flanges, and use with or without faceplates. Report this code for an ostomy pouch used on a barrier with a locking flange and two-piece filter.

A4424-A4427

A4424 Ostomy pouch, drainable, with barrier attached, with filter (one piece), each

A4425 Ostomy pouch, drainable; for use on barrier with nonlocking flange, with filter (two-piece system), each

A4426 Ostomy pouch, drainable; for use on barrier with locking flange (two-piece system), each

A4427 Ostomy pouch, drainable; for use on barrier with locking flange, with filter (two-piece system), each

These codes represent drainable ostomy pouches. Ostomy pouches are for use with patients who have had a surgically created opening for diversion of the urine. The ostomy pouch with barrier attached is a one-piece system in which a solid barrier serving to create an adhesive seal is part of the ostomy pouch. The barrier may be pectin-based or karaya-based for normal wear or pectin-based with special additives for extended wear. Filters prevent the buildup of gas trapped in the pouch by allowing the gas to be effectively expelled through a vent. A flange or plastic ring on both the pouch and skin barrier secures the barrier and the pouch.

A4428-A4434

A4428 Ostomy pouch, urinary, with extended wear barrier attached, with faucet-type tap with valve (one piece), each

A4429 Ostomy pouch, urinary, with barrier attached, with built-in convexity, with faucet-type tap with valve (one piece), each

A4430 Ostomy pouch, urinary, with extended wear barrier attached, with built-in convexity, with faucet-type tap with valve (one piece), each

A4431 Ostomy pouch, urinary; with barrier attached, with faucet-type tap with valve (one piece), each

A4432 Ostomy pouch, urinary; for use on barrier with nonlocking flange, with faucet-type tap with valve (two piece), each

A4433 Ostomy pouch, urinary; for use on barrier with locking flange (two piece), each

A4434 Ostomy pouch, urinary; for use on barrier with locking flange, with faucet-type tap with valve (two piece), each

These codes represent urinary ostomy pouches. Urinary ostomy pouches are for use with patients who have had a surgically created opening for diversion of the urine. The ostomy pouch with barrier attached is a one-piece system in which a solid barrier serving to create an adhesive seal is part of the ostomy pouch. The barrier may be pectin-based or karaya-based for normal wear or pectin-based with special additives for extended wear. The use of convexity is commonly indicated when a pouch seal is unable to fasten properly for an acceptable length of time or when persistent skin irritation occurs even without leakage. A flange or plastic ring on both the pouch and skin barrier secures the barrier and the pouch.

A4435

A4435 Ostomy pouch, drainable, high output, with extended wear barrier (one-piece system), with or without filter, each

An ostomy pouch is used for patients who have had a surgically created opening for diversion of stool. Ostomy pouches collect the stomal output, in this case feces, and can be drainable or closed. Drainable pouches have an opening at the bottom through which fecal contents can be emptied. There are also one-piece and two-piece systems. One-piece systems are supplied "with barrier attached" or "without barrier attached." Two-piece systems have a locking or nonlocking flange that is coupled to a skin barrier with flange. Skin barriers are an interface between the patient's skin and the pouching system and have a variety of different options, such as built-in convexity, filters, locking or nonlocking flanges, and use with or without faceplates.

A4436-A4437

A4436 Irrigation supply; sleeve, reusable, per month

A4437 Irrigation supply; sleeve, disposable, per month

Irrigation sets are used in the cleaning and maintenance of sigmoid colostomies. Full kits include all supplies necessary for proper irrigation of colostomies, such as a water bag regulator, cone, faceplate, belt, and sleeves. An irrigation sleeve allows for collection and drainage of irrigated contents to be directed into a toilet. Report A4436 for reusable sleeves; report A4437 for disposable sleeves.

A4450-A4452

A4450 Tape, nonwaterproof, per 18 sq in

A4452 Tape, waterproof, per 18 sq in

Tape is used to hold on a wound cover and can be an elastic roll gauze or non-elastic roll gauze. Additional tape is usually not required when a wound cover with an adhesive border is used. Tape change is determined by the frequency of wound cover change.

A4453

A4453 Rectal catheter for use with the manual pump-operated enema system, replacement only

This code reports the supply of a single use catheter for a transanal, manual irrigation system, consisting of an irrigation catheter with balloon for retention, leg straps, tubing, connectors, water bag, and a control unit with a manual switch that allows pressure to be added to the water bag and to inflate or deflate the balloon. The catheter is single use, but the other components are reusable. The system is designed to instill water or isotonic saline into the rectum and colon via a rectal catheter, which is held in place by an inflatable balloon. Warm water or saline is intermittently pulsed into the rectum/colon, stimulating the bowel and flushing out stool. Report A4453 for the single-use catheter.

A4455-A4456

A4455 Adhesive remover or solvent (for tape, cement or other adhesive), per oz

A4456 Adhesive remover, wipes, any type, each

Adhesives sometimes require adhesive remover or solvent for complete removal. They are usually petroleum based. Adhesive remover or solvent for removal of tape, cement, or other adhesive is reported per ounce.

A4458

A4458 Enema bag with tubing, reusable

This code reports the supply of a reusable enema bag and tubing. Traditionally, these are heavy gauge rubber bags that hold about two quarts of liquid. An enema bag is designed to hang about 18 inches above the patient in the SIMM's position (lying on the side). Tubing from the bag is inserted into the rectum. Fluid from the bag is allowed to drain into the colon. The fluid is retained for a short duration and the patient voids contents of the colon/rectum.

A4459

A4459 Manual pump-operated enema system, includes balloon, catheter and all accessories, reusable, any type

This code reports the supply of a transanal, manual irrigation system, consisting of tubing, straps, water bag, and a control unit with a pump. The system is designed to instill water into the rectum and colon via a rectal catheter, which is held in place by an inflatable balloon. Warm water is intermittently pulsed into the rectum/colon, stimulating the bowel and flushing out stool.

A4461-A4463

A4461 Surgical dressing holder, nonreusable, each

A4463 Surgical dressing holder, reusable, each

An abdominal dressing holder is usually a slightly elastic garment that may be worn over surgical dressings where adhesives might pose problems or among patients with limited mobility. The device typically opens from side panels, allowing for easy access to the dressings.

A4465

A4465 Nonelastic binder for extremity

A nonelastic extremity binder is used for the treatment of lymphedema. These binders apply a gentle, gradient pressure to the affected extremity by use of a sleeve in combination with adjustable straps that provide compression. The sleeve slides over the affected extremity and then the compression bands are adjusted. Some models have gauges that assess the pressure applied over any region of the extremity. These gauges ensure that compression applied to the patient's limb is consistently applied and in the proper range to provide optimal results.

A4467

A4467 Belt, strap, sleeve, garment, or covering, any type

Belts, straps, sleeves, garments, or coverings, any type, represent clothing created for medical purposes. One proprietary type of clothing is indicted for use by dialysis patients. These pants and shirts allow patients to get dressed for a treatment in the privacy of their own homes. The garments are treated with Triclosan, an antibacterial, antifungal, and antimicrobial agent. The manufacturer contends that the clothing serves a medical purpose in helping to prevent health care associated infections. The garments have zippers at the neck and down the sleeves and legs that provide easier access to medical sites. The manufacturer recommends that the garments be replaced every 90 days.

A4470

A4470 Gravlee jet washer

The Gravlee Jet Washer is a sterile, disposable, diagnostic device for detecting endometrial cancer by obtaining a tissue sample. The use of this device is indicated where the patient exhibits clinical symptoms or signs suggestive of endometrial disease, such as irregular or heavy vaginal bleeding. The tissue obtained is preserved by the addition of an equal amount of Papanicolaou fixative to the irrigation solution from which a cell block is prepared to give a histologic specimen. The use of the Gravlee jet washer should not be confused with a diagnostic curettage.

A4480

A4480 VABRA aspirator

The VABRA aspirator is a vacuum operated device designed to collect endometrial samples for biopsy. The cervix may be first accessed by a sounding device to assist in dilation. A pipette tip from the VABRA device is inserted into the vaginal canal, through the cervical os, and into the endometrial lining of the uterus. Retraction of an outer sleeve of the cannula creates a gentle suction to collect the specimen. The specimen is stabilized in neutral fluid and prepared for analysis. Collection of the endometrial tissues may be timed to a particular phase of the menstrual cycle for optimal results.

A4481

A4481 Tracheostoma filter, any type, any size, each

This code reports the supply of a filter designed to fit the opening of a tracheostomy. Typically, this device is a soft foam filter disk to cover the air entry of a tracheal stoma. The filter may be designed to interface with a silicon button fitted to the stoma.

A4483

A4483 Moisture exchanger, disposable, for use with invasive mechanical ventilation

Patients on mechanical ventilation lose the advantage of natural moisturizing effects of air flowing over the mucous membranes of the sinuses and nasopharynx. This code reports provision of a disposable moisture exchange device fitted to the mechanical ventilation system.

A4490-A4510

A4490 Surgical stockings above knee length, each

A4495 Surgical stockings thigh length, each

A4500 Surgical stockings below knee length, each

A4510 Surgical stockings full-length, each

Surgical compression stockings are designed to reduce edema and enhance circulation with graduated compression. Graduated compression means that each stocking has the greatest amount of compression at the ankle and gradually decreases as the garment comes up the leg toward the heart. Graduated compression ensures that the garment will not have a constricting or strangulation effect on the leg. Surgical stockings should be properly fit to the individual patient. A surgical compression stocking will have at least 20 mmHg of compression at the ankle, which is the minimum compression considered therapeutic. Ulcerations of the legs, edema of the legs, varicose veins, and lymphedema are some of the problems aided by surgical stockings. There are many different surgical stocking lengths available, such as above the knee, thigh length, below the knee, and full length. There are also many types of surgical stockings ranging in size and custom made. These HCPCS Level II codes do not include antiembolism stocking (TED hose) as these only have a minimal gradient compression.

A4520

A4520 Incontinence garment, any type, (e.g., brief, diaper), each

Incontinence garments may be disposable or reusable and may be a flat diaper or a brief. Disposable garments include those commonly found at supermarkets. Flat reusable cloth diapers are generally rectangular with the same thickness throughout. Fit is accomplished by folding. Reusable briefs come in many varieties and may vary from slightly contoured to fully fitted briefs. There are also fully fitted briefs made of patented materials that are designed to be used with internal pads.

A4550

A4550 Surgical trays

A surgical tray comprises procedure-specific instruments, devices, and dressings within a ready-to-use sterilized package. The trays are prepared and inventoried for any of a variety of anticipated procedures (e.g., suture removal). The instruments may be sterilized and repackaged; however, a recent trend is toward the use of disposable surgical trays.

A4553-A4554

A4553 Nondisposable underpads, all sizes

A4554 Disposable underpads, all sizes

Underpads are designed for incontinent patients to protect bedding and furniture from leakage. Most have a soft quick-drying cover layer, an absorbent center core, and a waterproof bottom layer. Disposable underpads are intended to be tossed out at every change. Non-disposable underpads are reusable and designed to be laundered.

A4555

A4555 Electrode/transducer for use with electrical stimulation device used for cancer treatment, replacement only

Electrically-insulated surface electrodes are applied to the head of the patient for the treatment of glioblastoma multiforme (GBM). These electrodes deliver alternating electric fields that are said to slow or stop the glioblastoma cells from dividing.

A4556-A4557

A4556 Electrodes (e.g., apnea monitor), per pair

A4557 Lead wires (e.g., apnea monitor), per pair

Electrodes for devices, such as apnea monitors or EKG units, are dispensed in pairs and may be stick-on electrodes or may be contained within an electrode belt. Electrodes are placed on the proper site to monitor breathing and/or electrical activity. Lead wires are also dispensed in pairs. They are typically color coded, as each wire must be attached to the correct electrode. For example, an apnea monitoring system usually has one black and one white lead wire. The white lead wire is attached to the electrode on the right side of the chest and the black one is attached to the electrode on the left. The lead wires are attached to the apnea monitor via a cable.

A4558-A4559

A4558 Conductive gel or paste, for use with electrical device (e.g., TENS, NMES), per oz

A4559 Coupling gel or paste, for use with ultrasound device, per oz

Conductive paste or gel may be used on the skin at the site where electrodes are placed to improve conduction of electrical impulses. Coupling gels and pastes are used with ultrasonic probes and devices. The gel and/or paste acts as an agent to keep the probe from sticking to the patient's skin, probe cover, or other covers. The probes temperature can range from cool to hot and may require specific, high-heat gels or pastes. Ultrasound conductive coupling gel may be covered and separately payable if an ultrasonic osteogenesis stimulator is covered.

A4561-A4562

A4561 Pessary, rubber, any type

A4562 Pessary, nonrubber, any type

A pessary is a hard rubber, plastic, or silicon device that is inserted into the vagina, often to support the uterus and/or bladder from prolapse. The device may be ring-shaped, similar to the outer structure of a cervical cap or diaphragm. Other designs are also seen. The device may be prescribed for extended use or for short-term treatment. Regardless, the device should be removed regularly for hygienic considerations.

A4563

A4563 Rectal control system for vaginal insertion, for long term use, includes pump and all supplies and accessories, any type each

Fecal incontinence is the uncontrollable discharge of stool from the rectum. A rectal control system consists of a vaginal insert and a pressure regulated pump. The vaginal insert includes a silicone covered stainless steel base and a posteriorly directed balloon. Once placed into the vagina, the balloon is inflated, reducing the size of the rectal lumen. When the patient needs to have a bowel movement, the balloon can be deflated. The vaginal insert requires a prescription and fitting during a physician office visit.

A4565

A4565 Slings

Typically constructed of canvas-type material or other materials such as cotton or nylon (including mesh-type products), an arm sling usually uses the shoulder/neck as the primary anchor, suspending the upper limb as needed, supporting the shoulder, upper arm, elbow, and, to a limited degree, the wrist and hand. Arm slings can be used with a cast or splint for any of these body areas, providing an added measure of support and protection. Arm slings may protect against reinjury.

A4566

A4566 Shoulder sling or vest design, abduction restrainer, with or without swathe control, prefabricated, includes fitting and adjustment

Abduction is a movement that draws a limb away from the median or sagittal plane of the body. An abduction restrainer is an immobilization device used to restrict movement in and around the shoulder by reducing movement and arm rotation. Most are figure eight designs that use a swathe that attaches to a sling or vest to position the arm.

A4570

A4570 Splint

A splint is an orthotic medical device used to immobilize a limb or the spine. A splint is usually composed of two pieces held in place by some type of cotton or nylon material. It may be used to temporarily immobilize a suspected fracture or dislocation until additional medical help can be obtained. Code A4570 is an undefined splint. Report this code only if a more appropriate HCPCS code is not available.

A4575

A4575 Topical hyperbaric oxygen chamber, disposable

A topical hyperbaric oxygen chamber is a device that applies oxygen at a high atmospheric pressure to a skin or surface wound. It is noninvasive and used in the home. The topical application of a limited supply of pressurized oxygen is purported to promote the healing of various acute and chronic wounds. The topical application has frequently been prescribed for decubitus ulcers and other chronic wounds of the skin and its underlying structures.

A4580-A4590

A4580 Cast supplies (e.g., plaster)

A4590 Special casting material (e.g., fiberglass)

Casting materials are made of plaster-imbedded strips or bandages or fiberglass wraps or strips, available in varieties pertinent to the type of fracture or post-surgical state requiring the support and protection of a cast. Some of these materials are initially dry and are water-activated, while others come pre-moistened for immediate application. Plaster varieties can be embedded with strength-adding chemical compounds such as polyurethane. Splints are used when a cast is not necessary but the injury or condition requires immobilization. Casts and casting materials support and protect fractured or strained extremities or other body areas. They hold manipulated (set) fractures in place or can assist other devices (pins, wires, screws) in doing so and protect against reinjury. These codes identify the different casting materials (e.g., fiberglass or plaster) for physicians, the type of immobilization provided (e.g., splint or cast for adult or pediatric patients), and the length or shape of casts for the different types of injuries or conditions (e.g., shoulder or body cast, long or short leg or arm cast).

A4595

A4595 Electrical stimulator supplies, 2 lead, per month, (e.g., TENS, NMES)

This code reports electrical stimulator supplies, two leads, per month (e.g., TENS, NMES). A transcutaneous electrical nerve stimulator (TENS) is a device that uses electrical current delivered through electrodes placed on the surface of the skin to decrease the patient's perception of pain by inhibiting the transmission of afferent pain nerve impulses and/or by stimulating the release of endorphins. The TENS unit can be applied in a variety of settings (in the patient's home, a physician's office, or in an outpatient clinic). A TENS unit alleviates or palliates acute postoperative pain, as well as chronic or intractable pain, depending on the etiology of the patient's condition. A four-lead TENS unit may be used with two leads or four leads, depending on the characteristics of the patient's pain. The leads direct the current from the stimulator to the electrodes to the area in which pain control is needed.

A4596

A4596 Cranial electrotherapy stimulation (CES) system supplies and accessories, per month

A cranial electrotherapy stimulation (CES) device delivers electronic microcurrent that is supposedly at a natural level. The current is delivered via small clips worn on the earlobes, and travels through the brain to stimulate specific groups of nerve cells. It is reportedly able to provide significant anxiety relief, mood normalization, pain relief, and better sleep. The device is controlled via two handheld probes. Accessories included in this code consist of the cranial electrotherapy stimulator, ear clip electrodes, electrode pads, and conductive solution. Accessories included in this code consist of the cranial electrotherapy stimulator, ear clip electrodes, electrode pads, and conductive solution. Report A4596 monthly.

A4600

A4600 Sleeve for intermittent limb compression device, replacement only, each

Intermittent limb compression devices are used to inflate and deflate a compression sleeve. The sleeve is inflated to apply compressive pressure gradient against the limb which will decrease from a lower to upper portion of the limb to enhance the acceleration of the flow of blood through the limb.

A4601

A4601 Lithium-ion battery, rechargeable, for nonprosthetic use, replacement

These battery systems fall into two major categories: primary or single-use batteries, which are cells containing lithium-metal anodes; and secondary or rechargeable batteries, which are systems utilizing lithium-ion chemistry. Primary lithium batteries have been used for implantable devices such as cardiac pacemakers, drug pumps, neurostimulators, and cardiac defibrillators. Rechargeable batteries have been used with left ventricular assist devices and total artificial hearts. All of these cells share the characteristics of high safety, reliability, energy density, and predictability of performance.

A4602

A4602 Replacement battery for external infusion pump owned by patient, lithium, 1.5 volt, each

This code reports the supply of a replacement 1.5 volt lithium battery for an external infusion pump that is owned by the patient. The battery is a standard, non-rechargeable lithium battery. A 3.6 volt replacement battery is reported with K0604. A 4.5 volt replacement battery is reported with K0605.

A4604

A4604 Tubing with integrated heating element for use with positive airway pressure device

Supply of tubing with an integrated heating element to be used with a positive airway pressure device is reported with A4604. The heating element is embedded in the outer spiral of the inspiratory limb of the tubing and has a smooth inner surface. This allows delivery of positive airway pressure with optimal humidity that does not condense in the tubing. This device is used primarily for individuals with obstructive sleep apnea who require heated humidification with positive airway pressure.

A4605

A4605 Tracheal suction catheter, closed system, each

A closed system tracheal suction catheter is designed to remove bronchial secretions in intubated patients. Closed suction catheters allow suctioning without requiring the patient to be disconnected from the ventilator. The advantage of a closed system is the prevention of hypoxemia during suctioning because ventilation is maintained during the suctioning process.

A4606

A4606 Oxygen probe for use with oximeter device, replacement

Oximetry is a noninvasive method to measure blood hemoglobin (Hb), usually to determine oxygen saturation. A probe is attached to the patient's earlobe or a fingertip. The probe emits a light source. The hemoglobin absorbs a percentage of the light, depending upon its oxygen saturation level, and the results are digitally recorded, sometimes in addition to other data, such as pulse. This code reports a replacement unit for the oxygen probe.

A4608

A4608 Transtracheal oxygen catheter, each

This code reports supply of a transtracheal oxygen (TTO) catheter, a small-diameter flexible tube that is fitted directly into the trachea. A stoma is surgically created to accommodate the catheter. The system is designed to directly deliver oxygen to the lungs at high efficiency. The catheter is inserted to a level several centimeters above the carinal junction. Compared to nasal cannulas, more oxygen is conserved, flow is largely uninterrupted, and arterial blood oxygen levels are better maintained. Additionally, speech is unimpeded and eating routines are unaffected. Generally, cleaning of the catheter is required several times per day. Durable catheters may require change-out about every 90 days, or earlier as needed. Other systems may feature disposable catheter components.

A4611-A4613

A4611 Battery, heavy-duty; replacement for patient-owned ventilator

A4612 Battery cables; replacement for patient-owned ventilator

A4613 Battery charger; replacement for patient-owned ventilator

This range of codes reports supply of batteries and related components for patient-owned ventilators. Patient-owned ventilators are likely to be conventional AC-powered devices with supplemental internal and external sealed lead acid (SLA) batteries for emergency use and portability. A 12 V or 24 V external battery and charging system with a direct current to alternating current inverter are common features of many ventilator systems. Typically, the external battery charges a 24 V internal battery, as does the AC system while in use. The internal battery always remains fully charged and is the power source of last resort. In emergencies, these systems can run on conventional 12 V car batteries. The SLA batteries are generally notable for price, reliability, charge retention, and relatively long life. Disadvantages include slow recharge time and the need to keep the charge topped off while the battery is not in use. Some patients prefer deep cycle marine batteries that stand up better to near-complete discharge and recharge. Most systems require special cables. Nickel cadmium (NiCad) batteries are usually acceptable for air travel and have other advantages, but they tend to lose charge over time while not in use.

A4614

A4614 Peak expiratory flow rate meter, hand held

A peak expiratory flow rate meter measures the maximum amount of air an individual can forcibly exhale. Hand held units are commonly used by asthmatics to determine a need for bronchodilation medications and to record regular readings in a daily journal. Hand held units vary in design, but many feature an air resistance cylinder that freezes a needle at the point of peak exhalation.

A4615

A4615 Cannula, nasal

A cannula is a hollow tube or sheath inserted into a vessel, duct, or cavity to facilitate passage of another instrument, such as a trocar or flexible tubing, fluid, or air. Report this code for a nasal cannula, one that sits in the nostrils to facilitate the delivery of therapeutic oxygen, also called nasal prongs.

A4616

A4616 Tubing (oxygen), per foot

Oxygen tubing is reported by the foot but is usually supplied in lengths of 25 and 50 feet. Tubing is crush resistant to prevent interruptions in the flow of oxygen and may be supplied with tubing connectors.

A4617

A4617 Mouthpiece

Mouthpieces for nebulizers may be purchased separately. They are available in pediatric and adult sizes. Mouthpieces are used to deliver inhalant medications dispensed via small volume nebulizers.

A4618

A4618 Breathing circuits

A breathing circuit is a component array used to connect an intubated patient's airway to a gas anesthesia delivery system. The circuit creates an artificial atmosphere that the patient both draws air from as well as breathes exhaled air into. Components include: a port to deliver various anesthetic and other gases to the breathing circuit; a port to the patient's intubated airway; a reservoir bag for gas; an expiration port to release and control exhaled gas into room air; a carbon dioxide absorbing system for total rebreathing circuit; and tubes to connect the various components. A breathing circuit can be set so that no rebreathing of air is allowed (fresh gas is not mixed with exhaled gas). A partial rebreathing setting allows for a portion of exhaled gas to be mixed with fresh gas. Total rebreathing settings require that exhaled gas be purged of carbon dioxide. A variety of breathing circuit features is available, including an interface with ventilation assist and alarms.

A4619

A4619 Face tent

A face tent is a soft plastic face mask type of device for the delivery of oxygen or combination of gases. The device differs from a face mask in that the perimeter of the device does not come in contact with the patient's skin. Face tents are useful for individuals who have had facial surgery or who otherwise cannot tolerate the contact of a face mask or nasal cannulas. Disadvantages include difficulty in delivering therapeutic quantities of gas due to the imperfect air seal.

A4620

A4620 Variable concentration mask

Variable concentration masks are also known as low flow masks and deliver oxygen at variable rates depending upon how the patient is breathing. The device is usually a simple face mask with tubing and is used in instances where a fixed concentration of oxygen is not required.

A4623

A4623 Tracheostomy, inner cannula

Inner cannulas are used inside of outer cannulas after a tracheostomy. A small opening is made through the stoma and a breathing tube is placed directly into the trachea (windpipe). There are three parts to the placement of a trach tube. The obturator is used to pass the trach tube into the trachea and a portion is removed leaving the outer cannula in place. The outer cannula has a plate that sits against the skin of the neck and holds the trach in place. The inner cannula fits inside the outer cannula and locks it into place.

A4624

A4624 Tracheal suction catheter, any type other than closed system, each

Tracheal suction catheters are used to clear the airways of excessive secretions. Catheters are made of soft rubber or hard plastic material. The diameter of each catheter is measured according to the French catheter scale, and they vary in length. Catheter tips may be a two-eye whistle tip design reducing the chance of damage to the mucosal tissue, or softer rounded style, which can be gentler on the mucosal lining. This code is for a tracheal suction catheter, any type.

A4625-A4626

A4625 Tracheostomy care kit for new tracheostomy

A4626 Tracheostomy cleaning brush, each

A tracheostomy care kit for a new tracheostomy is used following an open surgical tracheostomy that is expected to remain open for at least three months. These kits are composed of supplies that are used to routinely clean and care for tracheostomy tubes, accessories, and the area around the tracheostomy. Tracheostomy care is necessary to reduce the chance of inflammation and infection around the tracheostomy site. Cleaning the tracheostomy tube allows air to move freely through the tube.

A4627

A4627 Spacer, bag or reservoir, with or without mask, for use with metered dose inhaler

A spacer, bag, or reservoir used with a metered dose inhaler increases the space between the metered dose inhaler and the mouth. It helps the patient inhale more medication into the lungs and decreases the amount of medication that is deposited at the back of the throat. Spacers, bags, and reservoirs are particularly useful for children, particularly those with asthma, due to the difficulty some children have in inhaling slowly while depressing the inhaler at the same time.

A4628

A4628 Oropharyngeal suction catheter, each

An oropharyngeal suction catheter is used to remove secretions from the oral cavity and pharynx.

A4629

A4629 Tracheostomy care kit for established tracheostomy

A tracheostomy care kit for a new tracheostomy is used following an open surgical tracheostomy that is expected to remain open for at least three months. These kits are composed of supplies that are used to routinely clean and care for tracheostomy tubes, accessories, and the area around the tracheostomy. Tracheostomy care is necessary to reduce the chance of inflammation and infection around the tracheostomy site. Cleaning the tracheostomy tube allows air to move freely through the tube. Report this code for an established tracheostomy care kit.

A4630

A4630 Replacement batteries, medically necessary, transcutaneous electrical stimulator, owned by patient

Transcutaneous electrical nerve stimulator (TENS) units require the use of a 9-volt, standard battery or a rechargeable cell. The initial purchase of a TENS unit generally includes a battery. When the battery for a patient-owned, medically necessary TENS unit requires replacement, report this code.

A4633-A4634

A4633 Replacement bulb/lamp for ultraviolet light therapy system, each

A4634 Replacement bulb for therapeutic light box, tabletop model

Light box therapy is used in the treatment of seasonal affective disorder (SAD), diurnal disorders, or sometimes to mitigate the sedating effect of medications. Although bulbs are rated for 20,000 hours of use, they generally begin to lose intensity after four to five years of use and require replacement. When long-term ultraviolet light or light box therapy is required, the bulbs must be periodically replaced.

A4635-A4637

A4635 Underarm pad, crutch, replacement, each

A4636 Replacement, handgrip, cane, crutch, or walker, each

A4637 Replacement, tip, cane, crutch, walker, each

Underarm pads, hand grips, and tips for patient-owned crutches, canes, and walkers periodically require replacement.

A4638

A4638 Replacement battery for patient-owned ear pulse generator, each

This code reports a replacement battery for a patient-owned ear pulse generator used in the tympanic treatment of inner ear endolymphatic fluid, also known as Meniere's disease.

A4639

A4639 Replacement pad for infrared heating pad system, each

An infrared heating pad system consists of a pad or pads containing mechanisms (e.g., luminous gallium aluminum arsenide diodes) that generate infrared (or near infrared) light and a power source. Report this code for each replacement pad.

A4640

A4640 Replacement pad for use with medically necessary alternating pressure pad owned by patient

An alternating pressure pad is designed to distribute the patient's body weight more effectively, preventing pressure points from developing. The pressure pad is attached to a pump that alternately inflates and deflates air cells in the pressure pad. Air cycling through the air cells provides patient lift and pressure reduction that assists in reducing pressure on skin and tissues and facilitates blood flow to all areas of the body that come in contact with the mattress. Alternating pressure pads are used to prevent and/or treat pressure ulcers and lesions, such as decubitus ulcers.

A4641

A4641 Radiopharmaceutical, diagnostic, not otherwise classified

This code reports the supply of radiopharmaceutical diagnostic imaging agents that do not have a more specific HCPCS Level II code. Radiopharmaceuticals are radioactive isotopes, such as radioactive iodine or radioactive cobalt. They are often attached to carrier molecules and used in diagnostic nuclear medicine procedures.

A4642

A4642 Indium In-111 satumomab pendetide, diagnostic, per study dose, up to 6 mCi

Satumomab pendetide is a murine monoclonal antibody that binds to a glycoprotein, a cell surface antigen produced in large amounts by colorectal and ovarian tumors. This monoclonal antibody does not generally react with normal adult tissue, but it may react with salivary gland ducts, normal post-ovulatory endometria, some benign ovarian tumors, and fetal gastrointestinal tissue. Indium 111 is a radioactive form of the metallic element indium. It has a half-life of approximately 56 hours and decays by electron capture and gamma emission. The monoclonal antibody is combined with indium 111 chloride so that it can be readily identified in images. Indium 111 satumomab pendetide is administered intravenously. It rapidly attaches itself to colorectal adenocarcinomas and common epithelial ovarian carcinomas. Optimal images are obtained 48 to 72 hours following administration. Since satumomab pendetide may attach itself to nonmalignant tissue, use of this diagnostic agent is not recommended for screening purposes. Indium 111 satumomab pendetide is indicated for patients with known colorectal or ovarian cancer to determine the extent and location of disease.

A4648

A4648 Tissue marker, implantable, any type, each

An implantable tissue marker is a small, non-absorbable piece of material, usually metal, that is used to mark an area of concern within soft tissue. The tissue marker is usually visible with multiple types of imaging and can be used to mark an area that needs continued follow-up. The marker can also be used to indicate an area to be removed or biopsied.

A4649

A4649 Surgical supply; miscellaneous

This code reports miscellaneous surgical supplies and should only be reported if a more specific HCPCS Level II or CPT code is not available.

A4650

A4650 Implantable radiation dosimeter, each

An implantable radiation dosimeter is a permanent, small, non-absorbable device that is inserted into the target area that is to be irradiated with external beam ionizing radiation. The device measures the amount of radiation reaching the targeted area and serves as a marker. This allows the physician to better track and calibrate the location and amount of radiation delivered.

A4651

A4651 Calibrated microcapillary tube, each

This code reports the supply of each calibrated microcapillary tube. These are glass laboratory tubes designed to measure and contain extremely small quantities of liquid. Some may have a coating of heparin on the inside surface to maintain blood in liquid storage. Others may be tempered to withstand extreme temperature variations. Most can be sealed for centrifuging or mechanical agitation.

A4652

A4652 Microcapillary tube sealant

Microcapillary tubes are glass laboratory tubes used to measure and contain small quantities of liquid. Most can be sealed for centrifuging or mechanical agitation.

A4653

A4653 Peritoneal dialysis catheter anchoring device, belt, each

Peritoneal dialysis is an alternative to hemodialysis. Peritoneal dialysis requires that a peritoneal catheter be inserted into the abdominal (peritoneal) cavity. The catheter consists of a 15-inch tube with two cuffs in the middle of the catheter. One section of tubing is placed into the peritoneal cavity. The cuffs in the middle section are placed just outside the peritoneal cavity in the fatty tissue and protect the catheter site from infection and leakage. The outer portion of tubing is used to connect the dialysis solution. Dialysis solution is then instilled through the catheter into the peritoneal cavity where it removes impurities, waste products, and extra fluid when this function can no longer be performed by the kidneys due to disease or injury. Patients on peritoneal dialysis sometimes require additional supplies to protect the catheter, such as an anchoring device that helps to protect the catheter from becoming dislodged.

A4657

A4657 Syringe, with or without needle, each

A sterile syringe is used for injecting or withdrawing fluid from any vessel or cavity. Syringes may vary in size and may be supplied with or without a needle.

A4660

A4660 Sphygmomanometer/blood pressure apparatus with cuff and stethoscope

This code reports the supply of a sphygmomanometer with cuff and stethoscope, a traditional blood pressure measuring device still in common use. A cuff and rubber bag are wrapped around the upper arm and secured with Velcro. Tubing connects the bag to a mercury manometer, which measures pressure within the cuff. The bag is inflated, usually by squeezing an air bulb, until pressure on the arm exceeds arterial pressure. A stethoscope over the brachial artery below the cuff confirms that no blood movement is heard. A valve slowly releases pressure on the bag. The artery first emits sound upon peak pressure from the heart, or systolic pressure. This is noted by the observer and the manometer reading is taken. As pressure on the cuff continues to drop, arterial occlusion fails even upon lowest pressure from the heart, the diastolic pressure. This characteristic sound heard through the stethoscope is also noted by the trained observer and the second manometer reading is taken. The two pressures, systolic and diastolic, are recorded as the patient's blood pressure.

A4663

A4663 Blood pressure cuff only

This code reports the supply of a traditional sphygmomanometer blood pressure cuff only. The cuff is the portion of the apparatus that wraps around the upper arm and is secured with Velcro. The traditional cuff contains a rubber bag that is connected to a manometer or other device to measure pressure. The bag is inflated, usually by squeezing an air bulb, placing pressure on the arteries of the arm.

A4670

A4670 Automatic blood pressure monitor

An automatic blood pressure monitor consists of a digital gauge and a stethoscope in one unit. Automatic blood pressure monitors are powered by batteries. The cuff may be inflated manually or automatically depending on the model. The blood pressure recording is displayed on a digital screen that will also display error messages. The error messages help ensure accurate blood pressure readings. Deflation of the cuff is automatic. Some models of automatic blood pressure monitors will also provide a paper printout of blood pressure recordings.

A4671

A4671 Disposable cycler set used with cycler dialysis machine, each

During automated peritoneal dialysis, also called continuous cycling peritoneal dialysis (CCPD) or nocturnal cyclical peritoneal dialysis, a sterile mixture of sugar and minerals dissolved in water (dialysis solution) flows through a catheter into the peritoneal cavity using a cycler machine. Using osmosis, the solution draws wastes, impurities, chemicals, and extra water from the tiny blood vessels in the peritoneal membrane into the solution. The cycler machine automatically infuses the dialysis solution and then drains it several times during the night. Disposable cycler kits are available that contain supplies required for CCPD.

A4672-A4673

A4672 Drainage extension line, sterile, for dialysis, each

A4673 Extension line with easy lock connectors, used with dialysis

Extension lines for dialysis provide added length to catheters, which can assist in patient comfort and mobility.

A4674

A4674 Chemicals/antiseptics solution used to clean/sterilize dialysis equipment, per 8 oz

There are two types of dialysis, hemodialysis and peritoneal dialysis. Hemodialysis removes excess fluids, wastes, impurities, and chemicals from the blood by use of a dialyzer. Hemodialysis requires the use of a dialysis machine, dialyzer, dialysis solution, treated water, and disposable supplies. Peritoneal dialysis is an alternative to hemodialysis. Peritoneal dialysis uses the thin lining in the abdomen that coats the outer surface of the intestines (peritoneal membrane) to remove waste products and balance fluids. The dialysis solution is instilled through a catheter placed through the skin into the peritoneal cavity. The dialysis solution removes waste products and excess fluid and is then drained from the abdomen and discarded. Dialysis equipment must be properly cleaned and sterilized to prevent infection.

A4680

A4680 Activated carbon filter for hemodialysis, each

This code represents an activated carbon filter used for hemodialysis as a component of a water purification system to remove unsafe concentrations of chloride or chloramines.

A4690

A4690 Dialyzer (artificial kidneys), all types, all sizes, for hemodialysis, each

This code reports the supply of a dialyzer, the portion of a hemodialysis machine that cleanses blood in patients with end-stage renal disease (ESRD). Dialysis is a physicochemical and filtration process. The dialyzer portion of a hemodialysis unit is typically a two-chambered clear plastic cylinder. The cylinder is packed with hollow fiber strands that form a membrane between the chambers. One chamber circulates blood drawn from the patient. The second circulates a solution known as dialysate in the opposite direction from movement of the blood. This semipermeable membrane between the chambers allows accumulated uremic toxins, excess ions, and water in the blood to pass into the dialysate. A similar dialyzer design, known as the parallel plate process, separates the chambers by a cellophane-type membrane. With either process, cleansed blood is returned to the patient as the dialysate is constantly refreshed. The dialyzer is generally changed out between patients, although the same patient may use a single dialyzer repeatedly.

A4706-A4707

A4706 Bicarbonate concentrate, solution, for hemodialysis, per gallon

A4707 Bicarbonate concentrate, powder, for hemodialysis, per packet

These codes report the supply of bicarbonate concentrate for hemodialysis. Hemodialysis is a physicochemical and filtration process. The dialyzer portion of a hemodialysis unit is typically two-chambered. One chamber circulates blood drawn from the patient. The second circulates a solution known as dialysate in the opposite direction from movement of the blood. A semipermeable membrane between the chambers allows accumulated uremic toxins, excess ions, and water in the blood to pass into the dialysate. Cleansed blood is returned to the patient as the dialysate is constantly refreshed. Bicarbonate concentrate is added to treated water and acetic acid in a fixed proportion to form the dialysate base. Low concentrations of bicarbonate in the dialysate can result in metabolic acidosis. Ordinarily, a sensor and alarm on the hemodialysis unit alert the operator of an imbalance in the dialysate solution.

A4708-A4709

A4708 Acetate concentrate solution, for hemodialysis, per gallon

A4709 Acid concentrate, solution, for hemodialysis, per gallon

These codes report the supply of acetate concentrate and acid concentrate solutions for hemodialysis. Hemodialysis is a physicochemical and filtration process. The dialyzer portion of a hemodialysis unit is typically two chambered. One chamber circulates blood drawn from the patient. The second circulates a solution know as dialysate in the opposite direction from movement of the blood. A semipermeable membrane between the chambers allows accumulated uremic toxins, excess ions, and water in the blood to pass into the dialysate. Cleansed blood is returned to the patient as the dialysate is constantly refreshed. Acetate and/or acid concentrate, as well as bicarbonate concentrate, must be mixed with dialysate in specific ratios depending on the type of dialysis equipment being used to achieve the proper chemical balance in the dialysis solution.

A4714

A4714 Treated water (deionized, distilled, or reverse osmosis) for peritoneal dialysis, per gallon

Peritoneal dialysis is an alternative to hemodialysis. Peritoneal dialysis uses the thin lining in the abdomen that coats the outer surface of the intestines (peritoneal membrane) to remove waste products and balance fluids. The dialysis solution is instilled through a catheter placed through the skin into the peritoneal cavity. The dialysis solution removes waste products and excess fluid and is then drained from the abdomen and discarded. Treatments are generally performed by the patient. Peritoneal dialysis requires the use of dialysis solution, treated water, and disposable supplies.

A4719

A4719 "Y set" tubing for peritoneal dialysis

This code reports the supply of y-set tubing for peritoneal dialysis. Peritoneal dialysis (PD) is the main alternative to hemodialysis for patients with end-stage renal disease (ESRD). In PD, used dialysate is exchanged for fresh product, usually once or twice per day. The patient will have a surgically created stoma and an indwelling peritoneal catheter. A special y-tube with clamps is connected to the PD catheter. A clamp on the y-tube is opened and used dialysate is drained from the cavity and collected. Upon completion, the drain tube is clamped and about 1.5 to 3 liters of fresh dialysate is gravity infused through the other lead of the y-tube catheter into the peritoneal cavity. The dialysate may be left in place for one to eight hours, depending on the patient's requirements. Y-set tubing is reusable for up to several months.

A4720-A4726

A4720 Dialysate solution, any concentration of dextrose, fluid volume greater than 249 cc, but less than or equal to 999 cc, for peritoneal dialysis

A4721 Dialysate solution, any concentration of dextrose, fluid volume greater than 999 cc but less than or equal to 1999 cc, for peritoneal dialysis

A4722 Dialysate solution, any concentration of dextrose, fluid volume greater than 1999 cc but less than or equal to 2999 cc, for peritoneal dialysis

A4723 Dialysate solution, any concentration of dextrose, fluid volume greater than 2999 cc but less than or equal to 3999 cc, for peritoneal dialysis

A4724 Dialysate solution, any concentration of dextrose, fluid volume greater than 3999 cc but less than or equal to 4999 cc, for peritoneal dialysis

A4725 Dialysate solution, any concentration of dextrose, fluid volume greater than 4999 cc but less than or equal to 5999 cc, for peritoneal dialysis

A4726 Dialysate solution, any concentration of dextrose, fluid volume greater than 5999 cc, for peritoneal dialysis

This range of codes reports various sized supplies of dialysate solution for peritoneal dialysis. The codes are differentiated by volume of solution supplied. Peritoneal dialysis (PD) is the main alternative to hemodialysis for patients with end-stage renal disease

A

(ESRD). In PD, used dialysate is exchanged for fresh product, usually once or twice per day. The patient will have a surgically created stoma and an indwelling peritoneal catheter. A special y-tube with clamps is connected to the PD catheter. A clamp on the y-tube is opened and used dialysate is drained from the cavity and collected. Upon completion, the drain tube is clamped and about 1.5 to 3 liters of fresh dialysate is gravity infused through the other lead of the y-tube catheter into the peritoneal cavity. The fresh solution contains dextrose (sugar) that helps to withdraw wastes and excess fluids. This range of codes is independent of dextrose concentrations in the dialysate.

A4728

A4728 Dialysate solution, nondextrose containing, 500 ml

There are two types of dialysis, hemodialysis and peritoneal dialysis. Both make use of a solution called dialysate to draw waste products out of the blood. Hemodialysis removes excess fluids, wastes, impurities, and chemicals from the blood by use of a dialyzer. Hemodialysis requires the use of a dialysis machine, dialyzer, dialysis solution (dialysate), treated water, and disposable supplies. Peritoneal dialysis is an alternative to hemodialysis. Peritoneal dialysis uses the thin lining in the abdomen that coats the outer surface of the intestines (peritoneal membrane) to remove waste products and balance fluids. The dialysis solution (dialysate) is instilled through a catheter placed through the skin into the peritoneal cavity. The dialysis solution removes waste products and excess fluid and is then drained from the abdomen and discarded.

A4730

A4730 Fistula cannulation set for hemodialysis, each

This code reports the supply of each fistula cannulation set for hemodialysis. In most cases, patients will have had a surgically created arterial-venous fistula in the wrist or elbow region, and several configurations are seen. A synthetic graft of soft plastic tubing between the artery and the vein may be chosen. The plastic graft portion of the fistula, which may lie exteriorly, can then be repeatedly accessed for hemodialysis. The cannula set is designed to interface between the fistula and the hemodialysis unit.

A4736-A4737

A4736 Topical anesthetic, for dialysis, per g

A4737 Injectable anesthetic, for dialysis, per 10 ml

These codes report local anesthetics used during dialysis. Local anesthetics reduce sensation or feeling in the area of the body where they are applied or injected.

A4740

A4740 Shunt accessory, for hemodialysis, any type, each

A hemodialysis shunt is an artificial, external blood route that provides access to the blood supply. Shunt accessories such as connectors and adapters are attached to the hemodialysis shunt to perform dialysis. Examples of items that would be reported with this code include shunt connectors, universal connectors, Teflon connectors, shunt adapters, universal adapters, and Teflon adapters.

A4750-A4755

A4750 Blood tubing, arterial or venous, for hemodialysis, each

A4755 Blood tubing, arterial and venous combined, for hemodialysis, each

Hemodialysis tubing consists of a plastic tube or tubes that is attached to a fistula needle or shunt connector and allows blood to flow to and from the patient and dialyzer. Blood tubing for hemodialysis may be separate arterial and venous tubing or combined arteriovenous tubing.

A4760

A4760 Dialysate solution test kit, for peritoneal dialysis, any type, each

Dialysate is an electrolyte solution containing elements such as potassium, sodium, chloride, etc. Dialysate that is supplied in solution or powder concentrate form must be mixed with purified water prior to use. The mixed solution requires testing to verify that electrolyte levels are correct.

A4765-A4766

A4765 Dialysate concentrate, powder, additive for peritoneal dialysis, per packet

A4766 Dialysate concentrate, solution, additive for peritoneal dialysis, per 10 ml

Dialysate is an electrolyte solution containing elements such as potassium, sodium, chloride, etc. Dialysate that is supplied in solution or powder concentrate form must be mixed with purified water prior to use.

A4770-A4771

A4770 Blood collection tube, vacuum, for dialysis, per 50

A4771 Serum clotting time tube, for dialysis, per 50

These codes report blood collection tubes for dialysis. Vacuum tubes have a precisely controlled vacuum that allows the correct amount of blood to be collected for each specimen required. Serum clotting time tubes are designed specifically to test blood samples for clotting time.

A4772-A4774

A4772 Blood glucose test strips, for dialysis, per 50

A4773 Occult blood test strips, for dialysis, per 50

A4774 Ammonia test strips, for dialysis, per 50

These codes report test strips used to check blood glucose, occult blood, and ammonia levels in patients undergoing dialysis.

A4802

A4802 Protamine sulfate, for hemodialysis, per 50 mg

Protamine sulfate is used to neutralize the effects of heparin. Protamine sulfate is a strong basic polypeptide that when administered alone has an anticoagulant effect. However, when administered with heparin, protamine sulfate complexes with the strongly acidic heparin to form an inactive stable salt and the complex has no anticoagulant activity.

A4860

A4860 Disposable catheter tips for peritoneal dialysis, per 10

This code reports a supply of 10 disposable catheter tips used during peritoneal dialysis.

A4870-A4890

A4870 Plumbing and/or electrical work for home hemodialysis equipment

A4890 Contracts, repair and maintenance, for hemodialysis equipment

These codes report plumbing and electrical modifications required in the patient's home so that the dialysis equipment can be effectively and safely used, as well as contract work performed on hemodialysis equipment. Report A4870 for costs associated with plumbing and electrical modifications.

A4911-A4932

A4911 Drain bag/bottle, for dialysis, each

A4913 Miscellaneous dialysis supplies, not otherwise specified

A4918 Venous pressure clamp, for hemodialysis, each

A4927 Gloves, nonsterile, per 100

A4928 Surgical mask, per 20

A4929 Tourniquet for dialysis, each

A4930 Gloves, sterile, per pair

A4931 Oral thermometer, reusable, any type, each

A4932 Rectal thermometer, reusable, any type, each

These codes report additional supplies used during dialysis. All codes are for specific supplies except A4913, which should be used to report miscellaneous dialysis supplies when a more specific HCPCS Level II code is not available.

A5051-A5054

A5051 Ostomy pouch, closed; with barrier attached (one piece), each

A5052 Ostomy pouch, closed; without barrier attached (one piece), each

A5053 Ostomy pouch, closed; for use on faceplate, each

A5054 Ostomy pouch, closed; for use on barrier with flange (two piece), each

These codes represent ostomy pouches that are used with patients who have had a surgically created opening for diversion of stool. Ostomy pouches collect the stomal output, in this case feces, and can be drainable or closed. Drainable pouches have an opening at the bottom through which fecal contents can be emptied. Closed pouches have a sealed bottom with no outlet for feces. Drainable pouches have an opening at one end to allow the contents to be drained without removing the entire bag. There are also one-piece and two-piece systems. One-piece systems are supplied "with barrier attached" or "without barrier attached." Two-piece systems have a locking or non-locking flange that is coupled to a skin barrier with flange. Skin barriers are an interface between the patient's skin and the pouching system and have a variety of different options, such as built-in convexity, filters, locking or nonlocking flanges, and use with or without faceplates.

A5055

A5055 Stoma cap

Stoma caps are designed to retain discharge at the site of the stoma for patients with ostomies. A stoma is an artificial opening into a body passageway or organ. It is performed when the organ cannot function normally. Ostomies are usually permanent openings, created for drainage to the outside of the body, so that fecal or urinary materials can be eliminated. The stoma caps are extremely absorbent, flexible, waterproof covers that may also include odor control features.

A5056-A5057

A5056 Ostomy pouch, drainable, with extended wear barrier attached, with filter, (one piece), each

A5057 Ostomy pouch, drainable, with extended wear barrier attached, with built in convexity, with filter, (one piece), each

These codes represent ostomy pouches that are used with patients who have had a surgically created opening for diversion of stool. Ostomy pouches collect the stomal output, in this case feces, and can be drainable or closed. Drainable pouches have an opening at the bottom through which fecal contents can be emptied. Closed pouches have a sealed bottom with no outlet for feces. Drainable pouches have an opening at one end to allow the contents to be drained without removing the entire bag. There are also one-piece and two-piece systems. One-piece systems are supplied "with barrier attached" or "without barrier attached." Two-piece systems have a locking or non-locking flange that is coupled to a skin barrier with flange. Skin barriers are an interface between the patient's skin and the pouching system and have a variety of different options, such as built-in convexity, filters, locking or nonlocking flanges, and use with or without faceplates.

A5061-A5063

A5061 Ostomy pouch, drainable; with barrier attached, (one piece), each

A5062 Ostomy pouch, drainable; without barrier attached (one piece), each

A5063 Ostomy pouch, drainable; for use on barrier with flange (two-piece system), each

These codes represent drainable ostomy pouches. Ostomy pouches are used by patients who have had a surgically created opening for diversion of urine. The ostomy pouch with barrier attached is a one-piece system in which a solid barrier serving to create an adhesive seal is part of the ostomy pouch. The barrier may be pectin-based or karaya-based for normal wear, or pectin-based with special additives for extended wear. A flange or plastic ring on both the pouch and skin barrier secures the barrier and the pouch.

A5071-A5073

A5071 Ostomy pouch, urinary; with barrier attached (one piece), each

A5072 Ostomy pouch, urinary; without barrier attached (one piece), each

A5073 Ostomy pouch, urinary; for use on barrier with flange (two piece), each

These codes represent urinary ostomy pouches. Urinary ostomy pouches are for use with patients who have had a surgically created opening for diversion of the urine. There are one-piece and two-piece systems. In one-piece appliances, the collection pouch and barrier cannot be separated from one another, whereas the two-piece appliance is designed so that the barrier and collection pouch are separated by a locking mechanism. An ostomy faceplate is a solid interface between the patient's skin and the pouch. It is usually made of plastic, rubber, or encased metal. It can be taken off the skin and reattached repeatedly. It is held on by means of a separate adhesive and/or an elastic belt.

A5081-A5083

A5081 Stoma plug or seal, any type

A5082 Continent device; catheter for continent stoma

A5083 Continent device, stoma absorptive cover for continent stoma

These codes report specific supplies for continent stomas. A continent stoma usually involves a surgically fashioned "neobladder" that allows for natural voiding capability. In some instances the pouch is created from a section of ileum, cecum, or other portions of the colon. Part of the bladder may be preserved and the intestinal graft attached to it. Nerves and blood vessels of the graft are usually preserved. The ileocecal sphincter may be preserved and used as a valve. The stoma is managed by a plug and catheter system, and these codes report the supply of these products.

A5093

A5093 Ostomy accessory; convex insert

A convex insert is an ostomy accessory that fits between the ostomy pouch and the ostomy pad surrounding the stoma opening. The convex insert helps to provide the ostomy pouch with a tighter fit.

A5102

A5102 Bedside drainage bottle with or without tubing, rigid or expandable, each

Patients with urinary ostomies may use a bedside drainage bottle. The bedside drainage bottle is reusable and collects urinary output from a pouch. It is sometimes necessary, especially at night, for the bottle to be connected to the pouch to prevent urinary overflow and excessive weight in the pouch, which could cause urinary leakage and disruption of the pouch seal. The bottle is made of a high-density polyethylene and can hold up to 2,000 cc. Report this code for rigid or expandable bedside bottle with or without tubing.

A5105

A5105 Urinary suspensory with leg bag, with or without tube, each

This code reports the supply of an external urinary suspensory garment. This garment is usually designed for males and is worn like a jock strap. A urinal sheath is attachable to a portion that fits around the penis. This in turn is attachable to a tube and leg bag to drain urine.

A5112

A5112 Urinary drainage bag, leg or abdomen, latex, with or without tube, with straps, each

Urinary leg bags are used with male external urinary catheters. At the top is an anti-reflux flutter valve that attaches to the urinary catheter and allows urine to drain from the bladder into the leg bag. At the bottom is a drainage valve that allows the catheter to be emptied as needed. Leg bags may be constructed of a variety of materials.

A5113-A5114

A5113 Leg strap; latex, replacement only, per set

A5114 Leg strap; foam or fabric, replacement only, per set

These codes are for replacement leg straps used with a urinary leg bag. These codes are not reported for a leg strap for an indwelling catheter.

A5120

A5120 Skin barrier, wipes or swabs, each

Skin barrier wipes and swabs are used to clean and protect the stoma site. Wipes and swabs are formulated with soothing, non-sting cleanser that also provides a protective film around the stoma to prevent irritation of the stoma between pouch changes. Wipes and swabs may also be medicated to provide further protection to the stoma site.

A5121-A5122

A5121 Skin barrier; solid, 6 x 6 or equivalent, each

A5122 Skin barrier; solid, 8 x 8 or equivalent, each

Skin barriers are an interface between the patient's skin and the pouching system. They are used to create an adhesive seal between the skin and the pouch. Barriers can be curved with a built-in convexity creating a more adhesive bond to the patient's skin and better protrusion of the stoma. These codes represent solid ostomy skin barriers that are used independently, usually with a pouch that does not have its own integral skin barrier.

A5126

A5126 Adhesive or nonadhesive; disk or foam pad

Adhesive liquids are applied directly to the skin or to a protective barrier, such as a disk or foam pad, providing increased bonding of ostomy devices. These adhesives are in liquid form or are equal to a liquid available in bottles or spray cans. They are rubber based or acrylic based and non-toxic. Proper application of adhesives is a thin, light coat on the desired area. Adhesives can be removed with petroleum-based solvents. Report this code for the disk or foam pad utilized as a protective barrier.

A5131

A5131 Appliance cleaner, incontinence and ostomy appliances, per 16 oz

Appliance cleaners are used to deodorize, remove crystallized deposits, and clean the inside of rubber, latex, and plastic incontinence or ostomy collection devices. Report this code for every 16 oz. of cleaner.

A5200

A5200 Percutaneous catheter/tube anchoring device, adhesive skin attachment

A percutaneous catheter/tube anchoring device is a dressing with adhesive that is designed to be applied directly over the cutaneous opening through which the catheter/tube passes. This dressing has a hole through which the catheter/tube passes and a mechanism for firmly anchoring the catheter/tube to the dressing.

A5500-A5501

A5500 For diabetics only, fitting (including follow-up), custom preparation and supply of off-the-shelf depth-inlay shoe manufactured to accommodate multidensity insert(s), per shoe

A5501 For diabetics only, fitting (including follow-up), custom preparation and supply of shoe molded from cast(s) of patient's foot (custom molded shoe), per shoe

These items include fitting with follow-up, custom preparation, and supply of off-the-shelf or custom made shoes that accommodate various shoe inserts. Shoes and shoe inserts assist the diabetic patient with ambulation, decrease pressure points that may be present in non-prescription shoes, and help prevent ulcerative conditions of the feet. They are used in patients with partial or complete amputation (opposite foot). Previous foot ulcerations and current pre-ulcerative conditions may be present. Circulation may be impaired, and deformity and/or peripheral neuropathy may be present. Report A5500 for off-the-shelf depth shoes, which are custom prepared and have multi-density (varying depths) of insert. They usually are full-length. In A5501, a molded cast of the patient's foot may be performed or may be heat-molded to fit almost any foot. They also have removable inserts that can be altered, with some form of shoe closure. Each code is reported per shoe.

A5503-A5506

A5503 For diabetics only, modification (including fitting) of off-the-shelf depth-inlay shoe or custom molded shoe with roller or rigid rocker bottom, per shoe

A5504 For diabetics only, modification (including fitting) of off-the-shelf depth-inlay shoe or custom molded shoe with wedge(s), per shoe

A5505 For diabetics only, modification (including fitting) of off-the-shelf depth-inlay shoe or custom molded shoe with metatarsal bar, per shoe

A5506 For diabetics only, modification (including fitting) of off-the-shelf depth-inlay shoe or custom molded shoe with off-set heel(s), per shoe

These items include fitting with follow-up, custom preparation, and supply of off-the-shelf or custom made shoes with special added features. A molded cast of the patient's foot may be performed. Shoes and shoe inserts assist the diabetic patient with ambulation, decrease pressure points that may be present in non-prescription shoes, and help prevent ulcerative conditions of the feet. They are used in patients with partial or complete amputation (opposite foot). Previous foot ulcerations and current pre-ulcerative conditions may be present. Circulation may be impaired, and deformity and/or peripheral neuropathy may be present. Rigid rocker bottoms are exterior elevations. The apex (a narrowed or pointed end) is measured from the back end of the heel, positioned behind the metatarsal heads, and tapers off sharply to the front tip of the sole. Apex height helps to eliminate pressure at the metatarsal heads. The heel tapers off in back to cause the shoe heel to strike in the middle of the heel. The steel in a patient's shoe ensures rigidity. Roller bottoms (sole or bar) are the same as rocker bottoms, but the heel is tapered from the apex to the front tip of the sole. A shoe with wedges that are either of the hind foot, fore foot, or both and may be in the middle or to the side is reported with A5504. The function is to shift or transfer weight bearing upon standing or during ambulation to the opposite side for added support, stabilization, equalized weight distribution, or balance. An exterior bar is placed behind the metatarsal heads in order to remove pressure from the metatarsal heads. The bars are of various shapes, heights, and construction depending on the purpose it serves. Report A5506 for an offset heel flanged at its base either in the middle, to the side, or a combination, that is then extended upward to the shoe in order to stabilize extreme positions of the hind foot.

A5507

A5507 For diabetics only, not otherwise specified modification (including fitting) of off-the-shelf depth-inlay shoe or custom molded shoe, per shoe

This code reports therapeutic modifications to an off-the-shelf depth-inlay or custom-made shoe for a diabetic patient not identified with a more specific HCPCS Level II code.

A5508

A5508 For diabetics only, deluxe feature of off-the-shelf depth-inlay shoe or custom molded shoe, per shoe

Report this code for a deluxe feature of an off-the-shelf depth-inlay or custom-made shoe that does not contribute to the therapeutic function of the diabetic shoe. It may include, but is not limited to style, color, or type of leather.

A5510-A5514

A5510 For diabetics only, direct formed, compression molded to patient's foot without external heat source, multiple-density insert(s) prefabricated, per shoe

A5512 For diabetics only, multiple density insert, direct formed, molded to foot after external heat source of 230 degrees Fahrenheit or higher, total contact with patient's foot, including arch, base layer minimum of 1/4 inch material of Shore A 35 durometer or 3/16 inch material of Shore A 40 durometer (or higher), prefabricated, each

A5513 For diabetics only, multiple density insert, custom molded from model of patient's foot, total contact with patient's foot, including arch, base layer minimum of 3/16 inch material of Shore A 35 durometer (or higher), includes arch filler and other shaping material, custom fabricated, each

A5514 For diabetics only, multiple density insert, made by direct carving with CAM technology from a rectified CAD model created from a digitized scan of the patient, total contact with patient's foot, including arch, base layer minimum of 3/16 inch material of Shore A 35 durometer (or higher), includes arch filler and other shaping material, custom fabricated, each

A diabetic shoe insert is a total contact, removable inlay that is directly molded to the patient's foot or a model of the patient's foot and is made of a suitable material with regard to the patient's condition. There are several methods of fabrication including compression molded without the use of a heat source, direct formed with the use of a heat source, and custom molded from a model of the patient's foot. In

A5510, the insert is prefabricated, multiple density, and formed using a compression mold of the patient's foot without the use of a heat source. In A5512, the insert is prefabricated and direct formed to the foot using an external heat source and total contact with the patient's foot. In A5512, A5513, and A5514, the insert is custom-fabricated from a model of the patient's foot. These inserts must provide total contact including arch support with a base layer minimum of 1/4 inch material of Shore A durometer or 3/16 inch material of Shore A 40 durometer or higher.

A6000

A6000 Noncontact wound-warming wound cover for use with the noncontact wound-warming device and warming card

Wound healing occurs best in a warm, moist environment that enhances subcutaneous oxygen tension and increases blood flow to the wound. A noncontact wound warming device, also referred to as noncontact normothermic wound therapy (NNWT), is a wound treatment device designed to create an optimal environment to promote wound healing. A non-contact wound warming device includes a non-contact bandage and a warming unit designed to maintain 100 percent relative humidity and to produce optimal temperatures in the wound and surrounding tissues. The bandage consists of a sterile foam collar that adheres to the skin surrounding the wound and a sterile, transparent film that covers the top of the wound without touching it. An infrared warming card or flexible heat unit is inserted into a pocket in the film covering.

A6010-A6011

A6010 Collagen based wound filler, dry form, sterile, per g of collagen

A6011 Collagen based wound filler, gel/paste, per g of collagen

Collagen based wound filler is a natural hydrolyzed protein available in a dry powder or a gel/paste. Collagen based wound filler may be used for chronic wounds and dermal ulcers including pressure ulcers, stasis ulcers, diabetic ulcers, first- and second-degree burns, surgical wounds, and traumatic wounds. Collagen based wound fillers provide a platform for new cell growth, supply a nutritive protein to the wound site, and protect the wound from bacteria. The powder type forms a gel when it combines with the wound exudate to provide a moist healing environment. The gel/paste type is a hydrogel that contains collagen.

A6021-A6023

A6021 Collagen dressing, sterile, size 16 sq in or less, each

A6022 Collagen dressing, sterile, size more than 16 sq in but less than or equal to 48 sq in, each

A6023 Collagen dressing, sterile, size more than 48 sq in, each

Surgical dressings include both primary dressings (i.e., therapeutic or protective coverings applied directly to wounds or lesions on the skin) and secondary dressings (i.e., materials needed to secure a primary dressing). Collagen dressings are sterile dressings used for moderate to heavily draining wounds to enhance healing and tissue repair. These dressings can be used on burns, pressure ulcers, scrapes, cuts, and for dermatologic conditions. They also come in wet form for burns and other wounds. In general, these products are used for direct wound care, including protecting a wound from infection, absorbing wound exudate (drainage), filtering into the wound, and/or cleansing the wound. Dressings also reduce inflammation and edema and allow for gas exchange.

A6024

A6024 Collagen dressing wound filler, sterile, per 6 in

Usually made from a bovine collagen, sterile collagen dressing wound filler is a hydrolysate powder that interacts with the wound site and forms a gel that provides a moist wound-healing environment when mixed with the wounds exudate. Collagen promotes new cell growth and provides protein to the wound site. The collagen wound filler is typically used for the management of chronic wounds such as pressure ulcers, diabetic ulcers, and venous insufficiency ulcers, as well as surgically or trauma induced wounds.

A6025

A6025 Gel sheet for dermal or epidermal application, (e.g., silicone, hydrogel, other), each

Gel sheets help create and maintain a moist environment. Increasing moisture to a wound helps keep the wound clean and assists in debridement of necrotic tissue. Gel sheets are used mainly for wounds with minimal or no exudate.

A6154

A6154 Wound pouch, each

A wound pouch is a waterproof collection device with a drainable port that adheres to the skin around a wound. Report this code for each wound pouch supplied.

A6196-A6199

A6196 Alginate or other fiber gelling dressing, wound cover, sterile, pad size 16 sq in or less, each dressing

A6197 Alginate or other fiber gelling dressing, wound cover, sterile, pad size more than 16 sq in but less than or equal to 48 sq in, each dressing

A6198 Alginate or other fiber gelling dressing, wound cover, sterile, pad size more than 48 sq in, each dressing

A6199 Alginate or other fiber gelling dressing, wound filler, sterile, per 6 in

Alginate or other fiber gelling sterile dressing covers and fillers are used for moderately to highly exudative full thickness wounds (e.g., stage III or IV ulcers). Usual dressing change is up to once per day. One wound cover sheet of the approximate size of the wound or up to two units of wound filler (one unit = 6 inches of alginate or other fiber gelling dressing rope) is usually used at each dressing change. It is usually inappropriate to use alginates or other fiber gelling dressings in combination with hydrogels.

A6203-A6205

A6203 Composite dressing, sterile, pad size 16 sq in or less, with any size adhesive border, each dressing

A6204 Composite dressing, sterile, pad size more than 16 sq in, but less than or equal to 48 sq in, with any size adhesive border, each dressing

A6205 Composite dressing, sterile, pad size more than 48 sq in, with any size adhesive border, each dressing

Composite dressings are products combining physically distinct components into a single dressing that provides multiple functions. These functions must include, but are not limited to (a) a bacterial barrier, (b) an absorptive layer other than an alginate or other fiber gelling dressing, foam, hydrocolloid, or hydrogel, and (c) a semi-adherent or nonadherent property over the wound site. Usual composite dressing change is up to three times per week, one wound cover per dressing change.

A6206-A6208

A6206 Contact layer, sterile, 16 sq in or less, each dressing

A6207 Contact layer, sterile, more than 16 sq in but less than or equal to 48 sq in, each dressing

A6208 Contact layer, sterile, more than 48 sq in, each dressing

Contact layers are thin, non-adherent sheets placed directly on an open wound bed to protect the wound tissue from direct contact with other agents or dressings applied to the wound. They are porous to allow wound fluid to pass through for absorption by an overlying dressing. Contact layer dressings are used to line the entire wound; they are not intended to be changed with each dressing change. Usual dressing change is up to once per week.

A6209-A6215

A6209 Foam dressing, wound cover, sterile, pad size 16 sq in or less, without adhesive border, each dressing

A6210 Foam dressing, wound cover, sterile, pad size more than 16 sq in but less than or equal to 48 sq in, without adhesive border, each dressing

A6211 Foam dressing, wound cover, sterile, pad size more than 48 sq in, without adhesive border, each dressing

A6212 Foam dressing, wound cover, sterile, pad size 16 sq in or less, with any size adhesive border, each dressing

A6213 Foam dressing, wound cover, sterile, pad size more than 16 sq in but less than or equal to 48 sq in, with any size adhesive border, each dressing

A6214 Foam dressing, wound cover, sterile, pad size more than 48 sq in, with any size adhesive border, each dressing

A6215 Foam dressing, wound filler, sterile, per g

Foam dressings are used on full thickness wounds (e.g., stage III or IV ulcers) with moderate to heavy exudate. Usual dressing change for a foam wound cover used as a primary dressing is up to three times per week. When a foam wound cover is used as a secondary dressing for wounds with heavy exudate, dressing change may also be up to three times per week. Usual dressing change for foam wound fillers is up to once per day.

A6216-A6221

A6216 Gauze, nonimpregnated, nonsterile, pad size 16 sq in or less, without adhesive border, each dressing

A6217 Gauze, nonimpregnated, nonsterile, pad size more than 16 sq in but less than or equal to 48 sq in, without adhesive border, each dressing

A6218 Gauze, nonimpregnated, nonsterile, pad size more than 48 sq in, without adhesive border, each dressing

A6219 Gauze, nonimpregnated, sterile, pad size 16 sq in or less, with any size adhesive border, each dressing

A6220 Gauze, nonimpregnated, sterile, pad size more than 16 sq in but less than or equal to 48 sq in, with any size adhesive border, each dressing

A6221 Gauze, nonimpregnated, sterile, pad size more than 48 sq in, with any size adhesive border, each dressing

Usual non-impregnated gauze dressing change is up to three times per day for a dressing without a border and once per day for a dressing with a border. It is usually not necessary to stack more than two gauze pads on top of each other in any one area.

A6222-A6233

A6222 Gauze, impregnated with other than water, normal saline, or hydrogel, sterile, pad size 16 sq in or less, without adhesive border, each dressing

A6223 Gauze, impregnated with other than water, normal saline, or hydrogel, sterile, pad size more than 16 sq in but less than or equal to 48 sq in, without adhesive border, each dressing

A6224 Gauze, impregnated with other than water, normal saline, or hydrogel, sterile, pad size more than 48 sq in, without adhesive border, each dressing

A6228 Gauze, impregnated, water or normal saline, sterile, pad size 16 sq in or less, without adhesive border, each dressing

A6229 Gauze, impregnated, water or normal saline, sterile, pad size more than 16 sq in but less than or equal to 48 sq in, without adhesive border, each dressing

A6230 Gauze, impregnated, water or normal saline, sterile, pad size more than 48 sq in, without adhesive border, each dressing

A6231 Gauze, impregnated, hydrogel, for direct wound contact, sterile, pad size 16 sq in or less, each dressing

A6232 Gauze, impregnated, hydrogel, for direct wound contact, sterile, pad size greater than 16 sq in but less than or equal to 48 sq in, each dressing

A6233 Gauze, impregnated, hydrogel, for direct wound contact, sterile, pad size more than 48 sq in, each dressing

Impregnated gauze dressings are woven or non-woven materials into which substances such as iodinated agents, petrolatum, zinc paste, crystalline sodium chloride, chlorhexidine gluconate (CHG), bismuth tribromophenate (BTP), water, aqueous saline, hydrogel, or other agents have been incorporated into the dressing material by the manufacturer.

A6234-A6241

A6234 Hydrocolloid dressing, wound cover, sterile, pad size 16 sq in or less, without adhesive border, each dressing

A6235 Hydrocolloid dressing, wound cover, sterile, pad size more than 16 sq in but less than or equal to 48 sq in, without adhesive border, each dressing

A6236 Hydrocolloid dressing, wound cover, sterile, pad size more than 48 sq in, without adhesive border, each dressing

A6237 Hydrocolloid dressing, wound cover, sterile, pad size 16 sq in or less, with any size adhesive border, each dressing

A6238 Hydrocolloid dressing, wound cover, sterile, pad size more than 16 sq in but less than or equal to 48 sq in, with any size adhesive border, each dressing

A6239 Hydrocolloid dressing, wound cover, sterile, pad size more than 48 sq in, with any size adhesive border, each dressing

A6240 Hydrocolloid dressing, wound filler, paste, sterile, per oz

A6241 Hydrocolloid dressing, wound filler, dry form, sterile, per g

Hydrocolloid dressings are covered for use on wounds with light to moderate exudate. Usual dressing change for hydrocolloid wound covers or hydrocolloid wound fillers is up to three times per week.

A6242-A6248

A6242 Hydrogel dressing, wound cover, sterile, pad size 16 sq in or less, without adhesive border, each dressing

A6243 Hydrogel dressing, wound cover, sterile, pad size more than 16 sq in but less than or equal to 48 sq in, without adhesive border, each dressing

A6244 Hydrogel dressing, wound cover, sterile, pad size more than 48 sq in, without adhesive border, each dressing

A6245 Hydrogel dressing, wound cover, sterile, pad size 16 sq in or less, with any size adhesive border, each dressing

A6246 Hydrogel dressing, wound cover, sterile, pad size more than 16 sq in but less than or equal to 48 sq in, with any size adhesive border, each dressing

A6247 Hydrogel dressing, wound cover, sterile, pad size more than 48 sq in, with any size adhesive border, each dressing

A6248 Hydrogel dressing, wound filler, gel, per fl oz

Hydrogel dressings are used on full thickness wounds with minimal or no exudate (e.g., stage III or IV ulcers). Hydrogel dressings are not usually medically necessary for stage II ulcers.

A6250

A6250 Skin sealants, protectants, moisturizers, ointments, any type, any size

Skin sealants and protectants are liquid barrier films made of polymers and solvents. The solvent evaporates after the sealant or protectant is applied to the skin, leaving behind a protective film. A moisturizer is a water and oil mixture. Ointments are oil in water emulsions. This code reports any type or size of skin sealant, protectant, moisturizer, or ointment when a more specific code is not available.

A6251-A6256

A6251 Specialty absorptive dressing, wound cover, sterile, pad size 16 sq in or less, without adhesive border, each dressing

A6252 Specialty absorptive dressing, wound cover, sterile, pad size more than 16 sq in but less than or equal to 48 sq in, without adhesive border, each dressing

A6253 Specialty absorptive dressing, wound cover, sterile, pad size more than 48 sq in, without adhesive border, each dressing

A6254 Specialty absorptive dressing, wound cover, sterile, pad size 16 sq in or less, with any size adhesive border, each dressing

A6255 Specialty absorptive dressing, wound cover, sterile, pad size more than 16 sq in but less than or equal to 48 sq in, with any size adhesive border, each dressing

A6256 Specialty absorptive dressing, wound cover, sterile, pad size more than 48 sq in, with any size adhesive border, each dressing

Specialty absorptive dressings are unitized multi-layer dressings that provide either a semi-adherent quality or nonadherent layer and highly absorptive layers of fibers, such as absorbent cellulose, cotton, or rayon. These may or may not have an adhesive border.

A6257-A6259

A6257 Transparent film, sterile, 16 sq in or less, each dressing

A6258 Transparent film, sterile, more than 16 sq in but less than or equal to 48 sq in, each dressing

A6259 Transparent film, sterile, more than 48 sq in, each dressing

Transparent film dressings are used on closed wounds or open partial thickness wounds with minimal exudate. Usual dressing change is up to three times per week.

A6260

A6260 Wound cleansers, any type, any size

This code reports wound cleansers of any type and any size that do not a have more specific code listed. Wound cleansers remove wound debris as the wound is cleansed and washed. Wound cleansers are often over-the-counter products that can be used as a rinse or can be sprayed on the wound.

A6261-A6262

A6261 Wound filler, gel/paste, per fl oz, not otherwise specified

A6262 Wound filler, dry form, per g, not otherwise specified

Wound fillers are dressing materials that are placed into open wounds to eliminate dead space and absorb exudate or maintain a moist wound surface. Report these codes for wound fillers, gel/paste, or dry form not specifically listed elsewhere. Usual dressing change is performed once per day.

A6266

A6266 Gauze, impregnated, other than water, normal saline, or zinc paste, sterile, any width, per linear yd

Impregnated gauze dressings are woven or non-woven materials in which substances such as iodinated agents, petrolatum, zinc compounds, crystalline sodium chloride, chlorhexidine gluconate (CHG), bismuth tribromophenate (BTP), water, aqueous saline, or other agents have been incorporated into the dressing material by the manufacturer.

A6402-A6404

A6402 Gauze, nonimpregnated, sterile, pad size 16 sq in or less, without adhesive border, each dressing

A6403 Gauze, nonimpregnated, sterile, pad size more than 16 sq in but less than or equal to 48 sq in, without adhesive border, each dressing

A6404 Gauze, nonimpregnated, sterile, pad size more than 48 sq in, without adhesive border, each dressing

Usual non-impregnated gauze dressing change is up to three times per day for a dressing without a border and once per day for a dressing with a border. It is usually not necessary to stack more than two gauze pads on top of each other in any one area.

A6407

A6407 Packing strips, nonimpregnated, sterile, up to 2 in width, per linear yd

Packing strips are placed in open wounds and are often used in wet-to-dry type of wound treatment. They are sterile supplies that are usually made of fine mesh cotton gauze. Some are impregnated with antiseptics, such as iodoform.

A6410-A6412

A6410 Eye pad, sterile, each

A6411 Eye pad, nonsterile, each

A6412 Eye patch, occlusive, each

Eye pads are used to protect an injured eye from further injury by keeping the eyelid closed. Eye pads are usually constructed of soft absorbent cotton covered by fine mesh gauze and contoured to fit the eye. They may be sterile or nonsterile supplies. An occlusive eye patch may be used to protect an injured eye or to treat a condition such as amblyopia. Light occlusive eye patches, in addition to providing a soft absorbent pad, contain a film on the outer surface that blocks specific wavelengths of light.

A6413

A6413 Adhesive bandage, first aid type, any size, each

An adhesive bandage is a sterile piece of gauze or other absorptive material affixed to a fabric or film that has been coated with a pressure-sensitive adhesive.

A6441

A6441 Padding bandage, nonelastic, nonwoven/nonknitted, width greater than or equal to 3 in and less than 5 in, per yd

A nonelastic, nonwoven/nonknitted padding bandage is used to pad and protect the wound surface.

A6442-A6447

A6442 Conforming bandage, nonelastic, knitted/woven, nonsterile, width less than 3 in, per yd

A6443 Conforming bandage, nonelastic, knitted/woven, nonsterile, width greater than or equal to 3 in and less than 5 in, per yd

A6444 Conforming bandage, nonelastic, knitted/woven, nonsterile, width greater than or equal to 5 in, per yd

A6445 Conforming bandage, nonelastic, knitted/woven, sterile, width less than 3 in, per yd

A6446 Conforming bandage, nonelastic, knitted/woven, sterile, width greater than or equal to 3 in and less than 5 in, per yd

A6447 Conforming bandage, nonelastic, knitted/woven, sterile, width greater than or equal to 5 in, per yd

Nonelastic conforming bandages are made of a knitted, crocheted, or woven material that allows them to stretch. Nonelastic conforming bandages are supplied in rolls that are then used to wrap the wound. Other dressings such as 2 X 2's or 4 X 4's may be layered under and held in place by the conforming bandage.

A6448-A6452

A6448 Light compression bandage, elastic, knitted/woven, width less than 3 in, per yd

A6449 Light compression bandage, elastic, knitted/woven, width greater than or equal to 3 in and less than 5 in, per yd

A6450 Light compression bandage, elastic, knitted/woven, width greater than or equal to 5 in, per yd

A6451 Moderate compression bandage, elastic, knitted/woven, load resistance of 1.25 to 1.34 ft lbs at 50% maximum stretch, width greater than or equal to 3 in and less than 5 in, per yd

A6452 High compression bandage, elastic, knitted/woven, load resistance greater than or equal to 1.35 ft lbs at 50% maximum stretch, width greater than or equal to 3 in and less than 5 in, per yd

Elastic, knitted/woven compression bandages are used as support wraps for conditions such as sprains, strains, and venous ulcers. They come in a variety of types, including variable stretch, limited stretch, and high stretch, that provide varying degrees of compression. The type used depends on the condition or injury being treated.

A6453-A6455

A6453 Self-adherent bandage, elastic, nonknitted/nonwoven, width less than 3 in, per yd

A6454 Self-adherent bandage, elastic, nonknitted/nonwoven, width greater than or equal to 3 in and less than 5 in, per yd

A6455 Self-adherent bandage, elastic, nonknitted/nonwoven, width greater than or equal to 5 in, per yd

Elastic, self-adherent, nonknitted/nonwoven bandages are composed of laminated nonwoven and elastic materials. The wrap is made of a material that will stick to itself, but will not adhere to other fabrics, materials, or the skin. It is supplied in rolls in a variety of widths.

A6456

A6456 Zinc paste impregnated bandage, nonelastic, knitted/woven, width greater than or equal to 3 in and less than 5 in, per yd

A nonelastic, knitted/woven zinc paste-impregnated bandage may be used as a wrap for venous insufficiency or other conditions. Zinc oxide paste-impregnated bandages stay soft and flexible and conform to the leg to promote healing. A zinc oxide paste-impregnated bandage is typically used under a compression bandage, which is reported separately.

A6457

A6457 Tubular dressing with or without elastic, any width, per linear yd

Tubular dressing is a secondary dressing used to secure the primary dressing. It is used as an alternative to a gauze wrap or adhesive tape. Tubular dressings are available in a variety of materials, including synthetic materials such as nylon or natural materials such as cotton. Some types of tubular dressings require application using a metal cage device while others can be placed by hand.

A6460-A6461

A6460 Synthetic resorbable wound dressing, sterile, pad size 16 sq in or less, without adhesive border, each dressing

A6461 Synthetic resorbable wound dressing, sterile, pad size more than 16 sq in but less than or equal to 48 sq in, without adhesive border, each dressing

Resorbable wound dressings are used for a variety of wounds, including full and partial thickness, postsurgical, and traumatic wounds, as well as ulcers (e.g., diabetic, venous, pressure), and are designed to reduce adherence while managing wound exudate. Similar to a skin substitute, and comprised of synthetic biocompatible polymers, the dressing allows cell ingress and formation of soft tissue in the wound. After the wound site is prepared, the dressing is applied and does not require removal.

A6501-A6513

A6501 Compression burn garment, bodysuit (head to foot), custom fabricated

A6502 Compression burn garment, chin strap, custom fabricated

A6503 Compression burn garment, facial hood, custom fabricated

A6504 Compression burn garment, glove to wrist, custom fabricated

A6505 Compression burn garment, glove to elbow, custom fabricated

A6506 Compression burn garment, glove to axilla, custom fabricated

A6507 Compression burn garment, foot to knee length, custom fabricated

A6508 Compression burn garment, foot to thigh length, custom fabricated

A6509 Compression burn garment, upper trunk to waist including arm openings (vest), custom fabricated

A6510 Compression burn garment, trunk, including arms down to leg openings (leotard), custom fabricated

A6511 Compression burn garment, lower trunk including leg openings (panty), custom fabricated

A6512 Compression burn garment, not otherwise classified

A6513 Compression burn mask, face and/or neck, plastic or equal, custom fabricated

Compression burn garments are used to reduce hypertrophic scarring and joint contractures following a burn injury.

A6530-A6535

A6530 Gradient compression stocking, below knee, 18-30 mm Hg, each

A6531 Gradient compression stocking, below knee, 30-40 mm Hg, each

A6532 Gradient compression stocking, below knee, 40-50 mm Hg, each

A6533 Gradient compression stocking, thigh length, 18-30 mm Hg, each

A6534 Gradient compression stocking, thigh length, 30-40 mm Hg, each

A6535 Gradient compression stocking, thigh length, 40-50 mm Hg, each

This range of codes reports the supply of below-the-knee and thigh length compression stockings. These stockings may be prescribed for a variety of conditions, such as prevention of deep vein thrombosis (DVT) or postoperative prevention of venous thromboembolisms. Gradient compression refers to the difference in pressure exerted over the length of the stocking. For example, the squeezing pressure at the ankle is usually greatest, gradually diminishing proximally toward the calf area. The pressure is expressed in millimeters of mercury (mmHg). The patient's anatomical dimensions and the presence of edema can affect sizing of these stockings. Pressures less than 15 mmHg are generally considered less than therapeutic. Pressures in the 18 to 20 mmHg range are considered mildly therapeutic for minor varicosity. Pressures in the 20 to 30 mmHg range are considered firm while those above 30 mmHg are considered extra firm.

A6536-A6538

A6536 Gradient compression stocking, full-length/chap style, 18-30 mm Hg, each

A6537 Gradient compression stocking, full-length/chap style, 30-40 mm Hg, each

A6538 Gradient compression stocking, full-length/chap style, 40-50 mm Hg, each

This range of codes reports the supply of full length, chap style compression stockings. These stockings may be prescribed for a variety of conditions, such as prevention of deep vein thrombosis (DVT) or postoperative prevention of venous thromboembolisms. Gradient compression refers to the difference in pressure exerted over the length of the stocking. For example, the squeezing pressure at the ankle is usually greatest, gradually diminishing proximally toward the thigh and waist region. The pressure is expressed in millimeters of mercury (mmHg). The patient's anatomical dimensions and the presence of edema can affect sizing of these stockings. Pressures less than 15 mmHg are generally considered less than therapeutic. Pressures in the 18 to 20 mmHg range are considered mildly therapeutic for minor varicosity. Pressures in the 20 to 30 mmHg range are considered firm while those above 30 mmHg are considered extra firm.

A6539-A6544

A6539 Gradient compression stocking, waist length, 18-30 mm Hg, each

A6540 Gradient compression stocking, waist length, 30-40 mm Hg, each

A6541 Gradient compression stocking, waist length, 40-50 mm Hg, each

A6544 Gradient compression stocking, garter belt

This range of codes reports the supply of waist length compression stockings and related supplies for compression garments, as well as other supplies and accessories used with compression stockings. These stockings may be prescribed for a variety of conditions, such as prevention of deep vein thrombosis (DVT) or postoperative prevention of venous thromboembolisms. Gradient compression refers to the difference in pressure exerted over the length of the stocking. For example, the squeezing pressure at the ankle is usually greatest, gradually diminishing proximally toward the thigh and waist region. The pressure is expressed in millimeters of mercury (mmHg). The patient's anatomical dimensions and the presence of edema can affect sizing of these stockings. Pressures less than 15 mmHg are generally considered less than therapeutic. Pressures in the 18 to 20 mmHg range are considered mildly therapeutic for minor varicosity. Pressures in the 20 to 30 mmHg range are considered firm, while those above 30 mmHg are considered extra firm.

A6545-A6549

A6545 Gradient compression wrap, nonelastic, below knee, 30-50 mm Hg, each

A6549 Gradient compression stocking/sleeve, not otherwise specified

This code reports the supply of a below knee gradient compression wrap. It uses adjustable bands to provide therapeutic compression levels. Compression wraps may be prescribed for a variety of conditions, such as lymphedema, and to treat venous disease and active venous stasis ulcers. Surgical removal of lymph nodes can cause lymphedema, a condition hallmarked by fluid retention and swelling in the affected extremity. Gradient compression refers to the difference in pressure exerted over the length of the wrap. For example, the squeezing pressure at the ankle is usually greatest, gradually diminishing proximally toward the thigh and waist region. The pressure is expressed in millimeters of mercury (mmHg). The components of the gradient wrap are a nonelastic binder that is fitted at the prescribed compression level using markers on the neoprene strip and a built in pressure system that runs posterior length of the device.

A6550

A6550 Wound care set, for negative pressure wound therapy electrical pump, includes all supplies and accessories

Negative pressure wound therapy (NPWT), also called vacuum assisted closure (VAC), uses subatmospheric pressure to assist in treatment of acute, subacute, and chronic wounds. NPWT promotes healing by increasing local vascularity and oxygenation of the wound bed, evacuating wound fluid thereby reducing edema, and removing exudates and bacteria. The subatmospheric pressure is generated using an electrical pump that is reported as a separate supply (E2402). The electrical pump conveys intermittent or continuous subatmospheric pressure through connecting tubing to a specialized wound dressing. A specialized wound dressing includes porous foam dressing that covers the entire wound surface and an airtight adhesive dressing that seals the wound and contains the subatmospheric pressure at the wound site. Each wound care set inclusive of all supplies and accessories is reported with A6550.

A7000-A7002

A7000 Canister, disposable, used with suction pump, each

A7001 Canister, nondisposable, used with suction pump, each

A7002 Tubing, used with suction pump, each

Canisters to be used with suction pumps can be disposable or non-disposable. Canisters are made of a hard plastic and are used for collecting aspirated materials. Although they vary in size, they usually hold approximately 800 cc to 1200 cc and have a lid and splash guard. Tubing runs from the suction catheter to the canister to deliver the aspirated material.

A7003-A7006

A7003 Administration set, with small volume nonfiltered pneumatic nebulizer, disposable

A7004 Small volume nonfiltered pneumatic nebulizer, disposable

A7005 Administration set, with small volume nonfiltered pneumatic nebulizer, nondisposable

A7006 Administration set, with small volume filtered pneumatic nebulizer

Nebulizer base equipment is comprised of an air compressor for airflow nebulization or a generator for nebulization of liquid by means of ultrasonic vibrations. The actual nebulizer is the chamber in which the nebulization of the liquid medication or solution for inhalation occurs. The nebulizing chamber is attached to the aerosol compressor or an ultrasonic generator. Nebulization therapy is considered beneficial to patients with a variety of respiratory and/or pulmonary conditions and diseases, including cystic fibrosis, bronchiectasis, chronic obstructive pulmonary disease, emphysema, severe asthma (when metered dose inhalers are ineffective), as well as other conditions such as AIDS, which requires the administration of medications like pentamidine. Small volume nebulizers are designed primarily to deliver inhalation medications. Nebulization occurs when the medication and/or solution to be administered is vaporized and subsequently inspired by the patient via the lungs, through which the medication enters the patient's system, or the medication has a direct effect on mucus retained by the lungs and bronchi (known as mucolytic action). Various accessory supplies may be required for use with the nebulizer.

A7007-A7012

A7007 Large volume nebulizer, disposable, unfilled, used with aerosol compressor

A7008 Large volume nebulizer, disposable, prefilled, used with aerosol compressor

A7009 Reservoir bottle, nondisposable, used with large volume ultrasonic nebulizer

A7010 Corrugated tubing, disposable, used with large volume nebulizer, 100 ft

A7012 Water collection device, used with large volume nebulizer

Nebulizer based equipment is comprised of an air compressor for airflow nebulization or a generator for nebulization of liquid by means of ultrasonic vibrations. The actual nebulizer is the chamber in which the nebulization occurs. The nebulizing chamber is attached to the aerosol compressor or an ultrasonic generator. Large volume nebulizers are designed to deliver humidified gas, such as oxygen, in concentrations ranging from 28 percent to 98 percent along with medications. Large volume nebulizers are useful in the treatment of conditions such as cystic fibrosis, bronchiectasis, and tracheostomy where humidified gas assists in thinning respiratory secretions. Large volume nebulizers are also useful for administration of pentamidine in the treatment of HIV. Various accessory supplies may be required for use with the nebulizer.

A7013-A7016

A7013 Filter, disposable, used with aerosol compressor or ultrasonic generator

A7014 Filter, nondisposable, used with aerosol compressor or ultrasonic generator

A7015 Aerosol mask, used with DME nebulizer

A7016 Dome and mouthpiece, used with small volume ultrasonic nebulizer

Nebulizer base equipment is comprised of an air compressor for airflow nebulization or a generator for nebulization of liquid by means of ultrasonic vibrations. The actual nebulizer is the chamber in which the nebulization occurs. The nebulizing chamber is attached to the aerosol compressor or an ultrasonic generator. Various accessory supplies may be required for use with the nebulizer.

A7017

A7017 Nebulizer, durable, glass or autoclavable plastic, bottle type, not used with oxygen

A nebulizer is an apparatus for producing a fine spray or mist. This may be made by rapidly passing air through a liquid or by vibrating a liquid at a high frequency so that the particles produced are extremely small. Report this code for a durable, bottle-type nebulizer made of glass or plastic that can be sterilized in an autoclave and is not used with oxygen.

A7018

A7018 Water, distilled, used with large volume nebulizer, 1000 ml

Nebulizer base equipment is comprised of an air compressor for airflow nebulization or a generator for nebulization of liquid by means of ultrasonic vibrations. The actual nebulizer is the chamber in which the nebulization occurs. The nebulizing chamber is attached to the aerosol compressor or an ultrasonic generator. Large volume nebulizers are designed to deliver humidified gas, such as oxygen, in concentrations ranging from 28 percent to 98 percent along with medications. Large volume nebulizers are useful in the treatment of conditions such as cystic fibrosis, bronchiectasis, and tracheostomy where humidified gas assists in thinning respiratory secretions. Large volume nebulizers are also useful for administration of pentamidine in the treatment of HIV. Various accessory supplies may be required for use with the nebulizer.

A7020

A7020 Interface for cough stimulating device, includes all components, replacement only

Cough stimulating devices are used for people who are not able to cough to remove secretions from the lungs. Components for the cough stimulator should be replaced every two months to reduce the risk of infection and to ensure that the components are not worn out. This code represents a replacement patient interface device. Patient interface devices include a face mask, mouthpiece, or tracheal adapter.

A7025-A7026

A7025 High frequency chest wall oscillation system vest, replacement for use with patient-owned equipment, each

A7026 High frequency chest wall oscillation system hose, replacement for use with patient-owned equipment, each

These codes report replacement supplies that are used with a patient owned, high-frequency chest wall oscillation (HFCWO) system. The vest component consists of an inflatable vest connected by tubes to an air-pulse generator. The air-pulse generator rapidly inflates and deflates the vest, compressing and releasing the chest wall. HFCWO allows the patient to clear mucus by generating increased airflow velocities that create repetitive cough-like shear forces and decrease the viscosity of secretions.

A7027-A7039

A7027 Combination oral/nasal mask, used with continuous positive airway pressure device, each

A7028 Oral cushion for combination oral/nasal mask, replacement only, each

A7029 Nasal pillows for combination oral/nasal mask, replacement only, pair

A7030 Full face mask used with positive airway pressure device, each

A7031 Face mask interface, replacement for full face mask, each

A7032 Cushion for use on nasal mask interface, replacement only, each

A7033 Pillow for use on nasal cannula type interface, replacement only, pair

A7034 Nasal interface (mask or cannula type) used with positive airway pressure device, with or without head strap

A7035 Headgear used with positive airway pressure device

A7036 Chinstrap used with positive airway pressure device

A7037 Tubing used with positive airway pressure device

A7038 Filter, disposable, used with positive airway pressure device

A7039 Filter, nondisposable, used with positive airway pressure device

CPAP is a noninvasive method of providing air pressure through the patient's nostrils, usually through a nasal mask or flow generator system. These devices are used primarily in conservative therapy (vs. surgery) for patients with documented sleep apnea; however, not all patients benefit from this conservative approach because some cannot tolerate the CPAP device during sleep. The CPAP device assists the patient in nocturnal respiration (during sleep), particularly when the patient's oropharyngeal tissues relax, collapse, and/or otherwise obstruct the normal airflow during inspiration and expiration, causing a variety of symptoms including hypersomnolence during the day, loss of concentration, headache, agitation, depression, fatigue, and many others.

A7040-A7041

A7040 One way chest drain valve

A7041 Water seal drainage container and tubing for use with implanted chest tube

Chest tubes are inserted into the pleural space to drain blood, fluid, or air from the pleural cavity and to allow full expansion of the lungs. The chest tube is inserted through an incision between the ribs into the pleural space and connected to a water seal system to prevent air from being sucked into the chest cavity and to allow the continuous or intermittent removal of fluid. A water seal thoracic drainage unit for removal of fluids from the thoracic cavity of a patient can use one, two, or three containers. A single-container water seal consists of a drainage collection container that also serves as the water seal. The container is initially filled with 100 ml of sterile water to form the seal. A two-container water seal is comprised of a collection chamber for receiving fluids from the patient and a second container that provides the underwater seal. Generally, the water or other liquid for the seal is provided with the collection chamber and water seal container as a complete unit ready for use. A three-container water seal system uses a collection chamber, a water seal container, and a third container that provides suction control.

A7044

A7044 Oral interface used with positive airway pressure device, each

This code reports the supply of each oral interface used with a positive airway pressure (PAP) device. Such devices may also be prescribed for use on a continuous basis (CPAP). The oral interface may be a removable tube-like component that the patient uses during treatment.

A7045

A7045 Exhalation port with or without swivel used with accessories for positive airway devices, replacement only

Some masks used with positive pressure airway devices require the use of an accessory supply called an exhalation port to function properly. An exhalation port allows predetermined amounts of exhaled air to "leak" through the exhalation port. This is necessary to properly exhaust exhaled CO_2 from the mask so the patient does not rebreathe the CO_2. Some masks have a swivel device that allows the circuit tubing to move freely.

A7046

A7046 Water chamber for humidifier, used with positive airway pressure device, replacement, each

Some humidifiers used with positive airway pressure devices have separate water chambers. The water chamber holds the water used in the humidifier. Removable water chambers are more easily cleaned. This code reports replacement of a removable water chamber.

A7047

A7047 Oral interface used with respiratory suction pump, each

Oral interface used with respiratory suction pump is a replacement piece used with a portable home model respiratory suction pump. A portable home model respiratory suction pump is a lightweight, compact, electric aspirator designed for upper respiratory oral pharyngeal and tracheal suction to be used in the home.

A7048

A7048 Vacuum drainage collection unit and tubing kit, including all supplies needed for collection unit change, for use with implanted catheter, each

An implantable pleural catheter and drainage kit is used for long-term treatment of symptomatic, chronic/recurrent, malignant, pleural effusion. This type of implantable catheter allows intermittent drainage of the effusion. The small-bore catheter consists of three sections: internal, middle, and external. The internal section has a fenestrated end that is placed into the pleural space. The middle section is tunneled through the skin for several inches. The external section includes an exposed length of catheter with a one-way valve. A separate drainage kit is required that includes a lightweight, plastic, vacuum drainage bottle and tubing. Each day or as needed the patient or caregiver drains the pleural fluid by temporarily attaching the external length of catheter to the tubing, which is connected to the pre-evacuated (vacuum) drainage bottle.

A7501-A7502

A7501 Tracheostoma valve, including diaphragm, each

A7502 Replacement diaphragm/faceplate for tracheostoma valve, each

This code reports the supply of a tracheostoma valve, including diaphragm. These devices are typically used by laryngectomees who retain a level of potential voice function. Designs such as the prototypical Blom-Singer provide the user a means to speak without first manually occluding the stoma with a finger. Tracheostoma valves are often two-unit devices. A faceplate inserts over the tracheostoma. A disposable diaphragm in the valve can be adjusted to control airflow through the stomal opening. When the diaphragm is closed, or near closed, speech can be accomplished. The diaphragm may be set to allow one-way airflow upon expiration.

A7503-A7506

A7503 Filter holder or filter cap, reusable, for use in a tracheostoma heat and moisture exchange system, each

A7504 Filter for use in a tracheostoma heat and moisture exchange system, each

A7505 Housing, reusable without adhesive, for use in a heat and moisture exchange system and/or with a tracheostoma valve, each

A7506 Adhesive disc for use in a heat and moisture exchange system and/or with tracheostoma valve, any type each

A tracheostoma heat and moisture exchange system is used by some tracheostomy patients to add warmth and water vapor to the air when they inhale. A heat and moisture exchange system can retain up to 60 percent of the humidity in the patient's airway, greatly reducing coughing and mucus production. It consists of a reusable plastic holder or cap, also referred to as a cassette, that contains a filter made of foam, paper, or other material. The holder fits into reusable plastic housing that is held in place over the tracheostoma by an adhesive disc. A heat and moisture exchanger may be used by itself or in addition to a tracheostoma valve.

A7507-A7509

A7507 Filter holder and integrated filter without adhesive, for use in a tracheostoma heat and moisture exchange system, each

A7508 Housing and integrated adhesive, for use in a tracheostoma heat and moisture exchange system and/or with a tracheostoma valve, each

A7509 Filter holder and integrated filter housing, and adhesive, for use as a tracheostoma heat and moisture exchange system, each

A tracheostoma heat and moisture exchange system is used by some tracheostomy patients to add warmth and water vapor to the air when they inhale. A heat and moisture exchange system can retain up to 60 percent of the humidity in the patient's airway, greatly reducing coughing and mucus production. Some heat and moisture exchange systems use integrated components.

A7520-A7522

A7520 Tracheostomy/laryngectomy tube, noncuffed, polyvinyl chloride (PVC), silicone or equal, each

A7521 Tracheostomy/laryngectomy tube, cuffed, polyvinyl chloride (PVC), silicone or equal, each

A7522 Tracheostomy/laryngectomy tube, stainless steel or equal (sterilizable and reusable), each

A tracheostomy/laryngectomy tube, also called a trach tube, is a curved tube that is inserted into a tracheostomy stoma (the surgically created hole made in the neck and windpipe). Tracheostomy tubes can be made of a variety of materials including metal, plastic, or silicone. Plastic and silicone tubes have the advantage of being lighter weight with less crusting of secretions than with metal tubes. Tracheostomy tubes come in cuffed and uncuffed models. A cuff is a soft balloon around the distal (far) end of the tube. The cuff is inflated with air, foam, or sterile water to allow for mechanical ventilation in patients with respiratory failure. Cuffs can be low or high volume. The low volume cuff is round while a high volume cuff is barrel-shaped. The high volume cuff spreads the pressure out over a larger surface area and may be better at averting complications such as stenosis than the low volume cuff that tends to push on one spot in the airway. When the balloon is deflated, the tube allows air around the tube for vocalization.

A7523

A7523 Tracheostomy shower protector, each

A tracheostomy shower protector is used to protect the tracheostomy stoma (the surgically created hole made in the neck and windpipe) from water, soaps, and shampoos when showering. Tracheostomy shower protectors are made of waterproof materials such as latex and fit like a bib over the stoma site to shield and deflect the water from the stoma site when showering.

A7524

A7524 Tracheostoma stent/stud/button, each

A tracheostoma stent, stud, or button is a rigid cannula that is placed into the tracheostoma after removal of a tracheostomy tube. These devices are used primarily for conditions such as obstructive sleep apnea where the patient requires the tracheostoma for breathing at night, but does not need it for breathing during the day. A stent, stud, or button allows the stoma to be closed and the patient to breathe through the nose and mouth instead of through the tracheostoma site during the day. These devices do not extend into the tracheal lumen so patients are able to breathe and talk normally when these types of devices are in place.

A7525

A7525 Tracheostomy mask, each

Tracheostomy masks are used in conjunction with nebulizers. They are composed of a flexible, mask-shaped plastic covering that fits securely over the tracheostomy tube. The outer portion has an opening that connects with the nebulizer tubing. Masks are used for ventilation and to humidify inspired air.

A7526

A7526 Tracheostomy tube collar/holder, each

A tracheostomy tube collar or holder attaches to each side of the tracheostomy tube and loosely wraps around the back of the neck. A tracheostomy tube holder or collar is used to secure the tracheostomy tube in place. Collars and holders are made of a variety of materials that include stainless steel metal chains, laminates of foam and nylon, plastics, and other materials.

A7527

A7527 Tracheostomy/laryngectomy tube plug/stop, each

This code reports the specialized plug or stopper for use with a tracheostomy, fenestration, or laryngectomy tube, which the patient has in place. The plug, also called a decannulation plug, is used to obstruct the proximal end of the tube and permit breathing through the fenestration and the upper airway. Using the plug with the tube facilitates weaning in preparation for extubation and aids in speaking.

A8000-A8004

A8000 Helmet, protective, soft, prefabricated, includes all components and accessories

A8001 Helmet, protective, hard, prefabricated, includes all components and accessories

A8002 Helmet, protective, soft, custom fabricated, includes all components and accessories

A8003 Helmet, protective, hard, custom fabricated, includes all components and accessories

A8004 Soft interface for helmet, replacement only

Protective helmets are head coverings used to prevent or lessen injury or damage to the head. The helmets may be composed of hard material such as hard plastic or soft material such as nylon or fabric. Protective helmets may be used to protect patients prone to falling or hitting their head. Prefabricated helmets are pre-made and are usually purchased off the shelf. Custom-fabricated helmets are constructed specifically for a patient using the patient's physical measurements and needs. Helmets may contain straps or belts to hold the helmet on the head.

A9150

A9150 Nonprescription drugs

This code reports drugs that do not require a prescription, also referred to as over-the-counter (OTC) drugs. Identify the specific drug provided, as well as the strength, amount, and condition being treated.

A9152-A9153

A9152 Single vitamin/mineral/trace element, oral, per dose, not otherwise specified

A9153 Multiple vitamins, with or without minerals and trace elements, oral, per dose, not otherwise specified

Vitamins are organic substances found in small amounts within foods. Minerals are nonorganic solid substances found in the earth's crust. Trace mineral elements occur in very small amounts. These are essential nutrients needed by the body in varying, small amounts for proper metabolic function.

A9155

A9155 Artificial saliva, 30 ml

Natural saliva is more than 99 percent water, with some buffering agents, enzymes, and minerals. Saliva coats, lubricates, and helps cleanse the tissues in the mouth. It also begins the digestive process as we chew. When the saliva glands do not produce enough saliva, the mouth becomes dry. Artificial saliva is intended to replace natural saliva. Artificial saliva usually contains water, a mixture of buffering agents, cellulose derivatives, and flavoring agents. However, it does not contain the digestive and antibacterial enzymes, other proteins, or minerals present in real saliva. Artificial saliva is used to treat xerostomia, or dry mouth, which results from an inadequate flow of saliva. Drying irritates the soft tissues in the mouth, which can make them inflamed and more susceptible to infection.

A9180

A9180 Pediculosis (lice infestation) treatment, topical, for administration by patient/caretaker

A pediculicide is a topical medication applied to hair used to treat lice infestations. Pediculicides are available in both over-the-counter (OTC) formulas and by prescription. OTC formulas include pyrethrins, a natural extract from the chrysanthemum flower, sometimes in combination with piperonyl butoxide. Another OTC formula is permethrin. Treatment is the same regardless of whether an OTC or prescription medication is used. The pediculicide is applied to unwashed hair. After approximately eight to 12 hours, the hair should be checked for live lice. The hair should be combed to remove dead lice and any remaining live lice. The hair should be combed daily with a fine tooth or nit comb and checked every two to three days for the presence of live lice. The hair should be retreated seven to 10 days after the first treatment.

A9270

A9270 Noncovered item or service

Noncovered services are services that are billed to the patient. In many cases, the beneficiary is already aware that the services are noncovered because they are included in the information given in the Medicare handbook (e.g., oral medications, screening mammograms in less than the designated waiting period, etc.) or by their insurance provider. At other times, the services are listed as noncovered because they are considered either experimental or investigational in nature.

A9272

A9272 Wound suction, disposable, includes dressing, all accessories and components, any type, each

Wound suction devices are used to remove excess fluids such as blood, pus, serosanguineous fluid, and tissue secretions, from wounds. A buildup of fluids can cause infection and delay of healing. Mechanical suction uses nonelectrical powered methods, such as springs, to create suction around the wound to draw out the fluid. The fluid is collected in absorbent dressings. The device may have straps or belts to attach the device to the patient. The suction device can be left in place for several days. The system is disposable and is designed for single use. This code includes the cartridges, tubing, dressing, and any other accessories.

A9273

A9273 Cold or hot fluid bottle, ice cap or collar, heat and/or cold wrap, any type

An ice cap or collar is a cold therapy application to deliver treatment to affected tissues, usually following a surgical procedure or trauma. Cold therapy is generally used in the immediate postoperative or post-trauma period to reduce edema and control pain. An ice cap or collar is a passive method to deliver cold therapy. A water bottle is a container, usually made of plastic or rubber, that may be filled with hot or cold water and applied to an injured or painful body part.

A9274

A9274 External ambulatory insulin delivery system, disposable, each, includes all supplies and accessories

External ambulatory insulin delivery systems, also called insulin pumps, are computerized, battery-powered delivery devices with programming capabilities. These devices are used as a treatment for people with insulin-dependent diabetes mellitus. A sterile reservoir is filled with rapid-acting insulin. The sterile reservoir is connected to the patient by a thin plastic tube that has a small catheter needle attached. The needle is usually inserted into the subcutaneous tissue of the abdomen. The device continuously delivers micro-doses of insulin at a programmed rate.

A9275

A9275 Home glucose disposable monitor, includes test strips

Glucometers are used for patients with all types of diabetes mellitus to monitor blood glucose and are available in a variety of models with various features, including disposable home glucose monitors. Whether or not the patient is on insulin, many diabetics require frequent, if not daily, blood glucose monitoring. For Type I diabetes mellitus patients who require insulin (the patient's body does not manufacture insulin and therefore it must come from an external source, such as injections), blood glucose monitoring is a life-sustaining requirement. Disposable types of home glucose monitors are provided with test strips that are inserted into the monitor to provide a glucose reading. When all of the test strips have been used or upon the expiration date of the meter, whichever comes first, the patient discards the entire unit (meter and any remaining test strips).

A9276-A9278

A9276 Sensor; invasive (e.g., subcutaneous), disposable, for use with nondurable medical equipment interstitial continuous glucose monitoring system (CGM), one unit = 1 day supply

A9277 Transmitter; external, for use with nondurable medical equipment interstitial continuous glucose monitoring system (CGM)

A9278 Receiver (monitor); external, for use with nondurable medical equipment interstitial continuous glucose monitoring system (CGM)

Continuous glucose monitoring (CGM) systems make continuous measurements of glucose levels. Many of these devices take measurements from subcutaneous tissue rather than from blood. Most systems consist of a sensor that is attached to the back of the arm or abdomen. The sensor has a very thin wire that is inserted subcutaneously. The wire measures the glucose level in interstitial fluid that exits between the cells. The sensor is attached to a transmitter that sends the glucose readings to a wireless receiver. The receiver is a small, computerized device that records and stores the glucose readings. These HCPCS Level II codes represent replacement components for a nondurable medical equipment interstitial continuous glucose monitoring system.

A9279

A9279 Monitoring feature/device, stand-alone or integrated, any type, includes all accessories, components and electronics, not otherwise classified

This code may be applied to numerous technologies and is a nonspecific monitoring device. It represents an entire system, whether stand-alone or integrated into a delivery system. It includes all accessories, components, and electronics. Report a more specific code if there is one available.

A9280

A9280 Alert or alarm device, not otherwise classified

This code reports alert or alarm devices that do not have a more specific code available. A detailed description of the device may be required when reporting this code.

A9281

A9281 Reaching/grabbing device, any type, any length, each

A reaching/grabbing device is used to pick up objects without twisting the wrist. It typically lifts objects that are 5 pounds. or less. It is often used by people who have difficulty lifting objects due to arthritic conditions, small hands, or who have restrictive movement.

A9282

A9282 Wig, any type, each

A wig is hairpiece of human or artificial hair worn as personal adornment or to conceal baldness. A wig or hairpiece is a supply for hair loss.

A9283

A9283 Foot pressure off loading/supportive device, any type, each

This code reflects various devices used to reduce pressure on the foot to help prevent ulcers. The device usually has an antibacterial layer and an inner layer that may contain gel, foam, small beads, or other pressure reducing material that help support and redistribute the pressure of the foot. The patient can usually adjust the device as needed.

A9284

A9284 Spirometer, nonelectronic, includes all accessories

A spirometer measures pulmonary function. It measures the lung output on both inspiration and expiration and is used to track and diagnose a number of respiratory and cardiac conditions. It may also be used to keep the lungs clear and functioning.

A9285

A9285 Inversion/eversion correction device

This code represents a device that attaches to an orthosis and attempts to correct inversion and/or eversion of the foot. Eversion refers to the lifting up of the lateral (outside) edge of the foot and standing on the inside of the foot. Inversion refers to standing on the outside edge of the foot.

A9286

A9286 Hygienic item or device, disposable or nondisposable, any type, each

This is a catch-all code to be used for any type of hygienic item or device, disposable or non-disposable. Hygienic can be used to describe anything promoting health or cleanliness.

A9291

A9291 Prescription digital cognitive and/or behavioral therapy, FDA-cleared, per course of treatment

Used in conjunction with face-to-face therapy, digital behavioral or cognitive therapy, also known as prescription digital therapeutics (PDTs), delivers content directly to the patient when the clinician may not be available. Services are prescribed by clinicians, sent to a specialty pharmacy, and dispensed to the patient via a smartphone or tablet. PDTs are intended for the treatment of adults, ages 18 years and older, currently enrolled in an outpatient substance use disorder (SUD) program, who are not currently on opioid replacement therapy, do not abuse alcohol solely, or who do not abuse opioids as their primary substance of abuse. It is a 12-week (90 day) program, consisting of 62 interactive modules available 24/7, designed to increase abstinence from substances of abuse during treatment, and to increase retention in the outpatient treatment program. Patients can practice skills taught during face-to-face encounters and clinicians can customize treatment sessions based on patient-reported feelings, behavior, and activities during the week.

A9300

A9300 Exercise equipment

Report this code for exercise equipment used for rehabilitation therapy (e.g., stimulation balls, TheraPutty, and Thera-Bands).

A9500

A9500 Technetium Tc-99m sestamibi, diagnostic, per study dose

Sestamibi is a chemical complex that principally congregates in the heart, breast tissue, and parathyroid. Technetium is a radioactive metallic element that is a byproduct of uranium decay. It may also be produced by bombarding another metal, molybdenum, with specific atoms. Technetium 99m is a widely used radionuclide with a half-life of approximately six hours, which is long enough to examine metabolic processes but short enough to minimize the radiation dose received by the patient. It decays by gamma emission, which is measured by scintillation or gamma cameras. Sestamibi is combined with technetium 99m to produce functional and physiological images of the breast, heart, or parathyroid. The radiopharmaceutical is administered by intravenous injection. Technetium Tc-99m sestamibi is used to diagnose heart disease, parathyroid diseases, and thyroid disorders. It may also be used as a second-line diagnostic tool in breast imaging after a mammography to evaluate breast lesions in patients with an abnormal mammogram or a palpable breast mass.

A9501

A9501 Technetium Tc-99m teboroxime, diagnostic, per study dose

Teboroxime is a chemical complex that principally congregates in the heart. Technetium is a radioactive metallic element that is a byproduct of uranium decay. It may also be produced by bombarding another metal, molybdenum, with specific atoms. Technetium 99m is a widely used radionuclide with a half-life of approximately six hours, which is long enough to examine metabolic processes, but short enough to minimize the radiation dose received by the patient. It decays by gamma emission, which is then measured by scintillation or gamma cameras. Teboroxime is combined with technetium 99m to produce functional and physiological images of the heart. Technetium Tc-99m teboroxime is used to diagnose reversible myocardial ischemia in the presence or absence of an infarction, for myocardial perfusion studies in patients with known or suspected coronary artery disease, and for the assessment of patients being evaluated for heart disease.

A9502

A9502 Technetium Tc-99m tetrofosmin, diagnostic, per study dose

Tetrofosmin is a chemical complex that principally congregates in the heart. Technetium is a radioactive metallic element that is a byproduct of uranium decay. It may also be produced by bombarding another metal, molybdenum, with specific atoms. Technetium 99m is a widely used radionuclide with a half-life of approximately six hours, which is long enough to examine metabolic processes but short enough to minimize the radiation dose received by the patient. It decays by gamma emission, which is then measured by scintillation or gamma cameras. Tetrofosmin is combined with technetium 99m to produce functional and physiological images of the heart. The radiopharmaceutical is administered by intravenous injection. Technetium Tc-99m tetrofosmin is used to diagnose reversible myocardial ischemia in the presence or absence of an infarction, to study myocardial perfusion in patients with known or suspected coronary artery disease, and to assess left ventricular function (ejection fraction and wall motion) in patients being evaluated for heart disease.

A9503

A9503 Technetium Tc-99m medronate, diagnostic, per study dose, up to 30 mCi

Medronate is a chemical complex that principally congregates in the bone. Technetium is a radioactive metallic element that is a byproduct of uranium decay. It may also be produced by bombarding another metal, molybdenum, with specific atoms. Technetium 99m is a widely used radionuclide with a half-life of approximately six hours, which is long enough to examine metabolic processes but short enough to minimize the radiation dose received by the patient. It decays by gamma emission, which is then measured by scintillation or gamma cameras. Medronate is combined with technetium 99m to delineate areas of altered osteogenesis. The radiopharmaceutical is administered by intravenous injection. Optimal imaging is obtained from one to four hours after administration. Technetium Tc-99m medronate is used to diagnose disorders of bone formation.

A9504

A9504 Technetium Tc-99m apcitide, diagnostic, per study dose, up to 20 mCi

Apcitide is a synthetic peptide that binds to receptors on the surface of platelets. Technetium is a radioactive metallic element that is a byproduct of uranium decay. It may also be produced by bombarding another metal, molybdenum, with specific atoms. Technetium 99m is a widely used radionuclide with a half-life of approximately six hours, which is long enough to examine metabolic processes, but short enough to minimize the radiation dose received by the patient. It decays by gamma emission, which is then measured by scintillation or gamma cameras. Apcitide is combined with technetium 99m to locate areas of thrombus. The radiopharmaceutical is administered by intravenous injection. Optimal imaging is obtained from 10 to 60 minutes after administration.

A9505

A9505 Thallium Tl-201 thallous chloride, diagnostic, per mCi

Thallium is a toxic heavy metal found within various rare ores. It is usually recovered from the byproducts of lead and zinc ores by dissolving the ore in hydrochloric acid and precipitating out the thallous chloride. Thallium-201 is a radioactive isotope of thallous chloride that is used as a diagnostic imaging agent. It is administered by intravenous injection. Thallous chloride TL-201 is indicated for use in myocardial perfusion studies and localization of sites of parathyroid hyperactivity, as well as diagnosing and staging of head and neck cancer. Thallous chloride TL-201 has a half-life of 72 hours and decays by electron capture.

A9507

A9507 Indium In-111 capromab pendetide, diagnostic, per study dose, up to 10 millicuries

Capromab pendetide is a murine monoclonal antibody that binds to a glycoprotein, a cell surface antigen that attaches itself to the sites of prostate specific membrane antigen (PSMA). PSMA is associated with prostatic adenocarcinoma cells and is useful in diagnosing metastatic disease. Indium 111 is a radioactive form of the metallic element indium. It has a half-life of approximately 56 hours and decays by electron capture and gamma emission. The monoclonal antibody is combined with indium 111 chloride so that it can be readily identified in images. Indium In-III capromab pendetide is administered intravenously over five minutes. Optimal imaging is obtained from 72 to 120 hours after administration.

A9508

A9508 Iodine I-131 iobenguane sulfate, diagnostic, per 0.5 mCi

Iobenguane sulfate is an analogue of norepinephrine that binds to receptors in the sympathetic nervous system and to related tumors. Iodine 131 is a radioactive isotope of the common element iodine. Iodine 131 has a half-life of eight days and decays by beta and gamma emissions. Iobenguane sulfate combined with Iodine 131, also known as MIBG, is a radiopharmaceutical used as a diagnostic imaging agent for neuroendocrine tumors and disorders of the adrenal medulla. It is also used for local radiation therapy in the treatment of carcinoid syndrome, pheochromocytoma, and neuroblastoma. Iodine I-131 iobenguane sulfate is injected intravenously. Multiple scans are usually performed for up to four days post administration.

A9509

A9509 Iodine I-123 sodium iodide, diagnostic, per mCi

Iodine is a common nonmetallic element necessary for the proper function of the thyroid gland. Iodine 123 sodium iodide is a radioactive isotope of iodine produced in a cyclotron. It decays by electron capture and gamma emission with a half-life of 13 hours. Iodine 123 sodium iodide is administered orally in capsule form. It is readily absorbed from the gastrointestinal tract and congregates primarily in the thyroid gland. Optimal images may be initiated six hours after administration. Sodium iodide I-123 is indicated for diagnostic use in the evaluation of thyroid function and/or morphology.

A9510

A9510 Technetium Tc-99m disofenin, diagnostic, per study dose, up to 15 mCi

Disofenin is a derivative of an iminodiacetic acid that is a form of acetoacetic acid, a byproduct of metabolism that congregates in the gallbladder. Technetium is a radioactive metallic element that is a byproduct of uranium decay. It may also be produced by bombarding another metal, molybdenum, with specific atoms. Technetium 99m is a widely used radionuclide with a half-life of approximately six hours, which is long enough to examine metabolic processes but short enough to minimize the radiation dose received by the patient. It decays by gamma emission, which is then measured by scintillation or gamma cameras. Disofenin is combined with technetium 99m to provide images of the gallbladder and surrounding ducts. The radiopharmaceutical is administered by intravenous injection. Dosage is based upon the patient's body weight. Optimal imaging is obtained from one to four hours after administration. Technetium Tc-99m disofenin is used to diagnose acute cholecystitis and may be used to rule out this disease in patients with right upper quadrant pain or tenderness and jaundice.

A9512

A9512 Technetium Tc-99m pertechnetate, diagnostic, per mCi

Technetium Tc-99m pertechnetate is an ionized acid of technetium. Technetium is a radioactive metallic element that is a byproduct of uranium decay. It may also be produced by bombarding another metal, molybdenum, with specific atoms. Technetium 99m is a widely used radionuclide with a half-life of approximately six hours, which is long enough to examine metabolic processes but short enough to minimize the radiation dose received by the patient. It decays by gamma emission, which is then measured by scintillation or gamma cameras. The pertechnetate form of technetium rapidly diffuses into the blood stream and localizes in the thyroid gland, gastric mucosa, salivary glands, certain areas of the brain, sweat glands, and other mucosal tissues. The radiopharmaceutical is administered primarily by intravenous injection, but it may be administered orally as an ophthalmic solution or by instillation into the urinary bladder. The dosage administered depends upon the body area being imaged. Technetium Tc-99m pertechnetate is used to provide images of the thyroid, salivary glands, and nasolacrimal drainage system. It is also used for placental localization, brain imaging including cerebral angiography, blood pool imaging including angiography, and urinary bladder imaging for detection of vesicoureteral reflux. Technetium Tc-99m pertechnetate may also be used to prepare other technetium 99m imaging agents.

A9513

A9513 Lutetium Lu 177, dotatate, therapeutic, 1 mCi

Lutetium Lu 177 dotatate is a somatostatin analog utilized for the treatment of adult patients, 18 years of age or older, with somatostatin receptor-positive gastroenteropancreatic neuroendocrine tumors (GEP-NET), including tumors in the foregut, hindgut, and midgut. It binds to somatostatin receptors, including malignant somatostatin receptor positive tumors, inducing the formation of free radicals in somatostatin receptor-positive cells, causing damage in the tumor cells. It is supplied in a single dose vial. Recommended dose is 200 mCi (7.4 GBq) administered via intramuscular injection every eight weeks for a total of four doses. A 30 mg dose of a long-acting octreotide should be administered via intramuscular injection four to 24 hours after each lutetium Lu 177 dotatate dose every four weeks, until disease progression or up to 18 months after initiation of treatment. An amino acid solution should be started via intravenous infusion 30 minutes before lutetium Lu 177 dotatate infusion and should continue during and for three hours after the end of the lutetium Lu 177 dotatate infusion. Antiemetics should be administered 30 minutes prior to administration of the amino acid solution. Long-acting octreotides should be stopped for at least four weeks prior to initiation of treatment. A short-acting octreotide can be administered for management of symptoms, but must be discontinued for at least 24 hours prior to the start of treatment.

A9515

A9515 Choline C-11, diagnostic, per study dose up to 20 mCi

Choline C 11 is a radiopharmaceutical diagnostic imaging agent used in the positron emission tomography (PET) imaging of patients with suspected recurrence of cancer of the prostate, and who have had non-informative CT, MRI, or bone scintigraphy imaging. The drug helps identify sites for histological confirmation (biopsy). The patient should be fasting for at least six hours prior to administration. The dose is based on patient body size and the characteristics of the image acquisition system. Typically, 370 to 740 MBq (10 to 20 mCi) is given as a bolus intravenous injection and imaging from the base of the pelvis to the base of the skull is begun immediately following administration. Static emission images are obtained within 15 minutes of injection.

A9516

A9516 Iodine I-123 sodium iodide, diagnostic, per 100 mcCi, up to 999 mcCi

Iodine is a common nonmetallic element necessary for the proper function of the thyroid gland. Iodine 123 sodium iodide is a radioactive isotope of iodine produced in a cyclotron. It decays by electron capture and gamma emission with a half-life of 13 hours. Iodine 123 sodium iodide is administered orally in capsule form. It is readily absorbed from the gastrointestinal tract and congregates primarily in the thyroid gland. Optimal images may be initiated six hours after administration. Sodium iodide I-123 is indicated for diagnostic use in the evaluation of thyroid function and/or morphology.

A9517

A9517 Iodine I-131 sodium iodide capsule(s), therapeutic, per mCi

Iodine is a common nonmetallic element necessary for the proper function of the thyroid gland. Iodine 131 sodium iodide is a radioactive isotope of iodine produced in a cyclotron. It decays by beta and gamma emission with a half-life of eight hours. Iodine 131 sodium iodide is administered orally in capsule or solution form. It is readily absorbed from the gastrointestinal tract and congregates primarily in thyroid tissue. Therapeutic doses of sodium iodide I-131 capsules are indicated for the treatment of hyperthyroidism and selected cases of thyroid cancer. Palliative effects may be seen in patients with papillary and/or follicular carcinoma of the thyroid. Sodium iodide I-131 is not usually used for the treatment of hyperthyroidism in patients younger than 30 years of age unless circumstances preclude other methods of treatment.

A9520

A9520 Technetium Tc-99m, tilmanocept, diagnostic, up to 0.5 mCi

Tilmanocept is a diagnostic macromolecule composed of DTPA, mannose (CD-206), and dextran that selectively binds with mannose receptors on the surface of macrophages and dendrite cells. It accumulates in lymphatic tissue. Technetium is a radioactive metallic element that is a byproduct of uranium decay. It may also be produced by bombarding another metal, molybdenum, with specific atoms. Technetium 99m is a widely used radionuclide with a half-life of approximately six hours, which is long enough to examine metabolic processes but short enough to minimize the radiation dose received by the patient. It decays by gamma emission, which is measured by scintillation or gamma cameras. The radiopharmaceutical is administered by intradermal, subcutaneous, or peritumoral injection. Technetium Tc-99m tilmanocept is used for lymphatic mapping using a hand-held gamma counter. It is used for sentinel node mapping, the localization of lymph nodes that drain the primary tumor site, in patients with breast cancer, melanoma, and cancers of the head and neck. The recommended dosage is 0.5 mCi and should be administered at least 15 minutes prior to imaging. Each kit contains five vials that may be used for up to four patients.

A9521

A9521 Technetium Tc-99m exametazime, diagnostic, per study dose, up to 25 mCi

Exametazime, also known as hexamethylpropyleneamine oxime, is a chemical complex that is taken up by leukocytes and selectively retained in neutrophils. Technetium is a radioactive metallic element that is a byproduct of uranium decay. It may also be produced by bombarding another metal, molybdenum, with specific atoms. Technetium 99m is a widely used radionuclide with a half-life of approximately six hours, which is long enough to examine metabolic processes, but short enough to minimize the radiation dose received by the patient. It decays by gamma emission, which is then measured by scintillation or gamma cameras. Tc-99m exametazime is used to label autologous leukocytes. The labeled leukocytes are then used in imaging to localize or identify areas of intra-abdominal infection or inflammation. Optimal imaging with labeled leukocytes is two to four hours after administration. When technetium Tc-99m pertechnetate is added to the exametazime, the resulting radiopharmaceutical is taken up by lipids that can cross the blood-brain barrier. The technetium Tc-99m pertechnetate/exametazime is useful for only 30 minutes. Its useful life can be extended by the addition of methylene blue. Tc-99m pertechnetate/exametazime is used in cerebral perfusion imaging to detect regions altered by stroke. The radiopharmaceutical is administered by intravenous injection. Optimal imaging for cerebral perfusion studies may begin immediately after administration and can continue up to six hours after administration.

A9524

A9524 Iodine I-131 iodinated serum albumin, diagnostic, per 5 mcCi

Serum albumin is a protein component of blood. Iodine 131 is a radioactive isotope of the common element iodine. Iodine 131 has a half-life of eight days and decays by beta and gamma emissions. Serum albumin is combined with iodine 131 to provide images of the blood pool and its movement. The radiopharmaceutical is administered by intravenous injection and is dispersed within the intravascular pool within 10 minutes. Full distribution throughout the body takes from two to four days after administration. Dosage depends upon the imaging to be performed. Iodinated I-131 serum albumin is indicated for use in determinations of total blood and

A

plasma volumes, cardiac output, cardiac and pulmonary blood volumes and circulation times, and in protein turnover studies, heart and great vessel delineation, localization of the placenta, and localization of cerebral neoplasms.

A9526

A9526 Nitrogen N-13 ammonia, diagnostic, per study dose, up to 40 mCi

Nitrogen N-13 ammonia is a radioisotope composed of ammonia molecules combined with nitrogen N-13 that is widely used in cardiac imaging. Nitrogen N-13 is a radioactive isotope of nitrogen produced within a cyclotron. Nitrogen 13 has a half-life of approximately 10 minutes and decays by positron emission. The positrons are used to produce positron emission tomography (PET) images. Due to its short half-life, nitrogen N-13 ammonia must be produced shortly before use. Nitrogen N-13 ammonia is injected intravenously and is rapidly distributed to all organs of the body. Optimal imaging of the myocardium is generally obtained 15 to 20 minutes after administration. Nitrogen N-13 ammonia is currently approved only for myocardial perfusion for the diagnosis and management of patients with known or suspected coronary artery disease. The perfusion study may be performed at rest or with pharmacological stress.

A9527

A9527 Iodine I-125, sodium iodide solution, therapeutic, per mCi

Iodine 125 sodium iodide is a radioactive isotope of iodine produced by the neutron irradiation of xenon-124. It decays by electron capture and gamma emission with a half-life of 60 days. Therapeutic iodine 125 sodium iodide is administered in solution form. It is used to treat hyperthyroidism and prostate and brain cancers. This code represents one millicurie of I-125 sodium iodide solution used as a therapeutic dose.

A9528-A9531

A9528 Iodine I-131 sodium iodide capsule(s), diagnostic, per mCi

A9529 Iodine I-131 sodium iodide solution, diagnostic, per mCi

A9530 Iodine I-131 sodium iodide solution, therapeutic, per mCi

A9531 Iodine I-131 sodium iodide, diagnostic, per mcCi (up to 100 mcCi)

Iodine is a common nonmetallic element necessary for the proper function of the thyroid gland. Iodine 131 sodium iodide is a radioactive isotope of iodine produced in a cyclotron. It decays by beta and gamma emission with a half-life of eight hours. Iodine 131 sodium iodide is administered orally in capsule or solution form. It is readily absorbed from the gastrointestinal tract and congregates primarily in thyroid tissue. Therapeutic doses of sodium iodide I-131 capsules are indicated for the treatment of hyperthyroidism and selected cases of thyroid cancer. Palliative effects may be seen in patients with papillary and/or follicular carcinoma of the thyroid. Sodium iodide 1-131 is not usually used for the treatment of hyperthyroidism in patients younger than 30 years of age unless circumstances preclude other methods of treatment.

A9532

A9532 Iodine I-125 serum albumin, diagnostic, per 5 mcCi

Serum albumin is a protein component of blood. Iodine 125 is a radioactive isotope of the common element iodine. Iodine 125 has a half-life of 60 days and decays by beta and gamma emissions. Serum albumin is combined with iodine 125 to provide measures of the blood and plasma pool. The radiopharmaceutical is administered by intravenous injection. Dosage depends upon body weight and can vary from 5 to 50 microcuries. At five and 15 minutes after administration, blood samples are drawn from the arm that was not injected. The radioactivity of the blood samples is measured and a calculation of the patient's blood volume is determined. For plasma volume, the samples are first centrifuged and the red blood cells removed. Iodinated I-125 serum albumin is indicated for use in determinations of total blood and plasma volumes.

A9536

A9536 Technetium Tc-99m depreotide, diagnostic, per study dose, up to 35 mCi

Depreotide is a synthetic peptide that binds to somatostatin receptors in cells. Somatostatin is a peptide that regulates the release of hormones by many different neuroendocrine cells in the brain, pancreas, and gastrointestinal tract. Technetium is a radioactive metallic element that is a byproduct of uranium decay. It may also be produced by bombarding another metal, molybdenum, with specific atoms. Technetium 99m is a widely used radionuclide with a half-life of approximately six hours, which is long enough to examine metabolic processes, but short enough to minimize the radiation dose received by the patient. It decays by gamma emission, which is then measured by scintillation or gamma cameras. Depreotide is combined with technetium 99m to determine the nature of pulmonary masses in patients who have known or suspected malignancy. The radiopharmaceutical is administered by intravenous injection. Dosage is 15 to 20 mCi. Optimal imaging is obtained from two to four hours after administration.

A9537

A9537 Technetium Tc-99m mebrofenin, diagnostic, per study dose, up to 15 mCi

Mebrofenin is a derivative of an iminodiacetic acid that is a form of acetoacetic acid, a byproduct of metabolism that congregates in the gallbladder.

Technetium is a radioactive metallic element that is a byproduct of uranium decay. It may also be produced by bombarding another metal, molybdenum, with specific atoms. Technetium 99m is a widely used radionuclide with a half-life of approximately six hours, which is long enough to examine metabolic processes but short enough to minimize the radiation dose received by the patient. It decays by gamma emission, which is then measured by scintillation or gamma cameras. Mebrofenin is combined with technetium 99m to provide images of the gallbladder and surrounding ducts. Technetium Tc-99m mebrofenin is rapidly cleared and has a short useful life. The radiopharmaceutical is administered by intravenous injection. Dosage is based upon patient's body weight. Optimal imaging is obtained from 10 to 60 minutes after administration.

A9538

A9538 Technetium Tc-99m pyrophosphate, diagnostic, per study dose, up to 25 mCi

Pyrophosphate is a form of phosphorus formed by the breakdown of adenosine triphosphate (ATP) into adenosine monophosphate (AMP). Technetium is a radioactive metallic element that is a byproduct of uranium decay. It may also be produced by bombarding another metal, molybdenum, with specific atoms. Technetium 99m is a widely used radionuclide with a half-life of approximately six hours, which is long enough to examine metabolic processes but short enough to minimize the radiation dose received by the patient. It decays by gamma emission, which is then measured by scintillation or gamma cameras. Pyrophosphate combined with technetium 99m seems to be attracted to certain crystals found in bone and damaged heart cells. The radiopharmaceutical is administered by intravenous injection. Dosage and optimal imaging depend on the area being imaged. Technetium Tc-99m pyrophosphate is used in skeletal imaging to identify areas of altered bone, such as occurs in metastatic disease, Paget's disease, arthritis, osteomyelitis, and fractures. It is used in cardiac imaging to aid in the diagnosis of an acute myocardial infarction. Technetium Tc-99m pyrophosphate may also be used in conjunction with technetium Tc-99m pertechnetate for the labeling of red blood cells.

A9539

A9539 Technetium Tc-99m pentetate, diagnostic, per study dose, up to 25 mCi

The pentetate here refers to calcium trisodium pentetate, which is a chelating agent that forms stable bounds with metals, which are then excreted in the urine. Technetium is a radioactive metallic element that is a byproduct of uranium decay. It may also be produced by bombarding another metal, molybdenum, with specific atoms. Technetium 99m is a widely used radionuclide with a half-life of approximately six hours, which is long enough to examine metabolic processes, but short enough to minimize the radiation dose received by the patient. It decays by gamma emission, which is then measured by scintillation or gamma cameras. Pentetate combined with technetium 99m is rapidly distributed throughout the body and is excreted from the body by glomerular filtration. The images of the kidneys obtained in the first few minutes after administration will show the blood pool within the kidney. Subsequent images show kidney function. Technetium Tc-99m pentetate also tends to accumulate in intracranial lesions with many new blood vessels or with an altered blood-brain barrier. The radiopharmaceutical is administered by intravenous injection. Dosage and optimal imaging depend on the area being imaged. Technetium Tc-99m pentetate is used for kidney and brain imaging and to assess renal function and estimate the glomerular filtration rate. When in aerosol form, it is administered by inhalation. The aerosol form is used to assess airway patency, especially in conjunction with perfusion lung imaging to evaluate for a pulmonary embolism.

A9540

A9540 Technetium Tc-99m macroaggregated albumin, diagnostic, per study dose, up to 10 mCi

Macroaggregated albumin, also called aggregated albumin, is an unusually large amount of albumin, a protein component of blood. Technetium is a radioactive metallic element that is a byproduct of uranium decay. It may also be produced by bombarding another metal, molybdenum, with specific atoms. Technetium 99m is a widely used radionuclide with a half-life of approximately six hours, which is long enough to examine metabolic processes, but short enough to minimize the radiation dose received by the patient. It decays by gamma emission, which is then measured by scintillation or gamma cameras. Macroaggregated albumin combined with technetium 99m pertechnetate rapidly accumulates in pulmonary alveolar capillaries. The radiopharmaceutical is administered by intravenous injection. Dosage depends upon body weight. Optimal imaging can be obtained immediately after administration. Technetium Tc-99m macroaggregated albumin is used for a lung imaging agent and may be used as an adjunct in the evaluation of pulmonary perfusion in adults and pediatric patients. It may be used in adults for evaluation of peritoneovenous (LeVeen) shunt patency.

A9541

A9541 Technetium Tc-99m sulfur colloid, diagnostic, per study dose, up to 20 mCi

Sulfur colloid is suspension of very fine particles of sulfur, a nonmetallic element, in an isotonic saline liquid. Technetium is a radioactive metallic element that is a byproduct of uranium decay. It may also be produced by bombarding another metal, molybdenum, with specific atoms. Technetium 99m is a widely used radionuclide with a half-life of approximately six hours, which is long enough to examine metabolic processes but short enough to minimize the radiation dose received by the patient. It decays by gamma emission, which is then measured by scintillation or gamma cameras. Sulfur colloid combined with technetium 99m is rapidly eliminated by the reticuloendothelial system, which is a group of cells within the immune system. The radiopharmaceutical is administered orally or by intravenous or intra-peritoneal injection. Dosage and optimal imaging depends upon body weight and intended area study. Technetium Tc-99m sulfur colloid injected intravenously is used for imaging of the liver, spleen, and bone marrow. Administered orally, it is used for the evaluation of swallowing functions, gastroesophageal reflux studies, and the detection of pulmonary aspiration of gastric contents. Technetium Tc-99m sulfur colloid injected intra-peritoneally may be used in adults for evaluation of peritoneovenous (LeVeen) shunt patency.

A9542-A9543

A9542 Indium In-111 ibritumomab tiuxetan, diagnostic, per study dose, up to 5 mCi

A9543 Yttrium Y-90 ibritumomab tiuxetan, therapeutic, per treatment dose, up to 40 mCi

Ibritumomab is a murine monoclonal antibody produced in Chinese hamster ovary cells. This antibody is specifically directed against the CD20 antigen, which is found on the surface of normal and malignant B lymphocytes. Tiuxetan is a chelating agent that allows ibritumomab to form stable bonds with metals. Indium 111 is a radioactive form of the metallic element indium. It has a half-life of approximately 56 hours and decays by electron capture and gamma emission. Indium 111 ibritumomab tiuxetan is used to determine the biodistribution pattern in preparation for the administration of yttrium 90 of ibritumomab tiuxetan. The usual dose for diagnostic purposes is 5 millicuries injected intravenously. Yttrium 90 is a radioactive form of the metallic element yttrium found in rare earth minerals. Ibritumomab tiuxetan combined with yttrium 90 is used for the treatment of relapsed or refractory low-grade, follicular, or transformed B cell non-Hodgkin's lymphoma, including rituximab-refractory follicular non-Hodgkin's lymphoma. The dosage for therapeutic yttrium 90 ibritumomab tiuxetan depends upon body weight. It is administered by intravenous injection. Both forms of ibritumomab tiuxetan are administered in conjunction with rituximab.

A9546

A9546 Cobalt Co-57/58, cyanocobalamin, diagnostic, per study dose, up to 1 mcCi

Cyanocobalamin Co-57/58 is a radioactive form of vitamin B12 in which portions of the molecules contain cobalt 57 or cobalt 58. The drug is administered orally and used to diagnose pernicious anemia and intestinal defects of vitamin B12 absorption.

A9547

A9547 Indium In-111 oxyquinoline, diagnostic, per 0.5 mCi

Indium 111 oxyquinoline is a radioisotope used to label autologous white blood cells. These labeled cells are then administered intravenously and used to scan for abscesses and other inflammatory processes where the white cells would usually congregate. Indium 111 oxyquinoline is not the preferred technique for the initial evaluation of patients with a suspected abscess in an unknown location. It should be considered only if other methods prove unsuccessful or ambiguous. Imaging is performed approximately two hours postinjection. Indium 111 decays by electron capture with a half-life of 67.2 hours.

A9548

A9548 Indium In-111 pentetate, diagnostic, per 0.5 mCi

Pentetate, also known as pentetic acid or DTPA, is a chelating agent that binds with iron. Indium 111 is a radioactive form of indium, a metallic element. Indium 111 has a half-life of 2.8 days and decays by electron capture and gamma emission. Pentetate combined with indium In-111 is used to provide images of the cerebrospinal fluid (CSF) flow. It is indicated for use in radionuclide cisternography to study the flow of CSF in the brain for identification of CSF abnormalities and sites of CSF leakage, and for evaluation of CSF shunt patency. Indium In-111 pentetate is administered by intrathecal injection into the lumbar intrathecal space. It flows up the spinal canal with the CSF to the brain. Under normal flow patterns, it does not penetrate into the ventricles. Indium In-111 pentetate is supplied as a unit dose. Each unit dose vial contains 0.7 mCi of sterile indium In-111 pentetate. The maximum recommended dose for an adult (average weight 70 kg) is 10.5 mCi. Any unused portion must be discarded.

A9550

A9550 Technetium Tc-99m sodium gluceptate, diagnostic, per study dose, up to 25 mCi

Sodium gluceptate is a carbohydrate derivative. Technetium is a radioactive metallic element that is a byproduct of uranium decay. It may also be produced by bombarding another metal, molybdenum, with specific atoms. Technetium 99m is a widely used radionuclide with a half-life of approximately six hours, which is long enough to examine metabolic processes but short enough to minimize the radiation dose received by the patient. It decays by gamma emission, which is then measured by scintillation or gamma cameras. Sodium gluceptate combined with technetium 99m pertechnetate is rapidly eliminated from the body by the kidneys. It tends to accumulate in intracranial lesions with many new blood vessels or with an altered blood-brain barrier. Technetium 99m sodium gluceptate is used for kidney and brain imaging and to assess renal and brain perfusion. The radiopharmaceutical is administered by intravenous injection. The recommended adult dosage is 10 to 15 mCi for renal imaging and 15 to 20 mCi for brain imaging. Dynamic imaging may begin immediately after administration, and static images can be obtained up to several hours after administration.

A9551

A9551 Technetium Tc-99m succimer, diagnostic, per study dose, up to 10 mCi

Succimer, also known as DMSA, is a chelating agent that is similar to dimercaprol and is used in the treatment of heavy metal poisoning. Technetium is a radioactive metallic element that is a byproduct of uranium decay. It may also be produced by bombarding another metal, molybdenum, with specific atoms. Technetium 99m is a widely used radionuclide with a half-life of approximately six hours, which is long enough to examine metabolic processes, but short enough to minimize the radiation dose received by the patient. It decays by gamma emission, which is then measured by scintillation or gamma cameras. Succimer combined with technetium 99m pertechnetate is rapidly eliminated from the body by the kidneys. The radiopharmaceutical is administered by intravenous injection. Technetium 99m succimer is used in the evaluation of renal parenchymal disorders. The recommended adult dosage is 2 to 6 mCi. Optimal imaging may be obtained one to two hours after administration.

A9552

A9552 Fluorodeoxyglucose F-18 FDG, diagnostic, per study dose, up to 45 mCi

Glucose is a sugar actively taken up by cells. Fludeoxyglucose F18 (FDG) is a radioisotope widely used in positron emission tomography (PET imaging). FDG is a radioactive version of glucose that is administered intravenously. Peak imaging is at 30 to 40 minutes after injection. FDG is indicated for identifying regions of abnormal glucose metabolism that can be associated with foci of epileptic seizures or evaluation of malignancy in patients who have an existing diagnosis or who have known of or suspected abnormalities identified by other methods. FDG may also be used to assess coronary artery disease and left ventricular dysfunction when used together with myocardial perfusion. It must be produced from cyclotron bombardment of fluorine F18, which is itself produced from proton bombardment of enriched water. FDG decays by positron emission and has a half-life of 109.8 minutes.

A9553

A9553 Chromium Cr-51 sodium chromate, diagnostic, per study dose, up to 250 mcCi

Chromium CR 51 is a radioisotope of sodium chromate, which binds to red blood cells. Chromium 51 is used to label red blood cells and the labeled cells are administered intravenously. Labeled red blood cells are used for determining red blood cell volume or mass, evaluating blood loss, and studying red blood cell survival time for conditions such as hemolytic anemia. Chromium 51 decays by electron capture and gamma emission. It has a half-life of 27.7 days.

A9554

A9554 Iodine I-125 sodium iothalamate, diagnostic, per study dose, up to 10 mcCi

Sodium iothalamate is a solution of iodine and sodium hydroxide that is used as a contrast agent. Iodine I-125 is a radioactive version of iodine that has a half-life of 60 days and decays by electron capture and gamma emission. Sodium iothalamate combined with iodine I-125 is used to evaluate renal glomerular filtration when diagnosing and monitoring patients with renal disease. The compound is cleared by renal glomerular filtration without tubular secretion or reabsorption. The suggested dose range employed in an adult patient (average weight 70 kg) depends on the infusion method. For continuous intravenous infusion, the dose is 20 to 100 uCi. For single intravenous injection, the dose is 10 to 30 uCi. Blood and urine samples are collected from the patient at varying intervals post administration. The concentration of iodine I-125 in each specimen is then measured using scintillation counters. These figures are used to compute clearance factors, which provide an indication of renal function.

A9555

A9555 Rubidium Rb-82, diagnostic, per study dose, up to 60 mCi

Rubidium-82 is a radioisotope widely used in cardiac imaging, as it is a chemical analog to potassium. Potassium ions are metabolized by muscle tissue, including the heart. Once in the heart, the beta decay of the rubidium-82 is used to help produce a PET image. The half-life of rubidium-82 is 1.273 minutes. Due to its short half-life, rubidium-82 must be produced shortly before use by a rubidium-82 generator. Rubidium-82 is produced by the beta decay of strontium-82. Strontium-82 is an isotope that can readily be made in an accelerator and has a half-life of 25.5 days. The relatively long-lived strontium-82 in the form of a solution is loaded into the rubidium-82 generator. As the strontium-82 decays, rubidium-82 is produced. A solvent is then selectively used to remove the rubidium-82 from the solution. As the strontium-82 is continually decaying and producing rubidium-82, one can allow the rubidium to accumulate and remove the rubidium-82 as needed.

A9556

A9556 Gallium Ga-67 citrate, diagnostic, per mCi

Gallium is a rare metal that is liquid at room temperature. Gallium Ga 67 citrate is a radioactive version of gallium used to identify the presence and extent of Hodgkin's disease, lymphomas, and bronchogenic carcinomas. It may also be useful in detecting some inflammatory lesions. Gallium Ga 67 citrate is administered intravenously, and peak imaging is often 48 to 120 hours after injection. It must be produced from cyclotron proton bombardment of Zinc ZN 68 enriched metal. Gallium Ga 67 decays by electron capture and gamma emission. It has a half-life of 78.3 hours.

A9557

A9557 Technetium Tc-99m bicisate, diagnostic, per study dose, up to 25 mCi

Bicisate, also known as ethyl cysteinate dimer (ECD), is a lipophilic amine having the ability to cross the blood-brain barrier and localize in the brain. Technetium is a radioactive metallic element that is a byproduct of uranium decay. It may also be produced by bombarding another metal, molybdenum, with specific atoms. Technetium 99m is a widely used radionuclide with a half-life of approximately six hours, which is long enough to examine metabolic processes, but short enough to minimize the radiation dose received by the patient. It decays by gamma emission, which is then measured by scintillation or gamma cameras. Bicisate combined with technetium 99m pertechnetate is used in single photon emission computerized tomography (SPECT) imaging as an adjunct to conventional CT or MRI imaging in the localization of stroke in patients in whom stroke has already been diagnosed. The radiopharmaceutical is injected intravenously. The recommended adult dosage is 10 to 30 mCi. Optimal imaging may be obtained 30 to 60 minutes after administration.

A9558

A9558 Xenon Xe-133 gas, diagnostic, per 10 mCi

Xenon is a gaseous element that is not chemically reactive. Xenon Xe133 gas is a mixture of radioactive xenon gas and carbon dioxide inhaled by the patient for use in diagnostic evaluations of pulmonary functions, pulmonary imaging, and in the assessment of cerebral blood flow. The gas is a reactor-produced by-product of uranium U235 fission. Xenon Xe133 gas decays by beta and gamma emissions with a half-life of 5.245 days.

A9559

A9559 Cobalt Co-57 cyanocobalamin, oral, diagnostic, per study dose, up to 1 mcCi

Cyanocobalamin Co-57 is a radioactive forms of vitamin B12 in which portions of the molecules contain cobalt 57. The drug is administered orally and used to diagnose pernicious anemia and intestinal defects of vitamin B12 absorption.

A9560

A9560 Technetium Tc-99m labeled red blood cells, diagnostic, per study dose, up to 30 mCi

Technetium is a radioactive metallic element that is a byproduct of uranium decay. It may also be produced by bombarding another metal, molybdenum, with specific atoms. Technetium 99m is a widely used radionuclide with a half-life of approximately six hours, which is long enough to examine metabolic processes but short enough to minimize the radiation dose received by the patient. It decays by gamma emission, which is then measured by scintillation or gamma cameras. Technetium 99m pertechnetate is used to label autologous red blood cells, which are then injected intravenously. The recommended adult dosage is 10 to 20 mCi. Technetium Tc-99m labeled red blood cells are used for blood pool imaging, including cardiac first pass and gated equilibrium imaging, and for detection of sites of gastrointestinal bleeding.

A9561

A9561 Technetium Tc-99m oxidronate, diagnostic, per study dose, up to 30 mCi

Oxidronate, also known as HDP and HMDP, is a chemical compound that is attracted to sites of bone mineralization. Technetium is a radioactive metallic element that is a byproduct of uranium decay. It may also be produced by bombarding another metal, molybdenum, with specific atoms. Technetium 99m is a widely used radionuclide with a half-life of approximately six hours, which is long enough to examine metabolic processes, but short enough to minimize the radiation dose received by the patient. It decays by gamma emission, which is then measured by scintillation or gamma cameras. Oxidronate combined with technetium 99m is used for skeletal imaging to identify areas of altered bone growth. The radiopharmaceutical is injected intravenously. The recommended adult dosage is 10 to 20 mCi. Optimal imaging is three to four hours after administration.

A9562

A9562 Technetium Tc-99m mertiatide, diagnostic, per study dose, up to 15 mCi

Mertiatide is a chemical compound that binds to plasma protein. Technetium is a radioactive metallic element that is a byproduct of uranium decay. It may also be produced by bombarding another metal, molybdenum, with specific atoms. Technetium 99m is a widely used radionuclide with a half-life of approximately six hours, which is long enough to examine metabolic processes but short enough to minimize the radiation dose received by the patient. It decays by gamma emission, which is then measured by scintillation or gamma cameras. Mertiatide combined with technetium 99m pertechnetate is used for renal imaging to diagnose congenital and acquired abnormalities, renal failure, urinary tract obstruction, and calculi in adults and children. It is a diagnostic aid in providing renal function, split function, renal angiograms, and renogram curves for whole kidney and renal cortex. The radiopharmaceutical is injected intravenously. The recommended adult dosage is 5 to 10 mCi.

A9563

A9563 Sodium phosphate P-32, therapeutic, per mCi

Phosphorus is a common nonmetallic element essential to the human body. It is a major component of bone, is abundant in all tissues, and is involved in some form in almost all metabolic processes. Phosphorus 32 is a radioactive form of phosphorus. It has a half-life of approximately 14.28 days and decays by beta emission. Sodium is a common metallic element, an electrolyte necessary for the proper functioning of the body. Sodium phosphate P-32 is a compound of sodium and phosphorus P-32. It concentrates largely in rapidly proliferating tissue, accumulating in the liver, spleen, and bone marrow. Sodium phosphate P-32 is used for the therapeutic treatment of polycythemia vera, chronic myelocytic leukemia, and chronic lymphocytic leukemia. It may also be used for the palliative treatment of bone pain associated with multiple areas of skeletal metastases.

A9564

A9564 Chromic phosphate P-32 suspension, therapeutic, per mCi

Phosphorus is a common nonmetallic element essential to the human body. It is a major component of bone, is abundant in all tissues, and is involved in some form in almost all metabolic processes. Phosphorus 32 is a radioactive form of phosphorus. It has a half-life of approximately 14.28 days and decays by beta emission. Chromium is a metallic trace element used in glucose metabolism and is essential to the body in small amounts. Chromic phosphate P-32 is a compound of phosphorus 32 and chromium. It is administered by intraperitoneal or intrapleural instillation or interstitial injection. Chromic phosphate P-32 is used intraperitoneally or intrapleurally for the therapeutic treatment of effusions resulting from metastatic disease and interstitially in the treatment of certain ovarian and prostate carcinomas. Dosages vary from 0.1 to 20 millicuries depending on the disease being treated and method of administration.

A9566

A9566 Technetium Tc-99m fanolesomab, diagnostic, per study dose, up to 25 mCi

Fanolesomab is a murine monoclonal antibody that binds to the CD15 antigen. The CD15 antigen is found on the surface of some neutrophils, eosinophils, and monocytes, which are types of leukocytes or white blood cells. Technetium is a radioactive metallic element that is a byproduct of uranium decay. It may also be produced by bombarding another metal, molybdenum, with specific atoms. Technetium 99m is a widely used radionuclide with a half-life of approximately six hours, which is long enough to examine metabolic processes, but short enough to minimize the radiation dose received by the patient. It decays by gamma emission, which is then measured by scintillation or gamma cameras. Fanolesomab combined with technetium 99m pertechnetate labels the leukocytes or white blood cells. Leukocytes gather at the site of an infection. Technetium 99m fanolesomab is used to confirm appendicitis in patients with the signs and symptoms associated with appendicitis. The radiopharmaceutical is injected intravenously. The recommended adult dosage is 10 to 200 mCi. Imaging may begin immediately after administration.

A9567

A9567 Technetium Tc-99m pentetate, diagnostic, aerosol, per study dose, up to 75 mCi

The pentetate here refers to calcium trisodium pentetate, which is a chelating agent that forms stable bonds with metals, which are then excreted in the urine. Technetium is a radioactive metallic element that is a byproduct of uranium decay. It may also be produced by bombarding another metal, molybdenum, with specific atoms. Technetium 99m is a widely used radionuclide with a half-life of approximately six hours, which is long enough to examine metabolic processes but short enough to minimize the radiation dose received by the patient. It decays by gamma emission, which is then measured by scintillation or gamma cameras. Pentetate combined with technetium 99m is rapidly distributed throughout the body and is excreted from the body by glomerular filtration. The images of the kidneys obtained in the first few minutes after administration show the blood pool within the kidney. Subsequent images show kidney function. Technetium Tc-99m pentetate also tends to accumulate in intracranial lesions with many new blood vessels or with an altered blood-brain barrier. The radiopharmaceutical is administered by intravenous injection. Dosage and optimal imaging depend on the area being imaged. Technetium Tc-99m pentetate is used for kidney and brain imaging and to assess renal function and to estimate the glomerular filtration rate. When in aerosol form, it is administered by inhalation. The aerosol form is used to assess airway patency, especially in conjunction with perfusion lung imaging to evaluate for a pulmonary embolism.

A9568

A9568 Technetium Tc-99m arcitumomab, diagnostic, per study dose, up to 45 mCi

Arcitumomab is a murine monoclonal antibody directed to the carcinoembryonic antigen (CEA), a tumor-associated antigen whose expression is increased in various carcinomas, particularly of the gastrointestinal tract, and in certain inflammatory states (e.g., Crohn's disease, inflammatory bowel disease, post-radiation therapy to the bowel). Technetium is a radioactive metallic element that is a byproduct of uranium decay. It may also be produced by bombarding another metal, molybdenum, with specific atoms. Technetium 99m is a widely used radionuclide with a half-life of approximately six hours, which is long enough to examine metabolic processes but short enough to minimize the radiation dose received by the patient. It decays by gamma emission which is then measured by scintillation or gamma cameras. Arcitumomab combined with technetium 99m pertechnetate is indicated, in conjunction with standard diagnostic evaluations, for detection of the presence, location, and extent of recurrent and/or metastatic colorectal carcinoma involving the liver, extrahepatic abdomen, and pelvis in patients with a histologically confirmed diagnosis of colorectal carcinoma. The radiopharmaceutical is administered by intravenous injection. The recommended adult dosage is 1 mg labeled with 20-30 millicuries of technetium TC 99m arcitumomab. Optimal imaging is at two to five hours after administration.

A9569

A9569 Technetium Tc-99m exametazime labeled autologous white blood cells, diagnostic, per study dose

Exametazime, also known as hexamethylpropyleneamine oxime, is a chemical complex that is taken up by leukocytes and selectively retained in neutrophils. Technetium is a radioactive metallic element that is a byproduct of uranium decay. It may also be produced by bombarding another metal, molybdenum, with specific atoms. Technetium 99m is a widely used radionuclide with a half-life of approximately six hours, which is long enough to examine metabolic processes but short enough to minimize the radiation dose received by the patient. It decays by gamma emission, which is then measured by scintillation or gamma cameras. Tc-99m exametazime is used to label autologous leukocytes. The labeled leukocytes are then used in imaging to localize or identify areas of intra-abdominal infection or inflammation. Optimal imaging with labeled leukocytes is two to four hours after administration. When technetium Tc-99m pertechnetate is added to the exametazime, the resulting radiopharmaceutical is taken up by lipids that can cross the blood-brain barrier. The technetium Tc-99m pertechnetate/exametazime is useful for only 30 minutes. Its useful life can be extended by the addition of methylene blue. Tc-99m pertechnetate/exametazime is used in cerebral perfusion imaging to detect regions altered by stroke. The radiopharmaceutical is administered by intravenous injection. Optimal imaging for cerebral perfusion studies may begin immediately after administration and can continue up to six hours after administration.

A9570

A9570 Indium In-111 labeled autologous white blood cells, diagnostic, per study dose

Indium 111 is a radioactive form of indium, a metallic element. Indium 111 has a half-life of 2.8 days and decays by electron capture and gamma emission. Indium 111 is used to label autologous white blood cells. These labeled cells are then reinfused into the patient intravenously and used to scan for abscesses and other inflammatory processes where the white cells would usually congregate. Imaging is performed approximately two hours postinjection.

A9571

A9571 Indium In-111 labeled autologous platelets, diagnostic, per study dose

Indium 111 is a radioactive form of indium, a metallic element. Indium 111 has a half-life of 2.8 days and decays by electron capture and gamma emission. Indium 111 is used to label autologous platelets. These labeled cells are then reinfused into the patient intravenously. Platelets tend to aggregate at areas of thrombosis or active bleeding. Indium-labeled platelets are used to scan for deep vein thrombosis, vascular integrity, and platelet survival. Imaging is performed approximately two hours postinjection.

A9572

A9572 Indium In-111 pentetreotide, diagnostic, per study dose, up to 6 mCi

Pentetreotide is a mixture of pentetic acid and octreotide. Pentetic acid, also known as pentetate or DTPA, is a chelating agent that binds with iron. Octreotide is a synthetic version of somatostatin, which is a peptide that inhibits the release of growth hormone, thyrotropin, and corticotropin. Indium 111 is a radioactive form of indium, a metallic element. Indium 111 has a half-life of 2.8 days and decays by electron capture and gamma emission. Indium In-111 pentetreotide binds somatostatin receptors on cell surfaces throughout the body. After approximately an hour following intravenous injection most of the indium In-111 pentetreotide is distributed throughout the body and is seen concentrated in tumors containing a high density of somatostatin receptors. Indium In-111 pentetreotide allows imaging that identifies the presence and location of primary and metastatic neuroendocrine tumors bearing somatostatin receptors. Indium In-111 pentetreotide is administered by intravenous injection. The recommended dose for planar imaging is 3.0 mCi. The recommended dose for SPECT imaging is 6.0 mCi.

A9575

A9575 Injection, gadoterate meglumine, 0.1 ml

Magnetic resonance imaging (MRI) is a radiation-free, noninvasive technique used to produce high-quality sectional images of the inside of the body in multiple planes. MRI uses the natural magnetic properties of the hydrogen atoms in our bodies that emit radiofrequency signals when exposed to radio waves within a strong electromagnetic field. These signals are processed and converted by the computer into high-resolution, three-dimensional tomographic images. Gadolinium is a rare earth metal that is strongly magnetic at room temperature. Various forms of the metal are used to enhance an MRI. Gadoterate meglumine is a gadolinium-based contrast agent for use in MRI of the brain, spine, and associated tissues to detect and visualize areas with disruption of the blood brain barrier and/or abnormal vascularity. Gadoterate does not cross the intact blood-brain barrier (BBB) and, therefore, does not enhance normal brain or lesions that have a normal blood-brain barrier (e.g., cysts, mature postoperative scars). However, when there is a disruption of the BBB or abnormal vascularity gadoterate meglumine allows distribution of gadoterate in brain lesions such as neoplasms, abscesses, and infarcts. Dosage depends on patient body weight with a recommended dose of 0.2 ml per kg.

A9576-A9579

A9576 Injection, gadoteridol, (ProHance multipack), per ml

A9577 Injection, gadobenate dimeglumine (MultiHance), per ml

A9578 Injection, gadobenate dimeglumine (MultiHance multipack), per ml

A9579 Injection, gadolinium-based magnetic resonance contrast agent, not otherwise specified (NOS), per ml

Magnetic resonance imaging (MRI) is a radiation-free, noninvasive technique used to produce high-quality sectional images of the inside of the body in multiple planes. MRI uses the natural magnetic properties of the hydrogen atoms in our bodies that emit radiofrequency signals when exposed to radio waves within a strong electromagnetic field. These signals are processed and converted by the computer into high-resolution, three-dimensional tomographic images. Gadolinium is a rare earth metal that is strongly magnetic at room temperature. Various forms of the metal are used to enhance an MRI. The gadolinium is administered intravenously and circulates within the cardiovascular system allowing the MRI to capture greater detail. Gadolinium highlights disruptions of the blood-brain barrier and enhances areas of abnormal vascularization that is common in neoplasms, abscesses, or subacute infarcts. It is indicated for use in MRIs of the brain; spine; head and neck; thoracic, abdominal, and pelvic cavities; and retroperitoneal space. It is not indicated for use in cardiac imaging. Dosage depends on patient body weight with a recommended dose of 0.2 ml per kg.

A9580

A9580 Sodium fluoride F-18, diagnostic, per study dose, up to 30 mCi

Sodium fluoride F-18 is a radiopharmaceutical used with PET scans. It is a positron emitting substance used to detect abnormal bone activity in the patient. Abnormal activity can be a result of cancer, Paget's disease, or osteomyelitis. Sodium fluoride is injected through an IV line and allowed to circulate. It accumulates in the areas of bone activity. Those areas are visible with the PET scan. The normal dose of sodium fluoride F-18 is 5 mCi to 15 mCi.

A9581

A9581 Injection, gadoxetate disodium, 1 ml

Gadoxetate disodium is a paramagnetic, gadolinium-based contrast agent for MRI that creates a magnetic field. It provides a brightening of blood and tissue. It is used for liver MRIs to look for lesions or liver disease. The recommended dose of gadoxetate disodium is 0.1 mL/kg based on the patient's body weight. It is administered by IV injection.

A9582

A9582 Iodine I-123 iobenguane, diagnostic, per study dose, up to 15 mCi

Iobenguane sulfate is an analogue of norepinephrine that binds to receptors in the sympathetic nervous system and to related tumors. Iodine 123 is a radioactive isotope of the common element iodine produced in a cyclotron. It decays by electron capture and gamma emission with a half-life of 13 hours. Iobenguane sulfate combined with Iodine 123, also known as MIBG, is a radiopharmaceutical used as a diagnostic imaging agent for neuroendocrine tumors and disorders of the adrenal medulla. Iodine I-123 iobenguane sulfate is injected intravenously. Multiple scans are usually performed for up to four days post administration.

A9583

A9583 Injection, gadofosveset trisodium, 1 ml

Gadofosveset trisodium is a contrast agent used to evaluate vascular structures with magnetic resonance angiography (MRA). The recommended dose is based on body weight and is administered intravenously.

A9584

A9584 Iodine I-123 ioflupane, diagnostic, per study dose, up to 5 mCi

Iodine is a common, nonmetallic element necessary for the proper function of the thyroid gland. Iodine 123 is a radioactive isotope of iodine produced in a cyclotron. It decays by electron capture and gamma emission with a half-life of 13 hours. Ioflupane is a neuroimaging drug with an affinity for dopamine transporters in the striatal regions of the brain. Patients with Parkinson's disease have a marked reduction in dopaminergic neurons in the striatal regions of the brain. Once Iodine I-123 ioflupane has bound with the dopamine transporters, a quantitative measure and spatial distributions can be obtained. This radiopharmaceutical is used to diagnose Parkinson's disease and differentiate Parkinson's disease from other disorders that display similar symptoms.

A9585

A9585 Injection, gadobutrol, 0.1 ml

Gadobutrol is a paramagnetic macrocyclic contrast agent used for magnetic resonance imaging (MRI) procedures. The chemical name for gadobutrol is 10-[(lSR,2RS)-2,3-dihydroxy-l-hydroxymethylpropyl]-l,4,7,10-tetraazacyclododecane-l,4,7-triacetic acid, gadolinium complex. Gadobutrol is used to locate defects in the blood brain barrier (BBB) and abnormalities in the vascular structure of the central nervous system. When the gadobutrol is placed in the MRI machines, it shortens the relaxation time of the spin-lattice or longitudinal (T1) and the spin-spin or transverse (T2) relaxation times. Variations based on the relaxation times and the gadobutrol concentration can be identified during the scan. The recommended dose is 0.1 mL/kg body weight for children 2 years of age or older and adults. It is administered by intravenous injections prior to the MRI imaging.

A9586

A9586 Florbetapir F18, diagnostic, per study dose, up to 10 mCi

Florbetapir F-18 is a diagnostic radiopharmaceutical, used with positron emission tomography (PET) scans of the brain, that binds with Î^{2}-amyloid aggregates. This radiopharmaceutical uses fluorine (F-18) that decays by positron (Î^{2}+) emission and has a half-life of 109.77 minutes. The uptake of Florbetapir F-18 can be used to estimate Î^{2}-amyloid neuritic plaques in adult patients with cognitive impairment. This radiopharmaceutical does not establish a diagnosis of Alzheimer's disease or other cognitive disorders or predict development of dementia or other neurologic conditions.

A9587

A9587 Gallium Ga-68, dotatate, diagnostic, 0.1 mCi

Gallium is a rare metal that is liquid at room temperature. Gallium Ga 68 dotatate is a radioactive version of gallium used with positron emission tomography (PET) for the localization of somatostatin receptor positive neuroendocrine tumors (NET) in adult and pediatric patients. Recommended dose is 2 MBq/kg of body weight (0.054 mCi/kg) up to 200 MBq (5.4 mCi) administered as an intravenous bolus. Gallium Ga 68 dotatate is administered intravenously and peak imaging is often 40 to 90 minutes after injection. The acquisition must include a whole-body acquisition from skull to mid-thigh. It must be produced from germanium-68 and has a half-life of 68 minutes.

A9588

A9588 Fluciclovine F-18, diagnostic, 1 mCi

Fluciclovine F-18 is a synthetic amino acid analog, fluciclovine, radiolabeled with the radioactive fluorine 18 (F 18). It is indicated for positron emission tomography (PET) in men with suspected prostate cancer recurrence based on elevated blood prostate specific antigen (PSA) levels following prior treatment. Fluorine 18 (F 18) is a cyclotron produced radionuclide that decays by positron emission (ÃŸ+ decay) and orbital electron capture to stable oxygen 18. It has a half-life of 109.7 minutes. The recommended dose is 10 mCi administered as an intravenous bolus injection. PET scanning should begin three to five minutes after completion of the injection. It is recommended that image acquisition should start from mid-thigh and proceed to the base of the skull.

A9589

A9589 Instillation, hexaminolevulinate HCl, 100 mg

Hexaminolevulinate is an imaging drug used to identify bladder cancer. The medication is administered into the bladder where it collects in the neoplastic cells. A blue light cystoscope is used to view the areas of fluorescence. The abnormal cells appear bright red and the surrounding normal tissue appears blue. A blue light cystoscopy is performed in addition to the regular white light cystoscopy. The recommended dose is 50 mL administered into the bladder through a urinary catheter. The medication is instilled into the bladder approximately one hour before the start of the procedure.

A9590

A9590 Iodine I-131, iobenguane, 1 mCi

Therapeutic iodine I-131 iobenguane is a radioactive therapeutic agent indicated for the treatment of adult and pediatric patients older than age 12 with iobenguane scan positive, locally advanced, or metastatic pheochromocytoma or paraganglioma that requires systemic anticancer therapy. It has a half-life of eight days and decays by beta and gamma emissions. Iodine I-131 iobenguane is injected intravenously over 15 to 30 seconds. It is supplied in single-dose vials of 555 MBq/mL (15 mCi/mL) and is stored frozen. The product must be thawed in its leaded container for two to three hours prior to use. The recommend dosage is based on body weight. For dosimetric use, a dose of 185 to 222 MBq (5 or 6 mCi) should be administered for patients with a body weight greater than 50 kg. For patients with a body weight of 50 kg or less, the dosage is 3.7 MBq/kg (0.1 mCi/kg). For therapeutic use, a dose of 18,500 MBq (500 mCi) should be administered for patients with a body weight greater that 62.5 kg. For patients with a body weight of 62.5 kg or less, the dosage is 296 MBq/kg (8 mCi/kg). Antiemetics should be administered 30 minutes prior to each dose. The patient's thyroid should be blocked with inorganic iodine a day prior to administration and for 10 additional days following. A dosimetric dose is administered via intravenous injection over 60 seconds. Therapeutic doses are administered via intravenous infusion over 30 minutes at a rate of 100 mL/hour for adult patients, and over 60 minutes at a rate of 50 mL/hour for pediatric patients. Patients should receive two therapeutic doses 90 days apart.

A9591

A9591 Fluoroestradiol F-18, diagnostic, 1 mCi

Fluoroestradiol f 18, a radioactive diagnostic agent, is indicated for use with positron emission tomography (PET) imaging and as an adjunct to breast biopsy to detect estrogen receptor (ER)-positive lesions in patients with recurrent or metastatic breast cancer. The recommended dose is 6 millicurie (mCi) or 222 MBq, administered as an IV injection over one to two minutes. The recommended start time is 80 minutes following drug administration. This code reports 1 mCi.

A9592

A9592 Copper Cu-64, dotatate, diagnostic, 1 mCi

Copper Cu 64 dotatate, a positron emission tomography (PET) diagnostic agent, is indicated for the localization of somatostatin receptor-positive neuroendocrine tumors (NETs) in adult patients. This positron-producing radionuclide is administered as an intravenous (IV) bolus injection and adheres to the cells that express somatostatin receptors, particularly those that overexpress subtype 2 receptors (SSTR2) such as malignant neuroendocrine cells. The recommended dose is 148 MBq (4 mCi); images may be acquired 45 to 90 minutes following administration.

A9593-A9594

A9593 Gallium Ga-68 PSMA-11, diagnostic, (UCSF), 1 mCi

A9594 Gallium Ga-68 PSMA-11, diagnostic, (UCLA), 1 mCi

Gallium is a rare metal that is liquid at room temperature. Gallium Ga-68 PSMA-11 is a radioactive version of gallium used with positron emission tomography (PET) for the localization of prostate-specific membrane antigen (PSMA) positive lesions in adult male patients with prostate cancer who have a suspected recurrence based on serum prostate-specific antigen (PSA) levels, or who have suspected metastasis and are candidates for initial therapy. Recommended dose is 111 to 259 MBq (3 mCi to 7 mCi) administered as an intravenous bolus. The patient should be instructed to drink a sufficient amount of water, before and after administration, for hydration and to reduced radiation exposure. A diuretic may also be administered to potentially decrease the artifact from radiotracer accumulation in the bladder and ureters. Imaging should begin 50 to 100 minutes following administration and the patient should void immediately prior to the start of imaging. Report A9593 for Gallium Ga-68 PSMA-11 developed by the University of California San Francisco (UCSF). Report A9594 for Gallium Ga-68 PSMA-11 developed by the University of California, Los Angeles (UCLA).

A9595

A9595 Piflufolastat F-18, diagnostic, 1 mCi

Piflufolastat f-18 is a radiopharmaceutical diagnostic imaging agent used in the positron emission tomography (PET) imaging of patients with prostate cancer who have suspected metastasis and are candidates for initial definitive treatment or with suspected recurrence based on elevated serum prostate-specific antigen (PSA) level. The drug helps identify sites for histological confirmation (biopsy). The recommended dosage is 333 MBq (9 mCi) via single bolus intravenous (IV) injection. Imaging should be 60 minutes following administration. Patients should be advised to maintain adequate hydration before and after administration.

A9596

A9596 Gallium Ga-68 gozetotide, diagnostic, (Illuccix), 1 mCi

Gallium Ga-68 gozetotide is a diagnostic radiopharmaceutical used with positron emission tomography (PET) scans of prostate-specific membrane antigen (PSMA) positive lesions in adult males, ages 18 years and older, with prostate cancer with suspected metastasis who are candidates for initial definitive therapy or with suspected recurrence based on elevated prostate-specific antigen (PSA) level. It is supplied in two different three-vial kits configurations of cyclotron produce via GE FASTlab™ (configuration A) or IRE Galli EO ® Ge 68/Ga 68 generator (configuration B). The vials included contain gozetotide (Vial 1), acetate buffer (Vial 2), and a sterile vacuumed reaction vial (Vial 3). The recommended dosage is 111 MBq to 259 MBq (3 mCi to 7 mCi) administered via intravenous (IV) infusion. PET imaging should begin 50 to 100 minutes following administration. See full prescribing information for complete preparation, administration, imaging, and radiation dosimetry instructions.

A9597-A9598

A9597 Positron emission tomography radiopharmaceutical, diagnostic, for tumor identification, not otherwise classified

A9598 Positron emission tomography radiopharmaceutical, diagnostic, for nontumor identification, not otherwise classified

These codes represent diagnostic radiopharmaceuticals used in positron emission tomography (PET) that do not have specific HCPCS codes assigned. Report A9597 when the radiopharmaceutical is used for tumor identification. Report A9588 when the radiopharmaceutical is used for purposes other than tumor identification.

A9600

A9600 Strontium Sr-89 chloride, therapeutic, per mCi

Strontium is a metallic earth element that is similar to calcium, soft, and decomposes readily in water. Strontium 89 is a radioactive version of strontium. Strontium 89 has a half-life of 50.5 days and decays by beta emissions. Since strontium behaves like calcium, it is concentrated in the bone and in areas of calcium uptake. Strontium 89 is used as a source in radiation therapy. In the form of strontium 89 chloride, it is injected intravenously or delivered by catheter into a large vein. Strontium 89 chloride is indicated as a palliative treatment for debilitating bone pain in patients whose cancer has metastasized to bone. The bone metastasis should be confirmed prior to use of strontium 89. The recommended dosage is 4 mCi. Repeat treatments may be performed at 90-day intervals.

A9601

A9601 Flortaucipir F 18 injection, diagnostic, 1 mCi

Flortaucipir F 18 is a diagnostic radiopharmaceutical used with positron emission tomography (PET) scans of the brain for estimation of density and distribution of aggregated tau neurofibrillary tangles (NFTs) in adults with cognitive impairment being evaluated for Alzheimer's disease (AD). It should not be used for the evaluation of patients for chronic traumatic encephalopathy. It is supplied in a multiple-dose vial of 300 MBq/ml to 1,900 MBq/ml (8.1 mCi/ml to 51 mCi/ml). The recommended dosage is 370 MBq (10 mCi) administered via intravenous (IV) injection. PET imaging should begin 80 minutes following administration. See full prescribing information for complete preparation, administration, imaging, and radiation dosimetry instructions.

A9602

A9602 Fluorodopa F-18, diagnostic, per mCi

Fluorodopa f 18, a radioactive diagnostic agent, is indicated for use with positron emission tomography (PET) imaging of dopaminergic nerve terminals in the striatum to evaluate adults with suspected Parkinsonian syndromes (PS). The recommended dose is 185 MBq (5 mCi) administered via intravenous (IV) injection over one minute. Imaging should begin approximately 80 minutes following administration. See full prescribing information for complete administration instructions.

A9604

A9604 Samarium Sm-153 lexidronam, therapeutic, per treatment dose, up to 150 mCi

Samarium is a metallic rare earth element found in other rare earth mineral ores. Samarium 153 is a radioactive form of samarium that has a half-life of 46.7 hours and decays by beta and gamma emissions. Lexidronam, also known as ethylene diamine tetramethylene phosphonate or EDTMP, is a chemical complex that concentrates in the bone and in areas of calcium uptake. Samarium 153 lexidronam is indicated as a palliative treatment for debilitating bone pain in patients whose cancer has metastasized to bone. The bone metastasis should be confirmed prior to use of samarium 153. The recommended dosage is 1 mCi per kg of body weight. It is administered intravenously through an indwelling catheter.

A9606

A9606 Radium RA-223 dichloride, therapeutic, per UCI

Radium (RA) 223 dichloride is used for the treatment of castration resistant prostate cancer, symptomatic bone metastases, and unknown visceral metastatic disease. Radium 223 dichloride is an alpha emitting radiotherapeutic drug that mimics calcium and forms a mineral compound at areas of increased bone turnover, such as bone metastases. The recommended dosage is 50 kBq/kg of body weight (1.35 microcuries/kg) administered by slow intravenous (IV) injection over one minute every four weeks for six doses. Available in single use vials containing 6 ml of solution at a concentration of 1,000 kBq/ml (27 microcuries/ml) at the reference date with a total radioactivity of 3,000 kBq/vial (162 microcuries/vial) at the reference date. Six-stage decay is by predominantly alpha emissions with some beta and gamma emissions. The high linear energy transfer of alpha emitters leads to a high frequency of DNA breaks, resulting in cell death. Since alpha particle range is less than 100 micrometers, damage to adjacent tissue is limited.

A9607

A9607 Lutetium Lu 177 vipivotide tetraxetan, therapeutic, 1 mCi

Lutetium Lu 177 vipivotide tetraxetan is a radioligand therapeutic agent intended for the treatment of adult male patients with prostate-specific membrane antigen (PSMA)-positive metastatic castration-resistant prostate cancer (mCRPC) who have also been treated with androgen receptor (AR) pathway inhibition and taxane-based chemotherapy. Patients should be selected for treatment using an approved PSMA-11 imaging agent. It is supplied in single use vials of 1,000 MBq/ml (27 mCi/ml). The recommended dosage is 7.4 GBq (200 mCi) administered via intravenous (IV) infusion every six weeks up to six doses, or until disease progression or unacceptable toxicity. See full prescribing information for complete administration instructions.

A9698

A9698 Nonradioactive contrast imaging material, not otherwise classified, per study

Report this code when a HCPCS code for a contrast imaging material utilized has not been issued by CMS.

A9699

A9699 Radiopharmaceutical, therapeutic, not otherwise classified

This code reports the supply of radiopharmaceutical therapeutic imaging agents that do not have a more specific HCPCS Level II code. Radiopharmaceuticals are radioactive isotopes, such as radioactive iodine or radioactive cobalt. They are often attached to carrier molecules and used in therapeutic nuclear medicine procedures.

A9700

A9700 Supply of injectable contrast material for use in echocardiography, per study

This code reports the supply of injectable contrast material used in echocardiography that does not have a more specific HCPCS Level II code. There are HCPCS Level II codes for perflexane lipid microspheres, octafluoropropane microspheres, and perflutren lipid microspheres.

A9800

A9800 Gallium Ga-68 gozetotide, diagnostic, (Locametz), 1 mCi

Gallium is a rare metal that is liquid at room temperature. Gallium Ga-68 gozetotide is a radioactive version of gallium used with positron emission tomography (PET) for the localization of prostate-specific membrane antigen (PSMA) positive lesions in adult male patients with prostate cancer who have a suspected recurrence based on serum prostate-specific antigen (PSA) levels, or who have suspected metastasis and are candidates for initial therapy, and for selection of patients with metastatic prostate cancer for whom Lutetium Lu 177 vipivotide tetraxetan PSMA-directed therapy is indicated. Recommended dose is 111 to 259 MBq (3 mCi to 7 mCi) administered as a slow intravenous (IV) injection. The patient should be instructed to drink enough water, before and after administration, for hydration and to reduce radiation exposure. A diuretic may also be administered to potentially decrease the artifact from radiotracer accumulation in the bladder and ureters. Imaging should begin 50 to 100 minutes following administration and the patient should void immediately prior to the start of imaging.

A9900

A9900 Miscellaneous DME supply, accessory, and/or service component of another HCPCS code

Durable medical equipment includes any medical equipment used in the home to aid in a better quality of living. This code represents a miscellaneous DME supply, accessory, and/or service component of another HCPCS code.

A9901

A9901 DME delivery, set up, and/or dispensing service component of another HCPCS code

This code represents the delivery, set-up, and dispensing service component of another HCPCS code, such as hospital beds, wheelchairs, catheters, and glucose monitors.

A9999

A9999 Miscellaneous DME supply or accessory, not otherwise specified

This code is a catch all code for supplies, accessories, or services not covered in other DME HCPCS codes.

B

B4034-B4036

B4034 Enteral feeding supply kit; syringe fed, per day, includes but not limited to feeding/flushing syringe, administration set tubing, dressings, tape

B4035 Enteral feeding supply kit; pump fed, per day, includes but not limited to feeding/flushing syringe, administration set tubing, dressings, tape

B4036 Enteral feeding supply kit; gravity fed, per day, includes but not limited to feeding/flushing syringe, administration set tubing, dressings, tape

Patients with chronic illness or trauma cannot be sustained through oral feeding and must rely on enteral or parenteral therapy, depending upon the particular nature of the medical condition. Daily enteral nutrition is necessary for patients with a functioning gastrointestinal (GI) tract but nonfunctioning body structures for allowing food to reach the small bowel, or for patients with small bowel disease that impairs digestion and absorption of nutrients. Enteral nutrition is administered to a patient through a tube into the stomach or small intestine. The solutions may be administered by syringe, gravity, or infusion pump.

B4081-B4088

B4081 Nasogastric tubing with stylet

B4082 Nasogastric tubing without stylet

B4083 Stomach tube - Levine type

B4087 Gastrostomy/jejunostomy tube, standard, any material, any type, each

B4088 Gastrostomy/jejunostomy tube, low-profile, any material, any type, each

Patients with chronic illness or trauma cannot be sustained through oral feeding and must rely on enteral or parenteral therapy, depending upon the particular nature of the medical condition. Enteral nutrition is administered to a patient through a tube (nasogastric, jejunostomy, or gastrostomy) into the stomach or small intestine. There are several types of gastric tubes including Levin type stomach tube, gastric sump, Moss, Sengstaken Blakemore, and Miller-Abbott. Specifically, feeding tubes are generally referred to as G tubes, J tubes, NG tubes, or surgical feeding tubes. Surgical feeding tubes require intraoperative placement.

B4100

B4100 Food thickener, administered orally, per oz

Patients who have facial paralysis, due to a stroke, Parkinson's disease, multiple sclerosis, and other conditions, have difficulty swallowing liquids (dysphagia) and often benefit from the use of a food thickener. Thickened food has a pureed consistency necessary to help prevent choking. Commercial instant food thickener has no taste or aftertaste. It mixes with hot or cold foods and liquids and thickens in just 30 seconds. These products allow for normal hydration by releasing available fluid after consumption. The thickened food and liquid do not harden when chilled or cause constipation. Report this code per ounce of food thickener.

B4102-B4104

B4102 Enteral formula, for adults, used to replace fluids and electrolytes (e.g., clear liquids), 500 ml = 1 unit

B4103 Enteral formula, for pediatrics, used to replace fluids and electrolytes (e.g., clear liquids), 500 ml = 1 unit

B4104 Additive for enteral formula (e.g., fiber)

For patients who cannot be sustained through oral feedings, enteral nutrition is administered by means of a nasogastric, jejunostomy, or gastrostomy feeding tube directly into the stomach or small intestine. An enteral formula additive, such as fiber, is used to maintain normal bowel function and avoid constipation.

B4105

B4105 In-line cartridge containing digestive enzyme(s) for enteral feeding, each

For patients who cannot be sustained through oral feedings, enteral nutrition is administered by means of a nasogastric, jejunostomy, or gastrostomy feeding tube directly into the stomach or small intestine. For patients who also have fat malabsorption (inability to hydrolyze fats), a single use cartridge containing a digestive enzyme (iLipase or immobilized lipase) may be added to the enteral nutrition line. The iLipase mimics the function of the lipase that is normally secreted by the pancreas. When enteral formula flows through the in-line cartridge, the lipase binds to the fats in the formula, allowing for the fats to be digested and absorbed by the patient. Up to two cartridges can be used within a 24-hour period. The in-line cartridge should only be connected to enteral feeding pump tubing sets or enteral feeding sets, and should not be connected to an intravenous (IV) set up. Medications should not be administered through the cartridge or added to the enteral feed line between the enteral pump and the cartridge. The cartridge should be discarded once the feeding is complete and should not be stored or reused.

B4149

B4149 Enteral formula, manufactured blenderized natural foods with intact nutrients, includes proteins, fats, carbohydrates, vitamins and minerals, may include fiber, administered through an enteral feeding tube, 100 calories = 1 unit

For patients who cannot be sustained through oral feedings, enteral nutrition is administered by means of a nasogastric, jejunostomy, or gastrostomy feeding tube directly into the stomach or small intestine. Enteral formulas are composed of varying combinations of natural or semi-synthetic proteins, amino acids, fats, carbohydrates, vitamins, and minerals to fulfill different nutritional needs. A blenderized natural foods formula of intact nutrients includes proteins, fats, carbohydrates, vitamins and minerals, and possibly fiber per 100 cal unit. Intact nutrients are not already broken down and remain in a high molecular weight form, which require normal digestive and absorptive ability.

B4150-B4152

B4150 Enteral formula, nutritionally complete with intact nutrients, includes proteins, fats, carbohydrates, vitamins and minerals, may include fiber, administered through an enteral feeding tube, 100 calories = 1 unit

B4152 Enteral formula, nutritionally complete, calorically dense (equal to or greater than 1.5 kcal/ml) with intact nutrients, includes proteins, fats, carbohydrates, vitamins and minerals, may include fiber, administered through an enteral feeding tube, 100 calories = 1 unit

These codes report a nutritionally complete enteral formula or nutrient mixture administered to patients who cannot be sustained through oral feedings, given by means of a nasogastric, jejunostomy, or gastrostomy feeding tube directly into the stomach or small intestine. Tube feedings can be administered by bolus feedings, continuous drip feedings, or a combination of the two. Intact nutrients are not already broken down and remain in a high molecular weight form, which require normal digestive and absorptive ability.

B4153

B4153 Enteral formula, nutritionally complete, hydrolyzed proteins (amino acids and peptide chain), includes fats, carbohydrates, vitamins and minerals, may include fiber, administered through an enteral feeding tube, 100 calories = 1 unit

This code reports a nutritionally complete enteral formula or nutrient mixture administered to patients who cannot be sustained through oral feedings, given by means of a nasogastric, jejunostomy, or gastrostomy feeding tube directly into the stomach or small intestine. Tube feedings can be administered by bolus feedings, continuous drip feedings, or a combination of the two. This code reports a formula of hydrolyzed proteins of amino acids and peptide chain, including fats, carbohydrates, vitamins and minerals, and possibly fiber, per 100 cal unit. Hydrolyzed proteins have been split down into their smaller building-block forms of amino acids and peptide chains by enzymes, acids, or alkalis. They provide the same nutritive equivalent in a more easily digestible form.

B4154-B4155

B4154 Enteral formula, nutritionally complete, for special metabolic needs, excludes inherited disease of metabolism, includes altered composition of proteins, fats, carbohydrates, vitamins and/or minerals, may include fiber, administered through an enteral feeding tube, 100 calories = 1 unit

B4155 Enteral formula, nutritionally incomplete/modular nutrients, includes specific nutrients, carbohydrates (e.g., glucose polymers), proteins/amino acids (e.g., glutamine, arginine), fat (e.g., medium chain triglycerides) or combination, administered through an enteral feeding tube, 100 calories = 1 unit

A nutritionally complete enteral formula or nutrient mixture is administered to patients who cannot be sustained through oral feedings, given by means of a nasogastric, jejunostomy, or gastrostomy feeding tube directly into the stomach or small intestine. Tube feedings can be administered by bolus feedings, continuous drip feedings, or a combination of the two. These codes report a formula designed for special metabolic needs that are not a consequence of an inherited metabolism disorder. The formula may contain proteins, fats, and carbohydrates in altered composition, and possible fiber, per 100 cal unit. Nutritionally incomplete enteral formula of modular nutrients contains specific nutrient forms of carbohydrates, fats, or proteins to cover deficiency needs, such as glucose polymers, glutamine, arginine, and medium chain triglycerides.

B4157

B4157 Enteral formula, nutritionally complete, for special metabolic needs for inherited disease of metabolism, includes proteins, fats, carbohydrates, vitamins and minerals, may include fiber, administered through an enteral feeding tube, 100 calories = 1 unit

For patients who cannot be sustained through oral feedings, enteral nutrition is administered by means of a nasogastric, jejunostomy, or gastrostomy feeding tube directly into the stomach or small intestine. Enteral formulas are composed of varying combinations of natural or semisynthetic proteins, amino acids, fats, carbohydrates, vitamins, and minerals to fulfill different nutritional needs. This nutritionally complete formula is designed for the special metabolic needs of inherited metabolism disorders, per 100 cal unit.

B4158-B4159

B4158 Enteral formula, for pediatrics, nutritionally complete with intact nutrients, includes proteins, fats, carbohydrates, vitamins and minerals, may include fiber and/or iron, administered through an enteral feeding tube, 100 calories = 1 unit

B4159 Enteral formula, for pediatrics, nutritionally complete soy based with intact nutrients, includes proteins, fats, carbohydrates, vitamins and minerals, may include fiber and/or iron, administered through an enteral feeding tube, 100 calories = 1 unit

These codes report a pediatric enteral formula or nutrient mixture administered to patients who cannot be sustained through oral feedings, given by means of a nasogastric, jejunostomy, or gastrostomy feeding tube directly into the stomach or small intestine. Tube feedings can be administered by bolus feedings, continuous drip feedings, or a combination of the two in patients who require calorie and protein support. Intact nutrients are not already broken down and remain in a high molecular weight form, which require normal digestive and absorptive ability. The soy-based, pediatric enteral formula is used to avoid milk-protein sensitivity.

B4160

B4160 Enteral formula, for pediatrics, nutritionally complete calorically dense (equal to or greater than 0.7 kcal/ml) with intact nutrients, includes proteins, fats, carbohydrates, vitamins and minerals, may include fiber, administered through an enteral feeding tube, 100 calories = 1 unit

This code reports a pediatric enteral formula or nutrient mixture administered to patients who cannot be sustained through oral feedings, given by means of a nasogastric, jejunostomy, or gastrostomy feeding tube directly into the stomach or small intestine. Tube feedings can be administered by bolus feedings, continuous drip feedings, or a combination of the two in patients who require calorie and protein support. This code reports a calorically dense, nutritionally complete formula, with intact nutrients, greater than .7kcal/ml, and possibly including fiber, per 100 cal unit. Intact nutrients are not already broken down and remain in a high molecular weight form, which require normal digestive and absorptive ability.

B4161

B4161 Enteral formula, for pediatrics, hydrolyzed/amino acids and peptide chain proteins, includes fats, carbohydrates, vitamins and minerals, may include fiber, administered through an enteral feeding tube, 100 calories = 1 unit

This code reports a pediatric enteral formula or nutrient mixture administered to patients who cannot be sustained through oral feedings, given by means of a nasogastric, jejunostomy, or gastrostomy feeding tube directly into the stomach or small intestine. Tube feedings can be administered by bolus feedings, continuous drip feedings, or a combination of the two in patients who require calorie and protein support. This code reports a formula of hydrolyzed/amino acids and peptide chain proteins, including fats, carbohydrates, vitamins and minerals, and possibly fiber, per 100 cal unit. Hydrolyzed proteins have been split down into their smaller building-block forms of amino acids and peptide chains by enzymes, acids, or alkalis. They provide the same nutritive equivalent in a more easily digestible form.

B4162

B4162 Enteral formula, for pediatrics, special metabolic needs for inherited disease of metabolism, includes proteins, fats, carbohydrates, vitamins and minerals, may include fiber, administered through an enteral feeding tube, 100 calories = 1 unit

This code reports a pediatric enteral formula, or nutrient mixture administered to patients who cannot be sustained through oral feedings, given by means of a nasogastric, jejunostomy, or gastrostomy feeding tube directly into the stomach or small intestine. Tube feedings can be administered by bolus feedings, continuous drip feedings, or a combination of the two in patients who require calorie and protein support. This code reports a nutritionally complete pediatric formula designed for the special metabolic needs of inherited metabolism disorders, per 100 cal unit.

B4164-B4185

B4164 Parenteral nutrition solution: carbohydrates (dextrose), 50% or less (500 ml = 1 unit), home mix

B4168 Parenteral nutrition solution; amino acid, 3.5%, (500 ml = 1 unit) - home mix

B4172 Parenteral nutrition solution; amino acid, 5.5% through 7%, (500 ml = 1 unit) - home mix

B4176 Parenteral nutrition solution; amino acid, 7% through 8.5%, (500 ml = 1 unit) - home mix

B4178 Parenteral nutrition solution: amino acid, greater than 8.5% (500 ml = 1 unit) - home mix

B4180 Parenteral nutrition solution: carbohydrates (dextrose), greater than 50% (500 ml = 1 unit), home mix

B4185 Parenteral nutrition solution, not otherwise specified, 10 g lipids

Parenteral nutrition is administered to the patient intravenously. Since the alimentary tract of a patient with severe pathology does not function adequately for ingesting food normally, an indwelling catheter is placed percutaneously in the subclavian vein and advanced into the superior vena cava for infusing nutrients intravenously. Parenteral nutrition solutions are based on the composition of ingredients or nutrient source in each product, and whether it is supplied in a home mix or a premix. These codes report home mix solutions of 1 unit equaling 500 ml. Report B4185 when the parenteral solution is not otherwise specified by other HCPCS codes.

B4187

B4187 Omegaven, 10 g lipids

Omegaven is a fish oil triglyceride injectable emulsion indicated as a source of calories and fatty acids in pediatric patients with parenteral nutrition-associated cholestasis (PNAC). PNAC, defined as direct bilirubin greater than 2.0 mg/dL that is persistent for at least two consecutive tests during the administration of parenteral nutrition and not associated with other known causes of cholestasis, is a common complication of prolonged use of PN in very low birth weight infants. Administered via infusion into a central or peripheral vein, the recommended daily dose (and the maximum dose) in pediatric patients is 1 g/kg/day. The recommended duration of infusion is between eight and 24 hours, depending on the clinical situation.

B4189-B4216

B4189 Parenteral nutrition solution: compounded amino acid and carbohydrates with electrolytes, trace elements, and vitamins, including preparation, any strength, 10 to 51 g of protein, premix

B4193 Parenteral nutrition solution: compounded amino acid and carbohydrates with electrolytes, trace elements, and vitamins, including preparation, any strength, 52 to 73 g of protein, premix

B4197 Parenteral nutrition solution; compounded amino acid and carbohydrates with electrolytes, trace elements and vitamins, including preparation, any strength, 74 to 100 g of protein - premix

B4199 Parenteral nutrition solution; compounded amino acid and carbohydrates with electrolytes, trace elements and vitamins, including preparation, any strength, over 100 g of protein - premix

B4216 Parenteral nutrition; additives (vitamins, trace elements, Heparin, electrolytes), home mix, per day

Parenteral nutrition is administered to the patient intravenously. Since the alimentary tract of a patient with severe pathology does not function adequately for ingesting food normally, an indwelling catheter is placed percutaneously in the subclavian vein, and then advanced into the superior vena cava for infusing nutrients intravenously. Parenteral nutrition solutions are based on the composition of ingredients or nutrient source in each parenteral nutrient product, and whether it is supplied in a home mix or a premix. These codes report premix solutions, including preparation of any strength compounded amino acids and carbohydrates with electrolytes, trace elements, and vitamins.

B4220-B4224

B4220 Parenteral nutrition supply kit; premix, per day

B4222 Parenteral nutrition supply kit; home mix, per day

B4224 Parenteral nutrition administration kit, per day

Patients with chronic illness or trauma cannot be sustained through oral feeding and must rely on enteral or parenteral therapy, depending upon the particular nature of the medical condition. Parenteral nutrition is administered to the patient intravenously. These codes report the supply and administration kits for parenteral nutrition on a daily basis.

B5000-B5200

B5000 Parenteral nutrition solution: compounded amino acid and carbohydrates with electrolytes, trace elements, and vitamins, including preparation, any strength, renal - Amirosyn RF, NephrAmine, RenAmine - premix

B5100 Parenteral nutrition solution compounded amino acid and carbohydrates with electrolytes, trace elements, and vitamins, including preparation, any strength, hepatic-HepatAmine-premix

B5200 Parenteral nutrition solution compounded amino acid and carbohydrates with electrolytes, trace elements, and vitamins, including preparation, any strength, stress-branch chain amino acids-FreAmine-HBC-premix

Parenteral nutrition is administered to the patient intravenously. Since the alimentary tract of a patient with severe pathology does not function adequately for ingesting food normally, an indwelling catheter is placed percutaneously in the subclavian vein, and then advanced into the superior vena cava for infusing nutrients intravenously. Parenteral nutrition solutions are based on the composition of ingredients or nutrient source in each parenteral nutrient product and whether it is supplied in a home mix or a premix. These codes report premix solutions, including preparation of any strength compounded amino acids and carbohydrates with electrolytes, trace elements, and vitamins.

B9002

B9002 Enteral nutrition infusion pump, any type

Infusion pumps are available when enteral nutrition patients experience complications associated with syringe or gravity feedings. An enteral pump is ordered when feeding problems arise such as reflux and/or aspiration, severe diarrhea, dumping syndrome, an administration rate less than 100 ml/hr, blood glucose fluctuations, or circulatory overload.

B9004-B9006

B9004 Parenteral nutrition infusion pump, portable

B9006 Parenteral nutrition infusion pump, stationary

Permanent conditions of the alimentary tract cause the patient to be unable to maintain weight and strength through normal feeding and require parenteral therapy, the intravenous infusion of nutrients, with the use of a parenteral nutrition infusion pump. Report B9004 for a portable pump. Report B9006 for a stationary pump.

B9998-B9999

B9998 NOC for enteral supplies

B9999 NOC for parenteral supplies

Permanent conditions of the alimentary tract cause the patient to be unable to maintain weight and strength through normal feeding and require enteral therapy (nutrition administered through a feeding tube) or parenteral therapy (the intravenous infusion of nutrients with the use of a parenteral nutrition infusion pump). Report B9998 for enteral supplies, or B9999 for parenteral supplies, not captured with another valid code. These codes require a concise description of the supplies provided in Item 19 on the CMS-150 claim form or electronic equivalent. Supporting documentation may be required.

C

C1052

C1052 Hemostatic agent, gastrointestinal, topical

Gastrointestinal (GI) bleeding can occur in the upper GI tract (esophagus, stomach, or small intestine) or the lower GI tract (colon and rectum) as a result of artery or venous malformations, cancer, diverticulosis, gastric ulcers, or inflammatory bowel disease. An aerosolized spray, applied during an endoscopic procedure, delivers a mineral blend to the bleeding site in the upper and/or lower gastrointestinal tract that is intended to produce hemostasis to nonvariceal GI bleeds by absorbing fluids. Using an endoscope to access the gastrointestinal tract, a proprietary delivery system is passed through the accessory channel of the endoscope. Without contacting the GI tract wall, the delivery system is positioned just above the bleeding site. A bentonite powder is propelled through a polyethylene application catheter by releasing C02 from a cartridge located in the device handle and sprayed directly onto the bleeding site.

C1062

C1062 Intravertebral body fracture augmentation with implant (e.g., metal, polymer)

Osteoporosis, a condition that causes bones to gradually thin and weaken, often results in osteoporotic vertebral compression fractures (VCF). These fractures occur when the vertebral body in the spine collapses, leading to spinal deformity, loss of height, and exquisite pain. Although osteoporosis is the most common cause, compression fractures may also be caused by metastatic tumors or trauma. One proprietary fracture reduction system utilizes intravertebral body implants made of titanium. Under x-ray guidance, a slender, hollow needle is inserted through the skin and back muscles to the spine. Two implants are deployed, one in either side of the fractured vertebral body, and then expanded to restore it to its normal height. Once the desired position is achieved, the implants are locked and bone cement is injected to stabilize the restored vertebra. This treatment is appropriate for patients diagnosed with a VCF within the past four to six months.

C1713

C1713 Anchor/screw for opposing bone-to-bone or soft tissue-to-bone (implantable)

An implantable pin and/or screw is used to oppose soft tissue-to-bone, tendon-to-bone, or bone-to-bone. A screw opposes the tissue by means of drilling as follows: soft tissue-to-bone, tendon-to-bone, or bone-to-bone fixation. Pins are inserted or drilled into the bone with the intent to facilitate stabilization or oppose bone-to-bone. In many instances this may include orthopedic plates with accompanying washers and nuts.

C1714

C1714 Catheter, transluminal atherectomy, directional

This code represents a special type of catheter used in transluminal atherectomy procedures. Transluminal atherectomy procedures involve opening the patients blocked arteries or vein grafts by using specialized devices attached to the end of catheters, which assist in the removal of thrombi and plaque material. Rotational atherectomy involves a high speed rotational device that grinds up the plaque material being removed from the vessel. Directional atherectomy scrapes or directs the plaque into an opening on one side of the catheter. Transluminal extraction atherectomy uses a device that cuts plaque off vessel walls and then vacuums it into a bottle.

C1715

C1715 Brachytherapy needle

This code pertains to needles specifically used in brachytherapy and is utilized per needle not per procedure.

C1716-C1719

C1716 Brachytherapy source, nonstranded, gold-198, per source

C1717 Brachytherapy source, nonstranded, high dose rate iridium-192, per source

C1719 Brachytherapy source, nonstranded, nonhigh dose rate iridium-192, per source

Brachytherapy is a form of radiotherapy in which physicians place the source of irradiation close to the tumor or within a body cavity. Brachytherapy could include placing radioactive sources inside a body cavity (intracavitary brachytherapy) or putting radioactive material directly into body tissue using hollow needles (interstitial brachytherapy). Brachytherapy may be given in addition to external beam radiation, or it may be used as the only form of radiotherapy. In some cases, the radioactive sources may be permanently left in place; in other cases, they are removed after a specified time. Placement of radioactive sources may be repeated several times.

The isotope gold has a half-life of 2.7 days and is used in some cancer treatments and treatments for other diseases. There are two natural isotopes of iridium, and many radioisotopes, the most stable radioisotope being Ir-192 with a half-life of 73.83 days. Ir-192 beta decays into platinum-192, while most of the other radioisotopes decay into osmium.

C1721-C1722

C1721 Cardioverter-defibrillator, dual chamber (implantable)

C1722 Cardioverter-defibrillator, single chamber (implantable)

Implantable cardioverter defibrillators are used in patients at risk for recurrent, sustained ventricular tachycardia or fibrillation. The defibrillators are connected to leads that are positioned inside the heart or on the heart surface. These leads deliver electrical shocks, sense the heart's rhythm, and pace the heart as necessary. Various leads are tunneled to the pulse generator, which has been implanted in a pouch made in the skin of the abdomen or chest. When the defibrillator detects ventricular tachycardia or fibrillation, it will automatically shock the heart to restore normal rhythm.

C1724

C1724 Catheter, transluminal atherectomy, rotational

This code represents a special type of catheter used in transluminal atherectomy procedures. Transluminal atherectomy procedures involve opening the patient's blocked arteries or vein grafts by using specialized devices attached to the end of catheters, which assist in the removal of thrombi and plaque material. Rotational atherectomy involves a high speed rotational device that grinds up the plaque material being removed from the vessel. Directional atherectomy scrapes or directs the plaque into an opening on one side of the catheter. Transluminal extraction atherectomy uses a device that cuts plaque off vessel walls and then vacuums it into a bottle.

C1725

C1725 Catheter, transluminal angioplasty, nonlaser (may include guidance, infusion/perfusion capability)

A transluminal angioplasty nonlaser catheter is a small hollow tube that is inserted into the central space (or lumen) of an artery or vein .This code refers to a catheter that is not used with a laser, but is used with balloon or other device that is designed to be advanced through the blood vessels to the area of occlusion or blockage. When the catheter is in position, the device is used to compress, break up, or remove the obstruction.

C1726

C1726 Catheter, balloon dilatation, nonvascular

A nonvascular balloon dilatation catheter is a small hollow tube containing a deflated balloon that is inserted into body cavity, duct or other passageway. The catheter is advanced to the area of occlusion or blockage. When the catheter is in position, the balloon is inflated and used to dilate strictures or stenoses. Examples of common sites are the common bile duct, intestines, or ureter.

C1727

C1727 Catheter, balloon tissue dissector, nonvascular (insertable)

A balloon tissue dissector, nonvascular catheter is small hollow tube that contains a deflated balloon. The catheter is guided to the appropriate space; the balloon is inflated and sometimes elongated. It is used to create a space between soft tissues to improve operative vision and work space.

C1728

C1728 Catheter, brachytherapy seed administration

A brachytherapy seed administration catheter used to temporarily place encapsulated radioactive materials (seeds or sources) in or near the targeted tissue or tumor, or into a body cavity.

C1729

C1729 Catheter, drainage

A drainage catheter is a small hollow tube that is used to drain collected fluids from internal structures out through the skin and subcutaneous tissue. This category does not include Foley catheters or suprapubic catheters.

C1730-C1732

C1730 Catheter, electrophysiology, diagnostic, other than 3D mapping (19 or fewer electrodes)

C1731 Catheter, electrophysiology, diagnostic, other than 3D mapping (20 or more electrodes)

C1732 Catheter, electrophysiology, diagnostic/ablation, 3D or vector mapping

These codes describe catheters that assist in providing anatomic and physiologic information about the heart's electrical activity. Electrophysiology catheters are categorized into two main groups: (1) catheters used for mapping, pacing, and/or recording only, and (2) ablation (therapeutic) catheters that also have diagnostic capability. The electrophysiology ablation catheters are distinct from non-cardiac ablation catheters.

C1733

C1733 Catheter, electrophysiology, diagnostic/ablation, other than 3D or vector mapping, other than cool-tip

An electrophysiology, diagnostic/ablation catheter, other than 3D or vector mapping, other than cool-tip, is a small hollow tube that assists in providing anatomic and physiologic information about the cardiac electrical conduction system. Electrophysiology catheters are categorized into two main groups: 1) diagnostic catheters that are used for mapping, pacing, and/or recording only, and 2) ablation (therapeutic) catheters that also have diagnostic capability. The electrophysiology ablation catheters are distinct from noncardiac ablation catheters. Electrophysiology catheters designated as "cool-tip" refer to catheters with tips cooled by infused and/or circulating saline. Catheters designated as "other than cool-tip" refer to the thermistor tip catheter with temperature probe that measures temperature at the tissue catheter interface.

C1734

C1734 Orthopedic/device/drug matrix for opposing bone-to-bone or soft tissue-to bone (implantable)

An implantable orthopedic/device/drug matrix is used to oppose soft tissue-to-bone, tendon-to-bone, or bone-to-bone. A screw opposes the tissue by means of drilling as follows: soft tissue-to-bone, tendon-to-bone, or bone-to-bone fixation. Pins are inserted or drilled into the bone with the intent to facilitate stabilization or oppose bone-to-bone. In many instances, this may include orthopedic plates with accompanying washers and nuts.

C1747

C1747 Endoscope, single-use (i.e., disposable), urinary tract, imaging/illumination device (insertable)

An endoscope is a device consisting of a tube and optical system for viewing the inside of a hollow organ or cavity. This code reports a single-use, disposable endoscope indicated for urinary tract procedures that contains a camera and light source.

C1748

C1748 Endoscope, single-use (i.e. disposable), upper GI, imaging/illumination device (insertable)

This code reports a single-use, disposable endoscope for upper gastrointestinal (GI) procedures. An endoscope is a device consisting of a tube and optical system for viewing the inside of a hollow organ or cavity.

C1749

C1749 Endoscope, retrograde imaging/illumination colonoscope device (implantable)

A retrograde imaging/illumination colonoscope device is a J-shaped catheter that can be inserted into endoscope working channels. The rear-facing catheter contains an imaging device that provides illumination and a continuous retrograde view of the colon. It allows the physician to look behind the folds to find lesions. The device is intended for single patient use and is disposable.

C1750

C1750 Catheter, hemodialysis/peritoneal, long-term

This code describes a catheter that can be permanently placed with one or two cuffs. This catheter is surgically placed into the peritoneum in the abdomen via a small incision and works by permitting the exchange of fluid through the catheter, allowing dialysate in and out of the abdominal cavity.

C1751

C1751 Catheter, infusion, inserted peripherally, centrally or midline (other than hemodialysis)

An infusion catheter is a plastic catheter that may have multiple lumens that is inserted into a large vein and ends up in the subclavian, brachiocephalic, or iliac veins, the superior or inferior vena cava, or the right atrium. It can be inserted centrally into the jugular, subclavian, femoral vein or inferior vena cava or peripherally into the basilic or cephalic vein. It can be used to administer medication, hydration, nutrition, and for monitoring and withdrawing blood samples. There are two different types of catheters: tunneled and non-tunneled.

C1752

C1752 Catheter, hemodialysis/peritoneal, short-term

This code describes a catheter that can be temporary placed with one or two cuffs. This catheter is surgically placed into the peritoneum in the abdomen via a small incision and works by permitting the exchange of fluid through the catheter, allowing dialysate in and out of the abdominal cavity.

C1753

C1753 Catheter, intravascular ultrasound

This code describes a specially designed catheter with a very small ultrasound probe attached to the distal end of the catheter. The proximal end of the catheter is attached to computerized ultrasound equipment. It allows the application of ultrasound technology to see from inside blood vessels out through the surrounding blood column, allowing the visualization of the inner wall of blood vessels.

C1754

C1754 Catheter, intradiscal

An intradiscal catheter is a small hollow tube that is inserted into a vertebral disc through which therapeutic treatments are performed. The flexible catheter is threaded percutaneously using fluoroscopic guidance. The catheter may be used to deliver electrothermal therapy.

C1755

C1755 Catheter, intraspinal

An intraspinal catheter is small hollow tube that is inserted into the spinal column to deliver diagnostic or therapeutic substances within the central nervous system.

C1756

C1756 Catheter, pacing, transesophageal

A transesophageal pacing catheter is a small hollow tube that is inserted into the esophagus and positioned near the posterior aspect of the atria. The catheter contains an electrode that delivers electrical stimulation to the heart and usually includes a device to record an electrocardiogram. The catheter may be used for therapeutic purposes, such as converting an arrhythmia during an intraoperative procedure, or for diagnostic purposes, such as in evaluations of sinus node function.

C1757

C1757 Catheter, thrombectomy/embolectomy

A thrombectomy or embolectomy catheter is a small hollow tube that is inserted into a blood vessel and guided to the site of the embolism or thrombus. A device that breaks up or macerates the thrombus or embolus may be inserted through the catheter. Usually, the catheter is used to aspirate the thrombus or embolus.

C1758

C1758 Catheter, ureteral

Ureteral catheter is a small hollow tube that is inserted into the ureter to withdraw or introduce fluid. The catheter may be inserted either through the urethra and bladder or posteriorly via the kidney.

C1759

C1759 Catheter, intracardiac echocardiography

An intracardiac echocardiography (ICE) catheter is a small tube inserted into a blood vessel that contains an ultrasound device. It is maneuvered into the heart to provide anatomic and physiologic real time imaging within the heart walls. A Doppler device provides imaging of blood flow and velocity and of myocardial wall motion.

C1760

C1760 Closure device, vascular (implantable/insertable)

A vascular closure device seals femoral artery punctures caused by invasive or interventional procedures. The closure or seal is achieved by placing the vessel ends between the device's two primary structures, which are usually an anchor and a biologic substance (e.g., collagen) or suture through the tissue tract.

C1761

C1761 Catheter, transluminal intravascular lithotripsy, coronary

This code represents a special type of catheter used in transluminal intravascular lithotripsy (IVL). IVL delivers unfocused, circumferential, pulsatile mechanical energy to safely disrupt calcium deposits within the target lesion. The IVL catheter is guided to the target lesion and an integrated balloon is inflated to four atmospheres. Once the catheter is in place, an electrical discharge vaporizes fluid inside the balloon. This action creates a rapidly expanding and collapsing bubble, generating sonic pressure waves. The sonic pressure waves travel through soft vascular tissue, cracking the intimal and medial calcium within the vessel wall. The balloon may be used to dilate the target lesion at a low pressure to maximize luminal gain. Angioplasty is included, when performed.

C1762

C1762 Connective tissue, human (includes fascia lata)

Human connective tissue (includes fascia lata) is natural human cellular collagen or extracellular matrix obtained from autologous rectus fascia, decellularized cadaver fascia lata, or decellularized dermal tissue. The tissue is intended to repair or support damaged or inadequate soft tissue. They are used to treat urinary incontinence resulting from hypermobility or Intrinsic Sphincter Deficiency (ISD), pelvic floor repair, or for implantation to reinforce soft tissues where weakness exists in the urological anatomy. The category excludes those items that are used to replace skin.

C1763

C1763 Connective tissue, nonhuman (includes synthetic)

Nonhuman connective tissue (includes synthetic) is a natural collagen matrix typically obtained from porcine or bovine small intestinal submucosa, or pericardium. The material is acellular as all cells are removed leaving only a matrix or scaffold. This tissue is intended to promote the growth of the patient's cells within the implanted matrix. It is intended to repair or support damaged or inadequate soft tissue. Nonhuman connective tissue is used to treat urinary incontinence resulting from hypermobility or intrinsic sphincter deficiency (ISD), pelvic floor repair, or for implantation to reinforce soft tissues where weakness exists in the urological or musculoskeletal anatomy. This category excludes those items that are used to replace skin.

C1764

C1764 Event recorder, cardiac (implantable)

Event recorders are implanted in the left front of the chest in a pocket created in the skin. Once implanted, the patient's cardiac events are recorded. Implantable cardiac event monitors are for long-time use, enabling the recorder to capture more infrequent heart rhythms. The device can have auto activation or manual activation depending upon the needs of the patient. If the patient experiences syncopal episodes, the manual activation button can be pressed only after the patient is conscious again. If the device has auto activation, the device records rhythms automatically when the heart rate is in excess or under a preset limit.

C1765

C1765 Adhesion barrier

An adhesion barrier is a bioresorbable substance used on and around neural structures, minimizing the formation of scar tissue. It is mainly used in spinal surgeries, such as laminectomies and discectomies.

C1766

C1766 Introducer/sheath, guiding, intracardiac electrophysiological, steerable, other than peel-away

An intracardiac electrophysiological introducer or sheath, guiding, steerable, other than peel-away, is a small hollow tube that is inserted into the heart and guided to the target area. Electrophysiological devices and catheters are then passed through the introducer to the target area.

C1767

C1767 Generator, neurostimulator (implantable), nonrechargeable

An implantable nonrechargeable neurostimulator generator is a device that creates small electrical impulses that are transmitted to electrodes implanted near the spinal cord or a peripheral nerve. The small electrical impulses interrupt pain signals sent to the brain. This type of generator contains a battery that cannot be recharged, but must be removed and replaced.

C1768

C1768 Graft, vascular

A vascular graft uses material to patch a damaged, diseased, or injured area of an artery or for replacement of whole segments of vessels. Vascular grafts may be biological or synthetic. Biological grafts are generally taken from another site in the patient, also known as autografts. In a common autograft, the internal mammary artery is generally used in coronary artery bypass surgery. Other biological grafts can come from another member of the same species, such as the use of cadaver grafts. Synthetic grafts are usually made from Dacron or polytetrafluoroethylene (PTFE).

C1769

C1769 Guide wire

A guidewire is a thin piece of material that is guided into a desired blood vessel through a trocar. The trocar is then removed and the guidewire left in place. Catheters, cannulas, or other tubular devices can be inserted over the guidewire into the blood vessel and the guidewire is withdrawn.

C1770

C1770 Imaging coil, magnetic resonance (insertable)

An insertable magnetic resonance imaging coil is an intracavity probe that is placed in a relatively inaccessible or dense body area. The coil emits a magnetic signature that enhances images taken during the MRI.

C1771

C1771 Repair device, urinary, incontinence, with sling graft

A urinary incontinence repair device is used to attach or insert body tissue, synthetic material, or mesh for the purpose of strengthening the pelvic floor. The repair material is fashioned into a sling or hammock that supports the urethra. This code represents the device components used to deliver the sling graft and/or fixate (via permanent sutures or bone anchors) the sling graft. This code includes the sling graft.

C1772

C1772 Infusion pump, programmable (implantable)

An implantable programmable infusion pump is an electrical device that delivers drugs, nutrients, or fluids into the patient's body. It is surgically placed in a subcutaneous pocket with a catheter that is threaded into a desired position. This code represents a device that has a programmer that can be set to deliver the fluid continuously or at set intervals.

C1773

C1773 Retrieval device, insertable (used to retrieve fractured medical devices)

An insertable retrieval device is used to retrieve fractured medical devices that are lodged within the vascular system. This device can also be used to exchange intravascular introducers or sheaths.

C1776

C1776 Joint device (implantable)

A joint device is an artificial prosthetic device that is implanted in a patient as a replacement for a natural joint, such as a finger or toe. Generally a joint device is not used to oppose soft tissue-to-bone, tendon-to-bone, or bone-to-bone.

C1777

C1777 Lead, cardioverter-defibrillator, endocardial single coil (implantable)

An endocardial single coil cardioverter-defibrillator lead is an implanted wire with an electrode at its tip that connects a generator to the heart muscle. An electrode detects electrical changes in the heart which are recorded by the generator and transmits electrical charges created by the generator to the heart to correct and maintain a steady heart rhythm. A cardioverter-defibrillator is a device designed to detect ventricular tachycardia or fibrillation and to deliver an electrical shock to return the heart to normal rhythm. This is a lead that attaches to the heart wall of the heart muscle with the other end connected to a cardioverter-defibrillator.

C1778

C1778 Lead, neurostimulator (implantable)

An implantable neurostimulator lead is a wire with an electrode at its tip that connects a generator to the brain or nervous system. An electrode transmits electrical charges created by the neurostimulator. The electrical signal interrupts the brain function or nerve conduction. Neurostimulators can be used to reduce or eliminate pain, activate nerve responses, or control electrical brain discharges.

C1779

C1779 Lead, pacemaker, transvenous VDD single pass

A pacemaker is a device used to synchronize the beating of the heart. Single-pass VDD is a physiological stimulation mode that requires a single lead with a floating dipole to detect the atrial signal. A transvenous pacemaker lead senses and paces the ventricle and the atrium. The VDD pacemaker is used for AV nodal dysfunction with intact and appropriate sinus node behavior.

C1780

C1780 Lens, intraocular (new technology)

This code describes an artificial lens made of plastic, silicone, or acrylic that performs the function of the eye's natural lens, typically a quarter of an inch in diameter. The lens is usually soft enough that it can be folded and placed into the eye through a small incision. This code specifically refers to the intraocular lenses approved by CMS as "new technology IOL."

C1781

C1781 Mesh (implantable)

A mesh implant is a synthetic patch composed of absorbable or nonabsorbable material that is used to repair hernias, support weakened or attenuated tissue, cover tissue defects, etc.

C1782

C1782 Morcellator

A morcellator is a device that cuts, cores, and extracts tissue in laparoscopic procedures. The device uses suction to draw tissue into its tip where it is cut into small pieces by a rotating blade. The device removes the tissue from the field using suction.

C1783

C1783 Ocular implant, aqueous drainage assist device

Glaucoma is a group of ocular diseases that affect the optic nerve. High intraocular pressure frequently accompanies these diseases. This code describes a drain implanted into the anterior chamber of the eye that drains the aqueous humor to the outer eye. Drainage of the aqueous humor reduces intraocular pressure.

C1784

C1784 Ocular device, intraoperative, detached retina

An intraoperative ocular device for a detached retina is a carbon and fluorine (perfluorocarbon) gas that is instilled into the vitreous during a procedure to treat detached retina. The vitreous is a clear collagen gel that fills the eye that helps the retina lie smoothly and firmly against the back wall of the eyeball. The gas is injected to help return the retina to its normal position or to replace vitreous fluid removed during other retina repair procedures. The gas bubble eventually dissipates and may be replaced with body fluids.

C1785-C1786

C1785 Pacemaker, dual chamber, rate-responsive (implantable)

C1786 Pacemaker, single chamber, rate-responsive (implantable)

A pacemaker is a medical device that uses electrical impulses, delivered by electrodes contacting the heart muscles, to regulate the beating of the heart. The primary purpose of a pacemaker is to maintain an adequate heart rate. The dual chamber rate responsive pacemaker operates in an atrial synchronized modality when the sensed atrial rate is within a physiologic range and paces at a sensor determined rate when the atrial rate is above or below the physiologic range. The dual artificial pacemaker has two leads; one in the atrium and one in the ventricle, so electromechanical synchrony can be approximated and can deliver stimuli at a rate adjustable to some parameter independent of atrial activity. The single chamber pacemaker has only one lead in the atrium or ventricle. The pacemaker is placed beneath skin in the pectoral region.

C1787

C1787 Patient programmer, neurostimulator

A patient programmer is a handheld device that transmits operational commands to the neurostimulator. A patient may control the amplitude and rate of the electrical impulses delivered by the neurostimulator system

C1788

C1788 Port, indwelling (implantable)

An indwelling port (e.g., central venous access device) is a small medical appliance inserted subcutaneously that connects to a vein. The port contains a subcutaneous septum that allows blood to be withdrawn and drugs to be injected. The device consists of a reservoir (or portal) composed of a self-sealing silicone bubble and a catheter. The catheter runs from the port to a major vein (e.g., jugular, subclavian). Ideally it terminates in the superior vena cava near the right atrium. This position allows injected drugs to spread quickly and efficiently throughout the body.

C1789

C1789 Prosthesis, breast (implantable)

A breast implant is a prosthesis used to modify the size, form, and feel of a woman's breast in a post-mastectomy reconstruction; improve chest wall congenital deformities; augment the breast; or perform gender transition (male to female). Breast implants are surgically placed in anatomical relation to the pectoralis major muscle.

C1813

C1813 Prosthesis, penile, inflatable

The inflatable penile prosthesis is a medical device used for men with organic or psychogenic impotence who suffer from erectile dysfunction. This prosthesis is also used in the final stages of plastic surgery phalloplasty in gender reassignment surgery, as well as in total phalloplasty in males that need genital modification. The inflatable penile prosthesis is made of three components: cylinders, pump, and reservoir. It can be inflated and deflated upon demand.

C1814

C1814 Retinal tamponade device, silicone oil

Silicone oil is a silicon analogue of carbon based organic compounds that can form long and complex molecules based on silicon rather than carbon. This HCPCS Level II code represents silicone oil used as a permanent or prolonged retinal tamponade for the treatment of complex retinal detachments. The vitreous is a clear collagen gel that fills the eye and helps the retina lie smoothly and firmly against the back wall of the eyeball. Silicone oil is injected to help return the retina to its normal position or to replace vitreous fluid removed during other retina repair procedures. The silicone oil eventually dissipates and may be replaced with body fluids.

C1815

C1815 Prosthesis, urinary sphincter (implantable)

An artificial urinary sphincter (AUS) is a medical device that closely simulates the function of a biological urinary sphincter. A donut-shaped sac that circles the urethra, an AUS offers a competent bladder outlet during urinary storage and an open, unobstructed outlet to allow voiding. When the sac is filled with fluid, it squeezes the urethra closed. When a valve implanted under the skin is pressed, the fluid is released allowing the urethra to open and urine to flow.

C1816

C1816 Receiver and/or transmitter, neurostimulator (implantable)

A neurostimulator, also called an implanted pulse generator, is a battery powered medical device that delivers electrical impulses through a lead to electrodes implanted near the spinal cord or an affected peripheral nerve. The device is used to stimulate the spinal cord or peripheral nerve and block the transmission of pain to the brain. The neurostimulator system includes an integrated circuit, a radio-wave transceiver, a battery, and a connector block. There are two types of neurostimulation systems based on the location of the battery: a fully implanted system has an internal power source or one with an external power source.

C1817

C1817 Septal defect implant system, intracardiac

An intracardiac septal defect implant system is an implant placed within the heart for closure of a variety of defects that may occur in the dividing wall that separates the left and right sides of the heart. The septal defect implant system represented by this code includes a delivery catheter.

C1818

C1818 Integrated keratoprosthesis

An integrated keratoprosthesis is a flexible, one-piece biocompatible polymer lens. It is used to replace diseased native corneas in conditions where traditional corneal transplantation is not indicated or possible.

C1819

C1819 Surgical tissue localization and excision device (implantable)

A lesion localization device is an implantable radiofrequency guide that allows for stabilization, dissection, and excision of a lesion or foreign objects. Used with stereotactic, alphanumeric grid imaging techniques and ultrasound, this device may include radiofrequency, laser, or ultrasonic components. Implantation within the body proximate to the suspect tissue or object is done prior to surgery with one or more integrated transponder tags. At the time of surgery, scanning of the body with a radiofrequency scanner or reader activates the tag or tags and provides the surgeon with signals indicative of the location.

C1820

C1820 Generator, neurostimulator (implantable), with rechargeable battery and charging system

An implantable rechargeable neurostimulator generator is a device that creates small electrical impulses that are transmitted to electrodes implanted near the spinal cord or a peripheral nerve. The small electrical impulses interrupt pain signals sent to the brain. This type of generator contains a battery that can be recharged. This code represents a non-high-frequency system and includes the generator, rechargeable battery, and its charging system.

C1821

C1821 Interspinous process distraction device (implantable)

Interspinous process distraction implantable devices are implants placed between vertebral spinous processes. They aim to restrict painful motion while enabling normal motion. The implant is inserted between the spinous processes through a small incision and acts as a spacer between the spinous processes. After implantation, the device is opened or expanded to distract (open) the neural foramen and decompress the nerves. Reduction of vertebral motion may prevent pain caused by compression of blood vessels and nerves in the spine.

C1822

C1822 Generator, neurostimulator (implantable), high frequency, with rechargeable battery and charging system

An implantable rechargeable neurostimulator generator is a device that creates small electrical impulses that are transmitted to electrodes implanted near the spinal cord or a peripheral nerve. The small electrical impulses interrupt pain signals sent to the brain. This type of generator contains a battery that can be recharged. This code represents a high-frequency system and includes the generator, rechargeable battery, and its charging system.

C1823

C1823 Generator, neurostimulator (implantable), nonrechargeable, with transvenous sensing and stimulation leads

An implantable neurostimulator generator is a device that creates small electrical impulses that are transmitted to electrodes implanted near the spinal cord or a peripheral nerve. The small electrical impulses interrupt pain signals sent to the brain. This type of generator contains a battery that does not require recharging. This code includes the generator and battery.

C1824

C1824 Generator, cardiac contractility modulation (implantable)

A cardiac contractility modulation generator is a small implantable pulse generator (IPG), similar to a pacemaker, intended for the treatment of chronic heart failure in patients who are symptomatic despite appropriate medical treatment. In contrast to a pacemaker or a defibrillator, the system is designed to modulate the strength of contraction of the heart muscle rather than the rhythm. Typically implanted in the right pectoral region, the IPG is connected to two standard leads (electrodes) that are used to sense ventricular activity. Two electrodes in the right ventricular atrium ensure the precise timing of the cardiac contractility modulation (CCM) signals, delivering them just after the heart contracts (the absolute refractory period). The expected result is improvement in six-minute hall walking distance, quality of life, functional status, and exercise tolerance. In addition, the system contains an external charging device. The IPG unit should be recharged weekly for optimal device and battery performance. The U.S. Food and Drug Administration (FDA) granted breakthrough device exemption for the OPTIMIZER® Smart Implantable Pulse Generator (Impulse Dynamics, Orangeburg, NY) with approved use in the treatment of individuals with chronic, moderate-to-severe (New York Heart Failure [NYHA] Class III or ambulatory Class IV) heart failure (HF) who remain symptomatic despite guideline directed medical therapy (GDMT). Recipients must be in normal sinus rhythm with left ventricular ejection fraction (LVEF) from 25 to 45 percent and not considered a candidate for cardiac resynchronization therapy (CRT) to restore normal heart rhythm.

C1825

C1825 Generator, neurostimulator (implantable), nonrechargeable with carotid sinus baroreceptor stimulation lead(s)

A carotid sinus baroreflex activation system is implanted for the treatment of heart failure and resistant hypertension. This proprietary system sends electrical pulses to the baroreceptors (pressure sensors found within the walls of the carotid arteries that regulate heart rate and blood pressure) to restore balance to the automatic nervous system and improve the symptoms of heart failure. Consisting of an implantable pulse generator (IPG), a carotid sinus lead, and a wireless programmer system, the device prompts the body's natural reflexes to control blood pressure and the causal elements of heart failure progression. This code reports the nonrechargeable generator with carotid sinus baroreceptor stimulation leads.

C1826

C1826 Generator, neurostimulator (implantable), includes closed feedback loop leads and all implantable components, with rechargeable battery and charging system

An implantable rechargeable neurostimulator generator is a device that creates small electrical impulses that are transmitted to electrodes implanted near the spinal cord or a peripheral nerve. The small electrical impulses interrupt pain signals sent to the brain. This type of generator contains a battery that can be recharged. This code represents the implantable neurostimulator generator and includes closed feedback loop leads, all implantable components, a rechargeable battery, and its charging system.

C1827

C1827 Generator, neurostimulator (implantable), nonrechargeable, with implantable stimulation lead and external paired stimulation controller

An implantable nonrechargeable neurostimulator generator is a device that creates small electrical impulses that are transmitted to electrodes implanted near the spinal cord or a peripheral nerve. The small electrical impulses interrupt pain signals sent to the brain. This type of generator contains a battery that cannot be recharged but must be removed and replaced. This code represents the generator, implantable stimulation lead, and external paired stimulation controller.

C1830

C1830 Powered bone marrow biopsy needle

A bone marrow biopsy needle is a specialized stylus used to penetrate and withdraw bone marrow. This code represents a battery-powered rotary device that is similar to a hand held drill. The device drives a single lumen needle into the medullary cavity of an adult hip. The needle contains two parts: an outer cannula and an inner bevel-tipped stylet. The device appears to deliver larger volume bone marrow specimens in a more rapid fashion. Patients report less associated pain with the powered device.

C1831

C1831 Interbody cage, anterior, lateral or posterior, personalized (implantable)

An interbody cage is used to replace damaged spinal discs in spinal fusion procedures. The custom titanium cage is 3D printed for each patient after mapping the anatomy of the vertebral endplates and restores the correct height, angulation, and optimal surface contact between the interbody cage and the patient's vertebrae. The interbody cage is inserted into the disc space along with bone graft inserted in the hollow center, which allows fusion to occur between the two vertebra that surround the cage. This code reports an anterior, lateral, or posterior interbody cage only.

C1832

C1832 Autograft suspension, including cell processing and application, and all system components

RECELL® is an autologous cell harvesting device. It is a single use, stand-alone system containing needed actuators, enzymatic and delivery solutions, and sterile surgical instruments. The device processes a thin, split-thickness skin sample, obtained with the provider's preferred method, into a cell suspension for immediate application onto a prepared wound bed, in conjunction with a meshed autograft, that can cover a wound up to 1,920 cm^2. The cell suspension contains a mixed population of cells including fibroblasts, keratinocytes (activated, basal, and suprabasal) and melanocytes. These cells are critical for re-epithelialization and restoring natural pigmentation to the recipient area. RECELL® is indicated for the treatment of acute thermal burn wounds in adult patients ages 18 years and older. It should not be used for the treatment of infected or necrotic wounds or for patients with known hypersensitivity to adrenaline/epinephrine, anesthetics, chlorhexidine solutions, compound sodium lactate (Hartmann's Solution), povidone-iodine, or trypsin. See full instructions for use for complete information on device set-up, preparation of sterile and non-sterile work areas, and preparation of cell suspension.

C1833

C1833 Monitor, cardiac, including intracardiac lead and all system components (implantable)

An implantable cardiac monitor is a programmable device that monitors a patient's electrogram, vibrates to warn the patient of alarms and alerts, and stores electrogram data. It is indicated for use in patients with previous acute coronary syndrome (ACS) who remain at high risk for recurrent ACS events. The device detects sustained ST segment changes and alerts the patient to seek medical care for potential ACS events even in the absence of symptoms. The system consists of an implantable medical device (IMD) with a steroid-eluting endocardial pacing lead, a Programmer (computer) that allows the provider to establish parameters and alarm settings for each patient, and an external hand-held telemetry device that communicates with the Programmer and provides alarms and alerts based on programmed settings. The endocardial lead is implanted into the apex of the right ventricle using standard techniques and is attached to the IMD. A pocket for the IMD is created in the left pectoral region and any excess lead length is coiled behind the IMD with the header of the IMD proximal to the clavicle. Once implant verification is complete, the IMD should be secured, and the incision closed. A final communication session between the IMD and Programmer should be

C

established, and the post-implant setup procedure completed. The patient should be seen seven to 14 days later for initial IMD programming. See full instructions for use for complete implantation and set-up instructions.

C1834

C1834 Pressure sensor system, includes all components (e.g., introducer, sensor), intramuscular (implantable), excludes mobile (wireless) software application

An intramuscular pressure sensor system provides real-time continuous pressure measurements to assist in the diagnosis of acute compartment syndrome (ACS). ACS occurs when increased pressure inside the muscle compartment reduces blood supply to the surrounding tissue and causes severe pain. The condition is rare and difficult to diagnose. The pressure sensor system consists of a pressure sensor, introducer, lead-wire, and LCD screen. The pressure sensor is inserted into the muscle compartment. The sensor is attached to a lead wire that connects to an LCD screen that is adhered to the patient's skin. The device connects wirelessly to a mobile application via Bluetooth, transferring pressure data to provider cloud systems, allowing remote patient monitoring and timely monitoring of muscle pressure.

C1839

C1839 Iris prosthesis

Flexible, biocompatible, medical-grade silicone device indicated for use in adults or children, the prosthetic iris mimics the function of the natural iris (the colored part of the eye around the pupil) and creates an artificial pupil that reduces the amount of light entering the eye. Intended for those with congenital or traumatic aniridia (complete or partial absence of the iris), as well as iris defects due to conditions such as albinism or surgical removal due to melanoma, the device can be sized and colored for each individual patient. The artificial iris is implanted via a small incision and is held in place by the anatomical structures of the eye or by sutures if necessary.

C1840

C1840 Lens, intraocular (telescopic)

An intraocular lens is an artificial lens made of plastic, silicone, or acrylic that performs the function of the eye's natural lens. This code represents a miniature implantable telescope lens intended to improve visual acuity in patients with age-related macular degeneration. The device magnifies images onto the healthy areas of the retina to help improve central vision. The telescopic lens is implanted into the posterior chamber of the eye's anterior segment. It is held in place with haptic loops.

C1874

C1874 Stent, coated/covered, with delivery system

A stent with delivery system is a small hollow tube made of a biocompatible substance, such as phosphorylcholine, silicone, or metal, that is inserted into a natural body passage or conduit. The stent maintains the body passage or conduit allowing less restricted flow. This code represents a stent packaged with a delivery system that generally includes a stent mounted or unmounted on a balloon angioplasty catheter, introducer, and sheath.

C1875

C1875 Stent, coated/covered, without delivery system

A coated or covered stent without a delivery system is a small hollow tube made of a biocompatible substance, such as phosphorylcholine, silicone, or metal, that is inserted into a natural body passage or conduit. The stent maintains the body passage or conduit allowing less restricted flow. It is coated with a drug that helps prevent the conduit from becoming narrowed again. This code represents a stent packaged without a delivery system.

C1876-C1877

C1876 Stent, noncoated/noncovered, with delivery system

C1877 Stent, noncoated/noncovered, without delivery system

A stent is a small hollow tube made of stainless steel that is inserted into a natural body passage or conduit. The stent maintains the body passage or conduit allowing less restricted flow. These stents are not coated with any drugs or polymers. A delivery system is a method of delivering the device to its intended position in the body. Delivery systems can use balloon and guidewires or may be proprietary. These codes represent noncoated stents with and without a delivery system.

C1878

C1878 Material for vocal cord medialization, synthetic (implantable)

Material for vocal cord medialization is a synthetic implantable substance that is not absorbable. The substance is injected or implanted in a vocal cord to move the cord closer to midline to allow a greater strike with the opposite vocal cord.

C1880

C1880 Vena cava filter

A vena cava filter is a device that is inserted into the vena cava, the large vein that returns blood to the heart from the abdomen and legs (inferior vena cava). This filter is an umbrella-shaped barrier device that helps prevent blood clots that may form in the deep veins of the lower limbs from traveling to the lungs and heart where they may block blood flow. Vena cava filters are placed using a catheter inserted through a vein in the neck or groin. The device may be placed due to failure of anticoagulations, contraindications to anticoagulations, large clots in the vena cava or iliac veins, or for patients at high risk for having a pulmonary embolism.

C1881

C1881 Dialysis access system (implantable)

Hemodialysis requires access to the bloodstream or vascular access. The access is meant to be permanent so that it can be reused. The different types of access for hemodialysis include a fistula or a graft. A fistula is created by connecting one of the arteries to one of the veins in the lower arm. A graft uses a synthetic tube implanted under the skin of the arm to connect an artery and a vein. A temporary method using a venous catheter is usually used while permanent access develops. A catheter is placed in a vein in the neck, chest, or groin. Peritoneal dialysis access requires introduction of a catheter in the belly. Placement is usually done 10 to 14 days before dialysis starts. Because of a high risk of complications with prolonged use, these catheters are not commonly used.

C1882

C1882 Cardioverter-defibrillator, other than single or dual chamber (implantable)

A cardioverter-defibrillator is an electronic device that delivers an electric shock to the heart, helping re-establish normal contraction rhythms in a heart having dangerous arrhythmia or in cardiac arrest. An implantable cardioverter-defibrillator (ICD) has two components: a pulse generator and a defibrillator lead. The device is connected to leads positioned inside the heart or on its surface. These leads deliver electrical shocks, sense cardiac rhythm, and sometimes pace the heart, as needed. The various leads are connected to a pulse generator, which is implanted in a pouch beneath the skin of the chest or abdomen. The pulse generator's function is to generate energy, deliver defibrillating shocks, filter/analyze, and store electrical signals from the myocardium to distinguish normal from pathologic rhythms that require a response from the ICD. This code represents an implantable cardioverter-defibrillator, other than a single or dual chamber.

C1883

C1883 Adaptor/extension, pacing lead or neurostimulator lead (implantable)

A pacing or neurostimulator lead adaptor or extension is an implantable device that is placed in between an existing lead and a new generator. The end of the adaptor lead has the appropriate connector pin that enables the use of the existing lead with a new generator that has a different connecting receptacle. These are required when a generator is replaced or when two leads are connected to the same port in the connector block.

C1884

C1884 Embolization protective system

An embolization protective system is a system designed to trap, macerate, and remove atheromatous or thrombotic debris from the vascular system during an angioplasty, atherectomy, or stenting procedure.

C1885

C1885 Catheter, transluminal angioplasty, laser

A transluminal angioplasty laser catheter is a small hollow tube that is inserted into the central space (or lumen) of an artery or vein .This code refers to a catheter that has a laser at its tip. The catheter is advanced through the blood vessel to the area of occlusion or blockage. When the catheter is in position, the laser emits pulsating beams of light that break up or vaporize the obstruction.

C1886

C1886 Catheter, extravascular tissue ablation, any modality (insertable)

An ablation catheter is a long thin tube inside a sheath that is used to deliver destructive electrical or thermal energy to abnormal or problematic tissues. Electrodes are located in the catheter to generate the necessary energy. The catheter is inserted and maneuvered into the desired tissue Extravascular catheters are inserted into the body to treat the desired tissue. The catheter is designed to penetrate the tissue but not the vascular structure.

C1887

C1887 Catheter, guiding (may include infusion/perfusion capability)

A guiding catheter is a small hollow tube used to introduce interventional or diagnostic devices into the coronary or peripheral vascular system. It can be used to inject contrast material, function as a conduit through which other devices pass, and/or provide a mechanism for measuring arterial pressure, and maintain a pathway created by the guide wire during the performance of a procedure.

C1888

C1888 Catheter, ablation, noncardiac, endovascular (implantable)

A noncardiac endovascular ablation catheter is a small hollow tube containing a laser or radiofrequency tip that is inserted into a blood vessel. The catheter is advanced to the target area and a pulse from the laser or radiofrequency device is used to occlude or obliterate the blood vessel.

C1889-C1890

C1889 Implantable/insertable device, not otherwise classified

C1890 No implantable/insertable device used with device-intensive procedures

Report C1889 for a miscellaneous device that is implanted or inserted during a device-intensive OPPS procedure that is not described by a specific HCPCS Level II category C code. Report C1890 when a device is not implanted or inserted during a device-intensive OPPS procedure. Reporting these codes with a device intensive procedure satisfies the OPPS edit requiring a device code to be reported on a claim with a device-intensive procedure.

C1891

C1891 Infusion pump, nonprogrammable, permanent (implantable)

An implantable infusion pump is a medical device that delivers fluids, drugs, or nutrients into the patient's bloodstream in a consistent dose at a consistent rate with consistent pressure. The pump is intended to provide long-term, continuous, or intermittent drug infusion. Non-programmable pumps are used for fixed dosages of medication or fluids.

C1892

C1892 Introducer/sheath, guiding, intracardiac electrophysiological, fixed-curve, peel-away

A guiding, intracardiac electrophysiological, fixed-curve, peel-away introducer or sheath is a small hollow tube made of nonabsorbable material. The sheath or introducer that separates into two pieces is guided to the target area. A lead or catheter is then placed through the introducer and the sheath is removed.

C1893

C1893 Introducer/sheath, guiding, intracardiac electrophysiological, fixed-curve, other than peel-away

A guiding, intracardiac electrophysiological, fixed-curve, non peel-away introducer or sheath is a small hollow tube made of nonabsorbable material. The sheath or introducer, which separates into two pieces, is guided to the target area. The introducer or sheath is for cardiac use and measures the electrical activity within the heart while providing a conduit for the passage of a device. The lead or catheter is then placed through the introducer and the sheath is removed.

C1894

C1894 Introducer/sheath, other than guiding, other than intracardiac electrophysiological, nonlaser

An introducer or a sheath is a small hollow tube made of nonabsorbable material. The sheath or introducer, which separates into two pieces, is guided to the target area. This introducer or sheath is for anything other than cardiac electrophysiological use. The tube provides a conduit for the passage of a nonlaser device. The lead or catheter is then placed through the introducer and the sheath is removed.

C1895

C1895 Lead, cardioverter-defibrillator, endocardial dual coil (implantable)

A pacemaker/cardioverter-defibrillator combination is a specialized device composed of a cardiac defibrillator and a pacemaker. Pacemakers provide electrical stimulation when cardiac contractions are slow or absent. A defibrillator is designed to directly treat a cardiac tachydysrhythmia. Pacing systems consist of a pulse generator and pacing leads. A dual coil lead is a thin, flexible wire that is inserted transvenously and advanced to the right ventricle and/or atrium where it is implanted into the myocardial tissue. The pulse generator is placed subcutaneously or submuscularly in the chest wall. This code represents an endocardial dual coil that connects to a pacemaker/cardioverter-defibrillator combination (implantable).

C1896

C1896 Lead, cardioverter-defibrillator, other than endocardial single or dual coil (implantable)

A pacemaker/cardioverter-defibrillator combination is a specialized device composed of a cardiac defibrillator and a pacemaker. Pacemakers provide electrical stimulation when cardiac contractions are slow or absent. A defibrillator is designed to directly treat a cardiac tachydysrhythmia. Pacing systems consist of a pulse generator and pacing leads. A coil lead is a thin, flexible wire that is inserted transvenously and advanced to the right ventricle and/or atrium where it is implanted into the myocardial tissue. The pulse generator is placed subcutaneously or submuscularly in the chest wall. Report this code for a lead other than endocardial single or dual coil that connects to a pacemaker/cardioverter-defibrillator combination (implantable).

C1897

C1897 Lead, neurostimulator test kit (implantable)

Neurostimulators are medical devices that transmit electrical impulses to specified nerves through an implanted wire or lead. A neurostimulator test kit (implantable) allows for the temporary use of a neurostimulator and its leads to determine if the intended usage will be beneficial to the patient.

C1898

C1898 Lead, pacemaker, other than transvenous VDD single pass

A pacemaker is a device used to synchronize the beating of the heart. The lead is a small wire that conducts electrical impulses from the pacemaker to the heart. The lead is passed through a vein into the heart. The pacemaker is programmed to regulate the rhythm of the heart and the electronic impulses are conducted through the leads to the heart muscle.

C1899

C1899 Lead, pacemaker/cardioverter-defibrillator combination (implantable)

A pacemaker/cardioverter-defibrillator combination is a specialized device composed of a cardiac defibrillator and a pacemaker. Pacemakers provide electrical stimulation when cardiac contractions are slow or absent. A defibrillator is designed to directly treat a cardiac tachydysrhythmia. Pacing systems consist of a pulse generator and pacing leads. Endocardial leads are thin, flexible wires that are inserted transvenously and advanced to the right ventricle and/or atrium where they are implanted into the myocardial tissue. The pulse generator is placed subcutaneously or submuscularly in the chest wall.

C1900

C1900 Lead, left ventricular coronary venous system

A left ventricular coronary venous system lead is an implanted wire with an electrode at its tip that connects a generator to the left ventricle of the heart. It is intended to treat the symptoms associated with heart failure.

C1982

C1982 Catheter, pressure generating, one-way valve, intermittently occlusive

This code reports an intermittent occlusive catheter that has a pressure-generating, one-way valve. The catheter maintains a closed system, making it more difficult for bacteria to enter.

C2596

C2596 Probe, image guided, robotic, waterjet ablation

A single-use probe is utilized with a hand-piece in transurethral waterjet ablation of the prostate. This minimally invasive procedure employs an aquablation system to destroy prostatic glandular tissue using a high-speed solution of sodium chloride in water (saline) guided with exact electromechanical control using a real-time transrectal ultrasound image. The surgeon destroys the prostatic tissue by moving along a fixed, predetermined glandular tissue map, while at the same time collecting samples of prostatic tissue to analyze after the procedure has been completed. When needed, control of bleeding (hemostasis) is performed using a low power blue laser beam contained in a water column to cause coagulation. This procedure is performed for patients with symptomatic benign prostatic hyperplasia.

C2613

C2613 Lung biopsy plug with delivery system

A lung biopsy plug sealant system is a cylindrical, self-expanding hydrogel plug that establishes an airtight seal of the pleural space following a percutaneous, transthoracic lung biopsy. The sealant system is utilized for the prevention of biopsy-related pneumothorax, for biopsy paths between 1 cm and 7 cm long. The delivery system consists of the delivery device, a coaxial adapter, and a hydrogel plug. The coaxial adapter allows the plug to be delivered via the same needle introducer used for performing the biopsy. The coaxial adapter, containing the hydrogel plug, is attached to the needle introducer, the plug distance to be delivered is set and locked on the delivery device, and the delivery device is connected to the coaxial adapter. Upon delivery, the hydrogel plug swells to seal the biopsy site. The plug eventually resorbs into the body.

C2614

C2614 Probe, percutaneous lumbar discectomy

A percutaneous discectomy is the removal of a herniated intravertebral disc through a small incision. The probe is a small hollow tube that is inserted in the intervertebral disc. Tiny surgical instruments are inserted through the tube to cut and/or aspirate the disc material.

C2615

C2615 Sealant, pulmonary, liquid

Liquid pulmonary sealant is an absorbable hydrogel formed from two components. Human serum albumin is mixed with a synthetic cross-linking component of polyethylene glycol. It is indicated to seal visceral pleural air leaks during pulmonary resection. The liquid pulmonary sealant is intended for single use. It is not recommended that more than 30 ml be used per patient.

C2616

C2616 Brachytherapy source, nonstranded, yttrium-90, per source

Brachytherapy is a form of radiotherapy involving implantation of radioactive sources within the tumor bed, which allows delivery of high radiation doses to the tumor site, sparing adjacent normal tissue. This code reports radioactive isotope yttrium-90.

C2617

C2617 Stent, noncoronary, temporary, without delivery system

A noncoronary, temporary stent, without a delivery system is a small hollow tube made of a biocompatible substance, such as phosphorylcholine, silicone, or metal that is inserted into a natural body passage or conduit. The stent maintains the body passage or conduit allowing less restricted flow. This code represents a stent packaged without a delivery system. A temporary stent is designed to be removed and is placed for a period of less than one year.

C2618

C2618 Probe/needle, cryoablation

Cryoablation probes are hollow needles (cryoprobes) through which cooled, thermally conductive fluids are circulated. Cryoprobes are inserted into or placed adjacent to diseased tissue. Ablation occurs in tissue that has been frozen by at least three mechanisms: 1) formation of ice crystals within cells thereby disrupting membranes; 2) coagulation of blood thereby interrupting blood flow; 3) induction of apoptosis, the so-called programmed cell death cascade.

C2619-C2620

C2619 Pacemaker, dual chamber, nonrate-responsive (implantable)

C2620 Pacemaker, single chamber, nonrate-responsive (implantable)

A pacemaker is an electronic device that regulates contraction rhythms of the heart through electrical impulses. A pacemaker has two components: a pulse generator and lead(s). The pulse generator is connected to leads positioned inside the heart or on its surface. These leads are used to deliver electrical impulses, sense the cardiac rhythm, and pace the heart, as needed. The various leads are connected to a pulse generator, which is implanted in a pouch beneath the skin of the chest or abdomen. Dual chamber pacemakers can sense and pace in both heart chambers, atrium and ventricle. Single chamber pacemakers sense and pace in only one heart chamber, usually the ventricle. Rate responsive pacemakers sense both physiologic and nonphysiologic signals and adjust their output to meet patient needs. Nonrate-responsive pacemakers deliver a consistent fixed rate.

C2621

C2621 Pacemaker, other than single or dual chamber (implantable)

A pacemaker is an electronic system that monitors the electrical impulses of the heart and delivers an electrical charge when necessary to set normal heart rhythms. This code represents an implantable pacemaker that is neither a single nor dual chamber model.

C2622

C2622 Prosthesis, penile, noninflatable

A non-inflatable penile prosthesis consists of a pair of malleable cylinders that are surgically inserted into the penis. This prosthesis maintains the penis in a semi-rigid state. The penis must be manually positioned, up for intercourse or down for everyday activities.

C2623

C2623 Catheter, transluminal angioplasty, drug-coated, nonlaser

A transluminal angioplasty catheter is a small hollow tube that is inserted into the central space (or lumen) of an artery or vein. This code reports a catheter that has a drug-coated balloon. The catheter is advanced through the blood vessel to the area of occlusion or blockage. When the catheter is in position, the balloon is inflated, providing mechanical dilation of the lesion. The drug coating comes into contact with the targeted area, releasing the drug into the vessel wall, where it remains at a therapeutic dose for 180 days.

C2624

C2624 Implantable wireless pulmonary artery pressure sensor with delivery catheter, including all system components

An implantable wireless pulmonary artery pressure sensor system is designed to monitor pulmonary artery pressure and improve treatment of NYHA class III heart failure patients. A wireless sensor is permanently implanted into the pulmonary artery via a transluminal angioplasty delivery catheter. Pulmonary artery pressures are measured through a wireless electronics system. This code reports the pressure sensor and all related system components.

C2625

C2625 Stent, noncoronary, temporary, with delivery system

A noncoronary, temporary stent, with a delivery system is a small hollow tube made of a biocompatible substance, such as phosphorylcholine, silicone, or metal, that is inserted into a natural body passage or conduit. The stent maintains the body passage or conduit allowing less restricted flow. A temporary stent is designed to be removed and is placed for a period of less than one year. This code represents a stent packaged with a delivery system, generally including components such as a stent mounted or unmounted on a balloon angioplasty catheter, introducer, and sheath.

C2626

C2626 Infusion pump, nonprogrammable, temporary (implantable)

A nonprogrammable, temporary infusion pump is a short term pain management system which is a component of a permanent implantable system used for the management of chronic pain.

C2627

C2627 Catheter, suprapubic/cystoscopic

A suprapubic catheter is a flexible hollow tube that is inserted through the abdomen into the urinary bladder to drain urine. It is a popular method of long-term bladder drainage in voiding dysfunction. A cystoscopic catheter is a flexible hollow tube that is used in a cystoscopy.

C2628

C2628 Catheter, occlusion

An occlusion catheter is a flexible hollow tube with a balloon at the tip. The device is placed into an organ or blood vessel and the balloon is inflated. This blocks or occludes the vessel stopping blood flow.

C2629

C2629 Introducer/sheath, other than guiding, other than intracardiac electrophysiological, laser

An intracardiac, electrophysiological introducer or sheath is a small hollow tube made of nonabsorbable material that is used in the heart. The sheath or introducer, which separates into two pieces, is guided to the target area. A laser is placed through the introducer and the sheath is removed.

C2630

C2630 Catheter, electrophysiology, diagnostic/ablation, other than 3D or vector mapping, cool-tip

An electrophysiology, diagnostic or ablation, other than 3D or vector mapping, cool-tip catheter is a small hollow tube containing devices that aid in providing anatomic and physiologic information about the cardiac electrical conduction system. This device has temperature sensing capability also contains a cooling mechanism which is a tip cooled by infused, circulating saline.

C2631

C2631 Repair device, urinary, incontinence, without sling graft

A urinary incontinence repair device is used to attach or insert body tissue, synthetic material, or mesh for the purpose of strengthening the pelvic floor. The repair material is fashioned into a sling or hammock that supports the urethra. This code represents the device components used to deliver the sling graft and/or fixate (via permanent sutures or bone anchors) the sling graft, but does not include the sling graft.

C2634-C2645

C2634 Brachytherapy source, nonstranded, high activity, iodine-125, greater than 1.01 mCi (NIST), per source

C2635 Brachytherapy source, nonstranded, high activity, palladium-103, greater than 2.2 mCi (NIST), per source

C2636 Brachytherapy linear source, nonstranded, palladium-103, per 1 mm

C2637 Brachytherapy source, nonstranded, ytterbium-169, per source

C2638 Brachytherapy source, stranded, iodine-125, per source

C2639 Brachytherapy source, nonstranded, iodine-125, per source

C2640 Brachytherapy source, stranded, palladium-103, per source

C2641 Brachytherapy source, nonstranded, palladium-103, per source

C2642 Brachytherapy source, stranded, cesium-131, per source

C2643 Brachytherapy source, nonstranded, cesium-131, per source

C2644 Brachytherapy source, cesium-131 chloride solution, per mCi

C2645 Brachytherapy planar source, palladium-103, per sq mm

Brachytherapy is a form of radiotherapy in which physicians place the source of irradiation close to the tumor or within a body cavity. Brachytherapy could include placing radioactive sources inside a body cavity (intracavitary brachytherapy) or putting radioactive material directly into body tissue using hollow needles (interstitial brachytherapy). Brachytherapy may be given in addition to external beam radiation or it may be used as the only form of radiotherapy. In some cases, the radioactive sources may be permanently left in place; in other cases, they are removed after a specified time. Placement of radioactive sources may be repeated several times. The isotope gold-198 has a half-life of 2.7 days and is used in some cancer treatments and treatments for other diseases. There are two natural isotopes of iridium, and many radioisotopes, the most stable radioisotope being Ir-192 with a half-life of 73.83 days. Ir-192 beta decays into platinum-192, while most of the other radioisotopes decay into osmium.

C2698-C2699

C2698 Brachytherapy source, stranded, not otherwise specified, per source

C2699 Brachytherapy source, nonstranded, not otherwise specified, per source

Brachytherapy is a form of radiotherapy in which physicians place the source of irradiation close to the tumor or within a body cavity. Brachytherapy includes placing radioactive sources inside a body cavity (intracavitary brachytherapy) or putting radioactive material directly into body tissue using hollow needles (interstitial brachytherapy). Stranded sources are seeds or sources connected in a linear fashion using absorbable material.

C5271-C5278

C5271 Application of low cost skin substitute graft to trunk, arms, legs, total wound surface area up to 100 sq cm; first 25 sq cm or less wound surface area

C5272 Application of low cost skin substitute graft to trunk, arms, legs, total wound surface area up to 100 sq cm; each additional 25 sq cm wound surface area, or part thereof (list separately in addition to code for primary procedure)

C5273 Application of low cost skin substitute graft to trunk, arms, legs, total wound surface area greater than or equal to 100 sq cm; first 100 sq cm wound surface area, or 1% of body area of infants and children

C5274 Application of low cost skin substitute graft to trunk, arms, legs, total wound surface area greater than or equal to 100 sq cm; each additional 100 sq cm wound surface area, or part thereof, or each additional 1% of body area of infants and children, or part thereof (list separately in addition to code for primary procedure)

C5275 Application of low cost skin substitute graft to face, scalp, eyelids, mouth, neck, ears, orbits, genitalia, hands, feet, and/or multiple digits, total wound surface area up to 100 sq cm; first 25 sq cm or less wound surface area

C5276 Application of low cost skin substitute graft to face, scalp, eyelids, mouth, neck, ears, orbits, genitalia, hands, feet, and/or multiple digits, total wound surface area up to 100 sq cm; each additional 25 sq cm wound surface area, or part thereof (list separately in addition to code for primary procedure)

C5277 Application of low cost skin substitute graft to face, scalp, eyelids, mouth, neck, ears, orbits, genitalia, hands, feet, and/or multiple digits, total wound surface area greater than or equal to 100 sq cm; first 100 sq cm wound surface area, or 1% of body area of infants and children

C5278 Application of low cost skin substitute graft to face, scalp, eyelids, mouth, neck, ears, orbits, genitalia, hands, feet, and/or multiple digits, total wound surface area greater than or equal to 100 sq cm; each additional 100 sq cm wound surface area, or part thereof, or each additional 1% of body area of infants and children, or part thereof (list separately in addition to code for primary procedure)

These codes are designed to parallel the surgical procedures described by CPT codes under the heading in the CPT code book "Skin Replacement Surgery" and the subheading "Skin Substitute Grafts." OPPS considers that skin substitute products serve as a necessary supply for these surgical repair procedures. OPPS hospitals report these C codes when the skin substitute is considered the low-cost group. Report the appropriate code based on the area of the body and size of the wound surface. The following are currently considered low-cost skin substitutes: A2015-A2018, Q4100, Q4102, Q4111, Q4115, Q4117, Q4124, Q4134-Q4136, Q4165-Q4166, Q4170, Q4176, Q4179-Q4180, Q4199, Q4206, Q4208, Q4210, Q4212-Q4218, Q4220-Q4221, Q4235, Q4247-Q4248, Q4250-Q4255, and Q4259-Q4261. OPPS hospitals report CPT codes 15271-15278 when the skin substitute is in the high-cost group. CMS reviews costs and may revise them quarterly. There are a few skin substitute products that are applied as liquids or powders and are employed in procedures outside of the noted CPT code range. These products will not be classified as high cost or low cost but will be packaged into the surgical procedure in which they are used. The list of low-cost skin substitutes is updated on a quarterly basis.

C7500

C7500 Debridement, bone including epidermis, dermis, subcutaneous tissue, muscle and/or fascia, if performed, first 20 sq cm or less with manual preparation and insertion of deep (e.g., subfascial) drug-delivery device(s)

The physician surgically removes foreign matter and contaminated or devitalized bone (including epidermis, dermis, subcutaneous tissue, muscle, and/or fascia, if performed) caused by injury, infection, wounds, or chronic ulcers. Using the appropriate surgical instrument (i.e., scalpel) affected tissues are excised into the bone. This code represents the first 20 sq cm or less and includes manual preparation and insertion of a deep (subfascial) drug delivery system in which the physician or other qualified health care professional manually prepares and inserts a drug-delivery device that is not prefabricated into the deep tissues. Antibiotics or other therapeutic agents are mixed with a carrier substance, shaped into drug-delivery devices such as beads, nails, or spacers, and placed into the subfascial tissues.

C7501

C7501 Percutaneous breast biopsies using stereotactic guidance, with placement of breast localization device(s) (e.g., clip, metallic pellet), when performed, and imaging of the biopsy specimen, when performed, all lesions unilateral and bilateral (for single lesion biopsy, use appropriate code)

The physician performs breast biopsies (unilateral or bilateral) under stereotactic image guidance using a percutaneous needle core or automated vacuum assisted or rotating biopsy device and insertion of a localization device. Using image guidance, the physician places a metallic clip or pellet adjacent to the breast lesions to mark the sites. A large gauge (e.g., 14 gauge), hollow core biopsy needle or the biopsy device is inserted through the skin of the breast and into the suspicious breast tissue. The physician takes multiple core tissue samples from the lesions to obtain enough tissue for diagnosis. The needle or automated vacuum assisted or rotating biopsy device is withdrawn. Pressure and bandages are applied to the puncture sites. This code is not reported for biopsy of a single lesion.

C7502

C7502 Percutaneous breast biopsies using magnetic resonance guidance, with placement of breast localization device(s) (e.g., clip, metallic pellet), when performed, and imaging of the biopsy specimen, when performed, all lesions unilateral or bilateral (for single lesion biopsy, use appropriate code)

The physician performs breast biopsies (unilateral or bilateral) under magnetic resonance (MR) guidance using a percutaneous needle core or automated vacuum assisted or rotating biopsy device and insertion of a localization device. Using image guidance, the physician places a metallic clip or pellet adjacent to the breast lesions to mark the sites. A large gauge (e.g., 14 gauge), hollow core biopsy needle or the biopsy device is inserted through the skin of the breast and into the suspicious breast tissue. The physician takes multiple core tissue samples from the lesions to obtain enough tissue for diagnosis. The needle or automated vacuum assisted or rotating biopsy device is withdrawn. Pressure and bandages are applied to the puncture sites. This code is not reported for biopsy of a single lesion.

C7503

C7503 Open biopsy or excision of deep cervical node(s) with intraoperative identification (e.g., mapping) of sentinel lymph node(s) including injection of nonradioactive dye when performed

The physician performs an open biopsy or excision of one or more deep cervical lymph nodes. Following an incision through the skin overlying the lymph node, the physician incises the platysma, using sharp dissection to develop flaps underneath, and taking care to avoid the nearby cranial nerves and large caliber vessels. The deep cervical fascia overlying the targeted lymph node is incised, and the node is dissected free using appropriate methods (blunt, sharp, monopolar, and/or bipolar electrocautery dissection). Surrounding lymphatics and blood vessels are dissected and ligated with fine ties or cautery. The targeted node (or a portion) is removed and submitted to pathology for culture and histological examination. The wound is inspected and irrigated, the platysma is reapproximated with sutures, and the skin is closed. This procedure includes intraoperative identification/mapping of sentinel lymph nodes (the first to receive lymphatic drainage from a tumor) as well as the injection of nonradioactive dye, if performed.

C7504-C7505

C7504 Percutaneous vertebroplasties (bone biopsies included when performed), first cervicothoracic and any additional cervicothoracic or lumbosacral vertebral bodies, unilateral or bilateral injection, inclusive of all imaging guidance

C7505 Percutaneous vertebroplasties (bone biopsies included when performed), first lumbosacral and any additional cervicothoracic or lumbosacral vertebral bodies, unilateral or bilateral injection, inclusive of all imaging guidance

Percutaneous vertebroplasty is a minimally invasive, image-guided procedure performed by a one- or two-sided injection of a vertebral body. A local anesthetic is administered. A needle is guided into the fractured vertebra under imaging guidance through a small puncture in the patient's skin. Sterile biomaterial such as methyl methacrylate is injected from one or both sides into the damaged vertebral body and acts as a bone cement to reinforce the fractured or collapsed vertebra. The procedure does not restore the original shape to the vertebra, but it does stabilize the bone, preventing further fracture or collapse. Following the procedure, the patient may experience significant, almost immediate pain relief. These codes include a vertebral bone biopsy, if performed, during the same operative session. Report C7504 for percutaneous vertebroplasty of the first cervicothoracic and any additional cervicothoracic or lumbosacral vertebral bodies. Report C7505 for percutaneous vertebroplasty of the first lumbosacral and any additional cervicothoracic or lumbosacral vertebral bodies. All imaging guidance is included in these procedures.

C7506

C7506 Arthrodesis, interphalangeal joints, with or without internal fixation

The physician fuses one or more interphalangeal joints; internal fixation may be utilized. The physician incises the overlying skin and dissects to the interphalangeal joint. A wire may be used to stabilize the joint until fusion is complete. The incision is sutured in layers and the hand is splinted.

C7507-C7508

C7507 Percutaneous vertebral augmentations, first thoracic and any additional thoracic or lumbar vertebral bodies, including cavity creations (fracture reductions and bone biopsies included when performed) using mechanical device (e.g., kyphoplasty), unilateral or bilateral cannulations, inclusive of all imaging guidance

C7508 Percutaneous vertebral augmentations, first lumbar and any additional thoracic or lumbar vertebral bodies, including cavity creations (fracture reductions and bone biopsies included when performed) using mechanical device (e.g., kyphoplasty), unilateral or bilateral cannulations, inclusive of all imaging guidance

The physician performs a minimally invasive percutaneous kyphoplasty, a modification of the percutaneous vertebroplasty, to reduce the pain associated with osteoporotic vertebral compression fractures. This procedure has the added advantage of restoring or augmenting the vertebral body. The patient is placed in a prone, slightly flexed position. A 5 mm to 7 mm incision is made and small cannulae are inserted into the vertebral body from one or both sides. Balloon catheters, called "tamps," are inserted into the vertebra and inflated. Tamps create a void in the soft trabecular bone and restore vertebral alignment. Balloons are then deflated and high viscosity cement under direct image control is injected into the void previously created by the bone tamps. Report C7507 for a procedure performed on the first thoracic and any additional thoracic or lumbar vertebral bodies. Report C7508 if performed on the first lumbar and any additional thoracic or lumbar vertebral bodies. These codes include all imaging guidance, as well as any fracture reductions and bone biopsies, if performed.

C7509-C7510

C7509 Bronchoscopy, rigid or flexible, diagnostic with cell washing(s) when performed, with computer-assisted image-guided navigation, including fluoroscopic guidance when performed

C7510 Bronchoscopy, rigid or flexible, with bronchial alveolar lavage(s), with computer-assisted image-guided navigation, including fluoroscopic guidance when performed

The physician views the airway using a flexible fiberoptic or rigid bronchoscope that is introduced under appropriate anesthesia through the nasal or oral cavity with the use of computer-assisted, image-guided navigation. The bronchoscope is inserted and advanced past the larynx to inspect the bronchus. In C7509, after diagnostic visualization of the bronchus, cell washings may be obtained through the bronchoscope. In C7510, bronchoscopy includes bronchial alveolar lavage, which allows lung tissue to be sampled by irrigating with saline followed by suctioning the fluid. The bronchoscope is removed. These codes include fluoroscopic guidance, when performed.

C7511

C7511 Bronchoscopy, rigid or flexible, with single or multiple bronchial or endobronchial biopsy(ies), single or multiple sites, with computer-assisted image-guided navigation, including fluoroscopic guidance when performed

The physician views the airway using a flexible fiberoptic or rigid bronchoscope that is introduced under appropriate anesthesia through the nasal or oral cavity with the use of computer-assisted, image-guided navigation. The bronchoscope is inserted and advanced past the larynx to inspect the bronchus, including fluoroscopic guidance, if used. After diagnostic visualization of the bronchus, one or more samples of bronchial or endobronchial tissue is removed for study. More than one site may be biopsied. Bleeding is assessed and controlled, and the bronchoscope is removed.

C7512

C7512 Bronchoscopy, rigid or flexible, with single or multiple bronchial or endobronchial biopsy(ies), single or multiple sites, with transendoscopic endobronchial ultrasound (EBUS) during bronchoscopic diagnostic or therapeutic intervention(s) for peripheral lesion(s), including fluoroscopic guidance when performed

Endobronchial ultrasound (EBUS) is a minimally invasive technique utilizing ultrasound in conjunction with bronchoscopy to view the airway wall and adjacent structures. EBUS guidance and identification of lesions in peripheral (more distal) airways uses a radial ultrasound probe, which passes through the working channel of a bronchoscope without an integrated ultrasound-imaging component. This code reports a rigid or flexible bronchoscopy with one or more bronchial/endobronchial biopsies from one or more sites using EBUS for identification of peripheral lesions. Fluoroscopic guidance, when performed, is included.

C7513-C7514

C7513 Dialysis circuit, introduction of needle(s) and/or catheter(s), with diagnostic angiography of the dialysis circuit, including all direct puncture(s) and catheter placement(s), injection(s) of contrast, all necessary imaging from the arterial anastomosis and adjacent artery through entire venous outflow including the inferior or superior vena cava, fluoroscopic guidance, with transluminal balloon angioplasty of central dialysis segment, performed through dialysis circuit, including all required imaging, radiological supervision and interpretation, image documentation and report

C7514 Dialysis circuit, introduction of needle(s) and/or catheter(s), with diagnostic angiography of the dialysis circuit, including all direct puncture(s) and catheter placement(s), injection(s) of contrast, all necessary imaging from the arterial anastomosis and adjacent artery through entire venous outflow including the inferior or superior vena cava, fluoroscopic guidance, with all angioplasty in the central dialysis segment, and transcatheter placement of intravascular stent(s), central dialysis segment, performed through dialysis circuit, including all required imaging, radiological supervision and interpretation, image documentation and report

The physician inserts a needle or catheter into a dialysis circuit via a puncture in the skin overlying the circuit of a dialysis patient. The catheter is guided into the circuit and vessel to an area upstream of the site under investigation, and contrast material is injected into it. A catheter with a balloon attached is inserted into the central dialysis segment and fed into the narrowed portion, where its balloon may be inflated several times in order to stretch the diameter, allowing a more normal blood flow through the area. This code reports the initial access, including shunt access, contrast injections, and all fluoroscopic imaging deemed necessary from the arterial anastomosis and adjacent artery through the entire venous outflow (inferior and superior vena cava included). Report C7514 if transcatheter stent placement is also performed. A catheter with a stent-transporting tip is threaded over the guidewire into the central dialysis segment and the wire is extracted. The catheter travels to the point where the vessel needs additional support. The compressed stent is passed from the catheter out into the vessel, where it deploys, expanding to support the vessel walls. Once the procedure is complete, the catheter is removed and pressure is applied over the puncture site. All radiological supervision and interpretation, as well as image documentation and report, are included in these codes.

C7515

C7515 Dialysis circuit, introduction of needle(s) and/or catheter(s), with diagnostic angiography of the dialysis circuit, including all direct puncture(s) and catheter placement(s), injection(s) of contrast, all necessary imaging from the arterial anastomosis and adjacent artery through entire venous outflow including the inferior or superior vena cava, fluoroscopic guidance, with dialysis circuit permanent endovascular embolization or occlusion of main circuit or any accessory veins, including all required imaging, radiological supervision and interpretation, image documentation and report

The physician inserts a needle or catheter into a dialysis circuit via a puncture in the skin overlying the circuit of a dialysis patient. The catheter is guided into the circuit and vessel to an area upstream of the site under investigation, and contrast material is injected into it. Following diagnostic angiography, the physician performs embolization or occlusion of the dialysis circuit (main circuit or any accessory vein) due to complications or to assist in circuit maturity and/or patency. A guidewire is threaded through the needle into the vessel. The needle is removed. A catheter is threaded into the vessel and the wire is extracted. The catheter travels to the appropriate blood vessel and beads, coils, or other vessel-blocking devices are released. The catheter is removed and pressure is applied over the puncture site to stop bleeding. This code reports the initial access, including shunt access, contrast injections, and all fluoroscopic imaging deemed necessary from the arterial anastomosis and adjacent artery through the entire venous outflow (inferior and superior vena cava included). All radiological supervision and interpretation, as well as image documentation and report, is included.

C7516

C7516 Catheter placement in coronary artery(s) for coronary angiography, including intraprocedural injection(s) for coronary angiography, with endoluminal imaging of initial coronary vessel or graft using intravascular ultrasound (IVUS) or optical coherence tomography (OCT) during diagnostic evaluation and/or therapeutic intervention including imaging supervision, interpretation and report

The physician performs a catheter placement in one or more coronary arteries for coronary angiography, without concomitant left heart catheterization. The physician places an introducer sheath in an artery, typically the femoral artery, using percutaneous puncture; an angiography catheter is advanced through the introducer sheath into the ascending aorta, under fluoroscopic guidance, to the opening of the coronary artery. Radiopaque contrast material is injected through the catheter into the vessel while a cineangiogram is recorded. Intravascular ultrasound (IVUS) or optical coherence tomography (OCT) may be used for endoluminal imaging during diagnostic evaluation of a coronary vessel or graft. It may also be used before and after a therapeutic intervention on a coronary vessel or graft to assess patency and integrity of the vessel or graft. An intravascular ultrasound catheter is placed over a guidewire; the ultrasound probe is used to obtain images from inside the vessel to assess the area and extent of disease prior to interventional therapy, as well as adequacy of therapy after interventional therapy. The ultrasound probe provides a two-dimensional, cross-sectional view of the vessel or graft as the probe is advanced and withdrawn along the area of interest. When the ultrasound examination is complete, the catheter is removed. OCT utilizes light instead of sound to provide cross-sectional images in high resolution within the lumen. Following removal of catheters and sheaths, pressure is placed on the wound for 20 to 30 minutes to stem bleeding. This code includes imaging supervision and interpretation, as well as any required repositioning of catheters.

C7517

C7517 Catheter placement in coronary artery(s) for coronary angiography, including intraprocedural injection(s) for coronary angiography, with iliac and/or femoral artery angiography, nonselective, bilateral or ipsilateral to catheter insertion, performed at the same time as cardiac catheterization and/or coronary angiography, includes positioning or placement of the catheter in the distal aorta or ipsilateral femoral or iliac artery, injection of dye, production of permanent images, and radiologic supervision and interpretation

The physician performs a catheter placement in one or more coronary arteries for coronary angiography. The physician places an introducer sheath in an artery, typically the femoral artery, using percutaneous puncture. The physician advances an angiography catheter through the introducer sheath into the ascending aorta and advances it, under fluoroscopic guidance, to the opening of the coronary artery. Radiopaque contrast material is injected through the catheter into the vessel while a cineangiogram is recorded. The catheter is threaded over the guidewire from the access site, is positioned nonselectively in the distal aorta or iliac artery, and radiological examination of the iliac artery is performed. Contrast medium is injected, and a series of permanent images are taken to visualize the vessels and evaluate any abnormalities. Following removal of catheters and sheaths, pressure is placed on the wound for 20 to 30 minutes to stem bleeding. This code includes imaging supervision and interpretation, as well as any required repositioning of catheters.

C7518

C7518 Catheter placement in coronary artery(ies) for coronary angiography, including intraprocedural injection(s) for coronary angiography, imaging supervision and interpretation, with catheter placement(s) in bypass graft(s) (internal mammary, free arterial, venous grafts) including intraprocedural injection(s) for bypass graft angiography with endoluminal imaging of initial coronary vessel or graft using intravascular ultrasound (IVUS) or optical coherence tomography (OCT) during diagnostic evaluation and/or therapeutic intervention including imaging, supervision, interpretation and report

The physician performs a catheter placement in one or more coronary arteries and bypass grafts (i.e., internal mammary, free arterial, or venous grafts) for coronary and bypass graft angiography, without concomitant left heart catheterization. The physician places an introducer sheath in an artery, typically the femoral artery, using percutaneous puncture. The physician advances an angiography catheter through the introducer sheath into the ascending aorta and advances it, under fluoroscopic guidance, to the opening of the coronary artery or the bypass graft. The physician injects radiopaque contrast material through the catheter into the vessel while recording a cineangiogram. Intravascular ultrasound (IVUS) or optical coherence tomography (OCT) may be used for endoluminal imaging during diagnostic evaluation of a coronary vessel or graft. It may also be used before and after a therapeutic intervention on a coronary vessel or graft to assess patency and integrity of the vessel or graft. An intravascular ultrasound catheter is placed over a guidewire; the ultrasound probe is used to obtain images from inside the vessel to assess the area and extent of disease prior to interventional therapy, as well as adequacy of therapy after interventional therapy. The ultrasound probe provides a two-dimensional, cross-sectional view of the vessel or graft as the probe is advanced and withdrawn along the area of interest. When the ultrasound examination is complete, the catheter is removed. OCT utilizes light instead of sound to provide cross-sectional images in high resolution within the lumen. Following removal of catheters and sheaths, pressure is placed on the wound for 20 to 30 minutes to stem bleeding. This code includes imaging supervision and interpretation, as well as any required repositioning of catheters.

C7519

C7519 Catheter placement in coronary artery(ies) for coronary angiography, including intraprocedural injection(s) for coronary angiography, imaging supervision and interpretation, with catheter placement(s) in bypass graft(s) (internal mammary, free arterial, venous grafts) including intraprocedural injection(s) for bypass graft angiography with intravascular doppler velocity and/or pressure derived coronary flow reserve measurement (initial coronary vessel or graft) during coronary angiography including pharmacologically induced stress

The physician performs a catheter placement in one or more coronary arteries and bypass grafts (i.e., internal mammary, free arterial, or venous grafts) for coronary and bypass graft angiography, without concomitant left heart catheterization. The physician places an introducer sheath in an artery, typically the femoral artery, using percutaneous puncture. The physician places an angiography catheter through the introducer sheath into the ascending aorta and advances it, under fluoroscopic guidance, to the opening of the coronary artery or the bypass graft. Radiopaque contrast material is injected through the catheter into the vessel while a cineangiogram is recorded. During the angiography, the physician exchanges the guidewire through the balloon for the Doppler wire. The physician employs a miniaturized Doppler transducer mounted at the tip of a specialized guidewire and inserted through the diagnostic catheter to record intravascular coronary blood flow velocity measurement distal to a coronary lesion (both before and after administration of a pharmacologic stress agent such as adenosine). This device is small enough to be advanced beyond a coronary lesion without significantly increasing any occlusion; measurements are indicative of the hemodynamic significance of the stenosis and assist the practitioner in determining the benefit or necessity of a specific intervention, such as angioplasty or stents. Following removal of catheters and sheaths, pressure is placed on the wound for 20 to 30 minutes to stem bleeding. This code includes imaging supervision and interpretation, as well as any required repositioning of catheters.

C7520

C7520 Catheter placement in coronary artery(ies) for coronary angiography, including intraprocedural injection(s) for coronary angiography, imaging supervision and interpretation, with catheter placement(s) in bypass graft(s) (internal mammary, free arterial, venous grafts) includes intraprocedural injection(s) for bypass graft angiography with iliac and/or femoral artery angiography, nonselective, bilateral or ipsilateral to catheter insertion, performed at the same time as cardiac catheterization and/or coronary angiography, includes positioning or placement of the catheter in the distal aorta or ipsilateral femoral or iliac artery, injection of dye, production of permanent images, and radiologic supervision and interpretation

The physician performs a catheter placement in one or more coronary arteries for coronary angiography. An introducer sheath is placed into an artery, typically the femoral artery, using percutaneous puncture. The physician advances an angiography catheter through the introducer sheath into the ascending aorta and advances it, under fluoroscopic guidance, to the opening of the coronary artery. Radiopaque contrast material is injected through the catheter into the vessel while a cineangiogram is recorded. The catheter is threaded over the guidewire from the access site, is positioned nonselectively in the distal aorta or iliac artery, and radiological examination of the iliac artery is performed. Contrast medium is injected, and a series of permanent images are taken to visualize the vessels and evaluate any abnormalities. Following removal of catheters and sheaths, pressure is placed on the wound for 20 to 30 minutes to stem bleeding. This code includes imaging supervision and interpretation, as well as any required repositioning of catheters.

C7521

C7521 Catheter placement in coronary artery(ies) for coronary angiography, including intraprocedural injection(s) for coronary angiography with right heart catheterization with endoluminal imaging of initial coronary vessel or graft using intravascular ultrasound (IVUS) or optical coherence tomography (OCT) during diagnostic evaluation and/or therapeutic intervention including imaging supervision, interpretation and report

The physician performs a catheter placement in one or more coronary arteries for coronary angiography with concomitant right heart catheterization. An introducer sheath is placed into an artery, typically the femoral artery, using percutaneous puncture. The physician advances an angiography catheter through the introducer sheath into the ascending aorta and advances it, under fluoroscopic guidance, to the opening of the coronary artery. Radiopaque contrast material is injected through the catheter into the vessel while a cineangiogram is recorded. A right heart catheterization is also performed, in which the catheter is threaded into the right atrium, through the tricuspid valve into the right ventricle, and across the pulmonary valve into the pulmonary arteries. Intravascular ultrasound (IVUS) or optical coherence tomography (OCT) may be used for endoluminal imaging during the diagnostic evaluation of the coronary vessels or grafts. It may also be used before and after therapeutic interventions on coronary vessels or grafts to assess patency and integrity. An intravascular ultrasound catheter is placed over a guidewire; the ultrasound probe is used to obtain images from inside the vessel to assess area and extent of disease prior to interventional therapy, as well as adequacy of therapy after interventional therapy. The ultrasound probe provides a two-dimensional, cross-sectional view of the vessel or graft as the probe is advanced and withdrawn along the area of interest. When the ultrasound examination is complete, the catheter is removed. OCT utilizes light instead of sound to provide cross-sectional images in high resolution within the lumen. Following removal of catheters and sheaths, pressure is placed on the wound for 20 to 30 minutes to stem bleeding. This code includes imaging supervision, interpretation, and report.

C7522

C7522 Catheter placement in coronary artery(ies) for coronary angiography, including intraprocedural injection(s) for coronary angiography, imaging supervision and interpretation with right heart catheterization, with intravascular doppler velocity and/or pressure derived coronary flow reserve measurement (initial coronary vessel or graft) during coronary angiography including pharmacologically induced stress

The physician performs a catheter placement in one or more coronary arteries for coronary angiography with concomitant right heart catheterization. An introducer sheath is placed into an artery, typically the femoral artery, using percutaneous puncture. The physician advances an angiography catheter through the introducer sheath into the ascending aorta and advances it, under fluoroscopic guidance, to the opening of the coronary artery. Radiopaque contrast material is injected through the catheter into the vessel while a cineangiogram is recorded. A right heart catheterization is also performed, in which the catheter is threaded into the right atrium, through the tricuspid valve into the right ventricle, and across the pulmonary valve into the pulmonary arteries. During the angiography, the physician employs a miniaturized Doppler transducer mounted at the tip of a specialized guidewire and inserted through the diagnostic catheter to record intravascular coronary blood flow velocity measurement distal to a coronary lesion (both before and after administration of a pharmacologic stress agent such as adenosine). This device is small enough to be advanced beyond a coronary lesion without significantly increasing any occlusion; measurements are indicative of the hemodynamic significance of the stenosis and assist the practitioner in determining the benefit or necessity of a specific intervention, such as angioplasty or stents. Upon completion of the procedure, the physician removes the catheter and sheath from the artery of access. Pressure is placed on the wound for 20 to 30 minutes to stem bleeding. This code includes imaging supervision and interpretation.

C7523

C7523 Catheter placement in coronary artery(ies) for coronary angiography, including intraprocedural injection(s) for coronary angiography, imaging supervision and interpretation, with left heart catheterization including intraprocedural injection(s) for left ventriculography, when performed, with endoluminal imaging of initial coronary vessel or graft using intravascular ultrasound (IVUS) or optical coherence tomography (OCT) during diagnostic evaluation and/or therapeutic intervention including imaging supervision, interpretation and report

The physician places a catheter into one or more coronary arteries for coronary angiography. The physician threads a catheter to the heart, most frequently through an introducing sheath placed percutaneously into the femoral, brachial, or axillary artery using retrograde technique. The catheter passes through the aortic valve into the left ventricle. Intracardiac and intravascular pressures are recorded. Left ventricular injections may be performed for left ventriculography; the physician injects dye through a previously placed catheter threaded through a central line into the left ventricle or atrium to evaluate function with fluoroscopy. Intravascular ultrasound (IVUS) or optical coherence tomography (OCT) may be used for endoluminal imaging during diagnostic evaluation of a coronary vessel or graft. It may also be used before and after a therapeutic intervention on a coronary vessel or graft to assess patency and integrity of the vessel or graft. An IVUS catheter is placed over a guidewire; the ultrasound probe is used to obtain images from inside the vessel to assess the area and extent of disease prior to interventional therapy, as well as adequacy of therapy after interventional therapy. The ultrasound probe provides a two-dimensional, cross-sectional view of the vessel or graft as the probe is advanced and withdrawn along the area of interest. When the ultrasound

C

examination is complete, the catheter is removed. OCT utilizes light instead of sound to provide cross-sectional images in high resolution within the lumen. Following removal of catheters and sheaths, pressure is placed on the wound for 20 to 30 minutes to stem bleeding. This code includes imaging supervision and interpretation, as well as any required repositioning of catheters.

C7524

C7524 Catheter placement in coronary artery(ies) for coronary angiography, including intraprocedural injection(s) for coronary angiography, imaging supervision and interpretation, with left heart catheterization including intraprocedural injection(s) for left ventriculography, when performed, with intravascular doppler velocity and/or pressure derived coronary flow reserve measurement (initial coronary vessel or graft) during coronary angiography including pharmacologically induced stress

The physician places a catheter into one or more coronary arteries for coronary angiography. The physician threads a catheter to the heart, most frequently through an introducing sheath placed percutaneously into the femoral, brachial, or axillary artery using retrograde technique. The catheter passes through the aortic valve into the left ventricle. Intracardiac and intravascular pressures are recorded. Left ventricular injections may be performed for left ventriculography; the physician injects dye through a previously placed catheter threaded through a central line into the left ventricle or atrium to evaluate function with fluoroscopy. During the angiography, the physician employs a miniaturized Doppler transducer mounted at the tip of a specialized guidewire and inserted through the diagnostic catheter to record intravascular coronary blood flow velocity measurement distal to a coronary lesion (both before and after administration of a pharmacologic stress agent such as adenosine). This device is small enough to be advanced beyond a coronary lesion without significantly increasing any occlusion; measurements are indicative of the hemodynamic significance of the stenosis and assist the practitioner in determining the benefit or necessity of a specific intervention, such as angioplasty or stents. Upon completion of the procedure, the physician removes the catheter and sheath from the artery of access. Pressure is placed on the wound for 20 to 30 minutes to stem bleeding. This code includes imaging supervision and interpretation.

C7525

C7525 Catheter placement in coronary artery(ies) for coronary angiography, including intraprocedural injection(s) for coronary angiography, imaging supervision and interpretation, with left heart catheterization including intraprocedural injection(s) for left ventriculography, when performed, catheter placement(s) in bypass graft(s) (internal mammary, free arterial, venous grafts) with bypass graft angiography with endoluminal imaging of initial coronary vessel or graft using intravascular ultrasound (IVUS) or optical coherence tomography (OCT) during diagnostic evaluation and/or therapeutic intervention including imaging supervision, interpretation and report

The physician places a catheter into one or more coronary arteries (including catheter placement in internal mammary, free arterial, or venous bypass grafts) for coronary angiography. The physician threads a catheter to the heart, most frequently through an introducing sheath placed percutaneously into the femoral, brachial, or axillary artery using retrograde technique. The catheter passes through the aortic valve into the left ventricle. Intracardiac and intravascular pressures are recorded. Left ventricular injections may be performed for left ventriculography; the physician injects dye through a previously placed catheter threaded through a central line into the left ventricle or atrium to evaluate function with fluoroscopy. Endoluminal imaging of the initial coronary vessel or graft using intravascular ultrasound (IVUS) or optical coherence tomography (OCT) is performed during the diagnostic evaluation and/or any therapeutic intervention to assess patency and integrity of the vessel or graft. An IVUS catheter is placed over a guidewire; the ultrasound probe is used to obtain images from inside the vessel to assess area and extent of disease prior to interventional therapy, as well as adequacy of therapy after interventional therapy. The ultrasound probe provides a two-dimensional, cross-sectional view of the vessel or graft as the probe is advanced and withdrawn along the area of interest. When the ultrasound examination is complete, the catheter is removed. OCT utilizes light instead of sound to provide cross-sectional images in high resolution within the lumen. Following removal of catheters and sheaths, pressure is placed on the wound for 20 to 30 minutes to stem bleeding. This code includes imaging supervision, interpretation, and report.

C7526

C7526 Catheter placement in coronary artery(ies) for coronary angiography, including intraprocedural injection(s) for coronary angiography, imaging supervision and interpretation, with left heart catheterization including intraprocedural injection(s) for left ventriculography, when performed, catheter placement(s) in bypass graft(s) (internal mammary, free arterial, venous grafts) with bypass graft angiography with intravascular doppler velocity and/or pressure derived coronary flow reserve measurement (initial coronary vessel or graft) during coronary angiography including pharmacologically induced stress

The physician places a catheter into one or more coronary arteries for coronary angiography (including catheter placement in internal mammary, free arterial, or venous bypass grafts for bypass angiography). The physician threads a catheter to the heart, most frequently through an introducing sheath placed percutaneously into the femoral, brachial, or axillary artery using retrograde technique. The catheter passes through the aortic valve into the left ventricle. Intracardiac and intravascular pressures are recorded. Left ventricular injections may be performed for left ventriculography; the physician injects dye through a previously placed catheter threaded through a central line into the left ventricle or atrium to evaluate function with fluoroscopy. During the angiography, the physician employs a miniaturized Doppler transducer mounted at the tip of a specialized guidewire and inserted through the diagnostic catheter to record intravascular coronary blood flow velocity measurement distal to a coronary lesion (both before and after administration of a pharmacologic stress agent such as adenosine). This device is small enough to be advanced beyond a coronary lesion without significantly increasing any occlusion; measurements are indicative of the hemodynamic significance of the stenosis and assist the practitioner in determining the benefit or necessity of a specific intervention, such as angioplasty or stents. Upon completion of the procedure, the physician removes the catheter and sheath from the artery of access. Pressure is placed on the wound for 20 to 30 minutes to stem bleeding. This code includes imaging supervision and interpretation, as well as pharmacologically-induced stress.

C7527

C7527 Catheter placement in coronary artery(ies) for coronary angiography, including intraprocedural injection(s) for coronary angiography, imaging supervision and interpretation, with right and left heart catheterization including intraprocedural injection(s) for left ventriculography, when performed, with endoluminal imaging of initial coronary vessel or graft using intravascular ultrasound (IVUS) or optical coherence tomography (OCT) during diagnostic evaluation and/or therapeutic intervention including imaging supervision, interpretation and report

The physician places a catheter in one or more coronary arteries for coronary angiography; right and left heart function is evaluated. To accomplish right heart catheterization, the physician threads a catheter through an introducing sheath placed percutaneously into the femoral, subclavian, internal jugular, or antecubital vein. The catheter is threaded into the right atrium, through the tricuspid valve into the right ventricle, and across the pulmonary valve into the pulmonary arteries. Left heart catheterization is also performed, in this scenario using retrograde technique. The catheter is inserted through an introducing sheath placed percutaneously into the femoral, brachial, or axillary artery. The catheter is passed through the aortic valve into the left ventricle. Intracardiac and intravascular pressures are recorded. Left ventricular injections may be performed for left ventriculography; the physician injects dye through a previously placed catheter threaded through a central line into the left ventricle or atrium to evaluate function with fluoroscopy. Endoluminal imaging of the initial coronary vessel or graft using intravascular ultrasound (IVUS) or optical coherence tomography (OCT) is performed during the diagnostic evaluation and/or any therapeutic intervention to assess patency and integrity of the vessel or graft. An IVUS catheter is placed over a guidewire; the ultrasound probe is used to obtain images from inside the vessel to assess the area and extent of disease prior to interventional therapy, as well as adequacy of therapy after interventional therapy. The ultrasound probe provides a two-dimensional, cross-sectional view of the vessel as the probe is advanced and withdrawn along the area of interest. When the ultrasound examination is complete, the catheter is removed. OCT utilizes light instead of sound to provide cross-sectional images in high resolution within the lumen. Following removal of catheters and sheaths, pressure is placed on the wound for 20 to 30 minutes to stem bleeding. This code includes imaging supervision, interpretation, and report.

C

C7528

C7528 Catheter placement in coronary artery(ies) for coronary angiography, including intraprocedural injection(s) for coronary angiography, imaging supervision and interpretation, with right and left heart catheterization including intraprocedural injection(s) for left ventriculography, when performed, with intravascular doppler velocity and/or pressure derived coronary flow reserve measurement (initial coronary vessel or graft) during coronary angiography including pharmacologically induced stress

The physician places a catheter in one or more coronary arteries for coronary angiography; right and left heart function is evaluated. To accomplish right heart catheterization, the physician threads a catheter through an introducing sheath placed percutaneously into the femoral, subclavian, internal jugular, or antecubital vein. The catheter is threaded into the right atrium, through the tricuspid valve into the right ventricle, and across the pulmonary valve into the pulmonary arteries. Left heart catheterization is also performed, in this scenario using retrograde technique. The catheter is inserted through an introducing sheath placed percutaneously into the femoral, brachial, or axillary artery. The catheter is passed through the aortic valve into the left ventricle. Intracardiac and intravascular pressures are recorded. Left ventricular injections may be performed for left ventriculography; the physician injects dye through a previously placed catheter threaded through a central line into the left ventricle or atrium to evaluate function with fluoroscopy. During the angiography, the physician employs a miniaturized Doppler transducer mounted at the tip of a specialized guidewire and inserted through the diagnostic catheter to record intravascular coronary blood flow velocity measurement distal to a coronary lesion (both before and after administration of a pharmacologic stress agent such as adenosine). This device is small enough to be advanced beyond a coronary lesion without significantly increasing any occlusion; measurements are indicative of the hemodynamic significance of the stenosis and assist the practitioner in determining the benefit or necessity of a specific intervention, such as angioplasty or stents. Upon completion of the procedure, the physician removes the catheter and sheath from the artery of access. Pressure is placed on the wound for 20 to 30 minutes to stem bleeding. This code includes imaging supervision and interpretation.

C7529

C7529 Catheter placement in coronary artery(ies) for coronary angiography, including intraprocedural injection(s) for coronary angiography, imaging supervision and interpretation, with right and left heart catheterization including intraprocedural injection(s) for left ventriculography, when performed, catheter placement(s) in bypass graft(s) (internal mammary, free arterial, venous grafts) with bypass graft angiography with intravascular doppler velocity and/or pressure derived coronary flow reserve measurement (initial coronary vessel or graft) during coronary angiography including pharmacologically induced stress

The physician places a catheter in one or more coronary arteries for coronary angiography (including catheter placement in internal mammary, free arterial, or venous bypass grafts for bypass angiography); right and left heart function is evaluated. To accomplish right heart catheterization, the physician threads a catheter through an introducing sheath placed percutaneously into the femoral, subclavian, internal jugular, or antecubital vein. The catheter is threaded into the right atrium, through the tricuspid valve into the right ventricle, and across the pulmonary valve into the pulmonary arteries. Left heart catheterization is also performed, in this scenario using retrograde technique. The catheter is inserted through an introducing sheath placed percutaneously into the femoral, brachial, or axillary artery. The catheter is passed through the aortic valve into the left ventricle. Intracardiac and intravascular pressures are recorded. Left ventricular injections may be performed for left ventriculography; the physician injects dye through a previously placed catheter threaded through a central line into the left ventricle or atrium to evaluate function with fluoroscopy. During the angiography, the physician employs a miniaturized Doppler transducer mounted at the tip of a specialized guidewire and inserted through the diagnostic catheter to record intravascular coronary blood flow velocity measurement distal to a coronary lesion (both before and after administration of a pharmacologic stress agent such as adenosine). This device is small enough to be advanced beyond a coronary lesion without significantly increasing any occlusion; measurements are indicative of the hemodynamic significance of the stenosis and assist the practitioner in determining the benefit or necessity of a specific intervention, such as angioplasty or stents. Upon completion of the procedure, the physician removes the catheter and sheath from the artery of access. Pressure is placed on the wound for 20 to 30 minutes to stem bleeding. This code includes imaging supervision and interpretation, as well as pharmacologically-induced stress.

C7530

C7530 Dialysis circuit, introduction of needle(s) and/or catheter(s), with diagnostic angiography of the dialysis circuit, including all direct puncture(s) and catheter placement(s), injection(s) of contrast, all necessary imaging from the arterial anastomosis and adjacent artery through entire venous outflow including the inferior or superior vena cava, fluoroscopic guidance, with transluminal balloon angioplasty, peripheral dialysis segment, including all imaging and radiological supervision and interpretation necessary to perform the angioplasty and all angioplasty in the central dialysis segment, with transcatheter placement of intravascular stent(s), central dialysis segment, performed through dialysis circuit, including all imaging, radiological supervision and interpretation, documentation and report

The physician inserts a needle or catheter into a dialysis circuit via a puncture in the skin overlying the circuit of a dialysis patient. The catheter is guided into the circuit and vessel to an area upstream of the site under investigation, and contrast material is injected into it. A catheter with a balloon attached is inserted into the peripheral dialysis segment and fed into the narrowed portion, where its balloon may be inflated several times to stretch the diameter, allowing a more normal blood flow through the area. A catheter with a stent-transporting tip is threaded over the guidewire into the central dialysis segment and the wire is extracted. The catheter travels to the point where the vessel needs additional support. The compressed stent is passed from the catheter out into the vessel, where it deploys, expanding to support the vessel walls. Once the procedure is complete, the catheter is removed, and pressure is applied over the puncture site. This code reports the initial access, including shunt access, contrast injections, all fluoroscopic imaging deemed necessary from the arterial anastomosis and adjacent artery through the entire venous outflow (inferior and superior vena cava included), and angioplasty of the central dialysis segment. All radiological supervision and interpretation, as well as image documentation and report, is also included.

C7531

C7531 Revascularization, endovascular, open or percutaneous, femoral, popliteal artery(ies), unilateral, with transluminal angioplasty with intravascular ultrasound (initial noncoronary vessel) during diagnostic evaluation and/or therapeutic intervention, including radiological supervision and interpretation

The physician treats occlusive disease of a unilateral femoral or popliteal artery by endovascular revascularization (restoration of blood supply) using angioplasty. Access is gained using a femoral cutdown incision or a percutaneous sheath. Under local anesthesia, the physician accesses the femoral artery. After sheath or needle placement, intra-arterial heparin may be administered. A guidewire is inserted into the artery, followed by a catheter with an attached balloon. The catheter is advanced through the arterial system and into the narrowed portion of the targeted artery. There, the balloon is inflated to dilate the vessel to a larger diameter; several inflations may be necessary to achieve maximal results. An intravascular ultrasound catheter is placed over the guidewire before, during, and/or after the angioplasty to assess patency and integrity of the vessel or for diagnostic evaluation. The ultrasound catheter may be used to obtain images from inside the vessel to assess the area and extent of disease prior to interventional therapy, as well as adequacy of therapy after interventional therapy. The physician withdraws the catheter and guidewire and applies pressure to the puncture site to staunch the bleeding or closes the arteriotomy with suture. This code includes radiological supervision and interpretation.

C7532

C7532 Transluminal balloon angioplasty (except lower extremity artery(ies) for occlusive disease, intracranial, coronary, pulmonary, or dialysis circuit), initial artery, open or percutaneous, including all imaging and radiological supervision and interpretation necessary to perform the angioplasty within the same artery, with intravascular ultrasound (initial noncoronary vessel) during diagnostic evaluation and/or therapeutic intervention, including radiological supervision and interpretation

Transluminal balloon angioplasty is performed by open or percutaneous approach (except lower limb arterial occlusion, intracranial, coronary, pulmonary, or dialysis circuit). In an open procedure, the physician makes an incision in the skin overlying the initial artery. The vessel is dissected from adjacent critical structures, and vessel clamps are applied. The physician may nick the vessel to create an opening into which a catheter with a balloon attached is inserted into the vessel and threaded. The catheter is fed into the narrowed portion of the vessel, where its

C

balloon is inflated in the narrowed area. The blood vessel is stretched to a larger diameter, allowing a more normal outflow of blood through the area. Several inflations may be performed along the narrowed area. In a percutaneous approach, the physician isolates the initial artery and inserts a large needle through the skin and into the vessel. A guidewire is threaded through the needle into the vessel. The needle is removed. A catheter with a balloon attached follows the wire into the vessel. The wire is removed. The catheter is fed through the vascular system and into the narrowed portion of the affected vessel and the balloon is inflated. The blood vessel is stretched to a larger diameter, allowing a more normal outflow of blood through the area. Several inflations may be performed along the narrowed area. An intravascular ultrasound catheter is placed over the guidewire before, during, and/or after the angioplasty to assess patency and integrity of the vessel or for diagnostic evaluation. The ultrasound catheter may be used to obtain images from inside the vessel to assess area and extent of disease prior to interventional therapy, as well as adequacy of therapy after interventional therapy. The physician withdraws the catheter and guidewire and applies pressure to the puncture site to staunch the bleeding or closes the arteriotomy with suture. This code includes all imaging and radiological supervision and interpretation within the same artery.

C7533

C7533 Percutaneous transluminal coronary angioplasty, single major coronary artery or branch with transcatheter placement of radiation delivery device for subsequent coronary intravascular brachytherapy

The physician makes a small incision in the arm or leg to access a single major coronary artery or branch for placement of two catheters. A central venous catheter is inserted through the femoral or brachial artery and a second catheter with a balloon tip is threaded up to the heart and into an obstructed native coronary artery. The physician inflates the balloon at the tip of the second catheter to flatten plaque obstructing the artery against the walls of the coronary artery. If sufficient results are not obtained after the first inflation, the physician may reinflate the balloon for a longer period of time or at greater pressure. The physician places a delivery catheter in the coronary artery. The transfer delivery device is connected to the delivery catheter; the transfer delivery device is used to deliver the radioactive seeds to the location. There are various methods for transcatheter placement, but commonly the methods involve the use of a guiding catheter. The radioactive seeds are positioned by a radiation oncologist at the location for an appropriate length of time to administer radiation to the artery. At the completion of the radiation treatment, the radioactive seeds are returned to the transfer device. The catheters are removed. Pressure is placed over the incision for 20 to 30 minutes to stop bleeding.

C7534-C7535

C7534 Revascularization, endovascular, open or percutaneous, femoral, popliteal artery(ies), unilateral, with atherectomy, includes angioplasty within the same vessel, when performed with intravascular ultrasound (initial noncoronary vessel) during diagnostic evaluation and/or therapeutic intervention, including radiological supervision and interpretation

C7535 Revascularization, endovascular, open or percutaneous, femoral, popliteal artery(ies), unilateral, with transluminal stent placement(s), includes angioplasty within the same vessel, when performed, with intravascular ultrasound (initial noncoronary vessel) during diagnostic evaluation and/or therapeutic intervention, including radiological supervision and interpretation

The physician treats occlusive disease of a unilateral femoral or popliteal artery by endovascular revascularization (restoration of blood supply) using atherectomy in C7534. Access is gained using a femoral cutdown incision or a percutaneous sheath. Under local anesthesia, the physician accesses the femoral artery. After sheath or needle placement, intra-arterial heparin may be administered. The physician slides a guidewire through the atherectomy catheter or device and inserts the guidewire/atherectomy catheter combination through the introducer sheath. The atherectomy device is fluoroscopically positioned at the site of the stenosis. The physician activates the device to remove the stenotic tissue and rechecks the diameter of the lesion by angiography. Several passes with the atherectomy device may be required. In C7535, a catheter with a stent-transporting tip is threaded into the vessel. The catheter travels to the point where the vessel needs additional support, and the compressed stent is passed from the catheter into the vessel, where it deploys and expands to support the vessel walls. In C7534 and C7535, an intravascular ultrasound catheter is placed over the guidewire before, during, and/or after the therapeutic intervention to assess patency and integrity of the vessel or for diagnostic evaluation. The ultrasound catheter may be used to obtain images from inside the vessel to assess area and extent of disease prior to interventional therapy, as well as adequacy of therapy after interventional therapy. The physician withdraws the catheter and guidewire and applies pressure to the puncture site to staunch the bleeding or closes the arteriotomy with suture. These codes include all imaging and radiological supervision and interpretation. Angioplasty within the same vessel is included.

C7537-C7539

C7537 Insertion of new or replacement of permanent pacemaker with atrial transvenous electrode(s), with insertion of pacing electrode, cardiac venous system, for left ventricular pacing, at time of insertion of implantable defibrillator or pacemaker pulse generator (e.g., for upgrade to dual chamber system)

C7538 Insertion of new or replacement of permanent pacemaker with ventricular transvenous electrode(s), with insertion of pacing electrode, cardiac venous system, for left ventricular pacing, at time of insertion of implantable defibrillator or pacemaker pulse generator (e.g., for upgrade to dual chamber system)

C7539 Insertion of new or replacement of permanent pacemaker with atrial and ventricular transvenous electrode(s), with insertion of pacing electrode, cardiac venous system, for left ventricular pacing, at time of insertion of implantable defibrillator or pacemaker pulse generator (e.g., for upgrade to dual chamber system)

The physician inserts or replaces a permanent pacemaker with transvenous electrodes. Under appropriate anesthesia, the physician gains access to the central caval veins typically via a percutaneous approach through the subclavian vein or employing a cut-down technique to the cephalic vein. Less commonly, the axillary, internal jugular, or femoral vein may be used. The chosen vein is penetrated with a large needle and a wire is passed through it. A fluoroscope is used to guide the wire into the appropriate chamber of the heart. A pocket for the pacemaker generator is created and the wire is tested. The wire is connected to the generator. An additional electrode is placed in the left ventricle for biventricular pacing. A fluoroscope may be used for guidance and a pacing electrode is inserted in the left ventricular chamber of the heart, usually in the coronary sinus tributary. The generator is upgraded to a dual chamber system. The electrode is connected to the pulse generator and the pocket is closed. Report C7537 if the guide and pacemaker wires are placed in the right atrium only; C7538 if the guide and pacemaker wires are placed in the right ventricle only; and C7539 if the guide and pacemaker wires are placed into both the right atrium and right ventricle.

C7540

C7540 Removal of permanent pacemaker pulse generator with replacement of pacemaker pulse generator, dual lead system, with insertion of pacing electrode, cardiac venous system, for left ventricular pacing, at time of insertion of implantable defibrillator or pacemaker pulse generator (e.g., for upgrade to dual chamber system)

A permanent pacemaker pulse generator is removed and replaced. The pacemaker generator pocket is opened. The existing generator is disconnected from any existing wires and removed. The wires are left in place in the pocket and a new permanent pacemaker pulse generator dual lead system is inserted. The existing pacer wires are tested and connected to the generator. An additional electrode is placed in the left ventricle for biventricular pacing. A fluoroscope may be used for guidance and a pacing electrode is inserted in the left ventricular chamber of the heart, usually in the coronary sinus tributary. The generator is upgraded to a dual chamber system. The electrode is connected to the pulse generator and the pocket is closed.

C7541-C7542

C7541 Diagnostic endoscopic retrograde cholangiopancreatography (ERCP), including collection of specimen(s) by brushing or washing, when performed, with endoscopic cannulation of papilla with direct visualization of pancreatic/common bile ducts(s)

C7542 Endoscopic retrograde cholangiopancreatography (ERCP) with biopsy, single or multiple, with endoscopic cannulation of papilla with direct visualization of pancreatic/common bile ducts(s)

The physician performs an endoscopic retrograde cholangiopancreatography (ERCP) for diagnostic purposes. The physician passes the endoscope through the patient's oropharynx, esophagus, stomach, and into the small intestine. The ampulla of Vater is cannulated and filled with contrast. The common bile duct and the whole biliary tract, including the gallbladder, are visualized. Diagnostic brushing and washing may be performed and reported with C7541. Alternately, one or more biopsies may be performed and reported with C7542. During the same operative episode, the physician performs endoscopic cannulation of papilla with direct visualization of the pancreatic and/or common bile ducts. A catheter or papillotome is inserted through the channel of the ERCP scope. With or without the use of a guidewire, the pancreatic and/or common bile ducts are located and visually inspected.

C7543

C7543 Endoscopic retrograde cholangiopancreatography (ERCP) with sphincterotomy/papillotomy, with endoscopic cannulation of papilla with direct visualization of pancreatic/common bile ducts(s)

The physician performs an endoscopic retrograde cholangiopancreatography (ERCP) with a sphincter/papillotomy. The physician passes the endoscope through the patient's oropharynx, esophagus, stomach, and into the small intestine. The ampulla of Vater is cannulated and filled with contrast. The common bile duct and the whole biliary tract, including the gallbladder, are visualized. The sphincter is cannulated using a sphincterotome and divided using electrocautery to control bleeding. During the same operative episode, the physician performs endoscopic cannulation of papilla with direct visualization of the pancreatic and/or common bile ducts. A catheter or papillotome is inserted through the channel of the ERCP scope. With or without the use of a guidewire, the pancreatic and/or common bile ducts are located and visually inspected.

C7544

C7544 Endoscopic retrograde cholangiopancreatography (ERCP) with removal of calculi/debris from biliary/pancreatic duct(s), with endoscopic cannulation of papilla with direct visualization of pancreatic/common bile ducts(s)

The physician performs an endoscopic retrograde cholangiopancreatography (ERCP) to destroy or remove calculi or debris from the biliary and/or pancreatic ducts. The physician passes the endoscope through the patient's oropharynx, esophagus, stomach, and into the small intestine. The ampulla of Vater is cannulated and filled with contrast. The common bile duct and the whole biliary tract, including the gallbladder, are visualized. During the same operative episode, the physician performs endoscopic cannulation of papilla with direct visualization of the pancreatic and/or common bile ducts. A catheter or papillotome is inserted through the channel of the ERCP scope. With or without the use of a guidewire, the pancreatic and/or common bile ducts are located and visually inspected.

C7545

C7545 Percutaneous exchange of biliary drainage catheter (e.g., external, internal-external, or conversion of internal-external to external only), with removal of calculi/debris from biliary duct(s) and/or gallbladder, including destruction of calculi by any method (e.g., mechanical, electrohydraulic, lithotripsy) when performed, including diagnostic cholangiography(ies) when performed, imaging guidance (e.g., fluoroscopy), and all associated radiological supervision and interpretation

The physician exchanges a biliary drainage catheter using ultrasound and/or fluoroscopy to guide the process. A guidewire is inserted and advanced to the small bowel through the existing tube. The tube is removed, and a new tube is threaded over the guidewire. Fluoroscopy is used to assess the position of the catheter in the small bowel and within the bile ducts. Stones or debris are removed from the biliary duct and/or gallbladder. In one technique, a basket is used to capture the obstruction and break it up into fragments. The physician may also place a balloon catheter. After inflation, the balloon catheter is advanced over the guidewire multiple times until the stones or debris are cleared from the bile duct. Final adjustments are made for patient comfort, and the catheter may be sutured to the skin, capped, or a drainage bag may be attached. This code includes percutaneous exchange such as external, internal-external, or conversion of internal-external to external only. It also includes diagnostic cholangiography (when performed), imaging guidance, and all associated radiological supervision and interpretation.

C7546

C7546 Removal and replacement of externally accessible nephroureteral catheter (e.g., external/internal stent) requiring fluoroscopic guidance, with ureteral stricture balloon dilation, including imaging guidance and all associated radiological supervision and interpretation

The physician removes and replaces an externally accessible nephroureteral catheter under fluoroscopic guidance. A nephroureteral catheter is placed within the renal collecting system, through the renal pelvis and into the bladder; the other end remains outside the body for drainage. Contrast may be injected at the entry site to assess anatomy and positioning. The suture holding the pigtail in place is cut and a guidewire is threaded through the stent lumen until it exits the distal end. The original stent is removed over the guidewire. Diameter and length are noted for a new stent, which is threaded over the guidewire until the distal end forms within the bladder. Fluoroscopy is used to assess the proximal position of formation within the renal pelvis. A catheter containing a balloon is threaded over the guidewire to the ureteral stricture and the wire is removed. Balloon catheter sizes are determined based on normal ureter diameter as measured by radiological images. The balloon is inflated until stricture is minimalized; the process may be repeated until the desired result is achieved. Contrast may be injected to check position and function of the nephroureteral catheter and to determine adequate flow through the ureter. Final adjustments are made for patient comfort, and the catheter may be sutured to the skin, capped, or a drainage bag may be attached. This code includes imaging guidance and all associated radiological supervision and interpretation.

C7547

C7547 Convert nephrostomy catheter to nephroureteral catheter, percutaneous via pre-existing nephrostomy tract, with ureteral stricture balloon dilation, including diagnostic nephrostogram and/or ureterogram when performed, imaging guidance (e.g., ultrasound and/or fluoroscopy) and all associated radiological supervision and interpretation

A previously placed nephrostomy catheter is converted to a nephroureteral catheter via percutaneous approach along the current nephrostomy tract. The patient is placed face down and the conversion is performed over a stiff wire. Contrast is injected through the catheter to better visualize the kidneys and ureter. The wire is advanced, and the catheter is replaced over the wire and the wire removed. Imaging guidance assures proper placement. A catheter containing a balloon is threaded over the guidewire to a ureteral stricture and the wire is removed. Balloon catheter sizes are determined based on normal ureter diameter as measured by radiological images. The balloon is inflated until stricture is minimalized; the process may be repeated until the desired result is achieved. Contrast may be injected to check position and function of the nephroureteral catheter and to determine adequate flow through the ureter. The new nephroureteral catheter is secured to the skin with sutures. This code includes diagnostic nephrostogram and/or ureterogram, imaging guidance, and all associated radiological supervision and interpretation.

C7548

C7548 Exchange nephrostomy catheter, percutaneous, with ureteral stricture balloon dilation, including diagnostic nephrostogram and/or ureterogram when performed, imaging guidance (e.g., ultrasound and/or fluoroscopy) and all associated radiological supervision and interpretation

The physician changes a nephrostomy catheter by replacing the existing tube. Sutures holding an existing tube in place are removed. A guidewire is inserted, and the tube is pulled out over the wire. A new tube is threaded over the wire until proper placement is achieved. A catheter containing a balloon is threaded over the guidewire to a ureteral stricture and the wire is removed. Balloon catheter sizes are determined based on normal ureter diameter as measured by radiological images. The balloon is inflated until stricture is minimalized; the process may be repeated until the desired result is achieved. Contrast may be injected to check position and function of the nephrostomy catheter and to determine adequate flow through the ureter. The new nephrostomy catheter is secured to the skin with sutures. This code includes diagnostic nephrostogram and/or ureterogram, imaging guidance, and all associated radiological supervision and interpretation.

C7549

C7549 Change of ureterostomy tube or externally accessible ureteral stent via ileal conduit with ureteral stricture balloon dilation, including imaging guidance (e.g., ultrasound and/or fluoroscopy) and all associated radiological supervision and interpretation

The physician changes a ureterostomy tube or an externally accessible ureteral stent via an ileal conduit. Sutures holding an existing tube in place are removed. A guidewire is inserted, and the tube is pulled out over the wire. A new tube is threaded over the wire until proper placement is achieved and is secured to the skin with sutures. To change an externally accessible ureteral stent via an ileal conduit, a guidewire is inserted through the ileal conduit. An ileal conduit is an isolated loop of ileum to which the ureter has been anastomosed at one end with the opposite end exiting through the skin and attached to an ostomy bag. The existing stent is retrieved, and a new stent is placed. A catheter containing a balloon is threaded over the guidewire to a ureteral stricture and the wire is removed. Balloon catheter sizes are determined based on normal ureter diameter as measured by radiological images. The balloon is inflated until stricture is minimalized; the process may be repeated until the desired result is achieved. Contrast may be injected to determine adequate flow through the ureter. This code includes diagnostic imaging guidance and all associated radiological supervision and interpretation.

C7550

C7550 Cystourethroscopy, with biopsy(ies) with adjunctive blue light cystoscopy with fluorescent imaging agent

The physician examines the urinary collecting system with a cystourethroscope passed through the urethra and bladder. The physician first examines the urethra and bladder with a white light, then a blue light. Blue light cystoscopy increases tumor detection in nonmuscle invasive bladder cancer (NMIBC). Hexaminolevulinate HCL, an optical imaging agent, is instilled into the bladder one hour prior to the procedure via an intravesical catheter and retained in the bladder. This imaging agent causes cancerous cells to show up as fluorescent pink under the blue light. A cutting instrument is passed through the endoscope to the suspect tissue and traps a specimen of tissue. Multiple samples may be collected. The instrument and cystourethroscope are removed.

C7551

C7551 Excision of major peripheral nerve neuroma, except sciatic, with implantation of nerve end into bone or muscle

The physician excises a neuroma of a major peripheral nerve (excluding the sciatic nerve). A neuroma is a painful, benign tumor formed secondarily by trauma to the nerve when it is severed. The physician incises the area over the affected nerve. After locating the nerve with the symptomatic neuroma, the physician excises the tumor. The physician then implants the end of the affected nerve into a bone or muscle to prevent neuroma reformation following the excision. In bony implantation, the physician drills a small hole in the bone to implant the nerve end. The surrounding tissue is brought together around the nerve to secure the nerve to the bone. In muscle implantation, the nerve end is sutured into muscle bed. The surrounding tissue is brought together and sutured to secure the nerve in the muscle.

C7552

C7552 Catheter placement in coronary artery(s) for coronary angiography, including intraprocedural injection(s) for coronary angiography, imaging supervision and interpretation; with catheter placement(s) in bypass graft(s) (internal mammary, free arterial, venous grafts) including intraprocedural injection(s) for bypass graft angiography and right heart catheterization with intravascular doppler velocity and/or pressure derived coronary flow reserve measurement (coronary vessel or graft) during coronary angiography including pharmacologically induced stress, initial vessel

The physician places a catheter into one or more coronary arteries (including catheter placement in internal mammary, free arterial, or venous bypass grafts) for coronary and bypass graft angiography. An introducer sheath is placed into an artery, typically the femoral artery, using percutaneous puncture; an angiography catheter is advanced through the introducer sheath into the ascending aorta, under fluoroscopic guidance, to the opening of the coronary artery. Radiopaque contrast material is injected through the catheter into the vessel while a cineangiogram is recorded. Right heart catheterization is performed, in which the catheter is threaded into the right atrium, through the tricuspid valve into the right ventricle, and across the pulmonary valve into the pulmonary arteries. During the angiography, the physician employs a miniaturized Doppler transducer mounted at the tip of a specialized guidewire and inserted through the diagnostic catheter to record intravascular coronary blood flow velocity measurement distal to a coronary lesion (both before and after administration of a pharmacologic stress agent such as adenosine). This device is small enough to be advanced beyond a coronary lesion without significantly increasing any occlusion; measurements are indicative of the hemodynamic significance of the stenosis and assist the practitioner in determining the benefit or necessity of a specific intervention, such as angioplasty or stents. Upon completion of the procedure, the physician removes the catheter and sheath from the artery of access. Pressure is placed on the wound for 20 to 30 minutes to stem bleeding. This code includes all intraprocedural injections, imaging supervision and interpretation, and pharmacologically-induced stress.

C7553

C7553 Catheter placement in coronary artery(s) for coronary angiography, including intraprocedural injection(s) for coronary angiography, imaging supervision and interpretation; with right and left heart catheterization including intraprocedural injection(s) for left ventriculography, when performed, catheter placement(s) in bypass graft(s) (internal mammary, free arterial, venous grafts) with bypass graft angiography with pharmacologic agent administration (e.g., inhaled nitric oxide, intravenous infusion of nitroprusside, dobutamine, milrinone, or other agent) including assessing hemodynamic measurements before, during, after and repeat pharmacologic agent administration, when performed

The physician places a catheter in one or more coronary arteries for coronary angiography (including catheter placement in internal mammary, free arterial, or venous bypass grafts for bypass angiography); right and left heart function is evaluated. To accomplish right heart catheterization, the physician threads a catheter through an introducing sheath placed percutaneously into the femoral, subclavian, internal jugular, or antecubital vein. The catheter is threaded into the right atrium, through the tricuspid valve into the right ventricle, and across the pulmonary valve into the pulmonary arteries. Left heart catheterization is also performed, in this scenario using retrograde technique. The catheter is inserted through an introducing sheath placed percutaneously into the femoral, brachial, or axillary artery. The catheter is passed through the aortic valve into the left ventricle.

Intracardiac and intravascular pressures are recorded. Left ventricular injections may be performed for left ventriculography; the physician injects dye through a previously placed catheter threaded through a central line into the left ventricle or atrium to evaluate function with fluoroscopy. During this procedure, the physician administers a pharmacologic agent (inhaled nitric oxide or intravenous (IV) infusion of dobutamine, milrinone, nitroprusside, or other agent) to invoke stress on coronary vessels to measure blood flow through and around the heart. This produces the same result as physical exercise. Arteries become enlarged as the body increases physical activity that requires more oxygen. When plaque is present within a vessel, it does not allow for this enlargement. This slows the ability of the oxygenated blood to reach the necessary organs, which can lead to ischemia. Hemodynamic measurements are assessed before, during, and after administration. This code includes all intraprocedural injections, imaging supervision and interpretation, and repeat pharmacologic agent administration if performed.

C7554

C7554 Cystourethroscopy with adjunctive blue light cystoscopy with fluorescent imaging agent

The physician examines the urinary collecting system with a cystourethroscope passed through the urethra and bladder. The examination is performed with a white light followed by a blue light. Blue light cystoscopy increases tumor detection in nonmuscle invasive bladder cancer (NMIBC). Hexaminolevulinate HCl, an optical imaging agent, is instilled into the bladder one hour prior to the procedure via an intravesical catheter and retained in the bladder. This imaging agent will cause cancerous cells to show up as fluorescent pink under the blue light. No other procedure is performed at this time. The cystourethroscope is removed.

C7555

C7555 Thyroidectomy, total or complete with parathyroid autotransplantation

The physician removes all of the thyroid and excises and reimplants a portion of the parathyroid. The thyroid is exposed via a transverse cervical incision in the skin line. The platysmas are divided, and the strap muscles are separated in the midline. The thyroid gland is mobilized, and the superior and inferior thyroid vessels are ligated. The thyroid is resected free of the trachea and removed. All four parathyroid glands are completely removed. The platysmas and skin are closed. A separate incision is made at the site of the parathyroid reimplantation (e.g., arm or leg). After preparation and frozen section confirmation of the parathyroid tissue, segments are implanted into muscle pockets at the transplant site. The incision is closed. Remaining tissue may be prepared for cryopreservation.

C7900-C7902

C7900 Service for diagnosis, evaluation, or treatment of a mental health or substance use disorder, initial 15-29 minutes, provided remotely by hospital staff who are licensed to provide mental health services under applicable state law(s), when the patient is in their home, and there is no associated professional service

C7901 Service for diagnosis, evaluation, or treatment of a mental health or substance use disorder, initial 30-60 minutes, provided remotely by hospital staff who are licensed to provided mental health services under applicable state law(s), when the patient is in their home, and there is no associated professional service

C7902 Service for diagnosis, evaluation, or treatment of a mental health or substance use disorder, each additional 15 minutes, provided remotely by hospital staff who are licensed to provide mental health services under applicable state law(s), when the patient is in their home, and there is no associated professional service (list separately in addition to code for primary service)

Remote mental health services provided by hospital staff are reported by the hospital outpatient department for diagnosis, evaluation, or treatment of a mental health or substance use disorder. This code represents a telehealth visit while the patient is in the home and the hospital staff is located in the hospital at the time of the service. The patient is required to have an in-person service within 12 months of the remote visit. Beginning 152 days after the public health emergency (PHE), a patient who begins remote mental health treatment will also be required to have an in-person service within six months prior to the remote visit. The staff must be licensed to provide mental health services under state laws. The hospital must have the ability to furnish the service using two-way audio/video technology. The patient can choose audio-only if they do not consent to the video or if they are not capable of using video. No associated professional services can be reported under the physician fee schedule. These codes are time-based codes. Report C7900 for an initial visit lasting 15 to 29 minutes; C7901 for 30 to 60 minutes. Additional time is reported with C7902 for each additional 15 minutes.

C8900

C8900 Magnetic resonance angiography with contrast, abdomen

Magnetic resonance angiography (MRA) is an application of magnetic resonance imaging (MRI) that provides visualization of blood flow and images of normal and diseased blood vessels. MRA techniques typically are noninvasive because they do not require the use of contrast media. Contrast media may be used to enhance the images in MRA, but use of these agents is not necessary.

C8901

C8901 Magnetic resonance angiography without contrast, abdomen

Magnetic resonance angiography (MRA) is an application of magnetic resonance imaging (MRI) that provides visualization of blood flow and images of normal and diseased blood vessels. MRA techniques typically are noninvasive because they do not require the use of contrast media. Contrast media may be used to enhance the images in MRA, but use of these agents is not necessary.

C8902

C8902 Magnetic resonance angiography without contrast followed by with contrast, abdomen

Magnetic resonance angiography (MRA) is an application of magnetic resonance imaging (MRI) that provides visualization of blood flow and images of normal and diseased blood vessels. MRA techniques typically are noninvasive because they do not require the use of contrast media. Contrast media may be used to enhance the images in MRA, but use of these agents is not necessary.

C8903

C8903 Magnetic resonance imaging with contrast, breast; unilateral

Magnetic resonance imaging (MRI) is a noninvasive, painless test that assists the physician in diagnosing and treating certain medical conditions. MRI uses a powerful magnetic field, radio waves, and a computer to create detailed pictures of bone, organs, soft tissues, and other internal body structures. These detailed pictures allow the physician to better comprehend and evaluate the part of the body in question or diseased areas under scrutiny. An MRI of the breast assists in evaluating abnormalities detected via a mammography, evaluates the integrity of breast implants, differentiates between scar tissue and tumors, assesses multiple tumor locations, determines whether cancer detected by mammography or other radiological tests has spread further into the breast or chest wall pre- or post-surgery, assesses the effect of chemotherapy, and/or provides more information on a diseased breast to make medical treatment decisions.

C8905

C8905 Magnetic resonance imaging without contrast followed by with contrast, breast; unilateral

Magnetic resonance imaging (MRI) is a noninvasive, painless test that assists the physician in diagnosing and treating certain medical conditions. MRI uses a powerful magnetic field, radio waves, and a computer to create detailed pictures of bone, organs, soft tissues, and other internal body structures. These detailed pictures allow the physician to better comprehend and evaluate the part of the body in question or diseased areas under scrutiny. An MRI of the breast assists in evaluating abnormalities detected via a mammography, evaluates the integrity of breast implants, differentiates between scar tissue and tumors, assesses multiple tumor locations, determines whether cancer detected by mammography or other radiological tests has spread further into the breast or chest wall pre- or post-surgery, assesses the effect of chemotherapy, and/or provides more information on a diseased breast to make medical treatment decisions.

C8906

C8906 Magnetic resonance imaging with contrast, breast; bilateral

Magnetic resonance imaging (MRI) is a noninvasive, painless test that assists the physician in diagnosing and treating certain medical conditions. MRI uses a powerful magnetic field, radio waves, and a computer to create detailed pictures of bone, organs, soft tissues, and other internal body structures. These detailed pictures allow the physician to better comprehend and evaluate the part of the body in question or diseased areas under scrutiny. An MRI of the breast assists in evaluating abnormalities detected via a mammography, evaluates the integrity of breast implants, differentiates between scar tissue and tumors, assesses multiple tumor locations, determines whether cancer detected by mammography or other radiological tests has spread further into the breast or chest wall pre- or post-surgery, assesses the effect of chemotherapy, and/or provides more information on a diseased breast to make medical treatment decisions.

C8908

C8908 Magnetic resonance imaging without contrast followed by with contrast, breast; bilateral

Magnetic resonance imaging (MRI) is a noninvasive, painless test that assists the physician in diagnosing and treating certain medical conditions. MRI uses a powerful magnetic field, radio waves, and a computer to create detailed pictures of bone, organs, soft tissues, and other internal body structures. These detailed pictures allow the physician to better comprehend and evaluate the part of the body in question or diseased areas under scrutiny. An MRI of the breast assists in evaluating abnormalities detected via a mammography, evaluates the integrity of breast implants, differentiates between scar tissue and tumors, assesses multiple tumor locations, determines whether cancer detected by mammography or other radiological tests has spread further into the breast or chest wall pre- or post-surgery, assesses the effect of chemotherapy, and/or provides more information on a diseased breast to make medical treatment decisions.

C8909

C8909 Magnetic resonance angiography with contrast, chest (excluding myocardium)

Magnetic resonance angiography (MRA) is an application of magnetic resonance imaging (MRI) that provides visualization of blood flow and images of normal and diseased blood vessels. MRA techniques typically are noninvasive because they do not require the use of contrast media. This MRA procedure is designed to examine the heart and the blood vessels entering the lungs. Contrast media may be used to enhance the images in MRA, but use of these agents is not necessary.

C8910

C8910 Magnetic resonance angiography without contrast, chest (excluding myocardium)

Magnetic resonance angiography (MRA) is an application of magnetic resonance imaging (MRI) that provides visualization of blood flow and images of normal and diseased blood vessels. MRA techniques typically are noninvasive because they do not require the use of contrast media. This MRA procedure is designed to examine the heart and the blood vessels entering the lungs. Contrast media may be used to enhance the images in MRA, but use of these agents is not necessary.

C8911

C8911 Magnetic resonance angiography without contrast followed by with contrast, chest (excluding myocardium)

Magnetic resonance angiography (MRA) is an application of magnetic resonance imaging (MRI) that provides visualization of blood flow and images of normal and diseased blood vessels. MRA techniques typically are noninvasive because they do not require the use of contrast media. This MRA procedure is designed to examine the heart and the blood vessels entering the lungs. Contrast media may be used to enhance the images in MRA, but use of these agents is not necessary.

C8912-C8914

C8912 Magnetic resonance angiography with contrast, lower extremity

C8913 Magnetic resonance angiography without contrast, lower extremity

C8914 Magnetic resonance angiography without contrast followed by with contrast, lower extremity

Magnetic resonance angiography (MRA) is an application of magnetic resonance imaging (MRI) that provides visualization of blood flow and images of normal and diseased blood vessels. MRA techniques typically are noninvasive because they do not require the use of contrast media. This MRA procedure is designed to examine major blood vessels in the lower extremities. Contrast media may be used to enhance the images in MRA, but use of these agents is not necessary.

C8918-C8920

C8918 Magnetic resonance angiography with contrast, pelvis

C8919 Magnetic resonance angiography without contrast, pelvis

C8920 Magnetic resonance angiography without contrast followed by with contrast, pelvis

Magnetic resonance angiography (MRA) is an application of magnetic resonance imaging (MRI) that provides visualization of blood flow and images of normal and diseased blood vessels. MRA techniques typically are noninvasive because they do not require the use of contrast media. This MRA procedure is designed to examine major blood vessels in the pelvis. Contrast media may be used to enhance the images in MRA, but use of these agents is not necessary.

C8921-C8922

C8921 Transthoracic echocardiography (TTE) with contrast, or without contrast followed by with contrast, for congenital cardiac anomalies; complete

C8922 Transthoracic echocardiography (TTE) with contrast, or without contrast followed by with contrast, for congenital cardiac anomalies; follow-up or limited study

Transthoracic echocardiography is performed to detect congenital cardiac anomalies. Contrast is injected into the patient's vein. Transducers are placed on the patient's chest to record an echocardiograph, which uses ultrasound to visualize the heart's function, blood flow, valves, and chambers. Report contrast material separately.

C8923-C8924

C8923 Transthoracic echocardiography (TTE) with contrast, or without contrast followed by with contrast, real-time with image documentation (2D), includes M-mode recording, when performed, complete, without spectral or color doppler echocardiography

C8924 Transthoracic echocardiography (TTE) with contrast, or without contrast followed by with contrast, real-time with image documentation (2D), includes M-mode recording when performed, follow-up or limited study

A transthoracic echocardiography is performed with real-time image documentation (2D). Contrast material is injected into the vein. An ultrasound is used to visualize the heart's function, blood flow, valves, and chambers. Two-dimensional echocardiography, also referred to as real-time imaging, is performed using multiple transducers or a rotating transducer, and these images are recorded on videotape. Computer reconstruction provides the two-dimensional image of specific planes of the heart. M-mode, when performed, provides additional detail of specific portions of the heart. A stationary ultrasound beam is directed at the area of the heart requiring additional study. Report contrast material separately.

C8925-C8926

C8925 Transesophageal echocardiography (TEE) with contrast, or without contrast followed by with contrast, real time with image documentation (2D) (with or without M-mode recording); including probe placement, image acquisition, interpretation and report

C8926 Transesophageal echocardiography (TEE) with contrast, or without contrast followed by with contrast, for congenital cardiac anomalies; including probe placement, image acquisition, interpretation and report

Transesophageal echocardiography (TEE) is performed. TEE is an invasive technique whereby contrast material is injected into the vein. The transducer is placed at the tip of an endoscope and introduced into the patient's esophagus to record a two-dimensional echocardiograph. The codes include probe placement, image acquisition, interpretation, and report. Report contrast material separately.

C8927

C8927 Transesophageal echocardiography (TEE) with contrast, or without contrast followed by with contrast, for monitoring purposes, including probe placement, real time (2D) image acquisition and interpretation leading to ongoing (continuous) assessment of (dynamically changing) cardiac pumping function and to therapeutic measures on an immediate time basis

Transesophageal echocardiography (TEE) is performed to assess cardiac pumping function and for therapeutic measures on an immediate time basis. TEE is an invasive technique whereby contrast is injected into the vein. The transducer is placed at the tip of an endoscope and introduced into the patient's esophagus to record a two-dimensional echocardiograph. TEE provides high-quality, real-time images of the beating heart and mediastinal structures. This code reports ongoing hemodynamic monitoring using TEE. TEE may be used to monitor critically ill patients in the intensive care unit, as well as patients in certain operative settings. In both the intensive care unit and the operating room, it is used to monitor cardiac function including cardiac preload, contractility, and valve function in patients with acute hemodynamic decompensation. In addition, TEE may also be used to assess and monitor mediastinal, heart, lung, and aortic injury resulting from blunt chest trauma even in patients undergoing other life-saving procedures. Report contrast material separately.

C8928

C8928 Transthoracic echocardiography (TTE) with contrast, or without contrast followed by with contrast, real-time with image documentation (2D), includes M-mode recording, when performed, during rest and cardiovascular stress test using treadmill, bicycle exercise and/or pharmacologically induced stress, with interpretation and report

Transthoracic echocardiography (TTE) is performed while the patient is at rest and exercising on a treadmill or stationary bicycle with or without medication and includes M-mode recording, when performed. TTE is an invasive technique whereby contrast is injected into the vein. Transducers are placed on a patient's chest to record a two-dimensional echocardiograph, which uses ultrasound to visualize the heart's function, blood flow, valves, and chambers. Report contrast material separately.

C8929

C8929 Transthoracic echocardiography (TTE) with contrast, or without contrast followed by with contrast, real-time with image documentation (2D), includes M-mode recording, when performed, complete, with spectral doppler echocardiography, and with color flow doppler echocardiography

Transthoracic echocardiography (TTE) is performed. TTE is an invasive technique whereby contrast is injected into the vein. Transducers are placed on a patient's chest to record a two-dimensional echocardiograph, which uses ultrasound to visualize the heart's function, blood flow, valves, and chambers. This code reports a complete evaluation that includes spectral and color flow Doppler, which provides information regarding blood flow velocity, direction, type, and hemodynamics. Report contrast material separately.

C8930

C8930 Transthoracic echocardiography (TTE) with contrast, or without contrast followed by with contrast, real-time with image documentation (2D), includes M-mode recording, when performed, during rest and cardiovascular stress test using treadmill, bicycle exercise and/or pharmacologically induced stress, with interpretation and report; including performance of continuous electrocardiographic monitoring, with physician supervision

Transthoracic echocardiography (TTE) is performed. TTE is an invasive technique whereby contrast is injected into the vein. Transducers are placed on the patient's chest to record a two-dimensional echocardiograph, which uses ultrasound to visualize the heart's function, blood flow, valves, and chambers. This is completed while the patient is at rest and again while exercising on a treadmill or stationary bicycle, with or without medication, and includes M-mode recording, when performed. It also includes the performance of continuous electrocardiographic monitoring with physician supervision. Supply of the contrast agent and/or the drugs used in pharmacologic stress are reported separately.

C8931-C8936

C8931 Magnetic resonance angiography with contrast, spinal canal and contents

C8932 Magnetic resonance angiography without contrast, spinal canal and contents

C8933 Magnetic resonance angiography without contrast followed by with contrast, spinal canal and contents

C8934 Magnetic resonance angiography with contrast, upper extremity

C8935 Magnetic resonance angiography without contrast, upper extremity

C8936 Magnetic resonance angiography without contrast followed by with contrast, upper extremity

Magnetic resonance imaging uses the natural magnetic properties of the hydrogen atoms that emit radiofrequency signals when exposed to radio waves within a strong electromagnetic field. These signals are processed and converted by the computer into high-resolution, three-dimensional tomographic images. Magnetic resonance angiography (MRA) is magnetic resonance imaging (MRI) that specifically visualizes blood vessels and blood flow to evaluate vascular disorders within the structure being studied. Unlike conventional or CT images, MRIs/MRAs do not rely on the absorption of ionizing radiation. Patients with metallic or electronic implants or foreign bodies cannot be exposed to MRI. The patient must remain still while lying on a motorized table within the large, circular MRI tunnel. A sedative may be administered, as well as contrast material for image enhancement.

C8937

C8937 Computer-aided detection, including computer algorithm analysis of breast MRI image data for lesion detection/characterization, pharmacokinetic analysis, with further physician review for interpretation (list separately in addition to code for primary procedure)

Computer-aided detection (CAD) software is used with breast magnetic resonance imaging (MRI), a radiation-free, noninvasive technique that produces high-quality sectional images of the inside of the body in multiple planes. MRI uses the natural magnetic properties of the hydrogen atoms in the body that emit radiofrequency signals when exposed to radio waves within a strong electromagnetic field. These signals are processed and converted by the computer into high-resolution, three-dimensional, tomographic images. Patients with metallic or electronic implants or foreign bodies cannot be exposed to MRI. The patient must remain still while lying on a motorized table within the large, circular MRI tunnel. A sedative may be administered, as well as an IV injected contrast material for image enhancement. The use of a CAD system allows breast images to be converted into digital form. The software scans the images, looking for any areas of abnormality such as density, calcifications, or a mass, and alerts the radiologist who can then notify the referring physician of the need for additional evaluation.

C8957

C8957 Intravenous infusion for therapy/diagnosis; initiation of prolonged infusion (more than 8 hours), requiring use of portable or implantable pump

Intravenous infusion for therapy/diagnosis; initiation of prolonged infusion (more than 8 hours), requiring use of portable or implantable pump, is a route of administration in pharmacology and toxicology by which a path in a vein is made allowing the administration of a drug, fluid, or other substance for a period of more than 8 hours. An infusion pump is used for such prolonged infusions.

C9046

C9046 Cocaine HCl nasal solution for topical administration, 1 mg

Cocaine hydrochloride nasal solution is an ester local anesthetic that is indicated for the induction of local anesthesia of mucous membranes of the nasal cavities in adults, ages 18 years and older, during diagnostic or surgical procedures. It is intended for intranasal use only. Cocaine hydrochloride is supplied in a single use bottle of 160 mg/4 mL, equivalent to 142.4 mg/4 mL cocaine-free base. Prior to use, four cotton pledgets should be soaked in the full content of the vial until the solution has been completely absorbed. Once fully absorbed, two pledgets should be placed in each nasal cavity, against the nasal septum, and left in place for up to 20 minutes. Vital signs should be monitored. Cocaine hydrochloride is not recommended for use in patients with recent or active histories of congestive heart failure, coronary artery disease, myocardial infarction, uncontrolled hypertension, or unstable angina.

C9047

C9047 Injection, caplacizumab-yhdp, 1 mg

Caplacizumab-yhdp is a von Willebrand factor (VWF)-directed antibody fragment that is indicated for the treatment of adults, 18 years of age and older, with acquired thrombotic thrombocytopenic purpura (aTTP), a blood disorder that is characterized by low platelets, low red blood count, hemolytic anemia, as well as small areas of bleeding beneath the skin (purpura). Caplacizumab-yhdp is used in conjunction with immunosuppressive therapy and plasma exchange. It is supplied as a lyophilized powder in a single-use vial, as part of a single-use kit, and should be refrigerated in the original packaging. The kit contains an 11 mg vial of caplacizumab-yhdp and additional supplies for dilution. The recommended dosage for day 1 is an 11 mg bolus administered by intravenous injection at least 15 minutes before plasma exchange, then 11 mg administered by subcutaneous (SC) injection in the abdomen after plasma injection. During the plasma exchange period, 11 mg of caplacizumab-yhdp should be administered by SC injection in the abdomen once daily after plasma exchange. After the plasma exchange period, 11 mg of caplacizumab-yhdp should be administered by SC injection in the abdomen once daily for 30 days following the last plasma exchange. If signs of persistent underlying disease are present, treatment may be continued for an additional 28 days. Patients who have more than two recurrences of aTTP during treatment should discontinue use of caplacizumab-yhdp. Treatment with caplacizumab-yhdp is initiated in the inpatient setting and transitioned to self-administration at home.

C9067

C9067 Gallium Ga-68, Dotatoc, diagnostic, 0.01 mCi

Gallium Ga-68 Dotatoc is a diagnostic radiopharmaceutical used with positron emission tomography (PET) scans for localization of somatostatin receptor positive neuroendocrine tumors (NETs) in adult and pediatric patients. It is administered via intravenous (IV) infusion and is supplied in multiple dose vials containing 18.5 MBq/mL to 148 MBq/mL (0.5 mCi/mL to 4 mCi/mL). The recommended dosage for adult patients is 148 MBq (4 mCi) administered via an IV bolus injection. The recommended dosage for pediatric patients is 1.59 MBq/kg body weight (0.043 mCi/kg) with a range of 11.1 MBq (0.3 mCi) to 111 MBq (3 mCi) administered via an IV bolus injection. PET imaging should begin 55 to 90 minutes following administration. Short-acting somatostatin analogs should be discontinued 24 hours prior to imaging with Gallium Ga-68 Dotatoc. See full prescribing information for complete preparation, administration, imaging, and radiation dosimetry instructions.

C9088

C9088 Instillation, bupivacaine and meloxicam, 1 mg/0.03 mg

Bupivacaine and meloxicam is a combination of bupivacaine, an amide-type local anesthetic, and meloxicam, a nonsteroidal anti-inflammatory drug (NSAID). It is indicated for postoperative surgical site pain relief for up to 72 hours following bunionectomy, open inguinal herniorrhaphy, or total knee arthroplasty in adult patients, ages 18 years or older. It is supplied in four dosage strengths as a single dose kit and is applied into the surgical site, without a needle, following final irrigation and suction and prior to wound closure. See full prescribing information for complete administration instructions.

C9089

C9089 Bupivacaine, collagen-matrix implant, 1 mg

Bupivacaine collagen matrix implant is an amide-type local anesthetic. It is indicated for postoperative surgical site pain relief for up to 24 hours following open inguinal hernia repair in adult patients, ages 18 years and older. Bupivacaine collagen matrix implant is supplied as a single dose package of three implants (100 mg each) for a total dose of 300 mg bupivacaine HCl. Each implant should be cut in half, using aseptic technique. Three halves should be placed in the mesh placement site and the other three halves placed just below the skin closure. Additional local anesthetics should be avoided within 96 hours of use of bupivacaine collagen matrix implant. It should not be used for patients undergoing obstetrical paracervical block anesthesia.

C9101

C9101 Injection, oliceridine, 0.1 mg

Oliceridine is an opioid agonist that is indicated for the treatment of adults, ages 18 years and older, with acute pain severe enough to require treatment with an intravenous (IV) opioid analgesic but for whom alternative treatments are inadequate. Due to risks of addiction, misuse, or abuse, oliceridine should only be used to treat patients for whom alternative treatments have not been tolerated, are not expected to be tolerated, have not provided adequate analgesia, or are not expected to provide adequate analgesia. It is supplied in single dose vials of 1 mg/ml or 2 mg/2 ml and single-patient use vials of 30 mg/30 ml for patient controlled (PCA) analgesia. Recommended initial dosage is 1.5 mg administered via IV infusion. Subsequent doses of 0.75 mg can be administered by providers one hour following initial dose and hourly thereafter, as needed. For PCA analgesia, the initial recommended dosage is 1.5 mg followed by patient demand doses of 0.35 mg with a six-minute lock-out. Single doses of greater than 3 mg should not be administered. A cumulative total daily dose of 27 mg should not be exceeded. See full prescribing information for complete administration and dosage instructions.

C9113

C9113 Injection, pantoprazole sodium, per vial

Pantoprazole sodium is a compound that inhibits gastric secretions. Pantoprazole is a proton pump inhibitor (PPI) that suppresses the final step in gastric acid production by forming a covalent bond to two sites of the ATPase enzyme system at the secretory surface of the gastric parietal cell. This effect is dose-related and leads to inhibition of both basal and stimulated gastric acid secretion irrespective of the stimulus. This binding results in a period of antisecretory effect that persists longer than 24 hours for all doses tested. This drug is indicated for short-term treatment (seven to 10 days) for patients with gastroesophageal reflux disease (GERD) and a history of erosive esophagitis, and the hypersecretory conditions that may be associated with Zollinger-Ellison syndrome or other neoplastic conditions.

C9143

C9143 Cocaine HCl nasal solution (Numbrino), 1 mg

Cocaine HCl nasal solution is an ester local anesthetic that is indicated for use in adults, ages 18 years and older, for local anesthesia of the mucous membranes in diagnostic and surgical procedures of the nasal cavities. It is supplied as 4% nasal solution in bottles of 4 ml and 10 ml (40 mg/ml) and is administered via application of cotton or rayon pledgets applied to the nasal mucosa. The recommended dosage is 40 mg to 160 mg, depending on size of surface area treated. To prepare, 4 ml of the solution is drawn into a syringe and 2 ml is evenly applied to four stacked pledgets. The pledgets are turned over and the remaining 2 ml of solution is evenly applied. A maximum of two pledgets may be placed in each nasal cavity and can remain in place for up to 20 minutes. Cocaine HCl nasal solution should not be used in patients with epilepsy, hereditary pseudocholinesterase deficiency, or with concomitant use of cholinesterase inhibitors, alpha-modifying drugs, or tricyclic antidepressants. See full prescribing information for complete administration instructions. Report C9143 only for cocaine hydrochloride nasal solution manufactured by Lannett.

C9144

C9144 Injection, bupivacaine (Posimir), 1 mg

Bupivacaine is an amide local anesthetic indicated for the treatment of adults, ages 18 years and older, for postoperative surgical site pain relief for up to 72 hours following arthroscopic subacromial decompression. It is supplied in a single dose vial of 660 mg/5 ml (132 mg/ml) and is applied into an existing arthroscopic port prior to wound closure or through intact skin. Care should be taken to avoid intravascular injection. It should not be administered via epidural, intrathecal, intravascular, intra-articular, or regional nerve block injections. See full prescribing information for complete administration instructions.

C9248

C9248 Injection, clevidipine butyrate, 1 mg

Clevidipine butyrate is a channel blocker used to treat high blood pressure when other treatments are contraindicated. Channel blockers relax the blood vessels and allow more blood and oxygen to get to the heart. The dose varies depending on the patient's condition and blood pressure. Clevidipine butyrate is administered as an IV infusion.

C9250

C9250 Human plasma fibrin sealant, vapor-heated, solvent-detergent (Artiss), 2 ml

Human plasma fibrin sealant, vapor-heated, solvent-detergent (Artiss) is a two-component fibrin sealant used to adhere autologous skin grafts to surgically prepared wounds in burn patients. It is comprised of human sealer protein concentrate and human fibrin. When these two components are combined, the result is a fibrin that seals the graft to the prepared wound site. The solution is applied in a thin layer to the site and the graft is placed. A 2 ml package covers approximately 100 square centimeter surface area.

C9254

C9254 Injection, lacosamide, 1 mg

Lacosamide is a functional amino acid used as an adjunctive therapy in treating partial-onset seizures for patients 17 years of age or older who are diagnosed with epilepsy. The exact mechanism by which this drug controls seizures is unknown. The lacosamide is believed to act through voltage-gated sodium channels. Voltage-gated sodium channels help control the electrical activity of the neurons. Lacosamide targets neurons that are depolarized or active for long periods of time, typical of neurons at the focus of an epileptic seizure. The recommended dosage is from 100 mg to 400 mg per day, depending on the patient's response. The drug is administered as an IV infusion over 30 to 60 minutes.

C9257

C9257 Injection, bevacizumab, 0.25 mg

Bevacizumab is a monoclonal antibody produced by recombinant DNA technology in Chinese hamster ovaries. This monoclonal antibody binds to and inhibits the biologic activity of human vascular endothelial growth factor preventing the formation of new blood vessels. Bevacizumab, used in combination with intravenous 5-fluorouracil, is indicated for first-line treatment of patients with metastatic carcinoma of the colon or rectum. The recommended dose is 5 mg per kg of body weight administered once every 14 days disease progression is detected. Bevacizumab is administered by intravenous infusion. The initial dose infusion should be delivered over 90 minutes. If the first infusion is well tolerated, the second infusion may be administered over 60 minutes. If the 60-minute infusion is well tolerated, all subsequent infusions may be administered over 30 minutes.

C9285

C9285 Lidocaine 70 mg/tetracaine 70 mg, per patch

A lidocaine 70 mg/tetracaine 70 mg patch is a single-use topical anesthetic patch that delivers equal parts of lidocaine and tetracaine. The patch has a heat-assisted drug delivery device that enhances the delivery of the local anesthetic. The patch is indicated for use on intact skin to provide local dermal analgesia prior to painful procedures such as needle punctures and superficial dermatological procedures in adults and children 3 years of age or older. The patch should be applied 20 to 30 minutes prior to venipuncture or intravenous cannulation and 30 minutes prior to a superficial dermatological procedure.

C9290

C9290 Injection, bupivacaine liposome, 1 mg

Bupivacaine liposome is an amide-type local anesthetic used for postoperative surgical site pain relief. Liposomal encapsulated bupivacaine blocks the production and conduction of the nerve impulses to the brain. Bupivacaine liposome is injected into the soft tissue of the surgical site. Recommended dose varies depending on the surface area to be covered and the surgical site. The maximum dose should not exceed 266 mg.

C9293

C9293 Injection, glucarpidase, 10 units

Glucarpidase is an orphan drug that is an exogenous enzyme produced by recombinant DNA technology in *E. coli*. The enzyme is indicated as a treatment for toxic plasma methotrexate concentrations in patients with delayed clearance due to impaired kidney function. Glucarpidase converts methotrexate into its inactive components and provides a nonrenal path of elimination in patients with renal dysfunction. Recommended dose is a single injection of 50 units per kg. Glucarpidase is administered as an intravenous bolus over five minutes.

C

C9352

C9352 Microporous collagen implantable tube (NeuraGen Nerve Guide), per cm length

A microporous collagen implantable tube, trade name NeuraGen Nerve Guide, is an absorbable collagen tube intended to serve as an interface between a nerve and the tissue around it. The tube creates a channel for axonal growth across a nerve gap. This code specifies a size of per centimeter length.

C9353

C9353 Microporous collagen implantable slit tube (NeuraWrap Nerve Protector), per cm length

A microporous collagen implantable slit tube, trade name NeuraWrap Nerve Protector, is an absorbable collagen implant that provides a nontightening cover for peripheral nerves that are injure. This code specifies a size of per centimeter length.

C9354

C9354 Acellular pericardial tissue matrix of nonhuman origin (Veritas), per sq cm

Acellular pericardial tissue matrix of nonhuman origin, trade name Veritas, is a strong implantable tissue consisting of noncross linked bovine pericardium. This product is acellular meaning all cells have been removed leaving only a collagen matrix. The acellular pericardial tissue matrix is used as a scaffold for tissue repair. This code specifies a size of per square centimeter.

C9355

C9355 Collagen nerve cuff (NeuroMatrix), per 0.5 cm length

A collagen nerve cuff, trade name NeuroMatrix, is a resorbable, semipermeable, collagen tube intended to create a conduit for axon growth across a nerve gap of 2.5 cm or less. This code specifies a size of 0.5 centimeter length.

C9356

C9356 Tendon, porous matrix of cross-linked collagen and glycosaminoglycan matrix (TenoGlide Tendon Protector Sheet), per sq cm

A tendon, porous matrix of cross-linked collagen and glycosaminoglycan matrix, trade name TenoGlide Tendon Protector Sheet, is an absorbable implant made of a porous matrix of cross linked bovine collagen and glycosaminoglycan. This provides a nonconstricting, protective encasement for injured tendons. This item is intended to serve as an interface between the tendon and the tendon sheath or surrounding tissue. This code specifies a size of per square centimeter.

C9358

C9358 Dermal substitute, native, nondenatured collagen, fetal bovine origin (SurgiMend Collagen Matrix), per 0.5 sq cm

A dermal substitute, native, non-denatured collagen, fetal bovine origin, trade name SurgiMend Collagen Matrix, is an oval- or square-shaped, biocompatible, soft material made of an acellular collagen matrix. All cellular components are removed from fetal bovine dermis leaving a collagen matrix. This material is intended for soft tissue repair and reconstructive applications. This code specifies the size of 0.5 square centimeters.

C9359

C9359 Porous purified collagen matrix bone void filler (Integra Mozaik Osteoconductive Scaffold Putty, Integra OS Osteoconductive Scaffold Putty), per 0.5 cc

Porous purified collagen matrix is a synthetic type of bone void filler that is used for the treatment of gaps or osseous defects of the skeletal system in the extremities, spine, and pelvis. This filler is made from a purified collage matrix, and its chemical composition allows it to be absorbed and replaced with growing host bone during the healing process. The filler is supplied in powder form and mixed with the bone marrow of the host to form a putty-like substance. This putty is often used as a substitute for harvesting bone graft material from the patient's iliac crest.

C9360

C9360 Dermal substitute, native, nondenatured collagen, neonatal bovine origin (SurgiMend Collagen Matrix), per 0.5 sq cm

A dermal substitute, native, non-denatured collagen, neonatal bovine origin, trade name SurgiMend Collagen Matrix, is an oval- or square-shaped, biocompatible, soft material made of an acellular collagen matrix. All cellular components are removed from neonatal bovine dermis leaving a collagen matrix. This material is intended for soft tissue repair and reconstructive applications. This code specifies the size of 0.5 square centimeters.

C9361

C9361 Collagen matrix nerve wrap (NeuroMend Collagen Nerve Wrap), per 0.5 cm length

Collagen matrix nerve wrap (trade name NeuroMend Collagen Nerve Wrap) is a resorbable, collagen-based membrane matrix for use in the repair of crushed or severed peripheral nerves. The collagen wrap is designed to unroll and self-curl around the injured nerve. NeuroMend provides a protective setting to help the regeneration of the nerve across the injury or gap.

C9362

C9362 Porous purified collagen matrix bone void filler (Integra Mozaik Osteoconductive Scaffold Strip), per 0.5 cc

Porous purified collagen matrix bone void filler (trade name Integra Mozaik Osteoconductive Scaffold Strip and Scaffold Putty) is a resorbable bone filler designed to mimic the structure and composition of natural human bone. It is a highly purified bovine collagen that contains minerals and osteogenic protein-1. The bone filler is indicated as an alternative to autograft in long-bone nonunions, for spinal fusion where autograft is not possible, and for nonunions where alternative treatments failed.

C9363

C9363 Skin substitute (Integra Meshed Bilayer Wound Matrix), per sq cm

Integra Meshed Bilayer Wound Matrix is a biologic matrix that provides coverage for partial- and full-thickness wounds. It is used to treat chronic and traumatic wounds including pressure ulcers, venous ulcers, diabetic ulcers, chronic and vascular ulcers, tunneled or undermined wounds, surgical wounds, traumatic wounds abrasions, lacerations, and draining wounds. It is a two-layer material. It has a silicone outer layer and a second layer created of three-dimensional porous material made from the fibers of a cross-linked bovine tendon collagen. The silicone layer provides protection and moisture control. The matrix provides the framework for tissue and capillary growth. The physician completely debrides the wound site, and the wound matrix is applied. It is affixed to the wound site with sutures or staples. Within 14 to 21 days, the tissue is remodeled with the patient's own cells, and the silicone layer is removed.

C9364

C9364 Porcine implant, Permacol, per sq cm

A porcine collagen implant (trade name Permacol) is a dermal matrix from which cells, cell debris, DNA, and RNA are removed in a process that does not damage the 3D collagen matrix. This acellular collagen matrix is then cross-linked reportedly for better durability. A porcine collagen implant is indicated for abdominal wall repair.

C9399

C9399 Unclassified drugs or biologicals

This code should be used to report drugs and biologicals that have been approved by the FDA, but do not have a product-specific, drug/biological HCPCS Level II code assigned.

C9460

C9460 Injection, cangrelor, 1 mg

Cangrelor is a direct-acting P2Y12 platelet receptor inhibitor that blocks adenosine diphosphate (ADP)-induced platelet activation and aggregation. The drug binds selectively and reversibly to the P2Y12 receptor to prevent further platelet activation. Cangrelor is indicated as an adjunct to percutaneous coronary intervention (PCI) to reduce the risk of myocardial infarction, repeat coronary revascularization, and stent thrombosis in patients who have not been treated with a P2Y12 platelet inhibitor and are not being given a glycoprotein IIb/IIIa inhibitor. The recommended dosage is a 30 mcg/kg IV bolus followed immediately by a 4 mcg/kg/min IV infusion. The bolus infusion should be administered prior to the PCI. The maintenance infusion should ordinarily be continued for at least two hours or for the duration of PCI, whichever is longer.

C9462

C9462 Injection, delafloxacin, 1 mg

Delafloxacin is a fluoroquinolone antibacterial used for the treatment of acute bacterial skin and skin structure infections (ABSSSI) that are caused by indicated susceptible bacteria in adults 19 years of age and older. It is indicated for the treatment of the following organisms: *Escherichia coli, Enterobacter cloacae, Klebsiella pneumoniae, Pseudomonas aeruginosa, Staphylococcus aureus* (including methicillin-resistant [MRSA] and methicillin susceptible [MSSA] isolates), *Staphylococcus haemolyticus, Staphylococcus lugdunensis, Streptococcus agalactiae, Streptococcus anginosus* group (including *Streptococcus anginosus, Streptococcus intermedius,* and *Streptococcus constellatus*), *Streptococcus pyogenes,* and *Enterococcus faecalis.* The drug can be administered by intravenous infusion or orally. The dosage for intravenous infusion is 300 mg infused over 60 minutes every 12 hours. For oral administration, the dosage is 450 mg every 12 hours for five to 14 days.

C9482

C9482 Injection, sotalol HCl, 1 mg

Sotalol hydrochloride is an antiarrhythmic beta-blocker indicated for the treatment of patients with highly symptomatic heart rhythm disorders of the atrium, such as atrial fibrillation (AFIB) or atrial flutter (AFL), that are currently in sinus rhythm. It is administered in an effort to prolong the time the patient remains in normal sinus rhythm and to delay the recurrence of AFIB or AFL. The adult starting dosage is 75 mg administered once or twice daily by intravenous infusion over five hours, and can be titrated up to the maximum dosage of 150 mg once or twice daily, depending upon a creatinine clearance. If the creatinine is between 60 and 40 mL/min, it may be infused once daily; if less than 40 mg/mL, it should not be administered. The patient must remain under close ECG and QT interval monitoring. For pediatric patients 2 years of age or older, the starting dosage is 30 mg/m^2 administered three times daily by intravenous infusion, and can be titrated up to the maximum dosage of 60 mg/M^2. For pediatric patients younger than age 2, the dosage requires further reduction. Sotalol hydrochloride should not be confused with sotalol, as the two drugs are not used to treat the same conditions.

C9488

C9488 Injection, conivaptan HCl, 1 mg

Conivaptan hydrochloride is a dual arginine vasopressin (AVP) antagonist with nanomolar affinity for human V_{1A} and V_2 receptors. It is indicated for the treatment of hyponatremia, or low sodium levels, in adult patients. Vasopressin is a hormone produced by the posterior pituitary gland. Vasopressin has an antidiuretic effect causing the renal tubules to reabsorb water. High levels of vasopressin cause water retention and low sodium levels. Conivaptan hydrochloride reduces the level of vasopressin, and the body loses less sodium with urination. The recommended dose is a loading dose of 20 mg administered intravenously over 30 minutes, followed by continuous infusion of 20 mg per day over a 24-hour period for two to four days. After the loading dose, the subsequent doses may be increased up to 40 mg per day as needed. Conivaptan hydrochloride is not recommended for use in patients younger than age 18.

C9507

C9507 Fresh frozen plasma, high titer COVID-19 convalescent, frozen within 8 hours of collection, each unit

Plasma is the liquid portion of whole blood. Plasma is prepared by separating it from whole blood using a centrifuge, or by hemapheresis using centrifugation or filtration. The volume of plasma varies and appears on the label. One unit of fresh frozen plasma contains the plasma from one unit of whole blood, approximately 250 ml, separated and frozen within eight hours of collection. COVID-19 convalescent plasma is human plasma collected from patients who have recovered from COVID-19 and whose plasma contains high titers of anti-SARS-CoV02 antibodies and who meet all donor eligibility requirements and qualifications. COVID-19 convalescent plasma must be obtained from registered or licensed blood establishments from donors located in the United States. Donations must be tested for relevant transfusion-transmitted infections and for high titers of anti-SARS-CoV-2 antibodies prior to release. It is indicated for the treatment of COVID-19 in patients who are receiving immunosuppressive treatment or with immunosuppressive disease. It is administered via intravenous (IV) infusion over one to two hours and can be administered in the inpatient or outpatient setting.

C9600-C9601

C9600 Percutaneous transcatheter placement of drug eluting intracoronary stent(s), with coronary angioplasty when performed; single major coronary artery or branch

C9601 Percutaneous transcatheter placement of drug-eluting intracoronary stent(s), with coronary angioplasty when performed; each additional branch of a major coronary artery (list separately in addition to code for primary procedure)

A drug-eluting stent is coated with medication and used to hold open a blocked or collapsed native artery in the heart. The physician makes a small incision in the arm or leg to access the artery for placement of two catheters. A central venous catheter is inserted through the femoral or brachial artery and a second catheter is threaded up to the affected coronary artery. An obstruction may be treated first by inflating a balloon at the tip of the second catheter (PTCA) to flatten the obstruction. A stent is introduced through a catheter, placed under radiographic guidance, and expanded to fit the lumen of the artery by inflating the balloon on the second catheter. The catheters are removed. Pressure is placed over the incision for 20 to 30 minutes to stop the bleeding.

C

C9602-C9603

C9602 Percutaneous transluminal coronary atherectomy, with drug eluting intracoronary stent, with coronary angioplasty when performed; single major coronary artery or branch

C9603 Percutaneous transluminal coronary atherectomy, with drug-eluting intracoronary stent, with coronary angioplasty when performed; each additional branch of a major coronary artery (list separately in addition to code for primary procedure)

A drug-eluting stent is coated with medication and used to hold open a blocked or collapsed native artery in the heart. The physician makes a small incision in the arm or leg to access the artery for placement of two catheters. A central venous catheter is inserted through the femoral or brachial artery and a second catheter is threaded up to the affected coronary artery. Any obstruction is treated first by using a rotary cutter (atherectomy) to flatten or remove the obstruction. The obstruction may also be treated by inflating a balloon at the tip of the second catheter (PTCA). A stent is introduced through a catheter, placed under radiographic guidance, and expanded to fit the lumen of the artery by inflating the balloon on the second catheter. The catheters are removed. Pressure is placed over the incision for 20 to 30 minutes to stop the bleeding.

C9604-C9605

C9604 Percutaneous transluminal revascularization of or through coronary artery bypass graft (internal mammary, free arterial, venous), any combination of drug-eluting intracoronary stent, atherectomy and angioplasty, including distal protection when performed; single vessel

C9605 Percutaneous transluminal revascularization of or through coronary artery bypass graft (internal mammary, free arterial, venous), any combination of drug-eluting intracoronary stent, atherectomy and angioplasty, including distal protection when performed; each additional branch subtended by the bypass graft (list separately in addition to code for primary procedure)

The use of one or any combination of angioplasty, atherectomy, or drug-eluting stent placement is performed to restore a blocked coronary artery bypass graft (CABG). The physician makes a small incision in the arm or leg to access the artery for placement of two catheters. A central venous catheter is inserted through the femoral or brachial artery and a second catheter is threaded up to the affected graft. The obstruction may be treated by using a rotary cutter (atherectomy) to flatten or remove the obstruction, inflating a balloon at the tip of the second catheter (PTCA), or introducing a drug-eluting stent that is expanded to fit the lumen of the artery. The catheters are removed. Pressure is placed over the incision for 20 to 30 minutes to stop the bleeding.

C9606

C9606 Percutaneous transluminal revascularization of acute total/subtotal occlusion during acute myocardial infarction, coronary artery or coronary artery bypass graft, any combination of drug-eluting intracoronary stent, atherectomy and angioplasty, including aspiration thrombectomy when performed, single vessel

The use of one or any combination of angioplasty, atherectomy, or drug-eluting stent placement is performed to restore an acutely blocked coronary artery bypass graft (CABG) or native coronary artery during an acute myocardial infarction. The physician makes a small incision in the arm or leg to access the artery for placement of two catheters. A central venous catheter is inserted through the femoral or brachial artery and a second catheter is threaded up to the affected vessel or graft. The obstruction may be treated by using a rotary cutter (atherectomy) to flatten or remove the obstruction, inflating a balloon at the tip of the second catheter (PTCA), or introducing a drug-eluting stent that is expanded to fit the lumen of the artery. The catheters are removed. Pressure is placed over the incision for 20 to 30 minutes to stop the bleeding.

C9607-C9608

C9607 Percutaneous transluminal revascularization of chronic total occlusion, coronary artery, coronary artery branch, or coronary artery bypass graft, any combination of drug-eluting intracoronary stent, atherectomy and angioplasty; single vessel

C9608 Percutaneous transluminal revascularization of chronic total occlusion, coronary artery, coronary artery branch, or coronary artery bypass graft, any combination of drug-eluting intracoronary stent, atherectomy and angioplasty; each additional coronary artery, coronary artery branch, or bypass graft (list separately in addition to code for primary procedure)

The use of one or any combination of angioplasty, atherectomy, or drug-eluting stent placement is performed to restore a chronic totally blocked coronary artery bypass graft (CABG) or native coronary artery. The physician makes a small incision in the arm or leg to access the artery for placement of two catheters. A central venous catheter is inserted through the femoral or brachial artery and a second catheter is threaded up to the affected vessel or graft. The obstruction may be treated by using a rotary

C

cutter (atherectomy) to flatten or remove the obstruction, inflating a balloon at the tip of the second catheter (PTCA), or introducing a drug-eluting stent that is expanded to fit the lumen of the artery. The catheters are removed. Pressure is placed over the incision for 20 to 30 minutes to stop the bleeding.

C9725

C9725 Placement of endorectal intracavitary applicator for high intensity brachytherapy

An endorectal intracavitary applicator for high intensity brachytherapy is a disposable, flexible silicone tube developed to meet the criteria of the high dose rate of endorectal brachytherapy. This sphincter preservation surgery modality reduces treatment related toxicity associated with patients with locally advanced resectable rectal cancer. This possible complete sparing of the sphincter and surrounding healthy structures leads to a high sphincter preservation surgery rate and can decrease postoperative complication rates.

C9726

C9726 Placement and removal (if performed) of applicator into breast for intraoperative radiation therapy, add-on to primary breast procedure

An applicator for breast radiation therapy is a device for delivering high dose radiation to the tumor site while minimizing radiation exposure to surrounding tissue. Special catheters are used to deliver needles or a small sphere to the postsurgery cavity. This delivers radiation from the inside out and can save most of the normal breast tissue.

C9727

C9727 Insertion of implants into the soft palate; minimum of three implants

Vibrations and collapse of the soft palate contribute to snoring and sleep apnea. To prevent the collapse, implants are placed into the muscles of the soft palate. These implants stimulate fibrosis and overgrowth of fibrous tissue around the implant, which leads to a reduction in the soft palate leaving less to obstruct the airway.

C9728

C9728 Placement of interstitial device(s) for radiation therapy/surgery guidance (e.g., fiducial markers, dosimeter), for other than the following sites (any approach): abdomen, pelvis, prostate, retroperitoneum, thorax, single or multiple

The physician places one or more interstitial devices such as gold seeds (fiducial markers) for radiation therapy guidance or a dosimeter to gauge the amount of radiation received into the targeted soft tissue tumor. Allowing for precision in targeting radiation and/or for measuring the radiation doses received, a fiducial marker is visible by ultrasound and fluoroscopy and permits accurate triangulation of the tissue to be treated. A capsule dosimeter relays radiation dose information so that the clinical team can monitor for any deviation between the radiation plan and the actual radiation received. This code reports placement of the devices by any approach to areas other than abdomen, pelvis, prostate, retroperitoneum, or thorax.

C9733

C9733 Nonophthalmic fluorescent vascular angiography

Nonophthalmic fluorescent vascular angiography is an imaging procedure that uses a florescent agent, such as indocyanine green, and a low-power laser to visualize blood perfusion and/or flow. The technique is usually used as intraoperative imaging in conjunction with a surgical procedure that needs confirmation of site perfusion or blood flow.

C9734

C9734 Focused ultrasound ablation/therapeutic intervention, other than uterine leiomyomata, with magnetic resonance (MR) guidance

A focused ultrasound ablation or therapeutic intervention is a noninvasive procedure that uses high-intensity ultrasound waves targeted to a specific tissue. This heats the targeted tissue to temperatures of 65 to 100 degrees Celsius and creates local cavitation. Unlike other thermal therapies, high-intensity ultrasound waves heat only the targeted tissue with little heating of adjacent tissue. This code is reported for ablation of non-uterine leiomyomata and includes magnetic resonance (MR) guidance.

C9738

C9738 Adjunctive blue light cystoscopy with fluorescent imaging agent (list separately in addition to code for primary procedure)

Blue light cystoscopy increases tumor detection in nonmuscle invasive bladder cancer (NMIBC). It can be performed only after a white light cystoscopy has been completed. Hexaminolevulinate HCL, an optical imaging agent, is instilled into the bladder via an intravesical catheter and retained in the bladder for one hour. The bladder is evacuated and the blue light cystoscopy is performed. This code is an add-on code, and must be reported in conjunction with the appropriate CPT codes for cystourethroscopy.

C9739-C9740

C9739 Cystourethroscopy, with insertion of transprostatic implant; one to three implants

C9740 Cystourethroscopy, with insertion of transprostatic implant; four or more implants

Transprostatic implants are used to treat benign prostatic hypertrophy (BPH). A cystourethroscope is inserted and advanced to the area of the obstruction. The obstructing prostatic lobes are retracted away from the urethra. A portion of the lobe is compressed using a proprietary implant and, with the prostate held away from the urethra, flow is unobstructed. These implants are permanent and are composed of nitinol, stainless steel, and PET suture.

C9751

C9751 Bronchoscopy, rigid or flexible, transbronchial ablation of lesion(s) by microwave energy, including fluoroscopic guidance, when performed, with computed tomography acquisition(s) and 3D rendering, computer-assisted, image-guided navigation, and endobronchial ultrasound (EBUS) guided transtracheal and/or transbronchial sampling (e.g., aspiration[s]/biopsy[ies]) and all mediastinal and/or hilar lymph node stations or structures and therapeutic intervention(s)

Using a flexible catheter inserted through a bronchoscope, microwave energy is directed through a microwave antenna that has been placed inside a tumor. The microwave energy creates heat, destroying the diseased cells and tissue. This technique offers a cancer treatment option to those patients who are not surgical candidates.

C9756

C9756 Intraoperative near-infrared fluorescence lymphatic mapping of lymph node(s) (sentinel or tumor draining) with administration of indocyanine green (ICG) (List separately in addition to code for primary procedure)

A sentinel lymph node (SLN) is the first lymph node, or a group of lymph nodes, to which a tumor drains. The SLNs are the nodes most likely to contain metastatic disease. Intraoperative SLN lymphatic mapping is performed at the time of tumor excision and allows for the localization of lymph nodes that drain the primary tumor site. The SLNs undergo detailed pathologic examinations that are used to detect smaller metastases, develop appropriate treatment plans, and accurately stage the cancer. Near-infrared lymphatic mapping is performed by injecting indocyanine green (ICG), a fluorescent dye that rapidly localizes to the lymph nodes, near the tumor followed by manual massage of the tissue. A translucent image enhancer is used to compress subcutaneous tissue. The area of fluorescence is then marked for SLN biopsy. Once the biopsy is complete, a gamma probe is used to determine if any radioactive nodes remain.

C9757

C9757 Laminotomy (hemilaminectomy), with decompression of nerve root(s), including partial facetectomy, foraminotomy and excision of herniated intervertebral disc, and repair of annular defect with implantation of bone anchored annular closure device, including annular defect measurement, alignment and sizing assessment, and image guidance; 1 interspace, lumbar

A laminotomy (hemilaminectomy) is a type of spinal decompression surgery involving partial removal of the spine's lamina (bony protective covering at the back of the spinal canal). This procedure includes decompression of nerve roots, including removal of tiny bone growths that may be causing pain; enlarging of the opening through which the nerve root passes; and excision of herniated intervertebral discs. Report C9757 for the laminotomy/hemilaminectomy procedure and repair of annular defects with implantation of a bone-anchored annular closure device, including annular defect measurements, alignment, and sizing assessment. Image guidance is included. This code represents one lumbar interspace.

C9758

C9758 Blind procedure for NYHA Class III/IV heart failure; transcatheter implantation of interatrial shunt including right heart catheterization, transesophageal echocardiography (TEE)/intracardiac echocardiography (ICE), and all imaging with or without guidance (e.g., ultrasound, fluoroscopy), performed in an approved investigational device exemption (IDE) study

This HCPCS code was created to ensure that participants in a clinical trial for NYHA Class III/IV heart failure would be unable to discern which patient received an interatrial shunt or a placebo.

C9759

C9759 Transcatheter intraoperative blood vessel microinfusion(s) (e.g., intraluminal, vascular wall and/or perivascular) therapy, any vessel, including radiological supervision and interpretation, when performed

Transcatheter intraoperative blood vessel microinfusion therapy is intended for the infusion of diagnostic and therapeutic agents into the blood vessel wall, intraluminally, or in the perivascular area, into adventitial tissues (the fibrous connective tissue that surrounds an artery, vein, or organ). The

C

microinfusion device has a balloon-sheathed microneedle on the tip, which provides a protective covering for the small injection needle as it is passed through the vasculature to its intended target. Once the target is reached, the balloon is inflated to two atmospheres with saline and a radio-opaque contrast. This secures the device and allows the microneedle to slide through the vessel wall. The low-pressure inflation of the transcatheter intraoperative blood vessel microinfusion therapy device does not inflict trauma on the vessel wall. Standard angioplasty balloons operate between eight to 20 atmospheres.

C9760

C9760 Nonrandomized, nonblinded procedure for NYHA Class II, III, IV heart failure; transcatheter implantation of interatrial shunt, including right and left heart catheterization, transeptal puncture, transesophageal echocardiography (TEE)/intracardiac echocardiography (ICE), and all imaging with or without guidance (e.g., ultrasound, fluoroscopy), performed in an approved investigational device exemption (IDE) study

This HCPCS code was created for participants in a clinical trial for NYHA Class II/III/IV heart failure patients who are part of an approved investigational device exemption (IDE) study for the implantation of an interatrial shunt. The study is nonrandomized, or nonblinded, meaning the researchers and patients are aware of the procedures being performed. An interatrial shunt device provides continuous and dynamic compression of the left atrium, which may reduce symptoms and slow the progression of heart failure. The interatrial device is placed nonsurgically, via transcatheter implantation, by an interventional cardiologist, and creates a small opening between the left and right atria. This small opening allows for blood flow from the high pressure left atrium to the low pressure right atrium, and reduces pressure in the left side of the heart and in the lungs.

C9761

C9761 Cystourethroscopy, with ureteroscopy and/or pyeloscopy, with lithotripsy, and ureteral catheterization for steerable vacuum aspiration of the kidney, collecting system, ureter, bladder, and urethra if applicable (must use a steerable ureteral catheter)

The physician examines the urinary collecting system with endoscopes passed through the urethra into the bladder (cystourethroscope), ureter (ureteroscope), and renal pelvis (pyeloscope) and removes or manipulates a stone (calculus). To extract or manipulate a calculus, the physician passes the appropriate surgical instruments through an endoscope to fragment the calculus. An ultrasonic, electrohydraulic, or laser technique is used, and a single-use, steerable vacuum aspiration catheter is used to irrigate and collect remaining small stone fragments. A ureteral stent may be inserted to ensure adequate urine drainage and the endoscope and instruments are removed. Report C9761 only for a steerable vacuum aspiration catheter.

C9762-C9763

C9762 Cardiac magnetic resonance imaging for morphology and function, quantification of segmental dysfunction; with strain imaging

C9763 Cardiac magnetic resonance imaging for morphology and function, quantification of segmental dysfunction; with stress imaging

Cardiac magnetic resonance imaging (MRI) is a radiation-free, noninvasive technique that produces high quality, detailed, three-dimensional imaging of complex congenital heart defects, as well as functional cardiac analysis. MRI uses the natural magnetic properties of the hydrogen atoms in our bodies that emit radiofrequency signals when exposed to radiowaves within a strong electromagnetic field. These signals are processed and converted by the computer into high-resolution images. Patients with metallic or electronic implants or foreign bodies cannot be exposed to MRI. The patient must remain still while lying on a motorized table within a large, circular MRI tunnel. A sedative may be administered. Imaging is performed by obtaining tomographic cuts from the base to the apex and/or the interior to the posterior in order to interrogate the entire heart. Function studies may include observation of the atria and/or ventricles, qualitative and quantitative assessment of ventricular function, and obtaining numerical values for ejection fraction (EF) ventricular volumes, ventricular mass, and cardiac output. Strain imaging is used to determine left ventricular (LV) deformation: areas with blocks of 20 to 40 markers (pixels) that contain consistent patterns known as speckles. These markers or fingerprints are helpful in outlining irregularities by comprehensive assessment of regional myocardial function, specifically by discriminating between active and passive myocardial wall movement. Strain rate data assists in early detection of myocardial dysfunction and is beneficial in therapeutic decisions and follow-up of previous cardiac surgery. Stress imaging mimics the effects of exercise on the heart, including ischemia. Following a dobutamine injection, the physician evaluates the LV wall's ability to move during physical stress. Report C9762 for cardiac MRI with strain imaging. Report C9763 for cardiac MRI with stress imaging.

C9764-C9767

C9764 Revascularization, endovascular, open or percutaneous, lower extremity artery(ies), except tibial/peroneal; with intravascular lithotripsy, includes angioplasty within the same vessel(s), when performed

C9765 Revascularization, endovascular, open or percutaneous, lower extremity artery(ies), except tibial/peroneal; with intravascular lithotripsy, and transluminal stent placement(s), includes angioplasty within the same vessel(s), when performed

C9766 Revascularization, endovascular, open or percutaneous, lower extremity artery(ies), except tibial/peroneal; with intravascular lithotripsy and atherectomy, includes angioplasty within the same vessel(s), when performed

C9767 Revascularization, endovascular, open or percutaneous, lower extremity artery(ies), except tibial/peroneal; with intravascular lithotripsy and transluminal stent placement(s), and atherectomy, includes angioplasty within the same vessel(s), when performed

Intravascular lithotripsy (IVL) delivers unfocused, circumferential, pulsatile mechanical energy to safely disrupt calcium deposits within the target lesion. The IVL catheter is guided to the target lesion and an integrated balloon is inflated to four atmospheres. Once the catheter is in place, an electrical discharge vaporizes fluid inside the balloon. This action creates a rapidly expanding and collapsing bubble generating sonic pressure waves. The sonic pressure waves travel through soft vascular tissue, cracking the intimal and medial calcium within the vessel wall. The balloon may be used to dilate the target lesion at a low pressure to maximize luminal gain. Angioplasty is included, when performed. Report C9765 for IVL performed with transluminal stent placement. Report C9766 for IVL performed with atherectomy. Report C9767 for IVL performed with stent placement and atherectomy.

C9768

C9768 Endoscopic ultrasound-guided direct measurement of hepatic portosystemic pressure gradient by any method (list separately in addition to code for primary procedure)

The portosystemic pressure gradient measurement system provides access to the hepatic and portal veins to obtain local blood pressure measurements. The system consists of an endoscopic ultrasound needle, connecting tube, 10 mL syringe, stopcock, and a pressure transducer. See manufacturer instructions for system assembly and preparation instructions. The physician performs an esophagogastroduodenoscopy (EGD) with a concomitant ultrasound examination for diagnostic purposes. The patient is prepped for an upper gastrointestinal exam and the scope is advanced through the mouth into the stomach and duodenum or jejunum. An examination is carried out to determine if any bleeding, tumors, erosions, ulcers, or other abnormalities are present. Once the first desired vasculature is identified (hepatic and portal vein), the assembled and prepared device is advanced into the endoscope and fitted. The needle extension is set to the desired length and advanced into the target vein. Using the syringe, up to 0.5 mL of sterile fluid is instilled and time is allowed for the pressure reading to equilibrate. The instillation and obtaining pressure reading must be performed three times from the same vessel. The needle is completely retracted, the endoscope is repositioned, and the second vessel to be accessed is identified. The needle is advanced to the second target vessel and the instillation and pressure reading is performed three times. The needle is retracted, disconnected, and completely withdrawn from the endoscope. The endoscope is removed. This is an add-on code that represents the pressure measurement only and must be reported with the appropriate primary CPT endoscopic ultrasound procedure code.

C9769

C9769 Cystourethroscopy, with insertion of temporary prostatic implant/stent with fixation/anchor and incisional struts

The physician inserts a temporary prostatic implant that includes anchor fixation and incisional struts in a patient with lower urinary tract symptoms caused by benign prostatic hypertrophy (BPH) to improve voiding function and to allow for voluntary urination. Under appropriate anesthesia and with the patient in the lithotomy position, the physician performs routine cystoscopic inspection of the bladder and urethra. The temporary proprietary device, consisting of flexible nickel titanium alloy (nitinol) struts, is preloaded into a custom system, passed through the cystoscopic sheath, and deployed. The physician manipulates the device into the desired position with the anchoring leaflet situated under the bladder neck at the appropriate location. Once secured, the physician retracts the device so that the struts are positioned accurately and are in contact with the encroaching prostatic tissue. There, they will exert continuous pressure and result in ischemia and necrosis of the tissue, remodeling the prostatic urethra and bladder neck by creating channels or incisions through which urine can flow freely. Five to seven days postoperatively, the device is removed completely, and the newly formed incisions continue to provide relief.

C9770

C9770 Vitrectomy, mechanical, pars plana approach, with subretinal injection of pharmacologic/biologic agent

The physician performs a mechanical vitrectomy with subretinal injection of a pharmacologic or biologic agent utilizing a pars plana approach. This procedure is performed for the administration of a gene therapy product indicated for the treatment of adults and children, 12 months of age or older, with biallelic RPE65 mutation-associated retinal dystrophy. The physician applies a special contact lens to the cornea to better visualize the back of the eye. Three small incisions are made in the eyeball, each about 4 mm from the juncture of the cornea and sclera. One incision is for a light cannula, one for an infusion cannula, and one for the cutting or suction instruments. The physician extracts the vitreous, which is the clear gel filling the posterior cavity of the eyeball, using a mechanical cutting and suctioning process that may involve a roto extractor or vitreous infusion suction cutter (VISC). Following vitrectomy, prefilled syringes of the gene therapy product are mounted on high-pressure extension tubing with a subretinal injection cannula. The tip of the needle is placed into the vitreous cavity and an injection site is chosen using a high-magnification lens. The needle tip is placed in contact with the retinal surface and manual infusion is initiated. Once injection is confirmed with intraoperative optical coherence tomography (OCT) imaging, the needle is withdrawn.

C

C9771

C9771 Nasal/sinus endoscopy, cryoablation nasal tissue(s) and/or nerve(s), unilateral or bilateral

Chronic rhinitis, or inflammation of the nasal mucosa, causes excess mucus production, which is regulated by the nerves in the posterior nasal area. Symptoms include frequent sneezing, nasal congestion and itching, and postnasal drip. The physician performs cryotherapy treatment to ablate these nerves and disrupt the nerve signals that cause rhinitis. Using an endoscope, the physician performs a diagnostic evaluation of the nose and/or sinus cavities. An endoscope has a rigid fiberoptic telescope that allows the physician increased visualization and magnification of internal anatomy. Topical vasoconstrictive agents are applied to the nasal mucosa and nerve blocks with local anesthesia are performed. The endoscope is placed into the nose and a thorough inspection of the internal nasal or sinus structures is accomplished. A proprietary cryosurgical tool is then inserted under endoscopic guidance into the posterior nasal area at the targeted area of inflammation. Once precise placement is confirmed, the physician utilizes the cooling probe to freeze the mucosal lining at the site of the overstimulated nerves. Freezing continues for approximately 30 seconds, after which the cryoprobe is turned off. The ice crystals formed at the targeted area are allowed to thaw for approximately 30 seconds, and the cryoprobe is removed. This procedure may be repeated on the opposite side.

C9772-C9775

C9772 Revascularization, endovascular, open or percutaneous, tibial/peroneal artery(ies), with intravascular lithotripsy, includes angioplasty within the same vessel(s), when performed

C9773 Revascularization, endovascular, open or percutaneous, tibial/peroneal artery(ies); with intravascular lithotripsy, and transluminal stent placement(s), includes angioplasty within the same vessel(s), when performed

C9774 Revascularization, endovascular, open or percutaneous, tibial/peroneal artery(ies); with intravascular lithotripsy and atherectomy, includes angioplasty within the same vessel(s), when performed

C9775 Revascularization, endovascular, open or percutaneous, tibial/peroneal artery(ies); with intravascular lithotripsy and transluminal stent placement(s), and atherectomy, includes angioplasty within the same vessel(s), when performed

Intravascular lithotripsy (IVL), using technology similar to lithotripsy for renal calculi, is a new technology that uses intermittent lithotripsy pulsed soundwaves to disrupt high-density calcified plaque in patients with peripheral arterial disease in the tibial and/or peroneal arteries with minimal impact to soft tissue. The system consists of a generator, a connector cable, and a catheter that contains lithotripsy emitters enclosed within an integrated angioplasty balloon. The generator produces energy that travels through the connector cable and catheter to the lithotripsy emitters at one pulse per second. In C9772, the insertion site is prepared using standard sterile technique. Using an open or percutaneous approach, vascular access is achieved, and an introducer sheath is placed. An appropriate balloon catheter size is selected and prepared. A 20-cc syringe is filled with 5 cc of 50/50 saline/contrast medium. The syringe is attached to the inflation port on the catheter hub. The vacuum is pulled and released to allow the fluid to replace the air in the catheter. Under fluoroscopic guidance, the calcified arterial lesion is crossed with a 0.014-inch guidewire, and the over-the-wire lithotripsy catheter with an integrated balloon is advanced to the lesion and is positioned using radiopaque markers. With the integrated balloon expanded with the mixed saline and contrast solution, with sufficient diameter to achieve contact with the vessel wall, the generator is used to produce a small electrical discharge at the emitters that vaporizes the fluid and creates a rapidly expanding bubble within the balloon. The bubble generates a series of sonic pressure waves that travel through the fluid-filled balloon and pass through the soft vascular tissue, selectively cracking the hardened calcified plaque. The emitters positioned along the length of the device create a localized effect within the vessel to break up the calcium. The integrated balloon expands the blockages at low pressures to restore blood flow, provides circumferential pulsatile energy to ensure efficient energy transfer, and constrains the bubble expansion. Following the calcium disruption, the balloon is inflated and deflated as many times as needed to maximize the artery lumen until the desired diameter is achieved. An arteriogram may be performed to assess the results. Once the desired results are achieved, the device is deflated and the catheter with integrated balloon is removed intact. Pressure is placed over the access site for 20 to 30 minutes to stem bleeding or, if performed via open approach, the vessel may be repaired, and the skin incision closed by sutures. The patient is observed for a period afterward. In C9773, the physician places one or more transluminal stents percutaneously using a guidewire or by incision. A catheter with a stent-transporting tip is threaded into the vessel. The catheter travels to the point where the vessel needs additional support, and the compressed stent is passed from the catheter into the vessel, where it deploys and expands to support the vessel walls. The catheter is removed. In C9774, the physician performs atherectomy in conjunction with IVL. The physician slides a guidewire through the atherectomy catheter or device and inserts the guidewire/atherectomy catheter combination through the introducer sheath. The atherectomy device is fluoroscopically positioned at the site of the stenosis. The physician activates the device to remove the stenotic tissue and rechecks the diameter of the lesion by angiography. Several passes with the atherectomy device may be required. The physician removes the atherectomy catheter, guidewire, and introducer sheath. Report C9775 if the physician performs both stent placement and atherectomy in conjunction with IVL. Angioplasty within the same vessel is included in all codes.

C9776

C9776 Intraoperative near-infrared fluorescence imaging of major extra-hepatic bile duct(s) (e.g., cystic duct, common bile duct and common hepatic duct) with intravenous administration of indocyanine green (ICG) (list separately in addition to code for primary procedure)

Real-time intraoperative imaging is performed using near-infrared (NIR) light to visualize the extrahepatic bile ducts. Used in conjunction with injectable indocyanine green (ICG), a fluorescent dye that accumulates in the bile, imaging and identification of key vasculature and extrahepatic biliary structures can be accomplished during the separately reportable procedure.

C9777

C9777 Esophageal mucosal integrity testing by electrical impedance, transoral, includes esophagoscopy or esophagogastroduodenoscopy

This mucosal integrity testing system utilizes a balloon probe and proprietary software during routine endoscopy procedures to obtain real-time measurements of electrical properties in esophageal mucosa. Measuring conductivity of the esophageal epithelium directly, it provides the physician with a color contour map as well as predictive probability, allowing providers to rule out or to differentiate esophageal disorders such as gastroesophageal reflux disease (GERD) and eosinophilic esophagitis, as well as to monitor response to treatment. Mucosal integrity is measured at 180-degree intervals along a 10 cm section of the esophagus, providing real-time data. Esophagoscopy or esophagogastroduodenoscopy is included.

C9778

C9778 Colpopexy, vaginal; minimally invasive extraperitoneal approach (sacrospinous)

Colpopexy is performed by a minimally invasive transvaginal, extraperitoneal approach to restore the apex or vault of the vagina to its anatomic position in cases of prolapse. One version of this procedure utilizes a proprietary device mounted on the surgeon's index finger that is introduced into the vaginal cavity. The surgeon palpates the right ischial spine and the sacrospinous ligament (SSL) through the vaginal wall, then stabilizes the finger to the mid SSL. The device anchor is deployed and tested for adequate pull-out force. At the posterior vaginal wall, the surgeon makes a 1 cm incision. The anchor's suture is mounted on a needle. It is then inserted backward through the vaginal wall at the point of entry and passed under the vaginal wall, through the cervical isthmus, and out to the vaginal cavity, again through the posterior colpotomy. The surgeon repeats these steps on the left side, ties the suture, and closes the small posterior vaginal incision.

C9779

C9779 Endoscopic submucosal dissection (ESD), including endoscopy or colonoscopy, mucosal closure, when performed

Endoscopic submucosal dissection (ESD) is a surgical procedure performed via endoscopy to remove lesions or tumors from the gastrointestinal (GI) tract without removing the entire organ. The procedure is performed through an endoscope, a device consisting of a tube and optical system for viewing the inside of a hollow organ or cavity. Special instruments are passed through the endoscope, the lesion is highlighted with a special stain to distinguish it from surrounding healthy tissue, liquid is injected to lift the lesion and submucosal layer, and the lesion is dissected and removed in one piece through the endoscope. Closure of the mucosal layer may be required. This code reports the endoscopy, dissection, and mucosal closure, when required.

C9780

C9780 Insertion of central venous catheter through central venous occlusion via inferior and superior approaches (e.g., inside-out technique), including imaging guidance

A central venous access device (CVAD) or catheter is one in which the tip terminates in the subclavian, brachiocephalic, or iliac vein; the superior or inferior vena cava; or the right atrium. Access for these catheters are usually obtained through skin puncture and guidewire insertion through an access vein (i.e., subclavian, jugular). Because of multiple, failed venous access sites, patients often experience central venous occlusion. Venous occlusive disease develops over time and prevents patients from receiving lifesaving services such as chemotherapy and drug infusion, cardiac pacing, and hemodialysis. An inside-out access (IOA) technique allows for the placement of a CVAD catheter through femoral vein access, preserving and restoring access in chronically occluded veins. Using ultrasound guidance, vascular access is obtained through the right femoral vein and a guidewire is introduced and passed through the inferior vena cava and right atrium, into the superior vena cava (SVC), until it reaches the central venous occlusion. A transseptal sheath and dilator (workstation) is then passed over the guidewire to the occlusion site and the guidewire removed. The tip of the IOA device (a metal pole with needle-wire inside, attached to a handle) is advanced to and pushed through the occlusion under imaging guidance. The IOA tip is advanced to a target, placed on the right supraclavicular region prior to the procedure, just above the clavicle until the skin is tented. A small incision is made at the site of skin tenting and the needle-wire is retrieved from subcutaneous tissue. A sheath is locked onto the needle-wire, which becomes a guidewire, and is pulled into the right atrium. The desired tunneled catheter is then inserted and secured into position. Imaging guidance (ultrasound and/or fluoroscopy) for access and to check positioning of the catheter tip may be used and is included.

C9781

C9781 Arthroscopy, shoulder, surgical; with implantation of subacromial spacer (e.g., balloon), includes debridement (e.g., limited or extensive), subacromial decompression, acromioplasty, and biceps tenodesis when performed

The physician performs a surgical arthroscopy for the treatment of a massive irreparable rotator cuff tear (MIRCT). The patient is positioned side-lying with the arm suspended. Small, percutaneous poke hole incisions are made around the shoulder through which the arthroscopic instruments are inserted. A solution is pumped through one of these incisions to cleanse and expand the joint for better visualization. The physician first performs a diagnostic arthroscopic exam to assess the joint. A limited bursectomy may be performed with a subacromial decompression and/or acromioplasty, if necessary, but the spacer may be inserted as an isolated procedure. After measurement of the space is confirmed, a balloon-shaped spacer, made from a biodegradable polymer, is positioned in the subacromial space and inflated with normal saline. No sutures or other fixation devices are required. The spacer restores normal humeral head position and joint mechanics, allowing for improved function and decreased pain. The spacer biodegrades over approximately 12 months. The joint is irrigated, and a long-acting local anesthetic may be injected into the joint to help with postoperative pain. Sutures, band aids, or Steri-strips close the incisions. The area is covered with a dressing and a sling or a shoulder immobilizer is applied.

C9782

C9782 Blinded procedure for New York Heart Association (NYHA) Class II or III heart failure, or Canadian Cardiovascular Society (CCS) Class III or IV chronic refractory angina; transcatheter intramyocardial transplantation of autologous bone marrow cells (e.g., mononuclear) or placebo control, autologous bone marrow harvesting and preparation for transplantation, left heart catheterization including ventriculography, all laboratory services, and all imaging with or without guidance (e.g., transthoracic echocardiography, ultrasound, fluoroscopy), performed in an approved investigational device exemption (IDE) study

This HCPCS code was created for participants in a clinical trial for NYHA Class II or III heart failure, or Canadian Cardiovascular Society (CCS) Class III or IV chronic refractory angina patients who are part of an approved investigational device exemption (IDE) study for the transcatheter intramyocardial transplantation of autologous bone marrow cells. The study is blinded, meaning the patients are unable to discern whether they received the autologous bone marrow cells or a placebo. This code reports harvesting and preparation of bone marrow, left heart catheterization, ventriculography, laboratory services, and all imaging required.

C9783

C9783 Blinded procedure for transcatheter implantation of coronary sinus reduction device or placebo control, including vascular access and closure, right heart catherization, venous and coronary sinus angiography, imaging guidance and supervision and interpretation when performed in an approved investigational device exemption (IDE) study

This HCPCS Level II code was created for patients who are part of an approved investigational device exemption (IDE) study for transcatheter implantation of a coronary sinus reduction device. The study is blinded, meaning the patients are unable to discern whether they received the coronary sinus device or a placebo treatment. This code reports vascular access and closure, right heart catheterization, angiography, and all imaging guidance. Supervision and interpretation are required.

C9803

C9803 Hospital outpatient clinic visit specimen collection for severe acute respiratory syndrome coronavirus 2 (SARS-CoV-2) (coronavirus disease [COVID-19]), any specimen source

For hospital outpatient clinics, the Centers for Medicare and Medicaid Services (CMS) has created a code that may be reported to identify and reimburse specimen collection for COVID-19 testing under the Outpatient Prospective Payment System (OPPS). Specimens may be obtained through a variety of sources, such as nasopharyngeal or oropharyngeal swab, nasopharyngeal wash or aspirate, nasal aspirate, or sputum.

C9898

C9898 Radiolabeled product provided during a hospital inpatient stay

Hospitals are to report this code on outpatient claims for nuclear medicine procedures to indicate that a radiolabeled product that provides the radioactivity necessary for the reported diagnostic nuclear medicine procedure was provided during a hospital inpatient stay.

C9899

C9899 Implanted prosthetic device, payable only for inpatients who do not have inpatient coverage

This code is reported when an inpatient who does not have inpatient Part A coverage receives an implanted prosthetic device.

E

E0100-E0105

E0100 Cane, includes canes of all materials, adjustable or fixed, with tip

E0105 Cane, quad or three-prong, includes canes of all materials, adjustable or fixed, with tips

Walking canes provide the legs with some relief for weight bearing in conditions of impaired ambulation. Canes can be single, three, or four prongs and add another point or points of ground contact that alter the biomechanics of walking to affect balance, relieve pain, and provide stability. Canes are used on the opposite side of the injury or weakness, regardless of which hand is dominant. The patient puts all of their weight on the unaffected leg, then steps with the affected leg and cane at the same time. Tips provide traction.

E0110-E0117

E0110 Crutches, forearm, includes crutches of various materials, adjustable or fixed, pair, complete with tips and handgrips

E0111 Crutch, forearm, includes crutches of various materials, adjustable or fixed, each, with tip and handgrips

E0112 Crutches, underarm, wood, adjustable or fixed, pair, with pads, tips, and handgrips

E0113 Crutch, underarm, wood, adjustable or fixed, each, with pad, tip, and handgrip

E0114 Crutches, underarm, other than wood, adjustable or fixed, pair, with pads, tips, and handgrips

E0116 Crutch, underarm, other than wood, adjustable or fixed, with pad, tip, handgrip, with or without shock absorber, each

E0117 Crutch, underarm, articulating, spring assisted, each

Crutches (wood or aluminum), both standard underarm and forearm crutches that have cuffs encircling the lower portion of the arms, support the body during walking and help protect the injured body limb for patients with impaired ambulation.

E0118

E0118 Crutch substitute, lower leg platform, with or without wheels, each

A crutch substitute is a hands-free device that consists of a long metal bar with a platform attached at knee height at a 90-degree angle. The device has pads on the platform and straps to hold the leg. The patient places the bent knee on the platform and secures the upper leg to the metal bar and the knee to the platform. The device can have a rounded rubber foot or can have wheels attached to the distal end. The device can be used to replace a missing lower leg or to remove weight bearing from an injured lower leg.

E

E0130-E0144

E0130 Walker, rigid (pickup), adjustable or fixed height

E0135 Walker, folding (pickup), adjustable or fixed height

E0140 Walker, with trunk support, adjustable or fixed height, any type

E0141 Walker, rigid, wheeled, adjustable or fixed height

E0143 Walker, folding, wheeled, adjustable or fixed height

E0144 Walker, enclosed, four-sided framed, rigid or folding, wheeled with posterior seat

Walkers are used by patients with impaired ambulation when there is a need for greater stability and security than can be provided by a cane or crutches. Some walkers are simple "semi-cages," which look like two canes with supporting bars between them. Others are more complicated, and can be rigid or folding, with or without seating, with or without wheels, etc. Walkers may also include a device attached to the walker that provides trunk support. A trunk support device holds the patient upright in a standing position. The device may be flexible and soft padded or may be more rigid. The type of device depends upon the patient's medical condition. For example, a patient with cerebral palsy who has diminished muscle control of the trunk may need a rigid trunk support.

E0147-E0149

E0147 Walker, heavy-duty, multiple braking system, variable wheel resistance

E0148 Walker, heavy-duty, without wheels, rigid or folding, any type, each

E0149 Walker, heavy-duty, wheeled, rigid or folding, any type

Walkers are used by patients with impaired ambulation when there is a need for greater stability and security than can be provided by a cane or crutches. Some walkers are simple "semi-cages," which look like two canes with supporting bars between them. Others are more complicated, and can be rigid or folding, with or without seating, with or without wheels, etc. Heavy duty walkers are used by patients with severe neurological disorders or restricted use of one hand and those who exceed the weight limits of a standard wheeled walker.

E0153-E0159

E0153 Platform attachment, forearm crutch, each

E0154 Platform attachment, walker, each

E0155 Wheel attachment, rigid pick-up walker, per pair

E0156 Seat attachment, walker

E0157 Crutch attachment, walker, each

E0158 Leg extensions for walker, per set of four

E0159 Brake attachment for wheeled walker, replacement, each

These codes report the various attachments used with walkers and crutches.

E0160-E0175

E0160 Sitz type bath or equipment, portable, used with or without commode

E0161 Sitz type bath or equipment, portable, used with or without commode, with faucet attachment(s)

E0162 Sitz bath chair

E0163 Commode chair, mobile or stationary, with fixed arms

E0165 Commode chair, mobile or stationary, with detachable arms

E0167 Pail or pan for use with commode chair, replacement only

E0168 Commode chair, extra wide and/or heavy-duty, stationary or mobile, with or without arms, any type, each

E0170 Commode chair with integrated seat lift mechanism, electric, any type

E0171 Commode chair with integrated seat lift mechanism, nonelectric, any type

E0172 Seat lift mechanism placed over or on top of toilet, any type

E0175 Footrest, for use with commode chair, each

Commodes are generally portable toilets in a chair form that hold a pot under an open toilet seat. Some commodes, known as sitz baths, have large deep pans that also serve as a hip bath to soak the hips, buttocks, or perineal area wounds. There are many types/styles of commodes available on the market.

E0181-E0183

E0181 Powered pressure reducing mattress overlay/pad, alternating, with pump, includes heavy-duty

E0182 Pump for alternating pressure pad, for replacement only

E0183 Powered pressure reducing underlay/pad, alternating, with pump, includes heavy duty

These codes describe power pressure-reducing mattress overlays of alternating pressure or low air loss. These pressure reducing support devices consist of various pads that reduce the pressure of the patient's body weight on any area of the body. They are characterized by an air pump or blower that provides sequential inflation or deflation of air cells or a low interface pressure throughout the overlay. They have inflated cell height of the air cells through which air is being circulated of 2.5 inches or greater. The height of the air chambers, proximity of the air chambers to one another, frequency of air cycling (for alternating pressure overlays), and air pressure provide adequate patient lift, pressure reduction, and prevention of bottoming out. Typically used for patients who are fully or partially immobile (e.g., paraplegic patient), they assist in reducing the pressure on skin and tissues, allowing blood flow to the focal points in question, to prevent and/or treat pressure ulcers and lesions, such as decubitus ulcers.

E0184-E0187

E0184 Dry pressure mattress

E0185 Gel or gel-like pressure pad for mattress, standard mattress length and width

E0186 Air pressure mattress

E0187 Water pressure mattress

These codes report special mattresses that reduce the pressure of the patient's body weight on any particular area of the body. Generally used for patients who are fully or partially immobile (e.g., paraplegic patient), they assist in reducing the pressure on skin and tissues, allowing blood flow to the focal points in question, to prevent and/or treat pressure ulcers and lesions, such as decubitus ulcers. These codes describe non-powered pressure-reducing mattresses. A foam or dry pressure mattress is characterized by a height of 5 inches or greater, with a density and other qualities that provide adequate pressure reduction. It is durable, has a waterproof cover, and can be placed directly on a hospital bedframe. A gel or gel-like mattress overlay is characterized by a gel or gel-like layer contained within the pad reaching a height of 2 inches or greater. An air pressure or water pressure mattress is characterized by a height of 5 inches or greater of the air or water contained inside, has a durable, waterproof cover, and can be placed directly on a hospital bedframe.

E0188-E0189

E0188 Synthetic sheepskin pad

E0189 Lambswool sheepskin pad, any size

A decubitus ulcer is also known as a pressure ulcer, pressure sore, or bedsore. Bedsores can range from a mild erythema of the skin to a deep wound extending through bone. Pressure ulcers occur when an incapacitated, bedridden person has constant pressure against the skin, usually over a bony area, which decreases the blood supply, causing tissue death. Use of special pads or beds relieves pressure on the skin. Pads made of synthetic sheepskin or lambs wool with heel or elbow protectors prevent friction against thin fragile skin.

E0190

E0190 Positioning cushion/pillow/wedge, any shape or size, includes all components and accessories

Positioning cushions/pillows/wedges are typically made of foam or foam-like materials, and come in a variety of densities, shapes, and designs depending on the manufacturer. Most have anatomic-oriented designs so as to provide as much support as possible, although they somewhat limit range of motion. These cushions/pillows/wedges relieve and/or prevent neck tension and may protect against inadvertent reinjury during sleep.

E0191-E0194

E0191 Heel or elbow protector, each

E0193 Powered air flotation bed (low air loss therapy)

E0194 Air fluidized bed

A decubitus ulcer is also known as a pressure ulcer, pressure sore, or bedsore. Bedsores can range from a mild erythema of the skin to a deep wound extending through bone. Pressure ulcers occur when an incapacitated, bedridden person has constant pressure against the skin, usually over a bony area, which decreases the blood supply, causing tissue death. Use of special pads or beds relieves pressure on the skin. Pads made of synthetic sheepskin or lamb's wool with heel or elbow protectors prevent friction against thin fragile skin. Specialized beds, such as a powered air flotation bed or an air-fluidized bed, are often used for patients with stage three or four pressure sores that would otherwise require institutionalization.

E0196

E0196 Gel pressure mattress

A gel pressure mattress is a mattress with a top layer of gel that is enclosed in a durable, waterproof bladder. The gel layer must be at least a height of 5 inches. Some gel mattresses have a layer of soft or pillow-top material directly under the gel layer. This is a full mattress that can be placed directly on a bed frame. A gel pressure mattress is designed to distribute weight more evenly across the surface of the mattress and eliminate pressure points. When there is decreased pressure on skin at contact points, such as buttocks and ankles, skin and soft tissue is less likely to break down and form ulcers or other types of open wounds.

E0197-E0199

E0197 Air pressure pad for mattress, standard mattress length and width

E0198 Water pressure pad for mattress, standard mattress length and width

E0199 Dry pressure pad for mattress, standard mattress length and width

These codes, identified as "pressure pad for mattress," describe non-powered pressure reducing mattress overlays. These devices are designed to be placed on top of a hospital or home mattress of standard length and width. Pressure reducing support services consist of various pads for mattresses that reduce the pressure of the patient's body weight on any particular area of the body. Typically used for patient's that are fully or partially immobile (e.g., paraplegic patient), they assist in reducing the pressure on skin and tissues, allowing blood flow to the focal points in question, to prevent and/or treat pressure ulcers and lesions, such as decubitus ulcers. An air pressure pad is characterized by interconnected air cells having a cell height of 3 inches or greater. A water pressure mattress overlay (E0198) is characterized by a filled height of 3 inches or greater of water contained within the pads cells. A foam mattress overlay, or dry pressure pad, is characterized by a base thickness of 2 inches or greater and peak height of 3 inches or greater if it is a convoluted overlay (e.g., egg crate-type) or an overall height of at least 3 inches if it is a non-convoluted overlay.

E0200

E0200 Heat lamp, without stand (table model), includes bulb, or infrared element

Heat causes blood vessels to open, creating increased blood flow and allowing tissue purging of debris and by-products of injury. Heat therapy promotes relaxation of collagen tissues within muscle, tendons, and ligaments, which allow them to be stretched. Heat lamps provide dry heat to patients who cannot tolerate pressure of a directly applied heat source or who may have positioning needs. The heat from a lamp is controlled by the distance between the lamp and the patient. Report E0200 for a heat lamp without a stand.

E0202

E0202 Phototherapy (bilirubin) light with photometer

A phototherapy (bilirubin) light with photometer is used to treat infants with jaundice caused by elevated levels of bilirubin in the blood. Phototherapy lights provide a specific wavelength of blue fluorescent light that breaks down bilirubin into nontoxic water-soluble components that are excreted by the infant. The photometer or "blue meter" on the lamp measures the intensity of the light emission. Phototherapy lights are available in the form of a lamp, light panel, or special light blanket (wallaby blanket) and all are reported with this code.

E0203

E0203 Therapeutic lightbox, minimum 10,000 lux, table top model

A therapeutic lightbox with a minimum of 10,000 lux is used to treat seasonal affective disorder (SAD), which is a form of depression; diurnal disorders; or sometimes to mitigate the effects of medications. SAD occurs most frequently in the fall or winter as the daylight hours become shorter and shorter. Therapeutic lightboxes provide cool-white or full spectrum fluorescent light to treat this disorder. The light boxes deliver strong light near the intensity and wavelength of noontime during high summer. Patients expose themselves to the light for a prescribed amount of time per day at set times. Tabletop or desktop lightboxes that emit a minimum of 10,000 lux, which is a measurement of the light intensity, are reported with this code. Lightboxes that emit lower levels of lux (5,000 or 2,500) should not be reported.

E0205

E0205 Heat lamp, with stand, includes bulb, or infrared element

Heat causes blood vessels to open, creating increased blood flow and allowing tissue purging of debris and by-products of injury. Heat therapy promotes relaxation of collagen tissues within muscle, tendons, and ligaments, which allow them to be stretched. Heat lamps provide dry heat to patients who cannot tolerate pressure of a directly applied heat source or who may have positioning needs. The heat from a lamp is controlled by the distance between the lamp and the patient. Report E0205 for a heat lamp with a stand.

E0210-E0215

E0210 Electric heat pad, standard

E0215 Electric heat pad, moist

Heat causes blood vessels to open, creating increased blood flow and allowing tissue purging of debris and by-products of injury. Heat therapy promotes relaxation of collagen tissues within muscle, tendons, and ligaments, which allow them to be stretched. Electric heating pads are alternatives to hot packs. Because electric heating pads do not cool spontaneously, use should be limited to 20 minutes to avoid the risk of burns.

E0217-E0218

E0217 Water circulating heat pad with pump

E0218 Fluid circulating cold pad with pump, any type

Heat causes blood vessels to dilate, creating increased blood flow and allowing tissue purging of debris and by-products of injury. Heat therapy promotes relaxation of collagen tissues within muscle, tendons, and ligaments, which allows them to be stretched. Cold therapy is the application of cold treatment to affected tissues, generally used in the immediate postoperative or post-trauma period to reduce edema and enhance pain control. Pain sensations are inhibited by cold by reducing the speed of impulses conducted by nerve fibers. Cold therapy reduces muscle spasms and causes constriction of small arteries and veins, which reduces hemorrhage and swelling within injured tissues. A circulating heating pad with pump is a device that circulates heated water through the pad using a mechanical pump. A fluid or water circulating cold pad with pump consists of fluid or ice water placed into a reservoir that is circulated through a pad using a mechanical pump. Report E0217 for a water circulating pad with a pump. Report E0218 for a fluid circulating cold pad with a pump.

E0221

E0221 Infrared heating pad system

An infrared heating pad system consists of a pad or pads containing mechanisms, such as luminous gallium aluminum arsenide diodes, that generate infrared (or near infrared) light and a power source.

E0225

E0225 Hydrocollator unit, includes pads

Hydrocollator packs, also known as hot packs, warm tissue by conduction. Usually made of canvas bags filled with silicon dioxide, which absorbs many times its own weight in water, hydrocollator packs are immersed in a hot water bath, removed as needed, then wrapped in layered toweling or padding, or some kind of insulating cover, and applied to the patient. The packs cool slowly and can remain warm for around 30 minutes. The packs are stored in a hydrocollator unit where they are immersed in water of about 160 degrees. The tanks are fabricated from stainless steel and should be drained and cleaned every two weeks. The hydrocollator unit may be stationary or portable. Report this code for a stationary unit.

E0231-E0232

E0231 Noncontact wound-warming device (temperature control unit, AC adapter and power cord) for use with warming card and wound cover

E0232 Warming card for use with the noncontact wound-warming device and noncontact wound-warming wound cover

Wound healing occurs best in a warm, moist environment that enhances subcutaneous oxygen tension and increases blood flow to the wound. A noncontact wound warming device, also referred to as noncontact normothermic wound therapy (NNWT), is a wound treatment device designed to create an optimal environment to promote wound healing. A noncontact wound warming device includes a noncontact bandage and a warming unit designed to maintain 100 percent relative humidity and to produce optimal temperatures in the wound and surrounding tissues. The bandage consists of a sterile foam collar that adheres to the skin surrounding the wound and a sterile, transparent film that covers the top of the wound without touching it. An infrared warming card or flexible heat unit is inserted into a pocket in the film covering.

E0235

E0235 Paraffin bath unit, portable (see medical supply code A4265 for paraffin)

Paraffin baths are used mainly for treating contractures, occurring in patients with rheumatoid arthritis or scleroderma. The typical paraffin bath is a container that holds and heats a 1:7 mixture of mineral oil and paraffin, maintaining it at around 53°C into which the patient may either continuously immerse the treated part, such as the hand, for 20-30 minutes, or repetitively dip and remove the treated area from the paraffin. This code is for a portable paraffin bath unit, excluding the paraffin.

E0236

E0236 Pump for water circulating pad

Heat causes blood vessels to dilate, creating increased blood flow and allowing tissue purging of debris and by-products of injury. Heat therapy promotes relaxation of collagen tissues within muscle, tendons, and ligaments, which allows them to be stretched. Cold therapy is the application of cold treatment to affected tissues, generally used in the immediate postoperative or post-trauma period to reduce edema and enhance pain control. Pain sensations are inhibited by cold by reducing the speed of impulses conducted by nerve fibers. Cold therapy reduces muscle spasms and causes constriction of small arteries and veins, which reduces hemorrhage and swelling within injured tissues. A circulating heating pad with pump is a device that circulates heated water through the pad using a mechanical pump. A fluid or water circulating cold pad with pump consists of fluid or ice water placed into a reservoir that is circulated through a pad using a mechanical pump. Report this code for a water circulating pad.

E0239

E0239 Hydrocollator unit, portable

Hydrocollator packs, also known as hot packs, warm tissue by conduction. Usually made of canvas bags filled with silicon dioxide, which absorbs many times its own weight in water, hydrocollator packs are immersed in a hot water bath, removed as needed, then wrapped in layered toweling or padding, or some kind of insulating cover, and applied to the patient. The packs cool slowly and can remain warm for around 30 minutes. The packs are stored in a hydrocollator unit where they are immersed in water of about 160 degrees. The tanks are fabricated from stainless steel and should be drained and cleaned every two weeks. The hydrocollator unit may be stationary or portable. Report this code for a portable unit.

E0240

E0240 Bath/shower chair, with or without wheels, any size

A bath or shower chair is a seat designed to fit into a standard bathtub or walk-in shower that provides stable seating while bathing or showering for those people unsteady on their feet or those unable to stand.

E0241-E0244

E0241 Bathtub wall rail, each

E0242 Bathtub rail, floor base

E0243 Toilet rail, each

E0244 Raised toilet seat

Rails are safety items for home use to help a person get in and out of the bathtub or up and down from the toilet by providing a strong hold while securely stepping into the tub, or lowering or raising body weight.

E0245

E0245 Tub stool or bench

A tub stool or bench is a flat expanded surface, with or without a back, that provides stable seating while the person is bathing or showering. These benches may have arm rails that allow the person to more comfortably maneuver. The benches may be freestanding with legs or attachable to wall or tub. Stools or benches are intended for those people unsteady on their feet or those unable to stand. Heavy-duty benches are generally designed for people who weigh more than 300 pounds.

E0246

E0246 Transfer tub rail attachment

Rails are safety items for home use to help a person get in and out of the bathtub by providing a strong hold while securely stepping into the tub, or lowering or raising body weight. Report this code for a hand rail that attaches to the side of the bathtub.

E0247-E0248

E0247 Transfer bench for tub or toilet with or without commode opening

E0248 Transfer bench, heavy-duty, for tub or toilet with or without commode opening

A transfer bench for tub or toilet is a flat expanded surface without a back that provides stable seating while the person is bathing or showering. These benches may have a commode opening that allows the person to more comfortably maneuver and use a toilet. The benches may be freestanding with legs or attachable to wall or tub. Transfer benches are intended for those people unsteady on their feet or those unable to stand. Heavy-duty benches are generally designed for people who weigh more than 300 pounds.

E0249

E0249 Pad for water circulating heat unit, for replacement only

Heat causes blood vessels to dilate, creating increased blood flow and allowing tissue purging of debris and by-products of injury. Heat therapy promotes relaxation of collagen tissues within muscle, tendons, and ligaments, which allows them to be stretched. A circulating heating pad with pump is a device that circulates heated water through the pad using a mechanical pump. A fluid or water circulating cold pad with pump consists of fluid or ice water placed into a reservoir that is circulated through a pad using a mechanical pump. Report this code for the pad used with a water circulating heat unit.

E0250-E0251

E0250 Hospital bed, fixed height, with any type side rails, with mattress

E0251 Hospital bed, fixed height, with any type side rails, without mattress

Hospital beds for patient home use come in a variety of designs, with a multitude of features and accessories to assist and protect the patient. A hospital bed is generally needed when an ordinary (regular) bed is not suitable for the patient's medical needs. Hospital beds provide features such as head and leg elevation and height adjustment. Clinical cases generally requiring variable-height hospital bed use include severe arthritis and other injuries to lower extremities (e.g., fractured hip). Variable-height (hi-lo) feature beds assist patients to ambulate by enabling them to place their feet on the floor while sitting on the edge of the bed.

E0255-E0256

E0255 Hospital bed, variable height, hi-lo, with any type side rails, with mattress

E0256 Hospital bed, variable height, hi-lo, with any type side rails, without mattress

Hospital beds for patient home use come in a variety of designs, with a multitude of features and accessories to assist and protect the patient. A hospital bed is generally needed when an ordinary (regular) bed is not suitable for the patient's medical needs. Hospital beds provide features such as head and leg elevation and height adjustment. Clinical cases generally requiring variable-height hospital bed use include severe arthritis and other injuries to lower extremities (e.g., fractured hip). Variable-height (hi-lo) feature beds assist patients to ambulate by enabling them to place their feet on the floor while sitting on the edge of the bed.

E0260-E0266

E0260 Hospital bed, semi-electric (head and foot adjustment), with any type side rails, with mattress

E0261 Hospital bed, semi-electric (head and foot adjustment), with any type side rails, without mattress

E0265 Hospital bed, total electric (head, foot, and height adjustments), with any type side rails, with mattress

E0266 Hospital bed, total electric (head, foot, and height adjustments), with any type side rails, without mattress

Hospital beds for patient home use come in a variety of designs, with a multitude of features and accessories to assist and protect the patient. A hospital bed is generally needed when an ordinary, regular bed, is not suitable for the patient's medical needs. Hospital beds provide features such as head and leg elevation and height adjustment. Hospital beds with the semi-electric feature allow for head and foot adjustment, and are used by patients with congestive heart failure, chronic pulmonary disease, or problems with aspiration who require positioning of the body in ways not feasible with an ordinary flat bed.

E0270

E0270 Hospital bed, institutional type includes: oscillating, circulating and Stryker frame, with mattress

Standard institutional hospital beds typically include a frame for oscillating on a longitudinally extending axis and a patient support which is mounted on the oscillating frame, providing controlled pivoting of the patient support on a transverse axis. A Stryker bed consists of a bed frame that holds the patient and permits turning in various planes without individual motion of parts, allowing medical staff to turn a patient easily. These beds also include securing devices provided on the patient support to hold a patient in place. The mattress is typically made of water resistant vinyl and is durable for long term use while also being fire retardant.

E0271-E0272

E0271 Mattress, innerspring

E0272 Mattress, foam rubber

A foam rubber mattress is used to add comfort to a hospital bed. This device is commonly used in conjunction with other hospital bed components, such as bed boards and inner springs.

E0273

E0273 Bed board

A bed board is a device placed under a mattress to support the mattress and keep it firm by preventing the mattress from sagging. Bed boards usually consist of wood slats inside a canvas cover or are made of wood with hinges allowing the board to bend with the position of the bed.

E0274

E0274 Over-bed table

An over-bed table, board, or support device is a functional convenience item, adjustable in height, or angle, to allow the patient more comfort and ease while writing or eating in bed. An over-the-bed table has a laminate top affixed to a chrome-plated, height-adjustable bar, and casters to ease mobility of the table in any direction.

E0275-E0276

E0275 Bed pan, standard, metal or plastic

E0276 Bed pan, fracture, metal or plastic

Bedpans are used by patients whose conditions require them to remain in bed and not ambulate, even for the purpose of getting to the bathroom.

E0277

E0277 Powered pressure-reducing air mattress

This code describes a powered pressure-reducing mattress (alternating pressure, low air loss, or powered flotation without low air loss) that is characterized by the following: an air pump or blower that provides either sequential inflation and deflation of the air cells or a low interface pressure throughout the mattress; an inflated cell height of the air cells through which air is being circulated of 5 inches or greater; air chamber height and proximity and frequency of air circulation (for alternating pressure mattresses), which provides adequate patient lift and pressure reduction to prevent bottoming out; a surface designed to reduce friction; and the ability to be placed directly on a hospital bed frame.

E0280

E0280 Bed cradle, any type

A bed cradle is used for patients with acute gouty arthritis or burns for whom it is necessary to prevent contact with the bed coverings and any pressure applied to the area. Report this code for any type of bed cradle.

E0290-E0293

E0290 Hospital bed, fixed height, without side rails, with mattress

E0291 Hospital bed, fixed height, without side rails, without mattress

E0292 Hospital bed, variable height, hi-lo, without side rails, with mattress

E0293 Hospital bed, variable height, hi-lo, without side rails, without mattress

Hospital beds for patient home use come in a variety of designs, with a multitude of features and accessories to assist and protect the patient. A hospital bed is generally needed when an ordinary (regular) bed is not suitable for the patient's medical needs. Hospital beds provide features such as head and leg elevation and height adjustment. Clinical cases generally requiring variable-height hospital bed use include severe arthritis and other injuries to lower extremities (e.g., fractured hip). Variable-height (hi-lo) feature beds assist patients to ambulate by enabling them to place their feet on the floor while sitting on the edge of the bed.

E0294-E0297

E0294 Hospital bed, semi-electric (head and foot adjustment), without side rails, with mattress

E0295 Hospital bed, semi-electric (head and foot adjustment), without side rails, without mattress

E0296 Hospital bed, total electric (head, foot, and height adjustments), without side rails, with mattress

E0297 Hospital bed, total electric (head, foot, and height adjustments), without side rails, without mattress

Hospital beds for patient home use come in a variety of designs, with a multitude of features and accessories to assist and protect the patient. A hospital bed is generally needed when an ordinary, regular bed, is not suitable for the patient's medical needs. Hospital beds provide features such as head and leg elevation and height adjustment. Hospital beds with the semi-electric feature allow for head and foot adjustment, and are used by patients with congestive heart failure, chronic pulmonary disease, or problems with aspiration who require positioning of the body in ways not feasible with an ordinary flat bed.

E0300

E0300 Pediatric crib, hospital grade, fully enclosed, with or without top enclosure

A pediatric enclosed crib is an alternative bed for the pediatric patient. It allows the patient full range of motion with no traditional restraints. The crib consists of a mesh like screen that gently contains the patient and prevents wandering. Typically these cribs are available in different sizes and materials.

E0301-E0302

E0301 Hospital bed, heavy-duty, extra wide, with weight capacity greater than 350 pounds, but less than or equal to 600 pounds, with any type side rails, without mattress

E0302 Hospital bed, extra heavy-duty, extra wide, with weight capacity greater than 600 pounds, with any type side rails, without mattress

A hospital bed is generally needed when a home bed, sold as furniture, is not suitable for the patient's medical needs. Heavy duty, extra wide beds are available for individuals weighing more than 350 pounds. These beds have additional support in all parts, including the frame and legs. These beds include side rails as a safety feature.

E0303-E0304

E0303 Hospital bed, heavy-duty, extra wide, with weight capacity greater than 350 pounds, but less than or equal to 600 pounds, with any type side rails, with mattress

E0304 Hospital bed, extra heavy-duty, extra wide, with weight capacity greater than 600 pounds, with any type side rails, with mattress

A hospital bed is generally needed when a home bed, sold as furniture, is not suitable for the patient's medical needs. Extra-wide, heavy-duty hospital beds have side rails and a mattress that has additional support in all parts (e.g., legs) for an individual who weighs anywhere from 350-600 pounds or for an individual who weighs more than 600 pounds.

E0305-E0310

E0305 Bedside rails, half-length

E0310 Bedside rails, full-length

Bedside rails are used to protect the patient from injury. Full-length bedside rails, which run the entire length of the bed, are used when the patient has a higher risk of falling out of bed.

E0315

E0315 Bed accessory: board, table, or support device, any type

An over-bed table, board, or support device is a functional convenience item, adjustable in height, or angle, to allow the patient more comfort and ease while writing or eating in bed.

E0316

E0316 Safety enclosure frame/canopy for use with hospital bed, any type

A safety enclosure such as a frame or canopy is used to prevent a patient from leaving the bed. This item encloses the standard hospital bed with a netting attached to a frame and is designed for patients who would need to be restrained. This allows the patient to remain in a safe environment without the need for leg or wrist restraints.

E0325-E0326

E0325 Urinal; male, jug-type, any material

E0326 Urinal; female, jug-type, any material

A urinal is a hand-held container used to collect urine. Some urinals have handles. Urinals are usable in a variety of positions. Jug type urinals generally have a lid and can be used multiple times. Urinals provide an option for bed-confined people who cannot use a bedpan. Male urinals are designed to accommodate a penis. Female urinals have various designs that can be used by women to collect urine.

E

E0328-E0329

E0328 Hospital bed, pediatric, manual, 360 degree side enclosures, top of headboard, footboard and side rails up to 24 in above the spring, includes mattress

E0329 Hospital bed, pediatric, electric or semi-electric, 360 degree side enclosures, top of headboard, footboard and side rails up to 24 in above the spring, includes mattress

Pediatric hospital beds are surfaces for sleep or rest that are designed for non-adult patients. Different parts of the bed can be adjusted to different levels, angles, and configurations to provide physical relief or ease in comfort. Manual pediatric beds typically include manual cranks by which the patient can be raised or lowered in bed. Electric or semi-electric pediatric beds typically allow back and foot adjustment electronically. Some semi-electric beds allow manual height adjustment. Each type of bed usually includes removable bedside rails. The mattress used for these beds is typically made with a water resistant vinyl cover and is durable for long-term use while also being fire retardant.

E0350-E0352

E0350 Control unit for electronic bowel irrigation/evacuation system

E0352 Disposable pack (water reservoir bag, speculum, valving mechanism, and collection bag/box) for use with the electronic bowel irrigation/evacuation system

Pulsed irrigation bowel evacuation is used for bowel management of chronic constipation and fecal impaction in patients with neurogenic bowel dysfunction. Neurogenic bowel dysfunction may be present in patients with spinal cord injury, amyotrophic lateral sclerosis, spina bifida, multiple sclerosis, and diabetes mellitus. Pulsed irrigation bowel evacuation system is an electronic device that delivers small pulses of warm tap water into the rectum to rehydrate feces and promote peristalsis. The system consists of a speculum, tubing, water reservoir bag, valve, a disposable collection container, and an electrical unit that delivers positive and negative air pressure through the tubing.

E0370

E0370 Air pressure elevator for heel

Lower extremities are susceptible to pressure ulcers. The heel is a small area that receives a great deal of pressure as it rests on a surface. An air pressure elevator for a heel is a device consisting of one or more air filled chambers that surround the heel and raise it above a hard surface. It may be used with wheelchairs, day chairs, and in bed.

E0371

E0371 Nonpowered advanced pressure reducing overlay for mattress, standard mattress length and width

A nonpowered advanced pressure-reducing mattress overlay is a device composed of separate cells filled with air or fluid that is attached or laid on the top of a mattress. It generally has a height of three inches or more and is covered in a surface that reduces friction. This overlay is designed to raise pressure points. When there is decreased pressure on skin at contact points, such as buttocks and ankles, skin and soft tissue is less likely to break down and form ulcers or other types of open wounds.

E0372

E0372 Powered air overlay for mattress, standard mattress length and width

A powered pressure-reducing mattress overlay is a device filled with air or fluid that is attached to an electronic device that alternately raises and lowers the air pressure or circulates the air or fluid. The overlay is attached to or laid on top of a mattress. It generally has a height of 3 inches or more and is covered in a surface that reduces friction. This overlay is designed to raise pressure points. When there is decreased pressure on skin at contact points, such as buttocks and ankles, skin and soft tissue is less likely to break down and form ulcers or other types of open wounds.

E0373

E0373 Nonpowered advanced pressure reducing mattress

A nonpowered, advanced pressure-reducing mattress is a mattress composed of separate cells filled with air or fluid. It generally has a height of 5 inches or more and is covered in a surface that reduces friction. The mattress is designed to raise pressure points. When there is decreased pressure on skin at contact points, such as buttocks and ankles, skin and soft tissue is less likely to break down and form ulcers or other types of open wounds.

E0424-E0425

E0424 Stationary compressed gaseous oxygen system, rental; includes container, contents, regulator, flowmeter, humidifier, nebulizer, cannula or mask, and tubing

E0425 Stationary compressed gas system, purchase; includes regulator, flowmeter, humidifier, nebulizer, cannula or mask, and tubing

Oxygen is stored in several manners, one of which is as a compressed gas. The compression mandates use of heavy, reinforced tanks that constitute a stationary system. A regulator fits on top of the tank and is an adjustment device to control the flow of oxygen at the prescribed rate. A flow meter conserves the release of oxygen by turning on and shutting off the regulated flow as the patient inhales and exhales. A nasal cannula is common for lower delivery rates. A mask and/or nebulizer may be used for higher delivery rates and a catheter directly to the trachea is sometimes required. An in-line humidification system may also be used to modulate effects of higher flows.

E0430-E0431

E0430 Portable gaseous oxygen system, purchase; includes regulator, flowmeter, humidifier, cannula or mask, and tubing

E0431 Portable gaseous oxygen system, rental; includes portable container, regulator, flowmeter, humidifier, cannula or mask, and tubing

Portable gaseous oxygen systems are typically lightweight aluminum tanks (usually designated as C tanks) containing pressurized gaseous oxygen. The pressurized systems are stable and the product stores well up to time of use. In some instances, these units may be refilled from large stationary gas oxygen tanks. These systems are generally designed for emergency or occasional use. These codes include all delivery hardware associated with use of the system (regulator, flowmeter, mask, tubing, etc.).

E0433

E0433 Portable liquid oxygen system, rental; home liquefier used to fill portable liquid oxygen containers, includes portable containers, regulator, flowmeter, humidifier, cannula or mask and tubing, with or without supply reservoir and contents gauge

A portable liquid oxygen system is a cooling device that converts air into liquid oxygen by cooling it to -279 degrees Fahrenheit. The device is designed to store the liquid oxygen and allow patients to refill their portable oxygen containers.

E0434-E0435

E0434 Portable liquid oxygen system, rental; includes portable container, supply reservoir, humidifier, flowmeter, refill adaptor, contents gauge, cannula or mask, and tubing

E0435 Portable liquid oxygen system, purchase; includes portable container, supply reservoir, flowmeter, humidifier, contents gauge, cannula or mask, tubing and refill adaptor

Portable liquid oxygen tanks are insulated thermos-like units that store comparatively large quantities of oxygen at lower pressures than gaseous systems. Several hundred times more oxygen can be stored as liquid in the same amount of space than in its gaseous form. The liquid oxygen is stored cold and converted to gas as it is warmed through an apparatus at the reservoir. Portable units typically weigh eight to 10 pounds and are designed to be refillable from larger, stationary tanks. Portable liquid systems are prone to evaporation loss and the product should be used shortly after decanting. These codes include all oxygen delivery hardware associated with use of the system (regulator, flowmeter, mask, tubing, etc.), including refill adapters.

E0439-E0440

E0439 Stationary liquid oxygen system, rental; includes container, contents, regulator, flowmeter, humidifier, nebulizer, cannula or mask, & tubing

E0440 Stationary liquid oxygen system, purchase; includes use of reservoir, contents indicator, regulator, flowmeter, humidifier, nebulizer, cannula or mask, and tubing

Stationary liquid oxygen systems are insulated thermos-like units that store comparatively large quantities of oxygen at lower pressures than gaseous systems. (Several hundred times more oxygen can be stored as liquid in the same amount of space than in its gaseous form.) The liquid oxygen is stored cold and converted to gas as it is warmed through an apparatus at the reservoir. Stationary units may weigh 75 to 100 pounds and can contain enough liquid oxygen to last patients up to eight days, depending on level of use. In many instances, the stationary system is also used to decant liquid oxygen into smaller, portable systems. These codes include all oxygen delivery hardware associated with use of the stationary system (regulator, flowmeter, mask, tubing, etc.).

E0441-E0442

E0441 Stationary oxygen contents, gaseous, 1 month's supply = 1 unit

E0442 Stationary oxygen contents, liquid, 1 month's supply = 1 unit

Traditional oxygen systems are of two general varieties. Compressed gaseous systems, commonly known as "green tanks" or H tanks, are large stationary units that must be secured in place during use. These tanks may be steel, aluminum, or reinforced synthetic material. Smaller units, designated as E tanks and D tanks, are semi-portable units and, in some instances, may be refilled from a larger unit. Gaseous oxygen for stationary systems is typically sold in increments of 50 cubic feet. Report E0441 for a one-month supply of gaseous oxygen product for a purchased system, with or without refillable portable tanks. The second variety consists of liquid oxygen systems. Stationary liquid oxygen systems are insulated thermos-like units that store comparatively large quantities of oxygen at lower pressures than gaseous systems. (Several hundred times more oxygen can be stored as liquid in the same amount of space than in its gaseous form.) The liquid oxygen is stored cold and converted to gas as it is warmed through an apparatus at the reservoir. Stationary units may weigh 75 to 100 pounds and can contain enough liquid oxygen to last patients up to eight days, depending on level of use. In many instances, the stationary system is also used to decant liquid oxygen into smaller, portable systems. Liquid oxygen for stationary systems is typically sold in 10-pound increments.

E0443-E0444

E0443 Portable oxygen contents, gaseous, 1 month's supply = 1 unit

E0444 Portable oxygen contents, liquid, 1 month's supply = 1 unit

Traditional portable oxygen systems are of two general varieties. Smaller compressed gaseous systems are designated as E tanks and D tanks and are semiportable reinforced tanks. Fully portable gaseous oxygen systems are typically lightweight aluminum tanks (usually designated as C tanks) containing the pressurized gaseous oxygen. These pressurized systems are stable and the oxygen product stores well up to time of use. These systems are generally designed for emergency or occasional use. Gaseous oxygen for portable systems is typically sold in increments of five cubic feet. Report E0443 for a one-month supply of gaseous oxygen product for a portable system not refillable from a stationary tank. The second variety consists of liquid oxygen systems. Liquid oxygen is stored cold in low-pressure insulated tanks and converted to gas as it is warmed through an apparatus at the reservoir. Portable units may weigh eight to 10 pounds and can contain enough liquid oxygen to last patients up to four hours, depending on level of use. Liquid oxygen for portable systems is typically sold in one-pound increments. Report E0444 for a one-month supply of liquid oxygen product for a portable system.

E0445

E0445 Oximeter device for measuring blood oxygen levels noninvasively

Oximetry is a noninvasive method to measure blood hemoglobin (Hb) oxygen saturation. A probe is attached to the patient's earlobe or a fingertip. The probe emits a light source. The hemoglobin absorbs a percentage of the light, depending upon its oxygen saturation level, and the results are digitally recorded and displayed on a hand-held unit. Additional data, such as pulse, are sometimes recorded and displayed. This code reports supply of the oximeter unit itself.

E0446

E0446 Topical oxygen delivery system, not otherwise specified, includes all supplies and accessories

A topical oxygen delivery system supplies continuous oxygen therapy to wounds. The device converts room air to concentrated oxygen that is delivered directly to the wound. Components of the system include the oxygenation system, the battery charger, the protective covering, the oxygen delivery extension set, and the wound oxygen delivery cannula. This is used in conjunction with a moist dressing system.

E0447

E0447 Portable oxygen contents, liquid, 1 month's supply = 1 unit, prescribed amount at rest or nighttime exceeds 4 liters per minute (LPM)

Traditional portable oxygen systems are of two general varieties. Smaller compressed gaseous systems are designated as E tanks and D tanks and are semiportable reinforced tanks. Fully portable gaseous oxygen systems are typically lightweight aluminum tanks (usually designated as C tanks) containing the pressurized gaseous oxygen. These pressurized systems are stable and the oxygen product stores well up to time of use. These systems are generally designed for emergency or occasional use. Gaseous oxygen for a portable system is typically sold in increments of five cubic feet. The second variety consists of liquid oxygen systems. Liquid oxygen is stored cold in low-pressure insulated tanks and converted to gas as it is warmed through an apparatus at the reservoir. Portable units may weigh eight to 10 pounds and can contain enough liquid oxygen to last patients up to four hours, depending on level of use. Liquid oxygen for portable systems is typically sold in one-pound increments. Report E0447 for a one-month supply of liquid oxygen product for a portable system when the prescribed amount exceeds 4 liters per minute (LPM).

E0455

E0455 Oxygen tent, excluding croup or pediatric tents

An oxygen tent is a canopy placed over the head and shoulders or over the entire body of a patient to provide oxygen at a higher level than normal. They are made of plastic or other material through which oxygen cannot pass. Oxygen enters the tent through a hose. Physicians seldom use oxygen tents today as newer methods of oxygen delivery provide a better environment and easier patient access.

E0457-E0459

E0457 Chest shell (cuirass)

E0459 Chest wrap

A chest shell or cuirass is a rigid plastic or metal dome, similar to a tortoise shell, that surrounds the chest and abdomen. The shell has a rubber or foam seal that is attached to the edges of the shell to create a tight seal. A chest wrap is an impermeable nylon jacket suspended by a rigid chest piece that fits over the chest and abdomen. A hose is attached to the center or side of the shell or wrap. The other end of the hose is attached to the ventilator. The ventilator cycles air in and out, creating a vacuum. This causes the chest to raise and air to enter the nose and mouth. A cuirass and a chest wrap are non-invasive methods of negative pressure mechanical ventilation that assist people with paralyzed or weakened diaphragm or intercostal muscles. People with stable or slowly progressing neuromuscular diseases (such as polio or multiple sclerosis), central hypoventilation (e.g., apnea not due to airway obstruction), or chest wall deformities are candidates for the use of negative pressure ventilation.

E0462

E0462 Rocking bed, with or without side rails

A rocking bed is a bed mounted on a mechanized platform that moves the patient's upper body up and down. This change of positions promotes movement of the diaphragm and thus breathing, particularly for patients who are quadriplegic or have paralysis of the diaphragm. A rocking bed may also be used to improve blood circulation in the treatment of chronic occlusive arterial disease.

E0465-E0467

E0465 Home ventilator, any type, used with invasive interface, (e.g., tracheostomy tube)

E0466 Home ventilator, any type, used with noninvasive interface, (e.g., mask, chest shell)

E0467 Home ventilator, multi-function respiratory device, also performs any or all of the additional functions of oxygen concentration, drug nebulization, aspiration, and cough stimulation, includes all accessories, components and supplies for all functions

A home ventilator is a machine that supports breathing. The ventilator helps get oxygen into the lungs and removes carbon dioxide. Report E0465 when the interface is invasive, such as a tracheostomy tube. Report E0466 when the interface is noninvasive, such as a mask or chest shell. Report E0467 when the device also performs the function of aspiration, cough stimulation, drug nebulization, and/or oxygen concentration.

E

E0470-E0472

E0470 Respiratory assist device, bi-level pressure capability, without backup rate feature, used with noninvasive interface, e.g., nasal or facial mask (intermittent assist device with continuous positive airway pressure device)

E0471 Respiratory assist device, bi-level pressure capability, with back-up rate feature, used with noninvasive interface, e.g., nasal or facial mask (intermittent assist device with continuous positive airway pressure device)

E0472 Respiratory assist device, bi-level pressure capability, with backup rate feature, used with invasive interface, e.g., tracheostomy tube (intermittent assist device with continuous positive airway pressure device)

RADs are noninvasive, spontaneous respiratory assistance devices with positive pressure that use a nasal or facial mask interface, creating a seal. Some of these devices enable the treating physician to avoid the use of more invasive airway access, such as a tracheostomy, and some of these devices are used in conjunction with invasive therapies. A RAD without backup rate delivers adjustable, variable levels (within a single respiratory cycle) of positive air pressure by way of tubing and a nasal or oral facial mask to assist in the spontaneous respiratory efforts of the patient, and to supplement the volume of inspired air into the lungs. This is also called noninvasive positive pressure respiratory assistance or NPPRA. A RAD with backup rate has, in addition, a timed backup feature to deliver the air pressure whenever sufficient spontaneous patient respiratory efforts fail to occur (i.e., it has a trigger device to deliver a quantity of air into the patient's lungs whenever the patient's spontaneous respiration is insufficient). A RAD with backup rate used in conjunction with invasive therapy versus a noninvasive regimen, delivers adjustable, variable levels (within a single respiratory cycle) of positive air pressure to assist in the spontaneous respiratory efforts of the patient following invasive therapy or surgery, and to supplement the volume of inspired air into the lungs. Noninvasive RADs are different from invasive ventilation, which is administered through a securely intubated airway, generally in patients for whom interruption or failure of the ventilation support would lead to their imminent demise. These devices are not the same as the continuous positive airway pressure (CPAP) devices that are used primarily in the conservative therapy approach (versus surgery) for patients with documented sleep apnea. CPAP devices provide for continuous amounts of air pressure throughout the oropharynx to prevent the collapse of the oropharyngeal tissues during sleep.

E0480

E0480 Percussor, electric or pneumatic, home model

A pneumatic or electric percussor is typically a hand-held unit that mimics the hand percussion of the chest traditionally exercised by respiratory therapists to loosen and clear a patient's lungs of mucous and phlegm. Pneumatic models employ a gas driven cylinder to create pulses that reverberate into lung tissues. Electric models create a similar effect through vibration. Either variety will feature adjustments for pulse speed and intensity. Report E0480 for models designed for home use.

E0481

E0481 Intrapulmonary percussive ventilation system and related accessories

An intrapulmonary percussive ventilation system (IPV) is a device that delivers a series of very small bursts of pressurized gas at rates greater than 100 cycles per minute to the respiratory tract. IPV is a mechanized form of chest physical therapy. Instead of a therapist clapping or slapping the patient's chest wall, the IPV delivers small bursts of respiratory gases to the lungs via a mouthpiece. It is intended to mobilize endobronchial secretions and diffuse patchy atelectasis. The patient controls variables such as inspiratory time, peak pressure, and delivery rates. Code E0481 includes the compressor, hand held units, tubing, and all related accessories. This includes both systems in which the very small bursts of air are generated by the compressor and systems in which the very small bursts of air are generated by a hand-held percussive nebulizer used with a standard high-pressure compressor.

E0482

E0482 Cough stimulating device, alternating positive and negative airway pressure

This code reports supply of a specific variety of cough stimulating device. This type of device stimulates the cough reflex by providing alternating positive and negative airway pressure to loosen and clear a patient's lungs of mucous and phlegm. Peak cough ability is important to maintain in patients with diminished pulmonary function. These types of devices are designed to stimulate natural inspiratory and expiratory lung-clearing action. The units are non-invasive, using a mouthpiece or face mask.

E0483

E0483 High frequency chest wall oscillation system, with full anterior and/or posterior thoracic region receiving simultaneous external oscillation, includes all accessories and supplies, each

High frequency chest wall oscillation (HFCWO) is a therapy strategy to treat patients who suffer from excessive bronchial secretions. It may be used to treat patients with cystic fibrosis and other lung diseases where bronchial secretions can obstruct the airways. Treatments typically involve use of a vest, which is worn while the patient is in an upright position. Tubes connecting the vest to an air-pulse generator provide oscillations, which may be adjustable for intensity and duration. A patient can operate the equipment by use of hand or sometimes foot controls. Treatment intervals last about 10 minutes and may be repeated. The patient clears mobilized bronchial secretions by coughing. This code includes all accessories and supplies for the HFCWO system.

E0484

E0484 Oscillatory positive expiratory pressure device, nonelectric, any type, each

Oscillatory positive expiratory pressure devices create air vibrations to assist the patient in clearing the airway of mucous and secretions. Nonelectric devices are typically hand held units. They manipulate expired air by passing it through or over a vibration-creating apparatus. A vibrating metal ball within a cone is one method. Another involves use of a magnet and counterweight. The oscillation, or flutter, occurs as back pressure is created in the bronchial tract. The natural movement of secretions from the lungs and bronchial tract is assisted, similar to many tiny coughs.

E0485-E0486

E0485 Oral device/appliance used to reduce upper airway collapsibility, adjustable or nonadjustable, prefabricated, includes fitting and adjustment

E0486 Oral device/appliance used to reduce upper airway collapsibility, adjustable or nonadjustable, custom fabricated, includes fitting and adjustment

An oral device or appliance designed to reduce upper airway soft tissue collapse may be used to treat snoring and/or apnea during sleep. These devices increase the cross-sectional area of the upper airways by moving the mandible and/or the tongue forward. This helps to stabilize the upper airway in patients with obstructive sleep apnea syndrome (OSAS).

E0487

E0487 Spirometer, electronic, includes all accessories

A spirometer is a device used to measure pulmonary function. It measures the lung output on both inspiration and expiration. This is used to track and diagnose a number of respiratory and cardiac conditions. It may also be used to keep the lungs clear and functioning.

E0500

E0500 IPPB machine, all types, with built-in nebulization; manual or automatic valves; internal or external power source

This code reports the supply of any type of intermittent positive pressure breathing (IPPB) machine. These units will have a built-in reservoir for medications and neutral liquids. A nebulizer feature atomizes liquid to aerosol spray, which is inhaled by the patient. Control valves may be manual or automatic. Many units have a port to attach an oxygen supply to the mix. These units may be hand-held with a mouthpiece and are used with the nose occluded by a clip. Batteries, an external AC source, or both may power the unit. Although volume ventilators may deliver intermittent positive pressure treatments, these IPPB units are generally classified for use among patients with spontaneous breathing capabilities. The main use of an IPPB machine is for patients with atelectasis (inability to fully expand the lung) or for the delivery of aerosol medication, usually bronchodilators.

E0550-E0560

E0550 Humidifier, durable for extensive supplemental humidification during IPPB treatments or oxygen delivery

E0555 Humidifier, durable, glass or autoclavable plastic bottle type, for use with regulator or flowmeter

E0560 Humidifier, durable for supplemental humidification during IPPB treatment or oxygen delivery

Intermittent positive pressure breathing (IPPB) treatments may be used for a variety of respiratory conditions. During treatment, machine assisted pressure is delivered upon inspiration to help the patient take large, deep breaths. The IPPB unit features pressurized gas in tanks or an electric air compressor. Respiratory therapists usually provide treatments. The treatment may be used to deliver medication, to open air passages and loosen mucous, or to increase lung capacity. Humidification is often required for IPPB treatments, particularly when oxygen delivery is involved. Humidifiers reported by this range are durable, reusable containers and the connection devices for an IPPB treatment unit or oxygen system. The containers can be cleaned or autoclaved before refilling with distilled water.

E0561-E0562

E0561 Humidifier, nonheated, used with positive airway pressure device

E0562 Humidifier, heated, used with positive airway pressure device

A humidifier is a device that increases the amount of moisture in indoor air or in a stream of air. It operates by circulating air over a water-filled pan or wet surface. The water then evaporates and is incorporated into the air stream. Heated humidifiers gently heat the water and the air stream as it comes in contact with the device. This device is used in connection with a continuous positive airway pressure (CPAP) system.

E0565-E0585

E0565 Compressor, air power source for equipment which is not self-contained or cylinder driven

E0570 Nebulizer, with compressor

E0572 Aerosol compressor, adjustable pressure, light duty for intermittent use

E0574 Ultrasonic/electronic aerosol generator with small volume nebulizer

E0575 Nebulizer, ultrasonic, large volume

E0580 Nebulizer, durable, glass or autoclavable plastic, bottle type, for use with regulator or flowmeter

E0585 Nebulizer, with compressor and heater

Nebulizer base equipment is comprised of an air compressor for airflow nebulization or a generator for nebulization of liquid by means of ultrasonic vibrations. The actual nebulizer is the chamber in which the nebulization of the liquid (usually medication) occurs and is considered an accessory to the base equipment. The nebulizing chamber is attached to the aerosol compressor or an ultrasonic generator. Specific accessories, supplies, and medications are used with this equipment. Nebulization therapy is considered beneficial to patients with a variety of respiratory and/or pulmonary conditions and diseases, including cystic fibrosis, bronchiectasis, chronic obstructive pulmonary disease, emphysema, severe asthma (when metered dose inhalers are ineffective), as well as other conditions such as AIDS, which requires the administration of medications like pentamidine. Nebulization occurs when the medication and/or solution to be administered is vaporized and subsequently inspired by the patient via the lungs, through which the medication enters the patient's system, or the medication has a direct effect on mucus retained by the lungs and bronchi (known as mucolytic action). An aerosol compressor can be set for pressures above 30 pounds per sq inch (psi) at a flow of 6-8 L/m and is capable of continuous operation. A nebulizer with compressor is an aerosol compressor delivering a fixed low pressure, typically used with a small volume nebulizer. A portable compressor is an aerosol compressor that delivers a fixed low pressure, used with a small volume nebulizer. It must have battery or DC power capability, but may have an AC power option. The light duty adjustable pressure compressor is a pneumatic aerosol compressor that can be set for pressures above 30 psi at a flow of 6-8 L/m, but is only capable of intermittent operation.

E0600

E0600 Respiratory suction pump, home model, portable or stationary, electric

A portable home model respiratory suction pump is a lightweight, compact, electric aspirator designed for upper respiratory oral pharyngeal and tracheal suction to be used in the home. Use of the device does not require technical or professional supervision. Units are equipped with vacuum regulators to allow variation of vacuum values, varying lamp flow, overflow safety devices, and battery or AC power.

E0601

E0601 Continuous positive airway pressure (CPAP) device

A continuous airway pressure (CPAP) device is a noninvasive method of providing air pressure through the patient's nostrils, usually through a nasal mask or flow generator system. A CPAP device delivers single pressure continuously and assists the patient in nocturnal respiration (breathing during sleep), particularly when the patient's oropharyngeal tissues relax, collapse, and/or otherwise obstruct the normal airflow, causing a variety of symptoms including hypersomnolence during the day, loss of concentration, headache, agitation, depression, fatigue, and many others. These devices are used primarily in conservative therapy (vs. surgery) for patients with documented sleep apnea.

E0602-E0604

E0602 Breast pump, manual, any type

E0603 Breast pump, electric (AC and/or DC), any type

E0604 Breast pump, hospital grade, electric (AC and/or DC), any type

Breast pumps are available in a variety of configurations, all of which are designed to pump human breast milk for short- or long-term storage. Some models are simple cylinders that interface with a plastic cone that fits over the areola. A syringe-type piston can then be manually retracted by the user to create and release suction on the nipple. The pumped milk drains by gravity into an attached container. The milk can be decanted into plastic bags for refrigerated storage or freezing. Electric models work by creating pulsating suction, usually by pneumatic action against a diaphragm. Larger facilities may use hospital grade piston operated electric pumps. With the exception of disposable plastic storage containers, components to all models are generally cleanable and reusable.

E0605

E0605 Vaporizer, room type

This code reports the supply of a room type vaporizer. Humidifiers and moisturizers typically work by absorbing cool water through a wick, which is exposed to a fan. Some models vibrate the cool water (ultrasonic). These devices can effectively raise humidity to larger rooms. Vaporizers heat water to create steam and are usually used for individual treatment of respiratory illness. Extracts can be added to the heated water or steam. Vaporizers are not usually effective to humidify large cubic footage, although room-size models are available and are reported by this code.

E0606

E0606 Postural drainage board

Postural drainage uses the force of gravity to assist in effectively draining secretions from the lungs and into the central airway where they can be coughed up or suctioned out. The patient is placed in a head or chest down position and turned so that each lung segment can be drained. Percussion and vibration may be performed in conjunction with postural drainage. Postural drainage is used to assist patients with chronic pulmonary conditions or diseases that limit the ability to cough and eliminate secretions, such as cystic fibrosis. A postural drainage board is a smooth, flat, hard surface that supports the patient during postural drainage. Some boards may have foam or other padding that raises the patient's torso above the upper chest.

E0607

E0607 Home blood glucose monitor

Glucometers are used for patients with all types of diabetes mellitus to monitor blood glucose and are available in a variety of models with various features, including digital read-out, memory, result print-out, easy specimen capture, and many others. Glucometers with special features, such as voice-activated or voice-synthesized capabilities, are needed for patients with other concurrent conditions, such as patients with impaired vision. Whether or not the patient is on insulin, many diabetics require frequent, if not daily, blood glucose monitoring. For Type I diabetes mellitus patients who require insulin (the patient's body does not manufacture insulin and therefore it must come from an external source, such as injections), blood glucose monitoring is a life-sustaining requirement.

E0610-E0615

E0610 Pacemaker monitor, self-contained, (checks battery depletion, includes audible and visible check systems)

E0615 Pacemaker monitor, self-contained, checks battery depletion and other pacemaker components, includes digital/visible check systems

These codes report the supply of self-contained pacemaker monitors. A pacemaker is a device to control cardiac arrhythmias by programmed electrical stimulation of the heart. Pacemaker monitoring equipment detects impending battery failure and checks the overall performance of the pacemaker. Patients with pacemakers, whether permanent or temporary, require periodic examination of battery life and electrical functions. Self-contained units allow patients to perform the evaluation themselves. Some devices collect data that can be transmitted to a provider over a phone line. Battery life is a major factor in many pacemaker malfunctions and is monitored by these units. The conductivity of the pacemaker leads is another major consideration in monitoring.

E0616

E0616 Implantable cardiac event recorder with memory, activator, and programmer

Implantable event recorders are implanted in the left front of the chest in a pocket created in the skin. Once implanted, the patient's cardiac events are recorded. Implantable cardiac event monitors are used for long periods of time, which enables the recorder to capture more infrequent heart rhythms. The device can have autoactivation or manual activation depending upon the needs of the patient. If the patient experiences syncopal episodes, the manual activation button can be pressed after the patient is conscious again. If the device has an autoactivation, the device records rhythms automatically when the heart rate is in excess or under a preset limit.

E0617

E0617 External defibrillator with integrated electrocardiogram analysis

Automatic external defibrillators are compact and portable devices that deliver electrical shock to a person who has a sudden cardiac arrest. Automatic external defibrillator units use a microprocessor inside of a portable defibrillator to interpret a person's heart rhythm through electrodes. The computer recognizes ventricular fibrillation or ventricular tachycardia. Once recognized, the computer advises the operator/user that electrical defibrillation is needed or it will automatically deliver a countershock.

E0618-E0619

E0618 Apnea monitor, without recording feature

E0619 Apnea monitor, with recording feature

An apnea monitor is a device designed to detect cessation of breathing, either directly through measurement of respiration and/or indirectly through monitoring of physiological signs such as heart rate, pulse, or blood oxygen concentration. Devices typically feature both visual and audio alarm systems. Some models may differentiate between detection of obstructive apnea (such as is caused by mucous or oropharyngeal membrane) and central apnea (as may be caused by organ system failure). Models are typically connected to AC circuitry with battery power backup. Some may feature remote alarm systems, programmed software, and a monitor. An internal and/or hard copy recording system may also be featured.

E

E0620

E0620 Skin piercing device for collection of capillary blood, laser, each

A laser skin-piercing device is a low strength laser that is directed to one area, usually on a finger, and pierces the skin and subcutaneous tissue, allowing blood to be drawn from a capillary or surface blood vessel. This device is used in place of a lancet to draw blood for blood glucose monitoring or similar home blood testing.

E0621-E0625

E0621 Sling or seat, patient lift, canvas or nylon

E0625 Patient lift, bathroom or toilet, not otherwise classified

Patient lift mechanisms are hydraulic or motorized (electric) lifts that enable the patient to transfer from the bed to a chair or other sitting device, or vice versa. The electric patient lifts can be electric (AC) or battery powered (DC). These lift mechanisms assist patients with varying abnormalities that prevent them from being able to change, unassisted, from a lying down position (in a bed) to a seated position (in a chair, wheelchair, etc.), and vice versa. Trauma, stroke, and chronic diseases are the usual etiologies for the patient's inability to change in these positions. These devices can help during the convalescence period in posttraumatic or postoperative cases, and act as prevention against patient injury or reinjury. A seat or sling for a patient lift is a reinforced width of nylon or cloth that replaces a similar device used in a patient lift. A seat or sling is considered an accessory item. One type of device uses a manual pumping action to compress a cylinder filled with a fluid, usually oil. Since the oil is thick and molecule dense, it does not absorb the energy or force generated by the pumping action. Instead, the oil amplifies and transfers the energy to the lever used to raise the patient. The hydraulic action allows less energy to be used in the pumping action. Another type of device uses electricity to run a motor that raises and moves the patient from one surface (e.g., a bed, chair, or toilet) to another surface. The patient is positioned in a seat or sling and the device performs the work. Electric lifts can be freestanding or ceiling and wall mounted. One system raises and moves the patient using a hinged platform that can be manipulated into various positions. When laid flat and positioned close to the bed, the patient can roll or be lifted onto the platform. The platform can then be positioned so the patient is standing upright or in a seated position. The system can contain both hydraulic and electronic driven mechanisms. The system is padded or cushioned for patient comfort and may contain side rails or straps to securely hold the patient during transfer.

E0627-E0629

E0627 Seat lift mechanism, electric, any type

E0629 Seat lift mechanism, nonelectric, any type

Seat lift mechanisms are motorized seat lifts that enable the patient to change from a seated position to a standing position. The lifting mechanism is graded and not based on a catapult or other type of spring system. These mechanisms can be electric or battery powered. Some mechanisms can be used with the patient's own furniture; others are already built into specially designed chairs, sometimes incorporating the seat lift action with a more total patient lift action, including elevating and pushing the back and arms. Seat lift mechanisms assist patients with varying abnormalities that prevent them from being able to change, unassisted, from a seated to a standing position. Trauma and chronic diseases are the usual etiologies for the patient's inability to change in these positions. These devices can help in posttraumatic or postoperative convalescence, act as adjunctive treatment for chronic diseases, and act as prevention against patient injury or reinjury.

E0630-E0635

E0630 Patient lift, hydraulic or mechanical, includes any seat, sling, strap(s), or pad(s)

E0635 Patient lift, electric, with seat or sling

Please refer to codes E0621-E0625 for the description.

E0636-E0642

E0636 Multipositional patient support system, with integrated lift, patient accessible controls

E0637 Combination sit-to-stand frame/table system, any size including pediatric, with seat lift feature, with or without wheels

E0638 Standing frame/table system, one position (e.g., upright, supine or prone stander), any size including pediatric, with or without wheels

E0639 Patient lift, moveable from room to room with disassembly and reassembly, includes all components/accessories

E0640 Patient lift, fixed system, includes all components/accessories

E0641 Standing frame/table system, multi-position (e.g., 3-way stander), any size including pediatric, with or without wheels

E0642 Standing frame/table system, mobile (dynamic stander), any size including pediatric

A standing frame system is an assistive device that provides musculoskeletal support for disabled or injured individuals. This device allows an individual to move from a sitting to standing position and provides support when standing. Standing frame systems may include lift devices that assist the patient in moving from a sitting to standing position. Multi-position standing frames allow progressive levels of standing that gradually relieve contractures and spasticity. A standing frame system may be stationary or mobile. Patient lifts are mechanical devices that elevate and transfer patients from one point to another. The devices may be powered or manual. There are various designs based on the condition of the patient. The lift may be a flat litter, a chair, or other configuration. It usually has straps or restraints to hold the patient in place during the transfer. The lift may be fixed, such as a lift permanently anchored in the ceiling or on a wall, or may be moveable from one room to another with some disassembly and reassembly at each point.

E0650-E0673

E0650 Pneumatic compressor, nonsegmental home model

E0651 Pneumatic compressor, segmental home model without calibrated gradient pressure

E0652 Pneumatic compressor, segmental home model with calibrated gradient pressure

E0655 Nonsegmental pneumatic appliance for use with pneumatic compressor, half arm

E0656 Segmental pneumatic appliance for use with pneumatic compressor, trunk

E0657 Segmental pneumatic appliance for use with pneumatic compressor, chest

E0660 Nonsegmental pneumatic appliance for use with pneumatic compressor, full leg

E0665 Nonsegmental pneumatic appliance for use with pneumatic compressor, full arm

E0666 Nonsegmental pneumatic appliance for use with pneumatic compressor, half leg

E0667 Segmental pneumatic appliance for use with pneumatic compressor, full leg

E0668 Segmental pneumatic appliance for use with pneumatic compressor, full arm

E0669 Segmental pneumatic appliance for use with pneumatic compressor, half leg

E0670 Segmental pneumatic appliance for use with pneumatic compressor, integrated, two full legs and trunk

E0671 Segmental gradient pressure pneumatic appliance, full leg

E0672 Segmental gradient pressure pneumatic appliance, full arm

E0673 Segmental gradient pressure pneumatic appliance, half leg

Lymphedema is the swelling of subcutaneous tissue due to the accumulation of excessive lymph fluid from impairment in the normal clearing function of the lymphatic system and/or from excessive lymph production. Lymphedema pumps are segmental or nonsegmental long arm or leg sleeves (similar to a blood pressure cuff) that are placed up around the area of swelling. The device is turned on and the sleeve is periodically inflated to compress the tissues (in segments or in total length), and then deflated. A tube from the compression device (pump) that is attached to the sleeve allows air to be pumped into the sleeve (compression) or air to be removed from the sleeve (decompression). Pneumatic pumps mechanically assist blood and lymph flow through the extremities. This assistance lessens the accumulation of fluids in the affected limb and reduces associated complications such as thrombosis or vessel damage.

E0675

E0675 Pneumatic compression device, high pressure, rapid inflation/deflation cycle, for arterial insufficiency (unilateral or bilateral system)

Pneumatic compression devices, along with an electrical pneumatic pump, are used to pump compressed air into a garment placed on upper or lower extremities (including feet). The garment is intermittently inflated and deflated with pressure and various time cycles. The use of the pneumatic compression device can greatly reduce the risk of deep venous thrombosis (DVT) and pulmonary embolism (PE) by limiting venous stasis and increasing fibrinolytic activity at both the local and systemic levels.

E0676

E0676 Intermittent limb compression device (includes all accessories), not otherwise specified

An intermittent limb compression device inflates and deflates a compression sleeve that has multiple compression chambers encircling the limb of the patient. The sleeve inflates to apply compressive pressure gradient against the limb of the patient, which decreases from the lower to the upper portion of the limb to enhance the acceleration of blood flow through the limb.

E0691-E0694

E0691 Ultraviolet light therapy system, includes bulbs/lamps, timer and eye protection; treatment area 2 sq ft or less

E0692 Ultraviolet light therapy system panel, includes bulbs/lamps, timer and eye protection, 4 ft panel

E0693 Ultraviolet light therapy system panel, includes bulbs/lamps, timer and eye protection, 6 ft panel

E0694 Ultraviolet multidirectional light therapy system in 6 ft cabinet, includes bulbs/lamps, timer, and eye protection

An ultraviolet light therapy system is considered durable medical equipment typically consisting of a system panel, ultraviolet bulbs/lamp that emit UVB rays, a timer, and eye protection. It is commonly used for the treatment of skin conditions including psoriasis, pruritic eruptions of HIV, and acne.

E0700

E0700 Safety equipment, device or accessory, any type

Safety equipment such as a belts, harnesses, or vests are used to secure a patient's positioning when the patient is at risk for a fall that could lead to harm or injury. The equipment is comfortably secured around the patient and fastened to a bed or chair to prevent sliding or falling.

E0705

E0705 Transfer device, any type, each

A transfer board is used for ease of moving patients from one stable surface to another (i.e. bed to wheelchair, bed to portable toilet, wheelchair to toilet) and is primarily for seated type transports.

E0710

E0710 Restraints, any type (body, chest, wrist, or ankle)

Restraints are used to contain and control an individual who exhibits behavior that may be harmful to self or others, such as violent behavior or pulling at lifesaving treatments. This code includes body, chest, wrist, or ankle restraints. Each strap is designed with a cuff to be placed around the patient, and a strap that can be threaded through a U bar and secured. Report this code for any type of restraint.

E0720-E0730

E0720 Transcutaneous electrical nerve stimulation (TENS) device, two-lead, localized stimulation

E0730 Transcutaneous electrical nerve stimulation (TENS) device, four or more leads, for multiple nerve stimulation

A transcutaneous electrical nerve stimulator (TENS) is a device that uses electrical current delivered through electrodes placed on the surface of the skin to decrease the patient's perception of pain, by inhibiting the transmission of afferent pain nerve impulses and/or by stimulating the release of endorphins. The TENS unit can be applied in a variety of settings (in the patient's home, a physician's office, or in an outpatient clinic). This device alleviates or palliates acute postoperative pain, as well as chronic or intractable pain, depending on the etiology of the patient's condition. TENS therapy is typically not used for patients with visceral pain or headache, female patients with pelvic pain, and other types of pain considered unresponsive to TENS therapy.

E0731

E0731 Form-fitting conductive garment for delivery of TENS or NMES (with conductive fibers separated from the patient's skin by layers of fabric)

A form-fitting conductive garment has tiny electro-conductive leads and electrodes woven into a stretch fabric. The system offers a great many of easily accessible and interchangeable electrode sites throughout the fabric area. A second layer of conventional fabric lines the garment against the skin. The garment may be worn on an extremity alone or on part or the entire torso. The garment is designed to interface with a transcutaneous electrical nerve stimulation (TENS) generator. The system may be used for patients with conditions that require a great many TENS electrodes for effective therapy and for those with sensitive skin. The system is also sometimes used underneath plaster casting where conventional TENS therapy cannot reach.

E0740

E0740 Nonimplanted pelvic floor electrical stimulator, complete system

Pelvic floor stimulators are used for the treatment of urinary incontinence to strengthen and exercise the muscles of the pelvic floor. Electrical stimulations targeting the muscles involved are delivered via probes connected to an external pulse generator. The frequency and intensity of the electrical pulse varies based on the patient's needs. Report this code for a pelvic floor stimulator with a monitor, sensor, and/or trainer.

E0744

E0744 Neuromuscular stimulator for scoliosis

Neuromuscular stimulators are used to stimulate muscles into activity through an electrical impulse. These devices consist of superficial or implantable electrodes, a modulating output and control circuit, a signal generator, and a battery power supply.

E0745

E0745 Neuromuscular stimulator, electronic shock unit

Neuromuscular stimulation artificially stimulates muscles that may have atrophied because of damaged nerve pathways, often due to injury, surgery, or infarction. Computer-controlled sequential electrical stimulation of muscles simulates actual use, even when actual muscle contraction is not attained, and may result in a level of muscle tone and strength.

E0746

E0746 Electromyography (EMG), biofeedback device

An electromyography (EMG) biofeedback device consists of electrodes that are placed over specific muscles, and a recording unit that stores and displays the information from the physiological responses being monitored. Muscle activity can be displayed in real-time or an average over a period of time.

E0747-E0749

E0747 Osteogenesis stimulator, electrical, noninvasive, other than spinal applications

E0748 Osteogenesis stimulator, electrical, noninvasive, spinal applications

E0749 Osteogenesis stimulator, electrical, surgically implanted

An electrical osteogenesis stimulator is a device that provides electrical stimulation to augment bone repair by stimulating the production of osteocytes (bone cells) and can be invasive or noninvasive. A noninvasive electrical stimulator is characterized by an external power source, which is attached to a coil or electrodes placed on the skin, or placed on a cast or brace over a fracture or surgical bone fusion site. Invasive devices provide electrical stimulation directly at the fracture site, through percutaneous placement of cathodes or by implantation of a coiled cathode wire into the fracture site. The power pack is implanted into soft tissue near the fracture site and subcutaneously connected to the cathode, creating a self-contained system with no external components. With the noninvasive device, opposing pads, wired to an external power supply, are placed over the cast. An electromagnetic field is created between the pads at the fracture site. An ultrasonic osteogenic stimulator emits low intensity, pulsed ultrasound (as opposed to electricity) to stimulate bone repair. The ultrasound signal is applied to the skin surface at the fracture location via ultrasound conductive coupling gel to accelerate the healing time of the fracture. The device is intended for use with cast immobilization.

E0755

E0755 Electronic salivary reflex stimulator (intraoral/noninvasive)

An electronic salivary reflex stimulator is used to treat xerostomia (dry mouth). Chronic xerostomia may be caused by a number of conditions, including Sjogren's syndrome, certain medications, and radiation therapy. Xerostomia can cause difficulty in eating and swallowing. An electronic salivary reflex stimulator is an intraoral, noninvasive device that emits electrical impulses to the tongue and roof of the mouth. These electrical impulses are distributed to all residual salivary tissues in the oral and pharyngeal regions stimulating salivation.

E0760

E0760 Osteogenesis stimulator, low intensity ultrasound, noninvasive

An electrical osteogenesis stimulator is a device that provides electrical stimulation to augment bone repair by stimulating the production of osteocytes (bone cells) and can be invasive or noninvasive. A noninvasive electrical stimulator is characterized by an external power source, which is attached to a coil or electrodes placed on the skin, or placed on a cast or brace over a fracture or surgical bone fusion site. Invasive devices provide electrical stimulation directly at the fracture site, through percutaneous placement of cathodes or by implantation of a coiled cathode wire into the fracture site. The power pack is implanted into soft tissue near the fracture site and subcutaneously connected to the cathode, creating a self-contained system with no external components. With the noninvasive device, opposing pads, wired to an external power supply, are placed over the cast. An electromagnetic field is created between the pads at the fracture site. An ultrasonic osteogenic stimulator emits low intensity, pulsed ultrasound (as opposed to electricity) to stimulate bone repair. The ultrasound signal is applied to the skin surface at the fracture location via ultrasound conductive coupling gel to accelerate the healing time of the fracture. The device is intended for use with cast immobilization.

E0761

E0761 Nonthermal pulsed high frequency radiowaves, high peak power electromagnetic energy treatment device

A nonthermal pulsed high frequency radiowave, high peak power electromagnetic energy treatment device produces the energy used in electromagnetic therapy. The pulsed methodology allows treatment while allowing associated heat production to dissipate. Electromagnetic therapy is a distinct form of treatment using application of electromagnetic fields rather than direct electrical current for wound treatment.

E0762

E0762 Transcutaneous electrical joint stimulation device system, includes all accessories

A transcutaneous electrical joint stimulation device used to treat osteoarthritis of the knee and rheumatoid arthritis of the hands. This battery powered device consists of an electrical stimulator with electrical leads that are placed over the affected area. The leads are held in place with a lightweight, flexible wrap and Velcro fasteners. The device delivers electrical impulses of 0.0 to 12.0 volt output to the joint. The device is typically worn for at least six hours per day. The device appears to stimulate development of new hyaline cartilage. Patients using transcutaneous electrical joint stimulation devices report reduced pain and stiffness and improved range of motion and function of the treated joints. This code reports the electrical joint stimulation device and all accessories (wrap, fasteners) needed to use the device.

E0764

E0764 Functional neuromuscular stimulation, transcutaneous stimulation of sequential muscle groups of ambulation with computer control, used for walking by spinal cord injured, entire system, after completion of training program

This code reports a transcutaneous, functional neuromuscular stimulator with computer control used to stimulate muscles of ambulation, which aids patients with spinal cord injuries in walking. A functional neuromuscular stimulator provides sequential electrical stimulation of muscles in the spinal cord injured patient. Use of electrical stimulation to replace stimuli when the nerve pathway has been injured or destroyed may assist in maintaining healthy muscle tone and strength and may enable the spinal cord injured patient to stand or walk independently. Patients are required to complete a training program prior to receiving the device.

E0765

E0765 FDA approved nerve stimulator, with replaceable batteries, for treatment of nausea and vomiting

The FDA approved nerve stimulator for treatment of nausea and vomiting is a battery-powered, noninvasive, portable, stimulation device. It is a small, watch-like device with two metal electrodes that are placed in contact with the skin on the volar aspect of the wrist over the median nerve following application of a hypoallergenic conductive gel to the skin contact site. The device is held in place with a Velcro band. Nerve stimulation therapy is administered by direct skin contact via two metal electrodes. The device has five intensity levels that are controlled by the patient by means of a rotary dial. This device may be used to treat nausea and vomiting secondary to pregnancy, chemotherapy, anesthesia, and motion sickness.

E0766

E0766 Electrical stimulation device used for cancer treatment, includes all accessories, any type

Novo TTF-100A is a portable battery or power-supply operated system that produces changing electrical fields, called tumor treatment fields, within the human body. The complete system includes a portable electric field generator, transducer arrays, rechargeable batteries, and more. Electric fields are delivered through four transducer arrays that are placed directly on the scalp to target the tumor. The transducer array placement is determined based on each patient's MRI results to maximize the therapy's effect on the tumor. The electric fields stop the growth of tumor cells resulting in cell death of the rapidly dividing cancer cells. The geometrical shape and scattering of the electrical charges within the dividing tumor cells allows the electrical fields to physically break up the tumor cell membrane. The frequency of the fields used for a particular treatment is specific to the size of the cell type being treated. The system is intended as a treatment for adult patients (22 years of age or older) with confirmed glioblastoma multiforme (GBM), following confirmed recurrence in an upper region of the brain (supratentorial) after receiving chemotherapy. The device is intended to be used as a stand-alone treatment, and is an alternative to standard medical therapy for recurrent GBM after surgical and radiation options have been exhausted.

E0769

E0769 Electrical stimulation or electromagnetic wound treatment device, not otherwise classified

This code reports two different types of wound treatment devices that are not otherwise classified. The first type is an electrical stimulation wound treatment device. This type of device uses the application of electrical current through electrodes placed directly on the skin in close proximity to the wound. There are four categories of electrical

E

stimulation devices used for wound healing, including low intensity direct current (LIDC), high voltage pulsed current (HVPC), alternative current (AC), and transcutaneous electrical nerve stimulation (TENS). The second type of device described by this code is an electromagnetic wound treatment device. This type of device employs electromagnetic fields rather than a direct electrical current.

E0770

E0770 Functional electrical stimulator, transcutaneous stimulation of nerve and/or muscle groups, any type, complete system, not otherwise specified

This code reports a transcutaneous, functional electric stimulator for muscles or nerves not otherwise specified. A functional neuromuscular stimulator provides sequential electrical stimulation of muscles or nerves to help regain some function. Transcutaneous stimulation therapy is administered by direct skin contact via metal electrodes. Use of electrical stimulation to replace stimuli when the nerve pathway has been injured or destroyed may assist in maintaining healthy muscle tone and strength. This code should only be reported if there is not a more specific code for the device.

E0776

E0776 IV pole

An intravenous (IV) pole is generally a portable, adjustable stand designed primarily to hang IV solution bags. Most models are mounted on rollers and are adjustable from a base height of about 56 inches up to about 96 inches. Many also feature optional attachments such as urinary bag hooks and clamps to secure oxygen tanks.

E0779-E0781

E0779 Ambulatory infusion pump, mechanical, reusable, for infusion 8 hours or greater

E0780 Ambulatory infusion pump, mechanical, reusable, for infusion less than 8 hours

E0781 Ambulatory infusion pump, single or multiple channels, electric or battery operated, with administrative equipment, worn by patient

Ambulatory infusion pumps are portable devices that are typically carried or worn by the patient, often on a belt or strap, to directly infuse medications. The pumps reported by this code range may be electric or mechanical devices that feature reservoirs to hold liquid medication. Pressure is created, mechanically or electrically, to infuse a regulated flow of medication into the patient over a set period of time. Routes of administration are by cannula and may include intravenous, intra-arterial, intrathecal, or intraperitoneal, among others; however, subcutaneous delivery is perhaps most common. A multiple channel pump allows for several different infusions at one time and features a programmable display to enter the prescribed rates.

E0782

E0782 Infusion pump, implantable, nonprogrammable (includes all components, e.g., pump, catheter, connectors, etc.)

An implantable infusion pump is a device carried by the patient in a surgically created subcutaneous pocket to directly infuse medications. Implanted pumps contain a refillable reservoir to hold liquid medication. The units may be used to deliver chemotherapy medications, drugs to address chronic pain, anti-spasmodics, or heparin, among others. Routes may include intravenous, intra-arterial, intrathecal, or intraperitoneal, among others. The reservoir is refilled by needle injection through a self-sealing membrane.

E0783

E0783 Infusion pump system, implantable, programmable (includes all components, e.g., pump, catheter, connectors, etc.)

This code reports the supply of an implantable, programmable infusion pump system that can be programmed to deliver a prescribed quantity of medicine over a given period of time. These devices are subcutaneously implanted near the site where the infusion is needed. The system is designed for patients requiring regular or continuous intravenous or intra-arterial infusions of drugs. The system may be used to deliver any of a variety of medicines, particularly those for oncology therapy. Implantable infusion pumps are typically small, biocompatible stainless steel units that are surgically placed subcutaneously near the site of optimal drug delivery. The port and reservoir can be smaller in diameter than a nickel coin. A refillable reservoir delivers a constant, prescribed rate of liquid drug to the target site. Typically, the reservoir features a rubber diaphragm that can be penetrated by a non-coring needle to refill the drug.

E0784

E0784 External ambulatory infusion pump, insulin

An external ambulatory infusion pump, also known as continuous subcutaneous insulin infusion (CSII), is a portable, battery-powered device typically worn on a belt or strap. The device contains a reservoir to hold insulin. An infusion set comprised of catheter tubing and a needle delivers microdoses of insulin, usually into subcutaneous tissues of the abdomen. Delivery rates can be closely adjusted to meet changing background needs, such as during strenuous exercise or around meals.

E0785-E0786

E0785 Implantable intraspinal (epidural/intrathecal) catheter used with implantable infusion pump, replacement

E0786 Implantable programmable infusion pump, replacement (excludes implantable intraspinal catheter)

These codes report infusion pump systems that can be programmed to deliver a prescribed quantity of medicine over a given period of time. These devices are subcutaneously implanted near the site where the infusion is needed. The system is designed for patients requiring regular or continuous intravenous or intra-arterial infusions of drugs. The system may be used to deliver any of a variety of medicines, particularly those for oncology therapy. Implantable infusion pumps are typically small, biocompatible stainless steel units that are surgically placed subcutaneously near the site of optimal drug delivery. The port and reservoir can be smaller in diameter than a nickel coin. A refillable reservoir delivers a constant, prescribed rate of liquid drug to the target site. Typically, the reservoir features a rubber diaphragm that can be penetrated by a non-coring needle to refill the drug.

E0787

E0787 External ambulatory infusion pump, insulin, dosage rate adjustment using therapeutic continuous glucose sensing

An external ambulatory infusion pump, also known as continuous subcutaneous insulin infusion (CSII), is a portable, battery-powered device typically worn on a belt or strap. The device contains a reservoir to hold insulin. An infusion set comprised of catheter tubing and a needle delivers microdoses of insulin, usually into subcutaneous tissues of the abdomen. Delivery rates can be closely adjusted to meet changing background needs, such as during strenuous exercise or around meals. This code continuously measures insulin levels and adjusts the dosage based on its readings.

E0791

E0791 Parenteral infusion pump, stationary, single, or multichannel

A stationary parenteral infusion pump is used to deliver liquid nutritional emulsions to patients whose normal gastrointestinal functions are compromised, and for the delivery of certain medications such as chemotherapies and pain management drugs. Proteins, carbohydrates, lipids, and electrolytes are the main components of parenteral nutrition, usually in carefully balanced combinations. The pumps are programmable and multi-channel units allow for several different infusions at one time. Lipids may be introduced separately, for example. Routes of administration include the subclavian, jugular, and femoral veins, as well as smaller vessels and, in some instances, arterial vessels.

E0830

E0830 Ambulatory traction device, all types, each

An ambulatory traction device uses two supports positioned on the body in such a way that they can lift and provide a decompressive force to the affected body part. In addition to the two supports, a lifting or stretching mechanism must be employed to provide the traction. This code reports any type of ambulatory traction device. If multiple traction devices are employed, each device is reported separately.

E0840-E0860

E0840 Traction frame, attached to headboard, cervical traction

E0849 Traction equipment, cervical, free-standing stand/frame, pneumatic, applying traction force to other than mandible

E0850 Traction stand, freestanding, cervical traction

E0855 Cervical traction equipment not requiring additional stand or frame

E0856 Cervical traction device, with inflatable air bladder(s)

E0860 Traction equipment, overdoor, cervical

Cervical traction equipment extends the neck muscles, tissue, and ligaments of the upper portion of the spinal column through a gentle pulling action. Code E0840 reports a cervical traction frame designed to be attached to a headboard. Code E0849 reports cervical traction equipment inclusive of a freestanding stand or frame and pneumatic pump designed to apply traction force to the occiput or any site other than the mandible. Code E0850 reports a freestanding cervical traction stand. Code E0855 reports cervical traction equipment not requiring an additional stand or frame, which typically consists of a foam roll for under the neck, an adjustable head harness, and a weight bag. Code E0860 reports overhead cervical traction, which typically consists of a water-weighted bag suspended from a frame mounted on an overhead door. A cord is threaded through a pulley and attached to a stabilization harness on the patient's head. The traction is designed to relieve gravity pressure on a cervical injury. Code E0856 reports a cervical collar with inflatable air bladder is a bracing device made from plastic or another rigid material that surrounds and immobilizes the cervical spine and neck. The inflated air bladder assists in supporting the head, provides spacing between the cervical vertebrae, and helps to reduce intradiscal pressure. A cervical collar with an inflatable air bladder is indicated for short-term treatment of neck pain.

E0870-E0900

E0870 Traction frame, attached to footboard, extremity traction (e.g., Buck's)

E0880 Traction stand, free standing, extremity traction

E0890 Traction frame, attached to footboard, pelvic traction

E0900 Traction stand, freestanding, pelvic traction (e.g., Buck's)

Traction stands and frames are available in a variety of configurations, depending on the treatment desired. Perhaps most recognizable is the Buck's traction system, which applies gentle, but firm traction (pulling action) to the affected extremity to stabilize the injury. A floor stand or hospital bed is mounted with a frame that curves over the injured arm or leg like a gallows frame. The frame may be fitted with counterweights, pulleys, and cable that connect to traction pins transfixed to the fractured bone or to the casting. It can be a freestanding, floor mechanism or one that is attached using the support of another object for traction. Pelvic fractures may require supports at both ends of the bed or two floor stands at either end. These mechanisms usually comprise a padded sleeve or splint-type product that is applied to the affected extremity, as well as a metal or durable frame affixed to both the sleeve or splint and to the traction-exerting rope and pulley or other system. The benefits from traction use include better extremity circulation, pressure release, separation of bony components, support and protection, and prevention of surrounding ligament and myofascial contracture.

E0910-E0912

E0910 Trapeze bars, also known as Patient Helper, attached to bed, with grab bar

E0911 Trapeze bar, heavy-duty, for patient weight capacity greater than 250 pounds, attached to bed, with grab bar

E0912 Trapeze bar, heavy-duty, for patient weight capacity greater than 250 pounds, freestanding, complete with grab bar

A trapeze bar with a grab bar, also referred to as a Patient Helper, is used when a patient needs a device to assist with movement because of a respiratory condition, fracture, or other medical condition. The patient holds onto the bar to maintain control while lifting the body or changing position. Trapeze bars may be attached to the bed or freestanding.

E0920-E0930

E0920 Fracture frame, attached to bed, includes weights

E0930 Fracture frame, freestanding, includes weights

Fracture frames are over-the-bed support structures from which traction weights and pulley can be mounted for the treatment of serious fractures. The units are available in several configurations. One style attaches to brackets at either end of the bed and another is a freestanding unit, mounting on legged supports. Both feature a strong bar that bridges over the bed and connects to the brackets. Traction weights and pulleys are arrayed along the bar as needed. Most models are modular and can accommodate variations in prescribed traction and weights. Traction counterweights are suspended from an array of cables and pulleys and rarely exceed eight pounds. Fixed, balanced, and sliding traction may be prescribed for treatment.

E0935

E0935 Continuous passive motion exercise device for use on knee only

Passive motion exercise devices (also known as continuous passive motion or CPM) are rehabilitation treatment strategies that usually follow orthopedic surgery. The knee joint is treated to sessions of continuous motion provided by a mechanical device.

E0936

E0936 Continuous passive motion exercise device for use other than knee

A continuous passive motion (CPM) device is attached to the patient and moves the affected joint for flexion and/or extension continuously for extended periods of time without patient assistance. The power unit is used to set the variable range of motion and speed. The initial setting for range of motion is based on the patient's comfort level. There may also be other factors used to set motion and speed. Motion and stress play a key role in healing connective tissue. Motion enhances blood flow and decreases pain. CPM can used in postoperative patients to enhance pain relief, improve the circulation of the extremity, reduce edema, improve the cartilage of synovial joints, retard muscular atrophy, reduce stiffness, and prevent contractures and adhesions.

E0940

E0940 Trapeze bar, freestanding, complete with grab bar

A trapeze bar with a grab bar, also referred to as a Patient Helper, is used when a patient needs a device to assist with movement because of a respiratory condition, fracture, or other medical condition. The patient holds onto the bar to maintain control while lifting the body or changing position. Trapeze bars may be attached to the bed or freestanding. Report E0940 for a freestanding trapeze bar.

E0941

E0941 Gravity assisted traction device, any type

This code reports the supply of a specialized traction device. Gravity traction devices can range from so-called "tilt tables" to inversion racks and "gravity boots." All of the systems promote spinal or other orthopedic therapy by reversing gravitational forces. Inversion tables and racks turn the user upside-down for a period of time. Gravity boots work in a similar fashion to allow the user to stretch the spine and hips by hanging upside-down from specialized boots. Other gravity traction devices work in a similar fashion. Gravity traction devices may be used to relieve chronic back pain by offering the user a period of suspension from gravitational pressures on the vertebral disk spaces.

E0942

E0942 Cervical head harness/halter

This code reports the supply of a specialized head harness for rehabilitation therapy, usually for cervical injuries or disorders. A halo-type apparatus is fitted to the patient's head, sometimes in combination with a chinstrap. This halo is connected to a larger ring attached to a wall surface. Elastic resistance straps or springs connect the patient's halo apparatus to the larger, fixed ring. The patient goes through a variety of range of motion exercises designed to build strength and flexibility in the cervical spine and its supporting musculature.

E0944

E0944 Pelvic belt/harness/boot

This code reports the supply of a specialized orthopedic device known as a pelvic belt. This is a traction device that may be used intermittently by the patient, usually to relieve chronic pain of the lower back, sacrum, or pelvic regions, or to treat the effects of spondylosis. A wide, padded, form-fitting belt or harness is worn around the lower waist, often with Velcro closures. The belt is connected by elastic resistance straps to provide traction on the belt, relieving lumbosacral pressures.

E0945

E0945 Extremity belt/harness

This code reports supply of a specialized orthopedic device known as an extremity belt or harness. Extremity belts or harnesses are used with other traction devices to treat fractures of the extremities. The belt or harness is applied distal to the fracture site and is used to suspend the extremity so traction can be applied.

E0946

E0946 Fracture, frame, dual with cross bars, attached to bed, (e.g., Balken, four-poster)

A fracture frame with cross bars attached to a bed that consists of an overhead frame supported by upright bars attached to the bedposts or to a separate stand. The fractured limb may be splinted and suspended in a harness that is attached to a rope and pulley with a weight to provide the traction. This type of fracture frame may be referred to as a Balkan or four poster frame. This code reports the frame only.

E0947

E0947 Fracture frame, attachments for complex pelvic traction

Fracture and/or traction frames and related equipment are devices usually attached to a hospital bed. The unit uses free weights and/or pulleys to pull the injured body part by immobilizing, aligning, and reducing pain, inflammation, and muscle spasms. This code reports attachments for complex pelvic traction for fractures.

E0948

E0948 Fracture frame, attachments for complex cervical traction

A fracture frame for complex cervical traction describes cervical traction devices that provide traction for the cervical spine by the use of a free-standing frame or a headboard. Traction force is applied by means of pneumonic displacement to anatomical areas other than the mandible. The devices must be capable of generating traction forces greater than 20 pounds and the device permits traction to be applied with alternative vectors of force. This code reports attachments for complex cervical traction for fractures.

E0950

E0950 Wheelchair accessory, tray, each

Wheelchair accessory trays are attached securely to the side surface of a conventional wheelchair. There are different tray styles with different functionality, including concealed compartments beneath an extension of an armrest for holding personal items, a cane holder, and a table tray (usually a standard feature).

E0951

E0951 Heel loop/holder, any type, with or without ankle strap, each

A heel loop/holder is a wheelchair accessory used to position and hold the heel of the foot safely on the footrest and assist with maintaining proper foot alignment.

E0952

E0952 Toe loop/holder, any type, each

A toe loop/holder is a wheelchair accessory used to position and hold the toes of the foot safely on the footrest and assist with maintaining proper foot alignment.

E0953

E0953 Wheelchair accessory, lateral thigh or knee support, any type including fixed mounting hardware, each

This code reports a wheelchair positioning accessory for the lateral thigh or knee. These accessories are used to position a patient who is not able to shift weight or that has any significant postural asymmetries that are due to an absent or impaired sensation in the area of contact with the seating surface. These products pull the thighs together to stabilize sitting posture and prevent hip abduction.

E0954

E0954 Wheelchair accessory, foot box, any type, includes attachment and mounting hardware, each foot

This code reports a wheelchair positioning accessory for the foot. This accessory is used to position a patient who is not able to shift weight or that has any significant postural asymmetries that are due to an absent or impaired sensation in the area of contact with the seating surface. This product surrounds the lower extremity and protects the ankle, calves, and feet.

E0955

E0955 Wheelchair accessory, headrest, cushioned, any type, including fixed mounting hardware, each

A head rest is a wheelchair accessory that supports the head and neck muscles. This code represents any cushioned headrest of any type. It includes any fixed mounting hardware.

E0956

E0956 Wheelchair accessory, lateral trunk or hip support, any type, including fixed mounting hardware, each

A lateral trunk or a hip support is a wheelchair accessory used to position a patient who is not able to shift weight or that has any significant postural asymmetries that are due to an absent or impaired sensation in the area of contact with the seating surface. It provides positioning for proper body alignment.

E0957

E0957 Wheelchair accessory, medial thigh support, any type, including fixed mounting hardware, each

A medial thigh support is a wheelchair accessory used to position a patient who is not able to shift weight or that has any significant postural asymmetries that are due to an absent or impaired sensation in the area of contact with the seating surface. The medial thigh support separates the thighs for improved hip alignment.

E0958

E0958 Manual wheelchair accessory, one-arm drive attachment, each

A one-arm drive attachment is a manual wheelchair accessory that allows the patient to propel the wheelchair with only one hand. A patient with hemiplegia or an injury to one extremity might require this option.

E0959

E0959 Manual wheelchair accessory, adapter for amputee, each

This code is reported for any amputee adapter accessory that can be used on a manual wheelchair.

E0960

E0960 Wheelchair accessory, shoulder harness/straps or chest strap, including any type mounting hardware

This code reports a positioning accessory for the upper torso. The chest and shoulder harness/strap provides positioning for proper body alignment.

E0961

E0961 Manual wheelchair accessory, wheel lock brake extension (handle), each

This code is reported for an accessory for the rear wheel brakes in a manual wheelchair. The extension brake handle provides easier access to applying the brakes.

E0966

E0966 Manual wheelchair accessory, headrest extension, each

A headrest extension is an accessory for a manual wheelchair that allows the headrest to be raised to a higher position than standard headrest height. Patients requiring a headrest for support due to weak neck muscles and patients who require reclining back wheelchairs may also require a headrest extension for proper positioning of the headrest.

E0967

E0967 Manual wheelchair accessory, hand rim with projections, any type, replacement only, each

Hand rims are wheel attachments that allow the user to independently move the wheelchair. Hand rims have been found to reduce fatigue, stress in wrists and shoulders, and carpal tunnel syndrome. These rims are also known as push rims. Some have projections attached to the side for better grip. Report this code for a hand rim, with projections, for a manual wheelchair.

E0968

E0968 Commode seat, wheelchair

A wheelchair commode seat is a specialized seat that has cutouts that mimic a toilet seat. The entire wheelchair with the commode seat and a commode pail can be used as a bedside commode. It may also be positioned over an existing toilet for added user support or it can be used as a transport wheelchair inside the house.

E0969

E0969 Narrowing device, wheelchair

This code reports a wheelchair accessory device that permits a wheelchair to be made narrower temporarily by a few inches by using a crank and gear mechanism providing the force to begin the folding process. The narrowing device is usually left in place but the crank handle is removable for storage.

E0970

E0970 No. 2 footplates, except for elevating legrest

Footplates provide a flat surface on which to rest the foot. Footplates are generally a standard feature on a wheelchair. If a user has problems with the standard plates, an angle adjustable footplate may be used. Adjustability is limited to front to back and side to side. Footrests should not be lower than 2 1/2 inches from the ground to safeguard clearance.

E0971

E0971 Manual wheelchair accessory, antitipping device, each

Anti-tipping devices are common wheelchair accessory options, particularly for pediatric patients. The devices may be paired and clamped onto the front of the chair to prevent forward spills.

E0973

E0973 Wheelchair accessory, adjustable height, detachable armrest, complete assembly, each

An adjustable height, detachable armrest is a wheelchair accessory designed for patients who require an armrest height that is not available in standard nonadjustable armrests. This code reports a single armrest and all hardware required for complete assembly. For patients who require adjustable height, detachable armrests for both the right and left arms, the code is reported separately for each side.

E0974

E0974 Manual wheelchair accessory, antirollback device, each

Wheelchair anti-rollback devices prevent a manual wheelchair from rolling away when a person stands or lowers themselves into the chair. Most devices consist of breaking systems that automatically engage the tires when weight is removed from the wheelchair seat. One type uses a lever that makes direct contact with the seat. When the lever senses the patient's weight is removed from the seat, the brake arms automatically clamp down. The chair can be moved forwarded even with the device engaged, but cannot be rolled backward. The device is disengaged by weight placed on the seat.

E0978

E0978 Wheelchair accessory, positioning belt/safety belt/pelvic strap, each

A positioning belt, safety belt, or pelvic strap is a wheelchair accessory that helps maintain proper positioning in the wheelchair. One or more of these items may be required for a patient with weak upper body muscles, upper body instability, or muscle spasticity. If more than one positioning/safety belt/strap is required, each one is reported separately.

E0980

E0980 Safety vest, wheelchair

A safety vest is a restraint designed to securely hold a person in an upright position in a wheelchair. The vest prevents the patient from leaning forward or laterally. A patient that has weak upper body muscles, upper body instability, or muscle spasticity might need the safety vest for proper positioning.

E0981-E0982

E0981 Wheelchair accessory, seat upholstery, replacement only, each

E0982 Wheelchair accessory, back upholstery, replacement only, each

The life of a wheelchair seat cushion or back is usually five years or more. Upholstery is the covering and any underlying padding.

E0983-E0984

E0983 Manual wheelchair accessory, power add-on to convert manual wheelchair to motorized wheelchair, joystick control

E0984 Manual wheelchair accessory, power add-on to convert manual wheelchair to motorized wheelchair, tiller control

A wheelchair is a chair-like device that can be categorized as manual or as a power mobility device (e.g., power wheelchair [PWC] or power operated vehicle [POV]/scooter). There are options and accessories for wheelchairs that allow patients to function successfully in the home or to perform the usual activities of daily living. There are various types of power add-on attachments that convert a manual wheelchair into a power chair, including a master power switch that can be turned on and off. The majority of PWCs are controlled through a side-mounted joystick. The joystick can adjust up to five specific speed programs. A tiller is a lever that is pushed or pulled to control the PWC.

E0985

E0985 Wheelchair accessory, seat lift mechanism

Seat lifts are mechanisms that enable the patient to increase the seat height in their wheelchair. Some wheelchair seat lifts enable the patient to go from a sitting to standing position, allowing the patient to be in the most comfortable and functional position for his or her needs. The lifting mechanism is graded and not based on a catapult or other type of spring system.

These mechanisms can be manual, electric, or battery powered. These devices can help disabled patient's functionality and help with patient transfer.

E0986

E0986 Manual wheelchair accessory, push-rim activated power assist system

A push activated power assist accessory for a manual wheelchair is a device fitted to a rear wheel to sense the force exerted on the wheels. A battery-powered brake and/or propulsion system may then be activated to assist the patient in stopping or advancing the chair.

E0988

E0988 Manual wheelchair accessory, lever-activated, wheel drive, pair

A manual wheelchair is a chair-like device that grants the user some mobility when the user has limited or no control over the legs and/or spine. Manual wheelchairs are usually propelled by the use of a large wheel rotated by user movements. These movements put a great deal of stress and strain on the shoulder muscles. Lever activated wheel drives use pushing and pulling motion on the levers to move gears that propel the wheelchair.

E0990

E0990 Wheelchair accessory, elevating legrest, complete assembly, each

An elevating legrest is a wheelchair accessory required by patients who have musculoskeletal conditions, casts, or braces that prevent 90-degree flexion at the knee. It may also be required for patients with significant edema of the lower extremities requiring elevation of the legs and for patients who require a reclining back on the wheelchair. This code reports a single elevating legrest and all hardware required for complete assembly. For patients who require elevating legrests for both the right and left legs, the code is reported separately for each side.

E0992

E0992 Manual wheelchair accessory, solid seat insert

A solid seat insert is a wooden or plastic device to bridge the suspension-style seat that comes standard on collapsible wheelchairs.

E0994-E0995

E0994 Armrest, each

E0995 Wheelchair accessory, calf rest/pad, replacement only, each

Armrests are components of a wheelchair that support the arms and take the pull of gravity off user arms and shoulders. This straightens the spine and aids in keeping a person more upright in a wheelchair. The calf rests/pads are components of a wheelchair that support a person's calves when extended outward from the wheelchair.

E1002

E1002 Wheelchair accessory, power seating system, tilt only

This code reports a tilt power seating system, a wheelchair accessory that can be added to a power wheelchair. The tilt feature allows the wheelchair to be tilted backward to at least 45 degrees from horizontal. Tilting the chair can increase comfort, reduce fatigue, and relieve pressure points caused by sitting in the same position for long periods of time. Power tilt seating systems include a solid seat platform and solid back; any frame width and depth; armrests; fixed or swing-away detachable legrests; fixed or flip-up footplates; a motor and related electronics, with or without variable speed programmability; a switch control that is independent of the power wheelchair drive control interface; and any hardware required to attach the seating system to the wheelchair base. In addition to the tilt specifications, tilt systems must have a back height of at least 20 inches, the ability for the supplier to adjust the seat to back angle, and the ability to support a patient weighing up to 250 pounds.

E1003-E1008

E1003 Wheelchair accessory, power seating system, recline only, without shear reduction

E1004 Wheelchair accessory, power seating system, recline only, with mechanical shear reduction

E1005 Wheelchair accessory, power seating system, recline only, with power shear reduction

E1006 Wheelchair accessory, power seating system, combination tilt and recline, without shear reduction

E1007 Wheelchair accessory, power seating system, combination tilt and recline, with mechanical shear reduction

E1008 Wheelchair accessory, power seating system, combination tilt and recline, with power shear reduction

These codes report a recline power seating system and a combination tilt and recline power seating system, accessories that can be added to a power wheelchair. The tilt feature allows the wheelchair to be tilted to at least 45 degrees from horizontal. The recline feature allows the chair to recline to at least 150 degrees from horizontal. There are several types of systems, differing primarily in their ability to reduce the shearing forces that occur when the wheelchair is reclined. Shearing refers to the shifting of the torso in the chair as it is reclined or raised, causing the patient to slide along the back of the chair. Recline systems that reduce the shearing forces allow the patient's back to stay in contact with the chair without sliding. Wheelchair reclining systems that do not have shear reduction capabilities require that the wheelchair user be able to shift position to compensate for the 2- to 3-

inch shear that occurs when the wheelchair is reclined or raised. Reclining wheelchairs are categorized as those that do not provide shear reduction, those that provide mechanical shear reduction, and those that provide power shear reduction. A mechanical shear reduction feature consists of two separate back panels. As the posterior back panel reclines or rises, there is a mechanical linkage between the two panels that allows the patient's back to stay in contact with the anterior panel without sliding along that panel. A power shear reduction feature also consists of two back panels. As the posterior back panel reclines or rises, a separate motor controls the linkage between the two panels that allows the patient's back to stay in contact with the anterior panel without sliding along that panel. Power recline seating systems include a solid seat platform and solid back; any frame width and depth; arm rests; fixed or swing-away detachable leg rests; fixed or flip-up footplates; a motor and related electronics, with or without variable speed programmability; a switch control independent of the power wheelchair drive control interface; and any hardware required to attach the seating system to the wheelchair base. In addition to the recline specifications, recline systems must have a back height of at least 20 inches and the ability to support a patient weighing up to 250 pounds.

E1009-E1010

E1009 Wheelchair accessory, addition to power seating system, mechanically linked leg elevation system, including pushrod and legrest, each

E1010 Wheelchair accessory, addition to power seating system, power leg elevation system, including legrest, pair

A leg elevation system is a wheelchair accessory that can be added to a power seating system. Two types are available: a mechanically linked leg elevation system and a power leg elevation system. A mechanically linked system uses a pushrod that connects the leg rest to a power recline seating system. With such a leg elevation system, when the back reclines, the leg rest rises; when the back is raised, the leg rest lowers. A power leg elevation system uses a dedicated motor and related electronics, with or without variable speed programmability, that allows the leg rest to be raised and lowered independently of the recline and/or tilt of the seating system. It includes a switch control that may or may not be integrated with the power tilt or recline controls.

E1011

E1011 Modification to pediatric size wheelchair, width adjustment package (not to be dispensed with initial chair)

Some wheelchair companies offer "growth options" on pediatric wheelchairs since buying a new wheelchair each year would be very expensive. Growth kits or growth chairs allow adjustments to be made to the wheelchair. These replaceable components can be adjusted from smaller to larger to accommodate a growing child.

E1012

E1012 Wheelchair accessory, addition to power seating system, center mount power elevating leg rest/platform, complete system, any type, each

This code identifies a center mount, power elevating legrest/platform wheelchair accessory used in addition to a power seating system. It is a center mount, power elevating legrest/platform that uses mechanical levers, pulleys, and motors to raise, extend, and retract the leg and foot. This is a complete system of any type.

E1014

E1014 Reclining back, addition to pediatric size wheelchair

Reclining wheelchair backs are options that may be required for pediatric patients with certain medical conditions including quadriplegia, fixed hip angle, trunk or lower extremity casts/braces, excess extensor tone of the trunk muscles, or the need to rest in a recumbent position periodically during the day. A semi-reclining back is defined as one with a recline capability of greater than 15 degrees, but less than 80 degrees. A fully reclining back is one that can recline to greater than 80 degrees.

E1015-E1018

E1015 Shock absorber for manual wheelchair, each

E1016 Shock absorber for power wheelchair, each

E1017 Heavy-duty shock absorber for heavy-duty or extra heavy-duty manual wheelchair, each

E1018 Heavy-duty shock absorber for heavy-duty or extra heavy-duty power wheelchair, each

Wheelchair shock absorbers provide a smoother, less jarring ride for disabled patients. The shock absorbers are attached to the front wheels and include a suspension system with a hinge damper or a spring coil to absorb the impact of rough surfaces. The shock absorbers can be fit for manual or electric wheelchairs.

E1020

E1020 Residual limb support system for wheelchair, any type

A wheelchair residual limb support system is an attachment that provides a wheelchair patient a place to rest the stump of an amputated leg. This additional support allows the patient proper and comfortable positioning when seated in the wheelchair. The residual support device is similar to a leg rest but is shorter. It can be adjustable to allow for differences in the residual limb length and allow different positions.

E1028

E1028 Wheelchair accessory, manual swingaway, retractable or removable mounting hardware for joystick, other control interface or positioning accessory

Retractable or removable mounting hardware devices are used to attach wheelchair accessories that allow the accessory to be manually moved, either to the side or up and down, or removed from the wheelchair mount. This hardware is specific for a joystick, other control interface, or positioning accessory.

E1029-E1030

E1029 Wheelchair accessory, ventilator tray, fixed

E1030 Wheelchair accessory, ventilator tray, gimbaled

A ventilator tray is a platform attached to the wheelchair back that allows the patient's ventilator to be transported with the patient. A gimbaled tray remains horizontal when the seat back is raised or lowered.

E1031

E1031 Rollabout chair, any and all types with castors 5 in or greater

Rollabout chairs, any and all types that have casters of 5 inches or larger, are prescribed for ill, injured, or impaired individuals who require a level of mobility without standing and walking that may be met by the rollabout chair in lieu of a wheelchair. Rollabout chairs are not general use home or office chairs. Rollabout chairs are also referred to as mobile geriatric chairs and geri-chairs.

E1035-E1036

E1035 Multi-positional patient transfer system, with integrated seat, operated by care giver, patient weight capacity up to and including 300 lbs

E1036 Multi-positional patient transfer system, extra-wide, with integrated seat, operated by caregiver, patient weight capacity greater than 300 lbs

A multi-positional patient transfer system is a medical device, with an integrated seat, that allows positioning and adjustment of bed-bound people. The person can be transferred onto the device in a supine position. Once positioned, the device can be adjusted into chair-like positions. This device is not electric. It is operated by a caregiver.

E1037-E1039

E1037 Transport chair, pediatric size

E1038 Transport chair, adult size, patient weight capacity up to and including 300 pounds

E1039 Transport chair, adult size, heavy-duty, patient weight capacity greater than 300 pounds

Transport chairs come in a variety of sizes with multiple functions, also referred to as a companion wheelchair. Transport chairs are convenient for any type of travel. Transport chairs are usually light weight and can fit into the patient's back seat or trunk.

E1050-E1070

E1050 Fully-reclining wheelchair, fixed full-length arms, swing-away detachable elevating legrests

E1060 Fully-reclining wheelchair, detachable arms, desk or full-length, swing-away detachable elevating legrests

E1070 Fully-reclining wheelchair, detachable arms (desk or full-length) swing-away detachable footrest

Fully reclining wheelchairs are indicated for patients who are quadriplegic, have a fixed hip angle, may be currently wearing body or extremity casts or braces that necessitate a reclining position, and for patients who need to rest in their wheelchair in a recumbent position two or more times per day because transfer between wheelchair and bed is difficult. These wheelchairs include a fully reclining backrest with detachable armrests (desk arm or full-length) or fixed full-length armrests, and swing-away, detachable, elevating legrests with a pad used to support the calf when the legrest is in an elevated position.

E1083-E1086

E1083 Hemi-wheelchair, fixed full-length arms, swing-away detachable elevating legrest

E1084 Hemi-wheelchair, detachable arms desk or full-length arms, swing-away detachable elevating legrests

E1085 Hemi-wheelchair, fixed full-length arms, swing-away detachable footrests

E1086 Hemi-wheelchair, detachable arms, desk or full-length, swing-away detachable footrests

The hemi-wheelchair is indicated for patients requiring a lower seat height (17 to 18 inches) than the standard 19 to 21 inches from seat to floor because of short stature or the inability to place the feet on the ground for propulsion due to amputation, paralysis, or stroke. Hemi-wheelchairs have a fully reclining backrest.

E1087-E1090

E1087 High strength lightweight wheelchair, fixed full-length arms, swing-away detachable elevating legrests

E1088 High strength lightweight wheelchair, detachable arms desk or full-length, swing-away detachable elevating legrests

E1089 High-strength lightweight wheelchair, fixed-length arms, swing-away detachable footrest

E1090 High-strength lightweight wheelchair, detachable arms, desk or full-length, swing-away detachable footrests

The high-strength lightweight wheelchair is indicated for patients requiring a chair for self-propulsion and/or when the seat height, width, or depth measurements required cannot be accommodated by a standard, hemi, or lightweight wheelchair. This device weighs less than 34 pounds, is fully reclining, and has high-strength side frames and cross braces.

E1092-E1093

E1092 Wide heavy-duty wheel chair, detachable arms (desk or full-length), swing-away detachable elevating legrests

E1093 Wide heavy-duty wheelchair, detachable arms, desk or full-length arms, swing-away detachable footrests

A wide, heavy-duty wheelchair is indicated for obese patients when the seat measurements required cannot be accommodated by a standard wheelchair. This device is fully reclining and includes detachable desk or full-length arms.

E1100-E1110

E1100 Semi-reclining wheelchair, fixed full-length arms, swing-away detachable elevating legrests

E1110 Semi-reclining wheelchair, detachable arms (desk or full-length) elevating legrest

A semi-reclining wheelchair provides a backrest that tilts back from the upright position but not into a full-recumbent posture and swing-away, detachable elevating legrests that have a pad used to support the calf when the legrest is in an elevated position.

E1130-E1160

E1130 Standard wheelchair, fixed full-length arms, fixed or swing-away detachable footrests

E1140 Wheelchair, detachable arms, desk or full-length, swing-away detachable footrests

E1150 Wheelchair, detachable arms, desk or full-length swing-away detachable elevating legrests

E1160 Wheelchair, fixed full-length arms, swing-away detachable elevating legrests

A standard wheelchair generally has a seat width of 16, 18, or 20 inches, is 16 inches in depth, and 21 inches from seat to floor. It comes with a chrome-plated frame, 24 inch molded rear wheels, 8 inch molded casters, nylon or vinyl upholstery, and arm and footrests.

E1161

E1161 Manual adult size wheelchair, includes tilt in space

A tilt-in-space system in a standard wheelchair that changes a person's orientation in space while maintaining fixed hip, knee, and ankle angles. The system redistributes pressure from one area to another and maintains physical angles at the hips, knees, and ankles.

E1170-E1190

E1170 Amputee wheelchair, fixed full-length arms, swing-away detachable elevating legrests

E1171 Amputee wheelchair, fixed full-length arms, without footrests or legrest

E1172 Amputee wheelchair, detachable arms (desk or full-length) without footrests or legrest

E1180 Amputee wheelchair, detachable arms (desk or full-length) swing-away detachable footrests

E1190 Amputee wheelchair, detachable arms (desk or full-length) swing-away detachable elevating legrests

An amputee wheelchair is specially designed for patients missing one or both legs. When a patient has one or both legs amputated, the center of gravity and weight distribution changes. An amputee wheelchair is designed with large wheels and the rear axle placed further back on the chair to compensate for less weight at the front of the chair from the missing limb(s). Amputee wheelchairs are available with different options for patient need and comfort.

E1195

E1195 Heavy-duty wheelchair, fixed full-length arms, swing-away detachable elevating legrests

A heavy-duty wheelchair is designed to support larger people with weight capacities that begin at 500 pounds. Frames are usually reinforced. Seats are usually wider and deeper than non-heavy duty chairs.

E1200

E1200 Amputee wheelchair, fixed full-length arms, swing-away detachable footrest

An amputee wheelchair is specially designed for patients missing one or both legs. When a patient has one or both legs amputated, the center of gravity and weight distribution changes. An amputee wheelchair is designed with large wheels and the rear axle placed further back on the chair to compensate for less weight at the front of the chair from the missing limb(s). The swing away feature gets the attachment out of the way, allowing patients to be transferred in and out of the wheelchair and provides patients a fully adjustable amputee support.

E1220

E1220 Wheelchair; specially sized or constructed, (indicate brand name, model number, if any) and justification

A specially sized or constructed wheelchair is indicated for patients in cases when the measurements of a standard wheelchair will not accommodate the patient's needs. This wheelchair must be justified by reasons such as a patient's physical size or the specific requirements for wheelchair usage in the patient's place of residence, such as narrow doorways that prevent the passage of a standard wheelchair. Report the brand name and model number.

E1221-E1224

E1221 Wheelchair with fixed arm, footrests

E1222 Wheelchair with fixed arm, elevating legrests

E1223 Wheelchair with detachable arms, footrests

E1224 Wheelchair with detachable arms, elevating legrests

A wheelchair is a chair with wheels designed to provide mobility to people for whom walking is difficult or impossible. Armrests can be fixed to the chair or detachable. Footrests are usually attached to the chair. Elevating leg rests attach to the lower front of the chair and are used to support the legs. The elevating leg rest can be positioned to maintain the leg in an extended position or at varying angles.

E1225-E1226

E1225 Wheelchair accessory, manual semi-reclining back, (recline greater than 15 degrees, but less than 80 degrees), each

E1226 Wheelchair accessory, manual fully reclining back, (recline greater than 80 degrees), each

Manual semi-reclining or fully reclining wheelchair backs are options that may be required for patients with certain medical conditions including quadriplegia, fixed hip angle, trunk or lower extremity casts/braces, excess extensor tone of the trunk muscles, or the need to rest in a recumbent position periodically during the day. A semi-reclining back is defined as one with a recline capability of greater than 15 degrees, but less than 80 degrees. A fully reclining back is one that can recline to greater than 80 degrees.

E1227-E1228

E1227 Special height arms for wheelchair

E1228 Special back height for wheelchair

A specially sized or constructed wheelchair is indicated in cases where the measurements of a standard wheelchair do not accommodate the patient's needs. This wheelchair must be justified by reasons such as a patient's physical size or the specific requirements for wheelchair usage in the patient's place of residence, such as narrow doorways that prevent the passage of a standard wheelchair.

E1229

E1229 Wheelchair, pediatric size, not otherwise specified

Report this code for a pediatric sized wheelchair that is not otherwise specified in other HCPCS Level II codes.

E1230

E1230 Power operated vehicle (three- or four-wheel nonhighway), specify brand name and model number

A POV is a power-operated vehicle with three to four wheels. These may be indoor, outdoor, or both indoor/outdoor models. Indoor models are generally slow-speed with highly maneuverable mechanisms that assist the patient with mobility inside the home. Outdoor models can reach greater speeds and are more durable. POVs usually work from a battery power source. An indoor POV assists patients for whom a wheelchair is unsuitable in the activities of daily living, but POVs are not suited to all types of patients such as stroke victims or some quadriplegic and/or hemiplegic patients who cannot operate the controls nor be left alone while the vehicle is in operation. This code requires specifying the brand name and model number when reporting.

E1231-E1234

E1231 Wheelchair, pediatric size, tilt-in-space, rigid, adjustable, with seating system

E1232 Wheelchair, pediatric size, tilt-in-space, folding, adjustable, with seating system

E1233 Wheelchair, pediatric size, tilt-in-space, rigid, adjustable, without seating system

E1234 Wheelchair, pediatric size, tilt-in-space, folding, adjustable, without seating system

A tilt-in-space system in a standard wheelchair that changes a person's orientation in space while maintaining fixed hip, knee, and ankle angles. The system redistributes pressure from one area to another and maintains physical angles at the hips, knees, and ankles. This wheelchair provides positioning and is perfect for individuals who require tilt adjustment for pressure relief, digestion, and respiratory assistance. Pediatric wheelchairs are smaller in size to accommodate the smaller stature of a child. Rigid wheelchairs do not fold or collapse. Folding wheelchairs allow the chair to be folded for travel purposes. Seating systems include seat pads and back rests that can be customized to the user's needs.

E1235-E1238

E1235 Wheelchair, pediatric size, rigid, adjustable, with seating system

E1236 Wheelchair, pediatric size, folding, adjustable, with seating system

E1237 Wheelchair, pediatric size, rigid, adjustable, without seating system

E1238 Wheelchair, pediatric size, folding, adjustable, without seating system

Pediatric wheelchairs are smaller in size to accommodate the smaller stature of a child. Rigid wheelchairs do not fold or collapse. Folding wheelchairs allow the chair to be folded or collapsed for travel purposes. Seating systems include seat pads and back rests that can be customized to the user's needs.

E1239

E1239 Power wheelchair, pediatric size, not otherwise specified

A power wheelchair is a power-operated wheelchair with three to four wheels. These may be indoor, outdoor, or both indoor/outdoor models. Indoor models are generally slow-speed with highly maneuverable mechanisms that assist the patient with mobility inside the home. Outdoor models can reach greater speeds and are more durable. Power wheelchairs usually work from a battery power source. Pediatric wheelchairs are smaller in size to accommodate the smaller stature of a child. Report this code for a pediatric sized power wheelchair that is not otherwise specified by other HCPCS Level II codes.

E

E1240-E1270

E1240 Lightweight wheelchair, detachable arms, (desk or full-length) swing-away detachable, elevating legrest

E1250 Lightweight wheelchair, fixed full-length arms, swing-away detachable footrest

E1260 Lightweight wheelchair, detachable arms (desk or full-length) swing-away detachable footrest

E1270 Lightweight wheelchair, fixed full-length arms, swing-away detachable elevating legrests

Lightweight wheelchairs are designed for patients who spend a great deal of time in the unit and can take full advantage of the increased mobility a lighter chair offers. Most models weigh 26 to 34 pounds and the patient can mobilize it more effectively than conventional wheelchairs.

E1280-E1295

E1280 Heavy-duty wheelchair, detachable arms (desk or full-length) elevating legrests

E1285 Heavy-duty wheelchair, fixed full-length arms, swing-away detachable footrest

E1290 Heavy-duty wheelchair, detachable arms (desk or full-length) swing-away detachable footrest

E1295 Heavy-duty wheelchair, fixed full-length arms, elevating legrest

Heavy-duty wheelchairs may be called for to supply patients of extreme size or weight. Most models feature reinforced frames and wheels and can seat patients from 300 to 400 pounds or greater. Some models can accommodate up to 700 pounds. The unit itself may weigh up to 58 pounds.

E1296-E1298

E1296 Special wheelchair seat height from floor

E1297 Special wheelchair seat depth, by upholstery

E1298 Special wheelchair seat depth and/or width, by construction

A specially sized or constructed wheelchair component is indicated when the measurements of a standard wheelchair do not accommodate the patient's needs. This wheelchair must be justified by reasons such as a patient's physical size or the specific requirements for wheelchair usage in the patient's place of residence, such as narrow doorways that prevent the passage of a standard wheelchair. The standard seat height from the floor is 18 to 20 inches. The standard seat width and depth is 15 to 19 inches. When a deviation is more than 2 inches from the standard, the sizing is labeled "special."

E1300-E1310

E1300 Whirlpool, portable (overtub type)

E1310 Whirlpool, nonportable (built-in type)

A therapeutic bath device that uses circulating water and water jets to stimulate circulation, relieve pain, and massage the body. Whirlpools may have a single pump that circulates the water or multiple pumps—one to circulate the water and the others to drive the hydrotherapy jets.

E1352

E1352 Oxygen accessory, flow regulator capable of positive inspiratory pressure

The Noninvasive OPEN Ventilation System (NIOV™) by Breathe Technologies, Inc. provides positive pressure inspiratory support for patients using oxygen. This product consists of multiple components, including a control unit, flow regulator, connecting hose, and nasal interface (pillows).

E1353

E1353 Regulator

An oxygen regulator is a brass (or sometimes aluminum) device that governs the flow of gaseous oxygen from the tank. Some devices may feature an integrated pressure gauge and additional flow ports and safety relief valves.

E1354-E1355

E1354 Oxygen accessory, wheeled cart for portable cylinder or portable concentrator, any type, replacement only, each

E1355 Stand/rack

A wheeled cart is a device with a platform, straps, or hooks to secure the oxygen cylinder or concentrator and wheels. Using a wheeled cart facilitates traveling with oxygen. This cart falls into the category of additional oxygen related equipment. A stand or rack is a device with a platform, straps, or hooks to secure the oxygen cylinder or concentrator. Racks or stands can hold one or multiple cylinders. Some may attach to wheelchairs while others are freestanding. Stands and racks allow for easier movement of the oxygen equipment. This cart falls in the category of additional oxygen related equipment.

E1356

E1356 Oxygen accessory, battery pack/cartridge for portable concentrator, any type, replacement only, each

A battery pack or cartridge is an oxygen accessory that supplies power to a portable oxygen concentrator using AC/DC or lithium power cartridges. Batteries automatically charge if the units plugged into an AC source. These ambulatory systems make it easy for patients to go just about anywhere without the concern of running out of oxygen.

E1357

E1357 Oxygen accessory, battery charger for portable concentrator, any type, replacement only, each

A battery charger is a device used to put energy into rechargeable batteries by forcing an electric current through it. Simply insert the battery into the charger and it stops charging when the battery is fully charged.

E1358

E1358 Oxygen accessory, DC power adapter for portable concentrator, any type, replacement only, each

A direct current (DC) power adapter converts DC into the alternating current (AC) that a portable concentrator needs. Many DC adapters can power an oxygen concentrator from the "cigarette lighter" style sockets found in most vehicles.

E1372

E1372 Immersion external heater for nebulizer

An immersion external heater for a nebulizer is an accessory for a pneumatic nebulizer. It is an external slip-on heater that heats the aerosol mixture before inhalation. It is believed that the heating reduces the possibility of contamination.

E1390-E1392

E1390 Oxygen concentrator, single delivery port, capable of delivering 85 percent or greater oxygen concentration at the prescribed flow rate

E1391 Oxygen concentrator, dual delivery port, capable of delivering 85 percent or greater oxygen concentration at the prescribed flow rate, each

E1392 Portable oxygen concentrator, rental

An oxygen concentrator takes oxygen from room air and removes nitrogen, which comprises about 80 percent of room air. These units alternately compress ambient air through chambers containing zeolite granules, which absorb nitrogen. While one chamber is pressurized, the second rests and the zeolite release the absorbed nitrogen back into the room air. The concentrated oxygen is filtered and delivered at levels of about 5 liters per minute at levels approaching 95 percent pure oxygen.

E1399

E1399 Durable medical equipment, miscellaneous

Durable medical equipment is a diverse term used to describe any medical equipment used in the home to aid in a better quality of living where people can be more mobile and independent. The term "durable medical equipment" includes iron lungs, oxygen tents, nebulizers, continuous positive airway pressure devices, catheters, hospital beds, and wheelchairs, whether furnished on a rental basis or purchased. There are also other simple tools such as ramps that can help wheelchair users access steps and vehicles and highly specialized devices, such as hearing aids and a breathing apparatus. Report this code when a more specific HCPCS Level II code is not available for durable medical equipment.

E1405-E1406

E1405 Oxygen and water vapor enriching system with heated delivery

E1406 Oxygen and water vapor enriching system without heated delivery

Oxygen delivery systems are units of compressed gaseous, liquid, or concentrated O2 for home use, which are stationary or portable. In many cases, the units also include the system components required to administer the O2, such as the regulator, flowmeter, contents indicator, nebulizer, humidifier, cannula or mask, and the O2 tubing. The administration of O2 assists in oxygenation of tissues when the patient's cardiopulmonary system is unable to intake sufficient quantities of O2 or is unable to process outside or room air into its elemental components to use the O2 content. For instance, patients with severe chronic obstructive pulmonary disease and emphysema may require O2 therapy. Oxygen also aids in and/or expedites the healing of injured or diseased tissues or organs.

E1500-E1625

E1500 Centrifuge, for dialysis

E1510 Kidney, dialysate delivery system kidney machine, pump recirculating, air removal system, flowrate meter, power off, heater and temperature control with alarm, IV poles, pressure gauge, concentrate container

E1520 Heparin infusion pump for hemodialysis

E1530 Air bubble detector for hemodialysis, each, replacement

E1540 Pressure alarm for hemodialysis, each, replacement

E1550 Bath conductivity meter for hemodialysis, each

E1560 Blood leak detector for hemodialysis, each, replacement

E1570 Adjustable chair, for ESRD patients

E1575 Transducer protectors/fluid barriers, for hemodialysis, any size, per 10

E1580 Unipuncture control system for hemodialysis

E1590 Hemodialysis machine

E1592 Automatic intermittent peritoneal dialysis system

E1594 Cycler dialysis machine for peritoneal dialysis

E1600 Delivery and/or installation charges for hemodialysis equipment

E1610 Reverse osmosis water purification system, for hemodialysis

E1615 Deionizer water purification system, for hemodialysis

E1620 Blood pump for hemodialysis, replacement

E1625 Water softening system, for hemodialysis

These codes describe miscellaneous supplies and equipment needed to accomplish home dialysis. Dialysis is a filtration process that filters impurities from the blood. Dialysis assists malfunctioning kidneys and can replace nonfunctioning kidneys. The functioning of all body parts requires the removal of the various toxins and metabolic byproducts from the blood. If these impurities are allowed to accumulate, death will occur within days. Home dialysis allows the patient to perform this function in home rather than at a facility.

E1629

E1629 Tablo hemodialysis system for the billable dialysis service

Tablo hemodialysis system is an all-in-one dialysis system that can be operated from the patient's home when the patient can demonstrate time to obtain training, a clean and safe environment for treatment, storage space for the machine and supplies, and a trained caregiver. It is indicated for the treatment of patients with acute and/or chronic renal failure. The system is compact at 19 inches wide, is mobile, and needs only a power outlet connection, tap water, and a drain to perform dialysis. Tablo contains three components: 1) the Tablo Console, a single module of multiple fluidic systems that performs water purification and dialysis delivery; 2) the Tablo Cartridge, a single-use blood tubing set that is attached to an organizer; and 3) Tablo Connectivity and Data Ecosystem, a cloud-based monitoring system with patient analytics and clinical recordkeeping. A single-use cartridge is inserted into the front console panel for each dialysis treatment. The water purification system produces dialysis-quality water. The purified water is transferred to the dialysis delivery system where it is mixed with the correct proportion of dialysis concentrates. This dialysate passes through an ultrafilter and then into the dialyzer. The system has a touchscreen interface that provides 3D animation and conversational instruction to guide the patient and caregiver through set up, treatment, and troubleshooting, and it transmits treatment data to the provider and a remote diagnostic platform for service and support.

E1630-E1699

E1630 Reciprocating peritoneal dialysis system

E1632 Wearable artificial kidney, each

E1634 Peritoneal dialysis clamps, each

E1635 Compact (portable) travel hemodialyzer system

E1636 Sorbent cartridges, for hemodialysis, per 10

E1637 Hemostats, each

E1639 Scale, each

E1699 Dialysis equipment, not otherwise specified

These codes describe miscellaneous supplies and equipment needed to accomplish home dialysis. Dialysis is a filtration process that filters impurities from the blood. Dialysis assists malfunctioning kidneys and can replace nonfunctioning kidneys. The functioning of all body parts requires the removal of the various toxins and metabolic byproducts from the blood. If these impurities are allowed to accumulate, death will occur within days. Home dialysis allows the patient to perform this function in home rather than at a facility.

E

E1700

E1700 Jaw motion rehabilitation system

This code reports the supply of a rehabilitative device for disorders of the temporomandibular joint (TMJ) and restrictive jaw motion. These devices may feature a cushioned mouthpiece that the patient bites against. The patient then squeezes a lever that forces open the mouthpiece and the jaw. Adjustments on the device control the leverage action. The therapy works to improve the range of the TMJ. Patients who have undergone certain radiation treatments often suffer a restrictive and spastic jaw movement known as trismus. Rehabilitation for surgery of the jaw and treatment of conditions that cause "lockjaw" may also warrant use of this type of device.

E1701

E1701 Replacement cushions for jaw motion rehabilitation system, package of 6

Replacement cushions for a jaw motion rehabilitation system are padded bite plates attached to a scissor-like device that are intended to prevent hypomobility and gradually increase the range of jaw motion.

E1702

E1702 Replacement measuring scales for jaw motion rehabilitation system, package of 200

Replacement scales used in a jaw motion rehabilitation system are special disposable paper scale (measuring) devices that measure the opening, movement, and function of the mouth and jaw.

E1800-E1841

E1800 Dynamic adjustable elbow extension/flexion device, includes soft interface material

E1801 Static progressive stretch elbow device, extension and/or flexion, with or without range of motion adjustment, includes all components and accessories

E1802 Dynamic adjustable forearm pronation/supination device, includes soft interface material

E1805 Dynamic adjustable wrist extension/flexion device, includes soft interface material

E1806 Static progressive stretch wrist device, flexion and/or extension, with or without range of motion adjustment, includes all components and accessories

E1810 Dynamic adjustable knee extension/flexion device, includes soft interface material

E1811 Static progressive stretch knee device, extension and/or flexion, with or without range of motion adjustment, includes all components and accessories

E1812 Dynamic knee, extension/flexion device with active resistance control

E1815 Dynamic adjustable ankle extension/flexion device, includes soft interface material

E1816 Static progressive stretch ankle device, flexion and/or extension, with or without range of motion adjustment, includes all components and accessories

E1818 Static progressive stretch forearm pronation/supination device, with or without range of motion adjustment, includes all components and accessories

E1820 Replacement soft interface material, dynamic adjustable extension/flexion device

E1821 Replacement soft interface material/cuffs for bi-directional static progressive stretch device

E1825 Dynamic adjustable finger extension/flexion device, includes soft interface material

E1830 Dynamic adjustable toe extension/flexion device, includes soft interface material

E1831 Static progressive stretch toe device, extension and/or flexion, with or without range of motion adjustment, includes all components and accessories

E1840 Dynamic adjustable shoulder flexion/abduction/rotation device, includes soft interface material

E1841 Static progressive stretch shoulder device, with or without range of motion adjustment, includes all components and accessories

These codes report the supply of specific rehabilitation devices for the upper or lower limb. These devices are designed to be strapped onto the affected joint. The device may be dynamic, which allows a constant, slow stretch of the joint, or static, which is operated by the patient for intermittent use. The devices may include range of motion adjustment. Adjustable pads and cuffs are positioned to maximize function. The codes include supply of the soft material that interfaces between the skin and the hard structure of the device.

E1902

E1902 Communication board, nonelectronic augmentative or alternative communication device

An augmentative or alternative communication board is an umbrella term that encompasses methods of communication for people with impairments or restrictions on the production or comprehension of the spoken or written language. Augmentative or alternative communication board devices are therapeutically used to establish, develop, or maintain the ability to communicate functional needs. Low technology, non-electronic augmentative communication devices include boards that use letters, words, phrases, and/or symbols (communication boards); mini boards; schedule boards; and conversation books.

E2000

E2000 Gastric suction pump, home model, portable or stationary, electric

A gastric suction pump is an aspiration device used to remove gastrointestinal fluids under continuous or intermittent suction through a tube. It is generally used for patients who are unable to empty gastric secretions normally. This is a home model, portable or stationary, that is lightweight, compact and has an electric aspirator. Use of the device does not require technical or professional supervision.

E2100-E2101

E2100 Blood glucose monitor with integrated voice synthesizer

E2101 Blood glucose monitor with integrated lancing/blood sample

Glucometers are used for patients with all types of diabetes mellitus to monitor blood glucose and are available in a variety of models with various features, including digital read-out, memory, result print-out, easy specimen capture, and many others. Glucometers with special features, such as voice-activated or voice-synthesized capabilities, are needed for patients with other concurrent conditions, such as patients with impaired vision. Whether or not the patient is on insulin, many diabetics require frequent, if not daily, blood glucose monitoring. For Type I diabetes mellitus patients who require insulin (the patient's body does not manufacture insulin and therefore it must come from an external source, such as injections), blood glucose monitoring is a life-sustaining requirement.

E2102-E2103

E2102 Adjunctive, nonimplanted continuous glucose monitor (CGM) or receiver

E2103 Nonadjunctive, nonimplanted continuous glucose monitor (CGM) or receiver

Continuous glucose monitoring (CGM) systems make continuous measurements of glucose levels. Many of these devices take measurements from subcutaneous tissue rather than from blood. Most systems consist of a sensor that is attached to the back of the arm or abdomen. The sensor has a very thin wire that is inserted subcutaneously. The wire measures the glucose level in interstitial fluid that exits between the cells. The sensor is attached to a transmitter that sends the glucose readings to a wireless receiver. The receiver is a small, computerized device that records and stores the glucose readings. CGMs are classified as adjunctive (do not replace standard blood glucose monitors for treatment decisions) or nonadjunctive (can replace standard blood glucose monitors for treatment decisions). Report E2102 for the receiver/monitor component for an adjunctive, nonimplanted CGM system and E2103 for the receiver/monitor component for a nonadjunctive, nonimplanted CGM system.

E2120

E2120 Pulse generator system for tympanic treatment of inner ear endolymphatic fluid

A portable, low-pressure pulse generator system for tympanic treatment of inner ear endolymphatic fluid, also known as Meniere's disease, is reported with this code. Prior to application of the pulse generator, the patient undergoes a tympanostomy with ventilation tube insertion. The patient must then wait approximately two weeks before treatment with the pressure pulse generator can begin. The device delivers repeated pressure pulses to the ear canal using an air pressure generator and a close-fitting cuff in the ear canal. The treatment is performed several times a day for short intervals (approximately five minutes per treatment session).

E2201-E2204

E2201 Manual wheelchair accessory, nonstandard seat frame, width greater than or equal to 20 in and less than 24 in

E2202 Manual wheelchair accessory, nonstandard seat frame width, 24-27 in

E2203 Manual wheelchair accessory, nonstandard seat frame depth, 20 to less than 22 in

E2204 Manual wheelchair accessory, nonstandard seat frame depth, 22 to 25 in

A nonstandard seat frame for a manual wheelchair identifies seat supports that are different sizes. Such seats are required if the patient's physical dimensions justify the need for a nonstandard size.

E2205

E2205 Manual wheelchair accessory, handrim without projections (includes ergonomic or contoured), any type, replacement only, each

Handrims, also known as pushrims, are metal devices that attach to the wheels of a manual wheelchair. The user grips the handrim and turns the wheel, which propels the wheelchair. There are many types of handrims, including chrome, aluminum anodized, composite, vinyl coated, foam covered, projection, oblique projection, and natural fit.

E2206

E2206 Manual wheelchair accessory, wheel lock assembly, complete, replacement only, each

A wheel lock is a safety device that stops a wheelchair from moving. There are several different types of wheel locks, including push to lock, pull to lock, and an automatic wheel lock system. The automatic wheel

E

lock system helps prevent falls for people who cannot or do not consistently lock the manual brakes on their wheelchairs.

E2207

E2207 Wheelchair accessory, crutch and cane holder, each

A crutch and cane holder for a wheelchair is a clip device that attaches to a wheelchair to hold a crutch or a cane. This allows users to keep a cane or crutch handy. Gripping surfaces of the holder are soft plastic rollers and do not damage canes or crutches.

E2208

E2208 Wheelchair accessory, cylinder tank carrier, each

A cylinder tank carrier is a devise that attaches to a wheelchair to hold an oxygen tank. It offers increased mobility and freedom for individuals who are required to use oxygen and a wheelchair.

E2209

E2209 Accessory, arm trough, with or without hand support, each

An arm trough for a manual wheelchair is an accessory designed to support the arm in patients with quadriplegia, hemiplegia, or spasticity of the arms. The arm trough replaces the standard armrest.

E2210

E2210 Wheelchair accessory, bearings, any type, replacement only, each

A wheelchair bearing is a device that allows constrained motion between two parts of the wheelchair. There are three types. Stem bearings are located where the front fork attaches to the wheelchair frame. Caster bearings are located in the caster wheels. Rear bearings are located in the rear wheels.

E2211-E2212

E2211 Manual wheelchair accessory, pneumatic propulsion tire, any size, each

E2212 Manual wheelchair accessory, tube for pneumatic propulsion tire, any size, each

A pneumatic tire is a ring-shaped covering that fits around a wheel rim to protect it and to provide a cushion. These are commonly made of rubber and require an inner tube that is filled with air. Pneumatic tires are on most manual and power wheelchairs because they are lighter, shock-absorbing, and offer good traction. A propulsion tire is a large wheel that can be used by a person to propel the wheelchair with his/her arms.

E2213

E2213 Manual wheelchair accessory, insert for pneumatic propulsion tire (removable), any type, any size, each

A pneumatic tire is a ring-shaped covering that fits around a wheel rim to protect it and to provide a cushion. A pneumonic tire may come with an airless insert that is soft rubber or a latex gel that replaces the inner tube. This removable ring of firm material placed inside of a pneumatic tire allows a wheelchair to continue to move if the pneumatic tire is punctured. This type of tire insert is sometimes referred to as a flat free insert or a zero pressure tube. The ride is cushioned but it is a little heavier than the basic pneumonic tire. A propulsion wheel is a large wheel that can be used by a person to propel the wheelchair with his/her arms.

E2214-E2215

E2214 Manual wheelchair accessory, pneumatic caster tire, any size, each

E2215 Manual wheelchair accessory, tube for pneumatic caster tire, any size, each

A pneumatic caster tire is a ring-shaped device made of flexible fabric, such as India rubber, that contains an inner tube filled with compressed air. Pneumatic caster tires on a wheelchair are shock absorbing wheels that absorb vibrations thus providing a smooth cushioned ride and quiet operation. A caster tire is a small wheel that is in contact with the ground during normal operation of the wheelchair and cannot be used for arm propulsion.

E2216-E2219

E2216 Manual wheelchair accessory, foam filled propulsion tire, any size, each

E2217 Manual wheelchair accessory, foam filled caster tire, any size, each

E2218 Manual wheelchair accessory, foam propulsion tire, any size, each

E2219 Manual wheelchair accessory, foam caster tire, any size, each

A propulsion tire is a large wheel that allows the person in the wheelchair to move the chair with his or her arms. A caster tire is a small wheel that is in contact with the ground during normal operation of the wheelchair and cannot be used for arm propulsion. A foam tire made entirely of polyurethane. A foam filled tire is a rubber tire injected with polyurethane. These codes are reported for each tire.

E2220

E2220 Manual wheelchair accessory, solid (rubber/plastic) propulsion tire, any size, replacement only, each

A propulsion tire is a large wheel that allows the person in the wheelchair to move the chair with his or her arms. This code represents a propulsion tire made of hard plastic or rubber.

E2221

E2221 Manual wheelchair accessory, solid (rubber/plastic) caster tire (removable), any size, replacement only, each

A caster tire is a small wheel that is in contact with the ground during normal operation of the wheelchair and cannot be used for arm propulsion. This code is for a caster tire made of hard plastic or rubber.

E2222

E2222 Manual wheelchair accessory, solid (rubber/plastic) caster tire with integrated wheel, any size, replacement only, each

A caster tire is a smaller wheel that is in contact with the ground during normal operation of the wheelchair and cannot be used for arm propulsion. The integrated caster has the tire attached to the wheel as one unit. Report this code for an integrated caster tire made of hard plastic or rubber.

E2224

E2224 Manual wheelchair accessory, propulsion wheel excludes tire, any size, replacement only, each

A propulsion wheel is a large wheel that can be used by a person in a wheelchair to propel the chair with his or her arms. This code is for a propulsion wheel, excluding the tire.

E2225

E2225 Manual wheelchair accessory, caster wheel excludes tire, any size, replacement only, each

A caster wheel is a single, double, or compound wheel that is designed to be mounted to the bottom of a larger object to enable the object to be easily moved. Report this code for any size replacement caster wheel, tire not included.

E2226

E2226 Manual wheelchair accessory, caster fork, any size, replacement only, each

Wheelchair caster wheels are mounted using a caster fork assembly. A caster fork assembly consists of the fork, the caster stem bolt (the long bolt coming up from the top of the fork), caster stem bearings, and sometimes a spacer or spacers. This code is for any size replacement caster fork.

E2227

E2227 Manual wheelchair accessory, gear reduction drive wheel, each

A gear reduction drive wheel is a mechanical device that propels a manual wheelchair. The gear reduction device allows the user to slow down or speed up the motion. It provides a user with additional assistance by providing "leverage" through gearing (like a bicycle).

E2228

E2228 Manual wheelchair accessory, wheel braking system and lock, complete, each

Wheelchair locks prohibit motion of the wheels, keeping the wheelchair in "park" while the user transfers in or out of the chair. Wheelchair brakes help to slow or stop a wheelchair when descending or turning. There are different types of wheelchair brakes/locks, including manual, auto-lock, and disc brake systems. The push/pull style of lock is standard. The basic wheel lock is commonly known as a wheelchair brake.

E2230

E2230 Manual wheelchair accessory, manual standing system

A wheelchair standing system, also known as a standing chair or frame, is a mechanical device that allows the chair and the user to be moved into an upright standing position. A person can stand anywhere anytime.

E2231

E2231 Manual wheelchair accessory, solid seat support base (replaces sling seat), includes any type mounting hardware

Sling support seats are pieces of leather, plastic, or other material that are suspended loosely between two supports. The user sits in the sling, which conforms to his or her body. A solid seat support base provides a sturdy stiff pillow base that can improve posture and increase comfort.

E2291-E2292

E2291 Back, planar, for pediatric size wheelchair including fixed attaching hardware

E2292 Seat, planar, for pediatric size wheelchair including fixed attaching hardware

Planar systems are flat positioning components that allow a person to move. The planar system is composed of foam interfaced with a wood or plastic base. The simplest form of seating system is a linear seating system. A linear seating system refers to a planar seat and back with fixed angles and orientations. This solid base of support enhances posture and provides comfort for longer periods of sitting.

E2293-E2294

E2293 Back, contoured, for pediatric size wheelchair including fixed attaching hardware

E2294 Seat, contoured, for pediatric size wheelchair including fixed attaching hardware

A contoured cushion is shaped to the user's body helping bring the body back to the same place every time. The cushion helps support the correct positioning of the user's body.

E2295

E2295 Manual wheelchair accessory, for pediatric size wheelchair, dynamic seating frame, allows coordinated movement of multiple positioning features

A dynamic seating frame is a device that allows the wheelchair user's own body to initiate and control the level of seating movements. Benefits of such a system include relaxed overall muscle tone, increased muscle control, and the end or lessening of back/buttock pain and discomfort. This seat, which pivots, is connected to the wheelchair's frame and is attached to resilient supports. By various supports and attachments, a spring biases attaches to other components that enables the force of the spring to vary to alter resiliency of the support.

E2300

E2300 Wheelchair accessory, power seat elevation system, any type

A power seat elevation system allows the seat to be raised and lowered. The system should be able to raise the seat a minimum of 6 inches from its lowest point. A power seat elevation system consists of a motor and related electronics, with or without variable speed programmability; a switch control that is independent of the power wheelchair drive control interface; and hardware needed to attach the seating system to the wheelchair base.

E2301

E2301 Wheelchair accessory, power standing system, any type

A power standing system wheelchair accessory assists the patient in moving from a sitting to standing position. Power standing systems must have the ability to support a patient weight of at least 250 pounds. A power standing system consists of a solid seat platform and solid back; detachable or flip-up fixed height armrests; hinged legrests; anterior knee supports; fixed or flip-up foot plates; a motor and related electronics, with or without variable speed programmability; a basic switch control that is independent of the power wheelchair drive control interface; and any hardware that is needed to attach the seating system to the wheelchair base. A headrest is not included and should be reported additionally if supplied.

E2310-E2311

E2310 Power wheelchair accessory, electronic connection between wheelchair controller and one power seating system motor, including all related electronics, indicator feature, mechanical function selection switch, and fixed mounting hardware

E2311 Power wheelchair accessory, electronic connection between wheelchair controller and 2 or more power seating system motors, including all related electronics, indicator feature, mechanical function selection switch, and fixed mounting hardware

These codes describe electronic components that allow the patient to control two or more motors from a single interface using a proportional joystick, touchpad, or nonproportional interface. The motors that can be controlled from the electronic connection include power wheelchair drive, power tilt, power recline, power shear reduction, power leg elevation, power seat elevation, and power standing system. This type of wheelchair accessory includes a function selection switch that allows the patient to select the motor being controlled and an indicator feature to visually show which function has been selected. The indicator feature may also show the direction that has been selected (forward, reverse, left, right). The indicator feature may be in a separate display box or may be integrated into the wheelchair interface.

E2312

E2312 Power wheelchair accessory, hand or chin control interface, mini-proportional remote joystick, proportional, including fixed mounting hardware

A proportional interface is one in which the direction and amount of movement by the patient controls the direction and speed of the wheelchair. Mini proportional joysticks are small joysticks that require significantly less force and travel distance than a standard joystick. Joystick placement is typically by the hand, in line with an arm pad and parallel with the floor. When controlled by the chin, the gimbal is mounted on a swing-away mount of some sort and positioned slightly below and forward of the chin. Chin controls work much the same as conventional joysticks in that the user simply pushes the gimbal the direction he or she wants to go and controls speed by the distance the gimbal is pushed.

E2313

E2313 Power wheelchair accessory, harness for upgrade to expandable controller, including all fasteners, connectors and mounting hardware, each

A controller describes the microprocessor and related electronics that receive and interpret input from the drive control interface and converts that input into power output that controls speed and direction. The separate controller connects directly to the motors and batteries through a high power wire harness. An expandable controller is capable of accommodating one or more of the following additional functions: other types of proportional input devices, non-proportional input devices, and operation of three or more powered seating actuators through the drive control. It may also operate a separate display (i.e., for alternate control devices), some other electronic devices, and an attendant control. This code reports the harness, including wires, fuses, fuse boxes, circuits, switches, and similar items required for the operation of the expandable controller.

E2321-E2322

E2321 Power wheelchair accessory, hand control interface, remote joystick, nonproportional, including all related electronics, mechanical stop switch, and fixed mounting hardware

E2322 Power wheelchair accessory, hand control interface, multiple mechanical switches, nonproportional, including all related electronics, mechanical stop switch, and fixed mounting hardware

An interface is the mechanism for controlling the movement of the power wheelchair of which there are a number of different types. These codes describe a nonproportional hand control interface that uses a remote joystick (E2321) or multiple mechanical switches (E2322). A remote joystick is one that is separate from the box containing the electronics that connects the interface to the motor and gears (controller box). A mechanical switch system describes a system with three to five mechanical switches that require physical contact to be activated. The switch selected determines the direction of the wheelchair. A mechanical direction change switch, if provided, is included in E2322. A nonproportional interface is a type of interface that allows the patient to control the direction of the wheelchair, but the speed is pre-programmed and cannot be affected by the user. The two nonproportional interface mechanisms described by E2321 and E2322 include all related electronics, mechanical stop switch, and the fixed mounting hardware.

E2323

E2323 Power wheelchair accessory, specialty joystick handle for hand control interface, prefabricated

A prefabricated specialty joystick handle has a shape other than a straight stick. U-shaped and T-shaped handles are reported with this code. Joysticks that have some other nonstandard feature such as a flexible shaft are also reported with E2323.

E2324

E2324 Power wheelchair accessory, chin cup for chin control interface

Wheelchair users who do not have the ability to control a joystick using hand or upper extremity motion can have the joystick modified with a chin cup that allows movement of the wheelchair to be controlled with the chin. The chin cup is attached to the joystick and reported additionally with E2324.

E2325-E2326

E2325 Power wheelchair accessory, sip and puff interface, nonproportional, including all related electronics, mechanical stop switch, and manual swingaway mounting hardware

E2326 Power wheelchair accessory, breath tube kit for sip and puff interface

A sip and puff interface is a nonproportional interface in which the patient holds a tube in the mouth and controls the wheelchair by sucking in (sip) or blowing out (puff). A nonproportional interface is a type of interface that allows the patient to control the direction of the wheelchair, but the speed is pre-programmed and cannot be affected by the user. Code E2325 reports the nonproportional sip and puff interface, all related electronics, a mechanical stop switch, and manual swing-away mounting hardware. The breath tube kit for the sip and puff interface is reported additionally with E2326.

E2327-E2328

E2327 Power wheelchair accessory, head control interface, mechanical, proportional, including all related electronics, mechanical direction change switch, and fixed mounting hardware

E2328 Power wheelchair accessory, head control or extremity control interface, electronic, proportional, including all related electronics and fixed mounting hardware

An interface is the mechanism for controlling the movement of the power wheelchair of which there are a number of different types. Code E2327 describes a mechanical, proportional, head control interface, and E2328 describes an electronic, proportional, head or extremity control interface. A proportional interface is directly controlled by the patient such that both direction and speed is controlled by the patient. A mechanical, proportional, head control interface (E2327) is one in which a headrest is attached to a joystick-like device. The direction and amount of movement of the patient's head pressing on the headrest controls the direction and speed of the wheelchair. An electronic, proportional, head control interface (E2328) is one in which a patient's head movements are sensed by a box placed behind the patient's head, and the direction and speed of the wheelchair are controlled by the sensors. The box does not come into direct contact with the patient's head.

E

An electronic, proportional, extremity control interface, also reported with E2328, is one in which the direction and amount of movement of the patient's arm or leg control the direction and speed of the wheelchair. Interface mechanisms include all related electronics and the fixed mounting hardware. A mechanical direction control switch is included in E2327.

E2329-E2330

E2329 Power wheelchair accessory, head control interface, contact switch mechanism, nonproportional, including all related electronics, mechanical stop switch, mechanical direction change switch, head array, and fixed mounting hardware

E2330 Power wheelchair accessory, head control interface, proximity switch mechanism, nonproportional, including all related electronics, mechanical stop switch, mechanical direction change switch, head array, and fixed mounting hardware

An interface is the mechanism for controlling the movement of the power wheelchair of which there are a number of different types. Code E2329 describes a nonproportional, contact switch, head control interface, and E2330 describes a nonproportional, proximity switch, head control interface. A nonproportional interface is a type of interface that allows the patient to control the direction of the wheelchair, but the speed is preprogrammed and cannot be affected by the user. A nonproportional, contact switch, head control interface (E2329) is one in which the patient activates one of three mechanical switches placed around the back and sides of the head. These switches are activated by pressure of the head against the switch. The switch that is selected determines the direction of the wheelchair. A nonproportional, proximity switch, head control interface (E2330) is one in which the patient activates one of three switches placed around the back and sides of the head. These switches are activated by movement of the head toward the switch, though the head does not touch the switch. The switch that is selected determines the direction of the wheelchair. Both interface mechanisms include all related electronics, mechanical stop switch, mechanical direction change switch, head array, and the fixed mounting hardware.

E2331

E2331 Power wheelchair accessory, attendant control, proportional, including all related electronics and fixed mounting hardware

An attendant control for a power wheelchair allows a caregiver to drive the wheelchair instead of the patient. The attendant control is usually mounted on one of the rear canes of the wheelchair. Attendant control devices are proportional controls, allowing the attendant to control both the direction and the speed of the wheelchair, usually by means of a joystick. All related electronics and fixed mounting hardware are included.

E2340-E2343

E2340 Power wheelchair accessory, nonstandard seat frame width, 20-23 in

E2341 Power wheelchair accessory, nonstandard seat frame width, 24-27 in

E2342 Power wheelchair accessory, nonstandard seat frame depth, 20 or 21 in

E2343 Power wheelchair accessory, nonstandard seat frame depth, 22-25 in

A specially sized or constructed wheelchair component is indicated for patients when the measurements of a standard wheelchair do not accommodate the patient's needs. This wheelchair must be justified by reasons such as a patient's physical size or the specific requirements for wheelchair usage in the patient's place of residence, such as narrow doorways that prevent the passage of a standard wheelchair. The standard seat height from the floor is 18 to 20 inches. The standard seat width and depth is 15 to 19 inches. When a deviation is more than 2 inches from the standard, the sizing is nonstandard.

E2351

E2351 Power wheelchair accessory, electronic interface to operate speech generating device using power wheelchair control interface

An electronic interface is a device that allows the power wheelchair controls to operate a speech generating device. Speech generating devices are electronic systems that enable individuals with severe speech impairment to verbally communicate their needs. There are multiple methods of accessing messages on devices, which can be done directly, indirectly, and with specialized access devices. The method depends on the skills and abilities of the communicator.

E

E2358-E2365

E2358 Power wheelchair accessory, group 34 nonsealed lead acid battery, each

E2359 Power wheelchair accessory, group 34 sealed lead acid battery, each (e.g., gel cell, absorbed glass mat)

E2360 Power wheelchair accessory, 22 NF nonsealed lead acid battery, each

E2361 Power wheelchair accessory, 22 NF sealed lead acid battery, each (e.g., gel cell, absorbed glassmat)

E2362 Power wheelchair accessory, group 24 nonsealed lead acid battery, each

E2363 Power wheelchair accessory, group 24 sealed lead acid battery, each (e.g., gel cell, absorbed glassmat)

E2364 Power wheelchair accessory, U-1 nonsealed lead acid battery, each

E2365 Power wheelchair accessory, U-1 sealed lead acid battery, each (e.g., gel cell, absorbed glassmat)

Lead-acid batteries are physically large batteries that contain lead plates in a solution of acid to create electricity. During normal operation, water is lost from a non-sealed (or flooded) battery due to evaporation. They are also known as flooded, vented, or wet-cell batteries. Since they are not sealed, water must be frequently added. If inverted, the contents can spill out. These used to be the most common type of battery, but now they are seen as old fashioned and are becoming less common. Sealed batteries are known as maintenance free batteries. Sealed lead acid (SLA) batteries are valve-regulated, which fixes the acid electrolyte in a gel or in an absorptive fiberglass mat. The advantages of this design are that the battery needs no added water, can be operated in any position, and can be used in close proximity to people and sensitive equipment. Gelled batteries contain acid that has been "gelled" by the addition of Silica Gel, turning the acid into a solid mass that looks like gooey Jell-O. The advantage of these batteries is that it is impossible to spill acid even if they are broken. Absorbed glass mat is a very fine fiber Boron-Silicate glass mat. These type of batteries have all the advantages of gelled, but can take much more abuse.

E2366-E2367

E2366 Power wheelchair accessory, battery charger, single mode, for use with only one battery type, sealed or nonsealed, each

E2367 Power wheelchair accessory, battery charger, dual mode, for use with either battery type, sealed or nonsealed, each

A battery charger is a device that replenishes battery energy by forcing an electric current through it. There are three different main types of batteries: wet battery, gel battery, and the absorbed glass mat battery. A different battery charger is required for each model.

E2368

E2368 Power wheelchair component, drive wheel motor, replacement only

A motor is a machine that converts energy into useful mechanical motion. In a power wheelchair, motors provide the energy needed to propel the chair. Normally a motor is included in the purchase of a motored wheelchair.

E2369

E2369 Power wheelchair component, drive wheel gear box, replacement only

A gearbox is a protective casing for a system consisting of a collection of mechanical components that deliver maximum power from a motor by managing a series of gear ratios that in turn operate a transmission. These components include a gear selector, fork, collar, dog teeth, and a gear set.

E2370

E2370 Power wheelchair component, integrated drive wheel motor and gear box combination, replacement only

A motor is a machine that converts energy into useful mechanical motion. In a power wheelchair, motors provide the energy needed to propel the chair. A gearbox is a protective casing for a system consisting of a collection of mechanical components that deliver maximum power from a motor by managing a series of gear ratios that in turn operate a transmission. These components include a gear selector, fork, collar, dog teeth, and a gear set. Normally a motor and gearbox are included in the purchase of a motored wheelchair.

E2371-E2372

E2371 Power wheelchair accessory, group 27 sealed lead acid battery, (e.g., gel cell, absorbed glassmat), each

E2372 Power wheelchair accessory, group 27 nonsealed lead acid battery, each

Lead-acid batteries are physically large batteries that contain lead plates in a solution of acid to create electricity. During normal operation, water is lost from a non-sealed (or flooded) battery due to evaporation. They are also known as flooded, vented, or wet-cell batteries. Since they are not sealed, water must be frequently added. If inverted, the contents can spill out. These used to be the most common type of battery, but now they are seen as old fashioned and are becoming less common. Sealed batteries are known as maintenance free batteries. Sealed lead acid (SLA) batteries are valve-regulated, which fixes the acid electrolyte in a gel or in an absorptive fiberglass mat. The advantages of this design are that the battery needs no added water, can be operated in any position, and can be used in close proximity to people and sensitive equipment. Gelled batteries contain acid that has been "gelled" by the addition of Silica Gel, turning the acid into a solid mass that looks like gooey

Jell-O. The advantage of these batteries is that it is impossible to spill acid even if they are broken. Absorbed glass mat is a very fine fiber Boron-Silicate glass mat. These type of batteries have all the advantages of gelled, but can take much more abuse.

E2373-E2374

E2373 Power wheelchair accessory, hand or chin control interface, compact remote joystick, proportional, including fixed mounting hardware

E2374 Power wheelchair accessory, hand or chin control interface, standard remote joystick (not including controller), proportional, including all related electronics and fixed mounting hardware, replacement only

An interface is the mechanism for controlling the movement of the power wheelchair of which there are a number of different types. This code describes a proportional hand or chin control interface that uses a remote joystick or touchpad. A proportional interface is directly controlled by the patient such that both direction and speed is controlled by the patient moving the joystick or using the touchpad. A remote joystick is separate from the box containing the electronics that connects the interface to the motor and gears (controller box), and encompasses a standard joystick or one that can be controlled by small movements. The latter type may be mini-proportional, compact, or short throw joystick. The second type of interface described by this code is a touchpad similar to the pad-type mouse found on laptop computers. Interface mechanisms include all related electronics and the fixed mounting hardware. The chin cup is reported separately with E2324.

E2375-E2378

E2375 Power wheelchair accessory, nonexpandable controller, including all related electronics and mounting hardware, replacement only

E2376 Power wheelchair accessory, expandable controller, including all related electronics and mounting hardware, replacement only

E2377 Power wheelchair accessory, expandable controller, including all related electronics and mounting hardware, upgrade provided at initial issue

E2378 Power wheelchair component, actuator, replacement only

A controller describes the microprocessor and related electronics that receive and interpret input from the joystick (or some other drive control interface) and converts that input into power output that controls speed and direction. The separate controller connects directly to the motors and batteries through a high-power wire harness. A nonexpandable controller may have the ability to control up to two power seating actuators through the drive control and may allow for the incorporation of an attendant control. It is also capable of accommodating one or more other types of proportional input devices, nonproportional input devices, and operating three or more powered seating actuators through the drive control. A nonexpandable controller may also operate a separate display (i.e., for alternate control devices), some other electronic devices, and an attendant control.

E2381-E2382

E2381 Power wheelchair accessory, pneumatic drive wheel tire, any size, replacement only, each

E2382 Power wheelchair accessory, tube for pneumatic drive wheel tire, any size, replacement only, each

Drive wheels come in three positions on a power wheelchair: rear-wheel drive, mid-wheel drive, and front-wheel drive. A pneumatic tire is a rubber tire used in conjunction with a separate tube that is filled with air.

E2383

E2383 Power wheelchair accessory, insert for pneumatic drive wheel tire (removable), any type, any size, replacement only, each

A pneumonic tire comes with an airless insert that is soft rubber or a latex gel that replaces the inner tube. This is also known as a flat free insert. This removable ring of firm material placed inside of a pneumatic tire allows a wheelchair to continue to move if the pneumatic tire is punctured. This type of tire insert is sometimes referred to as a flat free insert or a zero pressure tube.

E2384

E2384 Power wheelchair accessory, pneumatic caster tire, any size, replacement only, each

A pneumatic caster tire is made of an annular tube of flexible fabric, such as India rubber, and filled with compressed air. A pneumatic caster tire is a shock absorbing wheel that absorbs vibrations thus providing a smooth cushioned ride and quiet operation. A caster is a smaller wheel that is in contact with the ground during normal operation of the wheelchair and that is not directly controlled by the motor. It may be in the front and/or rear, depending on the location of the drive wheel.

E2385

E2385 Power wheelchair accessory, tube for pneumatic caster tire, any size, replacement only, each

A caster is a smaller wheel that is in contact with the ground during normal operation of the wheelchair and is not directly controlled by the motor. It may be in the front and/or rear, depending on the location of the drive wheel. A pneumatic caster tire is formed of an annular tube of flexible fabric, such as India rubber, suitable to be inflated with air. A tube for a pneumatic tire is an inflatable rubber tube that fits inside the casing of a pneumatic tire. This inner tube keeps the tire airtight.

E2386

E2386 Power wheelchair accessory, foam filled drive wheel tire, any size, replacement only, each

Drive wheels come in three positions: rear-wheel drive, mid-wheel drive, and front-wheel drive on a power wheelchair. A foam filled drive wheel tire is a rubber tire shell that has been filled with foam that is nonremovable.

E2387

E2387 Power wheelchair accessory, foam filled caster tire, any size, replacement only, each

A caster tire is a smaller wheel that is in contact with the ground during normal operation of the wheelchair and is not directly controlled by the motor. It may be in the front and/or rear, depending on the location of the drive wheel. A foam filled caster tire is a rubber tire shell filled with foam that is nonremovable.

E2388

E2388 Power wheelchair accessory, foam drive wheel tire, any size, replacement only, each

Drive wheels come in three positions: rear-wheel drive, mid-wheel drive, and front-wheel drive on a power wheelchair. A foam tire is made entirely of self-skinning urethane.

E2389

E2389 Power wheelchair accessory, foam caster tire, any size, replacement only, each

A caster tire is a smaller wheel that is in contact with the ground during normal operation of the wheelchair and is not directly controlled by the motor. It may be in the front and/or rear, depending on the location of the drive wheel. A foam tire is made entirely of self-skinning urethane.

E2390

E2390 Power wheelchair accessory, solid (rubber/plastic) drive wheel tire, any size, replacement only, each

Drive wheels come in three positions: rear-wheel drive, mid-wheel drive, and front-wheel drive on a power wheelchair. This solid tire is made of hard plastic or rubber.

E2391

E2391 Power wheelchair accessory, solid (rubber/plastic) caster tire (removable), any size, replacement only, each

A caster is a smaller wheel that is in contact with the ground during normal operation of the wheelchair and is not directly controlled by the motor. It may be in the front and/or rear, depending on the location of the drive wheel. This solid caster tire is made of hard plastic or rubber. This code is for replacement of a solid (rubber/plastic) caster tire.

E2392

E2392 Power wheelchair accessory, solid (rubber/plastic) caster tire with integrated wheel, any size, replacement only, each

A caster is a smaller wheel that is in contact with the ground during normal operation of the wheelchair and is not directly controlled by the motor. It may be in the front and/or rear, depending on the location of the drive wheel. This solid caster tire is made of hard plastic or rubber. The integrated caster has the tire attached to the wheel as one unit. This code is for replacement of a solid (rubber/plastic) caster tire with an integrated wheel.

E2394

E2394 Power wheelchair accessory, drive wheel excludes tire, any size, replacement only, each

Drive wheel refers to the position of the wheels to which the motors are attached. In rear wheel drives wheelchairs, the drive wheels are located at the very back of the chair. In mid wheel drive wheelchairs, the drive wheels are located under the chair toward the center with smaller wheels (casters) in the front and behind. In front wheel drive wheelchairs, the drive wheels are located at the front of the chair with casters behind.

E2395

E2395 Power wheelchair accessory, caster wheel excludes tire, any size, replacement only, each

A caster wheel is a small wheel that is in contact with the ground during normal operation of the wheelchair and cannot be used for arm propulsion.

E2396

E2396 Power wheelchair accessory, caster fork, any size, replacement only, each

Wheelchair caster wheels are mounted to a caster fork assembly. A caster fork assembly consists of the fork, the caster stem bolt (the long bolt coming up from the top of the fork), caster stem bearings, and sometimes a spacer or spacers.

E2397

E2397 Power wheelchair accessory, lithium-based battery, each

Lithium-ion is a low maintenance battery made from chemicals. Lithium-ion batteries have no memory effect and do not use poisonous metals, such as lead, mercury, or cadmium. They require little to no maintenance, and can pack a lot of voltage into a small area. However, they are particularly fragile in nature and need to be protected from extreme temperatures.

E2398

E2398 Wheelchair accessory, dynamic positioning hardware for back

Accessories consisting of dynamic components, joints, linkages, and elastomers are designed to be attached to a wheelchair frame. The system is intended to accommodate the wheelchair user's flexion and extension with minimal displacement at the pelvis during movement. The variable spring resistance returns the individual to the initial posture.

E2402

E2402 Negative pressure wound therapy electrical pump, stationary or portable

Negative pressure wound therapy (NPWT) is controlled application of subatmospheric pressure to wounds. A pump continuously or intermittently carries subatmospheric pressure through connected tubes directly to a specialized wound dressing. A canister collects the drainage from the wound. NPWT promotes healing of chronic wounds and decubitus ulcers. Controlled pressure of the wound increases vascularity and oxygenation of the wound bed thus reducing edema by getting rid of the wound fluid and removing exudate and bacteria.

E2500-E2510

E2500 Speech generating device, digitized speech, using prerecorded messages, less than or equal to eight minutes recording time

E2502 Speech generating device, digitized speech, using prerecorded messages, greater than eight minutes but less than or equal to 20 minutes recording time

E2504 Speech generating device, digitized speech, using prerecorded messages, greater than 20 minutes but less than or equal to 40 minutes recording time

E2506 Speech generating device, digitized speech, using prerecorded messages, greater than 40 minutes recording time

E2508 Speech generating device, synthesized speech, requiring message formulation by spelling and access by physical contact with the device

E2510 Speech generating device, synthesized speech, permitting multiple methods of message formulation and multiple methods of device access

Speech generating devices, also called communication devices, enable an individual to communicate with others more effectively. There are many devices that assist individuals by using speech or voice output and other combinations of assistance. Speech generating devices have been created for individuals who cannot speak, are difficult to understand, or have language retrieval issues. Digitized speech devices are referred to as devices with "whole message" speech output. Digitized speech devices utilize words and phrases that have been pre-recorded by someone other than the user and used for playback by the user. Synthesized speech devices translate a user's input into device-generated speech. Users of synthesized speech devices are not limited to prerecorded messages but can independently create messages as their own communication needs arise. These devices require the user to use a keyboard, touch screen, or other display containing an alphanumeric display. Synthesized speech devices allow the user different methods of message formulation and many methods of access. These methods of message formulation must include the capability for message selection by two or more of the following methods: letters, words, pictures, or symbols. Multiple methods of access must include the capability to access the device by two or more of the following methods: entering information by a keyboard, touch screen, or indirect selection techniques via a specialized access device such as a joystick, a head-mouse, an optical head-pointer, a switch, a light pointer, an infrared pointer, a scanning device, or Morse code.

E2511

E2511 Speech generating software program, for personal computer or personal digital assistant

Speech generating software allows laptops and/or desktop computers or personal digital assistant (PDA) devices to function as a speech generating device. The information can be entered with a pen based system using a stylus and handwriting recognition software, keyboard, downloaded from a computer using special cables, and software.

E2512

E2512 Accessory for speech generating device, mounting system

A mounting system for a speech generating device is a mechanism for fastening the speech generating device to the wheelchair. Generally mounting systems consist of three parts: a mounting block, which attaches to the wheelchair frame; a tubing system, which provides the majority of positioning; and a mounting plate, which attaches to the device.

E2599

E2599 Accessory for speech generating device, not otherwise classified

Report this code for any accessory for a speech generating device that is not described in other HCPCS Level II codes.

E2601-E2602

E2601 General use wheelchair seat cushion, width less than 22 in, any depth

E2602 General use wheelchair seat cushion, width 22 in or greater, any depth

A general use wheelchair seat cushion is a static, prefabricated cushion. Several cushion types exist: planar, contoured, and molded. A planar surface offers the least support and pressure relief, but may require the least experience and is simplest to maintain. A contoured surface assumes contour with pressure through the use of foam, air, or gel within the cushion, or it may be preformed. It provides more support than the planar surface, and is more adjustable than the molded surface. A molded seat is created from liquid foam that follows the direct contours of the specific user. It offers the most support for an individual with reduced trunk control and may be formed to accommodate fixed deformities. Wheelchair seat cushions can provide leg positioning, pelvic stability, and pressure management for patients with postural asymmetry. A cushion may provide high-end protection for individuals considered prone to developing skin breakdown. The size of a standard adult wheelchair seat has a seat width of 18 inches, seat depth of 16 inches, and seat height of 20 inches.

E2603-E2604

E2603 Skin protection wheelchair seat cushion, width less than 22 in, any depth

E2604 Skin protection wheelchair seat cushion, width 22 in or greater, any depth

A skin protection wheelchair seat cushion is a static, prefabricated cushion. A skin protection seat cushion usually uses high-grade polyurethane foam and a gel solution or puffed layer to provide high-end protection for individuals considered prone to developing skin breakdown. A skin protection seat cushion is beneficial if a person has a past history of or current pressure ulcer on the area of contact with the seating surface, absent or impaired sensation in the area of contact with the seating surface, or significant postural asymmetries.

E2605-E2606

E2605 Positioning wheelchair seat cushion, width less than 22 in, any depth

E2606 Positioning wheelchair seat cushion, width 22 in or greater, any depth

A positioning seat cushion is a static, prefabricated cushion. Positioning seat cushions provide leg, hip, and pelvic positioning and stability, and pressure management for patients with postural asymmetry. A positioning seat cushion is beneficial to a person who has significant postural asymmetries, providing seat stabilization, positioning, pressure reduction, and correct seating posture.

E2607-E2608

E2607 Skin protection and positioning wheelchair seat cushion, width less than 22 in, any depth

E2608 Skin protection and positioning wheelchair seat cushion, width 22 in or greater, any depth

A skin protection positioning wheelchair seat cushion is a static, prefabricated cushion. A skin protection seat cushion usually uses high-grade polyurethane foam and a gel solution or puffed layer to provide high-end protection for individuals considered prone to developing skin breakdown while affording the positioning and stability necessary for the leg, hip, and pelvis. A skin protection positioning seat cushion is beneficial if a person has a past history of or current pressure ulcer on the area of contact with the seating surface, absent or impaired sensation in the area of contact with the seating surface, or significant postural asymmetries.

E2609

E2609 Custom fabricated wheelchair seat cushion, any size

Custom made seats for a wheelchair (e.g., custom fabricated from an impression or digital image of a specific body part) are indicated when the user has gross spinal deformities and/or severely impaired sitting ability.

E2610

E2610 Wheelchair seat cushion, powered

A powered wheelchair seat cushion is a prefabricated, battery-powered cushion in which an air pump provides sequential inflation and deflation of the air cells or a low interface pressure throughout the cushion. An alternating pressure cushion is one type of powered seat cushion.

E2611-E2612

E2611 General use wheelchair back cushion, width less than 22 in, any height, including any type mounting hardware

E2612 General use wheelchair back cushion, width 22 in or greater, any height, including any type mounting hardware

A general use wheelchair back is a static, prefabricated cushion that functions as a comfortable, supportive positioning device and provides pressure relief to the wheelchair user.

E2613-E2614

E2613 Positioning wheelchair back cushion, posterior, width less than 22 in, any height, including any type mounting hardware

E2614 Positioning wheelchair back cushion, posterior, width 22 in or greater, any height, including any type mounting hardware

A posterior positioning wheelchair back cushion aids in back support and is designed to provide posterior lateral pelvic stabilization, along with better trunk stability.

E2615-E2616

E2615 Positioning wheelchair back cushion, posterior-lateral, width less than 22 in, any height, including any type mounting hardware

E2616 Positioning wheelchair back cushion, posterior-lateral, width 22 in or greater, any height, including any type mounting hardware

A posterior-lateral positioning wheelchair back cushion aids in back support and is designed to provide posterior lateral pelvic stabilization, along with better trunk stability.

E2617

E2617 Custom fabricated wheelchair back cushion, any size, including any type mounting hardware

Custom-fabricated wheelchair back cushions provide positioning and/or pressure relief that cannot be met with a prefabricated cushion. They are fabricated using molded-to-patient-model techniques to create a configured cushion.

E2619

E2619 Replacement cover for wheelchair seat cushion or back cushion, each

A universal wheelchair cushion cover is made of durable material that is soft to the touch and is fluid-proof with a non-skid base material. A heavy duty cushion cover is made to protect the cushion from rough wear and tear and incontinence with fluid-resisting material and durable construction.

E2620-E2621

E2620 Positioning wheelchair back cushion, planar back with lateral supports, width less than 22 in, any height, including any type mounting hardware

E2621 Positioning wheelchair back cushion, planar back with lateral supports, width 22 in or greater, any height, including any type mounting hardware

A planar back with lateral supports on a positioning wheelchair refers to a modification in the back support to allow various lateral supports to be mounted.

E2622-E2623

E2622 Skin protection wheelchair seat cushion, adjustable, width less than 22 in, any depth

E2623 Skin protection wheelchair seat cushion, adjustable, width 22 in or greater, any depth

Adjustable wheelchair seat cushions provide skin protection and comfort for individuals who must sit for long periods of time. Adjustable cushions are those that can be adapted to conform to the specific requirements of the individual. Cushions can be constructed of a variety of materials including rubber, foam, gel-foam, and polyester fiber-filled cores with adjustable air pads that allow the user to control the cushion fit. Some cushions have dual air controls that allow the side and center to be inflated to differing levels.

E2624-E2625

E2624 Skin protection and positioning wheelchair seat cushion, adjustable, width less than 22 in, any depth

E2625 Skin protection and positioning wheelchair seat cushion, adjustable, width 22 in or greater, any depth

Adjustable positioning wheelchair seat cushions provide skin protection and positioning for individuals with paralysis, deformities, scoliosis, poor muscle control, or other conditions. Positioning seat cushions can aid in manipulation or control of objects, can assist in the performance of specific activities, and can provide added balance and support. Adjustable cushions are those that can be adapted to conform to the specific requirements of the individual. Cushions can be constructed of a variety of materials including rubber, foam, gel-foam, and polyester fiber-filled cores with adjustable air pads that allow the user to control the cushion fit. Some cushions have dual air controls that allow the sides and center to be inflated to differing levels.

E2626-E2632

E2626 Wheelchair accessory, shoulder elbow, mobile arm support attached to wheelchair, balanced, adjustable

E2627 Wheelchair accessory, shoulder elbow, mobile arm support attached to wheelchair, balanced, adjustable Rancho type

E2628 Wheelchair accessory, shoulder elbow, mobile arm support attached to wheelchair, balanced, reclining

E2629 Wheelchair accessory, shoulder elbow, mobile arm support attached to wheelchair, balanced, friction arm support (friction dampening to proximal and distal joints)

E2630 Wheelchair accessory, shoulder elbow, mobile arm support, monosuspension arm and hand support, overhead elbow forearm hand sling support, yoke type suspension support

E2631 Wheelchair accessory, addition to mobile arm support, elevating proximal arm

E2632 Wheelchair accessory, addition to mobile arm support, offset or lateral rocker arm with elastic balance control

A shoulder-elbow-wrist-hand orthosis (SEWHO) is used for the purpose of supporting injured, post-surgical, and/or weak or deformed areas of the shoulder, elbow, wrist, or hand. These codes may be similar in design, depending on the manufacturer and the intended application. These bracing devices are attached to wheelchairs, typically containing hardware such as aluminum or other lightweight arm supports for the desired degree of abduction, as well as plastic, polyethylene, or foam. These devices may use the patient torso or neck as an anchor, as well as the phalanges. There may be hinges at certain points in the device to allow for a certain degree of elbow or wrist motion. The treating provider must initially apply these items, but a person other than the patient can be instructed in the proper application when/if the patient removes the device during specified intervals. Sizes can vary according to the manufacturer (there may be pediatric sizes as well). The items are generally manufactured in right and left models. Shoulder braces with arm, elbow, and wrist immobilization support and control the range of motion of the upper extremity, including the upper arm, scapula, clavicle, elbow, forearm, and/or wrist. They also support most muscles and ligamentous tissues related to the movement of the upper extremity. They maintain a degree of abduction between the patient's torso and the affected upper limb, at the degree desired (usually 45-90 degrees). Each of these devices typically leaves the fingers free, but grasping heavy items is usually unable to be accomplished and is not advised. They are used posttraumatically for severe fractures and for certain types of surgical procedures, such as partial or total shoulder replacement. A prefabricated or custom fitted orthosis is one that the manufacturer has produced in quantity, without a specific patient in mind. A prefabricated orthosis may be trimmed, bent, molded (with or without heat), or otherwise modified for use by a specific patient (i.e., custom fitted). An orthosis that is assembled from prefabricated components is considered prefabricated. Any orthosis that does not meet the definition of a custom fabricated orthosis is considered prefabricated. A custom fabricated orthosis is one that is individually made for a specific patient, starting with basic materials including, but not limited to, plastic, metal, leather, or cloth in the form of sheets, bars, and so forth. It involves substantial work, such as cutting, bending, molding, sewing, and so forth. It may involve the incorporation of some prefabricated components. It involves more than trimming, bending, or making other modifications to a substantially prefabricated item. A molded-to-patient-model orthosis is a particular type of custom fabricated orthosis in which an impression of the specific body part is made (by means of a plaster cast, CAD-CAM technology, etc.). These codes describe shoulder-elbow-wrist-hand orthoses that are supports attached to a wheelchair.

E2633

E2633 Wheelchair accessory, addition to mobile arm support, supinator

An arm supinator is an accessory that attaches to a wheelchair and replaces the forearm swivel. It allows the patient's arm to be rotated to a palm up position.

E8000-E8002

E8000 Gait trainer, pediatric size, posterior support, includes all accessories and components

E8001 Gait trainer, pediatric size, upright support, includes all accessories and components

E8002 Gait trainer, pediatric size, anterior support, includes all accessories and components

A gait trainer is a device that allows patients to move about freely using their own legs. Each gait trainer should be specifically sized for the individual patient and is used in different therapy modalities for gait restoration. A gait trainer supports each patient according to ability and controls the center of mass in the vertical and horizontal directions.

E

G

G0008

G0008 Administration of influenza virus vaccine

This code is reported for the administration of an influenza virus vaccine. Do not report an office visit if the only reason for the visit was to receive a vaccination.

G0009

G0009 Administration of pneumococcal vaccine

This code is reported for the administration of a pneumococcal vaccine. Do not report an office visit if the only reason for the visit was to receive a vaccination.

G0010

G0010 Administration of hepatitis B vaccine

This code is reported for the administration of a hepatitis B vaccine. Do not report an office visit if the only reason for the visit was to receive a vaccination.

G0027

G0027 Semen analysis; presence and/or motility of sperm excluding Huhner

Semen analysis is the microscopic examination of semen for the presence, quality, and mobility of the sperm contained within the semen. This is usually performed to determine if this is the source of infertility.

G0068

G0068 Professional services for the administration of anti-infective, pain management, chelation, pulmonary hypertension, inotropic, or other intravenous infusion drug or biological (excluding chemotherapy or other highly complex drug or biological) for each infusion drug administration calendar day in the individual's home, each 15 min

Home infusion services, most often administered by a nurse, are provided to a patient under the care of a physician, nurse practitioner, or physician assistant. The drug is administered intravenously in the patient's home through a DME pump. Drugs include anti-infectives and those for chelation, pain management, pulmonary hypertension, and/or inotropic therapy for patients with heart failure. Do not report this code for the administration of chemotherapy or other highly complex drugs or biologicals. This code is reported for each 15 minutes of visits other than the initial visit.

G0069

G0069 Professional services for the administration of subcutaneous immunotherapy or other subcutaneous infusion drug or biological for each infusion drug administration calendar day in the individual's home, each 15 min

Home infusion services, most often administered by a nurse, are provided to a patient under the care of a physician, nurse practitioner, or physician assistant. The immunotherapy or other drug or biological is administered subcutaneously in the patient's home through a DME pump. This code is reported for each 15 minutes of visits other than the initial visit.

G0070

G0070 Professional services for the administration of intravenous chemotherapy or other intravenous highly complex drug or biological infusion for each infusion drug administration calendar day in the individual's home, each 15 min

Home infusion services, most often administered by a nurse, are provided to a patient under the care of a physician, nurse practitioner, or physician assistant. The chemotherapy or other highly complex drug or biological is administered subcutaneously in the patient's home through a DME pump. This code is reported for each 15 minutes of visits other than the initial visit.

G0071

G0071 Payment for communication technology-based services for 5 minutes or more of a virtual (nonface-to-face) communication between a rural health clinic (RHC) or federally qualified health center (FQHC) practitioner and RHC or FQHC patient, or 5 minutes or more of remote evaluation of recorded video and/or images by an RHC or FQHC practitioner, occurring in lieu of an office visit; RHC or FQHC only

A Federally Qualified Health Center (FQHC) or Rural Health Clinic (RHC) practitioner provides virtual communication services for a minimum of five minutes of technology-based services or remote evaluation of recorded video and/or images to a patient who has had a FQHC billable visit within the previous year. The medical discussion/remote evaluation is for a condition not related to a FQHC service provided within the prior seven days and does not lead to a FQHC visit within the next 24 hours or at the soonest available appointment.

G0088

G0088 Professional services, initial visit, for the administration of anti-infective, pain management, chelation, pulmonary hypertension, inotropic, or other intravenous infusion drug or biological (excluding chemotherapy or other highly complex drug or biological) for each infusion drug administration calendar day in the individual's home, each 15 min

Home infusion services, most often administered by a nurse, are provided to a patient under the care of a physician, nurse practitioner, or physician assistant. The drug is administered intravenously in the patient's home through a DME pump. Drugs include anti-infectives and those for pain management, pulmonary hypertension, and/or inotropic therapy for patients with heart failure. Chemotherapy or other highly complex drugs or biologicals are excluded. This code is reported for each 15 minutes of the initial visit.

G0089

G0089 Professional services, initial visit, for the administration of subcutaneous immunotherapy or other subcutaneous infusion drug or biological for each infusion drug administration calendar day in the individual's home, each 15 min

Home infusion services, most often administered by a nurse, are provided to a patient under the care of a physician, nurse practitioner, or physician assistant. The immunotherapy drug or other subcutaneous infusion drug/biological is administered subcutaneously in the patient's home through a DME pump. This code is reported for each 15 minutes of the initial visit.

G0090

G0090 Professional services, initial visit, for the administration of intravenous chemotherapy or other highly complex infusion drug or biological for each infusion drug administration calendar day in the individual's home, each 15 min

Home infusion services, most often administered by a nurse, are provided to a patient under the care of a physician, nurse practitioner, or physician assistant. The chemotherapy drug or other highly complex infusion drug/biological is administered intravenously in the patient's home through a DME pump. This code is reported for each 15 minutes of the initial visit.

G0101

G0101 Cervical or vaginal cancer screening; pelvic and clinical breast examination

This code reports a cervical or vaginal cancer screening and a pelvic and clinical breast examination. The specimen for cancer screening is collected by cervical, endocervical, or vaginal scrapings or by aspiration of vaginal fluid and cells. The pelvic and breast exams are done manually by the physician to check for abnormalities, pain, and/or any palpable lumps or masses.

G0102

G0102 Prostate cancer screening; digital rectal examination

This code reports a prostate cancer screening performed manually by the physician as a digital rectal exam in order to palpate the prostate and check for abnormalities.

G0103

G0103 Prostate cancer screening; prostate specific antigen test (PSA)

This code reports a total prostate specific antigen (PSA) test for cancer screening. The specimen collection is by venipuncture. Methods may include radioimmunoassay (RIA) and monoclonal two-site immunoradiometric assay. There are several forms of PSA present in serum. PSA may be complexed with the protease inhibitor alpha-1 antichymotrypsin (PSA-ACT) or found in a free form. Higher levels of free PSA are more often associated with benign conditions than with cancer. Total PSA measures both complexed and free levels to provide a total amount present in the serum. A percentage of each form is sometimes calculated to help distinguish benign from malignant conditions.

G0104

G0104 Colorectal cancer screening; flexible sigmoidoscopy

A flexible sigmoidoscopy is performed for colorectal cancer screening. After the patient's bowel has been prepped, the physician inserts the flexible sigmoidoscope through the anus and advances the scope into the sigmoid colon. The lumen of the sigmoid colon and rectum are visualized and brushings or washings may be obtained. The sigmoidoscope is withdrawn.

G0105

G0105 Colorectal cancer screening; colonoscopy on individual at high risk

A colonoscopy is performed on a high-risk patient for colorectal cancer screening. A high-risk patient is one with ulcerative enteritis or a history of malignant neoplasm of the lower gastrointestinal tract. After the patient's bowel has been prepped, the physician inserts the colonoscope through the anus and advances the scope through the colon past the splenic flexure. The lumen of the colon and rectum is visualized. Brushings or washings may be obtained. The colonoscope is withdrawn.

G0106

G0106 Colorectal cancer screening; alternative to G0104, screening sigmoidoscopy, barium enema

A colorectal screening for cancer is performed via barium enema as an alternative to a screening sigmoidoscopy (G0104). This is a radiological exam of the large intestine carried out after the administration of a barium enema to instill the contrast medium into the colon. Fluoroscopy and x-rays are used to observe the images as the contrast fills the colon and helps the physician to diagnose cancer, even colitis, and other diseases. After the patient has emptied the colon, more films are taken.

G0108-G0109

G0108 Diabetes outpatient self-management training services, individual, per 30 minutes

G0109 Diabetes outpatient self-management training services, group session (two or more), per 30 minutes

These codes are for diabetes self-management training services, either individually or in a group of two or more. Diabetes self-management training is done to teach the diabetic how to control and monitor blood glucose levels with the proper use of the monitoring device, dietary calculations and restrictions, and correct administration of diabetic medications. These codes are reported per 30 minute intervals.

G0117-G0118

G0117 Glaucoma screening for high risk patients furnished by an optometrist or ophthalmologist

G0118 Glaucoma screening for high risk patient furnished under the direct supervision of an optometrist or ophthalmologist

Glaucoma screening is performed on a high-risk patient. Glaucoma is a progressive eye disorder, without signs or symptoms in its earlier stages, that leads to irreversible vision loss. Aqueous pressure in the anterior chamber of a healthy eye remains constant even though it is continually being flushed and renewed. Too little or too much fluid can cause permanent damage. In a test for glaucoma, the patient drinks one quart of water after fasting and then the intraocular pressure of the eye is measured. The patient may also be placed in a dark room, where the eyes are rechecked once they have sufficiently dilated. This determines if fluids in the eyes are at proper levels. High risk factors are related to age, family history, and personal medical history, such as diabetes, previous eye injury, and use of certain medications such as steroids.

G0120

G0120 Colorectal cancer screening; alternative to G0105, screening colonoscopy, barium enema

A colorectal screening for cancer is performed via barium enema as an alternative to a screening colonoscopy on a high-risk individual (G0105). This is a radiological exam of the large intestine carried out after the administration of a barium enema to instill the contrast medium into the colon. Fluoroscopy and x-rays are used to observe the images as the contrast fills the colon and helps the physician to diagnose cancer, even colitis, and other diseases. After the patient has emptied the colon, more films are taken.

G0121

G0121 Colorectal cancer screening; colonoscopy on individual not meeting criteria for high risk

A colonoscopy is performed for colorectal cancer screening on a patient who does not meet high-risk criteria. This would be a patient without a diagnosis of ulcerative enteritis or without a history of malignant neoplasm of the lower gastrointestinal tract. After the patient's bowel has been prepped, the physician inserts the colonoscope through the anus and advances the scope through the colon past the splenic flexure. The lumen of the colon and rectum is visualized. Brushings or washings may be obtained. The colonoscope is withdrawn.

G0122

G0122 Colorectal cancer screening; barium enema

A colorectal screening for cancer is done via barium enema. This is a radiological exam of the large intestine carried out after the administration of a barium enema to instill the contrast medium into the colon. Fluoroscopy and x-rays are used to observe the images as the contrast fills the colon and helps the physician to diagnose cancer, even colitis, and other diseases. After the patient has emptied the colon, more films are taken.

G0123-G0124

G0123 Screening cytopathology, cervical or vaginal (any reporting system), collected in preservative fluid, automated thin layer preparation, screening by cytotechnologist under physician supervision

G0124 Screening cytopathology, cervical or vaginal (any reporting system), collected in preservative fluid, automated thin layer preparation, requiring interpretation by physician

These cervical or vaginal cytopathology screenings (any reporting system) of specimens collected in preservative fluid may be identified as 'thin prep." The specimen is collected by cervical, endocervical, or vaginal scrapings or by aspiration of vaginal fluid and cells. This method saves time by eliminating the need for the physician to prepare a smear; the specimen is placed in a preservative suspension instead. At the laboratory, special instruments take the cells in the preservative suspension and "plate-out" a monolayer for screening, which will carefully review the specimen for abnormal cells.

G0127

G0127 Trimming of dystrophic nails, any number

A physician trims fingernails or toenails usually with scissors, nail cutters, or other instruments when the nails are defective and dystrophic from nutritional or metabolic abnormalities. Report this code for any number of nails trimmed.

G0128

G0128 Direct (face-to-face with patient) skilled nursing services of a registered nurse provided in a comprehensive outpatient rehabilitation facility, each 10 minutes beyond the first 5 minutes

This code reports direct one-on-one skilled nursing services provided to the patient by a registered nurse in a comprehensive outpatient rehabilitation facility. Report this code as a unit of 10 minutes, for each 10 minutes beyond the initial 5 minutes.

G0129

G0129 Occupational therapy services requiring the skills of a qualified occupational therapist, furnished as a component of a partial hospitalization treatment program, per session (45 minutes or more)

Occupational therapy focuses on helping a person recovering from a serious illness or injury retain movement capabilities for independently managing the activities of daily life. Report this code per day that treatment was given.

G0130

G0130 Single energy x-ray absorptiometry (SEXA) bone density study, one or more sites; appendicular skeleton (peripheral) (e.g., radius, wrist, heel)

Bone mineral density studies are used to evaluate diseases of bone and/or the responses of bone disease to treatment. Densities are measured at the wrist, radius, hip, pelvis, spine, or heel. The studies assess bone mass or density associated with such diseases as osteoporosis, osteomalacia, and renal osteodystrophy. Single energy x-ray absorptiometry (SEXA) utilizes an x-ray tube as the radiation source that is pulsed at a certain energy level. SEXA is used to scan bone that is in a superficial location with little adjacent soft tissue, such as the wrist or heel. There is a differential attenuation between bone and soft tissue for the energy beam. Excessive soft tissue renders the measurement incorrect. An attenuation profile of the bony components is calculated and the results are given in two scores, which are reported as standard deviations from the normal bone density of a person the same sex, 30 years old, which is the age of peak bone mass, and from the normal bone density of an "age matched" that compares the patient's bone density to what is expected in someone the same age, sex, and size.

G0141

G0141 Screening cytopathology smears, cervical or vaginal, performed by automated system, with manual rescreening, requiring interpretation by physician

Cervical or vaginal cytopathology screenings are done on specimens prepared in a smear. The specimen is collected by cervical, endocervical, or vaginal scrapings or by aspiration of vaginal fluid and cells. The screening method is microscopy examination of a spray or liquid fixated smear prepared by the physician collecting the specimen. Screening, defined as the careful review of the specimen for abnormal cells, may then be accomplished by different methods that involve the use of automated systems.

G0143-G0145

G0143 Screening cytopathology, cervical or vaginal (any reporting system), collected in preservative fluid, automated thin layer preparation, with manual screening and rescreening by cytotechnologist under physician supervision

G0144 Screening cytopathology, cervical or vaginal (any reporting system), collected in preservative fluid, automated thin layer preparation, with screening by automated system, under physician supervision

G0145 Screening cytopathology, cervical or vaginal (any reporting system), collected in preservative fluid, automated thin layer preparation, with screening by automated system and manual rescreening under physician supervision

These cervical or vaginal cytopathology screenings (any reporting system) of specimens collected in preservative fluid may be identified as "thin prep." The specimen is collected by cervical, endocervical, or vaginal scrapings or by aspiration of vaginal fluid and cells. This method saves time by eliminating the need for the physician to prepare a smear; the specimen is placed in a preservative suspension instead. At the laboratory, special instruments take the cells in the preservative suspension and "plate-out" a monolayer for screening, which will carefully review the specimen for abnormal cells.

G0147-G0148

G0147 Screening cytopathology smears, cervical or vaginal, performed by automated system under physician supervision

G0148 Screening cytopathology smears, cervical or vaginal, performed by automated system with manual rescreening

Cervical or vaginal cytopathology screenings are done on specimens prepared in a smear. The specimen is collected by cervical, endocervical, or vaginal scrapings or by aspiration of vaginal fluid and cells. The screening method is microscopy examination of a spray or liquid fixated smear prepared by the physician collecting the specimen. Screening, defined as the careful review of the specimen for abnormal cells, may then be accomplished by different methods that involve the use of automated systems.

G0151-G0161

G0151 Services performed by a qualified physical therapist in the home health or hospice setting, each 15 minutes

G0152 Services performed by a qualified occupational therapist in the home health or hospice setting, each 15 minutes

G0153 Services performed by a qualified speech-language pathologist in the home health or hospice setting, each 15 minutes

G0155 Services of clinical social worker in home health or hospice settings, each 15 minutes

G0156 Services of home health/hospice aide in home health or hospice settings, each 15 minutes

G0157 Services performed by a qualified physical therapist assistant in the home health or hospice setting, each 15 minutes

G0158 Services performed by a qualified occupational therapist assistant in the home health or hospice setting, each 15 minutes

G0159 Services performed by a qualified physical therapist, in the home health setting, in the establishment or delivery of a safe and effective physical therapy maintenance program, each 15 minutes

G0160 Services performed by a qualified occupational therapist, in the home health setting, in the establishment or delivery of a safe and effective occupational therapy maintenance program, each 15 minutes

G0161 Services performed by a qualified speech-language pathologist, in the home health setting, in the establishment or delivery of a safe and effective speech-language pathology maintenance program, each 15 minutes

These codes report various services provided by different types of qualified professionals in a home health or hospice setting in 15-minute increments. Home health includes not only traditional private home settings, but also assisted living quarters, group homes, custodial care facilities, or similar type settings that constitute the patient's place of residence. Medicare requires that the discipline of the home health staff be reported using these codes. Check other payer requirements before using these codes on non-Medicare claims.

G0162

G0162 Skilled services by a registered nurse (RN) for management and evaluation of the plan of care; each 15 minutes (the patient's underlying condition or complication requires an RN to ensure that essential nonskilled care achieves its purpose in the home health or hospice setting)

This code represents skilled services by a registered nurse (RN) for management and evaluation of the plan of care; each 15 minutes. The patient's underlying condition or complication requires an RN to ensure that essential non-skilled care achieves its purpose in the home health or hospice setting. Time is reported in 15-minute increments. Home health includes not only traditional private home settings, but also assisted living quarters, group homes, custodial care facilities, or similar type settings that constitute the patient's place of residence. Medicare requires that the type of service be reported.

G0166

G0166 External counterpulsation, per treatment session

External counterpulsation is a therapy for relieving angina and is also beneficial for congestive heart failure patients. The treatment increases blood flow into the arteries and decreases the workload of the heart. The therapy is believed to work by stimulating the growth of new blood vessels around the arteries in the heart that are blocked. The patient has compressive cuffs wrapped around his/her calves and upper and lower thighs. The cuffs inflate when the heart is filling with blood and deflate when the heart is ejecting blood. Treatment sessions last one hour and are usually for a period of five times a week for seven weeks. This code reports one treatment session.

G0168

G0168 Wound closure utilizing tissue adhesive(s) only

Wound closure done by using tissue adhesive only, not any kind of suturing or stapling, is reported with this code. Tissue adhesives, such as Dermabond, are materials that are applied directly to the skin or tissue of an open wound to hold the margins closed for healing.

G0175

G0175 Scheduled interdisciplinary team conference (minimum of three exclusive of patient care nursing staff) with patient present

Report this code for an interdisciplinary team conference with a minimum of three care giving professionals present, not counting the patient care nursing staff. The patient is also present. An interdisciplinary team is composed of professionals who are specialists in different areas and who work together to coordinate the care of patients whose medical condition have multiple diagnoses that require more than one focus of care from different or related fields.

G0176

G0176 Activity therapy, such as music, dance, art or play therapies not for recreation, related to the care and treatment of patient's disabling mental health problems, per session (45 minutes or more)

Activity therapy is therapeutic activity such as music, dance, art, or play therapies not for recreation. The activities are related to the care and treatment of patient's disabling mental health problems and are intended to alter the thought process of a patient in a positive way. Each session should last 45 minutes or more.

G0177

G0177 Training and educational services related to the care and treatment of patient's disabling mental health problems per session (45 minutes or more)

Training and educational services are therapeutic procedures related to the care and treatment of a patient's disabling mental health problems. The goal is to alleviate patient discomfort and allow the patient to cope or control mental health issues. Each session should be 45 minutes or more.

G0179-G0180

G0179 Physician or allowed practitioner re-certification for Medicare-covered home health services under a home health plan of care (patient not present), including contacts with home health agency and review of reports of patient status required by physicians and allowed practitioners to affirm the initial implementation of the plan of care

G0180 Physician or allowed practitioner certification for Medicare-covered home health services under a home health plan of care (patient not present), including contacts with home health agency and review of reports of patient status required by physicians or allowed practitioners to affirm the initial implementation of the plan of care

These codes report one period of certification or recertification of a patient's qualifying status for Medicare-covered home health services under a home health plan of care by a physician, without the patient present. This includes all contacts made with the home health agency and reviewing of patient status reports required by physicians to affirm the initial implementation of the care plan designed to meet the patient's needs.

G0181-G0182

G0181 Physician or allowed practitioner supervision of a patient receiving Medicare-covered services provided by a participating home health agency (patient not present) requiring complex and multidisciplinary care modalities involving regular physician or allowed practitioner development and/or revision of care plans

G0182 Physician supervision of a patient under a Medicare-approved hospice (patient not present) requiring complex and multidisciplinary care modalities involving regular physician development and/or revision of care plans, review of subsequent reports of patient status, review of laboratory and other studies, communication (including telephone calls) with other health care professionals involved in the patient's care, integration of new information into the medical treatment plan and/or adjustment of medical therapy, within a calendar month, 30 minutes or more

These codes represent physician supervision of a patient receiving Medicare-covered services provided by a participating home health agency or of a patient under a Medicare-approved hospice. This includes complex and multidisciplinary care modalities involving regular physician development and/or revision of care plans, review of subsequent reports of patient status, review of laboratory and other studies, communication with other health care professionals involved in the patient's care, including all telephone calls, and integration of new information into the medical treatment plan and/or adjustment of medical therapy, within a calendar month. The patient is not present for the physician supervision.

G0186

G0186 Destruction of localized lesion of choroid (for example, choroidal neovascularization); photocoagulation, feeder vessel technique (one or more sessions)

The physician destroys a localized lesion of the choroid, such as choroidal neovascularization (CNV) due to age related macular degeneration, using extrafoveal laser photocoagulation of the feeder vessel providing blood supply to the CNV. The feeder vessel is identified by indocyanine green angiography and looks like a spot in the choroid that is seen to branch off into the CNV as a distinct blood vessel. The physician directs short spots of a laser's beam in a racquet-like pattern at the feeder vessel(s) that have grown beneath the macula to occlude or obliterate the vessel supplying blood flow to the lesion. One or two treatments may be necessary. The patient is followed-up with another angiography to determine that there has been closure of the feeder vessel after treatment.

G0219

G0219 PET imaging whole body; melanoma for noncovered indications

The whole body is imaged using data received from positron-emitting radionuclides administered to the patient in positron emission tomography (PET) imaging. The imaging relies upon capturing the gamma rays or the positively charged particles and photons, emitted by the decaying radionuclide. The collision of the positrons emitted by the radionuclide with the negatively-charged electrons normally present in body tissue is computer synthesized to produce an image, usually in vivid color, that shows the presence of cancer in tissue through the altered cell function caused by the disease and not simply from anatomical structure changes. PET imaging produces real time functional images of the metabolic processes of body tissue, such as glucose metabolism, and shows precisely where changes induced by a disease are taking place. This code is reported for whole body imaging of the entire body seeking regional lymph nodes with increased activity that may indicate that a diagnosed melanoma has metastasized.

G0235

G0235 PET imaging, any site, not otherwise specified

The whole body or body region is imaged using data received from positron-emitting radionuclides administered to the patient in positron emission tomography (PET) imaging. The imaging relies upon capturing the gamma rays or the positively charged particles, photons, emitted by the decaying radionuclide. This detection can be done by using stationary single or double-headed gamma cameras or by rotating a detector, or scanner, around the patient as is done with full and partial-ring bismuth germinate (BGO), sodium iodide (NAI), or crystal detector PET scanner systems. The collision of the positrons emitted by the radionuclide with the negatively-charged electrons normally present in body tissue is computer synthesized to produce an image, usually in vivid color, that shows the presence of cancer in tissue through the altered cell function caused by the disease and not simply from anatomical structure changes. PET imaging produces real time functional images of the metabolic processes of body tissue, such as glucose metabolism, and shows precisely where changes induced by a disease are taking place. This code is for PET imaging of any site not otherwise specified. Not otherwise specified codes are reported only when a more specific code is not available to describe the service.

G0237-G0239

G0237 Therapeutic procedures to increase strength or endurance of respiratory muscles, face-to-face, one-on-one, each 15 minutes (includes monitoring)

G0238 Therapeutic procedures to improve respiratory function, other than described by G0237, one-on-one, face-to-face, per 15 minutes (includes monitoring)

G0239 Therapeutic procedures to improve respiratory function or increase strength or endurance of respiratory muscles, two or more individuals (includes monitoring)

These codes report therapeutic procedures, performed under the supervision of a therapist, for the treatment of respiratory disorders. These may include proper breathing techniques, respiratory education, and specialized exercises. Code G0237 reports procedures or exercises intended to increase the strength or endurance of the respiratory muscles, while G0238 reports those intended to improve respiratory function. Both are reported once for each 15 minutes of individual, one-on-one, face-to-face therapy time. Code G0239 includes the previously mentioned procedural components when provided in a group setting of two or more individuals. All codes include monitoring.

G0245-G0246

G0245 Initial physician evaluation and management of a diabetic patient with diabetic sensory neuropathy resulting in a loss of protective sensation (LOPS) which must include: (1) the diagnosis of LOPS, (2) a patient history, (3) a physical examination that consists of at least the following elements: (a) visual inspection of the forefoot, hindfoot, and toe web spaces, (b) evaluation of a protective sensation, (c) evaluation of foot structure and biomechanics, (d) evaluation of vascular status and skin integrity, and (e) evaluation and recommendation of footwear, and (4) patient education

G0246 Follow-up physician evaluation and management of a diabetic patient with diabetic sensory neuropathy resulting in a loss of protective sensation (LOPS) to include at least the following: (1) a patient history, (2) a physical examination that includes: (a) visual inspection of the forefoot, hindfoot, and toe web spaces, (b) evaluation of protective sensation, (c) evaluation of foot structure and biomechanics, (d) evaluation of vascular status and skin integrity, and (e) evaluation and recommendation of footwear, and (3) patient education

Physician evaluation and management is given to a diabetic patient with diabetic sensory neuropathy resulting in a loss of protective sensation, including all of the following in addition to the initial diagnosis of lops: a patient history; patient education; and a physical examination consisting of at least visual inspection of the forefoot, hindfoot, and toe web spaces, evaluation of protective sensation, foot structure, and biomechanics, as well as vascular status and skin integrity, and evaluation and recommendation of footwear.

G0247

G0247 Routine foot care by a physician of a diabetic patient with diabetic sensory neuropathy resulting in a loss of protective sensation (LOPS) to include the local care of superficial wounds (i.e., superficial to muscle and fascia) and at least the following, if present: (1) local care of superficial wounds, (2) debridement of corns and calluses, and (3) trimming and debridement of nails

Routine foot care is provided by a physician to a diabetic patient with diabetic sensory neuropathy resulting in a loss of protective sensation and must include, when present, all of the following: local care of superficial wounds, debridement of corns and calluses, and trimming and debridement of nails.

G0248-G0250

G0248 Demonstration, prior to initiation of home INR monitoring, for patient with either mechanical heart valve(s), chronic atrial fibrillation, or venous thromboembolism who meets Medicare coverage criteria, under the direction of a physician; includes: face-to-face demonstration of use and care of the INR monitor, obtaining at least one blood sample, provision of instructions for reporting home INR test results, and documentation of patient's ability to perform testing and report results

G0249 Provision of test materials and equipment for home INR monitoring of patient with either mechanical heart valve(s), chronic atrial fibrillation, or venous thromboembolism who meets Medicare coverage criteria; includes: provision of materials for use in the home and reporting of test results to physician; testing not occurring more frequently than once a week; testing materials, billing units of service include four tests

G0250 Physician review, interpretation, and patient management of home INR testing for patient with either mechanical heart valve(s), chronic atrial fibrillation, or venous thromboembolism who meets Medicare coverage criteria; testing not occurring more frequently than once a week; billing units of service include four tests

Patients with a mechanical heart valve, chronic atrial fibrillation, or venous thromboembolism are at risk of developing intracardiac or intravascular thrombi and are frequently managed with long-term use of warfarin anticoagulation. Periodic monitoring is necessary to maintain a therapeutic effect of the anticoagulation treatment and reduce thromboembolic and hemorrhagic events. The use of the internationalized normalized ratio (INR) (rather than the prothrombin time) provides a result that is independent of the laboratory reagents used. The INR is the ratio of the patient's prothrombin time compared to the mean prothrombin time for a group of normal individuals. Patient self-testing and self-management through the use of a home INR monitor improve the time in therapeutic rate and hence clinical outcomes. Portable coagulometers that measure the prothrombin time and calculate the INR with the use of a drop of whole blood allow the patient to do self-testing.

G0252

G0252 PET imaging, full and partial-ring PET scanners only, for initial diagnosis of breast cancer and/or surgical planning for breast cancer (e.g., initial staging of axillary lymph nodes)

Positron emission tomography (PET) is a noninvasive diagnostic imaging procedure that assesses the level of metabolic activity and perfusion in various organ systems. Initial staging is when a cancer's stage remains in question after a standard diagnostic workup, including conventional imaging (computed tomography, magnetic resonance imaging, or ultrasound). PET is used to diagnose cancer when it is expected that conventional imaging is not sufficient for the patient's clinical management and when the patient's clinical management could differ depending on the cancer's stage. Report this code for PET imaging used for the initial diagnosis of breast cancer and/or surgical planning for breast cancer (e.g., initial staging of axillary lymph nodes).

G0255

G0255 Current perception threshold/sensory nerve conduction test, (SNCT) per limb, any nerve

A current perception threshold/sensory nerve conduction test (CPT/SNCT) is used to diagnose sensory neurological impairments caused by various pathological conditions or toxic substance exposures. It is a noninvasive test that uses transcutaneous electrical stimulus to evoke a sensation. CPT/SNCT methods quantitate the level of sensory deficit by comparing current output to the nerve conduction threshold. Sensory nerve conduction testing is based on the concept that nerves are voltage sensitive. It can be done to quantitate sensory function with an instrument that provides voltage mediated testing (V-SNCT). It painlessly gathers enough objective data so measurements of subtle changes preceding gross morbidity can be detected. This method measures the actual instigator of nerve conduction voltage and the results are independent of changes in skin resistance.

G0257

G0257 Unscheduled or emergency dialysis treatment for an ESRD patient in a hospital outpatient department that is not certified as an ESRD facility

Dialysis is a process to remove toxins from the blood and to maintain fluid and electrolyte balance when the kidneys no longer function. The patient's blood is removed through a previously placed catheter, pumped through a dialysis machine, and returned to the patient through a second catheter. This code is for an unscheduled or emergency dialysis treatment for a patient with end stage renal disease (ESRD) in a hospital outpatient department that has not been certified as an ESRD facility.

G0259-G0260

G0259 Injection procedure for sacroiliac joint; arthrography

G0260 Injection procedure for sacroiliac joint; provision of anesthetic, steroid and/or other therapeutic agent, with or without arthrography

The physician injects the sacroiliac joint for the purpose of arthrography, which is taking radiographic pictures of the joint internally to visualize the cartilage and ligaments, or for therapeutic treatment. The contrast material, anesthetic, steroid, or other therapeutic agent is drawn into a syringe and the target structure is localized. Through a posterior approach, the needle is inserted and advanced into the sacroiliac joint, the articulation between the sacrum and ilium in the pelvis, and the injection is visualized under the aid of separately reportable computerized tomography (CT) or fluoroscopic guidance. Report G0259 for injection for arthrography. Report G0260 for injection of anesthetic, steroid, or other therapeutic agent.

G0268

G0268 Removal of impacted cerumen (one or both ears) by physician on same date of service as audiologic function testing

Under direct visualization, the physician removes impacted cerumen (earwax) using suction, a cerumen spoon, or delicate forceps. If no infection is present, the ear canal may be irrigated. This is done on the same day that the physician performs an audiologic function test.

G0269

G0269 Placement of occlusive device into either a venous or arterial access site, postsurgical or interventional procedure (e.g., angioseal plug, vascular plug)

Incisions into arteries and veins must be closed by suture or a device to stem the loss of blood. Such incisions are frequently made during angioplasties and diagnostic radiological procedures. An occlusive device is a plug or stopper used to close an incision into an artery or vein. This code is intended only for devices such as an Angio-Seal or vascular plug. It should not be reported for procedures such as vascular or pseudoaneurysm repair.

G0270-G0271

G0270 Medical nutrition therapy; reassessment and subsequent intervention(s) following second referral in same year for change in diagnosis, medical condition or treatment regimen (including additional hours needed for renal disease), individual, face-to-face with the patient, each 15 minutes

G0271 Medical nutrition therapy, reassessment and subsequent intervention(s) following second referral in same year for change in diagnosis, medical condition, or treatment regimen (including additional hours needed for renal disease), group (two or more individuals), each 30 minutes

These codes report reassessment and interventions in a patient's medical nutrition therapy when a person has had a change in diagnosis or his/her medical condition and/or treatment regimen, following a second referral in the same year because of the change. Additional hours needed for renal disease cases are included.

G0276

G0276 Blinded procedure for lumbar stenosis, percutaneous image-guided lumbar decompression (PILD) or placebo-control, performed in an approved coverage with evidence development (CED) clinical trial

This code reports a percutaneous, image-guided lumbar decompression (PILD) performed in an approved coverage with evidence development (CED) blinded, randomized, and placebo-controlled clinical trial study. A posterior decompression of the lumbar spine is performed under indirect image guidance without any direct visualization of the surgical field. This procedure is proposed as a treatment for symptomatic lumbar spinal stenosis that is unresponsive to conservative therapy. The procedure is considered noninvasive, with specially designed instrumentation to percutaneously remove a portion of the lamina and debulk the ligamentum flavum. The procedure is performed under x-ray guidance (e.g., fluoroscopic, CT) with assistance of contrast media to identify and monitor the target area via an epidurogram.

G0277

G0277 Hyperbaric oxygen under pressure, full body chamber, per 30 minute interval

In hyperbaric oxygen (HBO) therapy, the patient is enclosed in a pressure chamber breathing oxygen at a pressure greater than one's atmosphere. The therapeutic result is hyperoxygenation, with extra oxygen dissolved into the blood plasma. Breathing pure oxygen at three times the normal pressure delivers 15 times as much dissolved oxygen to tissues than room air. This promotes formation of new capillaries into wound areas and sufficient oxygen tensions to meet the needs of the ischemic tissues. Anemias, ischemias, and certain poisonings are effectively treated using hyperoxygenation. HBO therapy also helps free gas bubbles that are trapped in the body. Hyperoxygenation reduces the size of gas bubbles by two-thirds and aids in successful reduction in gas volume to air embolisms and decompression sickness. There is also a "gas wash out" or mass action of gases. This is the flooding of the body with any one gas to wash out all other gases. This treatment occurs quickly under pressure and is excellent as a treatment for carbon monoxide poisoning/intoxication and acute cyanide poisoning. Vasoconstriction is also treated with HBO. High pressure oxygen causes the blood vessels to constrict without creating hypoxia, therefore decreasing edema in affected or injured tissues and decreasing intracranial pressure. This treatment is useful for interstitial bleeding, burns, and crash victims. HBO also restrains the growth of anaerobic and aerobic organisms called Bacteriosis and is useful in conditions where resistant elements are compromised, as in dysvascular conditions. This effect complements the improved action of host disease fighting components.

G0278

G0278 Iliac and/or femoral artery angiography, nonselective, bilateral or ipsilateral to catheter insertion, performed at the same time as cardiac catheterization and/or coronary angiography, includes positioning or placement of the catheter in the distal aorta or ipsilateral femoral or iliac artery, injection of dye, production of permanent images, and radiologic supervision and interpretation (List separately in addition to primary procedure)

An iliac artery is radiologically examined using contrast material at the same time as cardiac catheterization. The catheter that has been threaded over the guidewire from the access site is positioned nonselectively in the distal aorta or iliac artery. Contrast medium is injected and a series of permanent images are taken to visualize the vessels and evaluate any abnormalities. The catheter is removed and pressure applied to the site. Radiological supervision and interpretation is included. List this code separately in addition to the code for the main cardiac catheterization procedure.

G0279

G0279 Diagnostic digital breast tomosynthesis, unilateral or bilateral (list separately in addition to 77065 or 77066)

Digital breast tomosynthesis is an imaging modality that uses a limited number of projections from a narrow angular range that are combined to present a three-dimensional image of the breast.

G

G0281-G0283

G0281 Electrical stimulation, (unattended), to one or more areas, for chronic Stage III and Stage IV pressure ulcers, arterial ulcers, diabetic ulcers, and venous stasis ulcers not demonstrating measurable signs of healing after 30 days of conventional care, as part of a therapy plan of care

G0282 Electrical stimulation, (unattended), to one or more areas, for wound care other than described in G0281

G0283 Electrical stimulation (unattended), to one or more areas for indication(s) other than wound care, as part of a therapy plan of care

Electrical stimulation is the use of electric current that mimics the body's own natural bioelectric system's current when injured or impaired, and jumpstarts or accelerates the healing process by attracting the body's repair cells, changing cell membrane permeability and hence cellular secretion, and orientating cell structures. A current is generated between the skin and inner tissues when there is a break in the skin. The current is kept flowing until the open skin defect is repaired. There may be different types of electricity used, controlled by different electrical sources. A moist wound environment is required for capacitively coupled electrical stimulation, which involves using a surface electrode pad in wet contact (capacitively coupled) with the external skin surface and/or wound bed. Two electrodes are required to complete the electric circuit and are usually placed over a wet conductive medium in the wound bed and on the skin away from the wound. One of the most safe and effective wavelengths used is monophasic twin peaked high voltage pulsed current (HVPC), allowing for selection of polarity, variation in pulse rates, and very short pulse duration. Significant changes in tissue pH and temperature are avoided, which is good for healing. Codes G0281 and G0282 are reported for wound care. Code G0283 is reported for purposes other than wound care, such as nerve stimulation, pain reduction, and muscle contraction.

G0288

G0288 Reconstruction, computed tomographic angiography of aorta for surgical planning for vascular surgery

Report this code for the computer reconstruction of computerized tomography (CT) generated angiographic images of the aorta for the purpose of planning vascular surgery.

G0289

G0289 Arthroscopy, knee, surgical, for removal of loose body, foreign body, debridement/shaving of articular cartilage (chondroplasty) at the time of other surgical knee arthroscopy in a different compartment of the same knee

A surgical knee arthroscopy is done with removal of loose or foreign bodies and debridement of articular cartilage at the same surgical session as other arthroscopy done in a separate compartment of the knee. The physician makes 1.0 cm long portal incisions on either side of the patellar tendon for arthroscopic access into the knee joint. Any loose bodies (fragments of cartilage or bone) encountered are removed through the portal incisions. Small loose bodies are suctioned or irrigated from the joint. Larger loose or foreign bodies are grasped by a clamp and removed. A chondroplasty is done to debride or shave the partially fragmented or unstable articular cartilage with a motorized suction cutter. This smooths the roughened or damaged cartilage and promotes bleeding and regeneration of cartilage. The joint is thoroughly flushed. A temporary drain may be applied and incisions are closed with sutures.

G0293-G0294

G0293 Noncovered surgical procedure(s) using conscious sedation, regional, general, or spinal anesthesia in a Medicare qualifying clinical trial, per day

G0294 Noncovered procedure(s) using either no anesthesia or local anesthesia only, in a Medicare qualifying clinical trial, per day

Clinical trials are tests of a new procedure or drug using human patients to determine its effectiveness, side effects, and optimal dosage levels. These codes represent the use of the facility, staff time, and related supplies and drugs associated with an experimental procedure performed under regional, general, or spinal anesthesia, and the use of the facility, staff time, and related supplies and drugs associated with an experimental procedure performed without any type of anesthesia or under a local spinal anesthesia. These are daily charges and should not be reported more than once per calendar day.

G0295

G0295 Electromagnetic therapy, to one or more areas, for wound care other than described in G0329 or for other uses

Electromagnetic therapy is the application of low doses of electromagnetic current into the body. It is a form of electrical stimulation that is used for many different applications, including helping to heal wounds that have not been responding to conventional care. This code covers electromagnetic therapy applied for wound care that is not any type of chronic stage III or IV ulcer.

G0296

G0296 Counseling visit to discuss need for lung cancer screening using low dose CT scan (LDCT) (service is for eligibility determination and shared decision making)

In 2015, Medicare issued a national coverage determination (NCD) for the coverage of lung cancer screening with low-dose computed tomography (LDCT). This coverage includes lung cancer screening counseling and a shared decision-making visit, and, for appropriate beneficiaries, an annual screening for lung cancer with LDCT as an additional preventive service under Medicare if certain criteria are met. To meet the eligibility criteria for Medicare, the patient must be between ages 55 and 77 years; must be asymptomatic (no signs or symptoms of lung cancer); must have a tobacco smoking history of at least 30 pack-years (one pack-year equals smoking one pack per day for one year; one pack equals 20 cigarettes); must be a current smoker or one who has quit smoking within the last 15 years; and must have received a written order for a LDCT lung cancer screening. Note that the Medicare criteria differ slightly from the U.S. Preventive Services Task Force (USPSTF). This HCPCS code represents Medicare defined covered services.

G0299-G0300

G0299 Direct skilled nursing services of a registered nurse (RN) in the home health or hospice setting, each 15 minutes

G0300 Direct skilled nursing services of a licensed practical nurse (LPN) in the home health or hospice setting, each 15 minutes

These codes report services provided by nursing professionals in a home health or hospice setting. They are reported in 15-minute increments. Home health includes not only traditional private home settings, but also assisted living quarters, group homes, custodial care facilities, or similar type settings that constitute the patient's place of residence. Medicare requires that the discipline of the nursing staff be reported using these codes. Check other payer requirements before using these codes on non-Medicare claims.

G0302-G0305

G0302 Preoperative pulmonary surgery services for preparation for LVRS, complete course of services, to include a minimum of 16 days of services

G0303 Preoperative pulmonary surgery services for preparation for LVRS, 10 to 15 days of services

G0304 Preoperative pulmonary surgery services for preparation for LVRS, 1 to 9 days of services

G0305 Postdischarge pulmonary surgery services after LVRS, minimum of 6 days of services

Lung volume reduction surgery (LVRS) is an invasive procedure to reduce the volume of a hyperinflated lung, allowing the underlying lung to expand to improve respiratory function. LRVS may also be called reduction pneumoplasty, lung shaving, or lung contouring. The procedure may be performed on patients with severe upper lobe predominant emphysema or those with severe non-upper lobe emphysema with low exercise capacity.

G0306-G0307

G0306 Complete CBC, automated (HgB, HCT, RBC, WBC, without platelet count) and automated WBC differential count

G0307 Complete CBC, automated (HgB, HCT, RBC, WBC; without platelet count)

A complete blood count (CBC) is a series of tests of peripheral blood that measure the hematocrit, hemoglobulin, red blood cell count (RBC), white blood cell count (WBC), and the proportion of different white cells as they appear on a blood smear. The CBC may or may not include an enumeration of platelets within the specimen. A WBC differential count is an enumeration, expressed as a percentage, of the different types of white blood cells (e.g., leukocytes) that are present in a specific blood specimen. Both assays may be performed manually or automated.

G0310-G0315

G0310 Immunization counseling by a physician or other qualified health care professional when the vaccine(s) is not administered on the same date of service, 5-15 minutes time (This code is used for Medicaid billing purposes)

G0311 Immunization counseling by a physician or other qualified health care professional when the vaccine(s) is not administered on the same date of service, 16-30 minutes time (This code is used for Medicaid billing purposes)

G0312 Immunization counseling by a physician or other qualified health care professional when the vaccine(s) is not administered on the same date of service for ages under 21, 5-15 minutes time (This code is used for Medicaid billing purposes)

G0313 Immunization counseling by a physician or other qualified health care professional when the vaccine(s) is not administered on the same date of service for ages under 21, 16-30 minutes time (This code is used for Medicaid billing purposes)

G0314 Immunization counseling by a physician or other qualified health care professional for COVID-19, ages under 21, 16-30 minutes time (This code is used for the Medicaid Early and Periodic Screening, Diagnostic, and Treatment Benefit [EPSDT])

G0315 Immunization counseling by a physician or other qualified health care professional for COVID-19, ages under 21, 5-15 minutes time (This code is used for the Medicaid Early and Periodic Screening, Diagnostic, and Treatment Benefit [EPSDT])

Beginning in 2021, the Centers for Medicare and Medicaid Services (CMS) is requiring individual states to cover COVID-19 vaccine counseling visits without cost-sharing. These visits are for health care providers to discuss the importance of children's vaccinations, under 21 years old and eligible for the Medicaid Early and Periodic Screening, Diagnostic and Treatment (EPSDT) benefit, with their families. This action is intended to expand access to individualized medical advice and to address vaccine hesitancy issues by providing information from trusted health care providers. States are required to cover stand-alone vaccine counseling for all vaccines covered under the EPSDT benefit, regardless of any federal match for expenditures. Under the American Rescue Plan (ARP), CMS will match state expenditures for COVID-19 vaccine counseling services at 100 percent through the last day of the first quarter that begins one year following the end of the COVID-19 public health emergency, as part of the EPSDT benefit. This applies only when stand-alone COVID-19 vaccine counseling is covered for beneficiaries who are eligible for both EPSTD and the ARP COVID-19 vaccination coverage. These codes should only be reported for Medicaid beneficiaries. Report G0310-G0311 for non-COVID 19 vaccine counseling for patients ages 21 years and older. Report G0312-G0313 for non-COVID-19 vaccine counseling for patients under 21 years of age. Report G0314-G0315 for COVID-19 related vaccine counseling for EPSDT beneficiaries under 21 years of age.

G0316

G0316 Prolonged hospital inpatient or observation care evaluation and management service(s) beyond the total time for the primary service (when the primary service has been selected using time on the date of the primary service); each additional 15 minutes by the physician or qualified healthcare professional, with or without direct patient contact (list separately in addition to CPT codes 99223, 99233, and 99236 for hospital inpatient or observation care evaluation and management services). (Do not report G0316 on the same date of service as other prolonged services for evaluation and management codes 99358, 99359, 99418, 99415, 99416). (Do not report G0316 for any time unit less than 15 minutes)

The physician or qualified health care professional provides prolonged hospital inpatient or observation care (including partial hospitalization) evaluation and management (E/M) services, with or without direct patient contact. Report G0316 as an add-on code to represent each additional 15 minutes of services provided beyond the greatest amount of allowed time of the highest-level primary E/M service. These primary services include initial or subsequent inpatient or observation care, as well as that for patients whose admission and discharge occur on the same day, and do not differentiate between new or established patients. Note: G0316 has been added to the Medicare telehealth services list, effective through the end of calendar year 2023.

G

G0317

G0317 Prolonged nursing facility evaluation and management service(s) beyond the total time for the primary service (when the primary service has been selected using time on the date of the primary service); each additional 15 minutes by the physician or qualified healthcare professional, with or without direct patient contact (list separately in addition to CPT codes 99306, 99310 for nursing facility evaluation and management services). (Do not report G0317 on the same date of service as other prolonged services for evaluation and management codes 99358, 99359, 99418). (Do not report G0317 for any time unit less than 15 minutes)

The physician or qualified health care professional provides prolonged nursing facility evaluation and management (E/M) services, with or without direct patient contact. Report G0317 as an add-on code to represent each additional 15 minutes of services provided beyond the greatest amount of allowed time of the highest-level primary E/M service. These primary services include initial or subsequent nursing facility care that may be provided in nursing facilities and skilled nursing facilities, or for services in psychiatric residential treatment centers or immediate care facilities for patients with intellectual disabilities. They do not differentiate between new or established patients. Note: G0317 has been added to the Medicare telehealth services list, effective through the end of calendar year 2023.

G0318

G0318 Prolonged home or residence evaluation and management service(s) beyond the total time for the primary service (when the primary service has been selected using time on the date of the primary service); each additional 15 minutes by the physician or qualified healthcare professional, with or without direct patient contact (list separately in addition to CPT codes 99345, 99350 for home or residence evaluation and management services). (Do not report G0318 on the same date of service as other prolonged services for evaluation and management codes 99358, 99359, 99417). (Do not report G0318 for any time unit less than 15 minutes)

The physician or qualified health care professional provides prolonged evaluation and management (E/M) services, with or without direct patient contact, in a home or residence. Report G0318 as an add-on code to represent each additional 15 minutes of services provided beyond the greatest amount of allowed time of the highest-level primary E/M service. These primary services include the evaluation and management of a new or an established patient in a private residence or temporary lodging. Short-term accommodations such as a hotel, campground, hostel, or cruise ship are included, along with assisted living facility, group home, custodial care facility, or residential substance abuse treatment facility. Note: G0318 has been added to the Medicare telehealth services list, effective through the end of calendar year 2023.

G0320-G0321

G0320 Home health services furnished using synchronous telemedicine rendered via a real-time two-way audio and video telecommunications system

G0321 Home health services furnished using synchronous telemedicine rendered via telephone or other real-time interactive audio-only telecommunications system

Telemedicine services provided by home health providers can be included as part of a patient's plan of care. An initial comprehensive assessment is performed that indicates a need for the patient to continue services utilizing telemedicine technology to reach short- or long-term goals. This telemedicine visit does not replace a home visit ordered as part of the plan of care. Report G0320 for real-time, two-way audio and video technology; G0321 for audio only.

G0322

G0322 The collection of physiologic data digitally stored and/or transmitted by the patient to the home health agency (i.e., remote patient monitoring)

Remote therapeutic monitoring services are performed to assess and evaluate data related to the patient's adherence and response to therapies. Physiologic data may be objective, such as integrated data that is device-generated, or subjective, such as input reported by the patient. Examples include blood pressure or electrocardiogram data or glucose monitoring. This data can be stored digitally or sent to the home health agency by the patient or caregiver.

G0323

G0323 Care management services for behavioral health conditions, at least 20 minutes of clinical psychologist or clinical social worker time, per calendar month. (These services include the following required elements: initial assessment or follow-up monitoring, including the use of applicable validated rating scales; behavioral health care planning in relation to behavioral/psychiatric health problems, including revision for patients who are not progressing or whose status changes; facilitating and coordinating treatment such as psychotherapy, coordination with and/or referral to physicians and practitioners who are authorized by Medicare to prescribe medications and furnish E/M services, counseling and/or psychiatric consultation; and continuity of care with a designated member of the care team)

The clinical psychologist or clinical social worker provides at least 20 minutes per calendar month of care management services for behavioral health conditions. Required elements of these services include initial assessment or follow-up monitoring that incorporates the use of pertinent authorized rating scales; behavioral health care planning and appropriate revisions related to behavioral or psychiatric health problems; facilitation/coordination of such treatments as psychotherapy; coordination with/referral to Medicare-authorized physicians and practitioners who can furnish E/M services, counseling, psychiatric consultation, and medication prescription; and continuity of care with an assigned member of the patient's care team. The scope of services reported by this code does not include coordination of social care.

G0327

G0327 Colorectal cancer screening; blood-based biomarker

A blood-based biomarker, found in the patient's blood, is a measurable DNA (deoxyribonucleic acid), RNA (ribonucleic acid), or protein component that can be an indicator of a patient's disease risk or progression. Blood-based cancer biomarkers include, but are not limited to, specific gene mutations, methylation of genes, and antigens. This test screens for mutations of the Septin-9 protein that is associated with colorectal cancer (CRC). Aberrant hypermethylation of the SEPT9 gene increases methylated Septin9, or mSEPT9, a DNA methylation-based biomarker associated with CRC. The mSEPT9 gene DNA is released into the blood and can be detected in blood plasma. Risk of CRC can be estimated by determining how much DNA mSEPT9 is in the peripheral blood. The specimen is a real-time polymerase chain reaction (PRC) with a fluorescent hydrolysis probe for methylation specific detection of Septin-9 DNA target.

G0328

G0328 Colorectal cancer screening; fecal occult blood test, immunoassay, one to three simultaneous determinations

Colorectal cancer screening is a preventive measure to detect precancerous signs in the colon and rectum. A fecal-occult blood test is an examination that detects the presence of blood in the stool that cannot be seen with the naked eye. An immunoassay detects the presence of antigen or antibodies. Several methods of screening may be performed, including colonoscopy, barium enema, and fecal-occult blood tests. This code includes the use of a spatula or special brush to collect the appropriate number of samples.

G0329

G0329 Electromagnetic therapy, to one or more areas for chronic Stage III and Stage IV pressure ulcers, arterial ulcers, diabetic ulcers and venous stasis ulcers not demonstrating measurable signs of healing after 30 days of conventional care as part of a therapy plan of care

Electromagnetic therapy is a distinct form of treatment using application of electromagnetic fields rather than direct electrical current. Electromagnetic therapy is used for wound treatment for stage III and/or stage IV pressure ulcers, arterial ulcers, diabetic ulcers, and venous stasis ulcers. Electromagnetic therapy is only considered appropriate after standard wound therapy has been tried for a minimum of 30 days with documentation showing no measurable signs of healing.

G0330

G0330 Facility services for dental rehabilitation procedure(s) performed on a patient who requires monitored anesthesia (e.g., general, intravenous sedation (monitored anesthesia care) and use of an operating room

Facility services for procedures for dental rehabilitation are reported by the hospital outpatient department. These services require monitored anesthesia in the operating room. This level of dental care is often required for patients with disabilities or severe dental issues. This code is used for Medicare covered dental rehabilitation services only.

G0333

G0333 Pharmacy dispensing fee for inhalation drug(s); initial 30-day supply as a beneficiary

Medicare pays an initial dispensing fee to a pharmacy for the first 30-day period of inhalation drugs furnished through DME, regardless of the number of shipments or drugs dispensed during that time and regardless of the number of pharmacies a beneficiary uses during that time. This initial 30-day dispensing fee is a one-time fee applicable only to those who are using inhalation drugs for the first time as Medicare beneficiaries.

G0337

G0337 Hospice evaluation and counseling services, preelection

This code reports an evaluation of a terminally ill, Medicare beneficiary by a physician who is either the medical director or an employee of the hospice. This hospice consultation service is available to those who have not made a hospice election, nor received a previous hospice consultation. It includes an assessment of the patient's need for pain and symptom management, counseling regarding hospice and other care options, and may include advice regarding advanced care planning. The beneficiary or his or her physician must request this evaluation.

G0339-G0340

G0339 Image guided robotic linear accelerator-based stereotactic radiosurgery, complete course of therapy in one session or first session of fractionated treatment

G0340 Image guided robotic linear accelerator-based stereotactic radiosurgery, delivery including collimator changes and custom plugging, fractionated treatment, all lesions, per session, second through fifth sessions, maximum five sessions per course of treatment

Image-guided robotic linear accelerator-based stereotactic radiosurgery is treatment using a robotic device of a precisely defined area (stereotactic) with radiation generated by a linear accelerator. A linear accelerator is a device that increases the motion of ions to high energy or frequency levels. Electrodes are lined up with very small spaces between them creating very excited molecules that possess high levels of energy. The robotic device is guided by images taken during the course of treatment. This code includes collimator changes and custom plugging. This code represents all lesions treated in one treatment plan. When reporting fractionated treatments, the maximum number of fractionated treatments allowed is five.

G0341-G0343

G0341 Percutaneous islet cell transplant, includes portal vein catheterization and infusion

G0342 Laparoscopy for islet cell transplant, includes portal vein catheterization and infusion

G0343 Laparotomy for islet cell transplant, includes portal vein catheterization and infusion

Islets cells are found in clusters throughout the pancreas and can be taken from an organ donor and transferred into the pancreas of the patient. Once transplanted, the cells can take over the task of destroyed cells. For example, diabetic Type I patients have a pancreas that no longer makes insulin and must take insulin daily. Once implanted, the islet cells, which contain beta cells, begin to make insulin. Each approach requires access to the portal vein, commonly via a transhepatic approach.

G0372

G0372 Physician service required to establish and document the need for a power mobility device

A physician or treating nonphysician practitioner (a physician assistant, nurse practitioner, or clinical nurse specialist) must conduct a face-to-face examination of the patient and write a written order for a power mobility device (PMD). The written order must include the patient's name, the date of the face-to-face examination, the diagnoses and conditions that the PMD is expected to modify, a description of the item, the length of need, the physician or treating nonphysician practitioner's signature, and the date the order is written.

G0378

G0378 Hospital observation service, per hour

Observation in a hospital setting is the monitoring, testing, short term treatment, and assessment of a patient, to determine if the patient requires further treatment as a hospital inpatient or can be discharged from the hospital. Observation status is commonly assigned to patients who present to the emergency department and who then require a significant period of treatment or monitoring in order to make a decision concerning their admission or discharge.

G0379

G0379 Direct admission of patient for hospital observation care

Observation is commonly assigned to patients who present to the emergency department and who then require a significant period of treatment or monitoring in order to make a decision concerning their admission or discharge. The decision to admit a patient for observation care may sometimes be made in the physician office or other community setting. Report this code when a patient is admitted to observation directly from the community without being seen in the hospital's clinic or emergency department.

G0380-G0384

G0380 Level 1 hospital emergency department visit provided in a type B emergency department; (the ED must meet at least one of the following requirements: (1) it is licensed by the state in which it is located under applicable state law as an emergency room or emergency department; (2) it is held out to the public (by name, posted signs, advertising, or other means) as a place that provides care for emergency medical conditions on an urgent basis without requiring a previously scheduled appointment; or (3) during the calendar year immediately preceding the calendar year in which a determination under 42 CFR 489.24 is being made, based on a representative sample of patient visits that occurred during that calendar year, it provides at least one-third of all of its outpatient visits for the treatment of emergency medical conditions on an urgent basis without requiring a previously scheduled appointment)

G0381 Level 2 hospital emergency department visit provided in a type B emergency department; (the ED must meet at least one of the following requirements: (1) it is licensed by the state in which it is located under applicable state law as an emergency room or emergency department; (2) it is held out to the public (by name, posted signs, advertising, or other means) as a place that provides care for emergency medical conditions on an urgent basis without requiring a previously scheduled appointment; or (3) during the calendar year immediately preceding the calendar year in which a determination under 42 CFR 489.24 is being made, based on a representative sample of patient visits that occurred during that calendar year, it provides at least one-third of all of its outpatient visits for the treatment of emergency medical conditions on an urgent basis without requiring a previously scheduled appointment)

G0382 Level 3 hospital emergency department visit provided in a type B emergency department; (the ED must meet at least one of the following requirements: (1) it is licensed by the state in which it is located under applicable state law as an emergency room or emergency department; (2) it is held out to the public (by name, posted signs, advertising, or other means) as a place that provides care for emergency medical conditions on an urgent basis without requiring a previously scheduled appointment; or (3) during the calendar year immediately preceding the calendar year in which a determination under 42 CFR 489.24 is being made, based on a representative sample of patient visits that occurred during that calendar year, it provides at least one-third of all of its outpatient visits for the treatment of emergency medical conditions on an urgent basis without requiring a previously scheduled appointment)

G0383 Level 4 hospital emergency department visit provided in a type B emergency department; (the ED must meet at least one of the following requirements: (1) it is licensed by the state in which it is located under applicable state law as an emergency room or emergency department; (2) it is held out to the public (by name, posted signs, advertising, or other means) as a place that provides care for emergency medical conditions on an urgent basis without requiring a previously scheduled appointment; or (3) during the calendar year immediately preceding the calendar year in which a determination under 42 CFR 489.24 is being made, based on a representative sample of patient visits that occurred during that calendar year, it provides at least one-third of all of its outpatient visits for the treatment of emergency medical conditions on an urgent basis without requiring a previously scheduled appointment)

G0384 Level 5 hospital emergency department visit provided in a type B emergency department; (the ED must meet at least one of the following requirements: (1) it is licensed by the state in which it is located under applicable state law as an emergency room or emergency department; (2) it is held out to the public (by name, posted signs, advertising, or other means) as a place that provides care for emergency medical conditions on an urgent basis without requiring a previously scheduled appointment; or (3) during the calendar year immediately preceding the calendar year in which a determination under 42 CFR 489.24 is

G

being made, based on a representative sample of patient visits that occurred during that calendar year, it provides at least one-third of all of its outpatient visits for the treatment of emergency medical conditions on an urgent basis without requiring a previously scheduled appointment)

Type B emergency departments (ED) are areas within a hospital that provide emergency and urgent care to patients. Type B EDs meet the EMTALA definition of a dedicated ED, but do not meet the CPT definition of an ED. Hospitals that meet the CPT definition are labeled Type A EDs. Type B EDs most likely are not available 24 hours a day, seven days a week as required for the Type A designation. A Type B ED must be licensed by the state in which it is located under applicable state law as an ED, or be held out to the public (by name, posted signs, advertising, or other means) as a place that provides care for emergency medical conditions on an urgent basis without requiring a previously scheduled appointment, or provide one third of all its outpatient visits for the treatment of emergency medical conditions on an urgent basis without requiring a previously scheduled appointment. Hospitals may make their own determination as to the assignment of the various levels of care. Determination should be documented and consistently applied.

G0390

G0390 Trauma response team associated with hospital critical care service

Trauma response teams are specialized teams of key hospital personnel who respond to triage information from prehospital caregivers in advance of the patient's arrival. The trauma team designation may only be used by trauma center/hospitals as licensed or designated by the state or local government authority entitled to do so, or as verified by the American College of Surgeons. Patients can only be billed the trauma activation fee charge if there has been prehospital notification for them; they meet local, state, or American College of Surgeons field triage criteria; or they are delivered by inter-hospital transfers; and if they are given the appropriate team response.

G0396-G0397

G0396 Alcohol and/or substance (other than tobacco) misuse structured assessment (e.g., audit, dast), and brief intervention 15 to 30 minutes

G0397 Alcohol and/or substance (other than tobacco) misuse structured assessment (e.g., audit, dast), and intervention, greater than 30 minutes

Alcohol and substance misuse may be assessed by several different methods, including a drug abuse screening test (DAST) and an alcohol use disorder identification test (AUDIT).

G0398-G0400

G0398 Home sleep study test (HST) with type II portable monitor, unattended; minimum of 7 channels: EEG, EOG, EMG, ECG/heart rate, airflow, respiratory effort and oxygen saturation

G0399 Home sleep test (HST) with type III portable monitor, unattended; minimum of 4 channels: 2 respiratory movement/airflow, 1 ECG/heart rate and 1 oxygen saturation

G0400 Home sleep test (HST) with type IV portable monitor, unattended; minimum of 3 channels

Sleep apnea is a serious sleep disorder in which breathing repeatedly stops and starts. There are two main types of sleep apnea. Obstructive sleep apnea is the more common form that occurs when throat muscles relax. Central sleep apnea occurs when the brain doesn't send proper signals to the muscles that control breathing. Some people may have a complex sleep apnea, which is a combination of both. Medicare covers continuous positive airway pressure (CPAP) as a treatment for obstructive sleep apnea. Sleep studies, whether in a facility or performed at home, generally have the following components: electroencephalogram (EEG) to measure brain activity, electrooculogram (EOG) to monitor eye movements, electromyogram (EMG) to monitor muscle movements, electrocardiogram (EKG) to monitor heart rate and rhythm, blood oxygen saturation, breathing effort or respiratory disturbance index (RDI), and airflow monitors. Chest and abdomen movements are also sometimes monitored. Home sleep studies used to diagnose obstructive sleep apnea are reported with these codes.

G0402

G0402 Initial preventive physical examination; face-to-face visit, services limited to new beneficiary during the first 12 months of Medicare enrollment

An initial preventive physical examination is provided to a new beneficiary during the first 12 months of Medicare enrollment. It is also referred to as a "Welcome to Medicare" physical examination. The physician performs a thorough review of the patient's health. The physician takes a medical history on the patient and performs an exam that includes a blood pressure check, height and weight assessment, and a vision screen. Depending on the medical history information provided by the patient and the results of the physical examination, the physician orders or performs additional tests as medically necessary. The physician also provides preventive medicine education and counseling services based on the patient's medical history and examination results. The physician provides a written plan of care to the patient detailing any follow-up screening or preventive services that the patient should receive.

G0403-G0405

G0403 Electrocardiogram, routine ECG with 12 leads; performed as a screening for the initial preventive physical examination with interpretation and report

G0404 Electrocardiogram, routine ECG with 12 leads; tracing only, without interpretation and report, performed as a screening for the initial preventive physical examination

G0405 Electrocardiogram, routine ECG with 12 leads; interpretation and report only, performed as a screening for the initial preventive physical examination

Electrocardiogram (ECG) services are performed as a component of the initial preventive physical examination provided to a new beneficiary during the first 12 months of Medicare enrollment. Twelve electrodes are placed on a patient's chest to record electrical activity of the heart. A physician interprets the findings.

G0406-G0408

G0406 Follow-up inpatient consultation, limited, physicians typically spend 15 minutes communicating with the patient via telehealth

G0407 Follow-up inpatient consultation, intermediate, physicians typically spend 25 minutes communicating with the patient via telehealth

G0408 Follow-up inpatient consultation, complex, physicians typically spend 35 minutes communicating with the patient via telehealth

These codes report consultative visits or consultations that are furnished via telehealth in response to a request by the attending physician to follow up on an initial consultation or a subsequent consultative visit. Telehealth is the delivery of health-related services via telecommunications equipment. The initial inpatient visit may have also been made via telehealth. These services include following the progress and recommending modifications to the management of care or recommending a new plan of care as a result of changes in the patient's status or absence of changes in the health issue that required the consultation.

G0409

G0409 Social work and psychological services, directly relating to and/or furthering the patient's rehabilitation goals, each 15 minutes, face-to-face; individual (services provided by a CORF qualified social worker or psychologist in a CORF)

A comprehensive outpatient rehabilitation facility (CORF) is a facility established and operated at a single fixed location exclusively for the purpose of providing diagnostic, therapeutic, and restorative services to outpatients by or under the supervision of a physician. The CORF must provide at least the following three services: physicians' services, physical therapy, and social or psychological services. Social work and psychological services must be directly related to the patient's rehabilitation goal. .

G0410

G0410 Group psychotherapy other than of a multiple-family group, in a partial hospitalization setting, approximately 45 to 50 minutes

The psychiatric treatment provider conducts psychotherapy for a group of patients in one session. Group dynamics are explored. Emotional and rational cognitive interactions between individual persons in the group are facilitated and observed. Personal dynamics of any individual patient may be discussed within the group setting. Processes that help patients move toward emotional healing and modification of thought and behavior are used, such as facilitating improved interpersonal exchanges, group support, and reminiscing. The group may be composed of patients with separate and distinct maladaptive disorders or persons sharing some facet of a disorder. This code should be used for group psychotherapy with other patients, and not members of the patients' families.

G0411

G0411 Interactive group psychotherapy, in a partial hospitalization setting, approximately 45 to 50 minutes

A therapist provides therapeutic, interactive psychiatric services in a partial hospitalization setting to a group of individuals. The interactive method is most often used with individuals who are too young, or incapable, of developing expressive communication skills, or individuals who have lost that ability. This type of psychotherapy is often done with children. Toys, physical aids, and non-verbal play and interaction, including the use of interpreter skills, are employed to gain communication with a patient not capable of engaging with the clinician by using adult language skills.

G0412

G0412 Open treatment of iliac spine(s), tuberosity avulsion, or iliac wing fracture(s), unilateral or bilateral for pelvic bone fracture patterns which do not disrupt the pelvic ring, includes internal fixation, when performed

The physician performs open treatment of iliac spine(s), tuberosity avulsion, or iliac wing fracture(s) by making an incision overlying the site of injury. Dissection exposes the avulsion and/or fracture. For an avulsion, a screw(s) is drilled through the bone fragment, reattaching the tendon and bone fragment to the original positions. The physician stabilizes an iliac wing fracture with a plate and screws across the fracture. The incision is repaired in layers. Suction drains may be applied. This code reports unilateral or bilateral treatment for fracture patterns of the pelvic bone that do not disrupt the pelvic ring and includes internal fixation when performed.

G0413

G0413 Percutaneous skeletal fixation of posterior pelvic bone fracture and/or dislocation, for fracture patterns which disrupt the pelvic ring, unilateral or bilateral, (includes ilium, sacroiliac joint and/or sacrum)

The physician performs unilateral or bilateral percutaneous skeletal fixation of a posterior pelvic bone fracture (including ipsilateral ilium, sacroiliac joint, and/or sacrum) for fracture patterns that disrupt the pelvic ring. With the patient in a supine position, the physician inserts two to three pins through the skin and into the iliac crest. The pins are directed at specific angles. The physician attaches pin holders to each ring and curved ring segments to pin holders. The physician uses the rings to gently reduce (reposition) an unstable pelvic fracture or dislocation, if needed. Frame clamps are attached to the rings and tightened to secure fixation.

G0414

G0414 Open treatment of anterior pelvic bone fracture and/or dislocation for fracture patterns which disrupt the pelvic ring, unilateral or bilateral, includes internal fixation when performed (includes pubic symphysis and/or superior/inferior rami)

The physician performs unilateral or bilateral open treatment of an anterior pelvic bone fracture or dislocation (includes the pubic symphysis and/or superior/inferior rami). With the patient in a supine position, the physician makes a curvilinear, transverse incision above the superior pubic ramus. Dissection exposes the pubic symphysis and/or rami. The separation (fracture and/or dislocation) may be reduced by the physician by applying manual ilium-to-ilium compression. For internal fixation, a plate is applied with screws directed into the bone. The incision is repaired in layers with suction drains. This code is reported for fracture patterns that disrupt the pelvic ring and includes internal fixation when performed.

G0415

G0415 Open treatment of posterior pelvic bone fracture and/or dislocation, for fracture patterns which disrupt the pelvic ring, unilateral or bilateral, includes internal fixation, when performed (includes ilium, sacroiliac joint and/or sacrum)

The physician performs unilateral or bilateral open treatment of a posterior pelvic bone fracture or dislocation (includes ilium, sacroiliac joint, and/or sacrum). With the patient in a supine position, the physician makes an incision along the anterior iliac crest. The iliacus muscle is dissected and reflected medially with the abdominal contents to expose the injury. If needed, the physician manipulates the pelvis and leg to reduce (reposition) the fracture or dislocation. Compression plates and screws achieve internal fixation. In other approaches, reconstruction plates, transiliac rod fixators, or screws alone may be used for internal fixation of the ilium, sacroiliac joint, and/or sacrum. The incision is repaired in layers with suction drains. This code reports treatment for fracture patterns that disrupt the pelvic ring and include internal fixation when performed.

G0416

G0416 Surgical pathology, gross and microscopic examinations, for prostate needle biopsy, any method

An alternative technique to the transrectal ultrasound (TRUS) biopsy procedure, the prostate saturation biopsy (PSB) is used to help identify prostate cancer in high-risk patients. The procedure is especially helpful on patients who have high PSA levels and a history of negative biopsies or abnormal biopsies, or abnormal rectal exams. The PSB is usually done under general anesthesia and ultrasonic guidance. The physician can identify each specimen/biopsy and create a map of the cancer. Several biopsies are obtained, increasing the chances of detecting cancer. Report these codes for the pathology services.

G0420-G0421

G0420 Face-to-face educational services related to the care of chronic kidney disease; individual, per session, per 1 hour

G0421 Face-to-face educational services related to the care of chronic kidney disease; group, per session, per 1 hour

Face-to-face kidney disease education services provide patients with chronic kidney disease the information they need to manage concurrent health issues and to prevent complications. These services also include an explanation of the need to delay dialysis, as well as the treatment options available for renal replacement. These educational services may be done on an individual basis or in a group setting.

G0422-G0423

G0422 Intensive cardiac rehabilitation; with or without continuous ECG monitoring with exercise, per session

G0423 Intensive cardiac rehabilitation; with or without continuous ECG monitoring; without exercise, per session

Cardiac rehabilitation is a medically supervised program intended to help people with heart problems. The program includes training and education on the risk factors of heart disease, such as smoking, high blood pressure, and lack of exercise. Encouragement is given to adopt a healthy lifestyle by increasing physical activity, developing stress coping techniques, and adopting a healthy diet. The program may or may not include exercise and continuous ECG monitoring. Intensive cardiac rehabilitation (ICR) sessions are limited to 72 one-hour sessions, up to six sessions per day, over a period of up to 18 weeks.

G0425-G0427

G0425 Telehealth consultation, emergency department or initial inpatient, typically 30 minutes communicating with the patient via telehealth

G0426 Telehealth consultation, emergency department or initial inpatient, typically 50 minutes communicating with the patient via telehealth

G0427 Telehealth consultation, emergency department or initial inpatient, typically 70 minutes or more communicating with the patient via telehealth

These codes report an initial inpatient or emergency department consultative visit or consultations that are furnished via telehealth in response to a request by the attending physician. Telehealth is the delivery of health-related services via telecommunications equipment. These services include counseling and coordination of patient care with the other providers.

G0428

G0428 Collagen meniscus implant procedure for filling meniscal defects (e.g., CMI, collagen scaffold, Menaflex)

The meniscus collagen implant is designed to fill any meniscal defects that are still present after a partial meniscectomy. It cannot replace the entire meniscus since it requires a meniscal rim for attachment. The collagen implant works as a scaffold for new tissue growth in the meniscus. The implant is placed via arthroscopy and is sutured into position.

G0429

G0429 Dermal filler injection(s) for the treatment of facial lipodystrophy syndrome (LDS) (e.g., as a result of highly active antiretroviral therapy)

Facial lipodystrophy syndrome (LDS) is a condition that is characterized by localized loss of fat in the face. This loss of fat results in a facial abnormality, such as severely sunken cheeks. Patients with HIV can suffer from this condition due to antiviral treatment or the disease itself. Due to appearance, patients with LDS may discontinue treatment and feel depressed and stigmatized. Dermal filler injection gradually increases the fullness in the face to provide a more normal appearance. The treatment area is sterilely prepped and a series of injections are administered into the deep dermal, subcutaneous areas, or by depot technique. The areas are massaged periodically during the treatment to distribute the medication evenly. The patient may need additional injection sessions to obtain the desired result. This code includes the medication.

G0432-G0435

G0432 Infectious agent antibody detection by enzyme immunoassay (EIA) technique, HIV-1 and/or HIV-2, screening

G0433 Infectious agent antibody detection by enzyme-linked immunosorbent assay (ELISA) technique, HIV-1 and/or HIV-2, screening

G0435 Infectious agent antibody detection by rapid antibody test, HIV-1 and/or HIV-2, screening

These codes describe the screening tests used for early detection of HIV infection. The enzyme immunoassay (EIA) technique is the conventional test. The analysis is homogenous (no physical separation is done during the analysis). The enzyme-linked immunosorbent assay (ELIASA) is similar to the EIA but is heterogenous (the plate is washed before the reaction is allowed to be completed) and usually produces more accurate results. The HIV rapid antibody test can produce results in about 20 minutes and although it is usually done with oral fluids, it may also be done with blood from a finger stick.

G0438-G0439

G0438 Annual wellness visit; includes a personalized prevention plan of service (PPS), initial visit

G0439 Annual wellness visit, includes a personalized prevention plan of service (PPS), subsequent visit

The initial annual wellness visit (AWV) includes taking the patient's history; compiling a list of the patient's current providers; taking the patient's vital signs, including height and weight; reviewing the patient's risk factor for depression; identifying any cognitive impairment; reviewing the patient's functional ability and level of safety (based on observation or screening questions); setting up a written patient screening schedule; compiling a list of risk factors, and furnishing personalized health services and referrals, as necessary. Subsequent annual wellness visits (AWV) include updating the patient's medical and family history, updating the current provider list, obtaining the patient's vital signs and weight, identifying cognitive impairment, updating the screening schedule, updating the risk factors list, and providing personalized health advice to the patient.

G0442-G0443

G0442 Annual alcohol misuse screening, 5 to 15 minutes

G0443 Brief face-to-face behavioral counseling for alcohol misuse, 15 minutes

Screening and behavioral counseling interventions are used to identify and reduce alcohol misuse. Alcohol misuse includes risky/hazardous and harmful drinking that puts individuals at risk for future problems. Risky or hazardous drinking is defined by the United States Preventive Services Task Force (USPSTF) as "more than seven standard drinks per week or more than three drinks per occasion for women and anyone over the age of 65; more than 14 standard drinks per week or more than four drinks per occasion for men 65 years of age or younger; and alcohol use by pregnant women." Lower limits are recommended for patients taking medication that may interact with alcohol or who are performing activities that require attention, skill, or coordination, such as driving or operating heavy machinery or someone who has a medical condition that may be worsened by alcohol use. Harmful drinking is defined as anyone that is currently experiencing physical, social, or psychological harm from alcohol use but doesn't meet the criteria for dependence. Alcohol dependence can be defined as at least three of the following: tolerance; withdrawal symptoms; impaired control; preoccupation with acquisition or use; persistent desire or unsuccessful efforts to quit; sustains social, occupational, or recreational disability; or used continually despite adverse conditions. The face-to-face counseling code is reported for visits for patients, including pregnant women, who misuse alcohol but don't meet the criteria for alcohol dependence; who are competent and alert at the time counseling is provided; and whose counseling is furnished by a health care professional in the primary care setting. Report G0442 for an annual alcohol misuse screening lasting five to 15 minutes. Report G0443 for brief (15 minutes) face-to-face behavioral counseling for alcohol misuse.

G0444

G0444 Annual depression screening, 5 to 15 minutes

Annual depression screening services are used to identify depression in patients. There should be staff in place to ensure accurate diagnosis, effective treatment, follow-up, and coordinate referrals. There are various tools that can be used to determine the screening. Depression screening services do not include treatment options for depression or any diseases, complications, or chronic conditions that the patient may have due to the depression. It also doesn't include any therapeutic interventions, such as medication therapy, or a combination of drug and counseling to treat the depression. Report G0444 for an annual depression screening lasting from five to 15 minutes.

G0445

G0445 Semiannual high intensity behavioral counseling to prevent STIs, individual, face-to-face, includes education skills training & guidance on how to change sexual behavior

This code reports high intensity behavioral counseling to prevent sexually transmitted infections (STI) for sexually active and at risk patients. Risk reduction includes education, behavior modification, and skills training. The United States Preventive Services Task Force (USPSTF) considers patients at high or increased risk who have any of the following conducts: multiple sex partners, using barrier protection inconsistently, having sex under the influence of alcohol or drugs, having sex in exchange for money or drugs, age (24 years of age or younger and sexually active for women for chlamydia and gonorrhea), having an STI within the past year, and IV drug use (hepatitis B only). Men having sex with men (MSM) and engaged in high risk sexual behavior are also considered at risk. The health care provider should also determine risk factors not based on individual behavior, such as a high instance of sexually communicable diseases in the community. Behavioral counseling interventions should include the following Five A's approach that has been adopted by the (USPSTF): Assess: Ask about/assess behavioral health risk(s) and factors affecting choice of behavior and change goals/methods; Advise: Give clear, specific, and personalized behavior change advice, including information about personal health harms and benefits; Agree: Collaboratively select appropriate treatment goals and methods based on the patient's interest in and willingness to change the behavior; Assist: Using behavior change techniques (self-help and/or counseling), aid the patient in achieving agreed-upon goals by acquiring the skills, confidence, and social/environmental supports for behavior change, supplemented with adjunctive medical treatments when appropriate; Arrange: Schedule follow-up contacts (in person or by telephone) to provide ongoing assistance/support and to adjust the treatment plan as needed, including referral to more intensive or specialized treatment. The appropriate diagnosis code should be reported on the claim to indicate the risk factor.

G0446

G0446 Annual, face-to-face intensive behavioral therapy for cardiovascular disease, individual, 15 minutes

Annual intensive behavioral therapy for cardiovascular disease for risk reduction is reported with this code. Risk reduction includes encouraging aspirin therapy for the primary prevention of cardiovascular disease when the benefits outweigh the risks for men ages 45 to 70 years and women 55 to 79 years; screening for high blood pressure for patients 18 years and older; and intensive behavioral counseling to promote a healthy diet for adults with hyperlipidemia, hypertension, advancing age, and any other risk factors for cardiovascular and diet-related chronic disease. Behavioral counseling interventions should include the following Five A's approach that has been adopted by the United States Preventive Services Task Force (USPSTF): Assess: Ask about/assess behavioral health risk(s) and factors affecting choice of behavior and change goals/methods; Advise: Give clear, specific, and personalized behavior change advice, including information about personal health harms and benefits; Agree: Collaboratively select appropriate treatment goals and methods based on the patient's interest in and willingness to change the behavior; Assist: Using behavior change techniques (self-help and/or counseling), aid the patient in achieving agreed-upon goals by acquiring the skills, confidence, and social/environmental supports for behavior change, supplemented with adjunctive medical treatments when appropriate; Arrange: Schedule follow-up contacts (in person or by telephone) to provide ongoing assistance/support and to adjust the treatment plan as needed, including referral to more intensive or specialized treatment.

G0447

G0447 Face-to-face behavioral counseling for obesity, 15 minutes

Behavioral counseling for obesity is reported with this code. The United States Preventive Services Task Force (USPSTF) considers body mass index (BMI) a good indication of morbidity and mortality because of being overweight or obese. BMI is calculated using the following formula: BMI = (weight in pounds / (height in inches x height in inches)) x 703. Obese adults are considered those that have a BMI >=30 kg/m2. Behavioral counseling and behavior modification can be an effective combination to produce moderate, sustainable weight loss. The patients should have the following services: screening for obesity using BMI, assessment of food and nutritional intake, and counseling to include diet and exercise. Behavioral counseling interventions should include the following Five A's approach that has been developed by the United States Preventive Services Task Force (USPSTF): Assess: Ask about/assess behavioral health risk(s) and factors affecting choice of behavior and change goals/methods; Advise: Give clear, specific, and personalized behavior change advice, including information about personal health harms and benefits; Agree: Collaboratively select appropriate treatment goals and methods based on the patient's interest in and willingness to change the behavior; Assist: Using behavior change techniques (self-help and/or counseling), aid the patient in achieving agreed-upon goals by acquiring the skills, confidence, and social/environmental supports for behavior change, supplemented with adjunctive medical treatments when appropriate; Arrange: Schedule follow-up contacts (in person or by telephone) to provide ongoing assistance/support and to adjust the treatment plan as needed, including referral to more intensive or specialized treatment.

G0448

G0448 Insertion or replacement of a permanent pacing cardioverter-defibrillator system with transvenous lead(s), single or dual chamber with insertion of pacing electrode, cardiac venous system, for left ventricular pacing

This code is reported only by an ambulatory surgery center (ASC) when a permanent pacing cardioverter-defibrillator (ICD) system with transvenous lead(s), single or dual chamber, is inserted or replaced on the same date of service and at the same time as insertion of a pacing electrode, cardiac venous system, for left ventricular pacing (including upgrade to dual chamber system and pocket revision). Hospital outpatient departments and physicians continue to report the appropriate CPT codes. The physician inserts or replaces a permanent pacing cardioverter-defibrillator system, including the pulse generator with transvenous electrode placement. Transvenous placement is currently the most common technique for placing implantable cardioverter-defibrillator electrodes. An ICD is a device designed to administer an electric shock to control cardiac arrhythmias and restore a normal heartbeat. Local anesthesia is administered. An incision is made in the infraclavicular area. The subcutaneous tissue is opened and a pocket is created for the pulse generator. Transvenous electrode placement is performed under separately reportable fluoroscopic guidance. The electrode catheter is advanced through the superior vena cava into the heart and placed in the appropriate site in the right ventricle (single chamber system) or in the right ventricle and atrium (dual chamber system). Multiple leads may be required for single and dual chamber systems. When biventricular pacing is required, an additional electrode is placed in the left ventricle. A fluoroscope may be used for guidance and a pacing electrode is inserted in the left ventricular chamber of the heart, usually in the coronary sinus tributary. The electrode is connected to the generator and the generator pocket is closed.

G0451

G0451 Development testing, with interpretation and report, per standardized instrument form

Developmental testing is an assessment of the patient's mastery of developmental milestones. The assessment usually includes observation, interviews, and actual tests. The aim is to assess the person's current skills based on standardized criteria for each age group. This code represents testing using a standardized test form and includes the interpretation and a report prepared by a professional practitioner.

G0452

G0452 Molecular pathology procedure; physician interpretation and report

A molecular pathology procedure physician interpretation and report is used to report a medically necessary interpretation and written report of a molecular pathology test, above and beyond the report of laboratory results. This is a professional component only.

G0453

G0453 Continuous intraoperative neurophysiology monitoring, from outside the operating room (remote or nearby), per patient, (attention directed exclusively to one patient) each 15 minutes (list in addition to primary procedure)

Continuous intraoperative neurophysiology monitoring (IONM) is performed by a qualified health care provider other than the surgeon or anesthesiologist involved in the surgical procedure. IONM may include various electrophysiologic modalities, such as electroencephalography (EEG), electromyography (EMG), and evoked potentials. The provider must be solely dedicated to monitoring the neurophysiological tests and available to intervene if necessary.

G0454

G0454 Physician documentation of face-to-face visit for durable medical equipment determination performed by nurse practitioner, physician assistant or clinical nurse specialist

This HCPCS Level II code allows a physician who documents that a PA, NP, or CNS practitioner has performed a face-to-face encounter for the list of specified DME covered items to be paid for the service.

G0455

G0455 Preparation with instillation of fecal microbiota by any method, including assessment of donor specimen

Fecal microbiota transplantation (FMT) is the process of instilling fecal matter from a donor to a patient to treat a *Clostridium difficile* (*C. diff*) infection, most commonly. The donor stool is thinned using a normal saline solution and filtered for use in a nasogastric tube or an enema application. This code includes the screening protocol of the donor specimen for *C. diff* and other enteric bacterial pathogens and any ova or parasites.

G0458

G0458 Low dose rate (LDR) prostate brachytherapy services, composite rate

Low dose rate (LDR) brachytherapy is performed by inserting tiny permanent radioactive iodine (I-125) seeds into the prostate. The seeds are small enough that the patient does not feel their presence. The seeds emit a low dose radiation that is absorbed by the prostate gland. The treatment is customized to the patient based on the shape and size of the prostate. There are normally about 90 to 120 seeds implanted. The seeds deliver a radiation field capable of destroying the prostate cancer cells. The level of radiation gradually decreases over several months.

G0459

G0459 Inpatient telehealth pharmacologic management, including prescription, use, and review of medication with no more than minimal medical psychotherapy

Medication management is furnished via telehealth, which is the delivery of health-related services via telecommunications equipment.

G0460

G0460 Autologous platelet rich plasma for nondiabetic chronic wounds/ulcers, including phlebotomy, centrifugation, and all other preparatory procedures, administration and dressings, per treatment

Autologous platelet rich plasma (PRP) for nondiabetic chronic wounds/ulcers, including phlebotomy, centrifugation, and all other preparatory procedures, administration, and dressings, per treatment, is a biological prepared from the patient's blood that is used for nonhealing wounds. CMS covers autologous PRP only for the treatment of chronic, nondiabetic, venous, and/or pressure wounds when PRP is provided as a randomized clinical trial that meets specific requirements to assess the health outcomes of PRP for the treatment of chronic nondiabetic, venous, and/or pressure wounds.

G0463

G0463 Hospital outpatient clinic visit for assessment and management of a patient

OPPS hospitals are to report this code in place of CPT codes 99202–99205 and 99211–99215 for clinic visits. There is no distinction between new and established patients or levels of care.

G0465

G0465 Autologous platelet rich plasma (PRP) for diabetic chronic wounds/ulcers, using an FDA-cleared device (includes administration, dressings, phlebotomy, centrifugation, and all other preparatory procedures, per treatment)

Autologous platelet rich plasma (PRP) for chronic wounds/ulcers, including phlebotomy, centrifugation, and all other preparatory procedures, administration, and dressings, per treatment, is a biological prepared from the patient's blood that is used for nonhealing wounds. CMS covers autologous PRP only for the treatment of chronic, nonhealing diabetic wounds for up to 20 weeks when prepared by devices with FDA-cleared indications that include management of exuding cutaneous wounds, such as diabetic ulcers. Extension of coverage beyond 20 weeks is determined by local Medicare Administrative Contractors (MACs).

G0466-G0467

G0466 Federally qualified health center (FQHC) visit, new patient

G0467 Federally qualified health center (FQHC) visit, established patient

A new patient (G0466) or established patient (G0467) is seen in a federally qualified health center (FQHC). This service is payable under the FQHC prospective payment system (PPS). Code G0466 must be accompanied by qualifying visit code 92002, 92004, 97802, 99202-99205, 99324-99325, 99328, 99341-99345, 99381-99387, 99406, 99407,G0101, G0102, G0108, G0117, G0118, or G0442-G0447. Code G0467 must be accompanied by qualifying visit code 92012, 92014, 97802, 97803, 99211-99215, 99304-99310, 99315, 99316, 99318, 99334-99337, 99347-99350, 99391-99397, 99406, 99407, 99495, 99496, G0101, G0102, G0108, G0117, G0118, G0270, or G0442-G0447. Medical visit codes G0466-G0468 must be reported with revenue code 052X or 0519.

G0468

G0468 Federally qualified health center (FQHC) visit, initial preventive physical exam (IPPE) or annual wellness visit (AWV)

An initial preventive physical exam (IPPE) or an annual wellness visit (AWV) is performed in a federally qualified health center (FQHC). This service is payable under the FQHC prospective payment system (PPS). Code G0468 must be accompanied by qualifying visit code G0402, G0438, or G0439. Medical visit codes G0466–G0468 must be reported with revenue code 052X or 0519.

G0469-G0470

G0469 Federally qualified health center (FQHC) visit, mental health, new patient

G0470 Federally qualified health center (FQHC) visit, mental health, established patient

A new patient (G0469) or established patient (G0470) is seen for a mental health visit at a federally qualified health center (FQHC). This service is payable under the FQHC prospective payment system (PPS). Codes G0469 and G0470 must be accompanied by qualifying visit code 90791, 90792, 90832–90839, or 90845. Mental health visit codes G0469 and G0470 must be reported with revenue code 0900 or 0519.

G0471

G0471 Collection of venous blood by venipuncture or urine sample by catheterization from an individual in a skilled nursing facility (SNF) or by a laboratory on behalf of a home health agency (HHA)

This code reports the collection of venous blood by venipuncture or a urine sample by catheterization from an individual in a skilled nursing facility (SNF) or by a laboratory on behalf of a home health agency (HHA). This code should only be reported when the following statements apply. The sample is being collected by a laboratory technician that is employed by the laboratory performing the test or the sample is from an individual in an SNF or HHA.

G0472

G0472 Hepatitis C antibody screening for individual at high risk and other covered indication(s)

Hepatitis C virus (HCV) screenings test for HCV antibodies that indicate an infection with the hepatitis C virus. Results are usually reported as reactive or nonreactive. Screening for HCV is covered when ordered by the patient's primary care physician or practitioner within the context of a primary care setting, for the following patients. 1) Patients who are not high risk and are born between 1945 and 1965. A single screening test is covered for adults who do not meet the high risk criteria. HCV screening is limited to once per lifetime. 2) Adults at high risk for HCV infection. High risk is defined as persons with a current or past history of illicit injection drug use and persons who have a history of receiving a blood transfusion prior to 1992. Repeat screening for high-risk persons is covered annually only for persons who have had continued illicit injection drug use since the prior negative screening test. The determination of high risk for HCV is in the hands of the primary care physician or practitioner who assesses the patient's history, which is part of any complete medical history. The medical record should be a reflection of the service provided. 3) Beneficiaries determined to be high-risk. Initially ICD-10-CM diagnosis code Z72.89 (Other problems related to lifestyle) is required. For repeat annual testing, report ICD-10-CM diagnosis code F19.20 (Other psychoactive substance abuse, uncomplicated).

G0473

G0473 Face-to-face behavioral counseling for obesity, group (2-10), 30 minutes

Behavioral counseling for obesity in a group setting is reported with this code. The United States Preventive Services Task Force (USPSTF) considers body mass index (BMI) a good indication of morbidity and mortality. BMI is calculated using the following formula: BMI = (weight in pounds / (height in inches x height in inches)) x 703. Obese adults are considered those that have a BMI >=30 kg/m2. Behavioral counseling and behavior modification can be an effective combination to produce moderate, sustainable weight loss. The patients should have the following services: screening for obesity using BMI, assessment of food and nutritional intake, and counseling to include diet and exercise. Behavioral counseling interventions should include the following Five A's approach that has been developed by the United States Preventive Services Task Force (USPSTF): Assess: Ask about/assess behavioral health risk(s) and factors affecting choice of behavior and change goals/methods; Advise: Give clear, specific, and personalized behavior change advice, including information about personal health harms and benefits; Agree: Collaboratively select appropriate treatment goals and methods based on the patient's interest in and willingness to change the behavior; Assist: Using behavior change techniques (self-help and/or counseling), aid the patient in achieving agreed-upon goals by acquiring the skills, confidence, and social/environmental supports for behavior change, supplemented with adjunctive medical treatments when appropriate; Arrange: Schedule follow-up contacts (in person or by telephone) to provide ongoing assistance/support and to adjust the treatment plan as needed, including referral to more intensive or specialized treatment.

G0475

G0475 HIV antigen/antibody, combination assay, screening

These new combination assays allow for the testing of the HIV antibody, as well as antigen detection. This combination test is helpful in closing the window period (the time between HIV infection and appearance of antibodies to HIV) as HIV antigen is present in the blood before antibodies to HIV can be detected. Evaluation of testing kits by the WHO provided information on serum/plasma samples of various origins, seroconversion panels, and low titer panels.

G0476

G0476 Infectious agent detection by nucleic acid (DNA or RNA); human papillomavirus HPV), high-risk types (e.g., 16, 18, 31, 33, 35, 39, 45, 51, 52, 56, 58, 59, 68) for cervical cancer screening, must be performed in addition to pap test

Human papillomavirus detection by nucleic acid can be seen in biopsy samples taken in conjunction with a pap test for cervical cancer screening. In situ hybridization can visualize nucleic acid sequences within the cells to evaluate discrepancies pertaining to the lesion. Indicators may identify the form of the target DNA, while signal intensity may identify copy numbers. The assay can identify one to two copies of a target sequence per nucleus, which is more refined than the one- or three-step methods.

G0480-G0483

G0480 Drug test(s), definitive, utilizing (1) drug identification methods able to identify individual drugs and distinguish between structural isomers (but not necessarily stereoisomers), including, but not limited to, GC/MS (any type, single or tandem) and LC/MS (any type, single or tandem and excluding immunoassays (e.g., IA, EIA, ELISA, EMIT, FPIA) and enzymatic methods (e.g., alcohol dehydrogenase)), (2) stable isotope or other universally recognized internal standards in all samples (e.g., to control for matrix effects, interferences and variations in signal strength), and (3) method or drug-specific calibration and matrix-matched quality control material (e.g., to control for instrument variations and mass spectral drift); qualitative or quantitative, all sources, includes specimen validity testing, per day; 1-7 drug class(es), including metabolite(s) if performed

G0481 Drug test(s), definitive, utilizing (1) drug identification methods able to identify individual drugs and distinguish between structural isomers (but not necessarily stereoisomers), including, but not limited to, GC/MS (any type, single or tandem) and LC/MS (any type, single or tandem and excluding immunoassays (e.g., IA, EIA, ELISA, EMIT, FPIA) and enzymatic methods (e.g., alcohol dehydrogenase)), (2) stable isotope or other universally recognized internal standards in all samples (e.g., to control for matrix effects, interferences and variations in signal strength), and (3) method or drug-specific calibration and matrix-matched quality control material (e.g., to control for instrument variations and mass spectral drift); qualitative or quantitative, all sources, includes specimen validity testing, per day; 8-14 drug class(es), including metabolite(s) if performed

G0482 Drug test(s), definitive, utilizing (1) drug identification methods able to identify individual drugs and distinguish between structural isomers (but not necessarily stereoisomers), including, but not limited to, GC/MS (any type, single or tandem) and LC/MS (any type, single or tandem and excluding immunoassays (e.g., IA, EIA, ELISA, EMIT, FPIA) and enzymatic methods (e.g., alcohol dehydrogenase)), (2) stable isotope or other universally recognized internal standards in all samples (e.g., to control for matrix effects, interferences and variations in signal strength), and (3) method or drug-specific calibration and matrix-matched quality control material (e.g., to control for instrument variations and mass spectral drift); qualitative or quantitative, all sources, includes specimen validity testing, per day; 15-21 drug class(es), including metabolite(s) if performed

G0483 Drug test(s), definitive, utilizing (1) drug identification methods able to identify individual drugs and distinguish between structural isomers (but not necessarily stereoisomers), including, but not limited to, GC/MS (any type, single or tandem) and LC/MS (any type, single or tandem and excluding immunoassays (e.g., IA, EIA, ELISA, EMIT, FPIA) and enzymatic methods (e.g., alcohol dehydrogenase)), (2) stable isotope or other universally recognized internal standards in all samples (e.g., to control for matrix effects, interferences and variations in signal strength), and (3) method or drug-specific calibration and matrix-matched quality control material (e.g., to control for instrument variations and mass spectral drift); qualitative or quantitative, all sources, includes specimen validity testing, per day; 22 or more drug class(es), including metabolite(s) if performed

CPT codes reported for drug testing are grouped into drug classes and further broken down into therapeutic assays, presumptive testing, and definitive testing. Medicare is not prepared to accept and process the codes based on drug classes and has instead divided the procedures into presumptive and definitive categories only. Presumptive testing should be reported with the appropriate CPT code (80305-80307). Definitive testing may be reported once per day with one of the five definitive codes (G0480-G0483, G0659). Report G0659 for definitive testing of any number of drug classes, but without method or other drug-specific calibration. Report G0480 for definitive testing of one to seven drug classes; G0481 for eight to 14 drug classes; G0482 for 15 to 21 drug classes, and G0483 for 22 or more drug classes.

G0490

G0490 Face-to-face home health nursing visit by a rural health clinic (RHC) or federally qualified health center (FQHC) in an area with a shortage of home health agencies; (services limited to RN or LPN only)

A homebound patient located in areas with a shortage of home health agencies receives part-time or intermittent nursing care and supplies provided by a registered professional nurse (RN) or licensed practical nurse (LPN) under a written plan of treatment. This service is payable under the RHC all-inclusive rate payment system when reported on a RHC claim with revenue code 052X and modifier CG. This service is payable under the FQHC prospective payment system when reported on a FQHC claim with revenue code 052X and HCPCS Level II code G0466 (new patient) or G0467 (established patient).

G0491-G0492

G0491 Dialysis procedure at a Medicare certified ESRD facility for acute kidney injury without ESRD

G0492 Dialysis procedure with single evaluation by a physician or other qualified health care professional for acute kidney injury without ESRD

End stage renal disease (ESRD) facilities are able to furnish dialysis to acute kidney injury (AKI) patients. The AKI provision provides Medicare payment for renal dialysis services furnished to adult and pediatric patients beginning on dates of service January 1, 2017 and after to ESRD facilities, both hospital-based and freestanding. Medicare reimbursement for the dialysis treatment is based on the ESRD Prospective Payment System (PPS) base rate adjusted by the applicable geographic adjustment factor (wage index). The ESRD PPS base rate reimburses ESRD facilities for the items and services considered to be renal dialysis services; there is no separate payment for renal dialysis drugs, biologicals, laboratory services, or supplies when they are furnished by an ESRD facility to an individual with AKI. Code G0491 represents a dialysis procedure and G0492 represents a dialysis procedure with single evaluation by a physician or other qualified health care professional for acute kidney injury without ESRD.

G0493-G0496

G0493 Skilled services of a registered nurse (RN) for the observation and assessment of the patient's condition, each 15 minutes (the change in the patient's condition requires skilled nursing personnel to identify and evaluate the patient's need for possible modification of treatment in the home health or hospice setting)

G0494 Skilled services of a licensed practical nurse (LPN) for the observation and assessment of the patient's condition, each 15 minutes (the change in the patient's condition requires skilled nursing personnel to identify and evaluate the patient's need for possible modification of treatment in the home health or hospice setting)

G0495 Skilled services of a registered nurse (RN), in the training and/or education of a patient or family member, in the home health or hospice setting, each 15 minutes

G0496 Skilled services of a licensed practical nurse (LPN), in the training and/or education of a patient or family member, in the home health or hospice setting, each 15 minutes

These codes report services provided by nurses in a home health or hospice setting in 15-minute increments. Home health includes not only traditional private home settings, but also assisted living quarters, group homes, custodial care facilities, or similar type settings that constitute the patient's place of residence. Codes G0493 and G0494 represent the observation and assessment of the patient's condition; G0495 and G0496 represent the training and/or education of a patient or family member. For claims received on or after April 1, 2017, with dates of service on or after January 1, 2017, HHAs report visits previously reported with G0163 with one of the following codes: G0493 or G0494. HHAs report G0495 or G0496 in place of G0164.

G0498

G0498 Chemotherapy administration, intravenous infusion technique; initiation of infusion in the office/clinic setting using office/clinic pump/supplies, with continuation of the infusion in the community setting (e.g., home, domiciliary, rest home or assisted living) using a portable pump provided by the office/clinic, includes follow up office/clinic visit at the conclusion of the infusion

Home infusion therapy is intravenous (IV) administration of medication or fluids to patients in their own home. It is done as an alternative to receiving IV therapy in a clinical setting. Nurses and other specially trained individuals provide the insertion and management services of the IV and IV equipment, such as the IV pump. This code reports prolonged drug and biological infusions, continuing in the community setting, started incident to a physician service using a portable IV pump. Code G0498 is reported once per episode of care and includes the follow up office or clinic visit at the end of the infusion. Providers should continue to report the appropriate codes for drugs or biologicals as they are not included in the reimbursement for the pump administration.

G0499

G0499 Hepatitis B screening in nonpregnant, high-risk individual includes hepatitis B surface antigen (HBSAG), antibodies to HBSAG (anti-HBS) and antibodies to hepatitis B core antigen (anti-HBC), and is followed by a neutralizing confirmatory test, when performed, only for an initially reactive HBSAG result

CMS covers screenings for HBV infection with the appropriate FDA approved/cleared laboratory tests, used consistent with FDA approved labeling and in compliance with Clinical Laboratory Improvement Act (CLIA) regulations. The test must be ordered by the patient's primary care physician or practitioner within the context of a primary care setting, and performed by an eligible Medicare provider. The test is covered for patients that meet either of the following conditions: symptomatic, nonpregnant adolescents and adults at high risk for HBV infection; or at the first prenatal visit for pregnant women and then rescreening at time of delivery for those with new or continuing risk factors. High risk is defined as persons born in countries and regions with a high prevalence of HBV infection (i.e., ≥ 2%), US-born persons not vaccinated as infants whose parents were born in regions with a very high prevalence of HBV infection (i.e., ≥ 8%), HIV-positive persons, men who have sex with men, injection drug users, and household contacts or sexual partners of persons with HBV infection. CMS has determined that repeated screening is appropriate annually only for beneficiaries with continued high risk (i.e., men who have sex with men, injection drug users, household contacts or sexual partners of persons with HBV infection) who do not receive hepatitis B vaccination. In addition, CMS has determined that screening during the first prenatal visit is appropriate for each pregnancy, regardless of previous hepatitis B vaccination or previous negative hepatitis B surface antigen (HBsAg) test results.

G0500

G0500 Moderate sedation services provided by the same physician or other qualified health care professional performing a gastrointestinal endoscopic service that sedation supports, requiring the presence of an independent trained observer to assist in the monitoring of the patient's level of consciousness and physiological status; initial 15 minutes of intra-service time; patient age 5 years or older (additional time may be reported with 99153, as appropriate)

A physician or other trained health care provider administers medication that allows a decreased level of consciousness, but does not put the patient completely asleep, inducing a state called moderate (conscious) sedation. This allows the patient to breathe without assistance and respond to commands. This code is specific to gastrointestinal endoscopic services. This code reports sedation services provided by the same provider performing the primary procedure with the assistance of an independently trained health care professional to assist in monitoring the patient. Report CPT code 99153 separately in addition to this code for each additional 15 minutes of intra-service time.

G0501

G0501 Resource-intensive services for patients for whom the use of specialized mobility-assistive technology (such as adjustable height chairs or tables, patient lift, and adjustable padded leg supports) is medically necessary and used during the provision of an office/outpatient, evaluation and management visit (list separately in addition to primary service)

Code GO501 is an add-on code that represents the additional services furnished in conjunction with E/M services rendered to patients with mobility-related disabilities. When a person with a mobility-related disability goes to a physician or other practitioner's office for an E/M visit, the patient often requires resources that exceed the norm for the typical E/M visit. This code allows a payment adjustment for routine visits furnished to disabled patients for whom the use of specialized mobility-assistive technology is medically necessary, such as adjustable height chairs or tables, patient lifts, or adjustable padded leg supports. Code G0501 is not payable under the Medicare PFS for CY 2017, but practitioners may report the code, should they be inclined to do so.

G0506

G0506 Comprehensive assessment of and care planning for patients requiring chronic care management services (list separately in addition to primary monthly care management service)

This is an add-on code to be reported with another E/M service (the chronic care management initiating visit, which can be the AWV/IPPE or a qualifying face-to-face E/M visit). It cannot be an add-on code for a behavioral health initiative (BHI) initiating visit or BHI services. The care plan that the practitioner must create to report G0506 is subject to the same requirements as the care plan included in the monthly CCM services. It must be an electronic patient-centered care plan based on a physical, mental, cognitive, psychosocial, functional, and environmental (re)assessment and an inventory of resources and supports, a comprehensive care plan for all health issues. This distinguishes it from the more limited care planning included in the BHI codes, or the care planning included in G0505, which focuses on cognitive status. Work and time that is reported under G0506 should also not be reported under or counted toward the reporting of any other code reported, including any monthly CCM services codes. This code is reportable one time, at the outset of CCM services, WV/IPPE, or a qualifying face-to-face E/M visit.

G0508-G0509

G0508 Telehealth consultation, critical care, initial, physicians typically spend 60 minutes communicating with the patient and providers via telehealth

G0509 Telehealth consultation, critical care, subsequent, physicians typically spend 50 minutes communicating with the patient and providers via telehealth

Codes G0508 and G0509 represent professional consultations furnished via an interactive telecommunications system. An interactive telecommunications system is defined as multimedia communications equipment that includes, at a minimum, audio and video equipment permitting two-way, real-time interactive communication between the patient and distant site physician or practitioner. Code G0508 represents an initial 60-minute consultation for patients requiring critical care services, such as a stroke patient. Code G0509 represents a subsequent 50-minute consultation for critical care. The physician may communicate with the patient or a caregiver. In general, CMS feels that the overall work for G0508 is not as great as the critical care services of CPT code 99291, but that the service involves more work than G0427. Do not report G0508 or G0509 more than once per day.

G0511

G0511 Rural health clinic or federally qualified health center (RHC or FQHC) only, general care management, 20 minutes or more of clinical staff time for chronic care management services or behavioral health integration services directed by an RHC or FQHC practitioner (physician, NP, PA, or CNM), per calendar month

This code is intended to represent the care and management of Medicare patients with chronic care needs or behavioral health conditions that often require discussion, information-sharing, and planning between a primary care physician and a specialist. This code represents 20 minutes or more of clinical staff time for psychiatric collaborative care model (CoCM) services directed by a RHC or FQHC practitioner (physician, NP, PA, or CNM) per calendar month.

G0512

G0512 Rural health clinic or federally qualified health center (RHC/FQHC) only, psychiatric collaborative care model (psychiatric COCM), 60 minutes or more of clinical staff time for psychiatric COCM services directed by an RHC or FQHC practitioner (physician, NP, PA, or CNM) and including services furnished by a behavioral health care manager and consultation with a psychiatric consultant, per calendar month

Psychiatric collaborative care model (CoCM) is a specific, evidence-based model for behavioral health and psychiatric services. CoCM is typically provided by a primary care team consisting of a primary care provider and a care manager who works in collaboration with a consultant, such as a psychiatrist. Care is directed by the primary care team and includes structured care management with regular assessments of clinical status using validated tools and modification of treatment as appropriate. The psychiatric consultant provides regular consultations to the primary care team to review the clinical status and care of patients and to make recommendations. These codes are intended to represent the care and management for Medicare patients with behavioral health conditions that often require extensive discussion, information-sharing, and planning between a primary care physician and a specialist. This code represents 60 minutes or more of clinical staff time for psychiatric CoCM services directed by a RHC

G

or FQHC practitioner (physician, NP, PA, or CNM). It also includes services provided by a behavioral health care manager and consultation with a psychiatric consultant, per calendar month.

G0513-G0514

G0513 Prolonged preventive service(s) (beyond the typical service time of the primary procedure), in the office or other outpatient setting requiring direct patient contact beyond the usual service; first 30 minutes (list separately in addition to code for preventive service)

G0514 Prolonged preventive service(s) (beyond the typical service time of the primary procedure), in the office or other outpatient setting requiring direct patient contact beyond the usual service; each additional 30 minutes (list separately in addition to code G0513 for additional 30 minutes of preventive service)

The physician performs a thorough review of the patient's health. The physician takes a medical history on the patient and performs an exam that includes a blood pressure check, height and weight assessment, and a vision screen. Depending on the medical history information provided by the patient and the results of the physical examination, the physician orders or performs additional tests as medically necessary. The physician also provides preventive medicine education and counseling services based on the patient's medical history and examination results. The physician provides a written plan of care to the patient detailing any follow-up screening or preventive services that the patient should receive. These codes are add-on codes and must be reported along with the primary code for the preventive service. Report G0513 for the first 30 minutes of prolonged times and G0514 for each additional 30 minutes of time. Report G0514 in conjunction with G0513.

G0516-G0518

G0516 Insertion of nonbiodegradable drug delivery implants, four or more (services for subdermal rod implant)

G0517 Removal of nonbiodegradable drug delivery implants, four or more (services for subdermal implants)

G0518 Removal with reinsertion, nonbiodegradable drug delivery implants, four or more (services for subdermal implants)

A nonbiodegradable drug delivery implant is inserted to deliver a therapeutic dose of the drug continuously at a predetermined rate of release. One such system works via a semipermeable membrane at one end of the subcutaneous cylinder that permits the entrance of fluid; the drug is delivered from a port at the other end of the cylinder at a controlled rate appropriate to the specific therapeutic agent. The physician injects local anesthesia and makes a small incision in the skin with a scalpel to insert the miniature drug-containing cylinder, which is held in place with sutures tied by a knot or secured by a single running stitch. Various types of medications for different indications may be administered via a nonbiodegradable drug delivery implant system. In G0516, the physician inserts four or more drug delivery implants through a small incision. In G0517, the physician removes previously implanted drug delivery implants, four or more, through a small incision. In G0518, the physician removes previously implanted drug delivery implants, four or more, through a small incision and inserts four or more replacements. The wounds are sutured closed.

G0659

G0659 Drug test(s), definitive, utilizing drug identification methods able to identify individual drugs and distinguish between structural isomers (but not necessarily stereoisomers), including but not limited to, GC/MS (any type, single or tandem) and LC/MS (any type, single or tandem), excluding immunoassays (e.g., IA, EIA, ELISA, EMIT, FPIA) and enzymatic methods (e.g., alcohol dehydrogenase), performed without method or drug-specific calibration, without matrix-matched quality control material, or without use of stable isotope or other universally recognized internal standard(s) for each drug, drug metabolite or drug class per specimen; qualitative or quantitative, all sources, includes specimen validity testing, per day, any number of drug classes

CPT codes reported for drug testing are grouped into drug classes and further broken down into therapeutic assays, presumptive testing, and definitive testing. Medicare is not prepared to accept and process the codes based on drug classes and has instead divided the procedures into presumptive and definitive categories only. Presumptive testing should be reported with the appropriate CPT code (80305-80307). Definitive testing may be reported once per day with one of the five definitive codes (G0480-G0483, G0659). Report G0659 for definitive testing of any number of drug classes, but without method or other drug-specific calibration. Report G0480 for definitive testing of one to seven drug classes; G0481 for eight to 14 drug classes; G0482 for 15 to 21 drug classes, and G0483 for 22 or more drug classes.

G1028

G1028 Take-home supply of nasal naloxone; 2-pack of 8 mg per 0.1 ml nasal spray (provision of the services by a Medicare-enrolled Opioid Treatment Program); list separately in addition to code for primary procedure

This code reports the provision of a take-home supply of the drug naloxone indicated by an opioid treatment program (OTP). Report G1028 for nasal naloxone, two-pack of 8 mg per 0.1 ml nasal spray in addition to a code for the primary service. One add-on code (G1028) is allowed every 30 days; however, exceptions to this limit are allowed in cases in which the beneficiary overdoses and uses the initial supply of naloxone dispensed by the OTP to the extent that it is medically reasonable and necessary to furnish additional naloxone. If an additional supply is needed within 30 days of the original supply being provided, the OTP must document in the medical record the reason for the exception. These codes also include overdose education, and it is expected that when OTPs provide beneficiaries with a supply of naloxone, they will also inform them about how to use the medication they are being given.

G2000

G2000 Blinded administration of convulsive therapy procedure, either electroconvulsive therapy (ECT, current covered gold standard) or magnetic seizure therapy (MST, noncovered experimental therapy), performed in an approved IDE-based clinical trial, per treatment session

Electroconvulsive therapy (ECT) is used to treat mental illness. After the induction of general anesthesia and administration of a muscle relaxant, assisted ventilation with positive pressure oxygen is applied. A short electrical stimulus is applied to the scalp to induce a seizure of approximately one minute. The patient is monitored during the entire procedure. Magnetic Seizure Therapy (MST) uses high-frequency transcranial magnetic stimulation to induce therapeutic seizures. The electrical current used in MST can be targeted to avoid stimulation of the medial temporal lobe, which is thought to cause the cognitive impairments often associated with ECT.

G2010

G2010 Remote evaluation of recorded video and/or images submitted by an established patient (e.g., store and forward), including interpretation with follow-up with the patient within 24 business hours, not originating from a related E/M service provided within the previous 7 days nor leading to an E/M service or procedure within the next 24 hours or soonest available appointment

Physicians or other qualified practitioners review photos or video information submitted by the patient to determine if a visit is required. The service may be provided to an established patient when a related evaluation and management (E/M) service has not been provided in the previous seven days and may not lead to an E/M service within the next 24 hours or soonest available appointment.

G2011

G2011 Alcohol and/or substance (other than tobacco) misuse structured assessment (e.g., audit, dast), and brief intervention, 5-14 minutes

Assessment and brief intervention services lasting five to 14 minutes are directed at alcohol and substance misuse. Substance abuse screenings, utilizing instruments such as AUDIT and DAST, are used to determine the patient's opinion related to behavior change and provide input on a plan to change behavior with appropriate actions and motivation.

G2012

G2012 Brief communication technology-based service, e.g., virtual check-in, by a physician or other qualified health care professional who can report evaluation and management services, provided to an established patient, not originating from a related E/M service provided within the previous 7 days nor leading to an E/M service or procedure within the next 24 hours or soonest available appointment; 5-10 minutes of medical discussion

A physician or other qualified health care professional conducts a virtual check-in, lasting five to 10 minutes, for an established patient using a telephone or other telecommunication device to determine whether an office visit or other service is needed. The service may be provided when a related evaluation and management (E/M) service has not been provided in the previous seven days and it may not lead to an E/M service within the next 24 hours or soonest available appointment.

G2023-G2024

G2023 Specimen collection for Severe Acute Respiratory Syndrome Coronavirus 2 (SARS-CoV-2) (Coronavirus disease [COVID-19]), any specimen source

G2024 Specimen collection for severe acute respiratory syndrome coronavirus 2 (SARS-CoV-2) (coronavirus disease [COVID-19]) from an individual in a SNF or by a laboratory on behalf of a HHA, any specimen source

For clinical diagnostic laboratories, CMS has created codes that may be reported to identify and reimburse specimen collection for COVID-19 testing. Specimens may be obtained through a variety of sources, such as nasopharyngeal or oropharyngeal swab, nasopharyngeal wash or aspirate, nasal aspirate, or sputum.

G2025

G2025 Payment for a telehealth distant site service furnished by a Rural Health Clinic (RHC) or Federally Qualified Health Center (FQHC) only

A Federally Qualified Health Center (FQHC) or Rural Health Clinic (RHC) practitioner provides distant site telehealth services utilizing an interactive audio and video telecommunications system that allows for real-time communication between the patient and the provider. FQHCs and RHCs with these capabilities can immediately provide and be paid for distant site telehealth services to Medicare beneficiaries, for the duration of the COVID-19 Public Health Emergency (PHE). Services may be provided from any location, including the provider's home, during the period they are working for the FQHC or RHC, and can provide any telehealth service approved as distant site telehealth service under the Physician Fee Schedule (PFS). FQHCs and RHCs must report this code to identify services furnished via telehealth beginning January 27, 2020.

G2066

G2066 Interrogation device evaluation(s), (remote) up to 30 days; implantable cardiovascular physiologic monitor system, implantable loop recorder system, or subcutaneous cardiac rhythm monitor system, remote data acquisition(s), receipt of transmissions and technician review, technical support and distribution of results

Patients with a previously implanted cardiovascular physiologic monitor, loop recorder, or subcutaneous cardiac rhythm monitor system require periodic interrogation device evaluations. This code reports remote evaluation only and may be reported once per 30-day period. Evaluation includes the analysis of at least one recorded physiologic cardiovascular data element obtained from internal or external sensors. Report G2066 for the technical review, including technical support and distribution of results. The appropriate CPT code should be reported for the professional analysis of recorded heart rhythm data, including the provider's review and report. If the provider performs both the professional and technical components, report G2066 and the appropriate CPT code.

G2067-G2075

G2067 Medication assisted treatment, methadone; weekly bundle including dispensing and/or administration, substance use counseling, individual and group therapy, and toxicology testing, if performed (provision of the services by a Medicare-enrolled opioid treatment program)

G2068 Medication assisted treatment, buprenorphine (oral); weekly bundle including dispensing and/or administration, substance use counseling, individual and group therapy, and toxicology testing if performed (provision of the services by a Medicare-enrolled opioid treatment program)

G2069 Medication assisted treatment, buprenorphine (injectable); weekly bundle including dispensing and/or administration, substance use counseling, individual and group therapy, and toxicology testing if performed (provision of the services by a Medicare-enrolled opioid treatment program)

G2070 Medication assisted treatment, buprenorphine (implant insertion); weekly bundle including dispensing and/or administration, substance use counseling, individual and group therapy, and toxicology testing if performed (provision of the services by a Medicare-enrolled opioid treatment program)

G2071 Medication assisted treatment, buprenorphine (implant removal); weekly bundle including dispensing and/or administration, substance use counseling, individual and group therapy, and toxicology testing if performed (provision of the services by a Medicare-enrolled opioid treatment program)

G2072 Medication assisted treatment, buprenorphine (implant insertion and removal); weekly bundle including dispensing and/or administration, substance use counseling, individual and group therapy, and toxicology testing if performed (provision of the services by a Medicare-enrolled opioid treatment program)

G2073 Medication assisted treatment, naltrexone; weekly bundle including dispensing and/or administration, substance use counseling, individual and group therapy, and toxicology testing if performed (provision of the services by a Medicare-enrolled opioid treatment program)

G2074 Medication assisted treatment, weekly bundle not including the drug, including substance use counseling, individual and group therapy, and toxicology testing if performed (provision of the services by a Medicare-enrolled opioid treatment program)

G2075 Medication assisted treatment, medication not otherwise specified; weekly bundle including dispensing and/or administration, substance use counseling, individual and group therapy, and toxicology testing, if performed (provision of the services by a Medicare-enrolled opioid treatment program)

These codes represent a bundled episode of care payment for opioid use disorder services performed in an opioid treatment program (OTP). This provision requires that opioid use disorder treatment services include FDA-approved opioid agonist and antagonist treatment medications, the dispensing and administration of such medications (if applicable), substance use disorder counseling, individual and group therapy, toxicology testing, and other services determined appropriate. It does not include meals and transportation. For G2067 through G2073, report the code for the specific drug used in treatment. Report G2074 when the drug is not included in the bundled payment, and G2075 for medication not otherwise specified.

G2076-G2077

G2076 Intake activities, including initial medical examination that is a complete, fully documented physical evaluation and initial assessment by a program physician or a primary care physician, or an authorized health care professional under the supervision of a program physician qualified personnel that includes preparation of a treatment plan that includes the patient's short-term goals and the tasks the patient must perform to complete the short-term goals; the patient's requirements for education, vocational rehabilitation, and employment; and the medical, psycho-social, economic, legal, or other supportive services that a patient needs, conducted by qualified personnel (provision of the services by a Medicare-enrolled opioid treatment program); list separately in addition to code for primary procedure

G2077 Periodic assessment; assessing periodically by qualified personnel to determine the most appropriate combination of services and treatment (provision of the services by a Medicare-enrolled opioid treatment program); list separately in addition to code for primary procedure

These codes report initial intake (G2076) and periodic assessment (G2077) services rendered to each patient accepted for treatment at an opioid treatment program (OTP). Services should include initial and periodical assessments by qualified personnel to determine the most appropriate treatment plan and combination of services and treatment. These are add-on codes that are reported in addition to a code for the primary service.

G2078-G2079

G2078 Take home supply of methadone; up to 7 additional day supply (provision of the services by a Medicare-enrolled opioid treatment program); list separately in addition to code for primary procedure

G2079 Take home supply of buprenorphine (oral); up to 7 additional day supply (provision of the services by a Medicare-enrolled opioid treatment program); list separately in addition to code for primary procedure

These codes report the provision of a take-home supply of the indicated drug by an opioid treatment program (OTP). Report G2078 for methadone and G2079 for oral buprenorphine. Both codes report provision of drugs for up to a seven additional day supply and are reported in addition to a code for the primary service.

G2080

G2080 Each additional 30 minutes of counseling in a week of medication assisted treatment, (provision of the services by a Medicare-enrolled opioid treatment program); list separately in addition to code for primary procedure

Report G2080 in addition to a code for the primary service for each additional 30 minutes of counseling or group or individual therapy in a week of medication-assisted treatment when provided by a Medicare enrolled opioid treatment program (OTP).

G2082-G2083

G2082 Office or other outpatient visit for the evaluation and management of an established patient that requires the supervision of a physician or other qualified health care professional and provision of up to 56 mg of esketamine nasal self administration, includes 2 hours post administration observation

G2083 Office or other outpatient visit for the evaluation and management of an established patient that requires the supervision of a physician or other qualified health care professional and provision of greater than 56 mg esketamine nasal self administration, includes 2 hours post administration observation

Esketamine nasal spray is an N-methyl D-aspartate (NMDA) receptor antagonist. It is indicated for use in conjunction with an oral antidepressant for treatment-resistant depression (TRD) in adults. TRD is defined as a major depressive disorder (MDD) in adults who have not responded adequately to at least two different antidepressants of adequate dose and duration in the current depressive episode. It is administered under the direct supervision of a healthcare provider, with monitoring by the provider under a Risk Evaluation and Mitigation Strategy. Report G2082 for an office/outpatient visit for the evaluation and management (E/M) of an established patient in which up to 56 mg of esketamine is provided and G2083 if greater than 56 mg is provided. Both codes include two hours of observation post-administration.

G2086-G2088

G2086 Office-based treatment for opioid use disorder, including development of the treatment plan, care coordination, individual therapy and group therapy and counseling; at least 70 minutes in the first calendar month

G2087 Office-based treatment for opioid use disorder, including care coordination, individual therapy and group therapy and counseling; at least 60 minutes in a subsequent calendar month

G2088 Office-based treatment for opioid use disorder, including care coordination, individual therapy and group therapy and counseling; each additional 30 minutes beyond the first 120 minutes (list separately in addition to code for primary procedure)

These codes represent a bundled episode of care payment for opioid use disorder services performed in an office or via Medicare telehealth. This provision requires that opioid use disorder treatment services include FDA-approved opioid agonist and antagonist treatment medications, the dispensing and administration of such medications (if applicable), substance use disorder counseling, individual and group therapy, toxicology testing, and other services determined appropriate. It does not include meals and transportation.

G2168-G2169

G2168 Services performed by a physical therapist assistant in the home health setting in the delivery of a safe and effective physical therapy maintenance program, each 15 minutes

G2169 Services performed by an occupational therapist assistant in the home health setting in the delivery of a safe and effective occupational therapy maintenance program, each 15 minutes

These codes report various services provided by physical or occupational therapy assistants in a home health or hospice setting in 15-minute increments. Home health includes not only traditional private home settings, but also assisted living quarters, group homes, custodial care facilities, or similar type settings that constitute the patient's place of residence. Medicare requires that the discipline of the home health staff be reported using these codes. Check other payer requirements before using these codes on non-Medicare claims. Report G2168 for physical therapy assistants and G2169 for occupational therapy assistants.

G2212

G2212 Prolonged office or other outpatient evaluation and management service(s) beyond the maximum required time of the primary procedure which has been selected using total time on the date of the primary service; each additional 15 minutes by the physician or qualified healthcare professional, with or without direct patient contact (list separately in addition to CPT codes 99205, 99215, 99483 for office or other outpatient evaluation and management services.) (Do not report G2212 on the same date of service as codes 99358, 99359, 99415, 99416). (Do not report G2212 for any time unit less than 15 minutes)

Code G2212 reports prolonged total time (time with and without direct patient contact combined) that is provided by the physician or other qualified healthcare professional on the date of an office visit or other outpatient service. This code is assigned only when the code for the primary EM service has been selected based solely on total time, and only after exceeding by 15 minutes the maximum time that is required to report the highest-level service. For example, when reporting an established patient encounter (99215), code G2212 would not be reported until at least 15 minutes of time beyond 54 minutes has been accumulated (i.e., 69 minutes) on the day of the encounter.

G2213

G2213 Initiation of medication for the treatment of opioid use disorder in the emergency department setting, including assessment, referral to ongoing care, and arranging access to supportive services (list separately in addition to code for primary procedure)

This add-on code is reported in addition to evaluation and management (E/M) visit codes reported in the ED setting for treatment of opioid use disorder (OUD). It includes medication initiation (excluding the drug itself), follow-up care referral, post treatment follow-up, and access arrangement to supportive services. Practitioners should furnish activities that are clinically appropriate for the beneficiary that is being treated.

G2214

G2214 Initial or subsequent psychiatric collaborative care management, first 30 minutes in a month of behavioral health care manager activities, in consultation with a psychiatric consultant, and directed by the treating physician or other qualified health care professional

Psychiatric collaborative care management services describe care reported by a qualified clinician overseeing a behavioral health care manager and psychiatric consultant who provide a behavioral health assessment, including establishing, starting, revising, or monitoring a plan of care as well as providing brief interventions to a patient diagnosed with a mental health disorder. The psychiatric consultant contracts directly with the qualified clinician to render the consultation portion of the service. Patients are generally referred to a behavioral health care manager for assistance in receiving treatment for newly diagnosed conditions that have been unresponsive to traditional or standard care provided in a nonpsychiatric environment or who need additional examination and evaluation before a referral to a psychiatric care setting. The required elements include tracking patient follow-up and progress via registry; weekly caseload participation with a psychiatric consultant; working together and coordinating with the qualified clinician on a regular basis; additional ongoing review of the patient's progress and recommendations for treatment changes, including medications with the psychiatric consultant; provision of brief interventions with the use of evidence-based techniques; monitoring patient outcomes using validated rating scales; and relapse prevention planning. This code reports the first 30 minutes of initial or subsequent psychiatric collaborative care management in a month.

G2215-G2216

G2215 Take home supply of nasal naloxone; 2-pack of 4 mg per 0.1 ml nasal spray (provision of the services by a Medicare-enrolled Opioid Treatment Program); list separately in addition to code for primary procedure

G2216 Take home supply of injectable naloxone (provision of the services by a Medicare-enrolled opioid treatment program); list separately in addition to code for primary procedure

These codes report the provision of a take-home supply of the drug naloxone indicated by an opioid treatment program (OTP). Report G2215 for nasal naloxone and G2216 for that administered by injection. Both codes are reported in addition to a code for the primary service. One add-on code (G2215 or G2216) is allowed every 30 days; however, exceptions to this limit are allowed in cases in which the beneficiary overdoses and uses the initial supply of naloxone dispensed by the OTP to the extent that it is medically reasonable and necessary to furnish additional naloxone. If an additional supply is needed within 30 days of the original supply being provided, the OTP must document in the medical record the reason for the exception. These codes also include overdose education and it is expected that when OTPs provide beneficiaries with a supply of naloxone, they will also inform them about how to use the medication they are being given.

G2250

G2250 Remote assessment of recorded video and/or images submitted by an established patient (e.g., store and forward), including interpretation with follow-up with the patient within 24 business hours, not originating from a related service provided within the previous 7 days nor leading to a service or procedure within the next 24 hours or soonest available appointment

A nonphysician practitioner (NPP) reviews photos or video information submitted by the patient to determine if a visit is required. The service may be provided to an established patient when a related service has not been provided in the previous seven days and may not lead to a service or procedure within the next 24 hours or soonest available appointment. This code can be reported by practitioners who cannot independently bill for evaluation and management (EM) services; however, the service must be consistent with the scope of their benefit categories.

G2251

G2251 Brief communication technology-based service, e.g. virtual check-in, by a qualified health care professional who cannot report evaluation and management services, provided to an established patient, not originating from a related service provided within the previous 7 days nor leading to a service or procedure within the next 24 hours or soonest available appointment; 5-10 minutes of clinical discussion

A nonphysician practitioner (NPP) conducts a virtual check-in and clinical discussion, lasting five to 10 minutes, for an established patient using a telephone or other audio only telecommunication device to determine whether an office visit or other service is needed. The service may be provided when a related service has not been provided in the previous seven days and it may not lead to a service or procedure within the next 24 hours or soonest available appointment. Use of this code requires direct interaction between the NPP and the patient. This code is reported by practitioners who cannot independently bill for evaluation and management (EM) services; however, the service must be consistent with the scope of their benefit categories.

G2252

G2252 Brief communication technology-based service, e.g. virtual check-in, by a physician or other qualified health care professional who can report evaluation and management services, provided to an established patient, not originating from a related EM service provided within the previous 7 days nor leading to an EM service or procedure within the next 24 hours or soonest available appointment; 11-20 minutes of medical discussion

A physician or other qualified health care professional conducts a virtual check-in, lasting 11 to 20 minutes, for an established patient using a telephone or other telecommunication device to determine whether an office visit or other service is needed. The service may be provided when a related evaluation and management (EM) service has not been provided in the previous seven days and it may not lead to an EM service within the next 24 hours or soonest available appointment.

G3002-G3003

G3002 Chronic pain management and treatment, monthly bundle including, diagnosis; assessment and monitoring; administration of a validated pain rating scale or tool; the development, implementation, revision, and/or maintenance of a person-centered care plan that includes strengths, goals, clinical needs, and desired outcomes; overall treatment management; facilitation and coordination of any necessary behavioral health treatment; medication management; pain and health literacy counseling; any necessary chronic pain related crisis care; and ongoing communication and care coordination between relevant practitioners furnishing care e.g., physical therapy and occupational therapy, complementary and integrative approaches, and community-based care, as appropriate. Requires initial face-to-face visit at least 30 minutes provided by a physician or other qualified health professional; first 30 minutes personally provided by physician or other qualified health care professional, per calendar month. (When using G3002, 30 minutes must be met or exceeded)

G3003 Each additional 15 minutes of chronic pain management and treatment by a physician or other qualified health care professional, per calendar month. (List separately in addition to code for G3002. When using G3003, 15 minutes must be met or exceeded)

The physician or other qualified health care professional (QHP) provides monthly chronic pain management (CPM) and treatment. It is not required, when a beneficiary first presents for care, that there is an established history or diagnosis of chronic pain, or that the patient has been diagnosed with a condition that causes or involves chronic pain; rather, it is the clinician's responsibility to establish, confirm, or reject a chronic pain and/or pain-related diagnosis. When reporting G3002, an initial face-to-face visit of at least 30 minutes is required; this must be furnished in person, in a clinical setting such as a primary care practitioner's office or other applicable setting, without the use of telecommunications technology. Follow-up or subsequent visits may be non-face to face at the discretion and preference of the clinician and patient. The monthly bundle includes diagnosis, assessment/monitoring, and the administration of a pain rating scale or tool. An individual care plan must be developed, implemented, revised, and/or maintained that outlines the patient's strengths, goals, desired outcomes, and clinical needs. The coordination and facilitation of any needed behavioral health treatment as well as overall treatment management is included in the monthly bundle, as well as medication management. Pain/health literacy counseling must be provided to enable beneficiaries with chronic pain to make informed decisions about their care, increase pain knowledge, and strengthen self-management skills. In addition, any necessary chronic pain-related crisis care must be provided, as well as continuing communication and care coordination between pertinent practitioners. Care provided by these practitioners may include, as appropriate, physical/occupational therapy, community-based care, and complementary and integrative approaches. The CPM services reported by G3002 may not be rendered more than once per month by each individual practitioner billing the code for each beneficiary but may be rendered less than 12 times per year, depending on the specific needs of the chronic pain patient. Report add-on code G3003 for each additional 15 minutes of care beyond that reported by G3002. Code G3003 may be reported an unlimited number of times (as medically necessary) per calendar month, after HCPCS code G3002 has been billed. Note: these codes have been added to the Medicare telehealth services list, effective through the end of calendar year 2023.

G6001

G6001 Ultrasonic guidance for placement of radiation therapy fields

Ultrasound is used to place radiation therapy fields. Ultrasound is an imaging technique bouncing sound waves far above the level of human perception through interior body structures. The sound waves pass through different densities of tissue and reflect back to a receiving unit, which converts the waves to electrical pulses that are immediately displayed in picture form on screen. Images of normal and abnormal tissue structures are obtained and the treatment field area volume is determined. The normal tissues surrounding the treatment area are also defined. Acquiring this data is an important step in planning the patient's radiation treatment.

G6002

G6002 Stereoscopic x-ray guidance for localization of target volume for the delivery of radiation therapy

Radiation treatment delivery involves the transfer of a beam of high-energy radiation from a treatment machine distanced from the treatment area. Stereotactic body radiation therapy is a radiation therapy technique that uses special equipment to position a patient and precisely deliver a large radiation dose to discrete tumor sites while minimizing damage to healthy tissue. Stereoscopic x-ray guidance utilizes infrared and/or camera technology to precisely localize targets in conjunction with intensity modulated radiation therapy and stereotactic radiotherapy. This code reports the stereoscopic x-ray guidance only.

G6003-G6006

G6003 Radiation treatment delivery, single treatment area, single port or parallel opposed ports, simple blocks or no blocks: up to 5 mev

G6004 Radiation treatment delivery, single treatment area, single port or parallel opposed ports, simple blocks or no blocks: 6-10 mev

G6005 Radiation treatment delivery, single treatment area, single port or parallel opposed ports, simple blocks or no blocks: 11-19 mev

G6006 Radiation treatment delivery, single treatment area, single port or parallel opposed ports, simple blocks or no blocks: 20 mev or greater

Radiation treatment delivery involves the delivery of a beam of high-energy radiation from an external treatment machine distanced from the treatment area. External radiation is often delivered by linear accelerator, which can deliver x-rays (photons) or electrons to a targeted area. Cobalt teletherapy units and cesium teletherapy units are also used to direct gamma rays from a distance to the targeted area. Photons can target deeper lying tumor tissue, while electrons are used for the maximum dose of radiation near the skin surface, making the method suitable to treat skin, superficial lesions, and shallow tumor volumes where underlying tissues need to be protected. These codes are dependent upon the number and complexity of treatment areas, as well as the energy level, measured in megavolts (MeV). Report G6003 for a single treatment area, single port or parallel opposed ports, simple or no blocks, up to 5 MeV; G6004 for 6-10 MeV; G6005 for 11-19 MeV; and G6006 for 20 MeV or greater.

G6007-G6010

G6007 Radiation treatment delivery, two separate treatment areas, three or more ports on a single treatment area, use of multiple blocks: up to 5 mev

G6008 Radiation treatment delivery, two separate treatment areas, three or more ports on a single treatment area, use of multiple blocks: 6-10 mev

G6009 Radiation treatment delivery, two separate treatment areas, three or more ports on a single treatment area, use of multiple blocks: 11-19 mev

G6010 Radiation treatment delivery, two separate treatment areas, three or more ports on a single treatment area, use of multiple blocks: 20 mev or greater

Radiation treatment delivery involves the delivery of a beam of high-energy radiation from an external treatment machine distanced from the treatment area. External radiation is often delivered by linear accelerator, which can deliver x-rays (photons) or electrons to a targeted area. Cobalt teletherapy units and cesium teletherapy units are also used to direct gamma rays from a distance to the targeted area. Photons can target deeper lying tumor tissue, while electrons are used for the maximum dose of radiation near the skin surface, making the method suitable to treat skin, superficial lesions, and shallow tumor volumes where underlying tissues need to be protected. These codes are dependent upon the number and complexity of treatment areas, as well as the energy level, measured in megavolts (MeV). Report G6007 for two separate treatment areas, three or more ports on a single treatment area, multiple blocks, up to 5 MeV; G6008 for 6-10 MeV; G6009 for 11-19 MeV; and G6010 for 20 MeV or greater.

G6011-G6014

G6011 Radiation treatment delivery, three or more separate treatment areas, custom blocking, tangential ports, wedges, rotational beam, compensators, electron beam; up to 5 mev

G6012 Radiation treatment delivery, three or more separate treatment areas, custom blocking, tangential ports, wedges, rotational beam, compensators, electron beam; 6-10 mev

G6013 Radiation treatment delivery, three or more separate treatment areas, custom blocking, tangential ports, wedges, rotational beam, compensators, electron beam; 11-19 mev

G6014 Radiation treatment delivery, three or more separate treatment areas, custom blocking, tangential ports, wedges, rotational beam, compensators, electron beam; 20 mev or greater

Radiation treatment delivery involves the delivery of a beam of high-energy radiation from an external treatment machine distanced from the treatment area. External radiation is often delivered by linear accelerator, which can deliver x-rays (photons) or electrons to a targeted area. Cobalt teletherapy units and cesium teletherapy units are also used to direct gamma rays from a distance to the targeted area. Photons can target deeper lying tumor tissue, while electrons are used for the maximum dose of radiation near the skin surface, making the method suitable to treat skin, superficial lesions, and shallow tumor volumes where underlying tissues need to be protected. These codes are dependent upon the number and complexity of treatment areas, as well as the energy level, measured in megavolts (MeV). Report G6011 for three or more two separate treatment areas, custom blocking, tangential ports, wedges, rotational beam, compensators, electron beam, up to 5MeV; G6012 for 6-10 MeV; G6013 for 11-19 MeV; and G6014 for 20 MeV or greater.

G6015

G6015 Intensity modulated treatment delivery, single or multiple fields/arcs, via narrow spatially and temporally modulated beams, binary, dynamic MLC, per treatment session

Intensity modulated radiotherapy treatment (IMRT) is the use of varying intensities of radiation. A single dose is shaped by hundreds of beam-shaping devices called collimators. These collimators are calculated to hit tumors with high-dose radiation and sensitive normal tissues with modulated, lower-intensity beams, leaving them mostly unaffected. By dividing the radiation beam into multiple slices, the intensity of the beam in any slice can be varied by computer-controlled dynamic multileaf collimation (MLC) during the radiation exposure. MLC systems consist of multiple narrow leaves that are modulated under computer control and allow custom-shaped beam apertures without fabricated blocks. During IMRT delivery, the leaves of the MLC are adjusted while the beam is on to modify the delivery of radiation across the portal. This code reports IMRT delivery, single or multiple fields/arcs, via narrow spatially and temporally modulated beams, binary, dynamic MLC, per treatment session.

G6016

G6016 Compensator-based beam modulation treatment delivery of inverse planned treatment using three or more high resolution (milled or cast) compensator, convergent beam modulated fields, per treatment session

Compensator-based beam modulation treatment delivery of inversed planned treatment using three or more high-resolution (milled or cast) compensator convergent beam modulated fields is a method of delivering intensity modulated radiation therapy (IMRT). Prior to treatment delivery, a computerized planning system is used to calculate dose by inverse treatment planning method for IMRT optimization. The planner chooses beam angles and writes a prescription for targets identifying critical structures. The computerized planning system optimizes beam weights and modulation patterns and generates files for milling or casting of the required high-resolution compensators that are fabricated as prescribed and planned. During treatment delivery, solid filters modulate the beams. This code represents one treatment session.

G6017

G6017 Intra-fraction localization and tracking of target or patient motion during delivery of radiation therapy (e.g., 3D positional tracking, gating, 3D surface tracking), each fraction of treatment

Image-guided radiation therapy is a technique in which frequent imaging occurs during the course of a radiation therapy session (intra-fraction) in order to ensure that the radiation is delivered to the correct target location and spares surrounding tissues. Decisions regarding administration adjustments are made on the basis of the imaging results. Various methods of localization and tracking of patient or tumor motion may be used, including gating or 3D positional or surface tracking technology. In one method, an electromagnetic transponder is implanted into the prostate prior to external beam therapy for prostate cancer. This transponder transmits radiofrequency waves to a computerized system, which provides information regarding position and movement of the prostate. This motion data is used by clinicians to assist in radiation therapy setup and as a positional monitor during delivery of treatment, alerting the clinician if the tumor moves outside the pathway of the radiation beam. Report G6017 for each fraction of treatment.

G9143

G9143 Warfarin responsiveness testing by genetic technique using any method, any number of specimen(s)

This code was developed as a means of implementing Medicare's coverage policy for warfarin responsiveness testing, which is only covered by Medicare in the context of an approved, clinical study. This test is considered a once-in-a-lifetime procedure, unless there is a reason to think that the patient's genetics would change. Pharmacogenomics is a study of the response to drugs by a specific individual. The testing includes a study of the inherited components and gene variations that dictate the individual's response to drugs/medications. It also explores the ways that these individual variations can be used to predict a good, a bad, or no response to a drug. The influence of CYP2C9 and VKORC1 on warfarin dose, along with many other factors, has been used to partially predict an individual's response to warfarin.

G9147

G9147 Outpatient Intravenous Insulin Treatment (OIVIT) either pulsatile or continuous, by any means, guided by the results of measurements for: respiratory quotient; and/or, urine urea nitrogen (UUN); and/or, arterial, venous or capillary glucose; and/or potassium concentration

Medicare has determined that outpatient intravenous insulin treatment (OIVIT) is not reasonable and necessary since there is no evidence that it improves health outcomes in Medicare patients. The term OIVIT refers to an outpatient regimen that integrates pulsed or continuous intravenous infusion of insulin with the dosage depending on the results of measurement of respiratory quotient; urine urea nitrogen (UUN); arterial, venous, or capillary glucose; and/or potassium concentration. OIVIT is also known as cellular activation therapy (CAT), chronic intermittent intravenous insulin therapy (CIIT), hepatic activation therapy (HAT), intercellular activation therapy (iCAT), metabolic activation therapy (MAT), pulsatile intravenous insulin treatment (PIVIT), pulse insulin therapy (PIT), and pulsatile therapy (PT). This code is reported for noncovered OIVIT and any related services.

G9157

G9157 Transesophageal Doppler used for cardiac monitoring

Transesophageal Doppler is an ultrasound diagnostic procedure that uses low energy sound waves to provide noninvasive visualization. This code is specific to Medicare coverage of transesophageal Doppler monitoring of cardiac output for ventilated patients in the ICU and operative patients with a need for intraoperative fluid optimization. This service is only covered in a hospital setting or ambulatory surgical center and is included in the Inpatient Prospective Payment System payment.

G9473-G9479

G9473 Services performed by chaplain in the hospice setting, each 15 minutes

G9474 Services performed by dietary counselor in the hospice setting, each 15 minutes

G9475 Services performed by other counselor in the hospice setting, each 15 minutes

G9476 Services performed by volunteer in the hospice setting, each 15 minutes

G9477 Services performed by care coordinator in the hospice setting, each 15 minutes

G9478 Services performed by other qualified therapist in the hospice setting, each 15 minutes

G9479 Services performed by qualified pharmacist in the hospice setting, each 15 minutes

These codes indicate the type of professional rendering care in a hospice setting.

G

H

H0001

H0001 Alcohol and/or drug assessment

This code reports provision of alcohol and/or drug assessment services. A psychiatrist, clinical psychologist, or other specialized health care professional or team of professionals generally provides drug and/or alcohol assessments. Protocols vary, but an assessment is systematic and thorough and addresses all aspects of a patient's encounters with alcohol and/or drugs. A detailed family, social, and legal history is usually solicited and components may be verified independent of the patient interview. Quantity and frequency of alcohol and/or drug use is documented. Physical manifestations associated with alcohol or drug use or abuse may be noted if present, such as depression, mania, anxiety, etc. A physical medical examination may be a component of the assessment. Questionnaires and tests may be used as components of the assessment. A report is generally issued that characterizes the patient's contact with alcohol and/or drugs as casual, dependent, abusive, addictive, etc. Should alcohol or drug use be determined to have caused adverse effects in the life of the patient or others, a report is issued documenting abuse. In addition to a diagnostic status, an assessment of abuse can have legal repercussions. This assessment should be used to devise a plan of care in treating the patient effectively.

H0002

H0002 Behavioral health screening to determine eligibility for admission to treatment program

Behavioral health screening is done to determine a patient's eligibility for admission to a treatment program. Patients are screened for mental health conditions as well as substance use disorders and are medically assessed to ensure appropriate treatment is given.

H0003

H0003 Alcohol and/or drug screening; laboratory analysis of specimens for presence of alcohol and/or drugs

Alcohol and/or drug screening is performed through laboratory analysis of urine, blood, or hair specimens to determine the presence of alcohol and/or drugs in the patient's system.

H0004

H0004 Behavioral health counseling and therapy, per 15 minutes

This code reports provision of behavioral health counseling and therapy services. Behavioral health counseling and therapy provides individual counseling by a clinician for a patient in a private setting and is billed in 15-minute increments.

H0005

H0005 Alcohol and/or drug services; group counseling by a clinician

Alcohol and/or drug group counseling by a clinician provides the patient support in a group setting (two or more individuals) in abstaining from substance abuse and assisting the patient with sobriety maintenance. Group counseling focuses on cognitive or behavioral approaches that typically address triggers and relapse prevention, self-evaluation, the process of recovery, and issues pertaining to changes in lifestyle. Group sizes and treatment plans may vary according to the needs of the individual.

H0006

H0006 Alcohol and/or drug services; case management

Case management for patients needing services relating to alcohol or drug abuse provides assistance and care coordination based on the needs of the individual. The case manager assesses the needs of the patient, assists in developing plans to benefit the patient, as well as implementation of the plans, and reviews and evaluates the patient's status.

H0007

H0007 Alcohol and/or drug services; crisis intervention (outpatient)

Crisis intervention for alcohol and/or drug services is an emergency response by a clinician to provide immediate face-to-face support for an individual.

H0008-H0014

H0008 Alcohol and/or drug services; subacute detoxification (hospital inpatient)

H0009 Alcohol and/or drug services; acute detoxification (hospital inpatient)

H0010 Alcohol and/or drug services; subacute detoxification (residential addiction program inpatient)

H0011 Alcohol and/or drug services; acute detoxification (residential addiction program inpatient)

H0012 Alcohol and/or drug services; subacute detoxification (residential addiction program outpatient)

H0013 Alcohol and/or drug services; acute detoxification (residential addiction program outpatient)

H0014 Alcohol and/or drug services; ambulatory detoxification

These codes are for acute and subacute detoxification services in which the differentiating factor is the setting where the patient is monitored for the long-term symptoms associated with the withdrawal from alcohol and/or drugs. Subacute detoxification deals with severe symptoms, such as alcohol and drug cravings, that do not require immediate intervention. Acute detoxification services are those in which the patient is medically managed and stabilized on an inpatient hospitalization basis for severe withdrawal syndrome associated with the withdrawal from alcohol/drugs. Acute withdrawal begins within hours and includes severe physical and psychological symptoms that may require medical management with medications such as methadone.

H0015

H0015 Alcohol and/or drug services; intensive outpatient (treatment program that operates at least 3 hours/day and at least 3 days/week and is based on an individualized treatment plan), including assessment, counseling; crisis intervention, and activity therapies or education

This code reports alcohol and drug related services within an intensive outpatient treatment program requiring the patient to participate at least 3 hours per day for at least 3 days per week. The patient is assessed medically and psychologically, provided counseling, intervention, and activity therapy or education, according to the needs of the patient and the individual's treatment plan.

H0016

H0016 Alcohol and/or drug services; medical/somatic (medical intervention in ambulatory setting)

This service includes the supervision of medication, physical examinations, or other medical needs required to maintain the physical health of the patient receiving medical intervention treatment for alcohol and drug related problems in an ambulatory setting.

H0017

H0017 Behavioral health; residential (hospital residential treatment program), without room and board, per diem

Residential treatment on a per diem basis for behavior health issues in a hospital residential treatment program is designed to provide a 24-hour group living situation in which the patient receives treatment under the care of a physician. This code does not include daily room and board.

H0018

H0018 Behavioral health; short-term residential (nonhospital residential treatment program), without room and board, per diem

Short-term residential treatment is typically less than 30 days. This code applies to a residential treatment program for behavior health issues that is not part of a hospital but provides a 24-hour group living situation in which the patient receives treatment and does not include daily room and board.

H0019

H0019 Behavioral health; long-term residential (nonmedical, nonacute care in a residential treatment program where stay is typically longer than 30 days), without room and board, per diem

Long-term residential treatment is typically more than 30 days. This code applies to a residential treatment program for behavioral health issues that are neither medical nor acute in nature. This code is per diem, not including daily room and board.

H0020

H0020 Alcohol and/or drug services; methadone administration and/or service (provision of the drug by a licensed program)

Methadone administration and/or service programs provide opioid replacement treatment (ORT) or opioid maintenance treatment (OMT), including the administration of methadone to an individual for detoxification from opioids and/or maintenance treatment. Overall treatment must be delivered, which should include counseling/therapy, case review, and medication monitoring. ORT/OMT is delivered by providers functioning under a defined set of policies and procedures, including admission, discharge, and continued service criteria stipulated by state law and regulations, Substance Abuse and Mental Health Services Administration (SAMHSA) regulations, and Drug Enforcement Agency (DEA) regulations. The ORT must be licensed by the Drug Enforcement Agency. The ORT should also have accreditation from the Joint Commission on the Accreditation of Healthcare Organizations (JCAHO), Committee for Accreditation (COA), and/or the Commission on the Accreditation of Rehabilitation Facilities (CARF). The ORT/OMT must meet the requirements of the Substance Abuse and Mental Health Administration.

H0021

H0021 Alcohol and/or drug training service (for staff and personnel not employed by providers)

This code reports developing alcohol and/or drug service skills of staff and personnel that are not employed by an agency, such as training a counselor/clinician on proper techniques and approaches or sessions for clinicians on the effects of various types of drugs.

H0022

H0022 Alcohol and/or drug intervention service (planned facilitation)

Alcohol and drug intervention services provide treatment services and activities that assist the professionally trained interventionalist to pursue and detect alcohol and or drug addictions and to intercede to halt the progress of the addictions. These services also include early interventions.

H0023

H0023 Behavioral health outreach service (planned approach to reach a targeted population)

Behavioral health outreach is a service targeting specific, at-risk individuals in a given population who are in need of assistance with mental health issues. This may include mobile teams that contact at-risk individuals in the home, centers in which individuals can drop-in and obtain information regarding mental health treatment or social services, or other various methods of contact that are not represented by a more specific code.

H0024-H0025

H0024 Behavioral health prevention information dissemination service (one-way direct or nondirect contact with service audiences to affect knowledge and attitude)

H0025 Behavioral health prevention education service (delivery of services with target population to affect knowledge, attitude and/or behavior)

A behavioral health prevention information dissemination service is used to provide facts to individuals in the community or in at-risk populations on issues of mental health. This service includes any form of direct or non-direct contact with the targeted audience to increase their awareness and knowledge of the issues and to affect their attitude. A behavioral health prevention education service is used to deliver services to individuals of a target population on issues of mental health education and to affect their knowledge, attitude, and behavior. It may include screenings to assist individuals in obtaining appropriate treatment. Causes and symptoms of disorders are discussed so as to encourage early intervention and reduce severity of mental illness.

H0026

H0026 Alcohol and/or drug prevention process service, community-based (delivery of services to develop skills of impactors)

Community-based, alcohol and/or drug prevention process services enhance the ability of a community to provide violence, alcohol, and/or drug abuse prevention services. The activities include planning, interagency collaboration, coalition building, and networking. Examples include multi-agency coordination and collaboration, community and volunteer training, and systemic planning.

H0027

H0027 Alcohol and/or drug prevention environmental service (broad range of external activities geared toward modifying systems in order to mainstream prevention through policy and law)

Alcohol and/or drug prevention environmental services (broad range of external activities geared toward modifying systems in order to mainstream prevention through policy and law) establish or change written and unwritten community standards and postures that influence the incidence and prevalence of violence and/or the abuse of alcohol and/or drugs used in the general population.

H0028

H0028 Alcohol and/or drug prevention problem identification and referral service (e.g., student assistance and employee assistance programs), does not include assessment

This code reports alcohol and/or drug prevention problem identification and referral services (e.g., student assistance and employee assistance programs). Prevention strategies aim to identify individuals who have engaged in illegal and age-inappropriate use of tobacco, alcohol, and/or drugs. Services may include employee assistance programs (EAP), student assistance programs, and driving under the influence (DUI) education programs. Append modifier HA for 12 hours of education program within a community-based setting for youth younger than age 18 who are first-time offenders of alcohol or other drugs. Append modifier HB for 10 hours of education/diversion program within the circuit court districts for 19- to 20-year-olds who have been referred to the program due to an alcohol-related offense. Append modifier HK for 30 hours of IPP within a community based setting for adolescents who have multiple offenses of alcohol or other drug use.

H0029

H0029 Alcohol and/or drug prevention alternatives service (services for populations that exclude alcohol and other drug use e.g., alcohol free social events)

This code reports alcohol and/or drug prevention alternative services (services for populations that exclude alcohol and other drug use e.g., alcohol free social events). Service strategies provide for the participation of specific inhabitants of a community in activities free from violence and/or alcohol/drug use. This strategy is to create attractive, healthy, and safe activities that increase an individual's commitment to abstain from violence and/or alcohol and drugs. These activities provide opportunities for low-risk choices when it comes to alcohol use and/or violent behavior. Examples include leadership camps, chemical free events, social activities, recreational activities, cultural activities, and behavioral activities at local community centers and other like places.

H0030

H0030 Behavioral health hotline service

Behavioral health hotline is a telephone service that provides crisis intervention and emergency management such as mental health referrals, treatment information, and other verbal assistance.

H0031

H0031 Mental health assessment, by nonphysician

Mental health assessment is provided by someone other than a physician who is a trained staff member. The assessment identifies factors of mental illness, functional capacity, and gathers additional information used for the treatment of mental illness.

H0032

H0032 Mental health service plan development by nonphysician

A mental health service plan is developed for treating a patient, including modifying goals, assessing progress, planning transitions, and addressing other needs. This service is provided by someone other than a physician, who is a clinical, professional, or other specialist.

H0033

H0033 Oral medication administration, direct observation

Patients are assisted or observed by professional medical staff during the administration of oral medication. This is often used in the administration of drugs such as methadone when it must be established that the patient has received the medication.

H0034

H0034 Medication training and support, per 15 minutes

Medication training and support is an educational service to assist the patient, family, or other caretaker in the proper management of prescribed medication regimens, drug interactions, and side effects. This code is reported per 15 minutes.

H0035

H0035 Mental health partial hospitalization, treatment, less than 24 hours

Partial hospitalization for mental health services is a treatment period of less than 24 hours care in which the patient is assisted with issues related to the individual's reintegration into society. This code is not considered an inpatient service.

H0036-H0037

H0036 Community psychiatric supportive treatment, face-to-face, per 15 minutes

H0037 Community psychiatric supportive treatment program, per diem

Community psychiatric supportive treatment programs assist individuals with persistent and severe mental illness to gain and maintain independence in the community. This is done with ongoing assessments, crisis intervention, and support. These programs may include advocacy, family education, helping in the development of activities of daily living, and managing basic needs to assist with achieving independence. The treatment/service may be charged per 15 minutes of face-to-face increments or as a daily (per diem) charge.

H0038

H0038 Self-help/peer services, per 15 minutes

Self-help/peer services are specialized therapeutic interactions that are performed by individuals who are current or past recipients of behavioral health services. These individuals are trained and certified to provide support and assistance to individuals in their recovery and integration into the community. The goal is to provide understanding and coping skills and empowerment through mentoring and other supports so that individuals with severe and persistent mental disorders can cope with stress and achieve personal wellness.

H0039-H0040

H0039 Assertive community treatment, face-to-face, per 15 minutes

H0040 Assertive community treatment program, per diem

Assertive community treatment uses a team based, multidisciplinary approach. The goal is to reduce the extent of hospital admissions, to improve the individual's quality of life, and to function in social situations by providing focused, proactive treatments. These services are most appropriate for individuals with severe and persistent mental illness and the greatest level of functional impairment.

H0041-H0042

H0041 Foster care, child, nontherapeutic, per diem

H0042 Foster care, child, nontherapeutic, per month

Foster care is a service in which custodial care of a child under the age of 18 is assumed by someone outside the individual's family. The child is cared for and nurtured within a family context, nontherapeutically, per diem in H0041 and per month in H0042.

H0043-H0044

H0043 Supported housing, per diem

H0044 Supported housing, per month

Supported housing service provides individuals with assistance for the responsibilities of obtaining and maintaining independent living. Once housing is established, the clients are monitored through periodic visits to confirm the continued appropriateness of the living situation including affordability, and ensure that issues of independent living are addressed. This service does not include therapeutic aspects. Report H0043 for services performed per diem and code H0044 for services per month.

H0045

H0045 Respite care services, not in the home, per diem

Respite care services provided outside the home give assistance to clients in place of primary caregivers on a temporary per diem basis so the patient may be maintained at the current level of care required when the primary caregivers are temporarily absent.

H0046

H0046 Mental health services, not otherwise specified

Report this code for mental health services that are not described by any other HCPCS Level II code.

H0047

H0047 Alcohol and/or other drug abuse services, not otherwise specified

Report this code for alcohol and/or other drug abuse services that are not described by any other HCPCS Level II code.

H0048

H0048 Alcohol and/or other drug testing: collection and handling only, specimens other than blood

Collection of specimens for alcohol/drug analysis is dependent on the type of biological sample obtained. Samples typically include urine or hair. This code represents the collection and handling of specimens other than blood samples. The handling of specimens requires a chain of custody from the point of collection throughout the analysis process to ensure the integrity of the specimen.

H0049

H0049 Alcohol and/or drug screening

Patient screening is performed, annually or biannually, to identify possible high-risk behaviors such as alcohol and substance abuse. Standardized assessment tools, such as the World Health Organization's Alcohol Use Disorders Identification Test (AUDIT) and the Drug Abuse Screening Test (DAST), are used to identify the high-risk behavior and determine the appropriate intervention or treatment needed. Screening services do not include intervention, treatment, or therapeutic intervention, such as medication therapy or a combination of medication and counseling. This code is not widely used.

H0050

H0050 Alcohol and/or drug services, brief intervention, per 15 minutes

A brief intervention for a patient in a drug and/or alcohol treatment program is performed. Professionally trained interventionists who are experts in chemical dependency meet briefly with the patient and/or family members to discuss a current treatment issue. The service may be initiated by the patient or the interventionist in response to a specific issue. The purpose of the intervention is to provide support and feedback related to chemical dependency issues that are currently affecting the patient and/or family members. This code is reported per 15-minute time increments spent in the intervention service. This code is not widely used.

H1000

H1000 Prenatal care, at-risk assessment

A pregnancy is considered high risk when there are conditions that could affect the baby, the mother, or the baby and mother. Examples of risk factors for a high-risk pregnancy include the age of the mother (younger than 17 or older than 35 years of age when the baby is due); pre-pregnancy medical conditions such as STDs, diabetes, HIV, or other chronic infection; family history of genetic disorders; and a history of miscarriages. Medical conditions may occur during the pregnancy, including gestational diabetes and preeclampsia. Other pregnancy-related issues can classify a patient as high risk, including placenta previa, fetal problems, multiple births, and premature labor. Report this code for the at-risk assessment. This is usually done during the first trimester but may be done later if problems develop later in the pregnancy.

H1001-H1005

H1001 Prenatal care, at-risk enhanced service; antepartum management

H1002 Prenatal care, at risk enhanced service; care coordination

H1003 Prenatal care, at-risk enhanced service; education

H1004 Prenatal care, at-risk enhanced service; follow-up home visit

H1005 Prenatal care, at-risk enhanced service package (includes H1001-H1004)

A pregnancy is considered high risk when there are conditions that could affect the baby, the mother, or the baby and the mother. Examples of risk factors for a high-risk pregnancy include the age of the mother (younger than 17 or older than 35 years of age when the baby is due); pre-pregnancy medical conditions such as STD, diabetes, HIV, or other chronic infection;

family history of genetic disorders; and a history of miscarriages. Medical conditions may occur during the pregnancy, including gestational diabetes and preeclampsia. Other pregnancy-related issues can classify a patient as high risk, including placenta previa, fetal problems, multiple births, and premature labor. These codes report additional or enhanced services rendered that are required by the at-risk pregnancy. The physician in charge of the patient's care determines what additional services are required. These services can include the development and implementation of the plan of care for the specific patient, making referrals, monitoring the patient's progress, and assuring access to services required for a healthy pregnancy and birth. Enhanced education services include information to prepare the patient for the birth process, information to help the patient identify and try to prevent preterm labor, guidance for prenatal nutrition, and education on lifestyle and parenting support. The postpartum follow-up home visit is an additional and separate visit from the six week postpartum visit. It is usually done within the first two weeks post discharge of the mother. This visit is intended to provide special support by following up on the identified "at risk" medical conditions and addressing the stress involved with caring for the new baby.

H1010

H1010 Nonmedical family planning education, per session

Report this code for education of an individual or a couple in the methods of natural family planning.

H1011

H1011 Family assessment by licensed behavioral health professional for state defined purposes

This code reports, for Medicaid purposes, the assessment of a patient's family by a licensed behavioral health professional. Note that both the description of the service and the type of licensed professional are specific to each state.

H2000

H2000 Comprehensive multidisciplinary evaluation

A comprehensive multidisciplinary evaluation consists of a thorough investigation in several areas to provide an accurate representation of the individual's needs and strengths. This evaluates areas such as psychiatric, physical, psychosocial, family, recreational, and occupational therapy.

H2001

H2001 Rehabilitation program, per 1/2 day

The goal of a rehabilitation program is to enhance independent living, along with communication and social skills. The program may include training to develop skills in conflict resolution, problem solving, employment, and social interaction. Report this code for each half day of a rehabilitation program.

H2010

H2010 Comprehensive medication services, per 15 minutes

Comprehensive medication services are patient centered. They are provided by specially trained pharmacists who work with the patient to make sure that all drug therapies are effective for the intended use, appropriate for the patient's medical condition, able to be taken by the patient as intended, and are safe. The actual outcomes are recorded. These services are intended to improve the quality of patient care, reduce health care costs, and identify and resolve any problems with the drug therapy.

H2011

H2011 Crisis intervention service, per 15 minutes

Mental health crisis intervention provides immediate support for an individual in personal crisis with outpatient status. The aim of this service is to stabilize the individual during a psychiatric emergency and is billed in 15-minute increments.

H2012

H2012 Behavioral health day treatment, per hour

Day treatment for behavior health focuses on maintaining and improving functional abilities for the individual. Clients may participate in activities in a therapeutic and social environment several times per week for several hours per day to improve personal skills. This code is reported per hour of daytime behavioral health treatment.

H2013

H2013 Psychiatric health facility service, per diem

A psychiatric health facility is specifically licensed as such and is differentiated from a hospital with an inpatient psychiatric ward, psychiatric hospital, or crisis residential services. This facility provides services in an acute non-hospital inpatient setting, and includes appropriate care in psychiatry, clinical psychology, social work, rehabilitation, drug administration, and other basic needs, per diem.

H2014

H2014 Skills training and development, per 15 minutes

Skills training and development provides the patient with necessary abilities that will enable the individual to live independently and manage his/her illness and treatment. Training focuses on skills for daily living and community integration for patients with functional limitations due to psychiatric disorders, per 15 minutes.

H2015-H2016

H2015 Comprehensive community support services, per 15 minutes

H2016 Comprehensive community support services, per diem

Comprehensive community support services consist of mental health and substance abuse services. These services assist individuals in achieving their recovery and rehabilitation goals. The program aims to reduce psychiatric and addiction symptoms and to assist in developing community living skills. The services may include coordination of services, support during a crisis, development of system monitoring and management skills, monitoring medications, and help in developing independent living skills. Report H2015 for comprehensive community support services per each 15 minutes or H2016 for per diem.

H2017-H2018

H2017 Psychosocial rehabilitation services, per 15 minutes

H2018 Psychosocial rehabilitation services, per diem

Psychosocial rehabilitation services are intended to help individuals to compensate for or to eliminate functional deficits and environmental and interpersonal barriers associated with mental illness. The goal of the program is to help individuals achieve the fullest possible integration as an active and productive member of their family and community with the least possible ongoing professional intervention. Activities are done to achieve the goals for the individual. This is a face-to-face intervention and the services may be provided in a group or an individual setting. Report these codes for psychosocial rehabilitation services in 15-minute increments or a per diem charge.

H2019-H2020

H2019 Therapeutic behavioral services, per 15 minutes

H2020 Therapeutic behavioral services, per diem

Therapeutic behavioral services are treatments that attempt to change unhealthy, potentially dangerous, or self-destructive behaviors. It focuses on helping an individual understand how the behavior affects life and emotions. Behavioral therapy is usually action-based, using techniques of classical conditioning and operant conditioning. The behavior itself is the problem and the goal is to minimize or eliminate the problem. Each payer, agency, or organization has their own definition and categorization of therapeutic behavioral services. Consult the appropriate party for additional information.

H2021-H2022

H2021 Community-based wrap-around services, per 15 minutes

H2022 Community-based wrap-around services, per diem

Wrap-around community services are provided for a short period of time for seriously emotionally disabled youth. These services are provided for children/adolescents with a rate classification level (RCL) placement higher than 12. These codes include support and training for family members as an integral part of services provided.

H2023-H2024

H2023 Supported employment, per 15 minutes

H2024 Supported employment, per diem

Supported employment services are available to individuals with serious mental illness. Employment specialists assist in obtaining and maintaining employment in the community and in continuing treatment for the client to ensure rehabilitation and productive employment.

H2025-H2026

H2025 Ongoing support to maintain employment, per 15 minutes

H2026 Ongoing support to maintain employment, per diem

Ongoing support to maintain employment services are available to individuals with serious mental illness. Employment specialists provide supportive counseling and interventions within the work environment when needed to ensure the continued employment and self-sufficiency of the client.

H2027

H2027 Psychoeducational service, per 15 minutes

The National Library of Medicine, within the National Institutes of Health, defines a psychoeducational service as an item, action, or procedure "of or relating to the psychological aspects of education; specifically: relating to or used in the education of children with behavioral disorders or learning disabilities." Each payer, agency, or organization has its own definition and categorization of psychoeducational services. Consult the appropriate party for addition information.

H2028-H2029

H2028 Sexual offender treatment service, per 15 minutes

H2029 Sexual offender treatment service, per diem

Sexual offender treatment services provide rehabilitation services that vary depending on the type of treatment facility, security level, and staffing ratios available.

H2030-H2031

H2030 Mental health clubhouse services, per 15 minutes

H2031 Mental health clubhouse services, per diem

Mental health clubhouse is a community service provided for people with mental illness and promotes a structured environment in which individuals can improve interpersonal skills, and develop personal goals that will assist with success in the community. Participants are required to take part in the operations of the clubhouse.

H2032

H2032 Activity therapy, per 15 minutes

Activity therapy such as music, dance, creative art, or any type of play, not for recreation, but related to the care and treatment of the patient's disabling mental health problems is reported for services per 15 minutes.

H2033

H2033 Multisystemic therapy for juveniles, per 15 minutes

Multisystemic therapy uses the strengths found in key environmental settings of juveniles to promote and maintain positive behavioral changes. These services focus on individual, family, and extrafamilial (such as peer, school, and neighborhood) influences, reported in 15 minute increments.

H2034

H2034 Alcohol and/or drug abuse halfway house services, per diem

Halfway house services for alcohol and chemical dependency provide a transitional living environment. These services are structured to promote sobriety and independent living and to assist with continued treatment. Patients are free to work or attend classes during the day and return to the facility at night.

H2035-H2036

H2035 Alcohol and/or other drug treatment program, per hour

H2036 Alcohol and/or other drug treatment program, per diem

Outpatient services for alcohol and chemical dependency are structured to promote sobriety and independent living and to assist with continued treatment. Outpatient services allow patients to present for prescribed treatments and therapy and to maintain an otherwise routine home life. Code H2035 is for treatment billed per hour; H2036 is for treatment billed per diem.

H2037

H2037 Developmental delay prevention activities, dependent child of client, per 15 minutes

Developmental delay prevention activities are designed to reduce the occurrence of problems stemming from inhibited or suppressed development in children that can have effects carrying over into later years. The developmental activities promote the physical and mental well being of dependent children of patients in treatment for alcohol/drug abuse. These services focus on overall healthy development of the child, reported in 15-minute blocks.

H2038

H2038 Skills training and development, per diem

Skills training and development provides the patient with necessary abilities that will enable the individual to live independently and manage his/her illness and treatment. Training focuses on skills for daily living and community integration for patients with functional limitations due to psychiatric disorders, per diem.

J

J0120

J0120 Injection, tetracycline, up to 250 mg

Tetracycline is a broad-spectrum antibiotic prepared from cultures of certain species of streptomyces bacteria. It is thought to inhibit protein synthesis in bacteria, causing cell death. Many microorganisms have developed a resistance to tetracycline and related antibiotics. Susceptibility studies should be performed prior to administration. Tetracycline can be effective against gram-negative and gram-positive organisms. Susceptible organisms include *Rickettsiae, Mycoplasma pneumoniae, Borrelia recurrentis, Haemophilus ducreyi, Pasteurella pestis, Pasteurella tularensis, Bartonella bacilliformis, Bacteroides* species, *Vibrio comma, Vibrio fetus, Brucella* species (in conjunction with streptomycin), *Escherichia coli, Enterobacter aerogenes, Shigella* species, *Mima* species, *Herellea* species, *Haemophilus influenzae*, and *Klebsiella* species.

J0121

J0121 Injection, omadacycline, 1 mg

Omadacycline is a tetracycline class antibacterial used for the treatment of acute bacterial skin and skin structure infections (ABSSSI) and community-acquired bacterial pneumonia (CABP) in adult patients 18 years of age and older. It is indicated for the treatment of the following organisms: *Chlamydophila pneumoniae, Enterobacter cloacae, Haemophilus influenzae, Haemophilus parainfluenzae, Klebsiella pneumoniae, Legionella pneumophila, Mycoplasma pneumoniae, Staphylococcus aureus* (including methicillin-resistant [MRSA] and methicillin susceptible [MSSA] isolates),

Staphylococcus lugdunensis, Streptococcus anginosus group (including *Streptococcus anginosus, Streptococcus intermedius,* and *Streptococcus constellatus*), *Streptococcus pneumoniae, Streptococcus pyogenes*, and *Enterococcus faecalis.* It is supplied as a lyophilized powder in a single dose vial and requires reconstitution and further dilution. The recommended dosage for the treatment of ABSSSI and CABP is 200 mg administered via intravenous (IV) infusion over 60 minutes or 100 mg over 30 minutes twice on day one. The recommended maintenance dose for both conditions is 100 mg over 30 minutes once daily, or 300 mg tablets given orally, for a period of seven to 14 days.

J0122

J0122 Injection, eravacycline, 1 mg

Eravacycline is a tetracycline class antibacterial used for the treatment of complicated intra-abdominal infections in adult patients 18 years of age and older. It is indicated for the treatment of the following organisms: *Bacteroides* species, *Clostridium perfringens, Enterobacter cloacae, Enterococcus faecalis, Enterococcus faecium, Escherichia coli, Klebsiella oxytoca, Klebsiella pneumoniae, Parabacteroides distasonis, Staphylococcus aureus,* and *Streptococcus anginosus* group. It is supplied as a lyophilized powder in a single dose vial and requires reconstitution and further dilution. The recommended dosage is 1 mg/kg body weight administered via intravenous infusion over 60 minutes every 12 hours for a period of four to 14 days. For patients with severe hepatic impairment, the recommended dosage should be modified to 1 mg/kg body weight every 12 hours on day one, followed by 1 mg/kg body weight every 24 hours beginning on day two, and continued for a period of four to 14 days. For patients receiving a strong CYP3A inducer, the recommended dosage should be modified to 1.5 mg/kg body weight every 12 hours for a period of four to 14 days.

J0129

J0129 Injection, abatacept, 10 mg (code may be used for Medicare when drug administered under the direct supervision of a physician, not for use when drug is self-administered)

Abatacept is a protein combination of human cytotoxic T-lymphocyte-associated antigen 4 (CTLA-4) linked to a modified portion of human immunoglobulin G1 (IgG1). It is produced by recombinant DNA technology. Abatacept binds to specific receptor sites of T lymphocyte cells and inhibits their activation. Activated T lymphocytes are found in joint fluid of patients with rheumatoid arthritis. Abatacept is indicated for reducing signs and symptoms, slowing the progression of structural damage, and improving physical function of adult patients with moderately to severely active rheumatoid arthritis who have had an inadequate response to other drugs. The drug can be used singularly or in combination with other disease-modifying, anti-rheumatic drugs. The drug is administered by intravenous infusion over a 30-minute period. Dosage varies from 500 mg to 1 g depending on body weight.

J0130

J0130 Injection abciximab, 10 mg

Abciximab is a murine monoclonal antibody. It blocks certain glycoprotein receptors on platelets and prevents them from aggregating or sticking together. Abciximab also blocks receptors on vessel walls and smooth muscle cells preventing the platelets from aggregating in those sites. It is used as an adjunct with percutaneous transluminal coronary angioplasty (PTCA). Abciximab may be used to treat unstable angina when the patient is not responding to conventional therapy and PTCA is planned within 24 hours. The recommended dosage is 0.25 mg per kg of body weight. The drug is administered as an intravenous bolus 10 to 60 minutes prior to the PTCA, followed by continuous intravenous infusion for 12 hours. When given to unstable angina patients for whom PTCA is planned, a 0.25 mg bolus is administered followed by an 18 to 24 hour intravenous infusion.

J0131

J0131 Injection, acetaminophen, not otherwise specified, 10 mg

Acetaminophen is a nonsalicylate, antipyretic, and nonopioid analgesic agent. This code represents the intravenous formulation of acetaminophen. This drug is indicated for the management of mild to moderate pain, the management of moderate to severe pain with adjunctive opioid analgesics, and for fever reduction in adults and children 2 years of age or older. It is administered only as a 15-minute IV infusion and may be given as a single or repeated dose. The recommended dosage for adults and children weighing 50 kg or more is 1,000 mg every six hours or 650 mg every four hours to a maximum dose of 4,000 mg per day. For adults and children weighing less than 50 kg and for children 2 to 12 years of age, the recommended dosage is 15 mg/kg body weight every six hours or 12.5 mg/kg body weight every four hours to a maximum dose of 75 mg/kg body weight per day, with a minimum dosing interval of four hours. See full prescribing information for complete administration instructions.

J0132

J0132 Injection, acetylcysteine, 100 mg

Acetylcysteine is a derivative of the naturally occurring amino acid L-cysteine. It is used as an antidote for acetaminophen overdose to prevent life-threatening liver damage. Acetylcysteine reacts with the acetaminophen rendering some of the acetaminophen harmless. As an antidote for acetaminophen poisoning, acetylcysteine should be administered as soon as possible but within 24 hours after the overdose. Acetylcysteine is administered by intravenous infusion over 60 minutes.

J0133

J0133 Injection, acyclovir, 5 mg

Acyclovir injection is used to treat herpes infections, including herpes zoster and varicella (chickenpox). It does not cure the infection but does reduce pain and may promote faster healing. Acyclovir is given intravenously over at least an hour. This code reports a 5 mg injection.

J0134

J0134 Injection, acetaminophen (Fresenius Kabi) not therapeutically equivalent to J0131, 10 mg

Acetaminophen is a nonsalicylate, antipyretic, and nonopioid analgesic agent. This code represents the intravenous formulation of acetaminophen. It is indicated for the management of mild to moderate pain, the management of moderate to severe pain with adjunctive opioid analgesics, and for fever reduction in adults and children 2 years of age or older. It is administered only as a 15-minute intravenous (IV) infusion and may be given as a single or repeated dose. The recommended dosage for adults and children weighing 50 kg or more is 1,000 mg every six hours or 650 mg every four hours to a maximum dose of 4,000 mg per day. For adults and children weighing less than 50 kg and for children 2 to 12 years of age, the recommended dosage is 15 mg/kg body weight every six hours or 12.5 mg/kg body weight every four hours to a maximum dose of 75 mg/kg body weight per day, with a minimum dosing interval of four hours. See full prescribing information for complete administration instructions. Report J0134 only for acetaminophen manufactured by Fresenius Kabi.

J0135

J0135 Injection, adalimumab, 20 mg

Adalimumab is a human IgG1 monoclonal antibody that is specific for human tumor necrosis factor (TNF). It is produced by recombinant DNA technology. Adalimumab binds specifically to TNF-alpha, blocks its interaction with cell surface TNF receptors and lyses surface TNF expressing cells. Adalimumab also modulates biological responses that are induced or regulated by TNF, including changes in the levels of adhesion molecules responsible for leukocyte migration. Adalimumab is indicated for reducing signs and symptoms and inhibiting the progression of structural damage in adult patients with moderately to severely active rheumatoid arthritis who have had an inadequate response to one or more disease modifying antirheumatic drugs and patients with active arthritis with psoriatic arthritis. Adalimumab can be used alone or in combination with methotrexate or other disease modifying antirheumatic drugs. Adalimumab is administered by subcutaneous injection and can be self-administered.

J0136

J0136 Injection, acetaminophen (B. Braun) not therapeutically equivalent to J0131, 10 mg

Acetaminophen is a nonsalicylate, antipyretic, and nonopioid analgesic agent. This code represents the intravenous formulation of acetaminophen. It is indicated for the management of mild to moderate pain, the management of moderate to severe pain with adjunctive opioid analgesics, and for fever reduction in adults and children. It is administered only as a 15-minute intravenous (IV) infusion and may be given as a single or repeated dose. The recommended dosage for adults and children weighing 50 kg or more is 1,000 mg every six hours or 650 mg every four hours to a maximum dose of 4,000 mg per day. For adults and children weighing less than 50 kg and for children 2 to 12 years of age, the recommended dosage is 15 mg/kg body weight every six hours or 12.5 mg/kg body weight every four hours to a maximum dose of 75 mg/kg body weight per day, with a minimum dosing interval of four hours. For neonates and infants: neonates born at greater than or equal to 32 weeks gestational age to 28 days chronological age, the recommended dosage is 12.5 mg/kg body weight every six hours to a maximum of 50 mg/kg body weight per day with a minimum dosing interval of six hours; infants 29 days to 2 years of age, the recommended dosage is 15 mg/kg body weight every six hours to a maximum of 60 mg/kg body weight per day with a minimum dosing interval of six hours. See full prescribing information for complete administration instructions. Report J0136 only for acetaminophen manufactured by B. Braun.

J0153

J0153 Injection, adenosine, 1 mg (not to be used to report any adenosine phosphate compounds)

Adenosine is a nucleoside that is a component of RNA. Its nucleotides play major roles in the reactions and regulation of metabolism. Preparations of adenosine act as cardiac depressants, antiarrhythmics, and vasodilators. Adenosine is administered to convert paroxysmal supraventricular tachycardia (PSVT) to normal sinus rhythm. Diagnostic adenosine is administered to patients as an adjunct to a thallium myocardial perfusion scan for patients who are unable to adequately exercise. Recommended dose for therapeutic use is an initial 6 mg followed by 12 mg if the arrhythmia continues. Adenosine is administered via intravenous push injection.

J0171

J0171 Injection, adrenalin, epinephrine, 0.1 mg

Epinephrine hydrochloride (HCl), also known as adrenalin, is a synthetic version of a hormone secreted by the adrenal gland. Epinephrine is a potent stimulator of the sympathetic nervous system that increases blood pressure, stimulates the heart, and increases metabolic functions. Exogenous

J

epinephrine is used as a cardiac stimulant, to increase blood pressure, and to relax bronchial smooth muscles. The injectable version of epinephrine HCl is administered subcutaneously or intramuscularly and is used to treat serious hypersensitivity (allergic) reactions and anaphylaxis, and to restore cardiac rhythm in cardiac arrest.

J0172

J0172 Injection, aducanumab-avwa, 2 mg

Aducanumab-avwa is an amyloid beta-directed monoclonal antibody that is indicated for the treatment of adults, ages 18 years and older, with Alzheimer's disease. It is directed against aggregated soluble and insoluble forms of amyloid beta plaques in the brain, thought to be a defining pathophysiological feature of Alzheimer's disease. Treatment should be started in patients exhibiting mild cognitive impairment or mild dementia stage. It is supplied in single dose vials of 170 mg/1.7 mL and 300 mg/3 mL and requires dilution with 100 mL 0.9% sodium chloride prior to administration via intravenous (IV) infusion over one hour. Dosing must be titrated over the first six infusions until the recommended maintenance dosage of 10 mg/kg body weight is reached. Infusions should be administered every four weeks and at least 21 days apart, and MRIs are required prior to the seventh and twelfth infusions. See full prescribing information for complete administration instructions.

J0173

J0173 Injection, epinephrine (Belcher) not therapeutically equivalent to J0171, 0.1 mg

Epinephrine, also known as adrenalin, is a synthetic version of a hormone secreted by the adrenal gland. Epinephrine is an alpha- and beta-adrenergic agonist that is indicated for the treatment of adults, ages 18 years and older, to increase mean arterial blood pressure with hypotension associated with septic shock. It is supplied in a 2 ml ampule of 1 mg/1 ml (1:1,000 Injection, USP) and is administered via intravenous (IV) infusion. The recommended dosage is 0.05 mcg/kg body weight per minute to 2 mcg/kg body weight per minute, titrated to achieve desired mean arterial blood pressure. See full prescribing information for complete administration instructions. Report J0173 only for epinephrine manufactured by Belcher.

J0178

J0178 Injection, aflibercept, 1 mg

Aflibercept is a recombinant protein produced in Chinese hamster cells. The fused protein consists of portions of human vascular endothelial growth factor-A (VEGF) and placental growth factor (P1GF) receptors fused to human IgG1. VEGF and P1GF act on receptor sites to stimulate neovascularization and vascular permeability. Aflibercept is indicated as a treatment for neovascular (or wet) age-related macular degeneration (AMD). The recommended dose for aflibercept is 2 mg every four weeks for the first 12 weeks followed by 2 mg once every eight weeks. The drug is for intravitreal administration only.

J0179

J0179 Injection, brolucizumab-dbll, 1 mg

Brolucizumab-dbll is a human vascular endothelial growth factor (VEGF) inhibitor indicated for the treatment of neovascular (wet) age-related macular degeneration (AMD). It is administered by intravitreal injection. The recommended dose is 6 mg (0.05 mL of 120 mg/mL solution) monthly (approximately every 25 to 31 days) for the first three doses, followed by one dose of 6 mg (0.05 mL) every eight to 12 weeks.

J0180

J0180 Injection, agalsidase beta, 1 mg

Agalsidase beta is a recombinant human a-galactosidase A enzyme with the same amino acid sequence as the naturally occurring enzyme. It is produced by recombinant DNA technology in a Chinese hamster ovary. Agalsidase beta is an orphan drug specifically targeted to Fabry disease. Fabry disease is an X-linked genetic disorder of glycosphingolipid metabolism. A deficiency of enzyme a-galactosidase A leads to progressive accumulation of glycosphingolipids, predominantly GL-3, in many body tissues, occurring over a period of years or decades. Clinical manifestations of Fabry disease include renal failure, cardiomyopathy, and cerebrovascular accidents. Recommended dose is 1.0 mg per kg of body weight. Agalsidase beta is administered by intravenous infusion.

J0185

J0185 Injection, aprepitant, 1 mg

Aprepitant is a substance P/neurokinin-1 (NK1) receptor antagonist used for the treatment of adults to prevent acute and delayed nausea and vomiting associated with initial and repeat courses of highly emetogenic cancer chemotherapy (HEC), including high-dose cisplatin, as well as nausea and vomiting associated with moderately emetogenic cancer chemotherapy (MEC). NK1s are peptides found in the central and peripheral nervous systems involved in the transmission of a signal from outside the cell wall into the cell. Aprepitant blocks those transmissions. It is used in combination with a corticosteroid and a 5-HT3 antagonist. It is supplied as an injectable emulsion in a 100 mg single dose vial and is administered by intravenous infusion. For a single dose regimen, the dosage is 130 mg infused over 30 minutes approximately 30 minutes prior to chemotherapy administration on day one. For a three-day regimen, the dosage is 100 mg infused over 30 minutes approximately 30 minutes prior to chemotherapy administration on day one, followed by 80 mg aprepitant capsules given orally on days two and three. Aprepitant should not be used concurrently with pimozide.

J0190

J0190 Injection, biperiden lactate, per 5 mg

The injectable form of biperiden lactate has been discontinued.

J0200

J0200 Injection, alatrofloxacin mesylate, 100 mg

Per the FDA, this drug is no longer available in the United States.

J0202

J0202 Injection, alemtuzumab, 1 mg

Alemtuzumab is a monoclonal antibody produced by recombinant DNA technology in Chinese hamster ovaries. This monoclonal antibody is directed against the CD52 antigen, which is found on the surface of normal and malignant B and T lymphocytes, NK cells, monocytes, macrophages, and tissues of the male reproductive system. Alemtuzumab is indicated for the treatment of chronic B cell lymphocytic leukemia (CLL) in patients who have been treated with alkylating agents and who have failed fludarabine therapy. The drug is also indicated for the treatment of relapsing multiple sclerosis in patients who have had inadequate response to two or more drugs indicated for the treatment of multiple sclerosis. The recommended initial dose for the CLL is 3 mg rising to 30 mg as a maintenance dose. The drug is administered as a two-hour intravenous infusion. For the multiple sclerosis, the drug is administered in two courses by intravenous infusion over four hours. The first course is 12 mg/day on five consecutive days. The second course is 12 mg/day on three consecutive days, administered 12 months after the first.

J0205

J0205 Injection, alglucerase, per 10 units

Alglucerase is a modified form of beta-glucocerebrosidase prepared from pooled human placental tissue. It is an orphan drug used to treat Gaucher's disease caused by the lack of the enzyme glucocerebrosidase, which is crucial to the metabolism of fats. Alglucerase normalizes the pathway for membrane lipids. Dose is based on disease severity and individual patient response to treatment. Initial dosage may be as little as 2.5 units per kg of body weight three times a week up to as much as 60 units per kg administered as often as once a week or as infrequently as every four weeks. Alglucerase is administered by intravenous infusion over one to two hours.

J0207

J0207 Injection, amifostine, 500 mg

Amifostine is dephosphorylated in living tissue by an alkaline phosphate enzyme to become a biologically active form of free thiol in the body. Free thiol will bind to and detoxify the reactive metabolites of cisplatin, scavenges free radicals from tissues exposed to cisplatin. Amifostine is used to reduce the cumulative nephrotoxicity in patients who have received repeated doses of cisplatin because of advanced ovarian cancer, bladder cancer, testicular cancer, or non-small cell lung cancer. It is also newly used to reduce xerostomia in patients with head and neck cancer receiving postoperative radiation treatment. For patients on chemotherapy, it is injected over a 15-minute period one half hour before chemotherapy. For patients receiving radiation treatment, it is injected over a three minute period 15 to 30 minutes prior to radiation.

J0210

J0210 Injection, methyldopate HCl, up to 250 mg

Methyldopate hydrochloride is an aromatic-amino-acid decarboxylase inhibitor used primarily to treat hypertension or during a hypertensive crisis. It decreases the sympathetic outflow to the heart, kidneys, and peripheral vasculature. Decreased blood pressure may occur four to six hours after the administration of methyldopate hydrochloride and last 10 to 16 hours. The usual dose is 250 to 500 mg intravenously at six-hour intervals as required. The maximum recommended intravenous dose is 1 gram every six hours. Methyldopate hydrochloride is administered via intravenous infusion over 30 to 60 minutes.

J0215

J0215 Injection, alefacept, 0.5 mg

Alefacept is an injectable drug that suppresses the immune system and is used for the treatment of moderate to severe chronic plaque psoriasis. It interferes with lymphocyte activation by binding to the lymphocyte antigen and interfering with the human leukocyte function antigen-3 and the CD2 binding interaction. It is produced by recombinant DNA technology in a Chinese hamster ovary (CHO) mammalian cell expression system. The recommended dose is 7.5 mg given once weekly as an intravenous injection or 15 mg given once weekly as an intramuscular injection. The recommended regimen is a course of 12 weekly injections.

J0219

J0219 Injection, avalglucosidase alfa-ngpt, 4 mg

Avalglucosidase alfa-ngpt is an exogenous source of the human enzyme alpha-glucosidase (GAA) made from recombinant DNA technology using Chinese hamster ovaries. It is indicated for the treatment of patients, ages 1 year and older, with Pompe disease (GAA deficiency). Pompe disease is caused by the lack of the enzyme alpha-glucosidase, which is crucial to the metabolism of glycogen. A deficiency of GAA leads to a buildup of intralysosomal glycogen resulting in progressive muscle weakness. In infantile onset, Pompe disease may also lead to cardiomyopathy and impairment of respiratory function. For patients weighing 30 kg or less, the recommended dosage is 20 mg per kg body weight.

For patients weighing over 30 kg, the recommended dosage is 40 mg per kg body weight. It is administered by intravenous (IV) infusion, using an infusion pump, every two weeks. See full prescribing information for complete administration instructions.

J0220

J0220 Injection, alglucosidase alfa, 10 mg, not otherwise specified

Alglucosidase alfa is an exogenous source of the human enzyme alpha-glucosidase (GAA) made from recombinant DNA technology using Chinese hamster ovaries. It is an orphan drug used to treat infantile onset Pompe disease (GAA deficiency). Pompe disease is caused by the lack of the enzyme alpha-glucosidase, which is crucial to the metabolism of glycogen. A deficiency of GAA leads to a buildup of intralysosomal glycogen resulting in progressive muscle weakness. In infantile onset, Pompe disease may also lead to cardiomyopathy and impairment of respiratory function. The recommended dosage is 20 mg per kg of patient body weight. Alglucosidase alfa is administered by intravenous infusion, using an infusion pump, over four hours, every two weeks.

J0221

J0221 Injection, alglucosidase alfa, (Lumizyme), 10 mg

Alglucosidase alfa is an exogenous source of the human enzyme alpha-glucosidase made from recombinant DNA technology using Chinese hamster ovaries. It is an orphan drug used to treat non-infantile onset glycogen storage disease (GSD), type II or Pompe disease in patients 8 years of age and older who do not have cardiac hypertrophy. On August 1, 2014, Lumizyme was approved to also treat infantile onset Pompe's disease, including patients who are younger than 8 years of age. GSD II is caused by the lack of the enzyme alpha-glucosidase, which is crucial to the metabolism of glycogen. GSD II leads to a buildup of intralysosomal glycogen, resulting in progressive muscle weakness. In infantile onset, GSD II may also lead to cardiomyopathy and impairment of respiratory function. This code represents 1 mg of Lumizyme. The recommended dosage is 20 mg per kg of patient body weight. Alglucosidase alfa is administered by intravenous infusion, using an infusion pump, over four hours, every two weeks.

J0222

J0222 Injection, patisiran, 0.1 mg

Patisiran contains a transthyretin-directed double stranded siRNA that is indicated for the treatment of adults, ages 18 years and older, with polyneuropathy due to hereditary transthyretin-mediated (hATTR) amyloidosis. hATTR amyloidosis is caused by a gene mutation that affects the behavior of transthyretin (TTR), a protein that is made predominantly in the liver. TTR forms clusters, or amyloid deposits, that build up throughout the body and cause a range of symptoms. The siRNA in patisiran results in reduced serum TTR protein and reduced TTR protein deposits in the body. It is supplied in a single dose vial of 10 mg/5 ml and is administered by intravenous infusion over 80 minutes. The recommend dosage is 0.3 mg/kg every three weeks for patients weighing less than 100 kg and 30 mg for patients weighing 100 kg or more. Sixty minutes prior to infusion, oral acetaminophen, an intravenous corticosteroid, and H1 and H2 blockers should be administered.

J0223

J0223 Injection, givosiran, 0.5 mg

Givosiran is an aminolevulinate synthase 1-directed small interfering RNA that is indicated for the treatment of adults, ages 18 and older, with acute hepatic porphyria (AHP). AHP is a family of extremely rare genetic diseases that are characterized by potentially life-threatening attacks as well as chronic manifestations negatively affecting function and quality of life. The family of diseases include acute intermittent porphyria (AIP), ALA dehydratase-deficiency porphyria (ADP), hereditary coproporphyria (HCP), and variegate porphyria (VP). Symptoms may include server and diffuse abdominal pain, nausea and vomiting, dark or red urine, muscle weakness, numbness, respiratory failure, confusion, anxiety, seizures, hallucinations, and fatigue. Patients with VP and HCP may experience blistering lesions and erosions or ulcers of skin that has been exposed to sunlight. Givosiran is thought to degrade aminolevulinate synthase 1 (ALAS1) mRNA in hepatocytes through RNA interference and thereby reducing the circulating levels of neurotoxic intermediates aminolevulinic acid (ALA) and porphobilinogen (PBG). ALA and PGD are associated with acute attacks and other manifestations of AHP. It is supplied in a 189 mg/mL single dose vial. The recommended dosage is 2.5 mg per kg of body weight administered once monthly via subcutaneous injection. The required volume is calculated based on the recommended weight-based dosage and the indicated injection volume is withdrawn from the vial with a 21 gauge or larger needle. Doses requiring more than 1.5 mL should be divided equally into multiple syringes. Replace the needle with a 25- or 27-gauge needle with a ½-inch or 5/8-inch needle length. Administer subcutaneously into the abdomen, back of upper arms, or thighs. The injection site should be rotated for each administration.

J0224

J0224 Injection, lumasiran, 0.5 mg

Lumasiran is an HAO1-directed small interfering ribonucleic acid (siRNA) indicated for the treatment of adult and pediatric patients with primary hyperoxaluria type 1 (PH1). Primary hyperoxalurias are rare genetic diseases characterized by an overproduction of oxalate, a substance ingested in food and also produced by the body. PH1 is the most common and most severe type of primary hyperoxaluria. Lumasiran lowers urinary oxalate levels. The recommended dose is based on body weight and is administered by subcutaneous (SC) injection. See full prescribing information for complete administration instructions.

J0225

J0225 Injection, vutrisiran, 1 mg

Vutrisiran is a transthyretin-directed small interfering RNA that is indicated for the treatment of adults, ages 18 years and older, with polyneuropathy due to hereditary transthyretin-mediated amyloidosis (hATTR). hATTR amyloidosis is caused by a gene mutation that affects the behavior of transthyretin (TTR), a protein that is made predominantly in the liver. TTR forms clusters, or amyloid deposits, that build up throughout the body and cause a range of symptoms. The siRNA in vutrisiran can reduce serum TTR protein and TTR protein deposits in the body. It is supplied in a single dose prefilled syringe containing 25 mg/0.5 ml and is administered via subcutaneous (SC) injection by a health care professional. The recommended dosage is 25 mg once every three months. Patients receiving vutrisiran treatment may require vitamin A supplementation. See full prescribing information for complete administration instructions.

J0248

J0248 Injection, remdesivir, 1 mg

Remdesivir is a SARS-CoV-2 nucleotide analog RNA polymerase inhibitor that is indicated for the treatment of children and adults, ages 12 and older, weighing at least 40 kg, with coronavirus disease 2019 (COVID-19) that require hospitalization. In January 2022, additional EUA was granted for use in patients with positive SARS-CoV-2 viral testing, with mild-to-moderate COVID-19, are not hospitalized, and are at high-risk for progression to severe COVID-19 and hospitalization. Remdesivir is supplied in two formulas of 100 mg single-dose vials requiring dilution or reconstitution with 0.9% solidum chloride. The recommended dosage is a single loading dose of 200 mg on day one, administered via intravenous (IV) infusion over 30 to 120 minutes, followed by 100 mg administered daily via IV infusion beginning day two. The recommended total duration of treatment for patients not receiving extracorporeal membrane oxygenation (ECMO) or mechanical ventilation is five days. If clinical improvement is not demonstrated, treatment may be extended an additional five days. The recommended treatment duration for patients receiving ECMO or mechanical ventilation is 10 days. Remdesivir should only be administered in a health care setting that can provide acute care, similar to inpatient hospital care. See full prescribing information for complete administration instructions.

J0256

J0256 Injection, alpha 1-proteinase inhibitor (human), not otherwise specified, 10 mg

Alpha 1-proteinase inhibitor, human is a plasma product prepared from pooled human plasma of normal donors that contains high levels of purified human alpha 1-proteinase inhibitor (alpha1-PI) also known as alpha 1-antitrypsin. This is used to treat patients with alpha 1 antitrypsin deficiency (A1AD), a genetic protein deficiency that results in advanced emphysema showing up in young patients as an inherited disease, not related to smoking or environmental factors. It mimics COPD, asthma, and acquired emphysema and is therefore difficult to diagnose and rated as rare. Replacing the protein helps prevent the continued lung destruction caused by this deficiency. Recommended dose is 60 mg per kg of body weight once a week. Alpha 1-proteinase inhibitor is administered via intravenous infusion over 15 to 30 minutes.

J0257

J0257 Injection, alpha 1 proteinase inhibitor (human), (GLASSIA), 10 mg

Alpha 1-proteinase inhibitor (GLASSIA) human is a plasma product prepared from pooled human plasma of normal donors that contains high levels of purified human alpha 1-proteinase inhibitor (alpha1-PI), also known as alpha 1-antitrypsin. This is used to treat patients with alpha 1 antitrypsin deficiency (A1AD), also known as alpha1-antitrypsin (AAT) deficiency, a genetic protein deficiency that results in advanced emphysema showing up in young patients as an inherited disease, not related to smoking or environmental factors. It mimics COPD, asthma, and acquired emphysema and is therefore difficult to diagnose and rated as rare. Replacing the Alpha1-PI protein helps prevent the continued lung destruction caused by this deficiency. GLASSIA contains 2% active Alpha1-PI in a phosphate-buffered saline solution. Recommended dose is 60 mg per kg of body weight once a week. Alpha 1-proteinase inhibitor is administered via intravenous infusion over 60 to 80 minutes.

J0270-J0275

J0270 Injection, alprostadil, 1.25 mcg (code may be used for Medicare when drug administered under the direct supervision of a physician, not for use when drug is self-administered)

J0275 Alprostadil urethral suppository (code may be used for Medicare when drug administered under the direct supervision of a physician, not for use when drug is self-administered)

Alprostadil is a naturally occurring form of prostaglandin. It is a vasodilator that increases blood flow by expanding blood vessels. It is used for patients in need of palliative therapy for the temporary

J

maintenance of patency of ductus arteriosus who have congenital heart defects and who depend upon the patent ductus for survival. Studies have shown that alprostadil reopens a closing ductus arteriosus. It is also indicated in the treatment of erectile dysfunction. Alprostadil increases cavernous arterial blood flow and inhibits platelet aggregation. It induces erection by relaxing the trabecular smooth muscle and dilating the cavernosal arteries. This leads to expansion of lacunar spaces and entrapment of blood by compressing the venules against the tunica. This is also known as the corporal veno-occlusive mechanism. It also lowers the blood pressure and increases cardiac output. Alprostadil can be administered into a large vein or umbilical artery for infants with congenital heart defects. It is administered via injection into the corpora cavernosa or as a urethral suppository for erectile dysfunction. Both of the methods for treatment of erectile dysfunction can be self-administered.

J0278

J0278 Injection, amikacin sulfate, 100 mg

Amikacin sulfate is an antibiotic used to treat susceptible strains of Gram-negative bacteria. It binds to the RNA and will not allow the bacteria to synthesize protein that is essential to its growth. It is effective against *Pseudomonas* species, *E. coli, Proteus* species, *Klebsiella-Enterobacter-Serratia* species, *Providencia* species, *Salmonella* species, *Citrobacter* species, and *S. aureus*. Amikacin sulfate may be used to treat bacteremia, septicemia (including neonatal sepsis), osteomyelitis, septic arthritis, respiratory tract, urinary tract, intra-abdominal (including peritonitis) infections, and soft tissue abscesses. This medication is administered via intramuscular injection or intravenous infusion.

J0280

J0280 Injection, aminophyllin, up to 250 mg

Aminophylline is a bronchodilator that is used to treat breathing problems such as asthma, emphysema, and chronic bronchitis. It relaxes the smooth muscle in the bronchial airways and pulmonary blood vessels by interfering with phosphodiesterase, which is the enzyme that corrupts adenosine 3', 5'-cyclic monophosphate (cAMP).

J0282

J0282 Injection, amiodarone HCl, 30 mg

Amiodarone hydrochloride is an antiarrhythmic used in the treatment of ventricular fibrillation and hemodynamically unstable atrial fibrillation that do not respond to other treatment. It blocks the calcium channels and potassium channels and lengthens the cardiac action potential and slows the conduction and prolongation of refractoriness. It decreases the workload of the heart and the amount of oxygen it requires. Amiodarone hydrochloride can be administered orally or by intravenous push followed by intravenous infusion that may be continuous for several days.

J0283

J0283 Injection, amiodarone HCl (Nexterone), 30 mg

Amiodarone HCl is an antiarrhythmic agent used in the treatment and prophylaxis of ventricular fibrillation (VF) and hemodynamically unstable ventricular tachycardia (VT) that do not respond to other treatment in adults, ages 18 years and older. It blocks the calcium channels and potassium channels, lengthens the cardiac action potential, and slows the conduction and prolongation of refractoriness. It decreases the workload of the heart and the amount of oxygen it requires. It is supplied in single use, ready to use containers of 1.5 mg/ml (150 mg/100 ml) and 1.8 mg/ml (360 mg/200 ml) and is administered via intravenous (IV) infusion. No dilution is required. The recommended dosage is an initial loading dose of 150 mg in 100 ml infused over 10 minutes, followed by 1 mg/min for six hours, then 0.5 mg/min thereafter. For breakthrough VF or hemodynamically unstable VT, the recommended dosage is 150 mg in 100 ml infused over 10 minutes. It should not be used to treat patients with iodine sensitivity, cardiogenic shock, marked sinus bradycardia, or second- or third-degree atrioventricular (AV) block unless a pacemaker is available. See full prescribing information for complete administration instructions.

J0285-J0289

J0285 Injection, amphotericin B, 50 mg

J0287 Injection, amphotericin B lipid complex, 10 mg

J0288 Injection, amphotericin B cholesteryl sulfate complex, 10 mg

J0289 Injection, amphotericin B liposome, 10 mg

Amphotericin B is an antibiotic derived from a strain of *Streptomyces nodosus* that has antifungal properties. The drug is effective against a wide variety of fungi and some species of *Leishmania*. It binds to the fungus cell membrane and changes the permeability causing the cell contents to leak out, which causes cell death. Amphotericin B may be administered by intravenous infusion or intracavitary instillation over two to six hours. A topical version is used to treat superficial candidiasis. The cholesteryl complex version is administered by intravenous infusion to treat disseminated aspergillosis in patients refractory to or intolerant of conventional amphotericin B. The lipid complex is administered by intravenous infusion to treat invasive fungal infections in patients refractory to or intolerant of conventional amphotericin B. The liposome complex is administered by intravenous infusion to treat sever fungal infections and visceral leishmaniasis in patients refractory to or intolerant of conventional amphotericin B.

J0290

J0290 Injection, ampicillin sodium, 500 mg

Ampicillin is a form of penicillin used to treat respiratory or skin infections, urinary tract infections, bacterial meningitis, septicemia, and as a prophylaxis in dental procedures. It inhibits the formation of a cell wall during replication. It is effective against *E. coli, P. mirabilis*, enterococci, *Shigella, S. typh*osa and other Salmonella, non-penicillinase-producing *N. gonorrhoeae*, non-penicillinase-producing *H. influenzae* and staphylococci, and streptococci including *streptococcus pneumoniae, Shigella, S. typhosa* and other *Salmonella, E. coli, P. mirabilis*, and enterococci, and *O. Meningitides*. This drug may decrease the efficacy of oral contraceptives.

J0291

J0291 Injection, plazomicin, 5 mg

Plazomicin is an aminoglycoside antibiotic indicated for the treatment of adults,18 years of age and older, with complicated urinary tract infections (cUTI), including pyelonephritis, caused by the following organisms: *Escherichia coli, Klebsiella pneumoniae, Proteus mirabilis,* and *Enterobacter cloacae.* It is supplied in a single-dose vial of 500 mg/10 mL and is administered by intravenous infusion over 30 minutes every 24 hours for four to seven days. The recommended dosage is 15 mg/kg of body weight. Patients must have a creatinine clearance greater than or equal to 90 mL/min prior to start and daily during treatment. The dosage may need to be adjusted for patients with renal impairment and may need to be adjusted due to changes in renal function or results of daily creatinine clearance.

J0295

J0295 Injection, ampicillin sodium/sulbactam sodium, per 1.5 g

Ampicillin sodium and sulbactam sodium are used to treat gynecologic, intra-abdominal, and skin infections. Ampicillin inhibits the formation of a cell wall during replication and sulbactam inactivates the enzyme produced by the bacteria to make them resistant to the ampicillin. It is effective against *Staphylococcus aureus, Staphylococcus epidermidis, Staphylococcus saprophyticus, Streptococcus faecalis, Streptococcus pneumoniae, Streptococcus pyogenes, Streptococcus viridans, Haemophilus influenzae, Moraxella (Branhamella) catarrhalis, Escherichia coli, Klebsiella* species, *Proteus mirabilis, Proteus vulgaris, Providencia rettgeri, Providencia stuartii, Morganella morganii, Neisseria gonorrhoeae, Clostridium* species, *Peptococcus* species, *Peptostreptococcus* species, and *Bacteroides* species, including *B. fragilis*. Ampicillin sodium and sulbactam sodium are administered via intramuscular injection, which is given only to adults, and intravenous injection, which is given by slow infusion over 10 to 15 minutes.

J0300

J0300 Injection, amobarbital, up to 125 mg

Amobarbital is a barbiturate derivative that activates one of the major inhibitory neurotransmitters in the body, which reduces input resistance, depresses the electrical discharge along the cell and increases the conduction at the chloride channels, and increases the amplitude and decay time of inhibitory postsynaptic currents. Amobarbital, also known as truth serum, is indicated as a treatment for convulsions, anxiety, epilepsy, and as a short-term treatment of insomnia. The drug is also used for preoperative sedation. It is a schedule II drug with the suppository being a schedule III drug. This medication is administered orally, rectally, via intramuscular injection, and via intravenous push injection.

J0330

J0330 Injection, succinylcholine chloride, up to 20 mg

Succinylcholine chloride is skeletal muscle relaxant. It is used in combination with anesthesia to relax skeletal muscles for surgery, intubation, seizure control, and orthopedic manipulations. It reacts with cholinergic receptors of the motor end plates to create depolarization. Flaccid paralysis begins within one minute after administration and lasts approximately four to six minutes.

J0348

J0348 Injection, anidulafungin, 1 mg

Anidulafungin is a semisynthetic lipopeptide derived from the fungus *Aspergillus nidulans*. It is used as an antifungal drug. Anidulafungin disrupts the synthesis of a component of the fungal cell membrane. This component is not present in mammalian cells. Anidulafungin is indicated for the treatment of candidemia, intra-abdominal, peritoneal, and esophageal *Candida* infections. The drug may cause allergic reactions. Anidulafungin must be administered by intravenous infusion. Recommended dosage for esophageal candidiasis is an initial dose of 100 mg followed by 50 mg daily. The duration of treatment depends upon the patient's response, but should be for a minimum of 14 days or for at least seven days following resolution of symptoms. Recommended dosage for candidemia, intra-abdominal and peritoneal *Candida* infections is an initial dose of 200 mg followed by 100 mg daily. The duration of treatment depends upon the patient's response, but should continue for at least 14 days after the last positive culture.

J0350

J0350 Injection, anistreplase, per 30 units

Anistreplase is a complex composed of streptokinase and lys-plasminogen. It is also known as anisoylated plasminogen-streptokinase activator complex (APSAC). It is a thrombolytic agent used to dissolve blood clots that have formed in certain blood vessels.

It binds to fibrin, converts plasminogen into plasmin, and breaks down the thrombus into smaller components. Anistreplase is used primarily in the management of an acute myocardial infarction and should be administered as soon as possible after the onset of the heart attack symptoms. Anistreplase is administered via intravenous infusion.

J0360

J0360 Injection, hydralazine HCl, up to 20 mg

Hydralazine hydrochloride falls into a category of drugs known as antihypertensives. It works by exerting a vasodilating effect on vascular smooth muscle. It is used in combination with other drugs in treating a hypertensive crisis and eclampsia. Hydralazine hydrochloride can be administered by intramuscular injection, intravenous injection, or intravenous infusion.

J0364

J0364 Injection, apomorphine HCl, 1 mg

Apomorphine hydrochloride is a non-ergoline dopamine agonist. It is used for the acute, intermittent treatment of hypomobility, "off" episodes ("end-of-dose wearing off" and unpredictable "on/off" episodes) associated with advanced Parkinson's disease. Apomorphine should not be started without use of an associated antiemetic. Trimethobenzamide should be started three days prior to the initial dose of apomorphine and continued at least during the first two months of therapy. Ondansetron, granisetron, dolasetron, palonosetron, and alosetron should not be used as antiemetics due to reports of hypotension and loss of consciousness when given with apomorphine. The maximum recommended dose is 6 mg. Apomorphine is administered via subcutaneous injection.

J0365

J0365 Injection, aprotinin, 10,000 kiu

Aprotinin is broad-spectrum protease inhibitor obtained from a bovine lung that diminishes the inflammatory response in cardiopulmonary bypass surgery. It preserves glycoprotein in platelets. This reduces bleeding and decreases the need for allogenic blood transfusions. Patients receive a 1 milliliter test dose, for allergic reaction, intravenously at least 10 minutes prior to the loading dose. The loading dose is administered via intravenous infusion over 20 to 30 minutes after induction of anesthesia but prior to sternotomy. A dose is also added to the cardiopulmonary bypass circuit and a constant infusion is maintained until the end of surgery.

J0380

J0380 Injection, metaraminol bitartrate, per 10 mg

Metaraminol bitartrate is classified as an adrenergic agent, direct-acting vasopressor. It releases norepinephrine from storage sites and stimulates alpha-receptors, which causes an increase in blood pressure, venous tone, and pulmonary pressure. Metaraminol bitartrate is used in treating surgery related hypotension, trauma, adverse drug reactions, and spinal anesthesia. Metaraminol bitartrate can be administered via subcutaneous injection, intramuscular injection, intravenous push, or intravenous infusion.

J0390

J0390 Injection, chloroquine HCl, up to 250 mg

Chloroquine is an anti-infective used primarily in treating malaria and extraintestinal amebiasis. The mechanism of action is not fully understood but the drug does interfere with certain enzymes. It is effective against *Plasmodium vivax, Plasmodium malariae, P. ovale*, and susceptible strains of *Plasmodium falciparum* (but not the gametocytes of *P. falciparum*). It is not effective against exoerythrocytic forms of the parasite. Chloroquine is administered orally. The injectable form has been discontinued.

J0395

J0395 Injection, arbutamine HCl, 1 mg

Per the FDA, this drug is no longer available in the United States.

J0400-J0401

J0400 Injection, aripiprazole, intramuscular, 0.25 mg

J0401 Injection, aripiprazole, extended release, 1 mg

Aripiprazole is an antipsychotic medication used to treat schizophrenia and bipolar disorder. The precise mechanism of action of aripiprazole is not known. The drug has a strong attraction to dopamine and serotonin receptor sites and acts as an agonist to various dopamine and serotonin subtypes. Aripiprazole is indicated for: treatment of schizophrenia in patients age 13 years or older; acute and maintenance treatment of manic and mixed episodes of bipolar I disorder with or without psychotic features; adjunctive treatment of major depressive disorders; and treatment of agitation associated with schizophrenia or bipolar disorder, manic, or mixed. Aripiprazole is available in oral and injectable forms. The recommended oral dosage is 10 to 15 mg per day for schizophrenia, and 30 mg per day to treat bipolar disorder. When administered with an antidepressant, dosages may be as low as 2 mg per day. When aripiprazole is used to treat agitation associated with schizophrenia or bipolar mania, the dosage is usually 9.75 mg administered by intramuscular injection. The maximum daily dose is 30 mg/day.

J0456

J0456 Injection, azithromycin, 500 mg

Azithromycin is an antibiotic used in treating a wide range of bacterial infections including community acquired pneumonia, urethritis, and tonsillitis. It binds to the ribosomal subunit and disrupts microbial protein synthesis. It is effective against *Staphylococcus aureus, Streptococcus pneumoniae, Haemophilus influenzae, Moraxella catarrhalis, Neisseria gonorrhoeae, Chlamydia pneumoniae, Chlamydia trachomatis, Legionella pneumophila, Mycoplasma hominis, Mycoplasma pneumoniae, Streptococcus agalactiae, Streptococcus pyogenes*, and *Haemophilus ducreyi*. Recommended intravenous dose is 500 mg once a day for one or two days followed by an oral regimen. Azithromycin is administered orally or via intravenous infusion over one to three hours.

J0461

J0461 Injection, atropine sulfate, 0.01 mg

Atropine is an extract of an alkaloid from the plants belladonna, hyoscyamus, or stramonium. It is also made synthetically. Atropine sulfate is a highly toxic compound of atropine and sulfuric acid that has the same uses and effects as atropine. It blocks the neurotransmitter acetylcholine in muscarinic receptors of the parasympathetic system. Muscarinic receptors occur throughout the nervous system, including in the heart, smooth muscles of the blood vessels, lungs, salivary glands, gastrointestinal tract, and eye. Atropine sulfate in clinical doses counteracts the peripheral vessel dilatation and abrupt decrease in blood pressure produced by other drugs or biologicals. Systemic doses slightly raise systolic and lower diastolic pressures, slightly increase cardiac output, and decrease central venous pressure. Atropine is used as an antispasmodic to relax smooth muscles, to reduce secretions in the respiratory tract, and to temporarily increase heart rate or decrease AV-block until definitive treatment can take place, and as an antidote for cholinergic drugs toxins, poisoning from organophosphorus insecticides or certain toxic mushrooms. Since it counteracts the side effects of neuromuscular blockers and gases used in anesthesia, it may also be administered as a preanesthesia medication.

J0470

J0470 Injection, dimercaprol, per 100 mg

Dimercaprol, also known as BAL in oil, is a chemical compound dispersed in peanut oil used as a chelating agent. Certain heavy metals, especially arsenic, gold, lead, and mercury, bind with some of the pyruvate-oxidase enzymes and inhibit their normal functioning. Dimercaprol has a stronger attraction to the metal than the protein. It binds to the metal in a stable complex and carries it out of the body. It is indicated as a treatment for arsenic, gold, and mercury (soluble inorganic compounds) poisoning following ingestion, inhalation, or absorption through the skin of these metals or their salts, or following overdose of therapeutic agents containing these metals. Dimercaprol, in conjunction with edetate calcium disodium (calcium EDTA), is also used as a treatment for lead poisoning. Treatment should begin immediately after exposure. It is administered by intramuscular injection only and the drug needs to be administered repeatedly for several days. Dosages vary from 2.5 to 5 mg/kg of body weight every four to six hours depending on the metal that caused the poisoning. Pediatric dosages for lead poisoning vary from 50 to 75 mg per square meter of body surface area every four hours followed by calcium EDTA.

J0475-J0476

J0475 Injection, baclofen, 10 mg

J0476 Injection, baclofen, 50 mcg for intrathecal trial

Baclofen is a chemical analogue of y-aminobutyric acid, an amino acid also known as GABA that is used as a muscle relaxant and antispastic. GABA is the principal inhibitory neurotransmitter in the brain, but is also found in several extraneural tissues, including kidney and pancreatic islet cells. GABA modulates membrane chloride permeability and inhibits postsynaptic cell firing. Although baclofen is an analogue of GABA, its exact mechanism of action is not fully understood. It inhibits both monosynaptic and polysynaptic reflexes at the spinal level, possibly by decreasing excitatory neurotransmitter release. Baclofen is available in an oral self-administered version and in an intrathecal version. It is used intrathecally to treat spasticity of cerebral origin, including trauma to the brain or cerebral palsy. The intrathecal administration is a long-term infusion delivered by an implantable pump. Prior to the pump implantation, patients usually receive a test or trial dose of 50 mcg administered via an intrathecal injection.

J0480

J0480 Injection, basiliximab, 20 mg

Basiliximab is a chimeric (murine/human) monoclonal antibody produced by recombinant DNA technology that is an immunosuppressive agent. Basiliximab binds to certain interleukin-2, also as CD25 antigen, receptor sites on activated T lymphocytes. By blocking these receptor sites, it prevents the interleukin-2 from activating the immune response, preventing rejection of allogenic transplants. Basiliximab in combination with cyclosporine and corticosteroids is indicated for the prophylaxis of acute organ rejection in patients receiving renal transplants. It is administered by intravenous bolus or by infusion over a 20-30 minute period. The dosage varies from 10 -20 mg. Basiliximab should only be administered once prior to the transplant when it has been determined that the patient will have the transplant with the concomitant immunosuppression.

J0485

J0485 Injection, belatacept, 1 mg

Belatacept is an immunosuppressive drug that is a selective T-cell costimulation blocker. It is indicated for the prophylaxis of kidney transplant rejection in adult patients. Belatacept is used in combination with basiliximab induction, mycophenolate mofetil, and corticosteroids. The drug increases the risk for developing post-transplant lymphoproliferative disorder, mainly affecting the central nervous system. It has been found that patients without immunity to the Epstein-Barr virus (EBV) are at an increased risk and the manufacturer warns that belatacept should be used only in patients who are EBV seropositive. Belatacept is administered as an intravenous infusion with the total dosage dependent upon the patient's body weight.

J0490

J0490 Injection, belimumab, 10 mg

Belimumab is a human monoclonal antibody used to treat systemic lupus erythematosus (SLE). Lupus is an autoimmune disease in which a person's immune system attacks its own body systems. Belimumab is developed by recombinant DNA technology. Recombinant DNA technology combines two segments of DNA sections to create two or more DNA molecules. These newly created DNA molecules can be reproduced in mammal cells. In this type of technology, large quantities of a specific antibody component can be generated without creating the whole antibody. Recommended dose of belimumab is 10 mg/kg at two-week intervals for the first three doses and every four weeks after that. Administration is by IV infusion over a one-hour period.

J0491

J0491 Injection, anifrolumab-fnia, 1 mg

Anifrolumab-fnia is a human monoclonal antibody that binds to subunit 1 of the type 1 interferon receptor (IFNAR), inhibiting type 1 IFN signaling. It is indicated for the treatment of adult patients, ages 18 years and older, with systemic lupus erythematosus (SLE) who received standard therapy. SLE is an autoimmune disease in which a person's immune system attacks its own body systems. Anifrolumab-fnia is developed by recombinant DNA technology. Recombinant DNA technology combines two segments of DNA sections to create two or more DNA molecules. These newly created DNA molecules can be reproduced in mammal cells. In this type of technology, large quantities of a specific antibody component can be generated without creating the whole antibody. The recommended dosage is 300 mg administered via intravenous (IV) infusion over 30 minutes every four weeks. See full prescribing information for complete administration instructions.

J0500

J0500 Injection, dicyclomine HCl, up to 20 mg

Dicyclomine is a chemical compound that is an antispasmodic and anticholinergic (antimuscarinic) agent. It relieves smooth muscle spasms of the gastrointestinal tract. Dicyclomine appears to achieve this effect by inhibiting acetylcholine and by a direct effect on the smooth muscles. It is indicated for the treatment of irritable bowel syndrome. The injectable form is administered by intramuscular injection. Dosages are individualized to the patient depending upon response.

J0515

J0515 Injection, benztropine mesylate, per 1 mg

Benztropine mesylate is a chemical compound containing atropine and diphenhydramine. The drug has anticholinergic and antihistamine effects. Benztropine mesylate is indicated as an adjunct treatment of Parkinson's disease and as a treatment for extrapyramidal disorders except tardive dyskinesia due to neuroleptic drugs. The drug is available in injectable and oral forms. The injectable form is recommended when a rapid response is desired and is useful for psychotic patients with acute dystonic reactions or other reactions that make oral medication difficult or impossible. The injectable form is administered by intramuscular on intravenous injection. Dosages vary from 0.5 to 6 mg depending upon response.

J0517

J0517 Injection, benralizumab, 1 mg

Benralizumab is an interleukin-5 antagonist monoclonal antibody (IgG1 kappa) for the add-on maintenance treatment of severe asthma in patients age 12 years and older with an eosinophilic phenotype. Benralizumab should not be used for the treatment of other eosinophilic phenotypes or for the treatment of acute bronchospasm or status asthmaticus. Benralizumab is supplied in a 30 mg/mL prefilled, single dose syringe. The recommended dose is 30 mg every four weeks for the first three doses and 30 mg once every eight weeks thereafter. Benralizumab should not be used for patients who are hypersensitive to excipients.

J0520

J0520 Injection, bethanechol chloride, Myotonachol or Urecholine, up to 5 mg

Bethanechol chloride is a chemical compound that selectively stimulates the parasympathetic nervous system to release acetylcholine, a neurotransmitter. It stimulates the bladder muscles to contract and the motility of the gastric system. Bethanechol chloride is indicated for the treatment of acute postoperative and postpartum nonobstructive urinary retention and for neurogenic bladders with urinary retention. It is administered by subcutaneous injection. Dosages vary depending upon type and severity of the condition.

J0558

J0558 Injection, penicillin G benzathine and penicillin G procaine, 100,000 units

Penicillin G benzathine and penicillin G procaine is a suspension of equal amounts of each penicillin formulation. See the separate entries for penicillin G benzathine and penicillin G procaine for additional information. Penicillin G benzathine and penicillin G procaine is administered by deep intramuscular injection to the buttocks or thigh. The drug is slowly absorbed, released from the injection site. Once in the body, penicillin G benzathine and penicillin G procaine is hydrolyzed to penicillin G. The hydrolysis and slow absorption provide sustained, but lower blood levels of penicillin. Antibiotic action can be present for two to four weeks after a single injection. Susceptibility studies should be performed prior to the administration of this drug. Indications include severe upper respiratory tract infections of susceptible streptococci, scarlet fever, erysipelas, skin and soft tissue infections of susceptible streptococci, and severe pneumonia and otitis media due to susceptible pneumococci.

J0561

J0561 Injection, penicillin G benzathine, 100,000 units

Penicillin G benzathine, also known as benzathine benzylpenicillin, is a version of penicillin that contains dibenzylethylene diamine. Penicillins block the actions of transpeptidase, an enzyme needed to create the cell wall. This weakens the bacterial cell wall causing cellular death. This formulation is administered by deep intramuscular injection to the buttocks or thigh. The drug is slowly absorbed released from the injection site. Once in the body, penicillin G benzathine is hydrolyzed to penicillin G. The hydrolysis and slow absorption provide sustained, but lower blood levels of penicillin. Antibiotic action can be present for two to four weeks after a single injection. Susceptibility studies should be performed prior to the administration of penicillin G benzathine. Indications include mild to moderate upper respiratory tract infections of susceptible streptococci, syphilis, yaws, pinta, as a prophylaxis for rheumatic fever and chorea, and as a prophylactic follow-up for rheumatic heart disease and acute glomerulonephritis. Dosages vary from 300,000 units to 2,400,000 units depending upon the age of the patient and the disease being treated.

J0565

J0565 Injection, bezlotoxumab, 10 mg

Bezlotoxumab is a human monoclonal antibody indicated to reduce the risk of reoccurrence of clostridium difficile infections (CDI) for patients 18 years of age and older. It binds to CDI toxin B to neutralize its effects. Bezlotoxumab is not indicated for treatment of CDI and should only be administered with an antibacterial drug prescribed to treat the CDI. The recommended dosage is 10 mg/kg administered by intravenous infusion, through a central line or peripheral catheter, over 60 minutes.

J0567

J0567 Injection, cerliponase alfa, 1 mg

Cerliponase alfa is an enzyme replacement for the treatment of ceroid lipofuscinosis type 2 (CLN2) disease or tripeptidyl peptidase 1 (TPP1) deficiency, a form of Batten disease. Batten disease is one of approximately 50 diseases known as lysosomal storage disorders (LSD), in which genetic mutations disrupt the body's cells ability to dispose of wastes, causing a buildup of proteins and lipids. CLN2 disease typically occurs in infantile or late juvenile patients. Patients with this disease suffer gradually increasing neurological impairments, including cognitive disorders, loss of motor skills, personality and psychiatric disorders, seizures, and vision loss. Cerliponase alfa slows the loss of ambulation (crawling, walking) in symptomatic patients. It is indicated for patients 3 years of age or older. Recommended dosage is 300 mg administered by intraventricular infusion, followed by infusion of intraventricular electrolytes over 4.5 hours.

J0570

J0570 Buprenorphine implant, 74.2 mg

A buprenorphine implant is a partial opioid agonist indicated for the maintenance treatment of opioid dependence in patients who have achieved and sustained prolonged clinical stability on low-to-moderate doses of a transmucosal buprenorphine. This implant should be used as part of a complete treatment program to include counseling and psychosocial support. Four buprenorphine implants are inserted subdermally in the upper arm for six months. They should be removed by the end of the sixth month.

J0571

J0571 Buprenorphine, oral, 1 mg

Buprenorphine is a partial opioid antagonist for the treatment of opioid dependence. Buprenorphine is a Schedule III narcotic under the Controlled Substances Act. Because of the Drug Abuse Treatment Act, it is also one of the few drugs for the treatment of opiate dependence that can be prescribed through a doctor's office rather than an addiction treatment center. The drug is administered sublingually. The tablet is available in 2 mg and 8 mg dose strengths. Code J0571 is billed in 1 mg increments.

J0572-J0575

J0572 Buprenorphine/naloxone, oral, less than or equal to 3 mg buprenorphine

J0573 Buprenorphine/naloxone, oral, greater than 3 mg, but less than or equal to 6 mg buprenorphine

J0574 Buprenorphine/naloxone, oral, greater than 6 mg, but less than or equal to 10 mg buprenorphine

J0575 Buprenorphine/naloxone, oral, greater than 10 mg buprenorphine

Buprenorphine/naloxone is a fixed combination of buprenorphine, a partial antagonist at the mu-opioid receptor and an antagonist at the kappa-opioid receptor, as well as naloxone, an antagonist at the mu-opioid receptor. It is indicated for the treatment of opioid dependence. Buprenorphine is a Schedule III narcotic under the Controlled Substances Act. The drug is administered sublingually in buccal film or tablet form. The recommended dosage varies depending upon the patient's clinical condition (e.g., current opioid withdrawal, dependence, maintenance) and the brand and dosage prescribed by the clinician. For a dose less than or equal to 3 mg, report J0572. For a dose greater than 3 mg but less than or equal to 6 mg, report J0573. For a dose greater than 6 mg, but less than or equal to 10 mg, report J0574. For a dose greater than 10 mg, report J0575.

J0583

J0583 Injection, bivalirudin, 1 mg

Bivalirudin is a synthetic, 20 amino acid peptide that is a specific and reversible direct thrombin inhibitor. It binds to both circulating and clot-bound thrombin, which in turn prevents the thrombin from activating the coagulant cycle. Bivalirudin is indicated for use in conjunction with aspirin therapy as an anticoagulant in patients with unstable angina undergoing percutaneous transluminal coronary angioplasty (PTCA). The use of bivalirudin in conjunction with glycoprotein IIb/IIIa inhibitor is currently in clinical trials. Bivalirudin is also indicated for patients with or at risk for heparin-induced thrombocytopenia or heparin-induced thrombocytopenia with thrombosis syndrome who are undergoing percutaneous coronary interventions (PCI). Bivalirudin is not recommended for patients with acute coronary syndromes who are not undergoing PTCA or PCI. The drug is administered by intravenous injection and infusion. The recommended initial dosage is an intravenous bolus of 0.75 mg per kg of body weight. This is followed by an infusion of 1.75 mg per kg of body weight per hour for the duration of the procedure. Continued infusion of the drug after the procedure is left to the discretion of the treating physician.

J0584

J0584 Injection, burosumab-twza, 1 mg

Burosumab-twza is a fibroblast growth factor 23 (FGF23) blocking antibody that is indicated for the treatment of patients 1 year of age and older with X-linked hypophosphatemia (XLH). Hypophosphatemia is a low level of phosphorus in the blood. The most common form of hereditary hypophosphatemic rickets, XLH is due to genetic disorder carried on the X chromosome. The kidneys of patients with XLH treat phosphorus as a waste product rather than sending it back into circulation to be used by bones and teeth. Burosumab-twza works by binding to and inhibiting activity of FGF23, which restores renal phosphate reabsorption and increases the serum level of vitamin D. It is supplied in 10 mg/mL, 20 mg/mL, or 30 mg/mL single dose vials and is administered via subcutaneous injection. For pediatric patients, the recommended starting dose is 0.8 mg/kg of body weight, rounded to the nearest 10 mg, every two weeks. For adult patients, the recommended dose is 1 mg/kg body weight, rounded to the nearest 10 mg, up to a maximum dose of 90 mg, every four weeks.

J0585

J0585 Injection, onabotulinumtoxinA, 1 unit

Toxins are poisons, usually proteins produced by some higher plants, certain animals, and pathogenic bacteria, which are highly toxic for other living organisms. OnabotulinumtoxinA is a potent neurotoxin produced by the bacterium *Clostridium botulinum* type A. The toxin binds to sites on motor and sympathetic nerves and inhibits the release of acetylcholine. Injection of onabotulinumtoxinA produces partial chemical denervation at the injection site resulting in a localized reduction in muscular activity. OnabotulinumtoxinA is indicated as a cosmetic agent to provide temporary improvement in the appearance of moderate to severe glabellar lines associated with corrugator and/or procerus muscle activity. It may also be used as treatment for cervical dystonia in adults to decrease the severity of an abnormal head position and neck pain, severe primary axillary hyperhidrosis that is inadequately managed with topical agents, and strabismus and blepharospasm associated with dystonia in patients 12 years of age or older. OnabotulinumtoxinA is injected intramuscularly.

J0586

J0586 Injection, abobotulinumtoxinA, 5 units

AbobotulinumtoxinA is an acetylcholine release inhibitor and a neuromuscular blocker. It is used to treat adult cervical dystonia and the temporary treatment of glabellar lines in adults age 65 and over. It is a purified form of the Clostridium botulinum type A bacteria. The medication is injected into the affected muscles. The recommended dose is 500 units for patients who have not been treated before. They should be divided between the muscles being treated. The injections may be done with EMG guidance. In clinical studies, it appears that the peak affect is about two to four weeks. If any retreatments are need, there should be a span of at least twelve weeks. Retreatment dosage is between 250 and 1,000 units. The recommended dose for patients with glabellar lines is 50 units divided equally into the five areas. Retreatment should not be any more frequently than every three months.

J0587

J0587 Injection, rimabotulinumtoxinB, 100 units

Botulinum toxin type B is a purified form of the neurotoxin produced from fermentation of *Clostridium botulinum* type B. It inhibits acetylcholine release at the nerve and is used as a neuromuscular blocking agent. Botulinum toxin type B is indicated for the treatment of cervical dystonia to reduce the severity of abnormal head position and associated neck pain caused by cervical dystonia. Botulinum toxin type B is administered by injection directly into the muscles that are affected. The average dose of botulinum toxin type B in adults for the treatment of cervical dystonia and associated abnormal head position and neck pain is one or more injections up to a total of 2,500 to 5,000 units.

J0588

J0588 Injection, incobotulinumtoxinA, 1 unit

IncobotulinumtoxinA is a type of botulinum toxin that is purified and separated from other proteins, leaving a neurotoxin behind. It is used to treat adults with cervical dystonia to help alleviate the abnormal neck position. This may also be used to treat blepharospasm in patients who have previously received onabotulinumtoxinA. IncobotulinumtoxinA is administered by injection into the affected muscle. The recommended dose can vary from 1.25 units up to 150 units depending on the area being treated and the severity of the muscle spasm.

J0591

J0591 Injection, deoxycholic acid, 1 mg

Deoxycholic acid is a cytolytic drug indicated for the treatment of severe convexity (fullness) associated with submental fat in adults, ages 18 years and older. It is supplied in 2 mL single use vials and is administered via subcutaneous injection. Special care should be taken to avoid the marginal mandibular nerve, post-platysmal fat, dermis, muscle, salivary glands, lymph nodes, or into arteries or veins. A large bore needle is used to draw 1 mL of deoxycholic acid into a sterile 1 mL syringe; it is then injected into the preplatysmal fat using a 30-gauge or smaller 0.5-inch needle. The recommended dosage is 0.2 mL injections that are spaced 1 cm apart until the entire planned treatment area has been injected, not to exceed 50 injections/10 mL in a single treatment. Up to six single treatments can be administered at intervals of no less than one month apart. Treatment should not be injected into subcutaneous fat outside of the submental area.

J0592

J0592 Injection, buprenorphine HCl, 0.1 mg

Buprenorphine hydrochloride is a schedule V controlled substance. It is indicated for moderate to severe pain including postoperative pain and chronic pain of patients with terminal diseases. It is also used adjunctively with anesthesia as a means of providing postoperative pain relief. Although the action of the drug is not known, it binds with opiate receptors in the central nervous system and alters not only the perception of pain, but the emotional response as well. Buprenorphine hydrochloride is an injectable solution. It is administered by intramuscular, intravenous, or epidural injection. It may be administered by continuous intravenous infusion.

J0593

J0593 Injection, lanadelumab-flyo, 1 mg (code may be used for Medicare when drug administered under direct supervision of a physician, not for use when drug is self-administered)

Lanadelumab-flyo is a plasma kallikrein inhibitor (monoclonal antibody) indicated for prophylactic treatment of adults and children, 12 years and older, for the prevention of hereditary angioedema (HAE) attacks. HAE is a rare, but life-threatening genetic disorder of the immune system characterized by edema in various parts of the body, including the extremities, intestines, face, and airway. It is supplied in a 300 mg/2 ml ready-to-use solution in a single dose vial and is administered via subcutaneous injection into the abdomen, thigh, or upper arm. The vial should be removed from the refrigerator 15 minutes before injection. The recommended starting dose is 300 mg every two weeks. If HAE is well-controlled (patient has been attack-free for six months), the interval may be adjusted to every four weeks.

J0594

J0594 Injection, busulfan, 1 mg

Busulfan is a chemotherapeutic drug classified as a bifunctional alkylating agent that suppresses bone marrow function. Busulfan is used in combination with cyclophosphamide as a conditioning regiment prior to allogenic bone marrow or stem cell transplantation for chronic myelogenous leukemia. Injectable busulfan is administered as an intravenous infusion over two hours via a central venous catheter. The drug should be administered every six hours for four consecutive days for a total of 16 doses. The recommended dose is 0.8 mg per kg of adjusted ideal body weight.

J0595

J0595 Injection, butorphanol tartrate, 1 mg

Butorphanol tartrate is a schedule IV controlled substance. It is indicated for moderate to severe pain, including postoperative pain and labor. It is also used prior to the administration of anesthesia and adjunctively with anesthesia. Although the action of the drug is not known, it binds with opiate receptors in the central nervous system and alters not only the perception of pain, but the emotional response as well. Butorphanol tartrate is administered by intramuscular and intravenous push injection.

J0596

J0596 Injection, C1 esterase inhibitor (recombinant), Ruconest, 10 units

C-1 esterase inhibitor protein is one of nine complement proteins found in the blood that works with the body's immune system in coagulation, fighting disease and the development of inflammation. Hereditary angioedema (HAE) is a rare, but life-threatening genetic disorder of the immune system characterized by edema in various parts of the body, including the extremities, intestines, face, and airway. For adult and pediatric patients with HAE, C-1 esterase inhibitor (recombinant) lyophilized powder is used to treat acute attacks. Recommended dosage is 50 IU per kg with a maximum of 4,200 IU to be administered as a slow intravenous injection over a five-minute period. The drug is for intravenous use after reconstitution only. No more than two doses should be administered within 24 hours.

J0597-J0598

J0597 Injection, C1 esterase inhibitor (human), Berinert, 10 units

J0598 Injection, C1 esterase inhibitor (human), Cinryze, 10 units

C1 esterase inhibitor is a protein found in the blood that inactivates two components of C1 protease. Human plasma is used to develop the C1 esterase inhibitor protein. A deficiency of C1 esterase inhibitor gives rise to hereditary angioedema (HAE), a rare condition that affects the immune system and is passed down in families. HAE can cause sudden, severe swelling of arms, legs, lips, eyes, tongue, throat, or the intestinal tract. Berinert is used to treat acute attacks of abdominal or facial attacks HAE. Recommended dose is 20 units per kg body weight administered by slow intravenous injection at a rate of approximately 4 mL per minute. Cinryze is used as a prevention of the angioedema attacks. The recommended dose is 1,000 units every three or four days and is administered by IV infusion.

J0599

J0599 Injection, C1 esterase inhibitor (human), (Haegarda), 10 units

C1 esterase inhibitor (C1-INH) is a protein found in the blood that inactivates two components of C1 protease. A deficiency of C1-INH gives rise to hereditary angioedema (HAE), a rare condition that affects the immune system. HAE can cause sudden, severe swelling of arms, legs, lips, eyes, tongue, throat, or the intestinal tract. Haegarda, derived from human plasma, is indicated for patients 12 years of age and older to increase the body's level of C1-INH, reduce swelling, and prevent HAE attacks. Recommended dose is 60 units per kg body weight, after reconstitution with sterile water. It is administered by subcutaneous injection twice weekly.

J0600

J0600 Injection, edetate calcium disodium, up to 1,000 mg

Edetate calcium disodium is a chelating drug that is used as an antidote for lead poisoning and lead encephalopathy in adults and children. The mode of action of the drug is to form a stable chelate with any metal that has the ability to displace calcium, particularly lead. Edetate calcium disodium is used alone for patients with very high blood lead levels (>70 mcg/dl). When lead poisoning is present, the drug should be used in combination with dimercaprol. Therapy is administered over a five-day period, followed by an interruption of two to four days (to allow for redistribution of the lead, as well as to prevent depletion of other essential metals such as zinc), and then another treatment course is administered. Most often two courses of therapy are administered. Edetate calcium disodium is provided in injectable form only. The drug may be administered intramuscularly (preferred route for pediatric patients), as well as for all patients with lead encephalopathy. Intravenously, the drug is administered as a slow infusion over a period of eight to 12 hours.

J0604

J0604 Cinacalcet, oral, 1 mg, (for ESRD on dialysis)

Cinacalcet is a calcium sensing receptor agonist that is indicated for adult patients with secondary hyperparathyroidism (HPT) with chronic kidney disease (CKD), who are also on dialysis; hypercalcemia patients with parathyroid carcinoma (PC); and for hypercalcemia patients with primary HPT who are unable to undergo parathyroidectomy. Cinacalcet should not be used for CKD patients who are not on dialysis. The recommended dosage is based on clinical presentation. For secondary HPT with CKD on dialysis patients, a starting dose of 30 mg once daily is given, then the dose is titrated every two to four weeks through increased doses (30, 60, 90, 120, and 180 mg) once daily as indicated until the patient achieves targeted intact parathyroid hormone (iPTH) levels. For hypercalcemia with PC or hypercalcemia with primary HPT, a starting does of 30 mg twice daily is given, then the dose is titrated every two to four weeks through increased doses (60 mg twice daily, 90 mg twice daily, and 90 mg three or four times daily) as indicated to regulate serum calcium levels.

J0606

J0606 Injection, etelcalcetide, 0.1 mg

Etelcalcetide is a calcium sensing receptor agonist that is indicated for adult patients with secondary hyperparathyroidism (HPT) with chronic kidney disease (CKD), who are also on dialysis. Etelcalcetide should not be used for adult patients with parathyroid carcinoma, primary hyperparathyroidism, or CKD patients who are not on dialysis. The recommended starting dosage is 5 mg administered by intravenous bolus injections, three times per week, following the end of dialysis. It should be administered into the venous line of the dialysis circuit during rinse back, or intravenously after rinse back. The recommended maintenance dosage is titrated, from 2.5 mg to 15 mg, based on parathyroid hormone (PTH) and the corrected serum calcium response, three times per week. The dosage may be increased by increments of 2.5 mg or 5 mg every four weeks.

J0610

J0610 Injection, calcium gluconate (Fresenius Kabi), per 10 ml

Calcium gluconate is a form of calcium used to replace and maintain adequate levels of calcium. It is indicated for the treatment of adults and children, older than 28 days, with acute symptomatic hypocalcemia. It is supplied in single dose vials of 1,000 mg/10 ml (100 mg/ml), 5,000 mg/50 ml (100 mg/ml), and 10,000 mg/100 ml (100 mg/ml) requiring dilution with 5% dextrose or normal saline and is administered via bolus or continuous intravenous (IV) infusion. The recommended dosage varies based on severity of symptoms, serum calcium level, and onset acuity of hypocalcemia. Serum calcium should be measured during intermittent infusion every four to six hours and during continuous infusions every one to four hours. It should not be administered with fluids containing phosphate or bicarbonate. See full prescribing information for complete administration instructions. Report J0610 only for calcium gluconate manufactured by Fresenius Kabi.

J0611

J0611 Injection, calcium gluconate (WG Critical Care), per 10 ml

Calcium gluconate is a form of calcium used to replace and maintain adequate levels of calcium. It is indicated for the treatment of adults and children, 29 days and older, with acute symptomatic hypocalcemia. It is supplied in single dose bags of 1,000 mg/50 ml (20 mg/ml), 1,000 mg/100 ml (10 mg/ml), and 2,000 mg/100 ml (20 mg/ml) and is administered via intravenous (IV) infusion. No further dilution is required. The recommended dosage varies based on severity of symptoms, serum calcium level, and onset acuity of hypocalcemia. Serum calcium should be measured during intermittent infusion every four to six hours and during continuous infusions every one to four hours. It should not be administered with fluids containing phosphate or bicarbonate. See full prescribing information for complete administration instructions. Report J0611 only for calcium gluconate manufactured by WG Critical Care.

J0620

J0620 Injection, calcium glycerophosphate and calcium lactate, per 10 ml

Calcium is a metallic element that is the most abundant element in the human body. It is found in almost all organized tissues. Calcium, in combination with phosphorus, forms calcium phosphate, the dense, hard material of the teeth and bones. It is an essential dietary element, an electrolyte essential for the maintenance of normal heartbeat and functioning of nerves and muscles. Calcium also plays a role in multiple phases of blood coagulation and in many enzymatic processes. Calcium glycerophosphate and calcium lactate are electrolytes used to replace and maintain adequate levels of calcium. They are indicated for the prophylaxis and treatment of hypocalcemia. Calcium glycerophosphate and calcium lactate are administered by intramuscular or intravenous injection.

J0630

J0630 Injection, calcitonin salmon, up to 400 units

Calcitonin-salmon is a synthetic version of the hormone calcitonin originally obtained from salmon, but now produced by recombinant DNA technology. The salmon version has a slightly different amino acid sequence than the human form, but it produces the same effects. Calcitonin lowers plasma calcium and phosphate levels, inhibits bone resorption, and acts as an antagonist to the parathyroid hormone. Calcitonin-salmon is indicated for the treatment of symptomatic Paget's disease of bone, hypercalcemia, and postmenopausal osteoporosis. The drug is provided in injection solution for subcutaneous or intramuscular injection.

J0636

J0636 Injection, calcitriol, 0.1 mcg

Calcitrol is a form of cholecalciferol that is a parathyroid-like hormone. It increases the ability of the body to absorb vitamin D and to distribute calcium throughout the body. It is indicated for the treatment of hypocalcemia, hypophosphatemia, rickets, osteodystrophy associated with long-term dialysis, and such disorders as hypoparathyroidism and pseudo-hypoparathyroidism. It is available in oral and injectable forms. The injectable form is administered by intravenous injection. Dosages vary from 0.25 to 3 mcg depending upon the form and indication.

J0637

J0637 Injection, caspofungin acetate, 5 mg

Caspofungin acetate is an antifungal with the ability to inhibit one of the integral components of the cell wall of the fungus. It is indicated for treatment of presumed fungal infections in patients that are febrile and neutropenic, esophageal candidiasis, intra-abdominal candidiasis, pleural space candida infection, candida peritonitis, and for the treatment of invasive aspergillosis in patients who are intolerant of or refractory to other therapies. Caspofungin acetate is administered by slow intravenous infusion over one hour. It should not be mixed or infused with another drug. For the majority of indications, a 70 mg initial loading dose is administered on the first day, followed by 50 mg daily.

J0638

J0638 Injection, canakinumab, 1 mg

Canakinumab is a recombinant monoclonal antibody used to treat cryopyrin-associated periodic syndromes (CAPS), including familial cold autoinflammatory syndrome (FCAS), Muckle-Wells syndrome (MWS), and systemic juvenile idiopathic arthritis (SJIA). It is also used to treat tumor necrosis factor receptor associated periodic syndrome (TRAPS), familial Mediterranean Fever (FMF), and hyperimmunoglobulin D syndrome (HIDS)/Mevalonate kinase deficiency (MKD). CAPS and TRAPS are syndromes usually caused by a genetic mutation. The ultimate result of this mutation is increased interleukin-1 beta that stimulates inflammation. Canakinumab binds to the interleukin-1 beta, which counteracts its ability to bind with the receptors. SJIA is a severe autoinflammatory disease, driven by proinflammatory cytokines such as interleukin 1Î^{2} (IL-1Î^{2}). Recommended dose for CAPS, SJIA, or MWS is 150 mg for patients who weigh more than 40 kg every eight weeks. For patients under that weight or children, dose is based on body weight. The recommended dose for TRAPS, FMF, and HIDS/MKD patients with a body weight greater than 40 kg is 150 mg every four weeks. For patients under that weight or children, dose is based on body weight. Canakinumab is administered by subcutaneous injection.

J0640

J0640 Injection, leucovorin calcium, per 50 mg

Leucovorin calcium (folinic acid, citrovorum factor) is a form of folic acid. When used with the chemotherapy drug 5-fluorouraci (Adrucil, 5-FU), it increases the ability of that drug to reduce or stop cell growth in advanced colorectal cancer. Leucovorin calcium is also indicated as a treatment for or to prevent toxicities associated with folic acid antagonists including methotrexate (MTX, Rheumatrex), trimetrexate (Neutrexin), trimethoprim (Proloprim, Trimpex), trimethoprim/sulfamethoxazole (Bactrim, Septra), pyrimethamine (Daraprim), and pyrimethamine/sulfadoxine (Fansidar). Leucovorin calcium is also used for the treatment of folate-deficient megaloblastic anemias. Leucovorin calcium is available in injectable and oral forms. Doses and route of administration vary with regards to the condition being treated.

J0641

J0641 Injection, levoleucovorin, not otherwise specified, 0.5 mg

Levoleucovorin is similar to folate and used to reduce the toxicity in high-dose methotrexate therapy in osteosarcoma. Methotrexate is a folic acid antagonist. Folate is one of the B vitamins necessary for the production of DNA and RNA. Recommended dose is 7.5 mg administered as an IV infusion. It should not be mixed with other agents in the same mixture.

J0642

J0642 Injection, levoleucovorin (Khapzory), 0.5 mg

Levoleucovorin is a folate analog indicated for the treatment of metastatic colorectal cancer along with fluorouracil; to reduce the toxicity that is associated with an overdosage of folic acid antagonists or due to impaired elimination of methotrexate; and for rescue following high-dose methotrexate therapy in patients treated for osteosarcoma. It is supplied as a lyophilized powder in 175 mg and 300 mg single dose vials that require reconstitution with 0.9% sodium chloride and is administered via intravenous infusion. The recommended dosage is dependent upon the condition being treated. See full prescribing information for complete administration instructions. The drug should not be used to treat pernicious anemia or megaloblastic anemia due to lack of vitamin B12 and should not be used by patients that are hypersensitive to leucovorin products, folic acid, or folinic acid.

J0670

J0670 Injection, mepivacaine HCl, per 10 ml

Mepivacaine hydrochloride is a local anesthetic available in concentrations of 1%, 1.5%, and 2% for injection. As a local anesthetic, mepivacaine hydrochloride blocks the generation and conduction of nerve impulses. It may be administered by local infiltration, as a peripheral nerve block, or for caudal and lumbar epidural blocks. Dosages and concentrations of the drug vary with regards to how it is being administered.

J0689

J0689 Injection, cefazolin sodium (Baxter), not therapeutically equivalent to J0690, 500 mg

Cefazolin sodium is a semi-synthetic cephalosporin that inhibits synthesis of the cell wall used to prevent and treat a wide range of bacterial infections and is indicated for preoperative prophylaxis for adults ages 18 years and older. It is supplied in a single dose bag of 2 g/100 ml. Prior to treatment, a creatinine clearance greater than or equal to 35 ml/minute is required. The recommended dosage is 2 g administered via intravenous (IV) infusion over 30 minutes. See full prescribing information for complete administration instructions. Report J0689 only for cefazolin sodium manufactured by Baxter.

J0690

J0690 Injection, cefazolin sodium, 500 mg

Cefazolin sodium is a semi-synthetic cephalosporin that inhibits synthesis of the cell wall used to prevent and treat a wide range of bacterial infections. Susceptibility studies should be performed prior to the administration of cefazolin sodium. Susceptible bacteria include *S. pneumoniae*, *Klebsiella* species, *H. influenzae*, *S. aureus*, group A beta-hemolytic streptococci, *E. coli*, *P. mirabilis*, *S. aureus*, and some strains of *Enterobacter* and enterococci. Cefazolin sodium is available in an injectable form for intravenous and intramuscular injection or intravenous infusion. Dosages vary from 25 mg to 1 g depending on the indication and for children, their body weight.

J0691

J0691 Injection, lefamulin, 1 mg

Lefamulin is an antibiotic indicated for the treatment of adults, ages 18 years and older, with community-acquired bacterial pneumonia (CABP) caused by susceptible microorganisms such as *Streptococcus pneumoniae, Staphylococcus aureus* (methicillin-susceptible isolates), *Haemophilus influenzae, Legionella pneumophila, Mycoplasma pneumoniae,* and *Chlamydophila pneumoniae*. It is supplied in a 150 mL single dose vial and is administered via intravenous (IV) infusion and must be diluted with the supplied 250 mL solution of 10 mM citrate buffered 0.9% sodium chloride. The recommended adult dosage is 150 mg every 12 hours by IV infusion over 60 minutes for five to seven days, with the option to switch to 600 mg tablets every 12 hours to complete the treatment course. For patients with hepatic impairment, the dosage should be revised to 150 mg by IV infusion over 60 minutes every 24 hours. Tablets should not be used in patients with hepatic impairment.

J0692

J0692 Injection, cefepime HCl, 500 mg

Cefepime hydrochloride is a semi-synthetic, broad spectrum, fourth generation cephalosporin antibiotic that inhibits synthesis of bacterial cell walls. It is indicated for the treatment of adults and children with a wide range of bacterial infections caused by susceptible strains of organisms in the following: complicated intra-abdominal infections, complicated and uncomplicated urinary tract infections, empiric therapy for febrile neutropenic patients, pneumonia, and uncomplicated skin and skin-structure infections. Intramuscular (IM) administration is utilized only for infections caused by *Escherichia coli*. For all other infections, the drug is administered by intravenous (IV) infusion over a period of 30 minutes. Dosages and the form of administration depend on the type and severity of the infection being treated, as well as the patient's age and the weight of children. A reduced dosage may be required for patients with renal impairment. See full prescribing information for complete administration instructions.

J0694

J0694 Injection, cefoxitin sodium, 1 g

Cefoxitin sodium is a broad spectrum, third generation cephalosporin antibiotic. It works by inhibiting synthesis of the cell wall and is used to treat a wide range of bacterial infections. Cefoxitin sodium is administered by intravenous or intramuscular injection. Dosages vary from 80 mg to 2 g depending on the type and severity of the infection being treated and for children, their body weight.

J0695

J0695 Injection, ceftolozane 50 mg and tazobactam 25 mg

Ceftolozane/tazobactam is a fixed combination product that includes a cephalosporin-class antibacterial drug (ceftolozane) along with a beta-lactamase inhibitor (tazobactam). It is used for the treatment of complicated intraabdominal infections, along with metronidazole, and for complicated urinary tract infections, including pyelonephritis. Administered by intravenous infusion over one hour, the recommended dosage is 1.5 g every eight hours for adult patients 18 years and older who have a creatine clearance above 50 mL/min. For patients with renal function impairment, dosage must be titrated according to prescribing information based on the patient's creatine clearance.

J0696

J0696 Injection, ceftriaxone sodium, per 250 mg

Ceftriaxone sodium is a semisynthetic, third generation, broad-spectrum cephalosporin antibiotic that inhibits synthesis of bacterial cell walls. It is indicated for the treatment of adults and children with a wide range of bacterial infections caused by susceptible strains of organisms in the following: acute bacterial otitis media, bone and joint infections, gonorrhea, intra-abdominal infections, lower respiratory tract infections, meningitis, pelvic inflammatory disease, septicemia, skin and skin-structure infections, and urinary tract infections. It may also be used preoperatively for prevention. Dosages and the form of administration depend on the type and severity of the infection being treated, as well as the patient's age and the weight of children. See full prescribing information for complete administration instructions.

J0697

J0697 Injection, sterile cefuroxime sodium, per 750 mg

Cefuroxime sodium is a semisynthetic, second generation, broad-spectrum cephalosporin antibiotic that inhibits synthesis of bacterial cell walls. It is indicated for the treatment of adults and children, 3 months and older, with a wide range of bacterial infections caused by susceptible strains of organisms in the following: bone and joint infections, gonorrhea, lower respiratory tract infections, meningitis, septicemia, and skin and skin-structure infections. It may also be used preoperatively for prevention prior to open heart surgery. Dosages and the form of administration depend on the type and severity of the infection being treated, as well as the patient's age and the weight of children. A reduced dosage may be required for patients with renal impairment. See full prescribing information for complete administration instructions.

J0698

J0698 Injection, cefotaxime sodium, per g

Cefotaxime sodium is a semisynthetic, third generation, broad-spectrum cephalosporin antibiotic that inhibits synthesis of bacterial cell walls. It is indicated for the treatment of adults and children with a wide range of bacterial infections caused by susceptible strains of organisms in the following: bacteriemia, bone and joint infections, central nervous system infections, genitourinary and gynecologic infections, intra-abdominal infections, lower respiratory tract infections, meningitis, septicemia, and skin and skin-structure infections. It may also be used preoperatively for prevention. Dosages and the form of administration depend on the type and severity of the infection being treated, as well as the patient's age and the weight of children. A reduced dosage may be required for patients with renal impairment. See full prescribing information for complete administration instructions.

J0699

J0699 Injection, cefiderocol, 10 mg

Cefiderocol is a cephalosporin antibacterial indicated for the treatment of adults, ages 18 and older, with the following infections caused by susceptible gram-negative microorganisms: complicated urinary tract infections (including pyelonephritis), hospital-acquired bacterial pneumonia, and ventilator-associated bacterial pneumonia. In order to reduce the development of drug-resistant bacteria and to maintain the effectiveness of this and other antibacterial drugs, cefiderocol should only be used to treat or prevent infections that are proven or strongly suspected to be caused by bacteria. Recommended dosage is 2 grams for injection every eight hours by intravenous (IV) infusion over three hours in patients with creatinine clearance (CLcr) 60 to 119 mL/min; dose adjustments are required for patients with CLcr less than 60 mL/min or greater than 120 mL/min. See full prescribing information for complete administration instructions.

J0701

J0701 Injection, cefepime HCl (Baxter), not therapeutically equivalent to Maxipime, 500 mg

Cefepime HCl is a semi-synthetic, broad spectrum, fourth generation cephalosporin antibiotic that inhibits synthesis of bacterial cell walls. It is indicated for the treatment of adults and children with a wide range of bacterial infections caused by susceptible strains of organisms in the following: complicated intra-abdominal infections (in combination with metronidazole), complicated and uncomplicated urinary tract infections, empiric therapy for febrile neutropenic patients, pneumonia, and uncomplicated skin and skin-structure infections. It is supplied in single dose bags of 1 g/50 ml and 2 g/100 ml and is administered via intravenous (IV) infusion over 30 minutes. Duration and frequency of treatment varies based on the condition treated. The recommended dosage for children, ages 2 months to 16 years, with a creatinine clearance of 60 ml/minute, is 50 mg/kg body weight every 12 hours (every eight hours for febrile neutropenia). The recommended dosage of adults is a full 1 or 2 g dose. For adults with a creatinine clearance less than or equal to 60 ml/minute, dose adjustments are required. See full prescribing information for complete administration instructions. Report J0701 only for cefepime HCl manufactured by Baxter.

J0702

J0702 Injection, betamethasone acetate 3 mg and betamethasone sodium phosphate 3 mg

Betamethasone acetate and betamethasone sodium phosphate are injectable corticosteroid suspensions with anti-inflammatory and immunosuppressive abilities. The injectable corticosteroid suspensions are used to treat a wide variety of medical problems, including endocrine disorders, rheumatic disorders, collagen diseases, allergic states, ophthalmic diseases, gastrointestinal diseases, respiratory diseases, dermatologic diseases, hematologic disorders, neoplastic disorders, edematous states, nervous system disorders, tuberculous meningitis, and trichinosis with neurologic or myocardial involvement. The route of administration depends on the condition being treated. For most conditions, betamethasone acetate and betamethasone sodium phosphate are administered by intramuscular injection. For conditions such as bursitis, tenosynovitis, peritendinitis, ganglion cysts, or bone cysts, the injection is administered directly into the bursa, tendon sheath, or cystic lesions. For rheumatoid arthritis and osteoarthritis, administration is by intra-articular injection.

J0703

J0703 Injection, cefepime HCl (B. Braun), not therapeutically equivalent to Maxipime, 500 mg

Cefepime HCl is a semi-synthetic, broad spectrum, fourth generation cephalosporin antibiotic that inhibits synthesis of bacterial cell walls. It is indicated for the treatment of adults and children with a wide range of bacterial infections caused by susceptible strains of organisms in the following: complicated intra-abdominal infections (in combination with metronidazole), complicated and uncomplicated urinary tract infections, empiric therapy for febrile neutropenic patients, pneumonia, and uncomplicated skin and skin-structure infections. It is supplied in a single dose bag of 1 g/50 ml and 2 g/50 ml and is administered via intravenous (IV) infusion over 30 minutes. Duration and frequency of treatment varies based on the condition treated. The recommended dosage for children, ages 2 months to 16 years, with a creatinine clearance of 60 ml/minute, is 50 mg/kg body weight every 12 hours (every eight hours for febrile neutropenia). The recommended dosage of adults is a full 1 or 2 g dose. For adults with a creatinine clearance less than or equal to 60 ml/minute, dose adjustments are required. See full prescribing information for complete administration instructions. Report J0703 only for cefepime hydrochloride manufactured by B. Braun.

J0706

J0706 Injection, caffeine citrate, 5 mg

Caffeine is a methylxanthine that is a central nervous system stimulant, bronchial smooth muscle relaxant, cardiac stimulant, and a diuretic. Caffeine citrate is a compound of caffeine and citric acid. It is indicated for adjunct treatment of apnea in premature neonates between 28 to 33 weeks gestational age. The exact action of caffeine citrate is not known, but it is thought to stimulate the respiratory center; increase minute ventilate; diminish diaphragm fatigue; increase metabolic rate skeletal tone, and oxygen consumption response; and decrease the threshold to and increase the response to hypercapnia. A loading dose of 1 mg per kg of body weight is administered by intravenous infusion over a period of 30 minutes using an infusion pump followed by a maintenance dose of 5 mg per kg of body weight over a 10-minute period every 24 hours.

J0710

J0710 Injection, cephapirin sodium, up to 1 g

Per the FDA, this drug is no longer available in the United States.

J0712

J0712 Injection, ceftaroline fosamil, 10 mg

Ceftaroline fosamil is a semisynthetic, fourth generation, broad-spectrum, beta-lactamase resistant cephalosporin antibiotic that inhibits synthesis of bacterial cell walls. It is indicated for the treatment of adults and children with a wide range of gram-positive and gram-negative microorganisms in the following: acute bacterial skin and skin-structure infections (ABSSSI) and community-acquired bacterial pneumonia (CABP). Ceftaroline fosamil is the water-soluble prodrug of the bioactive ceftaroline. Dosages and the form of administration depend on the type and severity of the infection being treated, as well as the patient's age and the weight of children. See full prescribing information for complete administration instructions.

J0713

J0713 Injection, ceftazidime, per 500 mg

Ceftazidime is a cephalosporin, a bactericidal agent that prevents cell wall production, causing osmotic imbalance in cellular pressure, and leading to cell death. It is indicated for the treatment of adults and children with a wide range of bacterial infections caused by susceptible strains of organisms in the following: bacteriemia, bone and joint infections, central nervous system infections, genitourinary and gynecologic infections, intra-abdominal infections, lower respiratory tract infections, septicemia, and skin and skin-structure infections. Dosages and the form of administration depend on the type and severity of the infection being treated, as well as the patient's age and the weight of children. Chloramphenicol should not be administered concomitantly with ceftazidime. Concomitant use with aminoglycosides or potent diuretics produces an additive effect against some microorganisms and may increase nephrotoxicity and ototoxicity. A reduced dosage may be required for patients with renal impairment. See full prescribing information for complete administration instructions.

J0714

J0714 Injection, ceftazidime and avibactam, 0.5 g/0.125 g

Combination drug ceftazidime and avibactam is a cephalosporin antibacterial with in vitro activity against certain susceptible gram-negative and gram-positive bacteria. Ceftazidime is an antibiotic that attacks the bacteria, while avibactam is a beta-lactamase inhibitor that stops the bacteria from impairing the ceftazidime. It is indicated for the treatment of adults and children with the following: complicated urinary tract infections in adults and children, age 3 months and older; hospital-acquired bacterial pneumonia and ventilator-associated bacterial pneumonia (HABP/VABP) in adults, 18 years and older; and complicated intra-abdominal infections (cIAI) in adults and children, 3 months of age or older, and in combination with metronidazole. It is administered via intravenous (IV) infusion. Dosages depend on the type and severity of the infection being treated, as well as the patient's age and the weight of children. A reduced dosage may be required for patients with renal impairment. See full prescribing information for complete administration instructions.

J0715

J0715 Injection, ceftizoxime sodium, per 500 mg

Ceftizoxime sodium is a semisynthetic, third generation, broad-spectrum, beta-lactamase resistant cephalosporin antibiotic that inhibits synthesis of the bacterial cell walls. It is indicated for the treatment of adults and children with a wide range of bacterial infections caused by susceptible strains of organisms. Ceftizoxime sodium was discontinued in the United States on August 1, 2016.

J0716

J0716 Injection, Centruroides immune f(ab)2, up to 120 mg

Centruroides (scorpion) immune f(ab)2 (equine) is used to treat stings by Centruroides scorpions. Scorpion stings can cause serious reactions, such as loss of muscle control, roving or abnormal eye movements, slurred speech, respiratory distress, excessive salivation, frothing at the mouth, and vomiting. It is derived from horse plasma. The horses are immunized with the scorpion venom. The product is obtained by pepsin digestion of horse plasma and is fractionated and purified. The f(ab)2 fragments of immunoglobulin bind to the venom toxins to neutralize them. The recommended dose is three vials initially and additional doses if necessary. Centruroides (scorpion) immune f(ab)2 (equine) is administered by IV infusion over 10 minutes.

J0717

J0717 Injection, certolizumab pegol, 1 mg (code may be used for Medicare when drug administered under the direct supervision of a physician, not for use when drug is self-administered)

Certolizumab pegol is a tumor necrosis factor (TNF) blocker used to treat rheumatoid arthritis and the symptoms of Crohn's disease in patients who have not responded to conventional treatment. It is a recombinant humanized antibody Fab fragment that is manufactured in *E. coli*. For rheumatoid arthritis, the initial recommended dose is 400 mg (given as two subcutaneous injections of 200 mg). The same dose is given at weeks two and four. It is then reduced to 200 mg every other week. For maintenance, 200 mg may be given every four weeks. For Crohn's disease, the recommended initial adult dose is 400 mg (given as two subcutaneous injections of 200 mg). The same dose is given at weeks two and four. In patients who obtain a clinical response, the recommended maintenance regimen is 400 mg every four weeks. Certolizumab pegol is given as a subcutaneous injection.

J0720

J0720 Injection, chloramphenicol sodium succinate, up to 1 g

Chloramphenicol sodium is a potent antibiotic that is useful for, and should be reserved for, serious infections caused by organisms susceptible to its antimicrobial effects when other therapeutic agents that are potentially less hazardous are ineffective or contraindicated. The drug is able to inhibit bacterial protein synthesis and exert a bacteriostatic effect. Chloramphenicol is injected intravenously over a period of three to five minutes. Dosages depend on the type and severity of the infection being treated, as well as the patient's age, weight, and the presence of hepatic or renal function impairment. It should be used very cautiously in children and newborns with immature metabolic function. The adult dose is 50 to 100 mg/kg IV daily, divided into doses every six hours. For children, the dose is 50 mg/kg per day divided into four doses at six hour intervals. When cerebrospinal fluid concentrations of the drug are required, such as for meningitis, a dosage of up to 100 mg/kg a day can be administered. In newborns that are less than 2 weeks of age, a total of 25 mg/kg per day is administered in four equal doses at intervals of six hours.

J0725

J0725 Injection, chorionic gonadotropin, per 1,000 USP units

Chorionic gonadotropin is a hormone with actions nearly the same as luteinizing hormone (LH), which is produced by the pituitary gland and is the same as the hormone produced by the placenta during pregnancy. Indications for the use of chorionic gonadotropin vary with males and females. Used in many in vitro fertilization programs, chorionic gonadotropin is used to aid conception and is usually administered in combination with other drugs, including menotropins and urofollitropin. In male patients, LH and chorionic gonadotropin stimulate the testes to produce male hormones such as testosterone to treat cryptorchidism, male infertility, and hypogonadism. Although chorionic gonadotropin may be prescribed as a weight loss drug, it should not be used for this indication. It is available in an injectable form only. The dose and the frequency with which it is administered are determined based on the indication for its use. For the treatment of male patients with low male hormone levels, 1,000 to 4,000 units are provided intramuscularly (IM) two or three times weekly. Treatment may range from several weeks to several months. For women undergoing fertility treatment, 5,000 to 10,000 units are administered IM per the physician's instructions. Children being treated for cryptorchidism receive 1,000 to 5,000 units IM two or three times weekly for up to a total of 10 doses.

J0735

J0735 Injection, clonidine HCl, 1 mg

Clonidine hydrochloride is used in addition to opiates to treat severe pain caused by cancer. Although the action of the drug is not known, it is thought to stimulate alpha2 -adrenergic receptors and inhibit central vasomotor centers, which lowers sympathetic outflow to the kidneys, heart, and peripheral vascular system lowering vascular resistance, blood pressure, and heart rate.

J0739

J0739 Injection, cabotegravir, 1 mg

Cabotegravir is a long-acting HIV-1 integrase strand transfer inhibitor (INSTI) indicated for the treatment of adults and adolescents, ages 12 years and older and weighing at least 35 kg, for preexposure prophylaxis (PrEP) to reduce the risk of sexually acquired HIV-1 infection. All patients must be screened for HIV-1 infection immediately prior to initiating treatment and prior to each subsequent injection. Additionally, patients must be counseled regarding adherence to the administration schedule and safer sex practices. It is supplied in a single dose vial of 600 mg/3 ml (200 mg/ml) and is administered via gluteal intramuscular (IM) injection. The recommended initial dosage is 600 mg single injection followed by a 600 mg single injection one month later. Subsequent 600 mg injection should be administered every two months.

Prior to starting cabotegravir injections, patients may use an oral lead-in dosing for a month to determine drug tolerability. See full prescribing information for complete administration instructions.

J0740

J0740 Injection, cidofovir, 375 mg

Cidofovir is an injectable antiviral that is indicated for the treatment of cytomegalovirus (CMV) retinitis in patients with acquired immunodeficiency syndrome (AIDS). By selective inhibition of viral DNA synthesis, Cidofovir is able to suppress the replication of CMV. Dosage is based on the weight of the patient and is 5 mg/kg. It is administered by intravenous (IV) infusion over 60 minutes, every two weeks.

J0741

J0741 Injection, cabotegravir and rilpivirine, 2 mg/3 mg

Cabotegravir and rilpivirine, a co-packaged combination of cabotegravir, a human immunodeficiency virus type-1 (HIV-1) integrase strand transfer inhibitor (INSTI), and rilpivirine, an HIV-1 non-nucleoside reverse transcriptase inhibitor (NNRTI), is indicated for the treatment of HIV-1 infections in adults, ages 18 and older, who are virologically suppressed (HIV-1 RNA less than 50 copies per mL) and are currently on a stable antiretroviral regimen with no history of treatment failure and with no known or suspected resistance to cabotegravir or rilpivirine. It is supplied in two single dose kits. The 600 mg/900 mg kit for initial injection doses contains a single dose vial of 600 mg/2 mL (200 mg/mL) cabotegravir and a single dose vial of 900 mg/2 mL (300 mg/mL) rilpivirine. The 400 mg/600 mg kit for continued injections contains a single dose vial of 400 mg/2 mL (200 mg/mL) cabotegravir and a single dose vial of 600 mg/2 mL (300 mg/mL) rilpivirine. Patients should be treated with oral lead-in dosing (30 mg cabotegravir and 25 mg rilpivirine daily) for one month prior to initiating injectable treatment to assess tolerability. Individual intramuscular (IM) gluteal injections, on opposite sides or 2 cm apart, should begin on the last day of oral lead-in dosing and continue once every month thereafter. It must be administered by a health care professional. See full prescribing information for complete administration instructions.

J0742

J0742 Injection, imipenem 4 mg, cilastatin 4 mg and relebactam 2 mg

Imipenem (a penem antibacterial), cilastatin (a renal dehydropeptidase inhibitor), and relebactam (a beta-lactamase inhibitor) is indicated for the treatment of adults, ages 18 and older, who have limited or no other alternative treatment options for complicated urinary tract infections (cUTI) and complicated intra-abdominal infections (cIAI) caused by susceptible strains of organisms. The drug is supplied as a sterile powder for reconstitution in a single dose vial of imipenem 500 mg, cilastatin 500 mg, and relebactam 250 mg, and is administered via intravenous (IV) infusion. See full prescribing instructions for a complete list of appropriate diluents. The recommended dosage is 1.25 grams by IV infusion over 30 minutes every six hours for patients with a creatinine clearance of 90mL/min or greater. Dosage adjustments must be made for patients with renal impairment. It should not be administered to patients with a creatinine clearance of less than 15 mL/min unless hemodialysis is performed within 48 hours.

J0743

J0743 Injection, cilastatin sodium; imipenem, per 250 mg

Cilastatin sodium and imipenem injection is a potent, broad-spectrum antibiotic that inhibits synthesis of the bacterial cell walls. It is indicated for the treatment of adults and children, ages 3 months and older, with a wide range of bacterial infections caused by susceptible strains of organisms in the following: bone and joint infections, endocarditis, gynecologic infections, intra-abdominal infections, lower respiratory tract infections, skin and skin-structure infections, and urinary tract infections. Dosage and frequency of administration are determined by the type of infection, body area affected, the weight of the patient, and the age of the patient. A reduced dosage may be required for patients with renal impairment. See full prescribing information for complete administration instructions. Cilastatin sodium/imipenem should not be administered to patients with meningitis, pediatric patients with central nervous system (CNS) infections, or pediatric patients weighing less than 30 kg with renal impairment.

J0744

J0744 Injection, ciprofloxacin for intravenous infusion, 200 mg

Ciprofloxacin is a fluoroquinolone antibiotic that inhibits the synthesis of bacterial DNA. The broad-spectrum action of the drug makes it useful against a wide range of infections and organisms. Dosage, route, and frequency of administration depend on the type of infection, the age of patient (adult or child), and the weight of children.

J0745

J0745 Injection, codeine phosphate, per 30 mg

Codeine phosphate is an opioid analgesic indicated for the treatment of adults, ages 18 years and older, with mild to moderate pain and for control of nonproductive cough that does not respond to nonopioid antitussives. Although the action is unknown, it is known to bind with opiate receptors in the central nervous system and alter the perception of and response to pain. It is provided in an injectable form for subcutaneous (SC) or intramuscular (IM) injection. The dosage, route, and frequency of administration are determined by the degree of pain (e.g., mild to moderate). A reduced dosage may be required for patients with renal impairment. See full prescribing information for complete administration instructions.

J0770

J0770 Injection, colistimethate sodium, up to 150 mg

Colistimethate sodium is a polypeptide antibiotic that penetrates the bacterial cell membrane, causing its death. It is indicated for the treatment of adults and children with acute or chronic bacterial infections caused by susceptible organisms. It can be administered via intramuscular (IM) injection or intravenous (IV) infusion. The recommended dosage should be administered in two to four divided dose levels of 2.5 to 5 mg/kg per day for patients with normal renal function. A reduced dosage may be required for patients with renal impairment. See full prescribing information for complete administration instructions.

J

J0775

J0775 Injection, collagenase, clostridium histolyticum, 0.01 mg

Collagenase clostridium histolyticum is a purified form of the exotoxin collagenase produced by the bacteria *Clostridium histolyticum*. Collagenases are enzymes that break down collagen. This drug is indicated as a treatment for Dupuytren's contracture, which causes a buildup of collagen in tendon sheathes in the hands. This drug is administered as an injection directly into the collagen cord of the hand.

J0780

J0780 Injection, prochlorperazine, up to 10 mg

Prochlorperazine/prochlorperazine maleate is an antiemetic used for severe nausea and vomiting, such as that associated with the administration of chemotherapy and prior to induction of anesthesia to control nausea and vomiting during and after surgery. The drug inhibits nausea and vomiting by acting on the chemoreceptor trigger zone and partially depresses the vomiting center. Prochlorperazine is also indicated for treating adult psychiatric illnesses, including schizophrenia, nonpsychotic anxiety, and mild psychotic disorders. Prochlorperazine is available in injection form for intramuscular (IM) and intravenous (IV) administration. The dosage, route, and frequency of administration depends on the patient's diagnosis, severity of symptoms, and the patient's weight. The drug should be injected or infused slowly. Parenteral adult doses range from 2.5 to 10 mg at no more than 5 mg/minute IV injection for adults or 5 to 20 mg IM. For children, 0.132 mg/kg may be administered via IM injection. The maximum parenteral adult dose is 40 mg a day.

J0791

J0791 Injection, crizanlizumab-tmca, 5 mg

Crizanlizumab-tmca is a selectin blocker humanized monoclonal antibody (IgG2 kappa) produced by recombinant DNA technology using Chinese hamster ovaries. It binds to P-selectin and blocks interactions with its ligands, including P-selectin glycoprotein ligand 1, which then blocks interactions between endothelial cells, platelets, red blood cells, and leukocytes. Crizanlizumab-tmca is indicated in adults and children, ages 16 and older, with sickle cell disease to reduce the occurrence of vaso-occlusive crises (VOC). It is supplied in a 100 mg/10 mL (10 mg/mL) solution, single dose vial and is administered via intravenous (IV) infusion. It requires dilutions with 0.9% sodium chloride or 5% dextrose. The recommended dosage is 5 mg/kg of body weight by IV infusion over 30 minutes on week zero, week two, and every four weeks after.

J0795

J0795 Injection, corticorelin ovine triflutate, 1 mcg

Corticorelin ovine triflutate is used to differentiate pituitary and ectopic production of adrenocorticotropic hormone (ACTH) in Cushing's syndrome. After the hypercortisolism is determined to be caused from Cushing's syndrome and autonomous adrenal hyperfunction is eliminated as the cause, the corticorelin test is used to determine the source of the excessive ACTH. Blood samples are drawn 15 minutes before and immediately before the medication is administered. A baseline is determined by averaging the two samples. The corticorelin is administered by intravenous infusion over 30 to 60 second intervals at a dose of 1 mcg/kg body weight. Additional blood samples are drawn 15, 30, and 60 minutes after the patient receives the medication.

J0800

J0800 Injection, corticotropin, up to 40 units

Corticotropin is a pituitary hormone released in response to corticotrophin-releasing hormone (CRH), which is released by the hypothalamus. Corticotropin is administered as a diagnostic indicator or adrenocortical function, as well as an anti-inflammatory or immunosuppressant for conditions such as multiple sclerosis. Corticotropin replaces the body's own hormones and stimulates the adrenal cortex to secrete hormones. Corticotropin may be administered intravenously (IV), intramuscularly (IM), or subcutaneously (SC). Intravenously it is administered over a period of eight hours. Dosages, frequency, and method of administration vary according to the indication for the drug, as well as the age of the patient (adult or child). IV doses range from 10 to 25 units every 12 hours for one or two days. IM and SC doses range from 20 to 120 units every 24 to 72 hours.

J0834

J0834 Injection, cosyntropin, 0.25 mg

Cosyntropin is a synthetic version of adrenocorticotropic hormone (ACTH). It is a polypeptide that comprises the first 24 of the 39 amino acids of natural ACTH and has the same effect as natural ACTH. Cosyntropin is used as a diagnostic agent to screen patients with presumed adrenocortical insufficiency. Since it exerts a rapid effect on the adrenal cortex, it may be used to perform a 30-minute test of adrenal function (plasma cortisol response) as an office or outpatient procedure. Cosyntropin may be administered by intramuscular or intravenous injection for a rapid screening test of adrenal function. It may also be administered as an intravenous infusion over four to eight hours for greater stimulus to the adrenal glands. One of the rapid screening tests of adrenal function involves the collection of a control blood sample followed by an intramuscular injection of cosyntropin. A dose of 0.25 mg is provided to adults; for children 2 years of age or younger; a dose of 0.125 mg is adequate. A second blood sample is collected exactly 30 minutes after injection. When administered as an infusion, 0.25 mg is given over a six-hour period.

J0840

J0840 Injection, crotalidae polyvalent immune fab (ovine), up to 1 g

Crotalidae polyvalent immune fab is an antivenin used to treat the effects of venomous snake bites. The medication is created by immunizing sheep with one of four different venoms. The four different antivenins are extracted from the sheep serum and combined to create the final immunoglobulin product. The immunoglobulin binds to the toxins and neutralizes them. The recommended dose is based on the patient's response to treatment. Crotalidae polyvalent immune fab is administered by intravenous infusion.

J0841

J0841 Injection, crotalidae immune F(ab')2 (equine), 120 mg

Crotalidae immune F(ab')2 (equine) is an equine-derived antivenin that is indicated for the treatment of adult and pediatric patients with North American rattlesnake envenomation. It is manufactured from the plasma of horses immunized with venom of *Bothrops asper* and *Crotalus durissus*. It contains venom-specific F(ab')2 fragments of immunoglobulin G (IgG) that binds and neutralizes venom toxins as well as aiding in elimination of venom from the body. It is supplied as a sterile, lyophilize powder ready for dilution. The initial dose is 10 vials. Each vile must be reconstituted with 10 mL of normal sterile saline. The contents of each vial should then be combined and further diluted with normal sterile saline to a total volume of 250 mL. The solution is then administered via intravenous infusion. The infusion should begin at a rate of 250-50 mL/hour. If no reactions occur, the rate may be increased to the full 250 mL/hour until the infusion is complete. The infusion should be stopped at any time if allergic reactions occur. The patient should be monitored for 60 minutes following the infusion to determine if symptoms are progressing or resolved. An additional 10 vials may be administered if envenomation symptoms are progressing. Patients should be monitored for an additional 18 hours and an additional four vial doses may be administered if needed for symptom progression. The four vials should be diluted with 10 mL of normal sterile saline and then combined and further diluted to a total volume of 250 mL. This solution should be administered by intravenous infusion over 60 minutes.

J0850

J0850 Injection, cytomegalovirus immune globulin intravenous (human), per vial

Immune globulins are glycoproteins in the blood that function as antibodies. Immune globulins specific to a certain disease are antibodies with specific amino acid sequences that interact only with the antigen that stimulated its creation or with antigens that are closely related to the stimulating antigen. Immune globulins are usually derived from the pooled plasma of human donors who have antibodies to the specific disease. The antibodies from the exogenous immune globulin help the body to fight off a disease. Cytomegalovirus (CMV) is a virus of the subfamily Betaherpesvirinae that produces unique large cells with intranuclear inclusions. The majority of CMV infections are very mild. Depending on the age and immune status of the person, CMV infections can cause several serious diseases. CMV infections can include mononucleosis, encephalitis, retinitis, and pneumonia. In immunocompromised patients, CMV can cause a disseminated and sometimes fatal illness. In severely infected infants, CMV may cause hepatosplenomegaly, jaundice, retinitis, purpura, microcephaly, cerebral calcifications, blindness, deafness, quadriplegia, and mental retardation. CMV can be transmitted by respiratory droplets or from the mother to infant during birth or breast-feeding. CMV immune globulin is administered intravenously for the treatment and prophylaxis of CMV disease in transplant recipients and other immunocompromised patients.

J0875

J0875 Injection, dalbavancin, 5 mg

Dalbavancin is a glycopeptide antibiotic indicated for adults, ages 18 and older, with acute bacterial skin and skin structure infections (ABSSSI) caused by susceptible strains of gram-positive organisms. The recommended dosage is 1,000 mg followed by 500 mg one week later, administered via intravenous (IV) infusion over 30 minutes. A reduced dosage may be required for patients with renal impairment. See full prescribing information for complete administration instructions.

J0877

J0877 Injection, daptomycin (Hospira), not therapeutically equivalent to J0878, 1 mg

Daptomycin is a cyclic lipopeptide antibiotic that binds to the bacterial membrane, causing a rapid depolarization and leading to bacterial cell death. Daptomycin is indicated for the treatment of adults and children, ages 1 year and older, with bacteremia and complicated skin and skin-structure infections (cSSSI) caused by susceptible gram-positive bacteria. It should not be used for the treatment of pneumonia, left-sided infective endocarditis, or children under 1 year old. It is supplied in a single dose vial of 500 mg lyophilized powder for reconstitution in 0.9% sodium chloride and is administered by intravenous (IV) infusion over 30 minutes or injection over two minutes (adults only). Dosage and frequency of administration are determined by the type of infection, patient age, and creatinine clearance level. A modified dosage interval may be required for patients with renal impairment. See full prescribing information for complete administration instructions. Report J0877 only for daptomycin manufactured by Hospira.

J0878

J0878 Injection, daptomycin, 1 mg

Daptomycin is a cyclic lipopeptide antibiotic that binds to the bacterial membrane, causing a rapid depolarization and leading to bacterial cell death. Daptomycin is indicated for the treatment of adults, ages 18 and older, with bacteremia and complicated skin and skin-structure infections (cSSSI) caused by susceptible gram-positive bacteria. It should not be used for the treatment of pneumonia. It is administered by intravenous (IV) infusion and may be given in combination with other antibiotics. It should not be administered in conjunction with elastomeric infusion pumps. Dosage and the length and frequency of administration are determined by the type of infection. A reduced dosage may be required for patients with renal impairment. See full prescribing information for complete administration instructions.

J0879

J0879 Injection, difelikefalin, 0.1 mcg, (for ESRD on dialysis)

Difelikefalin is a kappa opioid receptor (KOR) agonist indicated for the treatment of patients, ages 18 years and older, with moderate to severe pruritus associated with chronic kidney disease (CKD) in adults undergoing hemodialysis (HD). The mechanism of action is not known. It is supplied in a single dose vial (65 mcg/1.3 ml). The recommended dose is 0.5 mcg/kg body weight administered via intravenous (IV) bolus injection into the venous line of the dialysis circuit following each HD treatment. See full prescribing information for complete administration instructions.

J0881-J0882

J0881 Injection, darbepoetin alfa, 1 mcg (non-ESRD use)

J0882 Injection, darbepoetin alfa, 1 mcg (for ESRD on dialysis)

Darbepoetin alfa is a drug used to stimulate red blood cell production. It is produced by recombinant DNA technology in Chinese hamster ovaries. Darbepoetin alfa contains more carbohydrate chains and sialic acid residues than epoetin alfa. This reduces the rate of clearance, extends the half-life, and allows for less frequent administration. It acts in the body similar to erythropoietin, which is produced by the kidneys. Erythropoietin is a hormone that is released into the blood system by the kidneys to prompt the production of red blood cells when low levels of oxygen are detected in the blood. Patients with chronic renal failure will not be able to produce adequate levels of erythropoietin in the kidneys. Darbepoetin alfa is used to treat patients with anemia due to chronic renal failure or due to chemotherapy for patients with nonmyeloid cancer. Dose is based on patient condition and indication. Darbepoetin alfa can be administered by subcutaneous or intravenous injection.

J0883-J0884

J0883 Injection, argatroban, 1 mg (for non-ESRD use)

J0884 Injection, argatroban, 1 mg (for ESRD on dialysis)

Argatroban is a synthetic direct thrombin inhibitor derived from the amino acid L-arginine. It binds to the active thrombin site and inhibits coagulation including fibrin formation, activation of coagulation factors and protein C, and platelet aggregation. Argatroban is indicated for use as an anticoagulant for prophylaxis and treatment of thrombosis in patients with heparin-induced thrombocytopenia. It is also indicated as an anticoagulant in patients with or at risk for heparin-induced thrombocytopenia undergoing percutaneous coronary interventions. Argatroban is supplied as a concentrate that must be diluted and administered via intravenous infusion.

J0885

J0885 Injection, epoetin alfa, (for non-ESRD use), 1000 units

Epoetin alfa is used to stimulate red blood cell production. It is produced by recombinant DNA technology in mammalian cells. It acts in the body similarly to erythropoietin, which is produced by the kidneys. Erythropoietin is a hormone the kidneys release into the blood system to prompt the production of red blood cells when low levels of oxygen are detected in the blood. Patients with chronic renal failure are not able to produce adequate levels of erythropoietin in the kidneys. Epoetin alfa is used to treat patients with anemia due to chronic renal failure due to chemotherapy for patients with nonmyeloid cancer, or anemia for HIV patients being treated with zidovudine. Epoetin alfa is also indicated in the preoperative treatment of anemic patients scheduled to undergo surgery with significant, anticipated blood loss who cannot donate autologous blood. The dose is based on the patient's condition and indication. Epoetin alfa can be administered by subcutaneous or intravenous injection.

J0887-J0888

J0887 Injection, epoetin beta, 1 mcg, (for ESRD on dialysis)

J0888 Injection, epoetin beta, 1 mcg, (for non-ESRD use)

Epoetin beta is used to stimulate red blood cell production. It is an erythropoietin receptor activator that acts in the body similarly to erythropoietin, which is produced by the kidneys. Erythropoietin is a hormone the kidneys release into the blood system to prompt the production of red blood cells when low levels of oxygen are detected in the blood. Patients with chronic renal failure are not able to produce adequate levels of erythropoietin in the kidneys. Epoetin beta is used to treat patients with anemia due to chronic renal failure for patients on dialysis and patients not on dialysis. It is not indicated for treatment of anemia due to cancer chemotherapy. The drug is formulated as a sterile, preservative free protein solution for intravenous (IV) or subcutaneous (SC) administration. IV administration is recommended for hemodialysis patients as it may be less immunogenic. The initial treatment is 0.6 mcg per kg body weight administered once every two weeks. When the drug is initiated or the dose adjusted, hemoglobin should be monitored every two weeks until stabilized, and every two to four weeks thereafter. The dose should be individualized to achieve and maintain hemoglobin levels within the range of 10.6 to 12 g/dL.

J0890

J0890 Injection, peginesatide, 0.1 mg (for ESRD on dialysis)

Peginesatide is an erythropoiesis-stimulating agent (ESA) used to treat anemia caused by chronic kidney disease (CKD) in adult patients, ages 18 and older, who are on dialysis. It binds with a hormone produced by the kidney to stimulate the formation of blood cells in bone marrow and increases the reticulocyte count, which are the young blood cells found in the blood. This elevation is an indicator that red cell production is increasing quickly in the blood. Peginesatide should not be administered to patients with uncontrolled hypertension or who have CKD but are not receiving dialysis. The recommended starting dose for patients not currently being treated with an ESA is 0.04 mg/kg body weight administered as a single intravenous (IV) or subcutaneous (SC) injection once monthly. The dose for patients currently being treated with an ESA is based on a conversion table. See full prescribing information for complete administration instructions.

J0891

J0891 Injection, argatroban (Accord), not therapeutically equivalent to J0883, 1 mg (for non-ESRD use)

Argatroban is a synthetic direct thrombin inhibitor derived from the amino acid L-arginine that binds to the active thrombin site and inhibits coagulation including fibrin formation, activation of coagulation factors and protein C, and platelet aggregation. Argatroban is indicated for use in adults, ages 18 years and older, as an anticoagulant for prophylaxis and treatment of thrombosis in patients with heparin-induced thrombocytopenia, and as an anticoagulant in patients with or at risk for heparin-induced thrombocytopenia undergoing percutaneous coronary interventions. Argatroban is supplied in a ready to use single dose vial of 50 mg/50 ml. The recommended dosage for heparin-induced thrombocytopenia is 2 mcg/kg body weight/minute administered via continuous intravenous (IV) infusion. The recommended dosage for patients undergoing coronary intervention is started at 25 mcg/kg body weight/minute administered via large bore IV line and a bolus of 350 mcg/kg body weight over three to five minutes. See full prescribing information for complete administration instructions. Report J0891 only for argatroban manufactured by Accord and administered for non-ESRD (end stage renal disease) use.

J0892

J0892 Injection, argatroban (Accord), not therapeutically equivalent to J0884, 1 mg (for ESRD on dialysis)

Argatroban is a synthetic direct thrombin inhibitor derived from the amino acid L-arginine that binds to the active thrombin site and inhibits coagulation including fibrin formation, activation of coagulation factors and protein C, and platelet aggregation. Argatroban is indicated for use in adults, ages 18 years and older, as an anticoagulant for prophylaxis and treatment of thrombosis in patients with heparin-induced thrombocytopenia, and as an anticoagulant in patients with or at risk for heparin-induced thrombocytopenia undergoing percutaneous coronary interventions. Argatroban is supplied in a ready to use single dose vial of 50 mg/50 ml. The recommended dosage for heparin-induced thrombocytopenia is 2 mcg/kg body weight/minute administered via continuous intravenous (IV) infusion. The recommended dosage for patients undergoing coronary intervention is started at 25 mcg/kg body weight/minute administered via large bore IV line and a bolus of 350 mcg/kg body weight over three to five minutes. See full prescribing information for complete administration instructions. Report J0892 only for argatroban manufactured by Accord and administered for ESRD (end stage renal disease) on dialysis use.

J0893

J0893 Injection, decitabine (Sun Pharma) not therapeutically equivalent to J0894, 1 mg

Decitabine is an antineoplastic drug that is an analogue of the nucleoside 2-deoxycytidine. It incorporates itself into cellular DNA suppressing methylation. It is thought that suppression of the methylation of DNA may restore normal function to genes. It is indicated as a treatment for adult patients, ages 18 years and older, with myelodysplastic syndromes (MDS), both previously treated and untreated. The drug may be used for newly diagnosed and secondary MDS. It is supplied in a single dose vial of 50 mg lyophilized powder that requires reconstitution with 0.9% sodium chloride or 5% dextrose. The three-day dosing regimen is 15 mg per m^2 of body surface administered by intravenous (IV) infusion over three hours, repeated every eight hours for three days in an inpatient setting. This cycle is repeated every six weeks. The five-day regimen is 20 mg/m^2 of body surface administered by IV infusion over one hour, repeated daily for five days in an outpatient setting. This regimen is repeated every four weeks. Patient response may take longer than four cycles and treatments may be continued as long as the patient benefits. See full prescribing information for complete administration instructions. Report J0893 only for decitabine manufactured by Sun Pharma.

J0894

J0894 Injection, decitabine, 1 mg

Decitabine is an antineoplastic drug that is an analogue of the nucleoside 2-deoxycytidine. It incorporates itself into cellular DNA suppressing methylation. It is thought that suppression of the methylation of DNA may restore normal function to genes. It is indicated as a treatment for adult patients, ages 18 and older, with myelodysplastic syndromes (MDS), both previously treated and untreated. The drug may be used for newly diagnosed and secondary MDS. The three-day dosing regimen is 15 mg per m^2 of body surface administered by intravenous (IV) infusion over three hours, repeated every eight hours for three days in an inpatient setting. This cycle is repeated every six weeks. The five-day regimen is 20 mg/m^2 of body surface administered by IV infusion over one hour, repeated daily for five days in an outpatient setting. This regimen is repeated every four weeks. Patient response may take longer than four cycles and treatments may be continued as long as the patient benefits. See full prescribing information for complete administration instructions.

J0895

J0895 Injection, deferoxamine mesylate, 500 mg

Deferoxamine mesylate is an iron-chelating agent that forms a stable complex with the iron and prevents it from being broken down any further in the body. It is indicated for the treatment of both acute iron intoxication and for chronic iron overload due to transfusion-dependent anemias. In acute iron intoxication, deferoxamine mesylate is administered along with standard measures for the treatment of acute iron intoxication. In patients with chronic iron overload secondary to multiple transfusions, deferoxamine mesylate can promote the excretion of iron. With long-term use, the drug can slow the accumulation of hepatic iron and slow or stop the progression of hepatic fibrosis. The action of the drug has been found to be poor in patients younger than 3 years of age without significant iron overload and should not be used unless the mobilization of 1 mg (or more) of iron per day can be demonstrated. This drug is not indicated for treating primary hemochromatosis. The drug is provided for intramuscular, subcutaneous, and intravenous administration.

J0896

J0896 Injection, luspatercept-aamt, 0.25 mg

Luspatercept-aamt is an erythroid maturation agent that is indicated for the treatment of adults, ages 18 and older, with anemia with beta thalassemia that requires regular red blood cell (RBC) transfusions, and with anemia failing an erythropoiesis stimulating agent and requiring two or more RBC units over eight weeks in patients with very low to intermediate risk myelodysplastic syndromes with ring sideroblasts (MDS-RS) or with myelodysplastic/myeloproliferative neoplasms with ring sideroblasts and thrombocytosis (MDS/MPN-RS-T). For the treatment of beta thalassemia, the recommended starting dosage is 1 mg/kg body weight once every three weeks by subcutaneous (SC) injection. After six weeks (two consecutive doses) at the starting dose, increase dose to the maximum of 1.25 mg/kg body weight every three weeks. If transfusion burden is not reduced after nine weeks (three doses), treatment should be discontinued. In absence of RBC transfusions, if hemoglobin rises to more than 2 g/dL within three weeks or predose hemoglobin is 11.5 g/dL or higher, the dose should be reduced, or treatment stopped. Hemoglobin results should be reviewed prior to each administration. For the treatment of MDS-RS or MDS/MPN-RS-T, the recommended starting dosage is 1 mg/kg body weight once every three weeks by SC injection. If the patient is not RBC transfusion-free after three weeks (two consecutive doses), increase dose to 1.33 mg/kg body weight every three weeks. If the patient is not RBC transfusion-free after six weeks (two consecutive doses) of 1.33 mg/kg, increase dose to 1.75 mg/kg every three weeks. If transfusion burden is not reduced after nine weeks (at least three consecutive doses of 1.75 mg/kg), discontinue treatment. It is supplied in 25 mg and 75 mg lyophilized powder single dose vials requiring reconstitution with sterile water. See full prescribing information for additional instructions for reconstitution and dosage adjustments. Luspatercept-aamt should not be used as a substitute for RBC transfusions needed for immediate correction of anemia.

J0897

J0897 Injection, denosumab, 1 mg

Denosumab is a monoclonal antibody used for the treatment of osteoporosis in postmenopausal women with a high risk of bone fractures that were not successful with other osteoporosis therapies. Denosumab reduces the possibility of fractures of the hip and vertebral and non-vertebral fractures because it is a RANK Ligand inhibitor. It works by binding to the Rank Ligand inhibiting osteoclast formation, function, and survival, therefore preventing the osteoclasts from resorbing bone. The recommended dose is 60 mg every six months. Denosumab is administered by subcutaneous injection.

J0898

J0898 Injection, argatroban (AuroMedics), not therapeutically equivalent to J0883, 1 mg (for non-ESRD use)

Argatroban is a synthetic direct thrombin inhibitor derived from the amino acid L-arginine that binds to the active thrombin site and inhibits coagulation including fibrin formation, activation of coagulation factors and protein C, and platelet aggregation. Argatroban is indicated for use in adults, ages 18 years and older, as an anticoagulant for prophylaxis and treatment of thrombosis in patients with heparin-induced thrombocytopenia, and as an anticoagulant in patients with or at risk for heparin-induced thrombocytopenia undergoing percutaneous coronary interventions. Argatroban is supplied in a ready to use single dose vial of 50 mg/50 ml. The recommended dosage for heparin-induced thrombocytopenia is 2 mcg/kg body weight/minute administered via continuous intravenous (IV) infusion. The recommended dosage for patients undergoing coronary intervention is started at 25 mcg/kg body weight/minute administered via large bore IV line and a bolus of 350 mcg/kg body weight over three to five minutes. See full prescribing information for complete administration instructions. Report J0898 only for argatroban manufactured by AuroMedics and administered for non-ESRD (end stage renal disease) use.

J0899

J0899 Injection, argatroban (AuroMedics), not therapeutically equivalent to J0884, 1 mg (for ESRD on dialysis)

Argatroban is a synthetic direct thrombin inhibitor derived from the amino acid L-arginine that binds to the active thrombin site and inhibits coagulation including fibrin formation, activation of coagulation factors and protein C, and platelet aggregation. Argatroban is indicated for use in adults, ages 18 years and older, as an anticoagulant for prophylaxis and treatment of thrombosis in patients with heparin-induced thrombocytopenia, and as an anticoagulant in patients with or at risk for heparin-induced thrombocytopenia undergoing percutaneous coronary interventions. Argatroban is supplied in a ready to use single dose vial of 50 mg/50 ml. The recommended dosage for heparin-induced thrombocytopenia is 2 mcg/kg body weight/minute administered via continuous intravenous (IV) infusion. The recommended dosage for patients undergoing coronary intervention is started at 25 mcg/kg body weight/minute administered via large bore IV line and a bolus of 350 mcg/kg body weight over three to five minutes. See full prescribing information for complete administration instructions. Report J0899 only for argatroban manufactured by AuroMedics and administered for ESRD (end stage renal disease) on dialysis use.

J0945

J0945 Injection, brompheniramine maleate, per 10 mg

Brompheniramine maleate is an antihistamine that blocks the effects of histamine in the body and provides relief of allergy symptoms including hives, rashes, itching, watery eyes, runny nose, and sneezing. It is also indicated for the treatment of motion sickness, anxiety or tension, and sleeplessness. Brompheniramine maleate is available in oral and injectable forms. The injectable form is administered by intramuscular injection.

J1000

J1000 Injection, depo-estradiol cypionate, up to 5 mg

Depo-estradiol cypionate is a long-acting estrogen in a sterile oil solution for intramuscular use. Depo-estradiol cypionate increases the synthesis of RNA, DNA and protein in tissues and inhibits the release of follicle stimulating and luteinizing hormones from the pituitary gland. Depo-estradiol cypionate is indicated for the treatment of atrophic vaginitis, the palliative treatment of inoperable breast and prostate cancer, severe vasomotor symptoms associated with menopause, and hypoestrogenism due to hypogonadism, castration, or primary ovarian failure. Dosage is based on the condition being treated as well as the patient's response to treatment and ranges from 10 mg every four weeks to 30 mg every week.

J1020-J1040

J1020 Injection, methylprednisolone acetate, 20 mg

J1030 Injection, methylprednisolone acetate, 40 mg

J1040 Injection, methylprednisolone acetate, 80 mg

Methylprednisolone is a corticosteroid used to treat a variety of conditions including allergic disorders, arthritis, blood diseases, certain cancers, endocrine disorders, eye diseases, intestinal disorders, renal diseases, respiratory diseases, rheumatic disorders, various skin diseases, as well as for the treatment of acute exacerbations of arthritis, bursitis, epicondylitis, and osteoarthritis. It may also be used with other medications as a replacement for certain hormones. Methylprednisolone works by decreasing the body's immune response to these diseases and reducing symptoms such as swelling and redness. Methylprednisolone may be administered by intra-articular, intralesional, or intramuscular (IM) injection. It should not be administered via epidural or intrathecal injection or used for the treatment of idiopathic thrombocytopenic purpura or systemic fungal infections. Dosage, frequency, and route of administration are determined by the type of disease/disorder treated and whether the disease/disorder is local or systemic. See full prescribing information for complete administration instructions.

J1050

J1050 Injection, medroxyprogesterone acetate, 1 mg

Medroxyprogesterone acetate is a progestin used in a variety of disorders and as a long-term injectable contraceptive. Medroxyprogesterone acetate suppresses ovulation by inhibiting the secretion of pituitary gonadotropin, which prevents maturation of follicles and causes thinning of the endometrial lining. It is indicated as antineoplastic treatment in endometrial, breast, and renal carcinoma. Medroxyprogesterone acetate is administered by subcutaneous or intramuscular injection.

J1071

J1071 Injection, testosterone cypionate, 1 mg

Testosterone cypionate is an anabolic steroid that stimulates the normal development of male sex organs and maintenance of secondary sex characteristics. It is indicated for the treatment of male patients, ages 18 and older, with an absence or deficiency of endogenous testosterone (hypogonadism). Hypogonadism may be congenital or acquired. Primary hypogonadism includes bilateral torsion, orchiectomy, orchitis, testicular failure due to cryptorchidism, and vanishing testis syndrome. Secondary hypogonadism includes idiopathic gonadotropin or luteinizing hormone-releasing hormone (LHRH) deficiency and pituitary-hypothalamic injury due to radiation, trauma, or tumors. Testosterone cypionate should not be administered to women or to children younger than 18 years of age. Administered via intramuscular (IM) injection, dosage and frequency of administration are determined by the disorder treated. It should not be administered via intravenous (IV) injection deep into the gluteal muscle. Testosterone cypionate cannot be used interchangeably with testosterone propionate. See full prescribing information for complete administration instructions.

J1094

J1094 Injection, dexamethasone acetate, 1 mg

Dexamethasone acetate is a synthetic corticosteroid similar to a natural hormone produced by the adrenal gland. It is 25 times as potent as cortisol. It has anti-inflammatory, antiemetic, and immunosuppressant properties and is used to treat a wide variety of disorders, as well as a diagnostic aid in the detection of Cushing's syndrome in dexamethasone suppression testing. Dexamethasone acetate is no longer available as stand-alone, FDA-approved product in the United States.

J1095

J1095 Injection, dexamethasone 9%, intraocular, 1 mcg

Dexamethasone 9% is a corticosteroid that is indicated for the treatment of intraocular postoperative inflammation in adult patients. Corticosteroids suppress inflammation by inhibiting inflammatory cytokines that cause an increase in edema and inflammatory cells. It is supplied in a kit with a single dose vial and is administered via injection. The recommended dose is 0.005mL injected into the posterior chamber behind the iris, at the end of ocular surgery. The postoperative injection replaces the need for patients to self-administer medicated drops following surgery. Patients should be monitored for an increase in intraocular pressure, delayed healing, cataract progression, as well as bacterial, fungal, and viral infections.

J1096

J1096 Dexamethasone, lacrimal ophthalmic insert, 0.1 mg

Dexamethasone ophthalmic insert is a corticosteroid indicated for the treatment of intraocular postoperative inflammation and pain in adult patients. Corticosteroids suppress inflammation by inhibiting inflammatory cytokines that cause an increase in edema and inflammatory cells. It is supplied as a fluorescent yellow, 3 mm cylindrical ophthalmic insert that is placed into the lower lacrimal punctum into the canaliculus. The provider dilates the punctum with an ophthalmic dilator and dries the punctal area. The insert is grasped with blunt forceps and inserted into the lower lacrimal canaliculus, just below the punctal opening. To further hydrate the insert, one to two drops of a balanced salt solution can be instilled into the punctum. The insert releases dexamethasone for up to 30 days. The insert is resorbable and does not require removal. If removal becomes necessary, it can be removed with manual expression or saline irrigation. Patients should be monitored for an increase in intraocular pressure, delayed healing, cataract progression, as well as bacterial, fungal, and viral infections.

J1097

J1097 Phenylephrine 10.16 mg/ml and ketorolac 2.88 mg/ml ophthalmic irrigation solution, 1 ml

Phenylephrine and ketorolac intraocular solution (1%/3%) is an alpha 1-adrenergic receptor agonist and nonselective cyclooxygenase inhibitor. It is used to maintain pupil size by preventing intraoperative miosis and for reducing postoperative pain in adults and children. The drug is added to irrigation solution used during cataract surgery or intraocular lens replacement. For irrigation purposes, 4 ml of the drug is diluted in 500 ml of ophthalmic irrigating solution and is used as needed during the surgical procedure.

J1100

J1100 Injection, dexamethasone sodium phosphate, 1 mg

Dexamethasone is a synthetic corticosteroid similar to a natural hormone produced by the adrenal gland. It is 25 times as potent as cortisol. Dexamethasone has anti-inflammatory, antiemetic, and immunosuppressant properties and is used to treat a wide variety of disorders, as well as a diagnostic aid in the detection of Cushing's syndrome in dexamethasone suppression testing. It is administered via intramuscular (IM) or intravenous (IV) injection. Dosage and frequency of administration are determined by the condition treated, age, weight, and other patient-specific factors. See full prescribing information for complete administration instructions.

J1110

J1110 Injection, dihydroergotamine mesylate, per 1 mg

Dihydroergotamine mesylate is indicated for acute treatment of migraine and cluster headaches. By stimulating alpha receptors, it causes peripheral vasoconstriction and may abort vascular headaches by direct vasoconstriction of the dilated carotid artery bed. It may be administered intravenously (IV), intramuscularly (IM), or subcutaneously (SC) with a dose of 1 mg that may be repeated every hour or two up to a maximum of 2 mg IV or 3 mg IM and SC in a 24-hour period. When administered by IV, it is given by a slow injection over three minutes. The weekly maximum is 6 mg.

J1120

J1120 Injection, acetazolamide sodium, up to 500 mg

Acetazolamide sodium is a carbonic anhydrase inhibitor that is intended for the treatment of adults, ages 18 and older, with edema caused by congestive heart failure or drugs, centrencephalic epilepsies (petit mal and unlocalized seizures), chronic simple (open-angle) glaucoma, secondary glaucoma, and preoperatively in acute angle-closure glaucoma to rapidly reduce intraocular pressure. Acetazolamide sodium is administered by intravenous (IV) injection after reconstitution with sterile water. Dosage and frequency of administration are determined by the disorder treated. See full prescribing information for complete administration instructions.

J1130

J1130 Injection, diclofenac sodium, 0.5 mg

Diclofenac sodium is an injectable nonsteroidal anti-inflammatory drug (NSAID) indicated for use in adults, ages 18 and older, for the management of mild-to-moderate pain as well as for the management of moderate-to-severe pain alone or in combination with opioid analgesics. The drug exhibits anti-inflammatory analgesic and antipyretic activities. The mechanism of action, like that of other NSAIDs, is not completely understood but may involve inhibition of the cyclooxygenase (COX-1 and COX-2) pathways. Its mechanism may also be related to inhibition of prostaglandin synthetase. Diclofenac sodium should not be used to treat perioperative pain following coronary artery bypass graft (CABG) surgery. Patients should be well hydrated prior to administration. The recommended dosage is 37.5 mg administered via intravenous (IV) injection over 15 seconds. Treatment may be repeated every six hours, not to exceed 150 mg/day.

J1160

J1160 Injection, digoxin, up to 0.5 mg

Digoxin is a cardiac glycoside extracted from the leaf of the digitalis (foxglove) plant. Digoxin acts directly on cardiac muscle and indirectly on the cardiovascular system and autonomic nervous system to strengthen heart contractions and slow the heart rate. It is intended for the treatment of adults with mild to moderate heart failure and control of resting ventricular rate in chronic atrial fibrillation. It is also used to treat myocardial contractility in children with heart failure. It is administered via intravenous (IV) injection over a period of five minutes or more and should not be given as a bolus injection. Digoxin should not be administered concomitantly with other drugs through the same IV line. Dosage and frequency of administration are determined by the condition treated, age, weight, renal function, and other patient-specific factors. A reduced dosage may be required for patients with renal impairment. See full prescribing information for complete administration instructions.

J1162

J1162 Injection, digoxin immune fab (ovine), per vial

Digoxin immune Fab (ovine) is an antigen-binding fragment (Fab) substance raised in sheep. Sheep are immunized with human antibodies specific to digoxin to produce antibodies specific for the antigenic determinants of the digoxin molecule. The antibody is then papain-digested and the digoxin-specific Fab fragments of the antibody are isolated and purified by affinity chromatography. Digoxin immune Fab is used to treat adults and children with life-threatening toxicity due to digoxin or digitoxin overdose. Life-threatening manifestations include severe ventricular arrhythmias, progressive bradyarrhythmias, or second- or third-degree heart block. The drug can be administered by intravenous (IV) infusion over 30 minutes. An IV bolus injection may be administered if cardiac arrest is imminent. Dosage and frequency will vary based on the amount of digoxin or digitoxin to be neutralized. See full prescribing information for complete administration instructions.

J1165

J1165 Injection, phenytoin sodium, per 50 mg

Phenytoin sodium is an anticonvulsant medication for the control of tonic-clonic and temporal lobe seizures. It can be taken daily as an oral medication for prophylactic treatment of seizures or be administered intravenously for treatment of acute episodes. Phenytoin sodium is somewhat related to barbiturates in chemical structure and acts upon the motor cortex to inhibit seizure activity. Therapeutic levels vary greatly among patients.

J1170

J1170 Injection, hydromorphone, up to 4 mg

Hydromorphone is a narcotic and opioid analgesic classified as a schedule II controlled substance. This drug binds to opiate nerve center receptors and alters the human pain response, as well as suppressing the cough reflex. It is available in oral and injectable forms. The injectable form can be administered by intramuscular, subcutaneous, and intravenous injection, or by intravenous infusion. Hydromorphone hydrochloride is indicated for the relief of moderate to severe pain.

J1180

J1180 Injection, dyphylline, up to 500 mg

Dyphylline is a derivative of theophylline. Theophylline is a xanthine compound that naturally occurs in tea leaves and can be made synthetically. Dyphylline acts directly on the bronchial smooth muscles as a bronchodilator. It is indicated to treat and prevent the symptoms of bronchial asthma, chronic bronchitis, and emphysema by relaxing the bronchial airways and improving the air flow through the lungs. The injectable form is administered by intramuscular injection for acute conditions. Dosage varies based on the severity of the condition and response.

J1190

J1190 Injection, dexrazoxane HCl, per 250 mg

Dexrazoxane hydrochloride is an intracellular chelating agent derived from ethylenediaminetetraacetic acid (EDTA). Dexrazoxane hydrochloride acts as a cardioprotective agent when used in conjunction with chemotherapeutic agents classified as anthracyclines. Anthracyclines, such as doxorubicin and daunorubicin, are known for their high rate of cardiotoxicity. The method of action is not entirely understood. However, in laboratory studies, dexrazoxane hydrochloride is converted intracellularly to a chelating agent that interferes with iron-mediated free radical generation thought to be responsible, in part, for anthracycline-induced cardiomyopathy. Dexrazoxane hydrochloride is supplied in 250 mg or 500 mg single use vials and is administered by intravenous infusion.

J1200

J1200 Injection, diphenhydramine HCl, up to 50 mg

Diphenhydramine hydrochloride is an antihistamine, a histamine receptor antagonist that has anticholinergic, antitussive, antiemetic, antivertigo, antipruritic, antidyskinetic, and sedative effects. It blocks the effects of histamine on the smooth muscle of the bronchial tubes, GI tract, uterus, and blood vessels. It also acts as a local anesthetic by preventing transmission of nerve impulses. Diphenhydramine hydrochloride is indicated for the treatment of anaphylaxis, Parkinsonism when the patient cannot tolerate other medications, drug-induced extrapyramidal disorders, motion sickness, allergies, vertigo, insomnia, and to suppress nausea and prevent vomiting. Its antiemetic effects allow it to be prescribed to treat nausea and vomiting associated with chemotherapy. Diphenhydramine hydrochloride is available in self-administrable oral forms and in an injectable form. The injectable form is administered by intramuscular or intravenous injection.

J1201

J1201 Injection, cetirizine HCl, 0.5 mg

Cetirizine HCl is a histamine-1 (H_1) receptor antagonist that inhibits peripheral H_1 receptors. The injected version is intended for the treatment of acute urticaria in adults and children, 6 months of age and older. It is supplied in 2 mL single use vials and is administered via intravenous (IV) push injection over one to two minutes. The recommended dosage for children 6 months to 5 years of age is 2.5 mg. For children 6 to 11 years of age, the recommended dosage is 5 mg or 10 mg, based on severity of symptoms. For adolescents and adults 12 years of age and older, the recommended dosage is 10 mg.

J1205

J1205 Injection, chlorothiazide sodium, per 500 mg

Chlorothiazide sodium is a thiazide diuretic. The mechanism of action of thiazides is unknown. They affect the distal renal tubular process of electrolyte reabsorption, increasing the excretion of sodium and chloride and, to a lesser extent, potassium and bicarbonate. Chlorothiazide sodium does not usually affect normal blood pressure. It is indicated, solely or in combination, for the treatment of edema associated with congestive heart failure, hepatic cirrhosis, diabetes insipidus, and renal dysfunction. It is administered by intravenous injection or infusion.

Dosages are dependent upon response and are individualized to the patient.

J1212

J1212 Injection, DMSO, dimethyl sulfoxide, 50%, 50 ml

Dimethyl sulfoxide, also known as DMSO, is an industrial solvent produced as a chemical byproduct of wood pulp in the production of paper. DMSO is FDA approved only as a preservative for transplant organs and for treating interstitial cystitis. It is also used as a preservative for stem cells collected from newborn umbilical cords, and has many off-label uses for medication delivery and pain control. DMSO has the ability to pass through membranes, including the skin barrier, carrying other drugs with it across those membranes. For interstitial cystitis, a 50 percent solution of DMSO is instilled in the bladder via catheter or syringe. The DMSO remains in the bladder for 15 minutes, when the patient is instructed to void.

J1230

J1230 Injection, methadone HCl, up to 10 mg

Methadone hydrochloride is a synthetic opioid analgesic with effects similar to those of morphine and heroin. It is a Schedule II controlled substance. Methadone hydrochloride is indicated for the treatment of severe pain and also as a substitute drug in the detoxification or maintenance in opioid addiction. It can be administered in an inpatient setting via intramuscular (IM), intravenous (IV), or subcutaneous (SC) injection. Dosage and frequency of administration depends on the goal of treatment and other patient-specific factors. The lowest effective dosage for the shortest duration to meet individual patient treatments goals should be used. See full prescribing information for complete administration instructions.

J1240

J1240 Injection, dimenhydrinate, up to 50 mg

Dimenhydrinate injection is a histamine receptor antagonist that has anticholinergic, antiemetic, antivertigo, and sedative effects. It is intended, in adults and children ages 12 and older, for the treatment and prevention of motion sickness or in cases of nausea and dizziness due to inner ear disturbances. It is thought that antihistamines may affect neural pathways that originate in the labyrinth, which inhibits nausea and vomiting. Dimenhydrinate injection should not be used in patients with chronic lung disease, narrow-angle glaucoma, or prostatic hypertrophy. It is administered via intramuscular (IM) injection but can be administered via slow intravenous (IV) injection (over two minutes) if diluted. It should not be injected arterially. Dosage, frequency, and route of administration are determined by the type of disorder treated and the age of the patient. See full prescribing information for complete administration instructions.

J1245

J1245 Injection, dipyridamole, per 10 mg

Dipyridamole inhibits platelet aggregation and is a coronary vasodilator. It is indicated as a prophylaxis to prevent thromboembolisms in patients with prosthetic heart valves, and to prevent additional events in patients who have had transient ischemic attacks or an ischemic stroke due to thrombosis. An infusion of dipyridamole may also be administered during diagnostic thallium myocardial perfusion imaging as an alternative to exercise. It is available in oral and injectable forms. The injectable form is administered by intravenous injection. The recommended dosage for prophylactic use is 75 to 100 mg. The recommended dosage for diagnostic testing is 0.142 mg/kg of body weight.

J1250

J1250 Injection, dobutamine HCl, per 250 mg

Dobutamine hydrochloride is a synthetic catecholamine that acts primarily on beta1 adrenergic receptors. It directly stimulates the heart muscle to increase its contractions and blood flow. Dobutamine hydrochloride is indicated for the treatment of cardiac decompensation in congestive heart failure or following cardiac surgery. It is administered by intravenous infusion through a central line or large peripheral vein. Dosage varies depending upon body weight and response.

J1260

J1260 Injection, dolasetron mesylate, 10 mg

Dolasetron mesylate is an antiemetic drug with a chemical compound that is a selective blocker of serotonin 5-HT3 receptors. Serotonin 5-HT3 receptors are present on the vagal nerve and at sensory nerve endings. Cytotoxic chemotherapy appears to trigger the release of serotonin in the small intestine, which may trigger the 5-HT3 receptors and initiate the vomiting reflex. It is indicated to prevent and treat nausea and vomiting associated with chemotherapy or surgery.

J1265

J1265 Injection, dopamine HCl, 40 mg

Dopamine hydrochloride (HCl) is a sympathomimetic amine vasopressor. This drug causes a release of norepinephrine and acts on the nerves in the central nervous system. It is a chemical naturally produced in the brain that increases heart rate and blood pressure. It is used to treat hemodynamic imbalances caused by myocardial infarction, trauma, endotoxic septicemia, open-heart surgery, renal failure, and chronic cardiac decompensation as in heart failure. Dopamine is administered via intravenous infusion.

J1267

J1267 Injection, doripenem, 10 mg

Doripenem is a synthetic, broad-spectrum carbapenem antibiotic structurally related to beta-lactam antibiotics. It inhibits bacterial cell wall synthesis by binding to penicillin binding proteins. It is used to treat complicated intraabdominal and urinary tract infections. The normal dose for doripenem is 500 mg administered by IV infusion over one hour.

J1270

J1270 Injection, doxercalciferol, 1 mcg

Doxercalciferol is a synthetic analogue of vitamin D that acts directly upon the parathyroid glands to suppress parathyroid hormone synthesis and secretion in order to control the levels of calcium and phosphate in the blood and bones. It is indicated in the treatment of secondary hyperparathyroidism in dialysis patients with chronic renal failure.

J1290

J1290 Injection, ecallantide, 1 mg

Ecallantide is a chemical compound that is a selective reversible inhibitor of plasma kallikrein. Kallikreins are enzymes that break peptide bonds in proteins. Ecallantide binds to the plasma kallikrein preventing the creation of bradykinin. Bradykinin is a vasodilator thought to be responsible for edema, inflammations, and pain. This medication is used to treat acute attacks of hereditary angioedema for patients who are 16 years of age or older. The recommended dosage is 30 mg administered subcutaneously in three injections.

J1300

J1300 Injection, eculizumab, 10 mg

Eculizumab is a monoclonal antibody produced from murine myeloma cell cultures. The antibody in the drug binds specifically to the complement protein C5, preventing the generation of a terminal complement complex that hemolyzes red blood cells. Eculizumab is indicated as a treatment for patients with paroxysmal nocturnal hemoglobinuria (PNH) to reduce hemolysis. PNH is a chronic acquired blood cell dysplasia with proliferation of a clone of stem cells producing erythrocytes, platelets, and granulocytes that are abnormally susceptible to lysis by complement. PHN patients have episodes of intravascular hemolysis causing hemolytic anemia, and venous thromboses, especially of the hepatic veins. Eculizumab is administered via intravenous infusion over 35 minutes. It should not be administered as a push or bolus. If an adverse reaction occurs during the administration, the infusion may be slowed, but total infusion time should not exceed two hours. The recommended dosage is 600 mg every seven days for the first four weeks, followed by 900 mg for the fifth dose seven days later, then 900 mg every 14 days thereafter. Since the use of this drug increases a patient's susceptibility to serious meningococcal infections (septicemia and/or meningitis), all patients without a history of prior meningococcal vaccination must receive the vaccine at least two weeks prior to receiving the first dose of eculizumab and be revaccinated according to current medical guidelines.

J1301

J1301 Injection, edaravone, 1 mg

Edaravone, a substituted 2-pyrazolin-5-one class, is a free radical scavenger (antioxidant) that works to remove oxygen-containing molecules that build up in patients with amyotrophic lateral sclerosis (ALS). This mechanism is thought to provide neuroprotective support to the nervous system, potentially slowing disease progression, or limiting additional damage by protecting motor neurons from oxidative trauma. Recommended dosage for adult patients is 60 mg administered by intravenous infusion as two consecutive 30 mg infusions over 60 minutes, daily, for 14 days. After a 14-day, drug-free period, subsequent treatments are administered daily for 10 days out of a 14-day period. All treatment cycles are separated by a 14-day, drug-free period.

J1302

J1302 Injection, sutimlimab-jome, 10 mg

Sutimlimab-jome is a complement inhibitor indicated to decrease the need for red blood cell (RBC) transfusions in adults, ages 18 years and older, with cold agglutinin disease or cold antibody hemolytic anemia. Cold agglutinin disease is a rare autoimmune disorder, triggered by cold temperatures, in which the body's immune system attacks and destroys RBCs. It is supplied in single dose vials of 1,100 mg/22 ml (50 mg/ml) and is administered via intravenous (IV) infusion. The recommended dosage for patients weighing less than 75 kg is 6,500 mg. For patients weighing 75 kg or more, the recommended dosage is 7,500 mg. Patients should be vaccinated against encapsulated bacteria at least two weeks prior to treatment. See full prescribing information for complete administration instructions.

J1303

J1303 Injection, ravulizumab-cwvz, 10 mg

Ravulizumab-cwvz is a complement inhibitor indicated as a treatment for adult patients, 18 years and older, with paroxysmal nocturnal hemoglobinuria (PNH) to reduce hemolysis. PNH is a chronic acquired blood cell dysplasia with proliferation of a clone of stem cells producing erythrocytes, platelets, and granulocytes that are abnormally susceptible to lysis by complement. PNH patients have episodes of intravascular hemolysis causing hemolytic anemia, and venous thromboses, especially of the hepatic veins. It is supplied in a single dose vial of 30 mg/30 ml (10 mg/ml) and the number of vials required is determined by the patient's weight and prescribed dose. The calculated volume of ravulizumab-cwvz must be withdrawn from the vials and diluted into an infusion bag of 0.9% sodium chloride to achieve a final concentration of 5 mg/ml and administered immediately via intravenous infusion through a 0.22 micron filter. The duration of the infusion is based on the total dosage volume. See the full prescribing information for maximum infusion rates. It should not be administered as a push or bolus. If an adverse reaction occurs during the administration, the infusion may be slowed. The recommended dosage consists of an initial loading dose followed by a maintenance dose every eight weeks; dosage is determined by body weight. See the full prescribing information for weight-based loading and maintenance dosages. For patients switching from eculizumab to ravulizumab-cwvz, the initial loading dose of ravulizumab-cwvz should be administered two weeks following the last eculizumab infusion. Since the use of this drug increases a patient's susceptibility to serious meningococcal infections (septicemia and/or meningitis), all patients without a history of prior meningococcal vaccination must receive the vaccine at least two weeks prior to receiving the first dose of ravulizumab-cwvz and be revaccinated according to current medical guidelines. If therapy must be started immediately, provide two weeks of antibacterial drug prophylaxis. Ravulizumab-cwvz should not be administered to patients with *Neisseria meningitidis* infections.

J1305

J1305 Injection, evinacumab-dgnb, 5 mg

Evinacumab-dgnb, an angiopoietin-like 3 (ANGPTL3) inhibitor, is indicated for the treatment of adults and children, ages 12 and older, with homozygous familial hypercholesterolemia (HoFH) in combination with other low-density lipoprotein-cholesterol (LDL-C) lowering therapies. It helps to reduce LDL-C, total cholesterol (TC), high-density lipoprotein-cholesterol (HDL-C), apolipoprotein B, and triglycerides (TG). It is supplied in 345 mg/2.3 mL (150 mg/mL) and 1,200/8 mL (150 mg/mL) single dose vials. The recommended dose is 15 mg/kg body weight administered once monthly by intravenous (IV) infusion over 60 minutes. Evinacumab-dgnb should not be administered concomitantly with other medications. See full prescribing information for complete administration instructions.

J1306

J1306 Injection, inclisiran, 1 mg

Inclisiran is a small interfering RNA (siRNA) directed to proprotein convertase subtilisin kexin type 9 (PCSK9) mRNA that is indicated for the treatment of adults, ages 18 years and older, with heterozygous familial hypercholesterolemia (HeFH) or clinical atherosclerotic cardiovascular disease (ASCVD) who require additional lowering of low-density lipoprotein cholesterol (LDL-C). It should be used as an adjunct to diet and maximally tolerated statin therapy. It is supplied in a single dose, prefilled syringe of 284 mg/1.5 ml (189 mg/ml) that is administered via subcutaneous (SC) injection by a health care professional. The recommended dose is 284 mg for the first injection, an additional SC injection at three months, and then every six months.

J1320

J1320 Injection, amitriptyline HCl, up to 20 mg

Amitriptyline is a tricyclic antidepressant, a dibenzocycloheptadiene derivative with additional sedative effects. It inhibits the membrane pump mechanism responsible for uptake of norepinephrine and serotonin. It is indicated for the treatment of depression, enuresis, and bulimia nervosa. The recommended dosage is 20 to 30 mg four times a day.

J1322

J1322 Injection, elosulfase alfa, 1 mg

Elosulfase alfa is an exogenous form of a human enzyme produced by recombinant DNA technology in a Chinese hamster ovary cell line. It is a hydrolytic lysosomal glycosaminoglycan-specific enzyme that hydrolyzes sulfate. The absence or a marked reduction in the activity of this enzyme, N-acetylgalactosamine-6-sulfatase, results in the accumulation of metabolic byproducts in the lysosomal compartment of cells throughout the body. The accumulation leads to widespread cellular, tissue, and organ dysfunction. Elosulfase alfa is intended to provide the exogenous enzyme that will be taken up into the lysosomes and help ready the cell of the protein byproducts. Elosulfase alfa is indicated for patients with Mucopolysaccharidosis type IVA (MPS IVA; Morquio A syndrome). The recommended dose is 2 mg per kg given intravenously over a minimum range of 3.5 to 4.5 hours, once every week.

J1324

J1324 Injection, enfuvirtide, 1 mg

Enfuvirtide is a synthetic peptide that inhibits the fusion of HIV, serotype 1 (HIV-1) into CD4+ cells. HIV-1 causes the majority of infections worldwide. Enfuvirtide, in combination with other antiretroviral agents, is indicated as a second-line therapy for the treatment of HIV-1 infections in patients who have evidence of continued HIV-1 replication despite ongoing antiretroviral therapy. The drug is administered by subcutaneous injection into the upper arm, anterior thigh, or abdomen. Recommended dosage is 90 mg twice a day. Enfuvirtide may be self-administered.

J1325

J1325 Injection, epoprostenol, 0.5 mg

Epoprostenol is a prostaglandin that acts as a direct vasodilator of pulmonary and systemic arteries and an inhibitor of platelet aggregation. It is usually administered parenterally through a permanent indwelling central venous catheter as a long-term medication to treat primary pulmonary hypertension and pulmonary hypertension secondary to scleroderma in NYHA Class III and IV patients. Initial administration may be through a peripheral intravenous infusion until a central venous catheter is established. It is manufactured as a powder that must be reconstituted with sterile diluent specific to the epoprostenol. Dosages vary dependent upon body weight and response. Once a regimen of epoprostenol has been established, it should never be stopped suddenly.

J1327

J1327 Injection, eptifibatide, 5 mg

Eptifibatide is an intravenous cyclical heptapeptide that prevents platelet aggregation and has a short half-life of 2.5 hours. It prevents the binding of fibrinogen, von Willebrand factor, and other ligands to glycoprotein IIb/IIIa stopping the platelets from joining. Eptifibatide is indicated as a treatment for acute coronary syndrome and to prevent thrombosis in patients undergoing percutaneous coronary interventions. Eptifibatide is administered by continuous intravenous infusion. Patients generally receive an infusion of eptifibatide for up to 96 hours following surgery or during medical hospitalization. Dosage is based on body weight.

J1330

J1330 Injection, ergonovine maleate, up to 0.2 mg

Ergonovine maleate is a natural or synthetic version of an ergot alkaloid. It is an oxytocic medication that acts to stimulate uterine and vascular smooth muscle contractions to reduce postpartum or post-abortion bleeding. It also is used to induce coronary artery spasms in diagnostic testing. Ergonovine maleate is available in oral and injectable forms. The injectable form is administered by intravenous or intramuscular injection.

J1335

J1335 Injection, ertapenem sodium, 500 mg

Ertapenem sodium is a carbapenem antibiotic that is structurally related to beta-lactam antibiotics. It works by prohibiting the creation of bacterial cell walls, causing cellular death. It is indicated for the treatment of adults and children, ages three months and older, with moderate to severe infections caused by susceptible bacteria in the following: acute pelvic infections, community-acquired pneumonia, complicated intra-abdominal infections, complicated urinary tract infections, and complicated skin and skin-structure infections, including diabetic foot infections without osteomyelitis. It may also be used prophylactically prior to elective colorectal surgery. Ertapenem sodium may be administered via intramuscular (IM) injection or intravenous (IV) infusion and should not be administered concomitantly with other drugs. Dosage, frequency, and route of administration are determined by age and other patient-specific factors. A reduced dosage may be required for patients with renal impairment. See full prescribing information for complete administration instructions.

J1364

J1364 Injection, erythromycin lactobionate, per 500 mg

Erythromycin lactobionate is a macrolide antibiotic produced by the bacterium *Streptomyces erythreus.* It inhibits protein synthesis causing cellular death. It is indicated for the treatment of adults and children with infections caused by susceptible bacteria in the following: acute pelvic inflammatory disease, diphtheria, erythrasma, Legionnaires' disease, lower and upper respiratory tract infections, prevention of bacterial endocarditis and rheumatic fever attacks in penicillin-allergic patients, and skin and skin-structure infections. Dosage and frequency are determined by the disease treated and body weight. See full prescribing information for complete administration instructions.

J1380

J1380 Injection, estradiol valerate, up to 10 mg

Estradiol valerate is an exogenous form of the natural hormone estrogen produced semisynthetically. Estradiol is produced naturally by the ovaries and placenta. It increases synthesis of DNA, RNA, and protein in responsive tissues and reduces the release of FSH from the pituitary gland. Estradiol valerate is a long-acting estrogen suspended in oil. It is indicated as a hormone replacement therapy for female hypogonadism, primary ovarian failure, absence of ovaries, postmenopausal osteoporosis, vasomotor menopausal symptoms, atrophic vaginitis, atrophic urethritis, and vulvar squamous metaplasia. It may also be used to treat advanced prostate cancer. Estradiol valerate is administered by deep intramuscular injection.

J1410

J1410 Injection, estrogen conjugated, per 25 mg

Estrogen conjugates are an exogenous form of the natural hormone estrogen. They may be derived from the urine of pregnant mares or produced synthetically. It increases synthesis of RNA, DNA, and protein in responsive tissue and inhibit release of FSH and luteinizing hormones from the pituitary gland. Estrogen conjugates are indicated as a hormone replacement therapy for female hypogonadism, primary ovarian failure, absence of ovaries, dysfunctional uterine bleeding, postmenopausal osteoporosis, vasomotor menopausal symptoms, atrophic vaginitis, atrophic urethritis, and vulvar squamous metaplasia. It may also be used to treat advanced prostate cancer.

J1426

J1426 Injection, casimersen, 10 mg

Casimersen is an antisense oligonucleotide (AO) used to potentially stop the disease process of genetic disorders by altering the synthesis of a particular protein. It is indicated for the treatment of adults and children with Duchenne muscular dystrophy (DMD) who have a confirmed mutation of the DMD gene that is responsive to exon 45 skipping. The synthetic AO binds to exon 45 of dystrophin pre-mRNA, allowing exon 45 to be ignored or skipped during mRNA processing. The cell can then generate the protein needed for muscular development. It is supplied in a 100 mg/2 mL (50 mg/mL) single dose vial requiring dilution. The volume of casimersen required should be withdrawn from the appropriate number of vials and diluted in 0.9% sodium chloride for a total volume of 100 to 150 mL. Once diluted, it should be administered immediately. The recommended dose is 30 mg/kg of body weight, administered once weekly via intravenous (IV) infusion over 35 to 60 minutes. See full prescribing information for complete administration instructions.

J1427

J1427 Injection, viltolarsen, 10 mg

Injectable drug indicated for the treatment of Duchenne muscular dystrophy (DMD) in patients who have a confirmed mutation of the DMD gene that is responsive to exon 53 skipping. This mutation affects approximately 8 percent of patients with DMD. DMD, a rare genetic disorder whose characteristics include progressive muscle deterioration and weakness, is the most common form of muscular dystrophy and occurs when one or more exons are deleted. This prevents the remainder of the gene being pieced together, which interferes with dystrophin protein production and results in the symptoms of DMD. Administered as an intravenous (IV) infusion over 60 minutes, the recommended dosage for this antisense oligonucleotide, also known as a molecular patch, is 80 milligrams per kilogram of body weight once weekly.

J1428

J1428 Injection, eteplirsen, 10 mg

Eteplirsen, an antisense oligonucleotide (AO), is a synthetic nucleic acid string used to potentially stop the disease process of genetic disorders by altering the synthesis of a particular protein. Eteplirsen is indicated for the treatment of adults and children with Duchenne muscular dystrophy (DMD) who have a confirmed mutation of the DMD gene that is responsive to exon 51 skipping. DMD is caused by a mutation of the dystrophin gene resulting in a break between exons 51 and 53. The synthetic AO targets that break, providing a molecular patch over the missing exon and allowing the break to be ignored or skipped. The cell can then generate the protein needed for muscular development. The recommended dose of eteplirsen is 30 milligrams per kilogram of body weight, administered once weekly via intravenous (IV) infusion over 35 to 60 minutes. Eteplirsen should not be administered with other medications through the same IV access.

J1429

J1429 Injection, golodirsen, 10 mg

Golodirsen is an antisense oligonucleotide (AO) used to potentially stop the disease process of genetic disorders by altering the synthesis of a particular protein. It is indicated for the treatment of adults and children with Duchenne muscular dystrophy (DMD) who have a confirmed mutation of the DMD gene that is responsive to exon 53 skipping. DMD is caused by a mutation of the dystrophin gene, resulting in a break between exons 51 and 53. The synthetic AO targets that break, providing a molecular patch over the missing exon and allowing the break to be ignored or skipped. The cell can then generate the protein needed for muscular development. It is supplied in a 100 mg/2 mL (50 mg/mL) single dose vial requiring dilution. The volume of golodirsen required should be withdrawn from the appropriate number of vials and diluted in 0.9% sodium chloride for a total volume of 100 to 150 mL. Once diluted, it should be administered immediately. The recommended dose is 30 mg/kg of body weight, administered once weekly via intravenous (IV) infusion over 35 to 60 minutes.

J1430

J1430 Injection, ethanolamine oleate, 100 mg

Ethanolamine oleate is a mild sclerosing agent consisting of ethanolamine combined with oleic acid in an aqueous solution. When injected intravenously for local use, it irritates the venous endothelium and produces an inflammatory response that results in fibrosis and potential occlusion of the vein. It is indicated as a treatment for varicose veins and esophageal varices.

J1435

J1435 Injection, estrone, per 1 mg

Estrone is the oxidation product of estradiol, a long-acting exogenous form of the natural hormone. Estrone may be produced synthetically or derived from human or animal urine, human ovarian fluid or placenta, or palm kernel oil. It is produced naturally by the ovaries and placenta. It is less potent than estradiol but more so than estriol and is metabolically convertible to estradiol. Estrone increases synthesis of DNA, RNA, and protein in responsive tissues and reduces the release of FSH from the pituitary gland. It is a long-acting estrogen and is given as an intramuscular injection. Estrone is indicated as a hormone replacement therapy for female hypogonadism, primary ovarian failure, absence of ovaries, dysfunctional uterine bleeding, postmenopausal osteoporosis, vasomotor menopausal symptoms, atrophic vaginitis, atrophic urethritis, and vulvar squamous metaplasia. It may also be used to treat advanced prostate cancer.

J1436

J1436 Injection, etidronate disodium, per 300 mg

Etidronate disodium is a diphosphate compound, also known as EHDP, that regulates bone metabolism. It inhibits formation and growth of hydroxyapatite crystals to calcium surfaces, and in so doing, slows resorption and accretion in abnormal bone turnover. Etidronate disodium is indicated as a treatment for osteitis deformans, heterotopic ossification, and hypercalcemia of malignancy. The drug is available in oral and injectable forms. The injectable form is administered by intravenous infusion over a two-hour period.

J1437

J1437 Injection, ferric derisomaltose, 10 mg

Ferric derisomaltose is an iron replacement for the treatment of iron deficiency anemia (IDA) in adult patients who have intolerance or poor response to oral iron products or who have nondialysis dependent chronic kidney disease. IDA etiologies may include cancer, gastrointestinal disorders, abnormal uterine bleeding, or chronic kidney disease. It is supplied in single dose vials of 100 mg iron/mL, 500 mg iron/5 mL, or 1,000 mg iron/10 mL each requiring dilution with 0.9% sodium chloride for a final concentration of 1 mg iron/mL. It is administered via intravenous (IV) infusion. The recommended dosage for patients weighing less than 50 kg is 20 mg/kg body weight via IV infusion over at least 20 minutes. The recommended dosage for patients weighing more than 50 kg is 1,000 mg via IV infusion over at least 20 minutes. Dosage may be repeated if IDA reoccurs.

J1438

J1438 Injection, etanercept, 25 mg (code may be used for Medicare when drug administered under the direct supervision of a physician, not for use when drug is self-administered)

Etanercept is an antirheumatic agent that binds to tumor necrosis factor, blocking its action and thereby causing a decrease in inflammation and autoimmune response. It is indicated for the treatment of juvenile rheumatoid arthritis, rheumatoid arthritis, psoriatic arthritis, ankylosing spondylitis, and chronic plaque psoriasis. Etanercept is administered by subcutaneous injection, typically the thigh, abdomen, or upper arm, once or twice weekly. The recommended adult dosage is 50 mg per week. The recommended dosage for patients 4 to 17 years of age is 0.8 mg/kg of body weight. The drug may be self-administered by the patient.

J1439

J1439 Injection, ferric carboxymaltose, 1 mg

Ferric Carboxymaltose is an iron replacement for the treatment of iron deficiency anemia (IDA) in adult patients who have intolerance or poor response to oral iron products or who have nondialysis dependent chronic kidney disease. IDA etiologies may include cancer, gastrointestinal disorders, abnormal uterine bleeding, or chronic kidney disease. The drug is administered intravenously by an undiluted slow push or by infusion. When administering as a slow intravenous push, it is given at the rate of approximately 100 mg (2 mL) per minute. For patients weighing 50 kg (110 lb) or more, it is administered in two doses separated by at least seven days. A dose of 750 mg for a total cumulative dose not to exceed 1,500 mg of iron is administered per course. For patients weighing less than 50 kg (110 lb), two doses are given separated by at least seven days. The dose should be 15 mg/kg body weight for a total cumulative dose not to exceed 1,500 mg of iron per course.

J1442

J1442 Injection, filgrastim (G-CSF), excludes biosimilars, 1 mcg

Filgrastim is a synthetic, human granulocyte colony stimulating factor (G-CSF). It is produced by recombinant DNA technology using *E. coli* bacteria. The drug binds to surface receptors on hematopoietic and stimulates neutrophil production, differentiation, maturation, and function. It is indicated as a treatment for neutropenia in patients receiving myelosuppressive therapy for nonmyeloid malignancies. Filgrastim is also used to mobilize hematopoietic progenitor cells for leukapheresis to be used for bone marrow transplants. The drug is administered by subcutaneous or intravenous injection and intravenous infusion. Recommended dosage varies from 5 to 10 mcg/kg of body weight per day depending on the indication.

J1443-J1444

J1443 Injection, ferric pyrophosphate citrate solution (Triferic), 0.1 mg of iron

J1444 Injection, ferric pyrophosphate citrate powder, 0.1 mg of iron

Ferric pyrophosphate citrate is an iron therapy for the treatment of anemia in adult patients with hemodialysis-dependent chronic kidney disease (HDD-CKD), and allows patients to maintain hemoglobin levels without intravenous (IV) iron and possible liver toxicity. It is supplied in a 5 mL ampule of solution equivalent to 27.2 mg of iron, a 50 mL ampule of solution equivalent to 272 mg of iron, or a packet of powder, also equivalent to 272 mg of iron. A 5 mL ampule is added to 2.5 gallons of bicarbonate concentrate, a 50 mL ampule is added to 25 gallons of bicarbonate concentrate for preparation of hemodialysate to achieve a concentration of Triferic iron (III) in the final hemodialysate of 2 uM (110/mcg/L). Report J1443 when administering a 5 mL or 50 mL ampule. Report J1444 when administering a powder packet. Report J1444 appended with modifier JE when administered via dialysate.

J1445

J1445 Injection, ferric pyrophosphate citrate solution (Triferic AVNU), 0.1 mg of iron

Ferric pyrophosphate citrate is an iron therapy for the treatment of anemia in adult patients with hemodialysis-dependent chronic kidney disease (HDD-CKD), and allows patients to maintain hemoglobin levels without intravenous (IV) iron and possible liver toxicity. It is supplied in a single dose luer lock ampule of 6.75 mg iron (III) per 4.5 mL solution (1.5 mg iron per mL). It is administered as a slow intravenous (IV) infusion over three to four hours through a pre-dialyzer infusion line, post-dialyzer infusion line, or through a separate venous blood line during dialysis. See full prescribing information for complete administration instructions.

J1447

J1447 Injection, tbo-filgrastim, 1 mcg

TBO-filgrastim is a non-glycosylated recombinant methionyl human granulocyte colony-stimulating growth factor (G-CSF) manufactured by recombinant DNA technology using the bacterium *E. coli*. It is composed of 175 amino acids. The endogenous human G-CSF is glycosylated and does not have the additional methionine amino acid residue. TBO-filgrastim is produced by recombinant DNA technology. It binds to G-CSF receptors and stimulates proliferation of neutrophils. G-CSF is known to stimulate differentiation and some end-cell functional activation, which increases neutrophil counts and activity. TBO-filgrastim is indicated for treatment of severe neutropenia in patients with nonmyeloid malignancies receiving myelosuppressive anticancer drugs. The product is available in prefilled syringes that contain 300 mcg or 480 mcg of TBO-filgrastim. The recommended dose is 5 mcg per kilogram of body weight per day administered as a subcutaneous injection.

J1448

J1448 Injection, trilaciclib, 1 mg

Trilaciclib is a kinase inhibitor indicated to decrease episodes of chemotherapy-induced myelosuppression in adult patients, ages 18 and older, when administered prior to a platinum/etoposide-containing regimen or topotecan-containing regimen for extensive-stage small cell lung cancer. When administered prior to chemotherapy, it arrests hematopoietic stem and progenitor cells (HSPC), protecting them during chemotherapy. It is supplied as a 300 mg lyophilized cake in a single dose vial. The recommended dose is 240 mg/m^2 administered via intravenous (IV) infusion over 30 minutes. It must be completed within four hours prior to chemotherapy for each day of chemotherapy. Trilaciclib should not be administered concomitantly with certain OCT2, MATE1, and MATE-2K substrates. See full prescribing information for complete administration instructions.

J1450

J1450 Injection, fluconazole, 200 mg

Fluconazole is a synthetic triazole antifungal agent. It is indicated as a treatment for vaginal, oropharyngeal, and esophageal candidiasis and cryptococcal meningitis. Fluconazole is also used as a prophylaxis for candidiasis in patients undergoing bone marrow transplantation, radiation therapy, or cytotoxic chemotherapy. It is available in oral and injectable forms. The injectable form is administered by intravenous infusion. Recommended dosage varies from 3 to 12 mg/kg of body weight depending on the indication.

J1451

J1451 Injection, fomepizole, 15 mg

Fomepizole is a competitive inhibitor of alcohol dehydrogenase, the enzyme that catalyzes the initial steps in the metabolism of ethylene glycol and methanol and prevents these two substances from forming the toxic metabolites that cause metabolic acidosis and renal damage. Fomepizole is indicated for use as an antidote in confirmed or suspected ethylene glycol (antifreeze) poisoning and methanol poisoning. It may be used alone or with hemodialysis. Fomepizole is administered by intravenous infusion. The usual initial dose is 15 mg/kg of body weight administered over 30 minutes. Subsequent doses are usually reduced to 10 mg/kg of body weight given every 12 hours over 30 minutes until ethylene glycol or methanol concentration decreases to less than 20 mg per dl.

J1452

J1452 Injection, fomivirsen sodium, intraocular, 1.65 mg

Fomivirsen sodium intravitreal injection is indicated for the local treatment of cytomegalovirus (CMV) retinitis in patients with acquired immunodeficiency syndrome (AIDS). Fomivirsen intravitreal injection is a local treatment that does not affect CMV infections of other sites. Treatment of bilateral CMV retinal infections requires injections in both eyes. Fomivirsen inhibits human cytomegalovirus (HCMV) replication by binding to the target mRNA and inhibiting IE2 protein synthesis, which prevents virus replication. Initial intravitreal injection for treatment of CMV retinitis is 330 mcg into the affected eye every other week for two doses. After the two initial doses, maintenance doses of 330 mcg are administered every four weeks.

J1453

J1453 Injection, fosaprepitant, 1 mg

Fosaprepitant, a prodrug of aprepitant, is a substance P/neurokinin-1 (NK_1) receptor antagonist. Once administered, it is quickly converted to aprepitant. Used in combination with other antiemetic drugs, it is indicated for the treatment of adults and children, ages 6 months and older, to prevent or reduce acute or delayed nausea and vomiting associated with chemotherapy. For adults, fosaprepitant is administered via an intravenous (IV) infusion. For children, it should be administered through a central venous catheter. Dosage and length of administration is based on patient's age. See full prescribing information for complete administration instructions.

J1454

J1454 Injection, fosnetupitant 235 mg and palonosetron 0.25 mg

Fosnetupitant/palonosetron is a fixed combination of fosnetupitant (a P/neurokinin 1 receptor antagonist) and palonosetron (a serotonin-3 receptor antagonist) that is used for the prevention of acute and delayed nausea and vomiting associated with cancer chemotherapy treatment in adult patients. Palonosetron inhibits the acute onset of nausea and vomiting while fosnetupitant inhibits nausea and vomiting during both the acute and delayed phase following chemotherapy. The drug is supplied in a single dose vial and contains 235 mg fosnetupitant and 0.25 mg palonosetron. The recommended dosage is one vial, reconstituted in 50 ml of 5% dextrose, administered via intravenous infusion over 30 minutes starting 30 minutes prior to chemotherapy. It should be administered in combination with dexamethasone.

J1455

J1455 Injection, foscarnet sodium, per 1,000 mg

Foscarnet sodium is an antiviral indicated for treatment of cytomegalovirus (CMV) retinitis in patients with acquired immune deficiency syndrome. It is also indicated for treatment of herpes simplex virus types 1 and 2 (HPV-1, HPV-2) mucocutaneous infections in immunocompromised patients. It works by inhibiting in vitro viral replication by binding to the pyrophosphate binding site on virus-specific DNA polymerases. Foscarnet sodium is administered by intravenous infusion over one to two hours. Dose is dependent on the specific viral infection being treated, as well as the patient's body weight.

J1456

J1456 Injection, fosaprepitant (Teva), not therapeutically equivalent to J1453, 1 mg

Fosaprepitant for injection, a prodrug of aprepitant, is a substance P/neurokinin-1 (NK_1) receptor antagonist. Once administered, it is quickly converted to aprepitant. Used in combination with other antiemetic drugs, it is indicated for the treatment of adults, ages 18 years and older, to prevent acute or delayed nausea and vomiting associated with highly emetogenic cancer chemotherapy (HEC). It is supplied in a single dose vial containing 150 mg fosaprepitant requiring reconstitution with 5 ml of 0.9% sodium chloride. Fosaprepitant for injection should not be administered concurrently with pimozide. The recommended dosage is 150 mg on day one administered via an intravenous (IV) infusion over 20 to 30 minutes, completing the infusion approximately 30 minutes prior to start of HEC treatment. See full prescribing information for complete administration instructions. Report J1456 only for fosaprepitant for injection manufactured by Teva.

J1457

J1457 Injection, gallium nitrate, 1 mg

Gallium is a rare metal that is liquid at room temperature. Gallium nitrate is a hydrated nitrate salt of gallium used in the treatment of symptomatic cancer-related hypercalcemia that has not responded to hydration therapy. Generally, patients should have serum calcium (corrected for albumin) equal to or greater than 12 mg/dl. The recommended usage for gallium nitrate is 200 mg per m2 of body surface daily infused over 24 hours for five consecutive days.

J1458

J1458 Injection, galsulfase, 1 mg

Galsulfase is a human enzyme produced by recombinant DNA technology in a Chinese hamster ovary. Galsulfase is an orphan drug used to treat the inherited metabolic disorder mucopolysaccharidosis VI (MPS VI or Maroteaux-Lamy Syndrome). Mucopolysaccharidosis VI is caused by a lack of the enzyme arylsulfatase B that normally breaks down certain carbohydrates known as glycosaminoglycans. While intelligence is not affected, MPS VI causes widespread cumulative organ and tissue damage. The drug is administered via a four-hour infusion every week.

J1459

J1459 Injection, immune globulin (Privigen), intravenous, nonlyophilized (e.g., liquid), 500 mg

Immune globulins are glycoproteins in the blood that function as antibodies. Immune globulins specific to a certain disease are antibodies with specific amino acid sequences that interact only with the antigen that stimulated its creation or with antigens that are closely related to the stimulating antigen. Immune globulins are usually derived from the pooled plasma of human donors who have antibodies to the specific disease. The antibodies from the exogenous immune globulin help the body to fight off a disease. The term intravenous immune globulin, IVIg, used with a qualifier generally refers to the full range of immunoglobulins contained within the blood. Immunoglobulins are divided into five classes, IgM, IgG, IgA, IgD, and IgE, on the basis of structure and biologic activity. IVIg is administered by intravenous injection or infusion. IVIg is indicated as a treatment for primary immune deficiency disorders, idiopathic thrombocytopenia purpura, autoimmune diseases, and as an adjunct treatment of Kawasaki disease. It is also indicated as a prophylaxis of infectious diseases associated with chronic lymphocytic leukemia, pediatric HIV infection, and bone marrow transplants. IVIg is available as a solution or in a lyophilized or freeze-dried form.

J1460

J1460 Injection, gamma globulin, intramuscular, 1 cc

Gamma globulins are serum globulins having the least rapid electrophoretic migration. Since the gamma globulin fractions are composed almost entirely of immune globulin, gamma globulin has come to be used as a synonym of immune globulin or immunoglobulin. Immune globulins are glycoproteins in the blood that function as antibodies. Immune globulins specific to a certain disease are antibodies with specific amino acid sequences that interact only with the antigen that stimulated its creation or with antigens that are closely related to the stimulating antigen. Immune globulins are usually derived from the pooled plasma of human donors who have antibodies to the specific disease. The antibodies from the exogenous immune globulin help the body to fight off a disease. The term immune globulin used with a qualifier generally refers to the full range of immunoglobulins contained within the blood. Immunoglobulins are divided into five classes, IgM, IgG, IgA, IgD, and IgE, on the basis of structure and biologic activity. Gamma globulins are administered by intramuscular injection. They are indicated as a treatment for primary immune deficiency disorders or as a prophylaxis after exposure to hepatitis A, measles, rubella, and varicella.

J1551

J1551 Injection, immune globulin (Cutaquig), 100 mg

Cutaquig (brand name) is a 16.5 percent immune globulin liquid indicated for the treatment of children and adults, ages 2 years and older, with primary humoral immunodeficiency (PI). Typically manifested by increased susceptibility to recurrent infections, PIs are rare deficiencies of the immune system, largely a dysfunction of antibody production. The humoral immune defect in congenital agammaglobulinemia, common variable immunodeficiency (CVID), X-linked agammaglobulinemia, Wiskott-Aldrich syndrome, and severe combined immunodeficiencies (SCID) are but a few examples of PI. Prior to treatment, the patient's IgG trough level should be obtained and then monitored regularly to guide subsequent dose adjustments. Administered by subcutaneous (SC) intravenous (IV) infusion, the recommended dosage varies depending on previous immune globulin treatments and serum Immunoglobulin G (IgG) trough levels. See full prescribing information for complete administration instructions.

J1554

J1554 Injection, immune globulin (Asceniv), 500 mg

Asceniv (brand name) is a 10 percent immune globulin liquid, indicated for the treatment of primary humoral immunodeficiency (PI) in adults and adolescents ages 12 to 17 years. Typically manifested by increased susceptibility to recurrent infections, PIs are rare deficiencies of the immune system, largely a dysfunction of antibody production. The humoral immune defect in congenital agammaglobulinemia, common variable immunodeficiency (CVID), X-linked agammaglobulinemia, Wiskott-Aldrich syndrome, and severe combined immunodeficiencies (SCID) are but a few examples of PI. Administered by intravenous (IV) infusion, the recommended dose of Asceniv for replacement therapy in PI is 300 to 800 mg/kg body weight administered every three to four weeks.

J1555

J1555 Injection, immune globulin (Cuvitru), 100 mg

Cuvitru is an immune globulin indicated for the treatment of patients, ages 2 and older, with primary humoral immunodeficiency (PI). Cuvitru is derived from human plasma and is intended to protect against infection by replacing antibodies that are not properly working or are missing. It is administered through subcutaneous (SC) infusion and infusion sites should be rotated with each administration. For the first two infusions, the recommended infusion rate is 10 to 20 mL/hr/site. For patients weighing <40 kg, the volume infused per site should be ≤20 mL. For patients weighing ≥40 kg, the volume per site should be ≤60 mL. If the first two infusions are tolerated well, the rate of subsequent infusions can be increased up to 60 mL/hr/site as tolerated. It may be infused simultaneously through up to four sites that are at least 4 inches apart. For infusion through four sites, the infusion rate for all sites combined should be no more than 240 mL/hr. The starting dosage varies depending on if patients are switching from IVIG, HYQVIA, or other SCIG treatments. If switching from HYQVIA or IVIG, the initial Cuvitru administration should begin one week after the last HYQVIA or IVIG treatment. The initial weekly dose is determined by dividing the previous HYQVIA or IVIG dose in grams by the number of weeks between HYQVIA or IVIG doses, then multiply by 1.30. If switching from SCIG, the dosage of Cuvitru would be the same. If the patient or physician wants infusions more frequently than weekly, divide the calculated weekly dose by the desired frequency per week. If biweekly administration is desired, multiply the weekly dose by two.

J1556

J1556 Injection, immune globulin (Bivigam), 500 mg

Bivigam is an exogenous source of human immunoglobulin G (IgG) antibodies used as replacement therapy. It is a concentrated human immunoglobulin purified from human plasma that undergoes rigorous testing. The drug is administered via intravenous infusion and is indicated for the treatment of primary humoral immunodeficiency. The recommended dosage is 300 mg to 800 mg per kg of body weight, which can be adjusted to achieve desired clinical response.

J1557

J1557 Injection, immune globulin, (Gammaplex), intravenous, nonlyophilized (e.g., liquid), 500 mg

Immune globulin (Gammaplex), intravenous, nonlyophilized (e.g., liquid) is an immune globulin liquid used in the treatment of replacement therapy of primary humoral immunodeficiency (PI). Gammaplex may also be used for treatment of a humoral immune defect in common variable immunodeficiency, Wiskott-Aldrich syndrome, X linked agammaglobulinemia, congenital agammaglobulinemia, and severe combined immunodeficiencies. Recommended dose is 300 to 800 mg/kg every three to four weeks. The dose and schedule may vary based on individual response to treatment. Gammaplex is administered by intravenous infusion.

J1558

J1558 Injection, immune globulin (xembify), 100 mg

Xembify (trade name) is an immune globulin indicated for the treatment of patients, ages 2 and older, with primary humoral immunodeficiency (PI). Xembify is derived from human plasma and is intended to protect against infection by replacing antibodies that are not properly working or are missing. Xembify is supplied as a 20% IgG (200 mg/mL; 0.2 g/mL) solution in a single use vial. It is administered through subcutaneous (SC) infusion into the abdomen, back, lateral hip, upper arm, or thigh. Up to six infusion sites may be administered simultaneously, allowing for at least two inches between infusion sites. Infusion sites should be rotated with each administration. The starting dosage varies depending on if patients are switching from immune globulin subcutaneous (human) treatment (IGSC) or immune globulin intravenous (human) (IVIG) treatments. If switching from IGSC, the weekly dose should remain the same. If switching from IVIG, the initial Xembify administration should begin one week after the last IVIG treatment. The initial weekly dose is determined by converting it from a monthly to a weekly dose. Divide the previous IVIG dose in grams multiplied by 1.37 by the number of weeks between IVIG doses. If the patient or physician wants infusions more frequently than weekly, divide the calculated weekly dose by the desired frequency per week. The recommended infusion rate is a maximum of 25 mL/hr/site. Dosage adjustments must be made by reviewing the patient's serum IgG trough level from the target IgG trough level. Using the table in the prescribing information, locate the amount to increase or decrease the weekly dose based on the patient's body weight. See full prescribing information for additional dosing adjustments.

J1559

J1559 Injection, immune globulin (Hizentra), 100 mg

Immune globulins are glycoproteins in the blood that function as antibodies. Immune globulins specific to a certain disease are antibodies with specific amino acid sequences that interact only with the antigen that stimulated its creation or with antigens that are closely related to the stimulating antigen. Immune globulins are usually derived from the pooled plasma of human donors who have antibodies to the specific disease. The antibodies from the exogenous immune globulin help the body to fight off a disease. It is indicated as a treatment for primary immune deficiency disorders. This includes, but is not limited to, the humoral immune defect in congenital agammaglobulinemia, common variable immunodeficiency, X-linked agammaglobulinemia, Wiskott-Aldrich syndrome, and severe combined immunodeficiencies. Subcutaneous injections are administered with the use of an infusion pump.

J1560

J1560 Injection, gamma globulin, intramuscular, over 10 cc

Gamma globulins are serum globulins having the least rapid electrophoretic migration. Since the gamma globulin fractions are composed almost entirely of immune globulin, gamma globulin has come to be used as a synonym of immune globulin or immunoglobulin. Immune globulins are glycoproteins in the blood that function as antibodies. Immune globulins specific to a certain disease are antibodies with specific amino acid sequences that interact only with the antigen that stimulated its creation or with antigens that are closely related to the stimulating antigen. Immune globulins are usually derived from the pooled plasma of human donors who have antibodies to the specific disease. The antibodies from the exogenous immune globulin help the body to fight off a disease. The term immune globulin used with a qualifier generally refers to the full range of immunoglobulins contained within the blood. Immunoglobulins are divided into five classes, IgM, IgG, IgA, IgD, and IgE, on the basis of structure and biologic activity. Gamma globulins are administered by intramuscular injection. They are indicated as a treatment for primary immune deficiency disorders or as a prophylaxis after exposure to hepatitis A, measles, rubella, and varicella.

J1561-J1569

J1561 Injection, immune globulin, (Gamunex/Gamunex-C/Gammaked), nonlyophilized (e.g., liquid), 500 mg

J1562 Injection, immune globulin (Vivaglobin), 100 mg

J1566 Injection, immune globulin, intravenous, lyophilized (e.g., powder), not otherwise specified, 500 mg

J1568 Injection, immune globulin, (Octagam), intravenous, nonlyophilized (e.g., liquid), 500 mg

J1569 Injection, immune globulin, (Gammagard liquid), nonlyophilized, (e.g., liquid), 500 mg

Immune globulins are glycoproteins in the blood that function as antibodies. Immune globulins specific to a certain disease are antibodies with specific amino acid sequences that interact only with the antigen that stimulated its creation or with antigens that are closely related to the stimulating antigen. Immune globulins are usually derived from the pooled plasma of human donors who have antibodies to the specific disease. The antibodies from the exogenous immune globulin help the body to fight off a disease. The term intravenous immune globulin, IVIg, used with a qualifier generally refers to the full range of immunoglobulins contained within the blood. Immunoglobulins are divided into five classes, IgM, IgG, IgA, IgD, and IgE, on the basis of structure and biologic activity. IVIg is administered by intravenous injection or infusion. IVIg is indicated as a treatment for primary immune deficiency disorders, idiopathic thrombocytopenia purpura, autoimmune diseases, and as an adjunct treatment of Kawasaki disease. It is also indicated as a prophylaxis of infectious diseases associated with chronic lymphocytic leukemia, pediatric HIV infection, and bone marrow transplants. IVIg is available as a solution or in a lyophilized or freeze-dried form.

J1570

J1570 Injection, ganciclovir sodium, 500 mg

Ganciclovir sodium is a synthetic guanine derivative active against cytomegalovirus (CMV). It is indicated for treatment and prevention of CMV in patients with acquired immunodeficiency syndrome (AIDS). It is also indicated for prevention of CMV in organ transplant patients. It works by inhibiting the replication of the virus. Ganciclovir is available as sterile lyophilized powder in 500 mg vials for intravenous administration. It is also available in 250 mg and 500 mg capsules for oral administration. For AIDS patients with CMV infection, initial treatment is by intravenous injection infused over one hour every 12 hours for 14 to 21 days. The dose depends on body weight. Following the intravenous course of treatment, maintenance therapy is administered by intravenous infusion once per day five to seven days per week or in oral capsule form. Maintenance intravenous therapy dose depends on body weight. Usual oral dose is 1,000 mg tid. Organ transplant patients typically receive initial intravenous therapy for up to 21 days, followed by maintenance doses given orally or by intravenous infusion.

J1571

J1571 Injection, hepatitis B immune globulin (Hepagam B), intramuscular, 0.5 ml

Immune globulins are glycoproteins in the blood that function as antibodies. Immune globulins specific to a certain disease are antibodies with specific amino acid sequences that interact only with the antigen that stimulated its creation or with antigens that are closely related to the stimulating antigen. Immune globulins are usually derived from the pooled plasma of human donors who have antibodies to the specific disease. The antibodies from the exogenous immune globulin help the body to fight off a disease. Hepatitis B is a viral infection of the liver. The virus is shed in all body fluids from infected individuals. While it is possible to become infected via oral transmission, it is more commonly transmitted by parenteral routes, such as blood transfusion, contaminated needles, and sexual contact. Hepatitis B has an incubation period of about 90 days with a range of 40 to 180 days. It can cause fever, malaise, anorexia, nausea and vomiting, jaundice, urticaria, angioedema, arthritis, and, rarely, glomerulonephritis or a serum sickness-like syndrome. Hepatitis B can cause massive liver necrosis. It is thought that the disease may be a cause of cirrhosis and primary liver cancer. Most patients recover completely. Some may remain chronic carriers or develop chronic active or persistent hepatitis. The disease is endemic worldwide. Hepatitis B immune globulin is derived from persons with high titers of antibodies against the hepatitis B surface antigen. It is administered by intramuscular injection for the prophylaxis of persons exposed to the virus or infants of mothers who test positive for the antigen.

J1572

J1572 Injection, immune globulin, (Flebogamma/Flebogamma Dif), intravenous, nonlyophilized (e.g., liquid), 500 mg

Immune globulins are glycoproteins in the blood that function as antibodies. Immune globulins specific to a certain disease are antibodies with specific amino acid sequences that interact only with the antigen that stimulated its creation or with antigens that are closely related to the stimulating antigen. Immune globulins are usually derived from the pooled plasma of human donors who have antibodies to the specific disease. The antibodies from the exogenous immune globulin help the body to fight off a disease. The term intravenous immune globulin, IVIg, used with a qualifier generally refers to the full range of immunoglobulins contained within the blood. Immunoglobulins are divided into five classes, IgM, IgG, IgA, IgD, and IgE, on the basis of structure and biologic activity. IVIg is administered by intravenous injection or infusion. IVIg is indicated as a treatment for primary immune deficiency disorders, idiopathic thrombocytopenia purpura, autoimmune diseases, and as an adjunct treatment of Kawasaki disease. It is also indicated as a prophylaxis of infectious diseases associated with chronic lymphocytic leukemia, pediatric HIV infection, and bone marrow transplants. IVIg is available as a solution or in a lyophilized or freeze-dried form.

J1573

J1573 Injection, hepatitis B immune globulin (Hepagam B), intravenous, 0.5 ml

Immune globulins are glycoproteins in the blood that function as antibodies. Immune globulins specific to a certain disease are antibodies with specific amino acid sequences that interact only with the antigen that stimulated its creation or with antigens that are closely related to the stimulating antigen. Immune globulins are usually derived from the pooled plasma of human donors who have antibodies to the specific disease. The antibodies from the exogenous immune globulin help the body to fight off a disease. Hepatitis B is a viral infection of the liver. The virus is shed in all body fluids from infected individuals. While it is possible to become infected via oral transmission, it is more commonly transmitted by parenteral routes, such as blood transfusion, contaminated needles, and sexual contact. Hepatitis B has an incubation period of about 90 days with a range of 40 to 180 days. It can cause fever, malaise, anorexia, nausea and vomiting, jaundice, urticaria, angioedema, arthritis, and, rarely, glomerulonephritis or a serum sickness-like syndrome. Hepatitis B can cause massive liver necrosis. It is thought that the disease may be a cause of cirrhosis and primary liver cancer. Most patients recover completely. Some may remain chronic carriers or develop chronic active or persistent hepatitis. The disease is endemic worldwide. Hepatitis B immune globulin is derived from persons with high titers of antibodies against the hepatitis B surface antigen. It is administered by intramuscular injection for the prophylaxis of persons exposed to the virus or infants of mothers who test positive for the antigen.

J1574

J1574 Injection, ganciclovir sodium (Exela) not therapeutically equivalent to J1570, 500 mg

Ganciclovir sodium is a nucleoside analogue cytomegalovirus (CMV) inhibitor indicated for the treatment of adults, ages 18 years and older, with CMV retinitis in immunocompromised patients, including acquired immunodeficiency syndrome (AIDS), as well as for prevention of CMV disease in transplant recipients at risk for CMV disease. It is supplied in a single dose bag of 500 mg/205 ml (2 mg/ml). The recommended dosage for treatment of CMV retinitis is induction of 5 mg/kg body weight administered at a constant rate via intravenous (IV) infusion over one hour every 12 hours for 12 to 21 days; maintenance dosage is 5 mg/kg body weight administered at a constant rate via intravenous (IV) infusion over one hour daily for seven days per week or 6 mg/kg body weight daily for five days per week. The recommended dosage for prevention of CMV disease is induction of 5 mg/kg body weight administered at a constant rate via intravenous (IV) infusion over one hour every 12 hours for seven to 14 days; maintenance dosage is 5 mg/kg body weight administered at a constant rate via intravenous (IV) infusion over one hour daily for seven days per week or 6 mg/kg body weight daily for five days per week until 100 to 120 days post-transplantation. See full prescribing information for complete administration instructions. Report J1574 only for ganciclovir sodium manufactured by Exela.

J1575

J1575 Injection, immune globulin/hyaluronidase, 100 mg immuneglobulin

Immune globulin used in combination with hyaluronidase can prevent and treat immunodeficiency in adults. Immune globulin increases the strength of the patient's immune system while hyaluronidase spreads to allow improved absorption of the immune globulin.

J1580

J1580 Injection, garamycin, gentamicin, up to 80 mg

Garamycin/gentamicin is an antibiotic indicated for the treatment of adults and children with a wide variety of primary and secondary bacterial infections caused by susceptible strains of gram-positive and gram-negative bacteria. Dosage is based on the disease being treated, age, and body weight. A reduced dosage may be required for patients with renal impairment. See full prescribing information for complete administration information.

J1595

J1595 Injection, glatiramer acetate, 20 mg

Glatiramer acetate is used in the treatment of relapsing-remitting multiple sclerosis (MS) and is indicated to reduce the frequency of relapses. The mechanism by which glatiramer acetate exerts its effects in patients with MS is not fully understood; however, it is thought that it has an effect on immune processes that are believed to be responsible for the origin and development of MS. Glatiramer acetate is available in 20 mg single dose, prefilled vials and is administered by subcutaneous injection. The recommended dose is 20 mg per day. Glatiramer acetate may be self-administered.

J1599

J1599 Injection, immune globulin, intravenous, nonlyophilized (e.g., liquid), not otherwise specified, 500 mg

Immune globulins are glycoproteins in the blood that function as antibodies. Immune globulins specific to a certain disease are antibodies with specific amino acid sequences that interact only with the antigen that stimulated its creation or with antigens that are closely related to the stimulating antigen. Immune globulins are usually derived from the pooled plasma of human donors who have antibodies to the specific disease. The antibodies from the exogenous immune globulin help the body to fight off a disease. Immune globulins may be administered intravenously or by subcutaneous injection. This code represents 500 mg of nonlyophilized (e.g., liquid) immunoglobulin, not otherwise specified in other HCPCS Level II codes.

J1600

J1600 Injection, gold sodium thiomalate, up to 50 mg

Gold sodium thiomalate is a gold salt indicated for the treatment of adult and juvenile rheumatoid arthritis. The mechanism of action in gold salts is not well understood. However, in patients with inflammatory arthritis, such as adult and juvenile rheumatoid arthritis, gold salts decrease the inflammation of the joint lining, preventing destruction of bone and cartilage. Gold salts, such as gold sodium thiomalate, are second-line drugs prescribed when anti-inflammatory drugs, such as nonsteroidal anti-inflammatory drugs (NSAID) and corticosteroids, are ineffective in preventing the progression of inflammatory arthritis. Gold sodium thiomalate is available as a 50 mg/ml injectable suspension to be administered by intramuscular injection

J1602

J1602 Injection, golimumab, 1 mg, for intravenous use

Golimumab is a human IgG1K monoclonal antibody specific for human tumor necrosis factor alpha. It was created using genetically engineered mice immunized with human TNF, resulting in a human-derived antibody produced by a recombinant cell line cultured by continuous perfusion and purified. Elevated TNF levels in the blood, synovium, and joints have been implicated in the pathophysiology of several chronic inflammatory diseases, such as rheumatoid arthritis, psoriatic arthritis, and ankylosing spondylitis. The specific mechanism by which golimumab treats ulcerative colitis is unknown. Golimumab is indicated for the treatment of adult patients in combination with methotrexate for moderately to severely active rheumatoid arthritis alone or in combination with methotrexate for active psoriatic arthritis, active ankylosing spondylitis, and for moderate to severe ulcerative colitis patients who have an inadequate response or intolerance to prior treatment or requiring continuous steroid therapy. Recommended dosage is 2 mg per kg administered as an intravenous infusion over 30 minutes. Each single use vial contains 50 mg of golimumab per 4 mL of solution (12.5 mg of golimumab per mL). A different formulation is available in prefilled syringes or autoinjectors of 50 and 100 mg and is administered by subcutaneous injection. It may be self-injected. There is no HCPCS code for the version that is injected subcutaneously.

J1610

J1610 Injection, glucagon HCl, per 1 mg

Glucagon hydrochloride is a synthetic polypeptide identical to human glucagon. It is produced by recombinant DNA technology using *E. coli* bacteria. An injection of glucagon stimulates the liver to release stored glycogen and convert it to glucose in order to raise blood glucose levels. It also relaxes smooth muscles of the gastrointestinal tract. Its principal use is in an emergency setting as a treatment for severe insulin reaction in which the patient is unconscious or otherwise unable to eat or drink. An emergency glucagon kit containing a vial of powdered glucagon and a syringe of sterile water is usually maintained in the homes of insulin-dependent diabetics. Glucagon is also useful as a diagnostic aid in radiological examination of the stomach and lower gastrointestinal tract when diminished motility would be advantageous, because glucagon acts as a smooth muscle relaxant. The diagnostic kit also contains a vial of powdered glucagon and a syringe of sterile water. Glucagon can be administered by subcutaneous, intravenous, or intramuscular injection. It can be administered in a nonmedical setting by nonmedical personnel.

J1611

J1611 Injection, glucagon HCl (Fresenius Kabi), not therapeutically equivalent to J1610, per 1 mg

Glucagon HCl is an antihypoglycemic agent and gastrointestinal (GI) motility inhibitor indicated for treatment of severe low blood sugar (hypoglycemia) in adults and children with diabetes, and as a diagnostic agent during radiologic examinations to inhibit movement of the GI tract in adults. For treatment of low blood sugar, it is supplied in an emergency kit as a sterile, lyophilized powder (1 mg vial glucagon and 1 ml single dose syringe sterile water for reconstitution). It is administered as an intramuscular (IM), intravenous (IV), or subcutaneous (SC) injection. For patients weighing more than 25 kg or pediatric patients with unknown weight, the recommended dosage is 1 mg (1 ml) administered by IM or SC injection into the upper arm, buttocks, or thigh, or by IV injection. If no response, an addition 1 mg (1 ml) may be administered while waiting for emergency assistance. For patients weighing less than 25 kg or pediatric patients younger than 6 years old, the recommended dosage is 0.5 mg (0.5 ml) administered by IM or SC injection into the upper arm, buttocks, or thigh, or by IV injection. If no response, an

J

additional 0.5 mg (0.5 ml) may be administered while waiting for emergency assistance. For use as a diagnostic aid, it is supplied in a pack of 10 single dose vials (1 mg/vial) and in a diagnostic kit (1 mg vial glucagon and 1 ml single dose syringe sterile water for reconstitution). The reconstituted solution should be used immediately. See full prescribing information for complete administration instructions. Report J1611 only for glucagon HCl manufactured by Fresenius Kabi.

J1620

J1620 Injection, gonadorelin HCl, per 100 mcg

Gonadorelin HCl is used primarily as a diagnostic agent for evaluating the functional capacity and response of the anterior pituitary gonadotropins. Side effects may include headache, abdominal discomfort, flushing, bronchospasm, and/or local swelling at the injection site. The use of gonadorelin is contraindicated in patients who are hypersensitive to gonadorelin hydrochloride or any of its components.

J1626

J1626 Injection, granisetron HCl, 100 mcg

Granisetron HCl is an antiemetic used to prevent postoperative and chemotherapy or radiation related nausea and vomiting. It is a selective antagonist of serotonin receptors located in the vagus nerve and in the central nervous system's chemoreceptor trigger zone. Granisetron hydrochloride may be administered orally in solution or tablets or by intravenous injection. It is usually given 30 minutes to one hour before chemotherapy, with a second oral dose often following 12 hours later.

J1627

J1627 Injection, granisetron, extended-release, 0.1 mg

Granisetron extended release is a serotonin-3 receptor antagonist that is used in combination with other antiemetics for the prevention of acute and delayed nausea and vomiting associated with moderately emetogenic chemotherapy (MEC) treatment or anthracycline and cyclophosphamide (AC) combination chemotherapy treatment. It is not recommended for use in patients younger than 18 years of age. The recommended adult dosage is 10 mg, administered through a slow subcutaneous injection 30 minutes prior to the start of chemotherapy treatment on day one. It should not be administered more than once every seven days and should not be used for chemotherapy cycles longer than six months.

J1628

J1628 Injection, guselkumab, 1 mg

Guselkumab is an interleukin-23 (IL-23) blocker indicated for the treatment of adults, 18 years of age and older, with moderate to severe plaque psoriasis and are candidates for systemic or phototherapy. IL-23 is a cytokine involved in the normal inflammatory and immune response. Guselkumab binds to IL-23, inhibiting the interaction with the IL-23 receptor, and blocks the release of inflammatory cytokines. Guselkumab is supplied in a single-dose, prefilled syringe of 100 mg/ml. It is administered by subcutaneous injection on weeks zero and four, and every eight weeks thereafter.

J1630-J1631

J1630 Injection, haloperidol, up to 5 mg

J1631 Injection, haloperidol decanoate, per 50 mg

Haloperidol and haloperidol decanoate are antipsychotics that are used in treating chronic psychosis due to schizophrenia, Tourette's syndrome, and other psychotic disorders. These drugs block the postsynaptic dopamine receptors in the brain. The injectable form is available in 5 mg/ml doses and may be administered by intravenous or intramuscular injection. Haloperidol decanoate is a long-acting form of haloperidol and is administered by intramuscular injection only. Haloperidol decanoate is available in 50 mg/ml and 100 mg/ml doses. Dosing is dependent on individual patient requirements and response to treatment.

J1632

J1632 Injection, brexanolone, 1 mg

Brexanolone is a neuroactive steroid gamma-aminobutyric acid (GABA) A receptor-positive modulator indicated for the treatment of postpartum depression (PPD) in adults. GABA is the body's principal inhibitory neurotransmitter. The mechanism of action of brexanolone in the treatment of PPD in adults is not fully understood but is thought to be related to its positive allosteric modulation of $GABA_A$ receptors. Administered as a continuous intravenous infusion over 60 hours, this drug requires that a healthcare provider must be available on site to continuously monitor the patient, and intervene as necessary, for the duration of the infusion. Recommended administration is as follows: zero to four hours initiate with a dosage of 30 mcg/kg/hour; four to 24 hours increase dosage to 60 mcg/kg/hour; 24 to 52 hours increase dosage to 90 mcg/kg/hour (alternatively consider a dosage of 60 mcg/kg/hour for those who do not tolerate 90 mcg/kg/hour); 52 to 56 hours decrease dosage to 60 mcg/kg/hour; and 56 to 60 hours decrease dosage to 30 mcg/kg/hour.

J1640

J1640 Injection, hemin, 1 mg

Hemin is an iron containing metalloporphyrin. It is an enzyme inhibitor derived from processed red blood cells and acts to limit the hepatic and marrow synthesis of porphyrin. Hemin is an orphan drug indicated for the treatment of acute intermittent porphyria, porphyria variegata, and hereditary coproporphyria. Hemin therapy must be administered under close supervision of a physician, and it is not curative. The drug is administered by an intravenous infusion of 10 to 15 minutes. Recommended dosage is 1 to 4 mg/kg of body weight daily. The infusions are given for three to 14 days depending on the clinical signs.

J1642

J1642 Injection, heparin sodium, (heparin lock flush), per 10 units

Heparin is an anticoagulant indicated for the treatment and prevention of blood clots, including pulmonary embolism and deep vein thrombosis. It is also used to ensure patency of indwelling intravenous catheters. Heparin inhibits reactions that lead to the clotting of blood and the formation of fibrin clots. It works by acting as an accelerant in forming antithrombin III-thrombin complex, which deactivates thrombin. This prevents the conversion of fibrinogen to fibrin. Heparin sodium is derived from bovine or porcine pulmonary or intestinal tissue and standardized for anticoagulant activity. It is administered by subcutaneous or intravenous injection. Heparin sodium is available in doses of 1,000, 5,000, and 10,000 units/ml. Heparin lock flush is available in 10 and 100 units/ml syringes or vials.

J1643

J1643 Injection, heparin sodium (Pfizer), not therapeutically equivalent to J1644, per 1000 units

Heparin sodium is an anticoagulant that inhibits reactions that lead to the clotting of blood and the formation of fibrin clots. It works by acting as an accelerant in forming antithrombin III-thrombin complex, which deactivates thrombin. This prevents the conversion of fibrinogen to fibrin. It is indicated for the treatment and prevention of blood clots, including venous thrombosis, as well as pulmonary and arterial embolism; treatment of thromboembolic complications from atrial fibrillation; treatment of acute/chronic consumption coagulopathies; anticoagulation in transfusion, extracorporeal circulation, and dialysis procedures; and prevention of clotting in arterial and cardiac surgeries. The preservative free formula is supplied in a single dose, 2,000 USP units/2 ml vial. Heparin sodium preserved with benzyl alcohol is available in multiple dose vials in various strengths. See full prescribing information for complete administration instructions. Report J1643 only for heparin sodium manufactured by Pfizer.

J1644

J1644 Injection, Heparin sodium, per 1000 units

Heparin is an anticoagulant indicated for the treatment and prevention of blood clots, including pulmonary embolism and deep vein thrombosis. It is also used to ensure patency of indwelling intravenous catheters. Heparin inhibits reactions that lead to the clotting of blood and the formation of fibrin clots. It works by acting as an accelerant in forming antithrombin III-thrombin complex, which deactivates thrombin. This prevents the conversion of fibrinogen to fibrin. Heparin sodium is derived from bovine or porcine pulmonary or intestinal tissue and standardized for anticoagulant activity. It is administered by subcutaneous or intravenous injection. Heparin sodium is available in doses of 1,000, 5,000, and 10,000 units/ml. Heparin lock flush is available in 10 and 100 units/ml syringes or vials.

J1645

J1645 Injection, dalteparin sodium, per 2500 IU

Dalteparin sodium is a low molecular weight heparin that is produced through controlled nitrous acid depolymerization of sodium heparin from porcine intestinal mucosa followed by a chromatographic purification process. It acts by enhancing the inhibition of Factor Xa and thrombin by antithrombin. Dalteparin sodium is an injected drug that is used for the prophylaxis of ischemic complications in unstable angina and non-Q-wave myocardial infarction when administered in conjunction with aspirin therapy. This drug is also indicated for the prophylaxis of deep vein thrombosis (DVT), which may lead to pulmonary embolism (PE) for patients who are undergoing hip replacement surgery or abdominal surgery and are at risk for thromboembolic complications or a patient who is at risk for thromboembolic complications due to severely restricted mobility during acute illness. The dosage recommended for patients with unstable angina or non-Q-wave myocardial infarction is 120 IU per kg of body weight (but not more than 10,000 IU) subcutaneously every 12 hours with concurrent oral aspirin therapy for a duration of five to eight days. Dosage for hip replacement therapy varies as to the regime, but the first dose of 2,500 or 5,000 IU is administered prior to surgery and follow-up administration of 2,500 to 5,000 IU is administered postoperatively. In patients undergoing abdominal surgery with a risk of thromboembolic complications, the recommended dosage is 2,500 IU once daily beginning one to two hours prior to surgery and then once daily for five to 10 days. If the patient is at high risk of thromboembolic complications, dosage is increased to 5,000 IU. Dosage for patients with severely restricted mobility is 5,000 IU administered once daily. Dalteparin sodium is administered by subcutaneous injection.

J1650

J1650 Injection, enoxaparin sodium, 10 mg

Enoxaparin sodium is a low molecular weight heparin that has antithrombotic properties. When given at a dose of 1.5 mg/kg, enoxaparin has a higher ratio of anti-Factor Xa to anti-Factor IIa activity when compared to the ratios observed for heparin. Enoxaparin sodium is used for the prophylaxis of ischemic complications in unstable angina and non-Q-wave myocardial infarction when administered in conjunction with aspirin therapy and for the prophylaxis of deep vein thrombosis (DVT), which may lead to pulmonary embolism (PE) for patients who are undergoing hip or knee replacement surgery or abdominal surgery and are at risk for thromboembolic complications. It is also prescribed to patients who are at risk for thromboembolic complications due to severely restricted mobility during acute illness. This drug is administered via subcutaneous injection. Dosage varies depending upon the clinical indication. When administered to patients undergoing abdominal surgery, the usual dosage is 40 mg once per day beginning two hours prior to surgery for a seven to 10 day duration. When administered to patients undergoing hip or knee replacement surgery, 30 to 40 mg is injected subcutaneously 12 to 24 hours prior to surgery and then once daily for seven to 10 days. When administered to patients who are at risk for thromboembolic complications due to severely restricted mobility during an acute illness, the recommended dosage is 40 mg per day for six to 11 days. An Injection of 1 mg/kg of enoxaparin sodium subcutaneously every 12 hours in conjunction with aspirin therapy is administered for treatment of unstable angina.

J1652

J1652 Injection, fondaparinux sodium, 0.5 mg

Fondaparinux sodium is a synthetic inhibitor of activated factor X (Xa). It has no known effect on platelet function because it does not affect thrombin (activated factor II). Fibrinolytic activity or bleeding times are not affected. Fondaparinux sodium is a low molecular weight heparin that has antithrombotic properties. It is indicated for the prophylaxis of deep vein thrombosis, which may lead to pulmonary embolism in patients undergoing hip fracture surgery, including extended prophylaxis, hip replacement surgery, knee replacement surgery, and abdominal surgery for patients who are at risk for thromboembolic complications. Fondaparinux sodium is also indicated for the treatment of acute deep vein thrombosis when administered in conjunction with warfarin sodium, and the treatment of acute pulmonary embolism when administered in conjunction with warfarin sodium when initial therapy is administered in the hospital. The dosage depends on the condition being treated and body weight.

J1655

J1655 Injection, tinzaparin sodium, 1000 IU

Tinzaparin sodium is a low weight heparin that is used to treat deep vein thrombosis with or without pulmonary embolism. Tinzaparin interferes with the body's natural blood clotting mechanism by inactivating thrombin. Thrombin is an important constituent in blood clot formation. Tinzaparin is available in multiple use 2 ml vials. Each ml contains 20,000 IU of tinzaparin for a total of 40,000 IU per vial. Tinzaparin is administered by subcutaneous injection. The recommended dosage for the treatment of deep vein thrombosis is 175 IU/kg of body weight once daily for at least six days.

J1670

J1670 Injection, tetanus immune globulin, human, up to 250 units

Immune globulins are glycoproteins in the blood that function as antibodies. Immune globulins specific to a certain disease are antibodies with specific amino acid sequences that interact only with the antigen that stimulated its creation or with antigens that are closely related to the stimulating antigen. Immune globulins are usually derived from the pooled plasma of human donors who have antibodies to the specific disease. The antibodies from the exogenous immune globulin help the body fight off a disease. Tetanus is an acute, often fatal, infectious disease caused by the bacterium Clostridium tetani. This bacterium produces a neurotoxin called tetanospasmin. Generalized tetanus is characterized by muscular contractions and hyperreflexia, resulting in trismus (lockjaw), glottal spasm, generalized muscle spasm, opisthotonos, respiratory spasm, seizures, and paralysis. Localized tetanus may be mild, with localized muscular twitching and spasm of muscle groups near the site of injury. Localized tetanus may progress to the generalized form. Tetanus usually enters the body through a puncture wound, such as a splinter or bite. It may also enter through a burn, surgical wound, skin ulcer, injection site of drug abusers, umbilical stump, or postpartum uterus. Tetanus immune globulin is administered by intramuscular injection. It is administered for the prophylaxis or treatment of tetanus.

J1675

J1675 Injection, histrelin acetate, 10 mcg

Histrelin acetate is the acetate salt of a synthetic nonapeptide that corresponds to a component of naturally occurring human growth hormone. Initially the drug stimulates release of human growth hormone-releasing hormone. However, chronic use desensitizes responsiveness of the pituitary gonadotropin, causing a reduction in ovarian and testicular steroidogenesis. Decreases in LH, FSH, and sex steroid levels are observed within three months of initiation of therapy. It is an orphan drug indicated for the treatment of children with central precocious puberty (idiopathic or neurogenic) occurring before 8 years of age in girls or 9.5 years of age in boys.

J1700-J1720

J1700 Injection, hydrocortisone acetate, up to 25 mg

J1710 Injection, hydrocortisone sodium phosphate, up to 50 mg

J1720 Injection, hydrocortisone sodium succinate, up to 100 mg

Hydrocortisone is a steroid hormone produced by the adrenal cortex. A preparation of this hormone may be obtained from natural sources or produced synthetically. It is a corticosteroid that decreases inflammation and suppresses the immune system. Hydrocortisone acetate, sodium phosphate, and sodium succinate are used to treat severe inflammation, shock reactions, adrenal insufficiency, ulcerative colitis, and other inflammatory processes.

J1726

J1726 Injection, hydroxyprogesterone caproate, (Makena), 10 mg

Hydroxyprogesterone caproate is a progestin medication used to treat women who have a history of delivering a single premature baby. It is not used to treat multiple gestation premature delivery or other risk factors for premature birth. Recommended dose is 250 mg once a week beginning between 16 weeks, zero days and 20 weeks, six days of gestation and continuing through delivery or 37 weeks (36 weeks, six days), whichever occurs first. Hydroxyprogesterone caproate is administered by IM injection.

J1729

J1729 Injection, hydroxyprogesterone caproate, not otherwise specified, 10 mg

Hydroxyprogesterone caproate is a progestational steroid ester that changes proliferative endothelium into secretory endothelium, encourages mammary gland duct development, and inhibits the production and/or release of gonadotropic hormone. It is used for the treatment of non-pregnant women with amenorrhea, for abnormal uterine bleeding due to hormonal imbalance, as a test for endogenous estrogen production, and for the treatment of stage III or IV adenocarcinoma of the uterine corpus. It is supplied in multiple dose 5 mL vials of 250 mg/mL and is administered via intramuscular (IM) injection. For stage III or IV adenocarcinoma of the uterine corpus, the recommended dosage is 1,000 mg or more administered one or more times per week, for a total of one to seven grams per week. Treatment should be stopped if relapse occurs or after 12 weeks without objective response. It should not be used for the treatment of stage I or II adenocarcinoma. Other conditions are treated with a cyclic therapy schedule: a 28-day cycle, repeated every four weeks. Day 1, 20 mg estradiol valerate is administered via IM injection. Two weeks after day, 1, 250 mg hydroxyprogesterone caproate and 5 mg estradiol valerate are administered via IM injection. Four weeks after day 1 is considered day 1 of the next cycle. The recommended dosage for other conditions varies. Refer to the product label for a complete therapy guide.

J1730

J1730 Injection, diazoxide, up to 300 mg

Diazoxide is a vasodilator when administered intravenously and a drug used to treat hypoglycemia when administered orally. Intravenous administration is indicated in the emergency reduction of blood pressure in severe nonmalignant and malignant hypertension. It is also used to reduce extremely high blood pressure caused by kidney disease where other medicines have not been effective. Diazoxide works by causing the muscle in the walls of the blood vessels to relax. This allows the arteries to widen rapidly and reduces blood pressure. Intravenous dose is dependent on body weight.

J1738

J1738 Injection, meloxicam, 1 mg

Meloxicam is an injectable nonsteroidal anti-inflammatory drug (NSAID). It is indicated for use in adults, ages 18 and older, for the treatment of moderate to severe pain. It may be used alone or in combination with non-NSAID analgesics. The drug exhibits anti-inflammatory analgesic and antipyretic activities. The mechanism of action, like that of other NSAIDs, is not completely understood but may involve inhibition of the cyclooxygenase (COX-1 and COX-2) pathways. Its mechanism may also be related to inhibition of prostaglandin synthetase. It is supplied in a single dose vial of 30 mg/mL and is administered via intravenous (IV) bolus injection over 15 seconds. Meloxicam should be used for the shortest duration required to reach specific patient treatment goals, and patients must be well hydrated prior to administration. It should not be used in patients with sensitivities to aspirin or other NSAIDS, in patients who have had coronary artery bypass graft (CABG) surgery, or in patients with moderate to severe renal insufficiency and/or renal failure due to volume depletion.

J1740

J1740 Injection, ibandronate sodium, 1 mg

Ibandronate sodium is a chemical compound that inhibits bone resorption. It binds to hydroxyapatite, which is part of the mineral matrix of bone. Ibandronate inhibits osteoclast activity reducing bone resorption and turnover. The drug is indicated for the prophylaxis and treatment of osteoporosis in postmenopausal women where it reduces the elevated rate of bone turnover, leading to a net gain in bone mass density.

J1741

J1741 Injection, ibuprofen, 100 mg

Injectable ibuprofen is a nonopioid, nonsteroidal anti-inflammatory drug (NSAID). This code represents the intravenous formulation of ibuprofen. This drug is indicated for the management of mild to moderate pain, the management of moderate to severe pain with adjunctive opioid analgesics, and for fever reduction. It is administered intravenously over 30 minutes. The recommended adult dosage varies from 100 to 800 mg depending on the indication and patient response. This code represents 100 mg of intravenous ibuprofen.

J1742

J1742 Injection, ibutilide fumarate, 1 mg

Ibutilide fumarate is an antiarrhythmic drug. Ibutilide fumarate is indicated for the rapid conversion of atrial fibrillation or atrial flutter of recent onset. It prolongs action potential duration in isolated adult cardiac myocytes and increases both atrial and ventricular refractoriness. This allows prolongation of atrial and ventricular action potential duration and refractoriness, aiding in a normal cardiac rhythm. It is supplied in single dose 10 ml vials containing 1 mg of ibutilide fumarate for intravenous injection. Usual adult dose is 1 mg administered by intravenous push over a 10-minute period.

J1743

J1743 Injection, idursulfase, 1 mg

Idursulfase is an exogenous, purified form of a human enzyme produced by recombinant DNA technology in a human cell line. Idursulfase is an orphan drug used to treat the inherited metabolic disorder mucopolysaccharidosis II (MPS II or Hunter's syndrome). MPS II is caused by a lack of the enzyme iduraonate-2-sulfase that normally breaks down certain carbohydrates known as glycosaminoglycans. MPS II causes widespread cumulative organ and tissue damage. The recommended dosage is 0.5 mg per kg of body weight. The drug is administered as an intravenous infusion every week over one to three hours.

J1744

J1744 Injection, icatibant, 1 mg

Icatibant is a synthetic chain of 10 amino acids that is a bradykinin B2 receptor antagonist indicated as a treatment for acute attacks of hereditary angioedema. Hereditary angioedema is caused by the absence or dysfunction of C1-esterase-inhibitor, which regulates a chain of reactions that lead to bradykinin production. Bradykinin is a vasodilator that is thought to cause hereditary angioedema. The drug may be self-administered. It is injected subcutaneously into the abdomen. The recommended dose is 30 mg, which can be repeated every six hours, up to three doses in a 24-hour period.

J1745

J1745 Injection, infliximab, excludes biosimilar, 10 mg

Infliximab is an injectable antibody that blocks the effects of tumor necrosis factor alpha (TNF alpha), a substance made by cells of the body that has an important role in promoting inflammation. Specifically, infliximab is used for treating the inflammation of Crohn's disease, rheumatoid arthritis, and psoriatic arthritis. Infliximab is administered by intravenous infusion, and dosage varies depending on the condition being treated. Dosage may range from 3 mg/kg of body weight (rheumatoid arthritis) to 5 mg/kg of body weight for moderate to severe Crohn's disease.

J1746

J1746 Injection, ibalizumab-uiyk, 10 mg

Ibalizumab-uiyk is a CD4-directed post-attachment HIV-1 inhibitor that is indicated for the treatment of human immunodeficiency virus type 1 (HIV-1). It is used in combination with other antiretroviral medications in adult patients older than 18 years of age who have taken multiple anti-HIV-1 regimens, have an HIV-1 virus that is resistant to many antiretroviral medications, and who are currently failing antiretroviral treatment. Supplied in a single dose vial, ibalizumab-uiyk is administered via intravenous (IV) injection. It should not be administered as an IV push or bolus. The recommended dosage is a single loading dose of 2,000 mg followed by an 800 mg maintenance dose every two weeks. The loading dose requires 10 vials that must be diluted in a 250 mL IV bag of 0.9% sodium chloride and administered over at least 30 minutes. The maintenance dose requires four vials that must be diluted in a 250 mL IV bag of 0.9% sodium chloride and administered over at least 15 minutes. The diluted solution should stand at room temperature for 30 minutes prior to administration.

J1750

J1750 Injection, iron dextran, 50 mg

Iron dextran is used to treat iron deficiency anemia. It is a complex of ferric hydroxide and dextran. It is absorbed from the injection site into the capillaries and the lymphatic system. The iron is bound to the protein and forms iron. This iron is used to resupply the body with iron. Recommended dose of iron dextran varies based on the patient's hemoglobin level. It is administered by IV or intramuscular injection.

J1756

J1756 Injection, iron sucrose, 1 mg

Iron sucrose is a form of iron that is safe for the treatment of iron deficiency anemias in patients with kidney disease. It is used primarily in patients receiving ongoing hemodialysis and patients who are taking the hormone erythropoietin to help balance the iron deficiency caused by hemodialysis. Iron sucrose provides elemental iron, which is essential in the formation of hemoglobin. Iron sucrose is administered by intravenous injection over a 15-minute period. The dosage varies dependent on the degree of iron deficiency and type of renal disease the patient suffers.

J1786

J1786 Injection, imiglucerase, 10 units

Imiglucerase is an enzyme used to treat and alleviate the symptoms of Gaucher's disease, a lysosomal storage disorder caused by a genetic lack of the enzyme glucocerebrosidase. Gaucher cells accumulate in the liver, spleen, and bone marrow, resulting in severe abdominal swelling, causing the spleen to break down red blood cells more rapidly than they are produced. Imiglucerase is a synthetic form of protein beta-glucocerebrosidase that works by catalyzing the hydrolysis of glucocerebrosidase to glucose and ceramide. Imiglucerase is used for the treatment of Type 1 Gaucher's disease that results in one or more of the following: anemia, thrombocytopenia, bone disease, hepatomegaly, or splenomegaly. Dosage is determined by body weight. The usual dose is 15 to 60 units/kg of body weight administered by intravenous injection over one to two hours.

J1790

J1790 Injection, droperidol, up to 5 mg

Droperidol is used as an adjunct to general or regional anesthesia or as a general anesthetic in diagnostic procedures. It also has an antiemetic effect and may be used prior to surgery or postoperatively to prevent nausea and vomiting. It is administered by intramuscular or intravenous injection. Dosage is dependent upon patient's age and weight.

J1800

J1800 Injection, propranolol HCl, up to 1 mg

Propranolol is a nonselective beta-blocker used to treat tremors, angina, heart rhythm disorders, hypertension, and other cardiac conditions. It has also been found to prevent myocardial infarction and lessen the severity of migraine headaches. It works by blocking catecholamine-induced increases in heart rate, blood pressure, and force of myocardial contraction, thereby reducing cardiac oxygen demand. It also depresses renin secretion and prevents vasodilation of the cerebral arteries. It may be administered orally by capsule, tablet, or oral suspension, or by intravenous injection or infusion. Intravenous administration is only used in life-threatening arrhythmias or those occurring under anesthesia. The usual dose ranges from 1 to 3 mg.

J1810

J1810 Injection, droperidol and fentanyl citrate, up to 2 ml ampule

Per the FDA, this drug is no longer available in the United States.

J1815-J1817

J1815 Injection, insulin, per 5 units

J1817 Insulin for administration through DME (i.e., insulin pump) per 50 units

Insulin is a hormone secreted by the beta cells of the pancreas that controls the metabolism and cellular uptake of sugars, proteins, and fats. As a drug, it is used principally to control Type I diabetes mellitus. Different forms of insulin may also be used to control blood sugar levels in patients with gestational diabetes to prevent fetal complications caused by maternal hyperglycemia. The use of insulin in Type II diabetes mellitus is typically only for patients who have failed to control their blood sugars with diet, exercise, and oral drugs. In the past, insulin for injection was obtained from beef or porcine pancreas. Most insulin now in use is made by recombinant DNA technology and is equivalent to human insulin from an immunological perspective. Dosage varies by the level of control of blood sugar needed. Insulin is administered by subcutaneous injection or by insulin pump.

J1823

J1823 Injection, inebilizumab-cdon, 1 mg

Inebilizumab-cdon is a humanized, afucosylated monoclonal antibody that targets CD19+ B-cells. It is indicated for the treatment of neuromyelitis optica spectrum disorder (NMOSD), a chronic disorder of the brain and spinal cord manifested by inflammation of the optic nerve and spinal cord, in adult patients who are anti-aquaporin-4 (AQP4) antibody positive. The recommended initial dose is 300 mg intravenous (IV) infusion followed two weeks later by a second 300 mg IV infusion. For subsequent doses (beginning six months from the first infusion), the recommendation is a single 300 mg IV infusion every six months. This code reports an injection of 1 mg.

J1826

J1826 Injection, interferon beta-1a, 30 mcg

Interferon beta-1a is a synthetic version of natural interferon beta-1a produced by recombinant DNA technology from Chinese hamster ovaries. Interferons are small, naturally occurring proteins that bind to specific cell membranes and initiate a series of events that include the inhibition of virus replication and the enhancement of macrophage and lymphocyte destruction of foreign cells. There are several types of interferons. Interferon beta-1a has been shown to control symptoms of muscular sclerosis, but its exact mechanism of action is unknown. Interferon beta-1a is indicated for the treatment of patients with relapsing forms of multiple sclerosis to decrease the frequency of clinical exacerbations and delay the onset of the physical disabilities associated with the disease. The drug may be self-administered as a subcutaneous injection. Interferon beta-1a is also available as an intramuscular injection.

J1830

J1830 Injection interferon beta-1b, 0.25 mg (code may be used for Medicare when drug administered under the direct supervision of a physician, not for use when drug is self-administered)

Interferon beta-1b is a biologic response modifier possessing both antiviral and immunoregulatory activities. Interferon beta-1b is indicated for the treatment of relapsing-remitting multiple sclerosis in ambulatory patients. The mechanisms by which interferon beta-1b exerts its actions in multiple sclerosis are not clearly understood. However, the biologic response-modifying properties are known to be mediated through its interactions with specific cell receptors found on the cell membrane, which cause cellular changes, including increased protein synthesis of human cells. The usual dosage is 0.25 mg self-injected subcutaneously every other day.

J1833

J1833 Injection, isavuconazonium, 1 mg

Isavuconazonium is an azole antifungal. It is utilized for the treatment of invasive aspergillosis and invasive mucormycosis in adult patients. Administration may be oral or via intravenous infusion. For oral dosing, 372 mg (two capsules) is taken every eight hours, in six doses, over a 48-hour period. A maintenance dose of 372 mg (two capsules) is taken once daily. For IV administration, 372 mg is administered intravenously, with an in-line filter, every eight hours, in six doses, over a 48-hour period. A maintenance dose of 372 mg is administered in the same way, once daily. Switching between oral and intravenous formulas is permissible.

J1835

J1835 Injection, itraconazole, 50 mg

Itraconazole is an antifungal used for the treatment of patients with aspergillosis, blastomycosis, histoplasmosis, esophageal and oropharyngeal candidiasis, and onychomycosis. It is also used to prevent fungal infections in patients with human immunodeficiency virus (HIV) or acquired immunodeficiency syndrome (AIDS). Itraconazole is in a class of antifungals called triazoles. It works by slowing the growth of fungi that cause infection. It may be administered orally as a capsule or oral solution or by intravenous (IV) infusion. Itraconazole administered by IV infusion is used primarily for immunocompromised patients with severe lung or systemic fungal infections at a recommended dosage of 200 mg administered over one hour. It should not be mixed or infused with any other medication.

J1840-J1850

J1840 Injection, kanamycin sulfate, up to 500 mg

J1850 Injection, kanamycin sulfate, up to 75 mg

Kanamycin sulfate is a bacterial antibiotic used to treat *E. coli, Proteus* species (both indole-positive and indole-negative), *Enterobacter aerogenes, Klebsiella pneumoniae, Serratia marcescens*, and *Acinetobacter* species. It inhibits the synthesis of protein in susceptible microorganisms. The recommended dose is 15 mg per kg per day divided equally for intramuscular injection and should not exceed 15 mg per kg per day for intravenous infusion. Kanamycin can be administered intramuscularly or intravenously over 30 to 60 minutes.

J1885

J1885 Injection, ketorolac tromethamine, per 15 mg

Ketorolac tromethamine is a nonsteroidal anti-inflammatory drug (NSAID) that is indicated for short-term (up to five days in adults) management of moderately severe acute pain that requires analgesia at the opioid level. Ketorolac tromethamine is available for intravenous (IV) or intramuscular (IM) administration as 15 mg in 1 mL (1.5%) and 30 mg in 1 mL (3%) in sterile solution; 60 mg in 2 mL (3%) of ketorolac tromethamine in sterile solution is available for IM administration only.

J1890

J1890 Injection, cephalothin sodium, up to 1 g

Cephalosporins are used in the treatment of infections caused by bacteria. They work by killing bacteria or preventing their growth. Cephalosporins are used to treat infections in many different parts of the body. They are sometimes given with other antibiotics. Some cephalosporins given by injection are also used to prevent infections before, during, and after surgery. Cephalothin will not work against infections caused by viruses such as colds or the flu. Per the FDA, this drug is no longer available for human use in the United States.

J1930

J1930 Injection, lanreotide, 1 mg

Lanreotide is an orphan drug used to treat acromegaly, often due to a benign pituitary gland tumor. It is a rare and potentially life-threatening disease in which abnormal growth hormone is secreted by the pituitary gland. This abnormal growth hormone can cause enlargement of the hands, feet, facial bones, and internal organs such as the heart and liver. Patients who are untreated may have a shortened life span from heart and respiratory diseases, diabetes mellitus, and colon cancer. Lanreotide is used to treat patients who are not able to undergo surgery or radiotherapy. The recommended dose is 90 milligrams. This medication is administered by deep subcutaneous injection every four weeks for three months.

J1931

J1931 Injection, laronidase, 0.1 mg

Laronidase is a polymorphic variant of the human enzyme L-iduronidase that is produced by recombinant DNA technology in a Chinese hamster ovary cell line. It is used to treat Hurler and Hurler-Scheie forms of mucopolysaccharidosis in patients who have moderate to severe symptoms. Laronidase has been shown to improve pulmonary function and walking capacity. Laronidase has not been evaluated for effects on the central nervous system manifestations of the disorder. The recommended dosage is 0.58 mg/kg of body weight administered once weekly as an intravenous infusion.

J1932

J1932 Injection, lanreotide, (Cipla), 1 mg

Lanreotide is a somatostatin analog used to treat acromegaly, often due to a benign pituitary gland tumor. It is a rare and potentially life-threatening disease in which abnormal growth hormone is secreted by the pituitary gland. This abnormal growth hormone can cause enlargement of the hands, feet, facial bones, and internal organs such as the heart and liver. Patients who are untreated may have a shortened life span from heart and respiratory diseases, diabetes mellitus, and colon cancer. Lanreotide is indicated for long-term treatment of acromegalic patients who cannot be treated with surgery or radiotherapy and for unresectable, well- or moderately-differentiated locally advance or metastatic gastroenteropancreatic neuroendocrine tumors (GEP-NETs) to improve progression-free survival. It is supplied in single-dose prefilled vials of 60 mg/0.2 ml, 90 mg/0.3 ml, and 120 mg/0.5 ml. The recommended dose for acromegaly is 90 milligrams every four weeks for three months. The recommended dose for GEP-NETs is 120 mg every four weeks. It is administered by deep subcutaneous (SC) injection. See full prescribing information for complete administration instructions. Report J1932 for lanreotide manufactured by Cipla.

J1940

J1940 Injection, furosemide, up to 20 mg

Furosemide is a diuretic that is an anthranilic acid derivative. It is used to treat edema, hypertension, and pulmonary edema. Dosage recommendations vary by the type of condition being treated, route of administration (oral, IV, or IM), and age and size of patient.

J1943

J1943 Injection, aripiprazole lauroxil, (Aristada Initio), 1 mg

Aripiprazole lauroxil (Aristada Initio) is an atypical antipsychotic medication used to treat schizophrenia. The precise mechanism of action of aripiprazole lauroxil is not known. The drug has a strong attraction to dopamine and serotonin receptor sites and acts as an agonist to various dopamine and serotonin subtypes. Aristada Initio, used in combination with oral aripiprazole, is indicated for the treatment of schizophrenia in patients aged 18 years and older. It should not be used for the treatment of patients with dementia-related psychosis. Aristada Initio and Aristada are not interchangeable due to their different pharmacokinetic profiles and care should be taken to ensure the correct product is administered. Aristada Initio is only for use as a single dose to begin treatment with Aristada, or to reinitiate treatment following a missed dose of Aristada. Aristada Initio should not be used for repeated doses. Aristada Initio is supplied in a single dose prefilled syringe of 675 mg. It is administered via intramuscular injection by a healthcare professional into the deltoid or gluteal muscle. For patients who have never taken Aristada, tolerability must be established with administration of oral aripiprazole (Abilify). Once tolerability has been established, the recommended dosage of Aristada Initio is a single 675 mg injection of Aristada Initio and one 30 mg dose of oral aripiprazole. The first Aristada injection may be administered on the same day or within 10 days. Aristada Initio and Aristada should not be administered into the same deltoid or gluteal muscle. For dosage recommendations following missed doses of Aristada, see full prescribing information.

J1944

J1944 Injection, aripiprazole lauroxil, (Aristada), 1 mg

Aripiprazole lauroxil (Aristada) is an atypical antipsychotic medication used to treat schizophrenia. The precise mechanism of action of aripiprazole lauroxil is not known. The drug has a strong attraction to dopamine and serotonin receptor sites and acts as an agonist to various dopamine and serotonin subtypes. Aristada is indicated for the treatment of schizophrenia in patients aged 18 years and older. It should not be used for the treatment of patients with dementia-related psychosis. Aristada and Aristada Initio are not interchangeable due to their different pharmacokinetic profiles and care should be taken to ensure the correct product is administered. Aristada is supplied in single dose prefilled syringes in four extended release dosages: 441 mg, 662 mg, 882 mg, or 1064 mg. It is administered via intramuscular injection by a healthcare professional. The 441 mg should be administered into the deltoid or gluteal muscle, while the 662 mg, 882 mg, and 1064 mg should be administered into the gluteal muscle. For patients who have never taken Aristada, tolerability must be established with administration of oral aripiprazole (Abilify). Once tolerability has been established, to initiate treatment, 21 consecutive days of oral aripiprazole may be administered along with the first Aristada injection, or one 675 mg injection of Aristada Initio and one 30 mg dose of oral aripiprazole can be administered together with the first Aristada injection. Maintenance doses can be administered with 441 mg, 662 mg, or 882 mg monthly; 882 mg every six weeks; or 1064 mg every eight weeks, depending upon patient needs. Aristada Initio and Aristada should not be administered into the same deltoid or gluteal muscle. For dosage recommendations following missed doses of Aristada, see full prescribing information.

J1945

J1945 Injection, lepirudin, 50 mg

Lepirudin is a bivalent direct thrombin inhibitor derived from yeast cells that reduces the risk of serious consequences of heparin-induced thrombocytopenia (HIT). It is indicated for anticoagulation in patients with HIT and associated thromboembolic diseases. The usual dosage is 0.4 mg/kg body weight (up to 110

J

kg) administered slowly intravenously (e.g., over 15 to 20 seconds) as a bolus dose, followed by 0.15 mg/kg body weight (up to 110kg/hour) as a continuous intravenous infusion for two to 10 days or longer if clinically needed.

J1950

J1950 Injection, leuprolide acetate (for depot suspension), per 3.75 mg

Leuprolide acetate is a synthetic analogue of the luteinizing hormone-releasing hormone (LHRH) that is used as an antineoplastic drug and a treatment for central precocious puberty, endometriosis, and uterine fibroids. It first stimulates and then suppresses follicle stimulating and luteinizing hormone release, resulting in suppression of testosterone and estrogen. A depot suspension is a drug that remains in the body long-term in storage and is slowly released into the blood. The leuprolide acetate depot suspension in dosages of 3.75 mg monthly and the 12.25 mg every three months are injected intramuscularly to treat endometriosis and uterine fibroids. When used to treat central precocious puberty, the dosage is individualized to the child and can range from 7.5 to 15 mg. Leuprolide acetate in doses of 7.5 mg and greater is injected subcutaneously and is used as a palliative treatment for advanced prostate cancer.

J1951

J1951 Injection, leuprolide acetate for depot suspension (Fensolvi), 0.25 mg

Leuprolide acetate is a gonadotropin releasing hormone (GnRH) agonist that is indicated for treatment of children, ages 2 and older, with central precocious puberty. It first stimulates and then suppresses follicle stimulating (FSH) and luteinizing hormone (LH) release, resulting in suppression of testosterone and estradiol. It is supplied in a two-syringe kit containing one syringe with the ARTIGEL Delivery System and one containing leuprolide acetate. The contents of the two syringes are mixed immediately prior to injection, creating a solid drug delivery depot. Once injected, the drug is delivered into the bloodstream at a controlled rate over a six-month period. The recommended dose is 45 mg administered by subcutaneous (SC) injection into an area with adequate amounts of subcutaneous tissue, once every six months. It must be administered by a health care professional. Response to the treatment should be monitored at one to two months following start of therapy and then as needed to confirm appropriate progression. Patient's height should be measured every three to six months and bone age should be measured periodically. See full prescribing information for complete administration instructions.

J1952

J1952 Leuprolide injectable, camcevi, 1 mg

Leuprolide is a gonadotropin-releasing hormone (GnRH) agonist that is indicated for the treatment of adult patients, ages 18 years and older, with advanced prostate cancer. Leuprolide inhibits gonadotropin secretion, reducing testosterone in prostatic cancer patients. It is supplied in a refrigerated, single dose prefilled syringe of 42 mg of leuprolide. The syringe must sit at room temperature prior to use. It is administered by a health care provider via subcutaneous (SC) injection in the upper- or mid-abdominal area. The formulation will deliver the medication over six months. See full prescribing information for complete administration instructions.

J1953

J1953 Injection, levetiracetam, 10 mg

Levetiracetam is an anticonvulsant indicated as an adjunctive therapy to help control partial onset seizures or myoclonic seizures in adults with juvenile myoclonic epilepsy. This injection is used when oral administration is not feasible. The precise mechanism by which levetiracetam controls seizure activity is unknown. The recommended dose is 500 milligrams twice a day. The dose can be increased every two weeks up to 3,000 milligrams. Levetiracetam is administered by IV injection over 15 minutes.

J1954

J1954 Injection, leuprolide acetate for depot suspension (Lutrate), 7.5 mg

Leuprolide acetate for depot suspension is a synthetic analogue of the gonadotropin releasing hormone (GnRH) that is indicated for the treatment of adults, ages 18 years and older, with advanced prostatic cancer. It inhibits gonadotropin secretion, growth of certain hormone-dependent tumors, and atrophy of the reproductive organs. A depot suspension allows a drug to be slowly released into the bloodstream. Leuprolide acetate for depot suspension is supplied in a prefilled, single dose administration kit containing a dual chamber syringe with the drug and the dilutant. The recommended dosage is 7.5 mg once every month administered as a single intramuscular (IM) injection under physician supervision. Fractional or combination doses should not be used concurrently. See full prescribing information for complete administration instructions.

J1955

J1955 Injection, levocarnitine, per 1 g

Levocarnitine is a naturally occurring substance required for energy metabolism. It has been shown to facilitate long-chain, fatty acid entry into cellular mitochondria, therefore delivering substrate for oxidation and subsequent energy production. With the exception of the brain, all tissues use fatty acids as an energy substrate and serve as a major fuel source in skeletal tissue and cardiac muscle. Levocarnitine is prescribed for the treatment of patients with an inherent error of metabolism that results in secondary carnitine deficiency. It is also used to prevent and treat carnitine deficiency in patients with end-stage renal disease who are on hemodialysis. The recommended dosage is a loading dose of 50 mg/kg given as a bolus injection over two to three minutes followed by 50 mg/kg daily by intravenous infusion.

J1956

J1956 Injection, levofloxacin, 250 mg

Levofloxacin is a quinolone antibiotic. It inhibits DNA synthesis causing cell death. Susceptibility studies should be performed prior to the administration of levofloxacin. Susceptible bacteria include *Streptococcus pneumoniae, Haemophilus influenzae, Moraxella catarrhalis, Staphylococcus aureus, Haemophilus parainfluenzae, Pseudomonas aeruginosa, Serratia marcescens, E. coli, Klebsiella pneumoniae, Chlamydia pneumoniae, Legionella pneumophila, Mycoplasma pneumoniae, Enterococcus faecalis, Streptococcus pyogenes, Proteus mirabilis, Staphylococcus epidermidis, Enterobacter cloacae, Staphylococcus saprophyticus*, and *Bacillus anthracis.*

J1960

J1960 Injection, levorphanol tartrate, up to 2 mg

Levorphanol tartrate is a potent synthetic opioid analgesic used to manage moderate to severe pain or as a pre- or postoperative medication where an opioid analgesic is appropriate. It may be administered by injection, intravenous infusion, or orally. The usual recommended starting dose for intravenous administration is up to 1 mg, given in divided doses, by slow push technique. This may be repeated every three to six hours as needed. The usual recommended starting dose administration by injection is 1 to 2 mg subcutaneously or intramuscularly repeated every six to eight hours as needed.

J1980

J1980 Injection, hyoscyamine sulfate, up to 0.25 mg

Hyoscyamine sulfate is a component of belladonna alkaloid and is used as an anticholinergic and antispasmodic. Hyoscyamine sulfate inhibits gastrointestinal propulsive motility and decreases gastric acid secretion. This drug also decreases pharyngeal, tracheal, and bronchial secretions. Hyoscyamine sulfate is used as an adjunct therapy for the treatment of peptic ulcer disease, to control gastric secretion or excessive saliva production, and to decrease visceral spasm and hypermotility in such conditions as spastic colitis, spastic bladder, cystitis, and pylorospasm. It may also be used to prevent drug induced bradycardia during surgery. Hyoscyamine sulfate may be administered by several forms including sublingual, oral, injection, or intravenously. Dosage varies depending upon the condition being treated, patient age, and the size and weight of the patient. It can range from 0.25 mg to 0.5 mg for adults.

J1990

J1990 Injection, chlordiazepoxide HCl, up to 100 mg

Chlordiazepoxide is a member of the benzodiazepine class of drugs. It acts on the gamma amino butyric acid (GABA) receptors in the brain resulting in the release of GABA and reducing the function of certain areas of the brain. GABA is a major inhibitory chemical in the brain that assists with inducing sleepiness and helps to control anxiety. Chlordiazepoxide is most commonly used to treat insomnia; however, it can also be used to relieve anxiety, particularly preoperative anxiety, and help alleviate alcohol withdrawal symptoms. It can be habit forming and is only used on a short-term basis. Dosage is dependent upon the condition being treated and the response of the individual patient.

J2001

J2001 Injection, lidocaine HCl for intravenous infusion, 10 mg

Lidocaine hydrochloride stabilizes the neuronal membrane by inhibiting the conduction of pain impulses, thereby providing local anesthesia. It also stabilizes heart rhythms when administered intravenously. Lidocaine hydrochloride is indicated for local or regional anesthesia by infiltration techniques, such as percutaneous injection and intravenous regional peripheral nerve block techniques, and for treatment of cardiac arrhythmias. The drug is available in topical and injectable forms. The injectable form can be administered by intravenous infusion, caudal, epidural, retrobulbar, peripheral nerve block, and sympathetic nerve block. Report J2001 for the intravenous infusion of lidocaine.

J2010

J2010 Injection, lincomycin HCl, up to 300 mg

Lincomycin hydrochloride (HCl) is an antibiotic used to treat serious, susceptible strains of streptococci, pneumococci, and staphylococci infections. It is specifically effective against the following organisms: *Streptococcus pyogenes, Viridans group, streptococci, Corynebacterium diphtheriae, Propionibacterium acnes, Clostridium tetani*, and *Clostridium perfringens*. It is used for patients who are allergic to penicillin or for whom penicillin treatment is inappropriate. Recommended dose is 600 mg intramuscularly every 24 hours and 600 mg to 1 gram via intravenous infusion every eight to 12 hours. Intravenous lincomycin should be infused over one hour or more.

J2020

J2020 Injection, linezolid, 200 mg

Linezolid is a synthetic antibacterial of the oxazolidinone class. This drug inhibits bacterial protein synthesis by binding to a specific site on RNA and preventing the translation process. This method of action is different from other antibacterials; cross-resistance between linezolid and other antibiotics is

J

unlikely. Susceptibility studies should be performed prior to the administration of linezolid. Susceptible bacteria include vancomycin-resistant *Enterococcus faecium*, methicillin-susceptible and resistant *Staphylococcus aureus, Streptococcus pneumoniae, Streptococcus pyogenes,* and *Streptococcus agalactiae*. Linezolid is available in injectable and oral forms. The injectable form is administered by intravenous infusion over a period of 30 to 120 minutes. The dosage varies by the route of administration, and by type and severity of the infection.

J2021

J2021 Injection, linezolid (Hospira) not therapeutically equivalent to J2020, 200 mg

Linezolid is a synthetic antibacterial of the oxazolidinone class. This drug inhibits bacterial protein synthesis by binding to a specific site on RNA and preventing the translation process. This method of action is different from other antibacterials; cross-resistance between linezolid and other antibiotics is unlikely. Susceptibility studies should be performed prior to the administration of linezolid. It is indicated for the treatment of adults and children for the treatment of community-acquired pneumonia; complicated skin and skin structure infections, including diabetic foot infections, without concomitant osteomyelitis; and vancomycin-resistant *Enterococcus faecium*. Linezolid is supplied in a single dose bag containing 600 mg/300 ml (2 mg/ml) and is administered by intravenous (IV) infusion. The recommended dosage for children 11 years and younger is 10 mg/kg body weight every eight hours. The recommended dosage for adults and children 12 years and older is 600 mg every 12 hours. The duration of treatment varies based on the condition treated. See full prescribing information for complete administration details. Report J2021 only for linezolid manufactured by Hospira.

J2060

J2060 Injection, lorazepam, 2 mg

Lorazepam is a psychotropic drug with potent hypnotic and sedative effects. Lorazepam injection may be prescribed as a preanesthetic medication. Lorazepam is also indicated for the management of anxiety disorders or for the short-term relief of symptoms of anxiety or anxiety associated with depressive symptoms. When administered by intramuscular injection, usual dosage is 0.05 mg/kg of body weight up to a maximum of 4 mg. For intravenous injection for the purposes of sedation or relief of anxiety, the usual dose is 0.02 mg/kg of body weight to a maximum of 2 mg.

J2062

J2062 Loxapine for inhalation, 1 mg

Loxapine inhalation powder is an inhaled form of a typical antipsychotic drug. It is indicated for the acute treatment of agitation associated with schizophrenia or bipolar I disorder in adults. Loxapine inhalation powder is a subclass of tricyclic agents whose mechanism of action is unknown. It is believed that it antagonizes central dopamine D2 and serotonin 5-HT2A receptors. Recommended dosage is 10 mg once in a 24-hour period. Loxapine inhalation powder is available only through a restricted program under a risk evaluation and mitigation strategy and must be administered in an enrolled facility.

J2150

J2150 Injection, mannitol, 25% in 50 ml

Mannitol is an osmotic diuretic that is readily diffused through the kidney. It is used to induce diuresis in the treatment and/or prevention of the oliguric phase of acute renal failure before irreversible damage is established. Mannitol is also used to reduce intracranial pressure and cerebral edema by reducing brain mass, to reduce elevated intraocular pressure, and to promote urinary excretion of toxic substances. Mannitol is administered by intravenous infusion. Dosage is dependent upon the condition being treated, with usual adult dosage ranging from 20 to 100 g in a 24-hour period.

J2170

J2170 Injection, mecasermin, 1 mg

Mecasermin is a synthesized version of human insulin-like growth factor-1 (IGF-1). It is produced by recombinant DNA technology using strains of *E. coli* bacteria. IGF-1 (formerly called somatomedin C) is a serum peptide formed within the liver and other tissues. IGF-1 in the human body is stimulated by human growth hormone and in turn stimulates cell growth and replication by increasing the metabolic uptake of glucose, fatty acids, and amino acids. Mecasermin is indicated for the long-term treatment of growth failure in children with severe primary IGF-1 deficiency or with genetic growth gene deletion that has developed neutralizing antibodies to growth hormone. The drug is not indicated for treatment of secondary forms of IGF-1 deficiency. Mecasermin should not be used in patients with closed epiphyses. Dosage is individualized for each patient and varies from an initial dose of 0.5 mg to 2 mg per kg of patient body weight. Mecasermin is administered subcutaneously and can be self-administered.

J2175

J2175 Injection, meperidine HCl, per 100 mg

Meperidine hydrochloride is a narcotic analgesic with similar effects as morphine. Meperidine hydrochloride is used for analgesia and sedation. It is primarily used to treat moderate to severe pain, as a preoperative medicate, and as a form of anesthesia.

J2180

J2180 Injection, meperidine and promethazine HCl, up to 50 mg

Meperidine and promethazine hydrochloride is a compound of a narcotic analgesic with similar effects as morphine (meperidine hydrochloride) and a phenothiazine derivative that provides antiemetic, sedative, and antihistaminic actions. It is primarily used to treat moderate to severe pain, as a preoperative medicate, and as a form of anesthesia. This drug is usually administered intramuscularly but the intravenous route may be employed. When used intravenously, it is preferable to use a push technique. Usual adult dosage is 50 mg every three to four hours; children's dosage is 0.5 mg/kg.

J2182

J2182 Injection, mepolizumab, 1 mg

Mepolizumab is an interleukin-5 antagonist monoclonal antibody (IgG1 kappa) for the add-on maintenance treatment of severe asthma patients aged 12 years and older and with an eosinophilic phenotype. Mepolizumab should not be used for the treatment of other eosinophilic phenotypes or for the treatment of acute bronchospasm or status asthmaticus. Mepolizumab is available in a single dose vial, with 100 mg of lyophilized powder, ready for reconstitution with 1.2 mL of sterile water. The dose is 100 mg, administered via subcutaneous injection into the abdomen, thigh, or upper arm, every four weeks.

J2184

J2184 Injection, meropenem (B. Braun) not therapeutically equivalent to J2185, 100 mg

Meropenem is a broad spectrum carbapenem antibiotic that is indicated for the treatment of adults and children, ages 3 months and older, with complicated skin and skin structure infections (cSSSI), complicated intra-abdominal infections, and bacterial meningitis (pediatric patients). Meropenem should only be used for children who require the full 500 mg or 1 g adult dose. It is supplied in a dual chamber, single dose container with both meropenem and a diluent. The diluent chamber contains 50 ml of 0.9% sodium chloride. Dual chamber vials are available in both 500 mg/50 ml and 1 g/50 ml strengths. It is administered via intravenous (IV) infusion over 15 to 30 minutes. The recommended dosage for patients with normal renal function for treatment of cSSSI is 500 mg every eight hours; for skin infections caused by *Pseudomonas aeruginosa* or intra-abdominal infections, 1 g every 8 hours. For pediatric patients with bacterial meningitis, the recommended dosage is 2 g every eight hours. Dose adjustments are required for adult patients with renal impairment. See full prescribing information for complete administration instructions. Report J2184 only for meropenem manufactured by B. Braun.

J2185

J2185 Injection, meropenem, 100 mg

Meropenem is a broad spectrum carbapenem antibiotic for intravenous administration. It is indicated for the treatment of infections of the skin, intra-abdominal infections such as peritonitis, and bacterial meningitis when caused by susceptible bacterial agents. Dosage varies depending upon the severity of the condition and the age and weight of the patient. In adults, the recommended dosage is 500 mg every eight hours for skin infections and 1 g given every eight hours for intra-abdominal infections. Pediatric patients receive doses of 10, 20, or 40 mg/kg every eight hours depending on the type of infection. The usual technique is intravenous infusion over 15 to 30 minutes; however, a bolus dose over three to five minutes may be prescribed.

J2186

J2186 Injection, meropenem, vaborbactam, 10 mg/10 mg, (20 mg)

Meropenem and vaborbactam is a combination of a penem antibacterial (meropenem) and a beta-lactamase inhibitor (vaborbactam) indicated for the treatment of complicated urinary tract infections (cUTI) caused by susceptible bacteria, including pyelonephritis, in adult patients 18 years of age and older. Meropenem breaches the cell wall of most gram-positive and gram-negative bacteria to bind penicillin-binding protein (PBP) targets. Vaborbactam protects meropenem from degradation by certain serine beta-lactamases (i.e., *Klebsiella pneumoniae* carbapenemase [KPC]). Susceptible bacteria include *Escherichia coli, Klebsiella pneumoniae,* and *Enterobacter cloacae* species complex. Meropenem and vaborbactam is supplied as a dry powder in a single dose vial that contains one gram of meropenem and one gram of vaborbactam. It must be constituted with 20 mL of 0.9% sodium chloride from an infusion bag. Once dissolved, the solution should be added immediately to a 0.9% sodium chloride infusion bag. The infusion must be completed within four hours of constitution. The recommended dosage is 4 grams (meropenem 2 grams and vaborbactam 2 gram) every eight hours administered by intravenous infusion over three hours for up to 14 days. Patients must have a glomerular filtration rate (eGFR) greater than or equal to 50 mL/min/1.73m^2. The eGFR should be monitored daily and the dosage adjusted for patients with changing renal function.

J2210

J2210 Injection, methylergonovine maleate, up to 0.2 mg

Methylergonovine maleate is a blood-vessel constrictor that is used to prevent or control postpartum hemorrhage caused by subinvolution or uterine atony. It works by causing the uterine muscles to contract, thereby reducing blood loss. Methylergonovine maleate is available in tablet and injectable forms. The injectable form can be

J

administered by intramuscular or intravenous injection; however, intravenous injection is administered only for life-threatening postpartum hemorrhage.

J2212

J2212 Injection, methylnaltrexone, 0.1 mg

Methylnaltrexone bromide is a peripheral acting mu-opioid receptor antagonist. The drug targets tissues such as those in the gastrointestinal tract and blocks the effects of opioids. Opioids slow gastrointestinal motility and transit, which creates constipation. Methylnaltrexone bromide is indicated for the treatment of constipation in patients receiving palliative care when constipation is not relieved by laxatives. The recommended dosage is 8 mg for patients weighing 38 to 62 kg or 12 mg for patients weighing 62 to 114 kg. The drug is given as a subcutaneous injection every other day. It should not be administered more than once every 24-hour period.

J2247

J2247 Injection, micafungin sodium (Par Pharm) not therapeutically equivalent to J2248, 1 mg

Micafungin sodium is a semisynthetic lipopeptide (echinocandin) that disrupts the synthesis of a component of the fungal cellular membrane. It is indicated for the treatment of adults and children, ages 4 months and older, with candidemia, acute disseminated candidiasis, *Candida* peritonitis and abscesses, esophageal candidiasis, and as a prophylactic therapy to prevent candida infections in patients undergoing hematopoietic stem cell transplants (HSCT). It may also be used for the treatment of candidemia, acute disseminated candidiasis, and *Candida* peritonitis and abscesses without meningoencephalitis and/or ocular dissemination in children younger than 4 months of age. Micafungin sodium is supplied as a lyophilized powder in single dose vials of 50 mg and 100 mg and is administered via intravenous (IV) infusion over one hour. It requires reconstitution with 5 ml 0.9% sodium chloride or 5% dextrose. It should not be mixed with or infused with any other medication. The recommended dosage varies based on patient age and condition. See full prescribing information for complete administration instructions. Report J2247 only for micafungin sodium manufactured by Par Pharm.

J2248

J2248 Injection, micafungin sodium, 1 mg

Micafungin sodium is a semisynthetic lipopeptide produced from Coleophoma empetri, a plant fungus. It is used as an antifungal drug. Micafungin sodium disrupts the synthesis of a component of the fungal cellular membrane. This component is not present in mammalian cells. Micafungin sodium is indicated for the treatment of esophageal candidiasis and as a prophylactic therapy to prevent candida infections in patients undergoing hematopoietic stem cell transplants. The drug may cause allergic reactions including anaphylaxis. Micafungin sodium must be administered via an intravenous infusion over one hour. It should not be mixed with or infused with any other medication.

J2250

J2250 Injection, midazolam HCl, per 1 mg

Midazolam hydrochloride is a benzodiazepine, a group of chemically similar psychotropic drugs. Because midazolam hydrochloride is associated with a high incidence of partial or complete recall impairment, it is used as preoperative sedation, sedation during diagnostic or therapeutic procedures, or for induction of general anesthesia. Dosage varies depending on the reason for administration and the age and weight of the patient.

J2251

J2251 Injection, midazolam HCl (WG Critical Care) not therapeutically equivalent to J2250, per 1 mg

Midazolam HCl is a benzodiazepine indicated for sedation of intubated and mechanically ventilated adults and children as a component of anesthesia or treatment in a critical care setting. It is supplied in a single dose bag of 50 mg/50 ml (1 mg/ml) or 100 mg/100 ml (1 mg/ml) and is administered via continuous intravenous (IV) injection. Care should be taken to avoid intra-arterial injection or extravasation. Dosing varies based on patient age and weight and reason for administration. See full prescribing information for complete administration instructions. Report J2251 only for midazolam HCl manufactured by WG Critical Care.

J2260

J2260 Injection, milrinone lactate, 5 mg

Milrinone lactate is a member of a class of bipyridine inotropic/vasodilator agents with phosphodiesterase inhibitor activity that is distinct from digitalis or catecholamines. Milrinone lactate is indicated for the short-term intravenous treatment of acute heart failure. It is administered intravenously with a loading dose of 50 mcg/kg followed by a maintenance dose of no more than 1.13 mg/kg/day.

J2265

J2265 Injection, minocycline HCl, 1 mg

Minocycline HCl is an antibiotic used to treat a wide variety of gram negative and gram positive infections. It is thought to inhibit the protein synthesis. The recommended adult dose of minocycline HCl is initially 200 mg and then 100 mg every 12 hours. For children, an initial dose of 4 mg/kg, then 2 mg/kg every 12 hours. It is administered by IV infusion.

J2270

J2270 Injection, morphine sulfate, up to 10 mg

Morphine sulfate is an opioid analgesic that principally affects the central nervous system and gastrointestinal tract. The drug increases the patient's tolerance for pain and decreases patient discomfort. The patient, however, may still recognize the presence of pain. Sedation also occurs. Dosage varies by route of administration, patient's age, weight, severity of illness, and comorbidities.

J2272

J2272 Injection, morphine sulfate (Fresenius Kabi) not therapeutically equivalent to J2270, up to 10 mg

Morphine sulfate is an opioid agonist that increases the patient's tolerance for pain and decreases patient discomfort. It is indicated for use in adults, ages 18 years and older, for the management of pain severe enough to require opioid analgesics and for which alternative treatments are inadequate. It is supplied in single dose prefilled syringes of 2 mg/ml, 4 mg/ml, 5 mg/ml, 8 mg/ml, and 10 mg/ml strengths. It can be administered via intramuscular (IM) or slow intravenous (IV) injections. The lowest effective dose for the shortest duration should be used. The recommended initial IM dose is 10 mg every four hours as needed. The recommended initial IV dose is 0.1 mg to 0.2 mg/kg body weight every four hours as needed. See full prescribing information for complete administration instructions. Report J2272 only for morphine sulfate manufactured by Fresenius Kabi.

J2274

J2274 Injection, morphine sulfate, preservative free for epidural or intrathecal use, 10 mg

Preservative-free morphine sulfate injection is a systemic narcotic analgesic for administration by epidural or intrathecal routes. It is used for the management of chronic, intractable pain not responsive to nonnarcotic analgesics. Morphine sulfate, administered epidurally or intrathecally, provides pain relief for extended periods without attendant loss of motor, sensory, or sympathetic function. The solution contains no antioxidant, bacteriostat, or antimicrobial agent and is intended as a single-dose injection to provide analgesia via the intravenous, epidural, or intrathecal routes. When the epidural route of administration is used, more time is required for the morphine to cross the dura and reach the dorsal horn in the spinal cord. In contrast, intrathecal morphine binds with opiate receptors in the spinal cord without having to cross the dura. Therefore, intrathecal delivery results in faster analgesic. Each ampul and vial is intended for single use only. Epidural adult dosage: Initial injection of 5 mg in the lumbar region may provide satisfactory pain relief for up to 24 hours. If adequate pain relief is not achieved within one hour, careful administration of incremental doses of 1 to 2 mg at intervals sufficient to assess effectiveness may be given. No more than 10 mg/24 hours should be administered. Intrathecal adult dosage: A single injection of 0.2 to 1 mg may provide satisfactory pain relief for up to 24 hours. Repeated intrathecal injections of preservative-free morphine sulfate injection are not recommended. A constant intravenous infusion of naloxone hydrochloride, 0.6 mg/hr, for 24 hours after intrathecal injection may be used to reduce the incidence of potential side effects. For aged or debilitated patients, administer with extreme caution. A lower dosage is usually satisfactory. Repeat dosage: If pain recurs, alternative routes of administration should be considered, since experience with repeated doses of morphine by the intrathecal route is limited. Pediatric use: No information on the use in pediatric patients is available.

J2278

J2278 Injection, ziconotide, 1 mcg

Ziconotide is a synthetic equivalent conopeptide produced from piscivorous marine snails. It binds to N-type calcium channels in the afferent nerves of the dorsal horn in the spinal column preventing the transmission of pain sensation. This drug must be administered intrathecally via an implanted variable-rate microinfusion device or an external microinfusion device and catheter. Ziconotide is indicated for the management of severe chronic pain in patients who are intolerant or refractory to other treatments. The effective dose of ziconotide is variable and the dose should be adjusted according to the patient's severity of pain, response to therapy, and the occurrence of adverse events.

J2280

J2280 Injection, moxifloxacin, 100 mg

Moxifloxacin hydrochloride is a synthetic, broad spectrum antibacterial agent. It is intended for the treatment of adults, ages 18 and older, with acute bacterial sinusitis, acute exacerbation of chronic bronchitis, community acquired pneumonia, plague, skin infections, and complicated intra-abdominal infections due to infections caused by susceptible strains of organisms. Moxifloxacin hydrochloride is administered via intravenous (IV) infusion over one hour. The recommended dosage is 400 mg daily. The duration of treatment depends upon the condition being treated.

J2281

J2281 Injection, moxifloxacin (Fresenius Kabi) not therapeutically equivalent to J2280, 100 mg

Moxifloxacin HCl is a synthetic, broad spectrum fluoroquinolone antibacterial agent intended for the treatment of adults, ages 18 years and older, with acute bacterial sinusitis, acute exacerbation of chronic bronchitis, community acquired pneumonia, plague, skin and skin structure infections, and complicated intra-abdominal infections due to infections caused by susceptible strains of organisms. It is supplied in a single use bag of 400 mg/250 ml and is administered via intravenous (IV) infusion over one hour. The recommended dosage is 400 mg daily and it should not be mixed with other medications. The duration of treatment depends upon the condition being treated. See full prescribing information for complete administration instructions. Report J2281 only for moxifloxacin HCL manufactured by Fresenius Kabi.

J2300

J2300 Injection, nalbuphine HCl, per 10 mg

Nalbuphine hydrochloride is a synthetic opioid analgesic that is chemically related to naloxone and oxymorphone. Nalbuphine hydrochloride is prescribed for the relief of moderate to severe pain or as a supplement to balanced anesthesia. It is also used for pre- and postoperative pain relief or obstetrical analgesia during labor and delivery. It may be administered by subcutaneous, intramuscular, or intravenous injection. The usual adult dose is 10 mg for every 70 kg every three to six hours as needed, adjusted according to the pain severity, condition of the patient, and other medications.

J2310

J2310 Injection, naloxone HCl, per 1 mg

Naloxone hydrochloride injection is indicated for the complete or partial reversal of narcotic depression induced by opioids, including natural and synthetic narcotics. Naloxone hydrochloride injection is also indicated for the diagnosis of suspected acute opioid overdosage. It may be administered intravenously, intramuscularly, or subcutaneously. The most rapid onset of action is achieved by intravenous administration, and this route is recommended in emergency situations. The usual intravenous dosage is 2 mg of naloxone hydrochloride in 500 mL of IV solution. Intramuscular or subcutaneous injection dosage varies depending upon patient's response.

J2311

J2311 Injection, naloxone HCl (Zimhi), 1 mg

Naloxone HCl is an opioid antagonist indicated for use in adults and children with known or suspected opioid overdose, as evidenced by respiratory and/or central nervous system depression. It is supplied in a single dose prefilled syringe of 5 mg/0.5 ml and is administered by intramuscular (IM) or subcutaneous (SC) injection. Emergency care should be obtained immediately following administration. See full prescribing information for complete administration instructions.

J2315

J2315 Injection, naltrexone, depot form, 1 mg

Naltrexone depot is an opioid antagonist. The drug binds to specific opioid receptors blocking the effects stimulated by alcohol ingestion. A depot suspension is a drug that remains in the body long term in storage and is slowly released into the blood. The depot form is indicated as a treatment of alcohol dependence in patients who are unable to abstain from alcohol consumption during outpatient therapy treatments. The drug should be a part of a comprehensive treatment management program. Patients should not actively consume alcohol during the initiation of naltrexone depot treatment. Naltrexone depot is administered by intramuscular injection into the gluteus once a month. The recommended dosage is 380 mg once a month. The depot form is not self-administrable.

J2320

J2320 Injection, nandrolone decanoate, up to 50 mg

Nandrolone decanoate is a long-acting synthetic version of testosterone that has strong anabolic properties and weak androgenic or masculinizing properties. Anabolic properties are any constructive metabolic process by which organisms convert substances into other components of the organism's chemical architecture. Nandrolone decanoate stimulates erythropoiesis, promotes tissue growth and building processes, and reverses tissue destruction. It is indicated as a treatment for chronic wasting diseases and anemia associated with renal insufficiency. Nandrolone decanoate is administered by intramuscular injection.

J2323

J2323 Injection, natalizumab, 1 mg

Natalizumab is a monoclonal antibody produced with recombinant DNA technology in murine myeloma cells. Natalizumab binds to the surface of leukocyte cells (except neutrophils) preventing their migration to the site of inflamed tissue. It is indicated as a monotherapy for the treatment of relapsing forms of multiple sclerosis in patients who cannot tolerate or have not adequately responded to other treatments. The recommended dose is 300 mg administered via intravenous infusion every four weeks. Note that this drug can only be prescribed, distributed and infused by providers, infusion centers and pharmacies registered with the manufacturer's TOUCH program. Patients must also be enrolled with the program.

J2325

J2325 Injection, nesiritide, 0.1 mg

Nesiritide is a human, B-type natriuretic peptide produced by recombinant DNA technology from *E. coli*. It has the same amino acid sequence as the endogenous peptide produced by the ventricular myocardium. Nesiritide binds to receptors of vascular smooth muscle and endothelial cells and increases intracellular concentrations of guanosine cyclic monophosphate (cGMP), which creates smooth muscle cell relaxation. Use of this drug should be strictly limited to patients with acutely decompensated heart failure with a clinical presentation severe enough to warrant hospitalization. The drug should be administered in a clinical setting where blood pressure can be closely monitored. Nesiritide is currently in a clinical trial to assess its use in intermittent and scheduled infusions to treat severely ill congestive heart failure patients in an outpatient setting. However, this setting and indication are not recommended and have not yet been approved. Nesiritide is not intended for use as a diuretic. The drug is administered by intravenous infusion, and the recommended dose is an initial intravenous bolus of 2 mcg/kg of body weight followed by a continuous infusion of 0.01 mcg/kg of body weight per minute.

J2326

J2326 Injection, nusinersen, 0.1 mg

Nusinersen is a survival motor neuron-2 (SMN2)-directed antisense oligonucleotide. Nusinersen is indicated for the treatment of spinal muscular atrophy (SMA) in pediatric and adult patients. Nusinersen is delivered by intrathecal injection. The recommended dose is 12 mg (5 mL) per administration. The patient is given four loading doses, with the first three administered at 14-day intervals; the fourth loading dose should be administered 30 days following the third dose. Maintenance doses should be administered once every four months. All intrathecal injections should be administered over one to three minutes through a spinal anesthesia needle. Prior to administration, 5 mL of cerebrospinal fluid should be removed from the patient. Sedation and ultrasound guidance may be needed to guide the injection, especially for pediatric patients.

J2327

J2327 Injection, risankizumab-rzaa, intravenous, 1 mg

Risankizumab-rzaa, an interleukin-23 (IL-23) antagonist, is a humanized immunoglobulin G1 (IgG1) monoclonal antibody, indicated for the treatment of adults, ages 18 years and older, with moderately to severely active Crohn's disease, active psoriatic arthritis, and moderate to severe plaque psoriasis. For the treatment of Crohn's disease, the recommended induction dosage is 600 mg administered via intravenous (IV) injection over a period of at least one hour at week zero, week four, and week eight and recommended maintenance dosage is 360 mg administered by subcutaneous (SC) injection at week 12, and every eight weeks thereafter. For the treatment of active psoriatic arthritis and moderate to severe plaque psoriasis, the recommended dosage is 150 mg administered via SC injection at week zero, week four, and every 12 weeks thereafter. It is supplied in a single dose vial of 600 mg/10 ml for IV infusion and prefilled, single dose pens (75 mg/ml, 150 mg/ml, 180 mg/1.2 ml, and 360 mg/2.4 ml) for SC injection. See full prescribing information for complete administration instructions.

J2350

J2350 Injection, ocrelizumab, 1 mg

Ocrelizumab is a recombinant humanized monoclonal antibody directed against CD20-expressing B-cells. CD20 is a cell surface antigen that is present on pre-B and mature B lymphocytes. Ocrelizumab binds to CD20 on B lymphocytes and causes antibody-dependent cellular cytolysis and complement-mediated lysis. It is for the treatment of adult patients with primary progressive or relapsing forms of multiple sclerosis (MS). Recommended dosage is 300 mg administered by intravenous infusion over 2.5 hours or longer. A second infusion of 300 mg is administered in two weeks. After the first two administrations, additional dosage is 600 mg administered by intravenous infusion, over 3.5 hours or longer, every six months. Patients should be premedicated with an antihistamine 30 to 60 minutes prior to each treatment and an intravenous corticosteroid 30 minutes prior to each administration; an antipyretic may also be administered.

J2353-J2354

J2353 Injection, octreotide, depot form for intramuscular injection, 1 mg

J2354 Injection, octreotide, nondepot form for subcutaneous or intravenous injection, 25 mcg

Octreotide is a synthetic analogue of the natural hormone somatostatin. It causes the same effects as somatostatin but has a prolonged duration. Somatostatin is a peptide produced by the hypothalamus gland and by pancreatic islet cells that inhibit the release of growth hormone, thyrotropin, corticotropin, insulin, glucagon, gastrin, renin, and secretin. The depot version is octreotide encased in biodegradable microspheres. The microspheres control the rate of drug release and allow it to be dispensed over longer periods of time. Both depot and non-depot formulations of octreotide are indicated as a treatment for acromegaly, as a symptomatic treatment for diarrhea, and flushing associated with metastatic carcinoid and vasoactive intestinal peptide tumors. Non-depot octreotide is administered by subcutaneous or intravenous injection. Dosages for the non-depot version vary from 50 to 600 mcg depending on the disease and response to treatment. Octreotide depot is administered by deep intramuscular injection into the buttocks every four weeks. The dosage for the depot version is usually 20 mg for patients who have been receiving the non-depot version.

J2355

J2355 Injection, oprelvekin, 5 mg

Oprelvekin is a synthetic interleukin-11 produced by recombinant DNA technology using *E. coli* bacteria. Interleukin-11 is a growth factor produced by bone marrow stromal cells that stimulates the production of hematopoietic stem cells and megakaryocyte progenitor cells and B cell differentiation. Oprelvekin is indicated for prevention of thrombocytopenia following myelosuppressive chemotherapy in patients with non-myeloid malignancies. It is administered by subcutaneous injection. The recommended dosage is 50 mg/kg of body weight.

J2356

J2356 Injection, tezepelumab-ekko, 1 mg

Tezepelumab-ekko is a thymic stromal lymphopoietin (TSLP) blocker, human monoclonal antibody (IgG2Λ) indicated for the treatment of children and adults, ages 12 years and older, with severe asthma. It is intended as an add-on maintenance treatment and should not be used for the treatment of acute bronchospasm or status asthmaticus. It is supplied in single dose vials or single dose, prefilled pens of 210 mg/1.91 ml. The recommended dosage is 210 mg administered by a health care provider via subcutaneous (SC) injection every four weeks. See full prescribing information for complete administration instructions.

J

J2357

J2357 Injection, omalizumab, 5 mg

Omalizumab is an anti-IgE monoclonal antibody produced by recombinant DNA technology using Chinese hamster ovaries. It binds specifically to human immunoglobulin E (IgE) and inhibits the binding of IgE to mast cells and basophils. The reduction in IgE binding limits the allergic response. Omalizumab is indicated for adults and children, 6 years or older, with moderate to severe persistent asthma who are reactive to air-borne allergens or have a positive skin test, and whose symptoms are not adequately controlled by inhaled corticosteroids; as an add-on treatment for adults, age 18 and older, with nasal polyps that are not adequately controlled by nasal corticosteroids; and for adults and children, age 12 and older, with chronic idiopathic urticaria not controlled despite H1 antihistamine treatment. Omalizumab should not be used for the treatment of acute bronchospasm, status asthmaticus, or for the treatment of other forms of urticaria. It is administered by subcutaneous injection. Dosages and frequency vary based on patient age, serum IgE level, body weight, and condition treated. See full prescribing information for complete administration instructions.

J2358

J2358 Injection, olanzapine, long-acting, 1 mg

Olanzapine is a psychotropic agent that belongs to the thienobenzodiazepine class. It is used to treat schizophrenia, acute mixed or manic episodes associated with bipolar disorder, agitation associated with schizophrenia, and bipolar disorder. Olanzapine is administered by deep intramuscular injection into the gluteal muscle.

J2360

J2360 Injection, orphenadrine citrate, up to 60 mg

Orphenadrine citrate is a synthetic analogue of diphenhydramine having analgesic, antihistaminic, anti-cholinergic, and antispasmodic properties. The drug acts on the brain stem selectively blocking facilitatory functions of the reticular formation. This produces a blocking of the pain transmission signals. Its therapeutic effects are not completely understood, but appear to be related to its analgesic properties. Orphenadrine is indicated for symptomatic relief of pain associated with acute musculoskeletal disorders. It can be used as an adjunct to rest, physical therapy, and other analgesic measures. Orphenadrine is available in an oral, self-administrable form and in an injectable form. The oral form is usually combined with aspirin and caffeine. Dosages of the oral form vary from 25 to 200 mg per day. Recommended dosage of the injectable form is 60 mg twice a day. The Injectable form is administered by intravenous or intramuscular injection.

J2370

J2370 Injection, phenylephrine HCl, up to 1 ml

Phenylephrine hydrochloride is an amine that is related to epinephrine and ephedrine. The drug is longer-acting than epinephrine or ephedrine. It affects the sympathetic nervous system by stimulating alpha adrenergic receptors. It functions predominately as a vasoconstrictor. Injectable phenylephrine hydrochloride is indicated for the treatment of hypotension, vascular failure in shock, and paroxysmal supraventricular tachycardia. The drug is also used to maintain adequate blood pressure during inhalation and spinal anesthesia and as a vasoconstrictor in regional analgesia. Injectable phenylephrine hydrochloride may be administered by intramuscular, subcutaneous, or intravenous injection and by intravenous infusion.

J2401

J2401 Injection, chloroprocaine HCl, per 1 mg

Chloroprocaine HCl is an ester local anesthetic for use as a spinal anesthesia in adults, ages 18 years and older, undergoing surgical procedures. It is supplied in a 5 ml glass ampule containing 50 mg (10 mg/ml) and is administered via intrathecal injection. It should not be administered via epidural injection and intravascular injection should be avoided. The recommended dose is 50 mg. See full prescribing information for complete administration instructions.

J2402

J2402 Injection, chloroprocaine HCl (Clorotekal), per 1 mg

Chloroprocaine HCl is an ester local anesthetic for use as a spinal anesthesia in adults, ages 18 years and older, undergoing surgical procedures. It is supplied in a 5 ml glass ampule containing 50 mg (10 mg/ml) and is administered via intrathecal injection. It should not be administered via epidural injection and intravascular injection should be avoided. The recommended dose is 50 mg. See full prescribing information for complete administration instructions. Report J2402 for chloroprocaine HCL, brand name Clorotekal, manufactured by B. Braun.

J2405

J2405 Injection, ondansetron HCl, per 1 mg

Ondansetron hydrochloride is a chemical compound that is a selective blocker of serotonin 5-HT3 receptors. It is an antiemetic drug available in oral and injectable forms. Serotonin 5-HT3 receptors are present on the vagal nerve and at sensory nerve endings. Cytotoxic chemotherapy appears to trigger the release of serotonin in the small intestine, which may trigger the 5-HT3 receptors and initiate the vomiting reflex. Ondansetron hydrochloride is indicated for the prevention of nausea and vomiting associated with surgery and antineoplastic drugs. The oral version is also indicated for the prevention of nausea and vomiting associated with radiation therapy. The drug is available in oral and injectable versions. The injectable version is administered by intravenous injection. When administered in conjunction with antineoplastic drugs, ondansetron hydrochloride should be diluted. The recommended dosage for this indication is a single 32 mg or three doses at 0.15 mg/kg of body weight infused over 15 minutes. Subsequent dosages may be infused at four and eight hours after the initial dose. When used to suppress postoperative vomiting, the drug does not need to be diluted. The recommended dose is 4 mg or 0.1 mg/kg of body weight administered by intravenous or intramuscular injection. Dosages for the oral version vary from 8 to 24 mg depending on the indication and patient.

J2406

J2406 Injection, oritavancin (Kimyrsa), 10 mg

Oritavancin (trade name Kimyrsa) is a lipoglycopeptide antibiotic indicated for the treatment of adult patients, ages 18 and older, with acute bacterial skin and skin structure infections (ABSSSI) caused by susceptible strains of gram-positive bacteria. The recommended dosage is a 1,200 mg single dose (one Kimyrsa vial) administered by intravenous (IV) infusion over three hours following reconstitution. Kimyrsa and Orbactiv, another oritavancin antibiotic, should not be used interchangeably as they have different preparation, infusion, and dosage instructions. See full prescribing information for complete administration instructions.

J2407

J2407 Injection, oritavancin (Orbactiv), 10 mg

Oritavancin (trade name Orbactiv) is a lipoglycopeptide antibiotic indicated for the treatment of adult patients, ages 18 and older, with acute bacterial skin and skin structure infections (ABSSSI) caused by susceptible strains of gram-positive bacteria. The recommended dosage is a 1,200 mg single dose (three Orbactiv vials) administered by intravenous (IV) infusion over three hours following reconstitution. Orbactiv and Kimyrsa, another oritavancin antibiotic, should not be used interchangeably as they have different preparation, infusion, and dosage instructions. See full prescribing information for complete administration instructions.

J2410

J2410 Injection, oxymorphone HCl, up to 1 mg

Oxymorphone hydrochloride is a semi-synthetic opioid substitute for morphine that is a potent analgesic and sedative. Oxymorphone hydrochloride exerts its effect on the central nervous system (CNS) and gastrointestinal tract. It binds to specific opiate receptors in the CNS providing an analgesic effect. The exact mechanism of action for its analgesic effect is unknown. Oxymorphone hydrochloride also produces respiratory depression; decreases gastric, biliary, and pancreatic secretions; and increases smooth muscle tone in the urinary tract. It is a schedule II controlled substance. Oxymorphone hydrochloride is indicated for the relief of moderate to severe pain, as an anesthetic premedication, and for the relief of anxiety related to dyspnea associated with pulmonary edema in patients with acute left ventricular dysfunction.

J2425

J2425 Injection, palifermin, 50 mcg

Palifermin is a human keratinocyte growth factor (KGF) produced by recombinant DNA technology in *Escherichia coli* (*E. coli*). It is different from endogenous human growth factor (EGF) in that the first 23 N-terminal amino acids have been deleted to improve protein stability. It stimulates the epithelial cells that line and protect the oral mucosa. It is used to treat severe oral mucositis that is often found as a side effect of high dose chemotherapy and/or radiation therapy in patients with hematologic malignancies. The recommended dose of palifermin is 60 mcg per kg per day. The medication is administered for three consecutive days prior to the myelotoxic therapy and three consecutive days after. Palifermin is administered by intravenous bolus injection.

J2426

J2426 Injection, paliperidone palmitate extended release, 1 mg

Paliperidone palmitate is a psychotropic agent used to treat schizophrenia in adults. The recommended dose is 234 mg on the first day of treatment and 156 mg one week later administered as an IM injection into the deltoid muscle. The recommended maintenance dose is 117 mg monthly administered as in IM injection in the deltoid or gluteal muscle. The maintenance dose may vary based on individual response to the treatment.

J

J2430

J2430 Injection, pamidronate disodium, per 30 mg

Pamidronate disodium is used to treat hypercalcemia from cancer, Paget's disease, osteolytic bone metastases of breast cancer, and osteolytic bone lesions of multiple myeloma. Pamidronate disodium acts as an antihypercalcemic, inhibiting the resorption of bone and blocking the formation of mature osteoclasts. Cardiovascular side effects of atrial fibrillation and tachycardia may occur, with hypertension a common side-effect as well as fatigue, abdominal pain, nausea, constipation, anorexia, and anemia.

J2440

J2440 Injection, papaverine HCl, up to 60 mg

Papaverine hydrochloride is an alkaloid extracted from opium or synthetically produced. The drug relaxes smooth muscles, especially when is has been contracted in spasm. The drug directly relaxes the cardiac and vascular systems, bronchial muscles, and gastrointestinal, biliary, and urinary tracts. Its effect on the vascular system includes coronary, cerebral, peripheral, and pulmonary arteries. It has minimal effect on the central nervous system, though large doses can cause some sedation. Papaverine hydrochloride is indicated in erectile dysfunction and various conditions where spasms occur, such as vascular spasm associated with acute myocardial infarction, angina pectoris, peripheral embolism, pulmonary embolism, and visceral spasms such as gastrointestinal colic and ureteral or biliary spasms. It may also be useful in peripheral vascular disease with vasospastic elements and certain cerebral angiospasms.

J2460

J2460 Injection, oxytetracycline HCl, up to 50 mg

Oxytetracycline hydrochloride is a broad-spectrum antibiotic of the tetracycline group produced by the bacterium *Streptomyces rimosus*. Its mechanism of action is not known, but it is thought to inhibit protein synthesis. It is indicated for the treatment of adults and children, ages 8 and older, with infections caused by a wide range of susceptible gram-positive and gram-negative organisms. Cross resistance among drugs in the tetracycline family is common. It may also be used in combination with amebicides to treat acute intestinal amebiasis. The recommend dosage for adults is 250 mg administered once every 24 hours or 300 mg administered every eight to 12 hours. For children, the recommended dosage is 15 to 25 mg/kg of body weight up to a maximum of 250 mg per injection daily. The dosage may also be divided and administered every eight to 12 hours.

J2469

J2469 Injection, palonosetron HCl, 25 mcg

Palonosetron hydrochloride is a chemical compound that is a selective blocker of serotonin 5-HT3 receptors. Serotonin 5-HT3 receptors are present on the vagal nerve and at sensory nerve endings. Cytotoxic chemotherapy appears to trigger the release of serotonin in the small intestine, which may trigger the 5-HT3 receptors and initiate the vomiting reflex. It is indicated to prevent and treat nausea and vomiting associated with chemotherapy. Palonosetron hydrochloride is administered by intravenous injection. The recommended dosage of the injectable form is 25 mcg.

J2501

J2501 Injection, paricalcitol, 1 mcg

Paricalcitol is a synthetic analogue of calcitriol, vitamin D. Vitamins are organic compounds necessary to the metabolic functioning of the body. Vitamin D is a fat-soluble vitamin that is a group of related compounds commonly called calciferol. Two common forms are cholecalciferol and ergocalciferol. Vitamin D is a steroid hormone precursor and helps to maintain calcium and phosphorus levels throughout the body. Human skin can produce vitamin D when exposed to sunlight, specifically UVB. Secondary hyperparathyroidism is characterized by an increase in parathyroid hormone to compensate for inadequate levels of active vitamin D hormone. Paricalcitol is indicated for the prevention and treatment of hyperparathyroidism secondary to chronic renal failure. The injectable form is administered by intravenous injection and is primarily used when the patient has stage 5 chronic renal disease.

J2502

J2502 Injection, pasireotide long acting, 1 mg

Pasireotide is a somatostatin analog. It is utilized for the treatment of acromegaly in patients who have an unsatisfactory response to surgery or where surgical intervention is not plausible. It is administered via intramuscular injection with an initial dose of 40 mg and repeated every four weeks (28 days). The subsequent doses should be adjusted based on treatment response and tolerance.

J2503

J2503 Injection, pegaptanib sodium, 0.3 mg

Pegaptanib sodium is a pegylated oligonucleotide for intravitreous injection. Pegylating is the addition of a polyethylene glycol (PEG) molecule, which allows a slow release of the carried substance. Pegaptanib sodium is a selective vascular endothelial growth factor antagonist that inhibits the growth of additional blood vessels. Pegaptanib sodium is indicated for the treatment of neovascular or wet age-related macular degeneration. The recommended dose is 0.3 mg administered by intravitreous injection to the affected eye once every six weeks.

J2504

J2504 Injection, pegademase bovine, 25 IU

Pegademase bovine is an orphan drug that provides an exogenous source for the enzyme adenosine deaminase. It is derived from bovine intestines. A deficiency of adenosine deaminase allows adenosine and some of its derivatives to accumulate in cells. This accumulation is toxic to lymphocytes, which are a main component of the immune system. Pegademase is indicated as a replacement enzyme in patients with severe combined immunodeficiency disease in whom the disease is due to the lack of adenosine deaminase. Pegademase is administered by intramuscular injection. Dosage needs to be individualized to the patient and varies from 10 to 30 IU/kg of body weight.

J2506

J2506 Injection, pegfilgrastim, excludes biosimilar, 0.5 mg

Pegfilgrastim is a pegylated form of filgrastim. Pegylated means that polyethylene glycol, a dispensing agent, has been added to the drug. Filgrastim is a synthetic human granulocyte colony-stimulating factor (G-CSF). Pegfilgrastim is produced by recombinant DNA technology using *E. coli* bacteria. The drug binds to surface receptors on hematopoietic cells and stimulates neutrophil production, differentiation, maturation, and function. Pegfilgrastim is longer acting than filgrastim. It is indicated as a treatment for neutropenia in patients receiving myelosuppressive therapy for nonmyeloid malignancies. The drug is administered by subcutaneous (SC) injection. Recommended dosage is 6 mg once each chemotherapy cycle. This code should be reported for the non-biosimilar formulation of pegfilgrastim.

J2507

J2507 Injection, pegloticase, 1 mg

Pegloticase is an exogenous source of the human enzyme uricase, which is recreated by recombinant DNA technology in *E. coli* bacteria. The enzyme is pegylated, attached to a polyethylene glycol molecule. Pegylation increases the molecular weight and stability of the enzyme and masks it from the patient's immune system. This uric acid specific enzyme is indicated as a treatment for chronic gout in patients who have not responded to other treatment. The medication stimulates the oxidation of uric acid to allantoin, which lowers the uric acid levels. The recommended dose of pegloticase is 8 mg every two weeks administered by IV infusion.

J2510

J2510 Injection, penicillin G procaine, aqueous, up to 600,000 units

Penicillin G procaine is a version of penicillin that contains procaine, a local anesthetic agent. Penicillins block the actions of transpeptidase, an enzyme needed to create the cell wall. This weakens the bacterial cell wall causing cellular death. The procaine provides a local anesthetic action and contributes to a slower release of the penicillin G from the injection site. Penicillin G procaine is not as long acting as penicillin G benzathine. Once in the body, penicillin G procaine is hydrolyzed to penicillin G. The hydrolysis and slow absorption provide sustained, but lower blood levels of penicillin. Susceptibility studies should be performed prior to the administration of penicillin G procaine. This formulation is administered by deep intramuscular injection. Dosage depends upon the bacterial infection being treated.

J2513

J2513 Injection, pentastarch, 10% solution, 100 ml

Pentastarch is a derivative of starch composed of 90 percent amylopectin. It is used in plasma volume expander. Intravenous infusion of pentastarch results in expansion of the plasma volume in excess of the volume infused. This expansion persists for approximately 18 to 24 hours and is expected to improve the hemodynamic status for 12 to 18 hours. It is indicated for plasma volume expansion when needed to manage shock due to hemorrhage, surgery, sepsis, burns, or other trauma. It is not a substitute for red blood cells or coagulation factors in plasma. Pentastarch is administered by intravenous infusion only. Total dosage and rate of infusion depend upon the amount of blood or plasma lost.

J2515

J2515 Injection, pentobarbital sodium, per 50 mg

Pentobarbital sodium is a short- to intermediate-acting barbiturate. Barbiturates are derivatives of barbituric acid that act as central nervous system depressants producing a wide variety of effects, from mild sedation to anesthesia. They enhance the neurotransmitter gamma aminobutyric acid (GABA), which inhibits the excitation of nerves. Pentobarbital sodium is indicated as a sedative, presurgical adjunct to anesthesia, as a short-term treatment for insomnia, and as an anticonvulsant.

J2540

J2540 Injection, penicillin G potassium, up to 600,000 units

Penicillin G potassium is a version of penicillin that contains potassium. Penicillins block the actions of transpeptidase, an enzyme needed to create the cell wall. This weakens the bacterial cell wall causing cellular death. Susceptibility studies should be performed prior to the administration of penicillin G potassium. The drug is available in oral and injectable forms. The injectable form can be administered by intramuscular, subcutaneous, intracavity, and intrathecal injection or continuous intravenous infusion. Dosage depends upon the bacterial infection being treated, as well as the form of the penicillin.

J2543

J2543 Injection, piperacillin sodium/tazobactam sodium, 1 g/0.125 g (1.125 g)

Piperacillin is a semisynthetic broad-spectrum penicillin. Penicillins block the actions of transpeptidase, an enzyme needed to create the cell wall. This weakens the bacterial cell wall causing cellular death. Many bacteria have developed a resistance to penicillin. Resistant bacteria produce an enzyme, penicillinase or beta-lactamase that protects it from the effects of penicillin. Tazobactam inhibits the penicillinase so the piperacillin is effective against a greater number of bacteria. Susceptibility studies should be performed prior to the administration of piperacillin. Susceptible bacteria include *E. coli,* Pseudomonas aeruginosa, enterococci, Clostridium spp., *Bacteroides* spp., *Klebsiella* spp., *Proteus* spp., *Neisseria gonorrhoeae, Enterobacter* spp., *Serratia* spp., *Streptococcus pneumoniae, Haemophilus influenzae, Acinetobacter* spp., *Morganella morganii*, and *Providencia rettgeri*. Piperacillin/tazobactam is administered by intramuscular injection or intravenous injection and infusion. Dosage varies from 2 to 6 g depending on the organism and extent of the infection.

J2545

J2545 Pentamidine isethionate, inhalation solution, FDA-approved final product, noncompounded, administered through DME, unit dose form, per 300 mg

Pentamidine isethionate is an aromatic diamidine that is an antimicrobial. Its mechanism of action is not completely known. It is thought the drug interferes with the synthesis of DNA, RNA, and protein, causing cell death. Pentamidine isethionate is indicated as a treatment for *Pneumocystis jirovecii* (previously classified as *P. carinii*), trypanosomiasis, and leishmaniasis. The drug may be administered by intramuscular injection, inhalation, or intravenous infusion over one hour. Dosage is usually 300 mg.

J2547

J2547 Injection, peramivir, 1 mg

Peramivir is an influenza virus neuraminidase inhibitor used for the treatment of acute, uncomplicated influenza in adult patients 18 years and older. Recommended dosage is 600 mg, administered by intravenous infusion over 15 to 30 minutes. A single dose should be administered within two days of the onset of influenza symptoms.

J2550

J2550 Injection, promethazine HCl, up to 50 mg

Promethazine hydrochloride is a phenothiazine derivative with antihistamine, sedative, antiemetic, and anticholinergic properties. The drug binds to histamine receptors preventing the histamine from dilating capillaries, constricting the bronchial smooth muscles, and increasing gastric secretions. Promethazine hydrochloride is indicated as an antiemetic, a sedative in anesthesia, as a treatment for motion sickness, and for allergic reactions, including rhinitis and pruritic skin reactions. The drug may be combined with other drugs in cough and cold preparations. Promethazine hydrochloride is available in injectable, oral, and rectal suppository forms. The injectable form is administered by intramuscular or intravenous injection although the preferred method is by IM injection. Dosage varies from 25 to 50 mg.

J2560

J2560 Injection, phenobarbital sodium, up to 120 mg

Phenobarbital sodium is a long-acting barbiturate. Barbiturates are derivatives of barbituric acid that act as central nervous system depressants that produce a wide variety of effects, from mild sedation to anesthesia. They enhance the neurotransmitter gamma aminobutyric acid (GABA), which inhibits the excitation of nerves. Phenobarbital sodium is indicated as a sedative, presurgical adjunct to anesthesia, as a short-term treatment for insomnia, and as an anticonvulsant. It is a schedule IV narcotic.

J2562

J2562 Injection, plerixafor, 1 mg

Plerixafor is a hematopoietic stem cell mobilizer that helps move hematopoietic stem cells to the peripheral blood for collection prior to autologous transplant in patients with non-Hodgkin's lymphoma and multiple myeloma (MM). It inhibits the CXCR4 chemokine receptor and blocks binding the stromal cell-derived factors. Those factors direct the hematopoietic stem cells to the bone marrow. Once the stem cells are circulating in the peripheral blood, they can be extracted and prepared for transplant. The recommended dose is 0.24 mg/kg body weight about 11 hours before starting the apheresis for up to four consecutive days. Plerixafor is given by subcutaneous injection.

J2590

J2590 Injection, oxytocin, up to 10 units

Oxytocin is an animal-derived or synthetic form of the hormone secreted by the hypothalamus and stored in the pituitary gland. Oxytocin promotes uterine contractions and stimulates milk secretion. It is indicated to induce labor, to promote uterine contractions after delivery of the placenta or abortion, and to control postpartum hemorrhage. Dosage depends upon uterine response.

J2597

J2597 Injection, desmopressin acetate, per 1 mcg

Desmopressin acetate, also known as DDAVP, is a potent synthetic analogue of the natural hormone vasopressin. Vasopressin is a hormone produced by the posterior pituitary gland. Vasopressin has an antidiuretic effect causing the renal tubules to reabsorb water. Desmopressin acetate is indicated for the treatment of diabetes insipidus, primary nocturnal enuresis, treatment of temporary polyuria and polydipsia secondary to trauma to or surgery in the pituitary region, and to increase coagulation factor VIII activity before surgical procedures in patients with hemophilia A and von Willebrand's disease.

J2650

J2650 Injection, prednisolone acetate, up to 1 ml

Prednisolone is a synthetic adrenal corticosteroid. Corticosteroids are natural substances produced by the adrenal glands located adjacent to the kidneys. Corticosteroids are widely used to treat allergies, inflammation, and many disease processes. Prednisolone is used to treat a wide variety of conditions. Oral and injectable prednisolone is used to suppress inflammation in many inflammatory and allergic conditions. Examples include rheumatoid arthritis, systemic lupus, acute gouty arthritis, psoriatic arthritis, ulcerative colitis, and Crohn's disease. Severe allergic conditions that fail conventional treatment may also be treated with prednisolone. Examples include bronchial asthma, allergic rhinitis, drug-induced dermatitis, and contact and atopic dermatitis. Prednisolone is also used in the treatment of leukemia and lymphomas, idiopathic thrombocytopenia purpura, and autoimmune hemolytic anemia. Other miscellaneous conditions treated with this medication include thyroiditis and sarcoidosis. Prednisolone is used as a hormone replacement in patients whose adrenal glands are unable to produce sufficient amounts of corticosteroids. Prednisolone injection or sterile suspension can be injected into a muscle, joint, lesion, or soft tissue. When used as an intra-articular injection, prednisolone is indicated as a treatment for joint pain and inflammation, epicondylitis, bursitis, and synovitis.

J2670

J2670 Injection, tolazoline HCl, up to 25 mg

Tolazoline hydrochloride is a chemical compound that is an adrenergic blocking agent and peripheral vasodilator. Per the FDA, this drug is no longer available in the United States for human use. It is still available for veterinary use.

J2675

J2675 Injection, progesterone, per 50 mg

Progesterone is an animal-derived or synthetic form of the natural human hormone produced by the adrenal cortex, ovaries, and placenta. The hormone prepares the uterus for the reception and development of the fertilized ovum and maintains an optimal intrauterine environment for pregnancy. Exogenous progesterone is used as a treatment for dysfunctional uterine bleeding, secondary amenorrhea, infertility, and as part of postmenopausal hormone replacement therapy.

J2680

J2680 Injection, fluphenazine decanoate, up to 25 mg

Fluphenazine decanoate is a phenothiazine derivative that blocks dopamine receptors in hypothalamus and pituitary glands. Fluphenazine decanoate has a slower release from the injection site than the fluphenazine hydrochloride, which results in a prolonged duration of action. The precise mechanism of action is not known, but it is believed to depress the reticular activating system. Fluphenazine decanoate is indicated in the management of manifestations of schizophrenia. Adult dosage varies from 1 to 10 mg daily depending on the severity and duration of symptoms. Fluphenazine decanoate is administered by intramuscular or subcutaneous injection.

J2690

J2690 Injection, procainamide HCl, up to 1 g

Procainamide hydrochloride is a benzoic acid derivative that depresses heart function. The drug increases the refractory period of the cardiac atria and ventricles. Procainamide hydrochloride is indicated as a treatment for documented life-threatening ventricular arrhythmias, such as sustained ventricular tachycardia. The drug is available in injectable and oral forms. The injectable form is administered by intramuscular or intravenous injection or intravenous infusion. Dosage varies from 100 to 1,000 mg depending upon response.

J2700

J2700 Injection, oxacillin sodium, up to 250 mg

Oxacillin sodium is a semi-synthetic penicillin that is penicillinase resistant. Penicillins block the actions of transpeptidase, an enzyme needed to create the cell wall. This weakens the bacterial cell wall causing cellular death. Many bacteria have developed a resistance to penicillin. Resistant bacteria produce an enzyme, penicillinase or beta-lactamase, that protects it from the effects of penicillin. Susceptibility studies should be performed prior to the administration of oxacillin sodium. Oxacillin sodium is indicated in the treatment of infections caused by penicillinase-producing staphylococci.

J2704

J2704 Injection, propofol, 10 mg

Propofol is a short-acting intravenous anesthetic agent suitable for induction and maintenance of general anesthesia and monitored anesthesia care sedation in adults, induction anesthesia in children at least 3 years of age, and maintenance anesthesia in children at least 2 months of age. It may also be used for sedation of ventilated patients receiving intensive care for up to three days. Induction of anesthesia with propofol is rapid and maintenance can be achieved with continuous infusion or intermittent bolus injections.

J2710

J2710 Injection, neostigmine methylsulfate, up to 0.5 mg

Neostigmine methylsulfate is a chemical that blocks the passage of nerve signals in the parasympathetic system. It competes with acetylcholine by attaching itself to the same receptors on a cell. Neostigmine methylsulfate is indicated for treatment of myasthenia gravis, prevention and postoperative treatment of distention and urinary retention, and reversal of the effects of nondepolarizing neuromuscular blocking agents, such as tubocurarine, metocurine, gallamine, or pancuronium following surgery. The recommended dose is dependent on the condition being treated. For myasthenia gravis, the recommended dose is 1:2000 solution (0.5 mg) administered by subcutaneous or intramuscular injection. For prevention and postoperative treatment of distention and urinary retention, the recommended dose is 1:4000 solution (0.25 mg) administered by subcutaneous or intramuscular injection. For reversal of the effects of nondepolarizing neuromuscular blocking agents, the recommended dose is 1:2000 solution (0.5 mg) administered by subcutaneous or intramuscular injection.

J2720

J2720 Injection, protamine sulfate, per 10 mg

Protamine sulfate is a simple protein with a low molecular weight. It occurs naturally in the sperm of salmon and certain other species of fish. When given alone, it has a weak anticoagulant effect. However, when given in the presence of heparin, a stable salt is formed and both drugs lose their anticoagulant effect. Protamine sulfate is indicated for the treatment of heparin overdose. Protamine sulfate is administered intravenously and has a rapid onset of action. Neutralization of heparin occurs within five minutes following intravenous administration. Each mg of protamine will neutralize approximately 90 USP units of heparin activity derived from beef lung tissue or about 115 USP units of heparin activity derived from porcine intestinal mucosa. Protamine sulfate is given by very slow intravenous injection in doses 50 mg or less over a 10-minute period.

J2724

J2724 Injection, protein C concentrate, intravenous, human, 10 IU

Protein C concentrate is used to replace congenitally deficient protein C. Protein C is a vitamin K-dependent plasma protein. When activated by thrombin, protein C inhibits the clotting mechanism by enzymatically breaking up the activated forms of clotting factors V and VIII. It also enhances fibrinolysis. Protein C concentrate is derived from pooled human plasma and uses a column of mouse monoclonal antibodies. It is indicated for the treatment of severe congenital protein C deficiency for the prevention and treatment of venous thrombosis and purpura fulminans. Protein C concentrate may be used for an acute episode, short-term prophylaxis, and long-term prophylaxis. The dosage, frequency, and duration of treatment depends on the severity of the patient's deficiency and the patient's age, clinical condition, and the plasma levels of protein C. Protein C concentrate is administered by intravenous infusion.

J2725

J2725 Injection, protirelin, per 250 mcg

Protirelin is a synthetic peptide similar to the endogenous thyrotropin releasing hormone produced by the hypothalamus. Thyrotropin releasing hormone stimulates the anterior pituitary gland to release thyroid stimulating hormone (TSH). Protirelin is indicated for diagnosis of mild hyperthyroidism, Graves' disease, and for differentiating between primary, secondary, and tertiary hypothyroidism. The drug is administered via an intravenous bolus with a recommended dosage of 500 mcg. TSH serum levels are then measured at different intervals.

J2730

J2730 Injection, pralidoxime chloride, up to 1 g

Pralidoxime chloride, also known as p2-PAM chloride, is a chemical that reactivates the parasympathetic nervous system. Pralidoxime chloride is indicated as an antidote in the treatment of poisoning due to pesticides and chemicals of the organophosphate class that block nerve signal transmission in the parasympathetic nervous system. Pralidoxime chloride is also indicated in the control of overdosage by some drugs used in the treatment of myasthenia gravis. The principal indications for the use of pralidoxime chloride are muscle weakness and respiratory depression. The principal action of pralidoxime chloride is to reactivate cholinesterase that has been inactivated by an organophosphate pesticide or related compound. This facilitates destruction of accumulated acetylcholine, which allows nerve signals to function normally. The most critical effect of pralidoxime chloride is in relieving paralysis of the respiratory muscles. Because pralidoxime chloride is less effective in relieving depression of the respiratory center, atropine is always administered concomitantly to block the effect of accumulated acetylcholine of the respiratory center. Pralidoxime chloride is administered by intravenous, intramuscular, or subcutaneous injection or infusion.

J2760

J2760 Injection, phentolamine mesylate, up to 5 mg

Phentolamine mesylate is a chemical compound that produces a short-term block of the adrenal hormones epinephrine and norepinephrine. It is indicated for the diagnosis of pheochromocytoma, the prophylaxis and treatment of hypertensive episodes in patients with pheochromocytoma, and the prophylaxis and treatment of dermal necrosis following intravenous administration or extravasation of norepinephrine. Pheochromocytoma is a neoplasm, usually benign, of the adrenal medulla or sympathetic paraganglia that results in increased secretion of epinephrine and norepinephrine. The drug is administered by intramuscular or intravenous injection. Dosage ranges from 5 to 10 mg.

J2765

J2765 Injection, metoclopramide HCl, up to 10 mg

Metoclopramide hydrochloride is a chemical compound that acts as a dopamine receptor antagonist. Dopamine produces nausea and vomiting by stimulating the chemoreceptor trigger zones. Metoclopramide hydrochloride blocks the stimulation of these zones. It stimulates upper gastrointestinal tract motility without stimulating the gastric, biliary, or pancreatic secretions. Metoclopramide hydrochloride is indicated for use as an antiemetic and in the treatment of gastroesophageal reflux and gastroparesis.

J2770

J2770 Injection, quinupristin/dalfopristin, 500 mg (150/350)

Quinupristin-dalfopristin is an antibiotic in the class known as streptogramins. The streptogramins are macromolecular antibiotics produced by *Streptomyces pristinaepiralis*. Quinupristin-dalfopristin is indicated for treatment of susceptible bacterial infections caused by antibiotic-resistant, gram-positive organisms, including severe infections caused by vancomycin-resistant *E. faecium*, nosocomial pneumonia, infections due to the use of intravascular catheters, and complicated skin and skin structure infections caused by methicillin-susceptible *Staphylococcus aureus* and *Streptococcus pyogenes* (group A streptococcus). The mechanism of action of quinupristin-dalfopristin is primarily inhibition of protein synthesis. Dalfopristin acts to block an early step in protein synthesis, forming a bond with a ribosome and preventing elongation of the peptide chain. Quinupristin acts to block a later step, preventing the extension of peptide chains and causing incomplete chains to be released. Quinupristin-dalfopristin is administered by intravenous injection or infusion.

J2777

J2777 Injection, faricimab-svoa, 0.1 mg

Faricimab-svoa is a bispecific immunoglobulin G1 (IgG1) antibody produced in Chinese hamster cells. It binds vascular endothelial growth factor A (VEGF-A) and angiopoietin-2 (Ang-2), suppressing endothelial cell proliferation, neovascularization, and vascular permeability; promoting vascular stability; and desensitizing blood vessels to the effects of VEGF-A. It is indicated for the treatment of adults, ages 18 years and older, with neovascular (wet) age-related macular degeneration (AMD) and for diabetic macular edema (DME). It is supplied in a single dose vial of 120 mg/ml and is administered via intravitreal injection. The recommended dosage varies based on the condition treated. See full prescribing information for complete administration instructions.

J2778

J2778 Injection, ranibizumab, 0.1 mg

Ranibizumab is a monoclonal antibody produced by recombinant DNA technology using a strain of *E. coli* bacteria. The drug binds to receptor sites of human vascular endothelial growth factor A (VEGF-A) and inhibits its activity. VEGF-A has been shown to cause new vascularization and leakage of blood vessels in the eye and contributes to the progression of age-related macular degeneration. Ranibizumab is indicated as a treatment for neovascular or wet, age-related macular degeneration. The drug is administered by intravitreal injection only. Recommended dosage is 0.5 mg once a month.

J2779

J2779 Injection, ranibizumab, via intravitreal implant (Susvimo), 0.1 mg

Ranibizumab sustained release intravitreal implant is a IgG1 kappa monoclonal antibody produced by recombinant DNA technology using a strain of *E. coli* bacteria. The drug binds to receptor sites of human vascular endothelial growth factor A (VEGF-A) and inhibits its activity. VEGF-A has been shown to cause new vascularization and leakage of blood vessels in the eye and contributes to the progression of age-related macular degeneration. Ranibizumab sustained release intravitreal implant is indicated as a treatment for adults, ages 18 years and older, with neovascular or wet, age-related macular degeneration who have responded to at least two previous intravitreal injections of a VEGF inhibitor. An ocular implant is surgically placed under aseptic technique in an operating room by a physician experienced in vitreoretinal surgery. Refill procedures must be performed under aseptic conditions by a physician experienced in ophthalmic surgery. The recommended dosage is 2 mg continuously delivered via ocular implant with implant refills every 24 weeks (six months). Supplemental treatment with 0.5 mg ranibizumab intravitreal injection may be administered into the affected eye if clinically necessary. If removal of the ocular implant is required, the procedure must be performed in an operating room by a physician experienced in vitreoretinal surgery. See full prescribing information for complete administration instructions.

J2780

J2780 Injection, ranitidine HCl, 25 mg

Ranitidine hydrochloride is a chemical compound that binds to histamine receptors preventing the histamine from increasing gastric acid secretions. Ranitidine hydrochloride, singularly or in combination, is indicated as a treatment and as maintenance therapy for gastric ulcers, duodenal ulcers, gastroesophageal reflex disease, pathological gastric hypersecretory conditions, and erosive esophagitis. Oral forms of ranitidine hydrochloride are available in smaller dosages over-the-counter. Larger dosages are prescription only and available in oral and injectable forms. The injectable form is administered by intramuscular or intravenous injection.

J2783

J2783 Injection, rasburicase, 0.5 mg

Rasburicase is a synthetic enzyme produced by recombinant DNA technology in Saccharomyces cerevisiae yeast. It catalyzes the oxidation of uric acid into an inactive and soluble metabolite. Rasburicase is indicated for the initial management of plasma uric acid levels in pediatric patients with leukemia, lymphoma, and solid tumor malignancies who are receiving antineoplastic therapy expected to result in tumor lysis and subsequent elevation of plasma uric acid. The drug is administered by intravenous infusion over 30 minutes. Recommended dosage is 0.15 or 0.20 mg/kg of body weight daily for five days.

J2785

J2785 Injection, regadenoson, 0.1 mg

Regadenoson is a vasodilator medication used as a cardiac stressing agent prior to myocardial perfusion imaging. This is an alternate to exercise stress when the patient is not a candidate for exercise stress. It is administered as a rapid IV push. The recommended dose is 0.4 mg of regadenoson.

J2786

J2786 Injection, reslizumab, 1 mg

Reslizumab is a humanized interleukin-5 antagonist (IgG4, kappa) monoclonal antibody that inhibits the IL-5 cytokine signal, reducing eosinophil production and survival, which contribute to inflammation. Inflammation is an essential element of the progression of asthma. Reslizumab is indicated for adult patients aged 18 or older for the treatment of severe asthma with an eosinophilic phenotype. Recommended dosage is 3 mg/kg administered once every four weeks by intravenous infusion.

J2787

J2787 Riboflavin 5'-phosphate, ophthalmic solution, up to 3 ml

Riboflavin 5'-phosphate is photo-enhancer that is indicated for the treatment of progressive keratoconus and corneal ectasia following refractive surgery in patients 14 years of age and older. It is a topical solution used as part of corneal collagen cross-linking with the KXL System. A photo-enhancer is thought to enhance refractive surgery procedures, restore corneal strength, halt the progression of keratoconus and ectasia, as well as slow the progression of acute keratoconus. Corneal ectasia is a group of conditions that can develop after refractive surgery. The most common is keratoconus (KC). KC is a condition where the normally dome-shaped cornea becomes progressively thin and weak, creating a cone-shaped bulge, causing optical distortion. Riboflavin 5'-phosphate is supplied in a 3 mL syringe and is administered via instillation into the eye. Once the epithelium of the cornea is debrided, one drop of riboflavin 5'-phosphate is instilled topically onto the eye every two minutes for a period of 30 minutes. After 30 minutes, the anterior chamber of the eye is examined under slit lamp for a yellow flare. If no flare is detected, one drop of Riboflavin 5'-phosphate is instilled every two minutes for an additional two to three drops and re-examined for a yellow flare. This process is repeated as necessary. Once yellow flare is detected, ultrasound pachymetry should be performed. If the corneal thickness is less than 400 microns, two drops are instilled every five to 10 seconds until the cornea reaches at least 400 microns. Once the 400 micron threshold is obtained, the eye is irradiated for 30 continuous minutes with the KXL System. During the 30-minute irradiation, riboflavin 5'-phosphate is instilled onto the eye every two minutes. Any remaining solution is discarded.

J2788-J2792

J2788 Injection, Rho D immune globulin, human, minidose, 50 mcg (250 IU)

J2790 Injection, Rho D immune globulin, human, full dose, 300 mcg (1500 IU)

J2791 Injection, Rho D immune globulin (human), (Rhophylac), intramuscular or intravenous, 100 IU

J2792 Injection, Rho D immune globulin, intravenous, human, solvent detergent, 100 IU

Rh factors are a group of antigens present on the membrane of erythrocytes. When a person who is Rh-negative receives an Rh-positive transfusion or becomes pregnant with an Rh-positive fetus, the person develops antibodies against Rh-positive blood. These antibodies will in future exposures attack and kill any Rh-positive erythrocytes. Rho (D) immune globulin suppresses the immune response of the Rh-negative person preventing antibody formation against the Rh-positive blood. Recommendations for administration during a pregnancy include a full dose of 300 mcg antepartum at 28 weeks and another full dose within 72 hours of delivery when there is known incompatibility between the mother and fetus. In cases of abortion, spontaneous or induced, of a fetus of less than 12 weeks, a mini-dose of 50 mcg is recommended. The mini-dose should be administered within three hours of the event. Dosages administered when an Rh incompatible blood transfusion occurs depend upon the volume of incompatible blood transfused and should be administered within 72 hours of the transfusion. Rho (D) immune globulin may be treated in several different ways to ensure that the pooled donor plasma has no pathogens. The immune globulin may be ultrafiltered, solvent washed, or detergent washed. It can be administered by intramuscular or intravenous injection.

J2793

J2793 Injection, rilonacept, 1 mg

Rilonacept is an interleukin 1 blocker used in the treatment and prevention of genetic conditions; cryopyrin associated periodic syndromes (CAPS), including Muckle Wells Syndrome (MWS); and familial cold auto inflammatory syndrome (FCAS) in adults and children age 12 or older. Although, used to treat and prevent these conditions, Rilonacept cannot cure these inherited conditions. Rilonacept is expressed in recombinant Chinese hamster ovary cells and comes in a sterile single use glass vial containing lyophilized powder for reconstitution. Recommended dose for adults is a loading dose of 320 mg administered by two separate subcutaneous injections. A maintenance dose of 160 mg is administered once a week by subcutaneous injection. Patients 12 to 17 years of age should receive a loading dose of 4.4 mg/kg with a maximum of 320 mg administered as one or two subcutaneous injections. Following that, the patient should receive 2.2 mg/kg with a maximum of 160 mg, once a week.

J2794

J2794 Injection, risperidone (RISPERDAL CONSTA), 0.5 mg

Risperidone is an antipsychotic drug of the class of benzisoxazole derivatives. The drug's mechanism of action is unknown. It is thought that the drug acts by mediating dopamine and serotonin levels. Long-acting risperidone is encased within microspheres so that the drug is slowly released over a two-week period. Risperidone is indicated for the treatment of schizophrenia. Long-acting risperidone is injected via deep muscular gluteal injection every two weeks with a recommended initial dosage of 25 mg. This drug should not be administered intravenously. If patients do not respond to the 25 mg injections, 37.5 mg or 50 mg injections may be administered every two weeks. Different strengths should not be combined within a single administration.

J2795

J2795 Injection, ropivacaine HCl, 1 mg

Ropivacaine hydrochloride is a chemical compound that is an amino amide local anesthetic agent. It locally blocks the generation and conduction of nerve transmissions. Ropivacaine hydrochloride is used as a peripheral nerve block, for percutaneous infiltration anesthesia, and as an epidural block. It may also be administered by continuous epidural infusion for acute postoperative pain management. Dosage varies by indication and extent of the anesthesia required.

J2796

J2796 Injection, romiplostim, 10 mcg

Romiplostim increases platelet production and is used to treat patients with idiopathic thrombocytopenic purpura (ITP) for whom other treatments have not been successful. It should be used for patients who have bleeding problems and not only for normalizing a patient's platelet count. Romiplostim is derived using DNA segments in *Escherichia coli (E. coli)*. Recommended dose is 1 mcg/kg based on the patient's weight. The dose is adjusted depending on the patient's platelet count. Romiplostim is administered by subcutaneous injection.

J2797

J2797 Injection, rolapitant, 0.5 mg

Rolapitant is a chemical complex used as an oral antiemetic drug. It seeks cell receptors of human substance P/neurokinin 1 (NK1). NK1s are peptides found in the central and peripheral nervous systems involved in the transmission of a signal from outside the cell wall into the cell. Rolapitant blocks those transmissions. It is used for adults to prevent delayed nausea and vomiting associated with initial and repeat courses of emetogenic cancer chemotherapy. It is supplied in 90 mg tablets and the recommended dosage is 180 mg, in combination with a corticosteroid and a 5-HT3 antagonist, administered one to two hours prior to chemotherapy administration. Rolapitant should not be used concurrently with thioridazine.

J2798

J2798 Injection, risperidone, (Perseris), 0.5 mg

Risperidone is an antipsychotic drug of the class of benzisoxazole derivatives, indicated for the treatment of schizophrenia in adults 18 years of age and older. It should not be used for the treatment of patients with dementia-related psychosis. The precise mechanism of action is unknown. It is thought that the drug acts by mediating dopamine and serotonin levels. It is supplied in a prefilled injection kit of dosages of 90 mg or 120 mg and should be injected monthly via subcutaneous injection into the abdomen. This drug should not be administered intravenously and should not be taken with oral risperidone. It should not be administered more than once per month. For patients who have never used risperidone, tolerability should be established with oral risperidone before administering risperidone injections. It should not be used in patients with dementia-related psychosis.

J2800

J2800 Injection, methocarbamol, up to 10 ml

Methocarbamol is a skeletal muscle relaxant, indicated for the treatment of muscle spasms and muscle pain and stiffness. Methocarbamol acts on the central nervous system to produce its muscle relaxant effects.

J

J

J2805

J2805 Injection, sincalide, 5 mcg

Sincalide is a gastrointestinal hormone peptide injected intravenously. It is used to stimulate gallbladder contractions for assessment via a cholecystogram or ultrasound; to stimulate pancreatic secretin prior to the obtaining of a duodenal aspirate; or to accelerate the transit of barium through the small bowel for fluoroscopic or x-ray examination of the intestinal tract.

J2810

J2810 Injection, theophylline, per 40 mg

Theophylline is a methylxanthine drug with structural and pharmacological similarity to caffeine. It is naturally found in black and green tea. Theophylline's exact mechanism of action is unknown. It is suggested that it is a nonspecific inhibitor of phosphodiesterase enzymes, which are enzymes that control the tissue concentration of various hormones and other enzymes. Inhibiting the phosphodiesterase enzymes would allow for increases in intracellular cyclic AMP. Cyclic AMP is a nucleotide involved in the activities of many hormones and cellular functions. Theophylline relaxes the smooth bronchial muscles and allows for easier breathing. It also increases the force of contraction of the diaphragmatic muscles. It is indicated for the prophylaxis and treatment of chronic asthma and COPD. Theophylline is also indicated as an emergency treatment in an acute severe asthma episode. Theophylline carries a high incidence of side-effects when used at its upper therapeutic range. The drug is also affected by many other drugs, including antibiotics, cimetidine, and phenytoin among others.

J2820

J2820 Injection, sargramostim (GM-CSF), 50 mcg

Sargramostim is a synthetic granulocyte-macrophage colony-stimulating factor (GM-CSF) produced by recombinant DNA technology in S. cerevisiae yeast. GM-CSF binds to receptor sites on stem cells and supports the survival, expansion, and differentiation of hematopoietic progenitor cells into granulocytes and macrophages. Sargramostim is indicated to stimulate hematopoiesis and decrease neutropenia as an adjunct to myelosuppressive cancer chemotherapy in patients with acute myelogenous leukemia and non-Hodgkin's lymphoma, to promote myeloid engraftment in bone marrow transplantation or hematopoietic stem cell transplantation, and to enhance peripheral progenitor cell yield in autologous hematopoietic stem cell transplantation. The drug is administered by intravenous infusion. Dosage varies from 250 mcg per m^2 of body surface per day.

J2840

J2840 Injection, sebelipase alfa, 1 mg

Sebelipase alfa is a hydrolytic lysosomal cholesteryl ester and triacylglycerol-specific enzyme used for the treatment of patients with lysosomal acid lipase deficiency (LAL-D). Patients with this condition are born without the LAL enzyme, which is important for breaking down fatty material. Sebelipase alfa provides the enzyme that is missing. Sebelipase alfa is administered via intravenous infusion over a period of at least two hours. The recommended dosage for pediatric and adult patients is 1 mg/kg body weight infused once every other week. For patients that are diagnosed within the first six months of life, the recommended starting dose is 1 mg/kg body weight once weekly. If optimal response is not obtained, the dosage can increase to 3 mg/kg once weekly.

J2850

J2850 Injection, secretin, synthetic, human, 1 mcg

Secretin is a synthetic version of the natural hormone secretin secreted by the mucosa of the duodenum and upper jejunum. Secretin stimulates the release of pancreatic juice by the pancreas and bile by the liver. Both bile and the pancreatic juices contain bicarbonate and change the pH of the duodenum from acid to alkaline which facilitates the action of intestinal digestive enzymes. Secretin is used in diagnostic tests for gastrinoma and pancreatic exocrine function, and to facilitate the identification of the ampulla of Vater and accessory papilla during endoscopic retrograde cholangiopancreatography (ERCP). Dosage is 0.2-0.4 mcg per kg of body weight depending on the indication. The drug is administered by intravenous injection.

J2860

J2860 Injection, siltuximab, 10 mg

Siltuximab is an interleukin-6 (IL-6) antagonist. It is utilized for the treatment of multicentric Castleman's disease (MCD). For this treatment, patients do not currently have the human immunodeficiency virus (HIV) or human herpes virus-8 (HHV-8). Administration is by intravenous infusion, 11 mg/kg over one hour, every three weeks.

J2910

J2910 Injection, aurothioglucose, up to 50 mg

Aurothioglucose is a gold salt used in treating inflammatory arthritis. The mechanism of action in gold salts is not well understood. However, in patients with inflammatory arthritis, such as adult and juvenile rheumatoid arthritis, gold salts decrease the inflammation of the joint lining, preventing destruction of bone and cartilage. Gold salts, such as aurothioglucose, are second-line drugs prescribed when anti-inflammatory drugs, such as nonsteroidal anti-inflammatory drugs (NSAID) and corticosteroids, are ineffective in preventing the progression of inflammatory arthritis. Aurothioglucose is available as a 50 mg/ml injectable suspension to be administered by intramuscular injection.

J2916

J2916 Injection, sodium ferric gluconate complex in sucrose injection, 12.5 mg

Sodium ferric gluconate is an iron oxide hydrate directly bound to sucrose and chelated with gluconate. The drug replenishes iron, which is critical for normal hemoglobulin synthesis to maintain oxygen transport. Iron is also required for the metabolism and synthesis of DNA and various enzymes. Sodium ferric gluconate is indicated for the treatment of iron deficiency in ESRD patients undergoing hemodialysis who are also receiving erythropoietin therapy. It is administered by intravenous infusion over one hour. The recommended dosage is 125 mg.

J2920-J2930

J2920 Injection, methylprednisolone sodium succinate, up to 40 mg

J2930 Injection, methylprednisolone sodium succinate, up to 125 mg

Methylprednisolone is a corticosteroid used to treat a variety of conditions. Indications include allergic disorders, arthritis, blood diseases, breathing problems, certain cancers, eye diseases, intestinal disorders, and collagen and skin diseases. Methylprednisolone may also be used with other medications as a replacement for certain hormones. Methylprednisolone works by decreasing the body's immune response to these diseases and reducing symptoms such as swelling and redness. Methylprednisolone may be administered orally, by intramuscular injection in the form of methylprednisolone acetate, or by intravenous infusion in the form of methylprednisolone sodium succinate.

J2940

J2940 Injection, somatrem, 1 mg

Somatrem is a version of human growth hormone (HGH) produced by recombinant DNA technology from a strain of *E. coli* bacteria. It contains the identical sequence of the 191 amino acids that compromise endogenous HGH. HGH has a direct effect on the metabolism of protein, carbohydrates, and fat and controls skeletal and visceral growth. Somatrem is indicated for the treatment of idiopathic HGH deficiency in children with growth failure. Treatment with somatrem should be discontinued when the epiphyses are fused. The drug is administered subcutaneously or intramuscularly at a dosage of 0.30 mg per body weight and may be self-administered.

J2941

J2941 Injection, somatropin, 1 mg

Somatropin is another name for human growth hormone (HGH). Most versions are produced by recombinant DNA technology from a strain of *E. coli* bacteria. It contains the identical sequence of the 191 amino acids that compromise endogenous HGH. HGH has a direct effect on the metabolism of protein, carbohydrates, and fat and controls skeletal and visceral growth. Somatrem is indicated for the treatment of growth failure in children born small for their gestational age, children with growth failure due to HGH deficiency, chronic renal insufficiency, Turner's syndrome, or Prader-Willi syndrome. Another indication is the treatment of adult patients with HGH deficiency, either primary or secondary to pituitary or hypothalamic diseases, radiation therapy, surgery, or trauma. The drug is administered subcutaneously or intramuscularly at a dosage of 0.30 mg per body weight and may be self-administered.

J2950

J2950 Injection, promazine HCl, up to 25 mg

Promazine hydrochloride belongs to a group of medications known as the phenothiazine antipsychotics. Promazine hydrochloride is indicated for the treatment of agitation alone and agitation and restlessness in the elderly. The mechanism of action involves blocking a variety of receptors in the brain, particularly dopamine receptors. Dopamine is a chemical that aids in transmission of signals between brain cells. An excess of dopamine in the brain can cause over-stimulation of dopamine receptors. Because dopamine receptors normally act to modify behavior, over-stimulation can result in psychotic illness. Promazine hydrochloride prevents over-stimulation by blocking these receptors, which then helps to control psychotic illness.

J2993

J2993 Injection, reteplase, 18.1 mg

Reteplase is a longer-acting derivative of alteplase, a synthetic tissue plasminogen activator. Reteplase is produced by recombinant DNA technology in *E. coli* bacteria. Tissue plasminogen activators are enzymes produced by endothelial cells that catalyze the breakdown of thrombi or blood clots. The drug is indicated as a treatment of acute myocardial infarction. Treatment should begin as soon as possible after the onset of symptoms. The drug is administered by two intravenous bolus injections. Each bolus should be 18.1 mg.

J2995

J2995 Injection, streptokinase, per 250,000 IU

Streptokinase is a protein produced by beta hemolytic streptococci bacteria that binds to plasminogen and breaks down thrombi or blood clots. Streptokinase is indicated as a treatment of acute myocardial infarction, acute pulmonary embolism, deep venous thrombosis, acute arterial thrombi or emboli, and occlusion of an arteriovenous shunt. Treatment of the acute myocardial infarction should begin within four hours of the onset of symptoms. Treatment of acute pulmonary embolism, deep venous thrombosis, and acute arterial thrombi or emboli should begin as soon as possible from onset of the event, preferably within seven days. The drug is administered by intravenous

J

infusion. Recommended dosage varies from 1,000,000 to 1,500,000 units depending upon the indication.

J2997

J2997 Injection, alteplase recombinant, 1 mg

Alteplase is a synthetic tissue plasminogen activator produced by recombinant DNA technology in Chinese hamster ovaries. Tissue plasminogen activators are enzymes produced by endothelial cells that catalyze the breakdown of thrombi or blood clots. Alteplase is indicated as a treatment of acute myocardial infarction, acute ischemic stroke, acute massive pulmonary embolism, or to restore the function of a thrombosed central venous access device. Treatment of the acute myocardial infarction should begin as soon as possible after the onset of symptoms. Treatment of acute ischemic stroke should begin within three hours of the onset of symptoms and after it has been determined that no intracranial hemorrhage has occurred. Treatment of acute massive pulmonary embolism should begin after objective confirmation of the diagnosis has been obtained. The drug is administered by intravenous injection and infusion. Recommended total dosage is based upon body weight, but should not exceed 100 mg.

J

J2998

J2998 Injection, plasminogen, human-tvmh, 1 mg

Plasminogen, human-tvmh, is plasma-derived human plasminogen that is intended for the treatment of children and adults, ages 11 months and older, with plasminogen deficiency type 1 (hypoplasminogenemia). Decreased plasminogen levels cause formation of fibrin-rich, ligneous pseudomembranous lesions on mucous membranes that can impair normal organ and tissue function. Replacement plasminogen therapy provides a temporary correction of plasminogen levels and reduction of fibrinous lesion formation. It is supplied in a 50 ml single dose vial of 68.8 mg of plasminogen requiring reconstitution with 12.5 ml sterile water, for a final volume of 5.5 mg/ml of plasminogen. The recommended dose is 6.6 mg/kg body weight administered via intravenous (IV) injection every two to four days. See full prescribing information for complete administration instructions.

J3000

J3000 Injection, streptomycin, up to 1 g

Streptomycin was the first of the aminoglycoside antibiotics. Aminoglycoside antibiotics are derived from various species of *Streptomyces* bacteria or produced synthetically. Aminoglycosides inhibit bacterial protein synthesis by binding with the 30S ribosomal subunit and are bactericidal. Streptomycin is derived from *Streptomyces griseus*. It inhibits protein synthesis, causing cell death. It is indicated for the treatment of adults and children with mycobacterium tuberculosis, as well as a wide variety of non-tuberculosis infections caused by gram-negative bacillary bacteria. For the treatment of mycobacterium tuberculosis, it should be used in combination with isoniazid (INH), rifampin, or pyrazinamide. Streptomycin is now in limited use due to the emergence of resistant bacterial strains. Susceptibility studies should be performed prior to the administration of streptomycin. It is administered by intramuscular (IM) injection to the buttocks or thigh. Dosages and frequency vary based on patient age, body weight, and disease treated, and should not be administered concomitantly with other drugs. A reduced dosage may be required for patients with renal impairment. See full prescribing information for complete administration instructions.

J3010

J3010 Injection, fentanyl citrate, 0.1 mg

Fentanyl is a schedule II, controlled substance pain medication in the narcotic and opioid analgesic class. Fentanyl is used as an adjunct to anesthesia, to manage chronic pain, and breakthrough persistent pain in cancer patients who have an increased physical tolerance to current opioid therapy. Fentanyl interacts primarily with the opioid mu-receptor. These mu-binding sites are distributed throughout the human brain, spinal cord, and other tissues. In clinical settings, fentanyl exerts its principal pharmacologic effects on the central nervous system. It is administered via intravenous push injection, intramuscular injection, transdermal patch, or transmucosal lozenges.

J3030

J3030 Injection, sumatriptan succinate, 6 mg (code may be used for Medicare when drug administered under the direct supervision of a physician, not for use when drug is self-administered)

Sumatriptan succinate is given to treat migraines and acute treatment of cluster headaches. It is thought to act by stimulating the specific serotonin receptors of the cranial arteries and the dura mater to cause vasoconstriction of the cerebral arteries, without affecting systemic vessels or blood pressure. Recommended injection dose is 6 mg. It can be administered by subcutaneous injection, through tablets, or nasal inhalation. The injection can be self-administered.

J3031

J3031 Injection, fremanezumab-vfrm, 1 mg (code may be used for Medicare when drug administered under the direct supervision of a physician, not for use when drug is self-administered)

Fremanezumab-vfrm is a calcitonin gene-related peptide (CGRP) antagonist, produced by recombinant DNA technology using Chinese hamster ovary cells, and is indicated for the prophylactic treatment of migraines in adults 18 years of age and older. It is thought to act by binding to CGRP ligand, which blocks it from binding to the receptor. Fremanezumab-vfrm is supplied as a single dose prefilled syringe of 225 mg/1.5 ml solution. Allow the prefilled syringe to sit at room temperature for 30 minutes. It should be protected from direct sunlight. There are two recommended doses: 225 mg monthly or 675 mg every three months (quarterly) administered via subcutaneous injection into the abdomen, thigh, or upper arm. The quarterly dose is administered as three consecutive injections of 225 mg each.

J3032

J3032 Injection, eptinezumab-jjmr, 1 mg

Eptinezumab-jjmr is a calcitonin gene-related peptide (CGRP) antagonist, produced by recombinant DNA technology using *Pichia pastoris* yeast cells, and is indicated for the prophylactic treatment of migraines in adults 18 years of age and older. It is thought to act by binding to the calcitonin gene related peptide (CGRP) ligand, which blocks it from binding to the receptor. The recommended dosage is 100 mg or 300 mg administered via intravenous (IV) infusion every three months over 30 minutes. It is supplied in a 100 mg/mL single dose vial that requires reconstitution in 100 mL of 0.9% sodium chloride. For the 100 mg dose, 1 mL of eptinezumab-jjmr should be withdrawn from the single dose vial by sterile needle and syringe and injected into a 100 mL bag of 0.9% sodium chloride. For the 300 mg dose, 1 mL from each of three single dose vials should be injected into a 100 mL bag of 0.9% sodium chloride.

J3060

J3060 Injection, taliglucerase alfa, 10 units

Taliglucerase alfa is a recombinant active form of the lysosomal enzyme beta-glucocerebrosidase, which is produced in a culture of genetically modified carrot plant root cells. It is an orphan drug used to treat Type 1 Gaucher's disease caused by a lack of the enzyme glucocerebrosidase, which is crucial to the metabolism of fats. Taliglucerase alfa assists in the breakdown of glucocerebroside to glucose and ceramide. The recommended dose is 60 units per kg of body weight administered once every two weeks as a 60 to 120 minute intravenous infusion. However, dosages can range from 11 units/kg to 73 units/kg every other week depending on disease severity and individual patient response to treatment.

J3070

J3070 Injection, pentazocine, 30 mg

Pentazocine is an opioid analgesic used for moderate to severe pain and during labor. It is thought that pentazocine HCl binds with opiate receptors in the central nervous system (CNS), which then alters both the emotional response to and perception of pain.

J3090

J3090 Injection, tedizolid phosphate, 1 mg

Tedizolid phosphate is an oxazolidinone-class antibiotic that is a phosphate prodrug that is converted to tedizolid in the presence of phosphates. Oxazolidine is an organic compound containing nitrogen and oxygen in a five-membered ring. The antibacterial effect of oxazolidinones works as a protein synthesis inhibitor. It is indicated for the treatment of adults, ages 18 and older, with acute bacterial skin and skin structure infections (ABSSSI) caused by designated gram-positive susceptible bacteria. The recommended dosage is 200 mg as an intravenous (IV) infusion over one hour, administered once daily for a period of six days. It should not be administered by IV push or bolus.

J3095

J3095 Injection, telavancin, 10 mg

Telavancin is a lipoglycopeptide antibacterial that is a synthetic derivative of vancomycin. It is indicated for the treatment of adults, ages 18 and older, with complicated skin and skin structure infections (cSSSI) and hospital-acquired and ventilator-associated bacterial pneumonia (HABP/VABP) caused by susceptible gram-positive bacteria. For the treatment of cSSSI, the recommended dosage is 10 mg/kg body weight by intravenous (IV) infusion over 60 minutes, every 24 hours for seven to 14 days. For the treatment of HABP/VABP, the recommended dosage is 10 mg/kg body weight by IV infusion over 60 minutes, every 24 hours for seven to 21 days. A reduced dosage may be required for patients with renal impairment. See full prescribing information for complete administration instructions.

J3101

J3101 Injection, tenecteplase, 1 mg

Tenecteplase is a thrombolytic enzyme used in treating the effects of a myocardial infarction. It is a tissue plasminogen activator (TPA) produced by recombinant DNA technology using Chinese hamster ovary cells. It binds with fibrin and converts plasminogen to plasmin. Tenecteplase is used to treat acute myocardial infarction and should be administered as soon as possible after the onset of symptoms. This medication is administered intravenously.

J3105

J3105 Injection, terbutaline sulfate, up to 1 mg

Terbutaline sulfate is a bronchodilator that relaxes both bronchial and uterine smooth muscle by stimulating beta2 receptors and is used primarily to treat bronchospasm in patients with reversible obstructive airway disease. It is available as tablets, aerosol inhaler, or subcutaneous injection. Side effects may include nervousness, palpitations, tachycardia, and/or diaphoresis.

J3110

J3110 Injection, teriparatide, 10 mcg

Teriparatide is a recombinant human parathyroid hormone (1-34) that has an identical structure to the naturally occurring hormone. Teriparatide is manufactured from a strain of *Escherichia coli*, and modified by recombinant DNA technology. Teriparatide is indicated for the treatment of postmenopausal women with osteoporosis who are at high risk for fracture. This includes women with a history of osteoporotic fracture, who have multiple risk factors for fracture, or who have failed or are intolerant of previous osteoporosis therapy. Teriparatide is also indicated to increase bone mass in men with primary or hypogonadal osteoporosis who are at high risk for fracture. This includes men with a history of osteoporotic fracture, who have multiple risk factors for fracture, or who have failed or are intolerant to previous osteoporosis therapy. Recommended dose is 20 mcg of teriparatide each day for up to 28 days. Teriparatide should be administered as a subcutaneous injection into the thigh or abdominal wall and can be self-administered.

J3111

J3111 Injection, romosozumab-aqqg, 1 mg

Romosozumab-aqqg is a sclerostin inhibitor, produced by recombinant DNA technology using Chinese hamster ovary cells, indicated for the treatment of osteoporosis in postmenopausal women with a high risk of bone fractures, multiple risk factors for fracture, or for women that were not successful or tolerant with other osteoporosis therapies. Romosozumab-aqqg inhibits the actions of sclerostin, increases bone formation, and decreases bone resorption, improving bone strength and structure. It is supplied as a solution of 105 mg/1.17 ml in a single use prefilled syringe. A full dose is comprised of two single use syringes. The recommended dose is two separate injections, one immediately following the other, for a total dose of 210 mg. The total dose of 210 mg should be administered subcutaneously in the abdomen, thigh, or upper arm once every month for a total of 12 doses. Administration must be performed by a healthcare provider. If the patient still requires treatment for osteoporosis after 12 doses, therapy with an antiresorptive agent should be considered. Therapy should be supplemented with calcium and vitamin D.

J3121

J3121 Injection, testosterone enanthate, 1 mg

Testosterone enanthate is a hormonal drug in the androgens grouping for injection. Testosterone is used in treating male hypogonadism and delayed puberty, as it stimulates the targeted gonadal tissue to develop normally. It is also used in treating some estrogen-dependent breast cancers as it has some counter-estrogenic action in women. Testosterone enanthate is absorbed more slowly so it can be given less often than free testosterone. Doses vary from 50 to 400 mg every two to four weeks. Testosterone enanthate is administered by intramuscular injection.

J3145

J3145 Injection, testosterone undecanoate, 1 mg

Testosterone undecanoate is a Schedule II controlled substance. It is an androgen used for replacement therapy in adult males for conditions associated with a deficiency or absence of natural testosterone in primary (congenital or acquired) hypogonadism, or congenital or acquired hypogonadotropic hypogonadism. Testosterone undecanoate is an ester of testosterone mixed with refined castor oil. These facts lead to a warning about the risks of pulmonary oil microembolism reactions (POME). The drug is available only under a risk evaluation and mitigation strategy (REMS). The recommended dosage is 750 mg (3 ml) at initiation, at four weeks, and then every 10 weeks, administered by intramuscular (IM) injection into the buttock. Patients with benign prostatic hyperplasia (BPH) should be monitored for worsening signs and symptoms.

J3230

J3230 Injection, chlorpromazine HCl, up to 50 mg

Chlorpromazine hydrochloride (HCl) is used in the treatment of manic psychosis, preoperative sedation, acute intermittent porphyria, an adjunct treatment for tetanus, intractable hiccups, some behavior problems in children, and nausea and vomiting. The main pharmacological actions are psychotropic. The mechanism of action is not known. It has a sedative and antiemetic effect.

J3240

J3240 Injection, thyrotropin alpha, 0.9 mg, provided in 1.1 mg vial

Thyrotropin alpha is indicated for use as an adjunctive diagnostic tool for serum thyroglobulin (Tg) testing in the follow-up of patients with well-differentiated thyroid cancer. This may be done with or without radioiodine imaging. It contains a highly purified recombinant form of human thyroid stimulating hormone (TSH), a glycoprotein that is produced by recombinant DNA technology in Chinese hamster ovaries. A dose of 0.9 mg can be administered every day for three days. Thyrotropin alpha is administered via intramuscular injection.

J3241

J3241 Injection, teprotumumab-trbw, 10 mg

Teprotumumab-trbw is an insulin-like growth factor 1 receptor inhibitor that is indicated for the treatment of thyroid eye disease (TED), also known as Grave's ophthalmopathy or Grave's eye disease, in adult patients ages 18 years and older. Grave's disease is an autoimmune disorder that typically results in overactivity of the thyroid gland (hyperthyroidism).

Antibodies directed against receptors that are present in the thyroid gland and on the surface of the cells behind the eyes cause inflammation, swelling, and the production of muscle and fat tissue behind the eyes. Teprotumumab-trbw is supplied as a lyophilized powder in a 500 mg single dose vial. It must be reconstituted with 10 mL of sterile water to create a volume of 10.5 mL. The reconstituted solution must be further diluted in a 0.9% sodium chloride infusion bag prior to administration. Using a sterile syringe and needle, the volume equivalent of the amount of reconstituted teprotumumab-trbw to be placed in the infusion bag should be removed and discarded. The required amount of teprotumumab-trbw required should be transferred into the infusion bag with a total volume of 100 mL (less than 1800 mg dose) or 250 mL (1800 mg and greater dose) and mixed by gentle inversion. It is administered via intravenous (IV) infusion over 90 minutes for the first two infusions. Subsequent infusions may be administered over 60 minutes if tolerated. It should not be administered concurrently with other medications. It may increase blood glucose levels, and diabetic patients should be monitored closely.

J3243

J3243 Injection, tigecycline, 1 mg

Tigecycline is an antibiotic of the class glycylcycline. The drug disrupts RNA protein synthesis in bacteria, causing cellular death. Tigecycline has proven effective in drug-resistant strains of many anaerobic and aerobic, gram-negative, and gram-positive microorganisms. It is indicated in the treatment of adults, ages 18 and older, with community-acquired bacterial pneumonia, complicated skin and skin-structure infections (cSSSI), and complicated intra-abdominal infections caused by susceptible strains of bacteria. Tigecycline may be used for children over the age of 8 when alternative antibacterial drugs are not available. It should not be used for the treatment of diabetic foot infections, hospital-acquired pneumonia, or ventilator-associated pneumonia. The recommended dosage is an initial 100 mg intravenous (IV) infusion, followed by 50 mg IV infusion every 12 hours, given over 30 to 60 minutes. Duration of therapy is between five to 14 days, depending upon the condition being treated. It should not be administered concomitantly with amphotericin B, amphotericin B lipid complex, diazepam, esomeprazole, or omeprazole. A reduced dosage may be required for patients with renal impairment. See full prescribing information for complete administration instructions.

J3244

J3244 Injection, tigecycline (Accord) not therapeutically equivalent to J3243, 1 mg

Tigecycline is an antibiotic of the class glycylcycline. The drug disrupts RNA protein synthesis in bacteria, causing cellular death. Tigecycline has proven effective in drug-resistant strains of many anaerobic and aerobic, gram-negative, and gram-positive microorganisms. It is indicated in the treatment of adults, ages 18 and older, with community-acquired bacterial pneumonia, complicated skin and skin-structure infections (cSSSI), and complicated intra-abdominal infections caused by susceptible strains of bacteria. It should not be used for the treatment of diabetic foot infections, hospital-acquired pneumonia, or ventilator-associated pneumonia. The recommended dosage is an initial 100 mg intravenous (IV) infusion, followed by 50 mg IV infusion every 12 hours, given over 30 to 60 minutes. Duration of therapy is between five to 14 days, depending upon the condition being treated. It should not be administered concomitantly with amphotericin B, amphotericin B lipid complex, diazepam, esomeprazole, or omeprazole. A reduced dosage may be required for patients with renal impairment. See full prescribing information for complete administration instructions. Report J3244 only for tigecycline manufactured by Accord.

J3245

J3245 Injection, tildrakizumab, 1 mg

Tildrakizumab is an interleukin-23 (IL-23) blocker indicated for the treatment of adults, 18 years of age and older, with moderate to severe plaque psoriasis who are candidates for systemic or phototherapy. IL-23 is a cytokine involved in the normal inflammatory and immune response. Tildrakizumab binds to IL-23, inhibiting the interaction with the IL-23 receptor, and blocks the release of inflammatory cytokines. Tildrakizumab is supplied in a single-dose, prefilled syringe of 100 mg/ml. It is administered by subcutaneous injection on weeks zero and four, and every 12 weeks thereafter.

J3246

J3246 Injection, tirofiban HCl, 0.25 mg

Tirofiban hydrochloride is an antiplatelet drug used to treat or prevent blood clots. It is used to treat certain types of angina, such as acute coronary syndrome, and may also be used prophylactically prior to angiography and angioplasty procedures. Tirofiban hydrochloride is a reversible antagonist of fibrinogen binding to the GP IIb/IIIa receptor, the major platelet surface receptor involved in platelet aggregation, thereby inhibiting ex vivo platelet aggregation. Tirofiban hydrochloride is administered by intravenous infusion at a recommended infusion rate of 0.4 mcg/kg/min initially for 30 minutes and then continuing at 0.1 mcg/kg/min for the duration of the infusion.

J3250

J3250 Injection, trimethobenzamide HCl, up to 200 mg

Trimethobenzamide hydrochloride (HCl) is an antiemetic used to alleviate nausea and vomiting. The mechanism of action is not known but it appears to act on the chemoreceptor trigger zone (CTZ) in the brain where vomiting impulses are transmitted. It can be administered via intramuscular injection. Trimethobenzamide HCl also comes in capsule and suppository forms.

J3260

J3260 Injection, tobramycin sulfate, up to 80 mg

Tobramycin is an aminoglycoside antibiotic. Aminoglycoside antibiotics are those derived from various species of *Streptomyces* bacteria or produced synthetically. Aminoglycosides inhibit bacterial protein synthesis by binding with the 30S ribosomal subunit and are bactericidal. Streptomycin is derived from *Streptomyces tenebrarius*. It inhibits protein synthesis, causing cell death. Susceptibility studies should be performed prior to the administration of tobramycin. It is indicated in the treatment of infections caused by susceptible strains of gram-negative bacillary bacteria. The injectable form is administered by intramuscular injection and intravenous infusion. Dosages vary depending on the form of administration, frequency of administration, and indication. See full prescribing information for complete administration information.

J3262

J3262 Injection, tocilizumab, 1 mg

Tocilizumab is a chemical compound that is an interleukin-6 receptor inhibitor. Interleukin-6 is a protein secreted by a variety of cells to stimulate immune response to trauma or other tissue damage leading to inflammation. Tocilizumab is indicated for adult patients with moderate to severe active rheumatoid arthritis who have had an inadequate response to one or more tumor necrosis factor inhibitors. This medication may be used as monotherapy or with methotrexate or other disease modifying antirheumatic drugs. The recommended dose is 4 mg to 8 mg per kg of patient weight. The drug is administered as a 60-minute intravenous (IV) infusion.

J3265

J3265 Injection, torsemide, 10 mg/ml

Torsemide is a diuretic that is used to treat patients with heart or liver failure, hypertension, or for those with hepatic cirrhosis. Torsemide acts on the loop of Henle by enhancing excretion of sodium, water, and chloride. Torsemide injection was moved to the "Discontinued Drug Product List" of the Federal Drug Administration's (FDA) Orange Book on June 16, 2008.

J3280

J3280 Injection, thiethylperazine maleate, up to 10 mg

Thiethylperazine maleate is indicated for the relief of nausea and vomiting. The exact mechanism of action is not known. However, it appears to have an effect on the vomiting center and the chemoreceptor trigger zone (CTZ) of the brain. Recommended oral dose is 10 to 30 mg a day. Thiethylperazine maleate can be administered orally or by intramuscular injection. Recommended intramuscular injection dose is 10 mg one to three times a day. Federal Drug Administration (FDA) approval was withdrawn on June 18, 2009.

J3285

J3285 Injection, treprostinil, 1 mg

Treprostinil is a prostacyclin, an analogue of prostaglandin that is a vasodilator. The drug directly dilates pulmonary and systemic arterial beds and inhibits platelet aggregation. Treprostinil is indicated for the treatment of pulmonary arterial hypertension (PAH) patients who have New York Heart Association Class II-IV symptoms. The drug may be administered via a continuous subcutaneous infusion. If the patient cannot tolerate subcutaneous infusion, the drug may be administered via continuous intravenous infusion by a central venous line. Treprostinil may be self-administered using an infusion pump. Dosage is dependent upon the patient's body weight and the relief of symptoms.

J3299

J3299 Injection, triamcinolone acetonide (Xipere), 1 mg

Triamcinolone acetonide is a synthetic corticosteroid indicated for the treatment of adults, ages 18 years and older, with macular edema associated with uveitis. It is contraindicated for patients with active or suspected ocular or periocular infections. It is supplied in a kit containing a single dose vial of triamcinolone acetonide, a syringe with attached vial adapter, and two 30-G needles. The recommended dose is 4 mg (0.1 ml) administered via suprachoroidal injection. See full prescribing information for complete administration instructions.

J3300-J3303

J3300 Injection, triamcinolone acetonide, preservative free, 1 mg

J3301 Injection, triamcinolone acetonide, not otherwise specified, 10 mg

J3302 Injection, triamcinolone diacetate, per 5 mg

J3303 Injection, triamcinolone hexacetonide, per 5 mg

Triamcinolone is a synthetic corticosteroid, which is analogous to corticosteroids produced by the adrenal cortex. The drug is one to two times more potent than prednisone. Its mechanism of action is not clearly defined. Triamcinolone does decrease inflammation by stabilizing leukocytes, suppress the chemicals normally released in immune response, and stimulate bone marrow. Triamcinolone acetonide is a more potent derivative of triamcinolone, approximately eight times more potent than prednisone. Triamcinolone acetonide is the version most commonly used in preparations. Diacetate and hexacetonide are different formulations of triamcinolone with hexacetonide having the longest acting effect. The drug has a number of uses, including hormone replacement when the adrenal gland does not produce adequate supplies. The injectable version may be administered intramuscularly, intra-articularly, intravitreally, or intralesionally. The injectable version is indicated for the treatment of a large number of symptoms and diseases. See full prescribing information for complete administration instructions.

J3304

J3304 Injection, triamcinolone acetonide, preservative-free, extended-release, microsphere formulation, 1 mg

Triamcinolone acetonide is an extended-release injectable synthetic corticosteroid for the treatment of adults with knee pain due to moderate to severe osteoarthritis. It is embedded in biodegradable microspheres that extend the amount of time the drug stays in the joint. Once injected, the microspheres lay on the synovium, where they slowly dissolve and release into the joint in liquid form. Triamcinolone acetonide is a corticosteroid that decreases inflammation by stabilizing leukocytes, suppressing the chemicals normally released in immune response, and stimulating bone marrow. It is administered intra-articularly and should not be administered through any other route. It is supplied in a single dose kit, with a vial of triamcinolone acetonide powder, a vial of 5 mL diluent, and a sterile vial adapter. The recommended dose is 32 mg administered as a single intra-articular injection in the knee.

J3305

J3305 Injection, trimetrexate glucuronate, per 25 mg

Trimetrexate glucoronate is a nonclassical folate antagonist. It is a synthetic inhibitor of the enzyme dihydrofolate reductase (DHFR) and is used as an alternative therapy for the treatment of moderate-to-severe *Pneumocystis jirovecii* pneumonia in immunocompromised patients. It interferes with the RNA, DNA, and protein synthesis, which results in cell death. Leucovorin calcium should be given with this medication to protect the patient from life-threatening toxicities. Trimetrexate glucoronate is administered by intravenous infusion over 60 minutes.

J3310

J3310 Injection, perphenazine, up to 5 mg

Perphenazine is used in treating psychosis and severe nausea and vomiting. The mechanism of action is not known. However, it does have an effect on the entire central nervous system particularly the hypothalamus. Dose is based on the condition and response of the patient. Perphenazine is administered orally. Per the FDA, the injectable form is no longer available in the United States.

J3315

J3315 Injection, triptorelin pamoate, 3.75 mg

Triptorelin pamoate is a synthetic decapeptide agonist analog of luteinizing hormone releasing hormone (LHRH or GnRH) with greater potency than the naturally occurring LHRH. It is used in the palliative treatment of advanced prostate cancer. This medication prevents gonadotropin secretion when given continuously in therapeutic doses. After the first dose there is an increase in the luteinizing hormone (LH), follicle-stimulating hormone (FSH), testosterone, and estradiol levels. Following continuous administration, there is a persistent decrease in LH and FSH secretion. There is also a significant decrease of testicular and ovarian steroidogenesis. The reduction of serum testosterone is that usually found in surgically castrated men. Recommended dose is 3.75 mg monthly. Triptorelin pamoate is administered by intramuscular injection.

J3316

J3316 Injection, triptorelin, extended-release, 3.75 mg

Triptorelin extended release is a gonadotropin releasing hormone (GnRH) agonist used to treat central precocious puberty (CPP) in pediatric patients 2 years of age and older. CPP is a condition where sexual development starts too early in children, typically younger than 9 years of age in boys and 8 years of age in girls. Triptorelin suppresses luteinizing hormone, gonadotropins, and sex steroids to prepubertal levels. It is supplied in a powder cake that must be reconstituted with sterile water immediately prior to use. The recommended dose is 22.5 mg, administered by intramuscular injections, once every 24 weeks.

J3320

J3320 Injection, spectinomycin dihydrochloride, up to 2 g

Spectinomycin dihydrochloride is an aminocyclitol antibiotic produced by the *Streptomyces spectabilis* species of soil microorganism. Spectinomycin dihydrochloride is indicated for treatment of susceptible, drug-resistant strains of acute *N. gonorrhea*. Spectinomycin dihydrochloride works by inhibiting protein synthesis in the bacterial cell. Spectinomycin dihydrochloride is administered by intramuscular injection.

J3350

J3350 Injection, urea, up to 40 g

Urea is an organic compound of carbon, nitrogen, oxygen, and hydrogen. It is the chief nitrogenous end-product from the metabolism of proteins. Intravenous infusions of urea are used as a diuretic and to lower intracranial pressure. Intravenous urea is indicated as a treatment for fluid accumulation in the brain, high intraocular pressure, or glaucoma.

J3355

J3355 Injection, urofollitropin, 75 IU

Urofollitropin is a highly purified, follicle stimulating hormone extracted from the urine of post-menopausal women. Follicle stimulating hormone is a gonadotropic hormone produced in the anterior pituitary gland. It stimulates the growth and maturation of follicles in the ovary. Urofollitropin is used to induce ovulation in polycystic ovary disease. It is administered by subcutaneous (SC) or intramuscular (IM) injection and dosage varies depending upon the condition being treated. See full prescribing information for complete administration instructions.

J3357

J3357 Ustekinumab, for subcutaneous injection, 1 mg

Ustekinumab is a human monoclonal antibody that is a human interleuken-12 and -23 antagonist. This drug is indicated as a treatment for adult patients diagnosed with moderate to severe plaque psoriasis. The recommended dose is based on the patient's body weight and is administered via subcutaneous (SC) injection. After initial administration, the second dose is given four weeks later and then every 12 weeks thereafter. See full prescribing information for complete administration instructions.

J3358

J3358 Ustekinumab, for intravenous injection, 1 mg

Ustekinumab is a human monoclonal antibody that is a human interleuken-12 and -23 antagonist. This drug is indicated as a treatment for adult patients, ages 18 and older, diagnosed with Crohn's disease. The recommended dose is based on the patient's body weight and is administered via intravenous (IV) infusion. The initial infusion is 260 mg up to 55 kg of body weight; 390 mg for 55 kg to 85 kg; or 520 mg for weight over 85 kg. The recommended maintenance dose is 90 mg intravenously every eight weeks following the initial dose. See full prescribing information for complete administration instructions.

J3360

J3360 Injection, diazepam, up to 5 mg

Diazepam is an antianxiety drug that acts on the central nervous system (CNS). This benzodiazepine produces anxiolytic effects by aiding the action of a specific inhibitory neurotransmitter in the brain, depressing the CNS in the limbic and subcortical areas, as well as seizure activity focused in the cortex and thalamus. Diazepam is used for anxiety, acute alcohol withdrawal, muscle spasm, and before endoscopic procedures. Dosages range from 2 to 20 mg based on patient condition. Diazepam can be administered via intramuscular injection or intravenous push.

J3364-J3365

J3364 Injection, urokinase, 5,000 IU vial

J3365 Injection, IV, urokinase, 250,000 IU vial

Urokinase is urokinase-type plasminogen activator (uPA) and is a serine protease. It is a thrombolytic agent obtained from human neonatal kidney cells grown in tissue culture. Urokinase is a thrombolytic enzyme used for treatment of acute pulmonary embolism, acute coronary arterial thrombosis, and to clear thrombi from intravenous catheters. Urokinase binds to fibrin, converts plasminogen into plasmin, and breaks down the thrombus into smaller components. Urokinase is administered via intravenous infusion.

J3370

J3370 Injection, vancomycin HCl, 500 mg

Vancomycin hydrochloride is a glycopeptide antibacterial used to treat serious infections in adult and pediatric patients, including septicemia, bone infections, endocarditis, lower respiratory tract infections, and skin and skin structure infections caused by susceptible strains of bacteria. It interferes with RNA synthesis and damages the bacterial cell's plasma membrane, making it susceptible to the forces of osmotic pressure. It is administered via intravenous (IV) infusion. Dosages and frequency vary based on patient age, body weight, and disease treated, and should not be administered concomitantly with other drugs. A reduced dosage may be required for patients with renal impairment. See full prescribing information for complete administration instructions.

J3371

J3371 Injection, vancomycin HCl (Mylan) not therapeutically equivalent to J3370, 500 mg

Vancomycin HCl is a glycopeptide antibacterial used to treat serious infections in adult and pediatric patients, including septicemia, bone infections, endocarditis, lower respiratory tract infections, and skin and skin structure infections caused by susceptible strains of bacteria. It interferes with RNA synthesis and damages the bacterial cell's plasma membrane, making it susceptible to the forces of osmotic pressure. It is supplied as a lyophilized powder requiring reconstitution in single dose vials of 250 mg, 750 mg, 1.25 g, and 1.5 g strengths, and is administered via intravenous (IV) infusion. Dosages and frequency vary based on patient age, body weight, and disease treated, and should not be administered concomitantly with other drugs. A reduced dosage may be required for patients with renal impairment. See full prescribing information for complete administration instructions. Report J3371 only for vancomycin HCl manufactured by Mylan.

J3372

J3372 Injection, vancomycin HCl (Xellia) not therapeutically equivalent to J3370, 500 mg

Vancomycin HCl is a glycopeptide antibacterial used to treat serious infections in adult and pediatric patients, including septicemia, bone infections, endocarditis, lower respiratory tract infections, and skin and skin structure infections caused by susceptible strains of bacteria. It interferes with RNA synthesis and damages the bacterial cell's plasma membrane, making it susceptible to the forces of osmotic pressure. It is supplied in single dose bags of 500 mg, 750 mg, 1.25 g, 1.5 g, and 1.75 g strengths, and is administered via intravenous (IV) infusion over 60 minutes. Dosages and frequency vary based on patient age, body weight, and disease treated, and should not be administered concomitantly with other drugs. A reduced dosage may be required for patients with renal impairment. See full prescribing information for complete administration instructions. Report J3372 only for vancomycin HCl manufactured by Xellia.

J3380

J3380 Injection, vedolizumab, 1 mg

Vedolizumab is a recombinant human IgG1 monoclonal antibody produced in Chinese hamster ovaries. It binds to a human alpha 4 beta 7 integrin site and blocks the interaction of this integrin with mucosal addressin adhesion molecules. This inhibits the migration of memory T-lymphocytes across the endothelium into the inflamed gastrointestinal tissue. This interaction is thought to be an important contributor to the chronic inflammation of ulcerative colitis and Crohn's disease. Vedolizumab is indicated for adult patients with moderate to severe active ulcerative colitis or Crohn's disease who have lost response or are intolerant of tumor necrosis factor (TNF) blockers, immunomodulation or corticosteroids. Recommended dosage is 300 mg infused intravenously over 30 minutes.

J3385

J3385 Injection, velaglucerase alfa, 100 units

Velaglucerase alfa is a hydrolytic lysosomal glucocerebroside specific enzyme used in the treatment of long-term enzyme replacement therapy (ERT) for adults or pediatric patients who are diagnosed with Type 1 Gaucher disease. Gaucher disease occurs in patients who do not produce an adequate amount of an enzyme called glucocerebrosidase, which can result in harmful amounts of lipid buildup in the spleen, bones, liver, nervous system, and bone marrow and may also prevent organs and cells from functioning properly. Velaglucerase alfa is used as a replacement for another enzyme replacement therapy, imiglucerase. Velaglucerase alfa comes in the form of a lyophilized powder to be reconstituted with diluted water and is administered by intravenous infusion.

J3396

J3396 Injection, verteporfin, 0.1 mg

Verteporfin is a benzoporphyrin derivative that is a photosensitizer or light-activated drug. Verteporfin is used together with a nonthermal red laser light to treat abnormal blood vessel formation in a part of the eye that, if left untreated, can lead to a loss of eyesight. Treatment with verteporfin and laser light occurs in two steps. First, verteporfin is administered via intravenous (IV) injection over 10 minutes. Second, 15 minutes later, a laser light is directed at the affected eye. Photodynamic therapy with verteporfin is approved to treat age-related macular degeneration (AMD) with neovascular changes, known as choroidal neovascularization (CNV). CNV can be described as classic or occult, based on appearance on fluorescein angiography. CNV can also be described by its location: extrafoveal, juxtafoveal, and subfoveal. Verteporfin is indicated for patients with predominately classic subfoveal CNV due to AMD, pathologic myopia, or presumed ocular histoplasmosis. Laser light treatment must follow verteporfin injection 15 minutes after the start of the injection. Once activated, the drug is thought to create free radical formation, causing cellular damage, eventually resulting in thrombosis of the vessels, and slowing of the progression of CNV. The patient should be evaluated three months following treatment. If choroidal neovascular leakage is detected, verteporfin treatment may be repeated.

J3397

J3397 Injection, vestronidase alfa-vjbk, 1 mg

Vestronidase alfa-vjbk is a recombinant human lysosomal beta glucuronidase that is indicated for pediatric and adult patients for the treatment of Mucopolysaccharidosis VII (MPS VII, Sly syndrome.) MPS VII is a condition in which patients are lacking the beta-glucuronidase enzyme essential to breaking down mucopolysaccharides heparan sulfate, chondroitin 4- and 6-sulfates, and dermatan sulfate. These materials remain in the body's tissues, causing progressive damage. Common presentation includes hydrops fetalis, where excess fluids build up prior to birth and may cause stillbirth or death soon after birth. Other patients show symptoms in early childhood, including macrocephaly, hepatosplenomegaly, hydrocephalus, umbilical or inguinal hernias, sleep apnea, and distinctive coarse facial features, including a large tongue. Patients can also develop skeletal abnormalities that include joint contractures and a short stature. Supplied in a single dose vial, vestronidase alfa-vjbk is administered via intravenous infusion every two weeks. The recommended dosage is 4 mg/kg of body weight infused over four hours. The first 2.5% of the total volume should be infused over the first hour. After the first hour, the infusion rate can be increased as tolerated to complete the infusion over the remaining three hours. The patient should be premedicated with a non-sedating antihistamine 30 to 60 minutes prior

J

to administration. An antipyretic may be administrated if needed. Patients should be observed for signs of anaphylaxis for at least 60 minutes following infusion.

J3398

J3398 Injection, voretigene neparvovec-rzyl, 1 billion vector genomes

Voretigene neparvovec-rzyl is an adeno-associated virus vector-based gene therapy that is indicated for the treatment of adults and children, 12 months of age or older, with biallelic RPE65 mutation-associated retinal dystrophy. To be considered for treatment, the physician must determine the patient has viable retinal cells. Mutations of the retinal pigment epithelial 65 kDa protein (RPE65) cause absent or reduced levels of RPE65 isomerohydrolase activity, which results in vision impairment. The therapy delivers a normal copy of the gene encoding the human RPE65 to cells in the retina of patients who have absent or reduced levels of biologically active RPE65. It is supplied in a single dose, 2 mL vial that requires a 1:10 dilution before administration. Recommended dose for each eye is $1.5 \times 10_{11}$ vector genomes (vg) administered via subretinal injection in a total volume of 0.3 mL. Administration should be performed on each eye on separate days, but no fewer than six days apart. Oral corticosteroids should be administered 1 mg/kg/day, with a maximum of 40 mg/day, for a total of seven days beginning three days prior to the first injection to each eye, followed by a tapering dose for the next 10 days.

J3399

J3399 Injection, onasemnogene abeparvovec-xioi, per treatment, up to 5x10^15 vector genomes

Onasemnogene abeparvovec-xioi is an adeno-associated virus vector-based gene therapy that is indicated for the treatment of adults and children, 2 years of age or older, with spinal muscular atrophy (SMA) with bi-allelic mutations in the *survival motor neuron 1 (SMN1)* gene. The therapy delivers a normal copy of the gene encoding the human SMN protein, allowing for sufficient SMN protein expression. It is supplied as a suspension in a customized kit that contains two to nine vials, with a combination of two vial fill volumes of 5.5 mL or 8.3 mL. All vials contain a concentration of 2.0×10^{13} vector genomes (vg) per mL. The customized kit is shipped frozen and may be kept refrigerated up to 14 days. The recommended dosage is 1.1×10^{14} vg/kg of body weight and is administered in a single dose intravenous (IV) infusion. Systemic corticosteroids should be administered beginning the day prior to infusion and continue for a total of 30 days. See full prescribing information for corticosteroid dose adjustments following the first 30 days. Liver function tests should be performed prior to start of treatment and for at least three months after treatment. Treatment should not be used for premature neonates until they have reached full term gestational age as the required corticosteroids may affect neurological development.

J3400

J3400 Injection, triflupromazine HCl, up to 20 mg

Per the FDA, this drug is no longer available in the United States.

J3410

J3410 Injection, hydroxyzine HCl, up to 25 mg

Hydroxyzine HCl is a piperazine derivative that has central nervous system depressant, antispasmodic, antihistamine, and antifibrillatory properties. It is used in adults and children, ages 6 and older, to treat a variety of conditions such as anxiety, pruritus from allergies, psychiatric and emotional emergencies, and nausea and vomiting. It tends to increase the effect of meperidine and barbiturates. It can be administered via intramuscular injection only. Dosages and frequency vary based on patient age, body weight, and condition treated. See full prescribing information for complete administration instructions.

J3411

J3411 Injection, thiamine HCl, 100 mg

Vitamins are organic compounds that are necessary for the metabolic functioning of the body. Thiamine, also known as vitamin B1, is a water-soluble vitamin that acts by binding with adenosine triphosphate to form a coenzyme needed for carbohydrate metabolism. It is found particularly in pork, organ meats, legumes, nuts, and whole grain or enriched cereals and breads. Thiamine hydrochloride is used to treat deficiency states including beriberi, alcoholic neuritis, and Wernicke-Korsakoff syndrome. It is available in injectable and oral forms. Oral forms are sold over-the-counter in singular or combined products and are self-administered. The injectable form can be administered by intramuscular or intravenous injection.

J3415

J3415 Injection, pyridoxine HCl, 100 mg

Pyridoxine is one of the forms of vitamin B6. Vitamins are organic compounds that are necessary for the metabolic functioning of the body. Vitamin B6 is a water-soluble vitamin used by the body in the metabolism of amino acids, in the degradation of tryptophan, and in the breakdown of glycogen to glucose-1-phosphate. Pyridoxine hydrochloride is used for patients with vitamin B6 deficiency, to prevent seizures during cycloserine therapy, and as an antidote for isoniazid and cycloserine poisoning.

J3420

J3420 Injection, vitamin B-12 cyanocobalamin, up to 1,000 mcg

Vitamin B12 cyanocobalamin is a coenzyme that stimulates metabolic cell function. It is required for cell replication, hematopoiesis, and nucleoprotein and myelin production. This medication is indicated for treatment of pernicious anemia, vitamin B12 malabsorption, and/or methylmalonic aciduria. Malabsorption can be caused by many conditions including neoplasms, AIDS, Crohn's disease, parasites, and tapeworms.

J3430

J3430 Injection, phytonadione (vitamin K), per 1 mg

Phytonadione (vitamin K injection) is given to prevent hemorrhagic conditions and promote liver formation of prothrombin. Hypoprothrombinemia occurs when the body lacks vitamin K, sometimes occurring secondary to malabsorption, oral anticoagulants, drug therapy, or too much vitamin A. Phytonadione is often used for pregnant women, those who are breast-feeding, and neonates who have hemorrhagic disease or vitamin K deficiency through breast milk. Phytonadione is administered by subcutaneous injection, intramuscular injection, intravenous infusion over two or three hours, or orally.

J3465

J3465 Injection, voriconazole, 10 mg

Voriconazole is an antifungal used to treat infections of the skin, abdomen, bladder wall, kidney, and esophageal candidiasis. It inhibits an essential protein found in the mitochondria of the cell that is needed for biosynthesis. This medication is effective against species of *Aspergillus* other than *A. fumigatus, Scedosporium apiospermum* (asexual form of *Pseudallescheria boydii*), and *Fusarium* species, including *Fusarium solani,* in patients intolerant of, or refractory to, other therapy. Voriconazole is administered via intravenous infusion over one to two hours or orally.

J3470

J3470 Injection, hyaluronidase, up to 150 units

Hyaluronidase is a protein enzyme produced from purified bovine testicular tissue. Hyaluronidase is a diffusing substance that modifies the permeability of connective tissue through the hydrolysis of hyaluronic acid, a polysaccharide. Hyaluronidase hydrolyzes hyaluronic acid by splitting the glucosaminidic bond between C1 of the glucosamine moiety and C4 of glucuronic acid. This temporarily decreases the viscosity of the cellular cement and promotes diffusion of injected fluids or of localized transudates or exudates facilitating their absorption. Hyaluronidase is indicated as an adjunct to increase the absorption and dispersion of other injected drugs, for hypodermoclysis, and as an adjunct in subcutaneous urography for improving resorption of radiopaque agents.

J3471-J3472

J3471 Injection, hyaluronidase, ovine, preservative free, per 1 USP unit (up to 999 USP units)

J3472 Injection, hyaluronidase, ovine, preservative free, per 1,000 USP units

Hyaluronidase is a protein enzyme. The ovine version is manufactured from purified testicular tissue and is preservative-free. Hyaluronidase is a diffusing substance that modifies the permeability of connective tissue through the hydrolysis of hyaluronic acid, a polysaccharide. Hyaluronidase hydrolyzes hyaluronic acid by splitting the glucosaminidase bond between C1 of the glucosamine moiety and C4 of glucuronic acid. This temporarily decreases the viscosity of the cellular cement and promotes diffusion of injected fluids or of localized transudates or exudates facilitating their absorption. Hyaluronidase is indicated as an adjunct to increase the absorption and dispersion of other injected drugs, for hypodermoclysis, and as an adjunct in subcutaneous urography for improving resorption of radiopaque agents.

J3473

J3473 Injection, hyaluronidase, recombinant, 1 USP unit

Hyaluronidase is a protein enzyme. The ovine version is manufactured from purified testicular tissue and is preservative free. The recombinant version is a purified protein produced by recombinant DNA technology in Chinese hamster ovaries. Hyaluronidase is a diffusing substance that modifies the permeability of connective tissue through the hydrolysis of hyaluronic acid, a polysaccharide. Hyaluronidase hydrolyzes hyaluronic acid by splitting the glucosaminidase bond between C1 of the glucosamine moiety and C4 of glucuronic acid. This temporarily decreases the viscosity of the cellular cement and promotes diffusion of injected fluids or of localized transudates or exudates facilitating their absorption. Hyaluronidase is indicated as an adjunct to increase the absorption and dispersion of other injected drugs, for hypodermoclysis, and as an adjunct in subcutaneous urography for improving resorption of radiopaque agents.

J3475

J3475 Injection, magnesium sulfate, per 500 mg

Magnesium sulfate is used to prevent or control seizures occurring in eclampsia or pre-eclampsia, for hypomagnesemia, acute nephritis in children, uterine tetany management of paroxysmal atrial tachycardia, and for constipation. Magnesium sulfate functions as an anticonvulsant and as a fluid and electrolyte replacement. Its anticonvulsant properties are thought to come by inhibiting the release of acetylcholine at the myoneural junction and thus reducing muscle contractions.

J3480

J3480 Injection, potassium chloride, per 2 mEq

Potassium chloride is an electrolyte that is used to prevent hypokalemia, digitalis intoxication, hypokalemic familial periodic paralysis, and to treat an acute myocardial infarction. Dose is based on age, weight, and clinical condition of the patient. Potassium ions are necessary for many essential physiological functions, including the maintenance of intracellular tonicity; the transmission of nerve impulses; the contraction of cardiac, skeletal, and smooth muscle; and the maintenance of normal renal function.

J3485

J3485 Injection, zidovudine, 10 mg

Zidovudine (formerly called azidothymidine or AZT) is a synthetic nucleoside analogue used as an antiviral for the treatment of human immunodeficiency virus (HIV) infection and to prevent maternal-fetal transmission of HIV. Zidovudine incorporates itself into the DNA chain preventing elongation and stopping DNA growth. Zidovudine can be administered via intravenous infusion over one hour or orally. Recommended dose is 1mg/kg given five to six times a day by IV infusion over one hour.

J3486

J3486 Injection, ziprasidone mesylate, 10 mg

Ziprasidone mesylate is used in the treatment of schizophrenia by inhibiting both the dopamine and serotonin-2 receptors, reducing schizophrenic symptoms. Some adverse reactions may include orthostatic hypotension, dry mouth, dysmenorrhea, rash, flu-like syndrome, and/or dyspepsia. Ziprasidone is contraindicated in patients who have experienced a recent myocardial infarction (MI) or have a history of long QT (time between the beginning of the QRS [ventricular depolarization] complex and the end of the T-wave) syndrome.

J3489

J3489 Injection, zoledronic acid, 1 mg

Zoledronic acid is a bisphosphate used to slow bone breakdown, decrease the amount of calcium released from the bones into the blood, and to treat hypercalcemia of malignancy. It is indicated as a treatment and prevention for postmenopausal osteoporosis and glucosteroid-induced osteoporosis, as a treatment of Paget's disease in men and women, and to increase bone mass in men with osteoporosis. It also appears to counteract the bone mineral density loss seen in patients with multiple myeloma and bone metastases from solid tumor cancers. Hypercalcemia is an abnormally high concentration of calcium in the bloodstream and results in malignancy cases from secretions by the cancer cells that promote the release of calcium stored in the bones into the bloodstream. Zoledronic acid is administered by intravenous infusion over no less than 15 minutes.

J3490

J3490 Unclassified drugs

Report this code to represent a drug that has been administered and that does not have any other specified level I or level II HCPCS code to represent it.

J3520

J3520 Edetate disodium, per 150 mg

Edetate disodium is indicated for the treatment of severe acute hypercalcemia and digitalis toxicity. It forms chelates, which displace calcium from molecules. A stable chelate will form with any metal that has the ability to displace calcium from the molecule, a feature shared by lead, zinc, cadmium, manganese, iron, and mercury. Edetate disodium is not well absorbed in the gastrointestinal tract. It does not seem to penetrate cells and is found mainly in the extracellular fluid. Edetate disodium is administered by intravenous infusion over three or more hours.

J3530

J3530 Nasal vaccine inhalation

Report this code to represent a drug that has been administered, when the route of administration is nasal, and it does not have any other specified level I or level II HCPCS code to represent it.

J3535

J3535 Drug administered through a metered dose inhaler

Report this HCPCS code to represent a drug that has been administered through a meter does inhaler and the drug does not have any other specified level I or level II HCPCS code to represent it.

J3570

J3570 Laetrile, amygdalin, vitamin B-17

Laetrile is a compound that contains a chemical called amygdalin. Amygdalin is found in the pits of many fruits, raw nuts, and plants. It is believed that the active anticancer ingredient in laetrile is cyanide. Laetrile has shown little anticancer effects in laboratory studies, animal studies, and human studies. The side effects of laetrile are like the symptoms of cyanide poisoning. Laetrile is not approved by the Food and Drug Administration (FDA). Laetrile is given by intravenous injection.

J3590

J3590 Unclassified biologics

Report this code to represent a biologic that has been administered and does not have any other specified level I or level II HCPCS code to represent it.

J3591

J3591 Unclassified drug or biological used for ESRD on dialysis

This code reports an unclassified drug or biologic that has been administered to patients with ESRD on dialysis and for which there is no more specific HCPCS Level I or Level II code to represent it.

J7030-J7040

J7030 Infusion, normal saline solution, 1,000 cc

J7040 Infusion, normal saline solution, sterile (500 ml=1 unit)

The infusion of normal saline solution replaces electrolytes and fluid loss in hyponatremia and/or severe salt depletion. Oral tablet form is also available. Normal saline solution may cause edema or pulmonary edema if administered too rapidly. Lab values may show electrolyte imbalance.

J7042

J7042 5% dextrose/normal saline (500 ml = 1 unit)

Dextrose/normal saline is a water-soluble sugar that minimizes glyconeogenesis and promotes anabolism in patients whose oral caloric intake is limited. It is used to provide fluid replacement and caloric supplementation for patients with cirrhosis, hepatitis, high metabolic stress, and for nutritional support for patients with renal failure. Some side effects may include fever, nausea, glycosuria, weight gain, and/or osteoporosis.

J7050

J7050 Infusion, normal saline solution, 250 cc

The infusion of normal saline solution replaces electrolytes and fluid loss in hyponatremia and/or severe salt depletion. Oral tablet form is also available. Normal saline solution may cause edema or pulmonary edema if administered too rapidly. Lab values may show electrolyte imbalance.

J7060

J7060 5% dextrose/water (500 ml = 1 unit)

A 5 percent dextrose/water solution is used to replace fluid and calories in patients that are not able to maintain adequate oral intake or are restricted from doing so. Side effects may include fever, confusion, hypertension, and/or pulmonary edema. Dextrose/water is contraindicated in patients with a known allergy to corn or corn related products.

J7070

J7070 Infusion, D-5-W, 1,000 cc

D5W is 5 percent dextrose in water. A 5 percent dextrose/water solution is used to replace fluid and calories in patients that are not able to maintain adequate oral intake or are restricted from doing so. This is also known as glucose, which is the main source of energy for all cells. D5W is administered via intravenous infusion.

J7100-J7110

J7100 Infusion, dextran 40, 500 ml

J7110 Infusion, dextran 75, 500 ml

Dextran is used as a hemodiluent in extracorporeal circulation, for plasma volume expansion, and in the prevention of venous thrombosis. It is made from glucose molecules and binds to platelets, red blood cells, and the lining of the vessel walls. This decreases their capability of binding together and forming clots. Dextran is administered by intravenous infusion.

J7120

J7120 Ringers lactate infusion, up to 1,000 cc

Ringer's lactate solution, or infusion, is a replacement solution for treating fluid and electrolyte imbalance. It contains sodium, potassium, calcium, chloride, and lactate in amounts that approximate the levels found in blood plasma. Ringer's lactate is administered by intravenous infusion.

J7121

J7121 5% dextrose in lactated ringers infusion, up to 1000 cc

Lactated ringers combined with 5% dextrose is administered intravenously to provide electrolyte and caloric supplement. The mixture contains sodium, potassium, calcium, chloride, and lactate.

J7131

J7131 Hypertonic saline solution, 1 ml

Hypertonic saline solution is a high concentration of sodium chloride and is approximately eight times saltier than physiologic saline used in most hospital IVs.

J7168

J7168 Prothrombin complex concentrate (human), Kcentra, per IU of Factor IX activity

Kcentra is a concentrate of human prothrombin complex derived from pooled plasma that has been purified, heat-treated, and nanofiltered. It is indicated for the urgent reversal of acquired coagulation factor deficiency induced by vitamin K antagonists (e.g., warfarin). It is indicated only for adult patients with acute major bleeding. It is NOT indicated for use in patients who do not have acute major bleeding. Kcentra contains factors II, VII, IX, and X, and antithrombin proteins C and S. The actual potency in each vial is listed on the carton. Actual dosage is dependent on the patient's body weight and the predose internal normalized ratio (INR) value. Vitamin K should be administered concurrently with Kcentra. Repeat dosing is not recommended. Kcentra is available as a single use vial of lyophilized concentrate. The potency is derived from the factor IX content. When reconstituted, the final factor IX concentration is from 20 to 31 units per mL.

J7169

J7169 Injection, coagulation Factor Xa (recombinant), inactivated-zhzo (Andexxa), 10 mg

Coagulation Factor Xa, inactivated-zhzo is a recombinant modified human Factor Xa (FXa) protein that is indicated for patients being treated with FXa inhibitors, apixaban and rivaroxaban, when anticoagulation reversal is indicated to treat life-threatening or uncontrolled bleeding. It is not indicated for the treatment of bleeding due to any FXa inhibitors other than apixaban and rivaroxaban. It binds and sequesters FXa inhibitors and inhibits the activity of tissue factor pathway inhibitor (TFPI). It is supplied as a lyophilized powder in single use vials of 100 mg that requires reconstitution with10 mL of sterile water. Treatment is available in low- or high-dose options. The dosage recommendation for the low-dose option is four vials (400 mg) for bolus administered by intravenous (IV) infusion over 30 minutes, and five vials administered by (IV) infusion for up to 120 minutes. The dosage recommendation for the high-dose option is eight vials (800 mg) for bolus administered by IV infusion over 30 minutes, and 10 vials administered by IV infusion for up to 120 minutes. Anticoagulant treatment should be resumed as soon as medically appropriate following treatment. Patients should be monitored for signs of cardiac arrest and ischemic or thromboembolic events.

J

J7170

J7170 Injection, emicizumab-kxwh, 0.5 mg

Emicizumab-kxwh is a bispecific Factor IXa- and Factor X-directed antibody, produced in Chinese hamster ovary cells, for use in adults and children with congenital Factor VIII deficiency (hemophilia A). The drug is used for routine prophylaxis to reduce the frequency of or prevent bleeding episodes. It works by restoring the missing activated Factor VIII needed to achieve hemostasis. Emicizumab-kxwh is supplied in 30, 60, 105, and 150 mg single dose vials. The recommended dosage is 3 mg/kg of body weight administered by subcutaneous injection once weekly for the first four weeks, followed by 1.5 mg/kg of body weight administered once weekly.

J7175

J7175 Injection, Factor X, (human), 1 IU

Coagulation Factor X (human) is a plasma-derived, sterile, purified concentrate of human coagulation Factor X. It is manufactured from plasma obtained from healthy donors who have passed viral screening tests. Coagulation Factor X (human) is a lyophilized powder to be reconstituted with sterile water for intravenous administration. It contains approximately 250 IU or 500 IU of Factor X activity and the exact potency is listed on the vial label. It is indicated for adults and children over the age of 12, with hereditary Factor X deficiency, for on-demand treatment and control of bleeding episodes, and perioperative management of bleeding in patients with mild hereditary Factor X deficiency. It is administered intravenously. The dosage and duration of treatment depend on the severity of the Factor X deficiency, on the location and extent of the bleeding, and on the patient's clinical condition. The recommended dosage in IU is equal to body weight (kg) x desired Factor X rise (IU/dL or % of normal) x 0.5.

J7177

J7177 Injection, human fibrinogen concentrate (Fibryga), 1 mg

Human fibrinogen concentrate is a lyophilized fibrinogen concentrate for the treatment of acute bleeding episodes and for perioperative prophylaxis in pediatric and adult patients 12 years of age and older with congenital afibrinogenemia and hypofibrinogenemia. Fibrinogen (Factor I) is a soluble plasma protein. During the coagulation process, Factor I is converted to fibrin, a key component of a blood clot. The target fibrinogen plasma level is 100 mg/dL for minor bleeding or surgery and 150 mg/dL for major bleeding or surgery. The recommended dosage for a patient with a known baseline fibrinogen level is calculated as: Dose (mg/kg body weight = [Target level (md/dL) — measured level (mg/dL)]/1.8 (mg/dL per mg/kg body weight). The dosage for a patient with an unknown baseline fibrinogen level is 60 mg per kg of body weight. Human fibrinogen concentrate is supplied in a single use bottle containing a sterile, freeze dried preparation of highly purified fibrinogen derived from human plasma. It is administered via slow intravenous infusion at a maximum rate of 5 ml per minute.

J7178

J7178 Injection, human fibrinogen concentrate, not otherwise specified, 1 mg

Fibrinogen (Factor I) is a component in the blood that helps with clotting and is used to treat patients with congenital fibrinogen deficiency, including afibrinogenemia and hypofibrinogenemia. It is a physiological substrate of three enzymes—thrombin, Factor XIIIa, and plasmin—and is manufactured from pooled human plasma that has been purified and concentrated. During the coagulation process, its molecules are used by the thrombin, Factor XIIIa, and plasmin to produce a fibrin monomer. This monomer, along with calcium ions and Factor XIII, makes the clot stronger and more elastic. The dose is dependent on the patient's body weight, condition, and blood levels. The solution is administered by intravenous injection.

J7179

J7179 Injection, von Willebrand factor (recombinant), (Vonvendi), 1 IU VWF:RCo

Von Willebrand factor is a recombinant von Willebrand factor (VWF) indicated for treatment and control of bleeding episodes in adults diagnosed with von Willebrand disease. It is administered intravenously. For each bleeding episode, the first dose is administered with an approved recombinant (non-von Willebrand factor containing) factor VIII if factor VIII baseline levels are below 40 percent or are unknown. The recommended initial dose is 40 to 80 IU per kg of body weight. The dosage should be adjusted based on the extent and location of bleeding.

J7180

J7180 Injection, Factor XIII (antihemophilic factor, human), 1 IU

Antihemophilic factor XIII injection is used to treat a rare genetic bleeding disorder. Factor XIII is usually found in the blood platelets, monocytes, and macrophages. It helps stabilize the blood clot, give it strength, and make it more pliable and resistant to fibrinolysis. It is made from heat treated pooled human plasma and the factor XIII is concentrated. It is then sterilized and purified. Recommended dose is 40 units per kg body weight administered by IV injection every 28 days.

J7181

J7181 Injection, Factor XIII A-subunit, (recombinant), per IU

Factor XIII A-subunit (antihemophilic factor, recombinant) is a recombinant human factor XIII-A2 composed of two factor XIIIA-subunits. It is manufactured as a soluble protein in yeast, extracted and purified. No human or animal products are used in its manufacture. Factor XIII is the final enzyme in the blood coagulation process. When activated by thrombin at the site of a vessel injury, it crosslinks fibrin and other proteins in the fibrin clot. Factor XIII A-subunit is indicated for routine prophylaxis for bleeding in patients with congenital factor XIII A-subunit deficiency. The dose for routine prophylaxis is 35 IU per kilogram of body weight administered once a month.

J7182

J7182 Injection, Factor VIII, (antihemophilic factor, recombinant), (NovoEight), per IU

Turoctocog alfa (trade name NovoEight Factor VIII) is an antihemophilic factor VIII used for the treatment of adult and pediatric patients with Hemophilia A. The treatment is aimed at the control and prevention of bleeding, perioperative management, and routine prophylactic treatment to reduce bleeding episodes by replacing missing factor VIII. The dosage of turoctocog alfa varies depending upon the severity of factor VIII deficiency, location and extent of bleeding, and the clinical condition of the patient. The formula for the recommended dosage is Dosage (IU) = Body Weight (kg) x Desired Factor VIII Increase (IU/dL or % normal) x 0.5. The final dose calculated is expressed as IU/kg per IU/dL. The drug is administered by slow intravenous infusion push over two to five minutes.

J7183

J7183 Injection, von Willebrand factor complex (human), Wilate, 1 IU VWF:RCO

Von Willebrand's factor complex is a concentrated blood-clotting factor extracted from human blood, pasteurized and used to treat hemophilia A. It contains highly concentrated levels of antihemophilic/von Willebrand factors and ristocetin cofactor (vWF:RCo). It is indicated for use in adult and pediatric patients for treatment of spontaneous and trauma-induced bleeding episodes in severe von Willebrand's disease and in mild to moderate von Willebrand's disease where use of desmopressin is known or suspected to be inadequate. Other indications include the treatment of adult patients with hemophilia A (classic hemophilia). Von Willebrand's factor complex is administered by intravenous injection and can be self-administered.

J7185

J7185 Injection, Factor VIII (antihemophilic factor, recombinant) (Xyntha), per IU

Antihemophilic factor recombinant is used as a preventive measure before a surgical procedure for patients with hemophilia A (congenital factor VIII deficiency). XYNTHA does not contain plasma or albumin. The antihemophilic factor is secreted by Chinese hamster ovary cells and is grown in a culture medium that contains recombinant insulin. It does not contain von Willebrand factor and is not appropriate for patients with von Willebrand's disease. It is used as a short-term, routine prophylaxis to reduce bleeding incidences during surgery. Dose and length of treatment is based on the patient's body weight, condition, the procedure being performed, and the extent of bleeding. Antihemophilic factor recombinant is administered by IV infusion. The medication can be self-administered.

J7186

J7186 Injection, antihemophilic Factor VIII/von Willebrand factor complex (human), per Factor VIII IU

Von Willebrand's factor complex is a concentrated blood-clotting factor extracted from human blood and pasteurized. It contains highly concentrated levels of antihemophilic/von Willebrand factors. It is indicated for use in adult and pediatric patients for treatment of spontaneous and trauma-induced bleeding episodes in severe von Willebrand's disease and in mild to moderate von Willebrand's disease where use of desmopressin is known or suspected to be inadequate. Other indications include the treatment of adult patients with hemophilia A (classic hemophilia).Von Willebrand's factor complex is administered by intravenous injection and can be self-administered.

J7187

J7187 Injection, von Willebrand factor complex (Humate-P), per IU VWF:RCO

Von Willebrand's factor complex is a concentrated blood-clotting factor extracted from human blood and pasteurized used to treat hemophilia A. It contains highly concentrated levels of antihemophilic/von Willebrand factors and ristocetin cofactor (VWF:RCo). It is indicated for use in adult and pediatric patients for treatment of spontaneous and trauma-induced bleeding episodes in severe von Willebrand's disease and in mild to moderate von Willebrand's disease where use of desmopressin is known or suspected to be inadequate. Other indications include the treatment of adult patients with hemophilia A (classic hemophilia). Von Willebrand's factor complex is administered by intravenous injection and can be self-administered.

J7188

J7188 Injection, Factor VIII (antihemophilic factor, recombinant) (Obizur), per IU

This drug is a recombinant DNA derived antihemophilic factor used to treat bleeding in adults with acquired hemophilia A. Recently drugs are being introduced as a preventive treatment allowing for the preservation of normal joint function in boys and young men. Hemophilia A typically affects the male gender due to having one X chromosome while women can be carriers passing the disease on to the sons.

J7189

J7189 Factor VIIa (antihemophilic factor, recombinant), (NovoSeven RT), 1 mcg

Factor VIIa recombinant is an antihemophilic drug that is a purified protein produced by recombinant DNA technology in baby hamster kidney cells. It is a vitamin K-dependent glycoprotein that is involved in the extrinsic pathway of blood coagulation. In conjunction with tissue factor, it activates coagulation Factor X and Factor IX to Factor IXa. These factors then assist in the conversion of prothrombin to thrombin and fibrinogen to fibrin inducing local hemostasis. Factor VIIa recombinant is indicated for the treatment of bleeding episodes in hemophilia A or B patients with inhibitors to Factor VIII or Factor IX. The drug is available only in an injectable form. It should be administered as an intravenous bolus only under the direct supervision of a physician experienced in the treatment of hemophilia. The recommended dosage for hemophilia A or B patients with inhibitors varies from 35 to 120 Î¼g/kg of body weight every two hours until hemostasis is achieved, or until the treatment has been judged to be inadequate. Dosage and administration intervals are dependent upon the severity of the bleeding and patient response.

J7190-J7192

J7190 Factor VIII (antihemophilic factor, human) per IU

J7191 Factor VIII (antihemophilic factor (porcine)), per IU

J7192 Factor VIII (antihemophilic factor, recombinant) per IU, not otherwise specified

Factor VIII, antihemophilic factor is used to replace deficient clotting factor and treat bleeding in patients with hemophilia A or to prevent bleeding when surgery is needed. The desired level of factor VIII to be given is calculated from a formula multiplying body weight in kilograms by the level of desired factor VIII increase (or the percent of normal) by 0.5. The percent of normal used depends on the purpose of administration: to prevent spontaneous hemorrhage, 5 percent of normal is used; for moderate hemorrhage and minor surgery, 30 to 50 percent of normal is used. Severe hemorrhage requires 80 to 100 percent of normal antihemophilic factor. Factor VIII is administered by intravenous injection and can be self-administered.

J7193

J7193 Factor IX (antihemophilic factor, purified, nonrecombinant) per IU

Factor IX nonrecombinant is an antihemophilic drug. Factor IX nonrecombinant is a sterile, stable, lyophilized concentrate of factor IX prepared from pooled human plasma and is indicated for treatment of factor IX deficiency, also known as hemophilia B or Christmas disease. Factor IX is isolated from the source material by use of a murine monoclonal antibody, and extraneous plasma-driven proteins, including factors II, VII, and X, are removed by use of immunoaffinity chromatography. Once factor IX has been isolated and other proteins removed, the factor IX is dissociated from the monoclonal antibody and further purified, resulting in a highly purified form of factor IX. Each vial of factor IX nonrecombinant, which is administered by intravenous infusion, contains the labeled amount of factor IX activity expressed in international units (IU). One IU represents the activity of factor IX present in 1 ml of normal, pooled plasma.

J7194

J7194 Factor IX complex, per IU

Factor IX complex is an antihemophilic drug that is a sterile, dried, plasma fraction containing coagulation factors II, IX, X, and low levels of factor VII. Factors II, VII, IX, and X are the vitamin K dependent coagulation factors synthesized in the liver. Factor IX complex is indicated for treatment of factor IX deficiency, also known as hemophilia B or Christmas disease, in patients with current or impending bleeding episodes. It is also indicated for treatment of bleeding episodes in patients with hemophilia A (factor VIII deficiency) who have inhibitors to factor VIII. Factor IX complex is also used in emergency situations, usually as a secondary measure following the administration of fresh frozen plasma, to treat patients with Coumadin-induced hemorrhage when prompt reversal is required. Factor IX complex administered for these indications raises the plasma level of factor IX and restores hemostasis in patients with the listed conditions. Each vial of factor IX complex, which is administered by intravenous infusion, contains the labeled amount of factor IX activity expressed in international units (IU). One IU represents the activity of factor IX present in 1 ml of normal, pooled plasma.

J7195

J7195 Injection, Factor IX (antihemophilic factor, recombinant) per IU, not otherwise specified

Factor IX recombinant is an antihemophilic drug. Factor IX recombinant is a purified protein produced by recombinant DNA technology and indicated in the treatment of factor IX deficiency, also known as hemophilia B or Christmas disease. Indications also include control or prevention of bleeding during surgery in factor IX deficient individuals. Recombinant DNA technology involves the use of a genetically engineered animal cell line that secretes recombinant factor IX into a cell culture medium. It uses a genetically engineered Chinese hamster ovary (CHO) cell line shown to be free of infectious agents. The stored cell banks are also free of blood or plasma products. The CHO cell line secretes recombinant factor IX into a defined cell culture medium that does not contain any proteins derived from animal or human sources. The recombinant factor IX is then purified by a chromatography purification process without the use of a monoclonal antibody yielding a high-purity, active product. The potency is verified by use of in vitro clotting assay. Factor IX recombinant is administered by intravenous infusion. Each vial of factor IX recombinant contains the labeled amount of factor IX activity expressed in international units (IU).One IU represents the activity of factor IX present in 1 ml of normal, pooled plasma.

J7196

J7196 Injection, antithrombin recombinant, 50 IU

Antithrombin III is a sterile, nonpyrogenic, stable, lyophilized preparation of purified recombinant human antithrombin. Antithrombin III is normally present in human plasma and is the major plasma inhibitor of thrombin. It is produced by introducing the DNA coding sequence for human antithrombin and mammary gland DNA sequence into a genetically engineered goat and is expressed in the goat's milk. Antithrombin III is indicated for the treatment of patients with hereditary antithrombin III deficiency in connection with surgical or obstetrical procedures or when they suffer from thromboembolism. Antithrombin III is prepared from pooled units of human plasma from normal donors. Antithrombin III is administered by intravenous infusion. Each vial of antithrombin III contains the labeled amount of antithrombin III activity expressed in international units (IU).

J7197

J7197 Antithrombin III (human), per IU

Antithrombin III is a sterile, nonpyrogenic, stable, lyophilized preparation of purified human antithrombin III. Antithrombin III is normally present in human plasma and is the major plasma inhibitor of thrombin. Antithrombin III is indicated for the treatment of patients with hereditary antithrombin III deficiency in connection with surgical or obstetrical procedures or when they suffer from thromboembolism. Antithrombin III is prepared from pooled units of human plasma from normal donors. Antithrombin III is administered by intravenous infusion. Each vial of antithrombin III contains the labeled amount of antithrombin III activity expressed in international units (IU).

J7198

J7198 Antiinhibitor, per IU

Anti-inhibitor is a sterile product prepared from pooled human plasma. Anti-inhibitor contains, in concentrated form, variable amounts of activated and precursor vitamin K-dependent clotting factors. Factors of the kinin generating system are also present. The product is standardized by its ability to correct the clotting time of Factor VIII deficient plasma or Factor VIII deficient plasma that contains inhibitors to Factor VIII. Anti-inhibitor is indicated for use in patients with Factor VIII or Factor IX inhibitors who are bleeding or are to undergo surgery. Anti-inhibitor is intended to control bleeding episodes in such patients. Anti-inhibitor is administered by intravenous infusion. Anti-inhibitor is labeled with the number of Hyland Factor VIII Correctional Units that it contains. One Hyland Factor VIII Correctional Unit is that quantity of activated prothrombin complex that, upon addition to an equal volume of Factor VIII deficient or inhibitor plasma, will correct the clotting time to a normal time of 35 seconds. The recommended dosage depends on the severity of hemorrhage and ranges from 25 to 100 Hyland Factor VIII Correctional Units per kg of body weight. The dose may be repeated if no improvement is observed approximately six hours following the initial administration.

J7199

J7199 Hemophilia clotting factor, not otherwise classified

Use this code to represent a hemophilia clotting factor that has been administered and does not have any other specified level I or level II HCPCS code to represent it.

J7200

J7200 Injection, Factor IX, (antihemophilic factor, recombinant), Rixubis, per IU

Factor IX recombinant is produced from a genetically engineered Chinese hamster ovary (CHO) cell line with no human or animal proteins. The CHO cell line secretes the factor IX protein, which is then purified by chromatography. Deficiencies of factor IX, called hemophilia B or Christmas disease, is an inherited blood clotting disorder mainly affecting males. It is caused by mutations in the factor IX gene and leads to deficiency of factor IX. Factor IX recombinant, trade name Rixubis, is indicated for use in people with hemophilia B who are 16 years of age and older. It is indicated for the control and prevention of bleeding episodes, perioperative (period extending from the time of hospitalization for surgery to the time of discharge) management, and routine prophylactic use to prevent or reduce the frequency of bleeding episodes. Factor IX recombinant is administered by intravenous injection after reconstitution with sterile water. When used for the routine prevention of bleeding episodes, it is administered twice weekly.

J7201

J7201 Injection, Factor IX, Fc fusion protein, (recombinant), Alprolix, 1 IU

Factor IX (antihemophilic factor, recombinant), trade name Alprolix, is a recombinant coagulation factor IX protein that has a primary amino acid sequence identical to the human plasma derived factor IX. It is produced from a human embryonic kidney cell line that contains no animal or human protein. The drug has no human blood or preservatives. Factor IX is indicated for adults and children with hemophilia B for the control of bleeding episodes, perioperative management, or routine prophylaxis. Dosage and the duration of treatment depend upon the severity of the Factor IX deficiency, the patient's clinical condition, and the location and extent of bleeding. Recombinant antihemophilic factor IX is administered intravenously.

J7202

J7202 Injection, Factor IX, albumin fusion protein, (recombinant), Idelvion, 1 IU

Coagulation Factor IX (recombinant), albumin fusion protein (rIX-FP), is a recombinant coagulation factor IX protein that has a primary amino acid sequence identical to the human plasma derived factor IX. It is produced from a genetically engineered Chinese hamster ovary cell line that contains no animal or human protein. The drug has no human blood or preservatives. Factor IX is indicated for adults and children with hemophilia B for the control of bleeding episodes, perioperative management, or routine prophylaxis. Dosage and the duration of treatment depend upon the severity of the Factor IX deficiency, the patient's clinical condition, and the location and extent of bleeding. Recombinant antihemophilic factor IX is administered intravenously.

J7203

J7203 Injection Factor IX, (antihemophilic factor, recombinant), glycoPEGylated, (Rebinyn), 1 IU

Factor IX (antihemophilic factor, recombinant), glycopegylated, is a recombinant DNA-derived coagulation Factor IX concentrate for use in adults and children with hemophilia B for the control of bleeding episodes and perioperative management. It should not be used for routine prophylaxis. It is produced from a genetically engineered Chinese hamster ovary cell line that contains no animal or human protein. The drug has no human blood or preservatives. It is supplied as a lyophilized powder in single use vials of 500, 1,000, and 2,000 IU and is administered intravenously. For control of bleeding episodes, the recommended dose is 40 IU/kg body weight for minor and moderate bleeds, and 80 IU/kg body weight for major bleeds. Additional doses of 40 IU/kg body weight can be administered. For perioperative management, the recommended dose is 40 IU/kg body weight for minor surgery and 80 IU/kg body weight for major surgery. Repeated doses of 40 IU/kg body weight during the first week following major surgery may be given in one- to three-day intervals. After the first week, it can be extended to one dose per week until bleeding is controlled.

J7204

J7204 Injection, Factor VIII, antihemophilic factor (recombinant), (Esperoct), glycopegylated-exei, per IU

Antihemophilic factor (recombinant), glycopegylated-exei, is a recombinant DNA-derived coagulation Factor VIII concentrate indicated for use in children and adults with hemophilia A for on demand control of bleeding episodes, perioperative bleeding management, and routine prophylaxis to reduce bleeding episodes. It temporarily replaces the missing coagulation Factor VIII that is required for hemophilia A patients and should not be used for the treatment of von Willebrand disease. It is produced in Chinese hamster ovary (CHO) cells line that is purified with a series of chromatographic steps. The drug is supplied as a lyophilized powder in single use vials of 500, 1,000, 2,000, and 3,000 IU that require reconstitution with the included saline diluent. The reconstituted solutions contain 125, 250, 375, 500, or 750 IU per mL, respectively. Once reconstituted, the solution should be administered immediately via intravenous (IV) infusion over two minutes and should not be administered with any other medicinal products. For on demand control of bleeding, the recommended dosage for adolescents and adults is 40 IU/kg body weight for minor or moderate bleeds and 50 IU/kg body weight for major bleeds; for children younger than 12 years of age, 65 IU/kg for minor, moderate, or major bleeds. For perioperative bleeding management, the recommended dosage for adolescents and adults is a preoperative dose of 50 IU/kg body weight; for children younger than 12 years of age, 65 IU/kg body weight. For routine prophylaxis, the recommended dosage for adolescents and adults is 50 IU/kg body weight every four days; for children younger than 12 years of age, 65 IU/kg body weight twice weekly. Frequency of administration for all treatments is determined by the treating physician.

J7205

J7205 Injection, Factor VIII Fc fusion protein (recombinant), per IU

Factor VIII (Recombinant) Fc Fusion is a recombinant DNA derived antihemophilic factor for adult and pediatric patients with Hemophilia A. The treatment is aimed at the control and prevention of bleeding, perioperative management, and routine prophylactic treatment to reduce bleeding episodes by replacing missing factor VIII. The dosage of factor VIII (Recombinant) Fc Fusion varies depending upon the severity of factor VIII deficiency, location and extent of bleeding, and the clinical condition of the patient. The formula for the recommended dosage for bleeding episodes or perioperative management is as follows: Estimated Increment of Factor VIII (IU/dL or % of normal) = [Total Dose (IU)/body weight (kg)] x 2 (IU/dL per IU/kg) or Required Dose (IU) = Body Weight (kg) x Desired Factor VIII Rise (IU/dL or % of normal) x 0.5 (IU/kg per IU/dL). The recommended dosage for routine prophylaxis is 50 IU/kg every four days. This may be adjusted based on the patient's clinical response with a dose in the range of 25 to 65 IU/kg at three- to five-day intervals. Pediatric patients younger than 6 years may require more frequent or higher doses, up to 80 IU/kg. The drug is administered by intravenous infusion, with a bolus given first and then infusion at a rate no greater than 10 ml per minute.

J7207

J7207 Injection, Factor VIII, (antihemophilic factor, recombinant), PEGylated, 1 IU

Factor VIII (antihemophilic factor, recombinant) PEGylated is an antihemophilic factor VIII used for the treatment of adult patients and children 12 years and older with Hemophilia A. The treatment is aimed at routine prevention of bleeding episodes, reduction in number of bleeding episodes, and on demand treatment of bleeding episodes. Factor VIII (antihemophilic factor, recombinant) PEGylated should not be used for treatment of patients with von Willebrand disease. The dosage varies depending upon the severity of factor VIII deficiency, location and extent of bleeding, and the clinical condition of the patient. To determine the correct dosage, first an estimate of the increase of factor VIII (desired factor VIII rise) level must be calculated: total dose (IU)/body weight (kg) x 2 (IU/dL per IU/kg). The formula for the recommended final dosage is then calculated: dosage (IU) = Body Weight (kg) x Desired Factor VIII Increase x 0.5. The final dose calculated is expressed as IU/kg per IU/dL. The drug is administered by intravenous (IV) infusion.

J7208

J7208 Injection, Factor VIII, (antihemophilic factor, recombinant), PEGylated-aucl, (Jivi), 1 IU

Factor VIII (antihemophilic factor, recombinant), pegylated-aucl (trade name Jivi) is an antihemophilic factor VIII used for the treatment of adult and pediatric patients, ages 12 and older, with Hemophilia A (congenital Factor VIII deficiency). The treatment is aimed at the control and prevention of bleeding, perioperative management, and routine prophylactic treatment to reduce bleeding episodes by replacing missing factor VIII. It should not be used for the treatment of von Willebrand disease or in previously untreated patients (PUP). It is supplied as a lyophilized powder in single-use vials of 500, 1000, 2000, or 3000 IU and requires reconstitution with sterile water. The dosage varies depending upon the severity of factor VIII deficiency, location, and extent of bleeding, and the clinical condition of the patient. To determine the correct dosage for control of bleeding and perioperative management, first an estimate of the increase of factor VIII (desired factor VIII rise) level must be calculated: total dose (IU)/body weight (kg) x 2 (IU/dL per IU/kg). The formula for the recommended final dosage is then calculated: dosage (IU) = body weight (kg) x desired factor VIII increase (% of normal or IU/dL). The final dose calculated is expressed as IU/kg per IU/dL. The maximum recommended total dose is approximately 6000 IU per infusion. For routine prophylaxis, the initial recommended regimen is 30 to 40 IU/kg twice weekly. Based on the patient's bleeding episodes, the regimen may be adjusted to 45 to 60 IU/kg every five days. The drug is administered by intravenous infusion over one to 15 minutes, with a maximum infusion rate of 2.5 mL/min.

J7209

J7209 Injection, Factor VIII, (antihemophilic factor, recombinant), (Nuwiq), 1 IU

Factor VIII (antihemophilic factor, recombinant) is an antihemophilic factor VIII used for the treatment of adult patients, and children aged 2 years and older, with Hemophilia A. The treatment is aimed at routine prevention of bleeding episodes, reduction in number of bleeding episodes, on demand treatment of bleeding episodes, and perioperative bleeding management. Factor VIII (antihemophilic factor, recombinant) should not be used for treatment of patients with von Willebrand disease. The dosage of factor VIII varies depending upon the severity of factor VIII deficiency, location and extent of bleeding, and the clinical condition of the patient. For on-demand treatment, to determine the correct dosage, first an estimate of the increase of factor VIII (desired factor VIII rise) level must be calculated: Total dose (IU)/body weight (kg) x 2 (IU/dL per IU/kg). The formula for the recommended final dosage is then calculated: Dosage (IU) = Body Weight (kg) x Desired Factor VIII Increase x 0.5. The final dose calculated is expressed as IU/kg per IU/dL. The dosage for prophylaxis is 20 to 40 IU/kg given at two to three day intervals. The drug is administered by intravenous infusion.

J7210

J7210 Injection, Factor VIII, (antihemophilic factor, recombinant), (Afstyla), 1 IU

AFSTYLA is a purified Factor VIII protein produced in Chinese hamster ovary (CHO) cells using recombinant DNA. It replaces the missing coagulation Factor VIII needed for effective hemostasis. AFSTYLA is indicated for adults and children with hemophilia A (congenital Factor VIII deficiency) for the control and treatment of bleeding episodes, routine prophylaxis, and for perioperative management of bleeding. For adults and adolescents (≥12 years), the recommended starting regimen is 20 to 50 IU per kg administered two to three times weekly. The dosage may be adjusted based on patient response.

J7211

J7211 Injection, Factor VIII, (antihemophilic factor, recombinant), (Kovaltry), 1 IU

KOVALTRY is a recombinant, full length Factor VIII protein derived from human DNA sequence. It replaces the missing coagulation Factor VIII needed for effective hemostasis. It is indicated for adults and children with hemophilia A (congenital Factor VIII deficiency) for the control and treatment of bleeding episodes, routine prophylaxis, and for perioperative management of bleeding. It should not be used for the treatment of von Willebrand disease. KOVALTRY is supplied as lyophilized powder in single use vials, and must be reconstituted with the prefilled solution in the package. For routine prophylaxis in adults and adolescents (≥12 years), the recommended starting regimen, administered through intravenous infusion, is 20 to 40 IU per kg administered two to three times weekly. For children ≤12 years, 25 to 50 IU per kg is administered two to three times weekly. For the control of bleeding episodes and perioperative management: Required dose (IU) = body weight (kg) x desired Factor VIII rise (% of normal or IU/dL) x reciprocal of expected/observed recovery (e.g., 0.5 for a recovery of 2 IU/dL per IU/kg). Required dose (IU) = body weight (kg) x desired Factor VIII rise (% of normal or IU/dL) x reciprocal of expected/observed recovery (e.g., 0.5 for a recovery of 2 IU/dL per IU/kg).

J7212

J7212 Factor VIIa (antihemophilic factor, recombinant)-jncw (Sevenfact), 1 mcg

Factor VIIa (antihemophilic factor, recombinant)-jncw is indicated for the treatment and control of bleeding episodes occurring in adults and adolescents, 12 years of age and older, with hemophilia A or B with inhibitors. Indicated for intravenous (IV) use and dosed according to the severity of the bleeds, its active ingredient is a recombinant analog of human coagulation factor VIIa. Treatment should be initiated as soon as a bleeding event occurs; frequency and duration are based on the patient's clinical response and evaluation of hemostasis. This code reports 1 microgram.

J7294-J7295

J7294 Segesterone acetate and ethinyl estradiol 0.15 mg, 0.013 mg per 24 hours; yearly vaginal system, ea

J7295 Ethinyl estradiol and etonogestrel 0.015 mg, 0.12 mg per 24 hours; monthly vaginal ring, ea

These codes report the contraceptive supply of a hormone containing vaginal ring. Unlike the daily contraceptive pill, hormone containing vaginal rings are used on a monthly basis. The ring is inserted once a month in the vaginal wall and stays in place for about three weeks depending on the product used. During this time, the contraceptive medication releases a dose of hormones needed to prevent pregnancy. The patient usually takes a week break before inserting a new ring. The hormones released from the ring prevent the ovaries from producing mature eggs. The hormones are absorbed by the vaginal walls and distributed in the bloodstream. Report J7294 for the supply of segesterone acetate/ethinyl estradiol (0.15 mg/0.013 mg). Report J7295 for ethinyl estradiol/etonogestrel (0.015 mg/0.12 mg).

J7296

J7296 Levonorgestrel-releasing intrauterine contraceptive system, (Kyleena), 19.5 mg

Levonorgestrel-releasing intrauterine contraceptive system consists of a T-shaped polyethylene frame, or T-body, and a steroid reservoir with 19.5 mg of levonorgestrel (LNG). The reservoir is attached to the vertical arm of the device and is covered with a membrane that allows release of levonorgestrel at a rate of approximately 17.5 mcg per day after 24 days. The release rate progressively decreases to 9.8 mcg/day after one year and 7.4 mcg/day after five years. The device is distinguished by blue removal threads and a silver ring that is visible on ultrasound. A physician must fit the device into the uterus. It is an effective, long-acting, reversible contraceptive with an effective life span of five years. After five years, it must be removed and replaced if continued contraception via the device is desired. Report this code for Kyleena.

J7297-J7298

J7297 Levonorgestrel-releasing intrauterine contraceptive system (Liletta), 52 mg

J7298 Levonorgestrel-releasing intrauterine contraceptive system (Mirena), 52 mg

Levonorgestrel-releasing intrauterine contraceptive system consists of a Nova T-device and a Silastic rod impregnated with 52 mg of levonorgestrel. The silastic rod is attached to the vertical arm of the device and is covered with a rate limiting silastic membrane that allows release of progestin levonorgestrel at a constant rate of 20 mcg per day directly to the lining of the uterus. The device is a combination hormonal and intrauterine method of birth control. The device appears to work by suppressing the production of human chorionic gonadotropin, thereby preventing fertilization. A physician must fit the device into the uterus. It is an effective, long-acting, reversible contraceptive, with an effective life span of three to five years. After five years, it must be removed and replaced. Report J7297 for the Liletta device and J7298 for the Mirena device.

J7300

J7300 Intrauterine copper contraceptive

An intrauterine copper contraceptive, also called the copper IUD, is a long-term, reversible, method of birth control that is comparable to oral contraceptives and tubal ligation in efficacy. This is an alternative choice for women who do not use hormonal contraceptives due to smoking or other conditions that contraindicate their use. The contraceptive device is about the size of a quarter in a T-shape, made of soft, flexible plastic with copper, and is designed to fit in the uterus. The physician inserts in the device, which requires no further attention outside of monthly chain checks and may be left in for continuous use up to 10 years. The copper IUD may be removed at any time. Use of this device is contraindicating in women with pelvic inflammatory disease (PID) or any history of PID.

J7301

J7301 Levonorgestrel-releasing intrauterine contraceptive system (Skyla), 13.5 mg

A levonorgestrel-releasing intrauterine contraceptive system contains 13.5 mg of levonorgestrel, a progestin, in a T-shaped polyethylene frame, or T-body, with a steroid reservoir that provides an initial release rate of about 14 mcg/day of LNG after 24 days. The rate decreases to 5 mcg/day after three years, its expected life. Use this code for SKYLA.

J7304

J7304 Contraceptive supply, hormone containing patch, each

A birth control patch is applied to the skin and releases hormones through the skin into the bloodstream to prevent pregnancy. The progesterone and estrogen prevents ovulation (mature eggs are not produced). The patch will also thicken the mucus produced in the cervix making it difficult for sperm to enter and reach an egg that may have been released. The hormones may also affect the lining of the uterus so that if an egg is fertilized it may have a hard time attaching itself to the wall of the uterus. The patch must be placed on the skin on the first day of the menstrual cycle (there may be differences with difference suppliers of birth control patches). The patch should only be applied to one of four areas: abdomen, buttocks, upper arm, or upper torso, except for the breasts. The patch is worn for three weeks and no patch for the fourth week. Follow all manufacturers' instructions.

J7306

J7306 Levonorgestrel (contraceptive) implant system, including implants and supplies

Levonorgestrel is a synthetic hormone used as contraception in females. A long-term administration is available as an implant system. Typically, the contraceptive is available as a kit of soft plastic capsules, which are imbedded under the skin of the upper arm. Depending on the kit selected, one, two, or up to six rods may be inserted. A small subdermal incision is made and a trocar is used to deliver each matchstick-sized capsule. The six capsules are arranged in a fanlike manner to facilitate drug dispersion and later removal of the capsules. The drug diffuses gradually through the walls of the capsule into the bloodstream. Protection can last up to five years with the six-capsule system. Fertility is restored within weeks upon removal of the implants.

J7307

J7307 Etonogestrel (contraceptive) implant system, including implant and supplies

An etonogestrel implant system is a progestin-only female contraceptive that is implanted under the skin. Once the rod is implanted under the skin, it slowly releases the hormone that can prevent pregnancy for a period of up to 3 years. This is a completely reversible method of contraception. The implant system works in three ways: first, it suppresses ovulation; second, the hormone increases the thickness of the cervical mucus in order to prevent the egg from implanting itself into the uterine wall; third, the hormone alters that inner lining of the uterus also in an effort to prevent the egg from implanting itself.

J7308

J7308 Aminolevulinic acid HCl for topical administration, 20%, single unit dosage form (354 mg)

Aminolevulinic acid hydrochloride is a topical solution that photosensitizes the skin to which it is applied. It is applied topically, directly on the individual lesions. Aminolevulinic acid hydrochloride is used in conjunction with blue light photodynamic therapy applied 14 to 18 hours later. This photodynamic therapy is indicated as a treatment for nonhyperkeratotic actinic keratoses of the face or scalp. This drug should not be applied to the eyes or mucous membranes. Actinic keratoses are precancerous skin lesions, appearing as scaly red or brown patches of skin, which if left untreated may become malignant.

J7309

J7309 Methyl aminolevulinate (MAL) for topical administration, 16.8%, 1 g

Methyl aminolevulinate (MAL) is a topical cream that is used in addition to red light photodynamic therapy. Photodynamic therapy is used to treat nonhyperkeratotic, nonpigmented actinic keratoses of the face and scalp. The treatment sessions are provided once a week for two weeks. Recommended dose of MAL is not more than 1 gram per treatment session. The lesion is prepped by removing scales and crust with a dermal curette and the cream is applied about 1 mm thick to the lesion and surrounding normal tissue. The lesion is covered with an occlusive dressing for three hours prior to the light treatment. The photodynamic illumination is targeted at the treated lesion for about seven to 10 minutes. Nitrile gloves should be worn when handling the cream.

J7310

J7310 Ganciclovir, 4.5 mg, long-acting implant

Ganciclovir implant is an antiviral indicated for the treatment of cytomegalovirus (CMV) retinitis in individuals with acquired immune deficiency syndrome (AIDS). The ganciclovir implant does not cure the CMV retinitis; however, it does keep the infection under control and can help to prevent the CMV retinitis from worsening. The implant is surgically inserted. The ganciclovir is released into the eye over a five to eight month period after which it is surgically removed. At the time of removal, another ganciclovir implant may be inserted to provide ongoing treatment for the CMV retinitis. The implants contain a minimum of 4.5 mg of ganciclovir.

J7311

J7311 Injection, fluocinolone acetonide, intravitreal implant (Retisert), 0.01 mg

The fluocinolone acetonide intravitreal implant is a tablet designed to slowly release the synthetic corticosteroid fluocinolone to the posterior segment of the eye. It must be placed via a surgical incision into the ciliary disk or pars plana. Each tablet contains 0.59 mg of fluocinolone acetonide. The implant is indicated for the treatment of chronic noninfectious uveitis affecting the posterior segment of the eye. It is contraindicated in most viral diseases, vaccina, varicella, mycobacterial and fungal eye infections. The fluocinolone acetonide implant has a life of approximately 30 months. If uveitis recurs, the implant may be replaced.

J7312

J7312 Injection, dexamethasone, intravitreal implant, 0.1 mg

Dexamethasone intravitreal implant is a corticosteroid indicated for the treatment of macular edema following branch retinal vein occlusion or central retinal vein occlusion, and for the treatment of noninfectious uveitis affecting the posterior segment of the eye. Each intravitreal implant contains 0.7 mg of dexamethasone.

J7313

J7313 Injection, fluocinolone acetonide, intravitreal implant (Iluvien), 0.01 mg

Fluocinolone acetonide intravitreal implant is a non-bioerodible synthetic corticosteroid delivered by intravitreal injection inferior to the optic disc and posterior to the equator of the eye. This drug implant is used to treat diabetic macular edema in patients who have had prior treatment with corticosteroids and did not have a substantial rise of intraocular pressure. The implant contains 0.19 mg of fluocinolone acetonide, and is designed to release the drug over the course of three years. This code reports 0.01 mg of the drug; therefore, 19 units should be reported per implant. Per CMS, this code is to be used specifically for Iluvien (trade name) and should not be used to report any other brand of fluocinolone acetonide implant.

J7314

J7314 Injection, fluocinolone acetonide, intravitreal implant (Yutiq), 0.01 mg

Fluocinolone acetonide intravitreal implant is indicated for the treatment of adults, 18 years of age and older, with chronic noninfectious uveitis affecting the posterior segment of the eye. It is supplied as a nonbioerodible tablet, in a preloaded applicator that is designed to slowly release a synthetic corticosteroid fluocinolone. The implant must be placed via an intravitreal injection under adequate anesthesia. Each tablet contains 0.18 mg of fluocinolone acetonide. It is contraindicated in most viral diseases, vaccinia, varicella, mycobacterial, and fungal eye infections. The fluocinolone acetonide implant initially delivers 0.25 mcg per day and has a life of approximately 36 months. Patients should be monitored for increased intraocular pressure and signs of endophthalmitis. If uveitis recurs, the implant may be replaced.

J7315

J7315 Mitomycin, opthalmic, 0.2 mg

Mitomycin is an antibiotic isolated from the bacterium *Streptomyces verticillus Yingtanensis.* It selectively inhibits DNA synthesis. Ophthalmic mitomycin is an antimetabolite indicated for use as an adjunct to glaucoma surgery. It is not intended for intraocular administration, which can severely damage the eye. The ophthalmic mitomycin is intended for topical application at the site of glaucoma filtration surgery.

J7316

J7316 Injection, ocriplasmin, 0.125 mg

Ocriplasmin is a proteolytic enzyme (or proteinase) that breaks down the long chain proteins into peptides and eventually into amino acids. Its activity is directed against the protein components of the vitreous body and the vitreoretinal interface where it dissolves the vitreomacular adhesions. Ocriplasmin is a truncated version of human plasmin produced by recombinant DNA technology created in yeast *Pichia pastoris.* Ocriplasmin is indicated for the treatment of symptomatic vitreomacular adhesion, which is a progressive sight-threatening condition. It is for intravitreal injection only. Recommended dosage is 0.125 mg as a single dose to the affected eye.

J7318

J7318 Hyaluronan or derivative, Durolane, for intra-articular injection, 1 mg

Hyaluronan, also known as hyaluronic acid or hyaluronate, is a glycosaminoglycan, a high-molecular-mass polysaccharide found in the extracellular matrix that is widely distributed throughout connective, epithelial, and neural tissues. Hyaluronan has various physiological functions in the intercellular matrix, providing a significant contribution to cell proliferation and migration. Hyaluronan is anchored firmly in the plasma membrane or bound via hyaluronan-specific binding proteins (receptors). These receptors have been identified on many different cells. Hyaluronan is a major component of synovial fluid and articular cartilage. In the cartilage, it coats each chondrocyte cell providing resilience. Hyaluronan is injected directly into the knee joint to supplement the knee joint's natural synovial fluid, relieving pain and improving use of the knee. This treatment is also called viscosupplementation. Hyaluronan is used to treat osteoarthritis of the knee that has not improved with other treatments, such as analgesics and physical therapy. Hyaluronan described by J7318 is for a single, intra-articular injection of the knee. It is supplied in a single use, 3 ml syringe.

J7320-J7325

J7320 Hyaluronan or derivative, GenVisc 850, for intra-articular injection, 1 mg

J7321 Hyaluronan or derivative, Hyalgan, Supartz or Visco-3, for intra-articular injection, per dose

J7322 Hyaluronan or derivative, Hymovis, for intra-articular injection, 1 mg

J7323 Hyaluronan or derivative, Euflexxa, for intra-articular injection, per dose

J7324 Hyaluronan or derivative, Orthovisc, for intra-articular injection, per dose

J7325 Hyaluronan or derivative, Synvisc or Synvisc-One, for intra-articular injection, 1 mg

Hyaluronan, also known as hyaluronic acid or hyaluronate, is a glycosaminoglycan, which is a high-molecular-mass polysaccharide found in the extracellular matrix that is widely distributed throughout connective, epithelial, and neural tissues. Hyaluronan has various physiological functions in the intercellular matrix, providing a significant contribution to cell proliferation and migration. Hyaluronan is anchored firmly in the plasma membrane or bound via hyaluronan-specific binding proteins (receptors). These receptors have been identified on many different cells. Hyaluronan is a major component of synovial fluid and articular cartilage. In the cartilage, it coats each chondrocyte cell providing resilience. Hyaluronan described by J7320, J7322, J7323, and J7324 is derived from purified bacterial cells. Hyaluronan described by J7321 and J7325 is derived from avian hyaluronan. Hyaluronan is injected directly into the knee joint to supplement the knee joint's natural synovial fluid, relieving pain and improving use of the knee. This treatment is also called visco supplementation. Hyaluronan is used to treat osteoarthritis of the knee that has not improved with other treatment, such as analgesics and physical therapy. Treatment includes three or five shots into the knee joint over three to five weeks. Some study results have indicated improved symptoms of osteoarthritis and joint function, while other studies have been inconclusive about the effectiveness of hyaluronan injections.

J7326

J7326 Hyaluronan or derivative, Gel-One, for intra-articular injection, per dose

Hyaluronan, also known as hyaluronic acid or hyaluronate, is a glycosaminoglycan, which is a high-molecular-mass polysaccharide found in the extracellular matrix that is widely distributed throughout connective, epithelial, and neural tissues. Hyaluronan has various physiological functions in the intercellular matrix providing a significant contribution to cell proliferation and migration. Hyaluronan is anchored firmly in the plasma membrane or bound via hyaluronan-specific binding proteins (receptors). These receptors have been identified on many different cells. Hyaluronan is a major component of synovial fluid and articular cartilage. In the cartilage, it coats each chondrocyte cell providing resilience. This code describes a derivative from avian hyaluronan. In this product, strands of hyaluronan are cross-linked or bound to each other with cinnamic acid, which increases its viscoelasticity. Hyaluronan is injected directly into the knee joint to supplement the knee joint's natural synovial fluid, relieving pain and improving use of the knee. This treatment is also called visco supplementation. Hyaluronan is used to treat osteoarthritis of the knee that has not improved with other treatment, such as analgesics and physical therapy. Treatment is one injection into the knee joint. Some study results have indicated improved symptoms of osteoarthritis and joint function, while other studies have been inconclusive about the effectiveness of hyaluronan injections.

J7327

J7327 Hyaluronan or derivative, Monovisc, for intra-articular injection, per dose

Monovisc is a high molecular weight hyaluronic acid. It is intended to deliver a single injection to supplement the synovial fluid of an osteoarthritic knee joint. This injection treats the pain and improves joint stability. The hyaluronic acid is derived from bacterial fermentation in *Streptococcus equi* cells and is ultra-purified. The drug is supplied in prefilled 5 ml syringes containing 4 ml of Monovisc. Recommended dosage is one syringe.

J7328

J7328 Hyaluronan or derivative, GELSYN-3, for intra-articular injection, 0.1 mg

Hyaluronan, also known as hyaluronic acid or hyaluronate, is a glycosaminoglycan or a high-molecular-mass polysaccharide found in the extracellular matrix that is widely distributed throughout connective, epithelial, and neural tissues. Hyaluronan has various physiological functions in the intercellular matrix, providing a significant contribution to cell proliferation and migration. Hyaluronan is anchored firmly in the plasma membrane or bound via hyaluronan-specific binding proteins (receptors). These receptors have been identified on many different cells. Hyaluronan is a major component of synovial fluid and articular cartilage. In the cartilage, it coats each chondrocyte cell providing resilience. Hyaluronan is injected directly into the knee joint to supplement the knee joint's natural synovial fluid, relieving pain and improving use of the knee. This treatment is also called visco supplementation. Hyaluronan is used to treat osteoarthritis of the knee that has not improved with other treatments, such as analgesics and physical therapy. Treatment includes three or five shots into the knee joint over three to five weeks. Some study results have indicated improved symptoms of osteoarthritis and joint function, while other studies have been inconclusive about the effectiveness of hyaluronan injections.

J7329

J7329 Hyaluronan or derivative, Trivisc, for intra-articular injection, 1 mg

Hyaluronan, also known as hyaluronic acid or hyaluronate, is a glycosaminoglycan, a high-molecular-mass polysaccharide found in the extracellular matrix widely distributed throughout connective, epithelial, and neural tissues. Hyaluronan has various physiological functions in the intercellular matrix, providing a significant contribution to cell proliferation and migration. Hyaluronan is anchored firmly in the plasma membrane or bound via hyaluronan-specific binding proteins (receptors). These receptors have been identified on many different cells. Hyaluronan is a major component of synovial fluid and articular cartilage. In the cartilage, it coats each chondrocyte cell providing resilience. Hyaluronan is injected directly into the knee joint to supplement the knee joint's natural synovial fluid, relieving pain and improving use of the knee. This treatment is also called viscosupplementation. Hyaluronan is used to treat osteoarthritis of the knee that has not improved with other treatments, such as analgesics and physical therapy. Hyaluronan described by J7329 is for a single, intra-articular injection of the knee. It is supplied in a single use, 2.5 ml syringe.

J7330

J7330 Autologous cultured chondrocytes, implant

Autologous cultured chondrocytes, also known as Carticel, are a type of cartilage tissue graft indicated for the repair of cartilage defects of the knee, including meniscal knee injuries, osteochondritis dissecans, chondromalacia, and other disorders of cartilage of the knee. Autologous cultured chondrocytes are derived from healthy cartilage tissue cells that are harvested from the patient. The harvested cells are sent to a laboratory and grown in a tissue culture. The cultured chondrocytes are then implanted into the patient's knee at the site of the injury or defect by periosteal injection. The amount of autologous cultured chondrocytes needed to repair damaged knee cartilage varies and is dependent on the size of the damaged area. Most patients receive between 0.64 million and 3.3 million cells for each square centimeter of damaged area.

J7331

J7331 Hyaluronan or derivative, SYNOJOYNT, for intra-articular injection, 1 mg

Hyaluronan, also known as hyaluronic acid or hyaluronate, is a glycosaminoglycan, a high-molecular-mass polysaccharide found in the extracellular matrix that is widely distributed throughout connective, epithelial, and neural tissues. Hyaluronan has various physiological functions in the intercellular matrix, providing a significant contribution to cell proliferation and migration. Hyaluronan is anchored firmly in the plasma membrane or bound via hyaluronan-specific binding proteins (receptors). These receptors have been identified on many different cells. Hyaluronan is a major component of synovial fluid and articular cartilage. In the cartilage, it coats each chondrocyte cell providing resilience. Hyaluronan is injected directly into the knee joint to supplement the knee joint's natural synovial fluid, relieving pain and improving use of the knee. This treatment is also called viscosupplementation. Hyaluronan is used to treat osteoarthritis of the knee that has not improved with other treatments, such as analgesics and physical therapy. Hyaluronan described by J7331 is for a single, intra-articular injection of the knee (trade name SYNOJOYNT). It is supplied in a single use, 3 ml syringe, containing 2 ml of hyaluronan. A series of injections should be administered one week apart for a total of three injections.

J7332

J7332 Hyaluronan or derivative, Triluron, for intra-articular injection, 1 mg

Hyaluronan, also known as hyaluronic acid or hyaluronate, is a glycosaminoglycan, a high-molecular-mass polysaccharide found in the extracellular matrix that is widely distributed throughout connective, epithelial, and neural tissues. Hyaluronan has various physiological functions in the intercellular matrix, providing a significant contribution to cell proliferation and migration. Hyaluronan is anchored firmly in the plasma membrane or bound via hyaluronan-specific binding proteins (receptors). These receptors have been identified on many different cells. Hyaluronan is a major component of synovial fluid and articular cartilage. In the cartilage, it coats each chondrocyte cell providing resilience. Hyaluronan is injected directly into the knee joint to supplement the knee joint's natural synovial fluid, relieving pain and improving use of the knee. This treatment is also called viscosupplementation. Hyaluronan is used to treat osteoarthritis of the knee that has not improved with other treatments, such as analgesics and physical therapy. Hyaluronan described by J7332 is for a single, intra-articular injection of the knee (trade name Triluron). It is supplied in a single use syringe or single uses vials of 2 ml of hyaluronan. A series of injections should be administered one week apart for a total of three injections.

J7336

J7336 Capsaicin 8% patch, per sq cm

A capsaicin patch is a localized dermal delivery system. It is a synthetic version of the natural occurring substance found in chili peppers. Capsaicin is an irritant that causes sensation of heat and pain. The capsaicin selectively binds to a protein known as TRPV1 (i.e., capsaicin receptor) that resides on pain and heat sensing neurons. When capsaicin binds to TRPV1, it overwhelms the neuron and depletes one of the neurotransmitters for pain and heat. Neurons that do not contain TRPV1 are unaffected. The capsaicin patch is indicated to relieve the pain of postherpetic neuralgia caused by shingles.

J7340

J7340 Carbidopa 5 mg/levodopa 20 mg enteral suspension, 100 ml

Parkinson's disease is thought to be caused by a depletion of dopamine in brain tissue. On its own, dopamine cannot cross the blood-brain barrier. Levodopa, a precursor to dopamine, can cross the blood-brain barrier and is presumably converted to dopamine in the brain. Carbidopa inhibits the breakdown of the levodopa. The combination of carbidopa and levodopa is indicated for treatment of the symptoms of idiopathic Parkinson's disease, postencephalitic Parkinsonism, and symptomatic parkinsonism. This code represents an enteral suspension of 5 mg carbidopa and 20 mg levodopa.

J7342

J7342 Instillation, ciprofloxacin otic suspension, 6 mg

Ciprofloxacin otic suspension is a fluoroquinolone antibacterial used for the treatment of pediatric patients with bilateral otitis media with effusion who are undergoing tympanostomy tube placement. The drug is administered through intratympanic instillation via a 20 to 24 gauge, 2 to 3 inch, blunt, flexible needle. The recommended dosage is 0.1 ml (6 mg) into each affected ear, following the suctioning of middle ear effusion.

J7345

J7345 Aminolevulinic acid HCl for topical administration, 10% gel, 10 mg

Aminolevulinic acid hydrochloride is a topical solution that photosensitizes the skin to which it is applied. It is applied topically, directly on the individual lesions. Aminolevulinic acid hydrochloride is used in conjunction with red light photodynamic therapy, which is applied three hours later. This photodynamic therapy is indicated as a treatment for non-hyperkeratotic actinic keratoses of the face or scalp. This drug should not be applied to the eyes or mucous membranes. Actinic keratoses are precancerous skin lesions, appearing as scaly red or brown patches of skin, which if left untreated may become malignant.

J7351

J7351 Injection, bimatoprost, intracameral implant, 1 mcg

Bimatoprost intracameral implant is a prostaglandin analog that is indicated for the treatment of intraocular pressure (IOP) in patients with open angle glaucoma (OAG) or ocular hypertension (OHT). The implant contains 10 mcg bimatoprost and is designed to release the drug over the course of several months and slowly biodegrades in the eye. It is supplied in a prefilled applicator. It is administered via intracameral implant performed under magnification. The eye should not be dilated prior to the procedure. The needle of the applicator should be advanced through the cornea and into the anterior chamber with the needle bevel, parallel to the iris plane and adjacent to the limbus, visible through clear cornea into the superotemporal quadrant. The needle should be inserted two bevel lengths and the bevel should be completely within the anterior chamber. Placement directly over the pupil should be avoided. Once the needle is in place, the back half of the actuator button should be firmly pressed until and audible or palpable click in noted to release the implant. After release, the needle should be withdrawn via the same track it was inserted and tamponade the opening. Ensure the implant is not in the corneal injection track. The injection site should be checked for leaks and to ensure it has self-sealed. The patient must remain upright for at least one hour following the procedure. A bimatoprost intracameral implant should not be readministered to an eye that has received a previous bimatoprost intracameral implant.

J7352

J7352 Afamelanotide implant, 1 mg

The afamelanotide implant, a hormonal therapy intended for subcutaneous/intradermal administration, is a melanocortin 1 receptor (MC1-R) agonist. It is indicated to increase pain-free light exposure in adult patients with a history of phototoxic reactions from erythropoietic protoporphyria (EPP), a rare inherited metabolic disorder whose major symptom is hypersensitivity of the skin to sunlight and some types of artificial light, such as fluorescent lights. Using an implantation cannula, a single implant is inserted subcutaneously above the anterior supra-iliac crest every two months.

J7402

J7402 Mometasone furoate sinus implant, (Sinuva), 10 mcg

The Sinuva (brand name) sinus implant is a treatment for nasal polyps with resultant congestion and nasal obstruction in adult patients, 18 years and older, who have previously undergone ethmoid sinus surgery. The device is implanted via a delivery system through the nasal opening under endoscopic visualization and local anesthesia during a routine office visit. The implant expands in the ethmoid sinus. It contains 1,350 mcg of mometasone furoate and delivers a sustained release of this corticosteroid directly to the nasal polyps over a 90-day period. The implant may be removed using surgical instruments on or before day 90.

J7500-J7501

J7500 Azathioprine, oral, 50 mg

J7501 Azathioprine, parenteral, 100 mg

Azathioprine is an immunosuppressant used to prevent rejection of kidney transplants. It is also indicated to treat severe rheumatoid arthritis when other medications and treatments have not helped. Less frequently, azathioprine is used to treat ulcerative colitis. Azathioprine is available in oral and injectable forms. Its mechanism of action is not known. The drug suppresses hypersensitivities of the cell-mediated type and causes variable alterations in antibody production.

J7502

J7502 Cyclosporine, oral, 100 mg

Cyclosporine is used to prevent rejection of skin, pancreas, kidney, liver, heart, small intestine, and bone marrow transplants. When a patient receives an allogenic tissue or organ transplant, lymphocytes in the allograft recipient recognize the foreign tissue and attack the transplanted tissue or organ. Cyclosporine can also be used to treat rheumatoid arthritis that is not responding to methotrexate and severe psoriasis. The exact mechanism of action is not known. T-lymphocytes are preferentially inhibited. The 1-helper cell is the primary target, but the 1-suppressor cell may also be suppressed. Cyclosporine also inhibits lymphokine production and release, including interleukin-2 or 1-cell growth factor (TCGF). It should be administered with adrenal corticosteroids but not with other immunosuppressive agents.

J7503

J7503 Tacrolimus, extended release, (Envarsus XR), oral, 0.25 mg

Tacrolimus is used to reduce the risk of rejection by the body of liver and kidney allogeneic transplants and of bone marrow transplants, usually used with corticosteroids. Recent trials show it to be effective in managing heart, pancreas, pancreatic island cell transplants, and small bowel disease patients. Tacrolimus prevents rejection by impeding T lymphocyte cells, cells that are in the immune system. A lower dose can be used than with cyclosporine because of its potency. Tacrolimus should not be used at the same time as cyclosporine. The current drug should be stopped at least 24 hours before beginning the other one. Tacrolimus can be administered orally, topically, or via intravenous infusion.

J7504

J7504 Lymphocyte immune globulin, antithymocyte globulin, equine, parenteral, 250 mg

Lymphocyte immune globulin, antithymocyte globulin helps to prevent organ rejection in renal allograft transplant patients. It is given at the time of rejection or as an adjunct with other immunosuppressants to delay onset of the first rejection episode. It reduces the number of thymus-dependent lymphocytes and changes the T lymphocyte immunity, which is partially responsible for cell-mediated immunity. Other medications may be prescribed to help prevent rejection of the transplanted kidney (e.g., corticosteroids, azathioprine) and/or prevent infection (e.g., antibiotics, antifungals, antivirals). Lymphocyte immune globulin, antithymocyte globulin is also used for the treatment of moderate to severe aplastic anemia in patients who cannot undergo bone marrow transplantation. It is administered via intravenous infusion over at least four hours.

J7505

J7505 Muromonab-CD3, parenteral, 5 mg

Muromonab-CD3 is a murine monoclonal antibody specific to the CD3 antigen of human T cells. It inhibits the functioning of T cells, which play a major role in acute allograft rejection. It is an immunosuppressant. Muromonab is a monoclonal antibody used to prevent organ transplant rejection in patients who have received kidney, heart, and liver transplants. It blocks the function of the T cells, which play a major role in organ transplant rejection. Recommended adult dose is 5 mg per day in an intravenous injection.

J7507-J7508

J7507 Tacrolimus, immediate release, oral, 1 mg

J7508 Tacrolimus, extended release, (Astagraf XL), oral, 0.1 mg

Tacrolimus is used to reduce the risk of rejection by the body of liver and kidney allogeneic transplants and of bone marrow transplants, usually used with corticosteroids. Recent trials show it to be effective in managing heart, pancreas, pancreatic island cell transplants, and small bowel disease patients. Tacrolimus prevents rejection by impeding T lymphocyte cells, cells that are in the immune system. A lower dose can be used than with cyclosporine because of its potency. Tacrolimus should not be used at the same time as cyclosporine. The current drug should be stopped at least 24 hours before beginning the other one. Tacrolimus can be administered orally, topically, or via intravenous infusion.

J7509

J7509 Methylprednisolone, oral, per 4 mg

Methylprednisolone is a corticosteroid used to treat a variety of conditions. Indications include allergic disorders, arthritis, blood diseases, breathing problems, certain cancers, eye diseases, intestinal disorders, and collagen and skin diseases. Methylprednisolone may also be used with other medications as a replacement for certain hormones. Methylprednisolone works by decreasing the body's immune response to these diseases and reducing symptoms such as swelling and redness. Methylprednisolone may be administered orally, by intramuscular injection in the form of methylprednisolone acetate, or by intravenous infusion in the form of methylprednisolone sodium succinate.

J7510

J7510 Prednisolone, oral, per 5 mg

Prednisolone is a synthetic adrenal corticosteroid. Corticosteroids are natural substances produced by the adrenal glands located adjacent to the kidneys. Corticosteroids are widely used to treat allergies, inflammation, and many disease processes. Prednisolone is used to treat a wide variety of conditions. Oral and injectable prednisolone is used to suppress inflammation in many inflammatory and allergic conditions. Examples include rheumatoid arthritis, systemic lupus, acute gouty arthritis, psoriatic arthritis, ulcerative colitis, and Crohn's disease. Severe allergic conditions that fail conventional treatment may also be treated with prednisolone. Examples include bronchial asthma, allergic rhinitis, drug-induced dermatitis, and contact and atopic dermatitis. Prednisolone is also used in the treatment of leukemia and lymphomas, idiopathic thrombocytopenia purpura, and autoimmune hemolytic anemia. Other miscellaneous conditions treated with this medication include thyroiditis and sarcoidosis. Prednisolone is used as a hormone replacement in patients whose adrenal glands are unable to produce sufficient amounts of corticosteroids. Prednisolone injection or sterile suspension can be injected into a muscle, joint, lesion, or soft tissue.

J7511

J7511 Lymphocyte immune globulin, antithymocyte globulin, rabbit, parenteral, 25 mg

Lymphocyte immune globulin, antithymocyte globulin helps prevent organ rejection in renal allograft transplant patients. It is given at the time of rejection or as an adjunct with other immunosuppressants to delay onset of the first rejection episode. It reduces the number of thymus-dependent lymphocytes and changes the T lymphocyte immunity, which is partially responsible for cell-mediated immunity. Other medications may be prescribed to help prevent rejection of the transplanted kidney (e.g., corticosteroids, azathioprine) and/or prevent infection (e.g., antibiotics, antifungals, antivirals). Lymphocyte immune globulin, antithymocyte globulin is also used for the treatment of moderate to severe aplastic anemia in patients who cannot undergo bone marrow transplantation. It is administered via intravenous infusion over at least four hours.

J7512

J7512 Prednisone, immediate release or delayed release, oral, 1 mg

Prednisone is a corticosteroid. Corticosteroids are widely used in medicine to control allergies, inflammation, and many disease processes. Prednisone is similar to a natural hormone produced by the adrenal glands. It is often used to replace this chemical when the body does not make enough. It relieves inflammation and is used to treat certain forms of arthritis; skin, blood, kidney, eye, thyroid, and intestinal disorders; severe allergies; and asthma. Prednisone also is used with other drugs to prevent rejection of transplanted organs and to treat certain types of cancer.

J7513

J7513 Daclizumab, parenteral, 25 mg

Daclizumab is an immunosuppressive agent indicated to prevent organ rejection in kidney transplant patients. Immunosuppressive agents work to lower the body's natural immunity in patients who receive tissue and organ transplants. When a patient receives a kidney transplant, lymphocytes in the allograft recipient recognize the foreign tissue and attack the transplanted kidney. Daclizumab works by preventing lymphocytes from rejecting the allograft. More specifically, daclizumab works by inhibiting IL2 mediated activation of lymphocytes, a critical pathway in the cellular immune response involved in allograft rejection. The dose of daclizumab varies, but the recommended dose is 1 mg per kg (0.45 mg per

J

pound) of body weight. Daclizumab is administered by intravenous infusion.

J7515-J7516

J7515 Cyclosporine, oral, 25 mg

J7516 Cyclosporine, parenteral, 250 mg

Cyclosporine is used to prevent rejection of skin, pancreas, kidney, liver, heart, small intestine, and bone marrow transplants. When a patient receives an allogenic tissue or organ transplant, lymphocytes in the allograft recipient recognize the foreign tissue and attack the transplanted tissue or organ. Cyclosporine can also be used to treat rheumatoid arthritis that is not responding to methotrexate and severe psoriasis. The exact mechanism of action is not known. T-lymphocytes are preferentially inhibited. The 1-helper cell is the primary target, but the 1-suppressor cell may also be suppressed. Cyclosporine also inhibits lymphokine production and release including interleukin-2 or 1-cell growth factor (TCGF). It should be administered with adrenal corticosteroids but not with other immunosuppressive agents.

J7517

J7517 Mycophenolate mofetil, oral, 250 mg

Mycophenolate mofetil is an immunosuppressive agent indicated to prevent organ rejection in kidney, heart, and liver transplant patients. Immunosuppressive agents work to lower the body's natural immunity in patients who receive tissue and organ transplants. When a patient receives an allogenic tissue or organ transplant, lymphocytes in the allograft recipient recognize the foreign tissue and attack the transplanted tissue or organ. Mycophenolate mofetil works in two ways to prevent rejection. First, it inhibits rejection by preventing the production of T-cells, lymphocytes, and development of antibodies from B-cells that stimulate rejection. Second, mycophenolate mofetil inhibits mobilization of leukocytes to inflammatory sites. It is generally used in conjunction with cyclosporin and corticosteroids to prevent rejection. Mycophenolate mofetil may be administered orally by tablet (available in 250 mg or 500 mg doses) or in a liquid suspension (available in a dose of 200 mg/ml). This agent may also be administered by intravenous infusion in the form of mycophenolate mofetil hydrochloride (available in 500 mg vials) at a suggested rate not to exceed 500 mg over a two-hour period.

J7518

J7518 Mycophenolic acid, oral, 180 mg

Mycophenolic acid is a formulation of mycophenolate sodium. It acts by inhibiting lymphocyte proliferation and antibody production and is an immunosuppressive agent indicated to prevent organ rejection in kidney transplant patients. Mycophenolic acid is generally used in conjunction with cyclosporine and corticosteroids to prevent rejection. The recommended dose of mycophenolic acid is 720 mg orally twice a day on an empty stomach.

J7520

J7520 Sirolimus, oral, 1 mg

Sirolimus is an immunosuppressive agent formerly known as rapamycin. It is a macrocyclic lactone found in the soil of Easter Island. Sirolimus resembles tacrolimus and binds to the same intracellular binding protein or immunophilins known as FKBP-12. Sirolimus, in combination with cyclosporine or tacrolimus and steroids, is used for the prevention of acute kidney allograft rejection. Sirolimus is administered orally.

J7525

J7525 Tacrolimus, parenteral, 5 mg

Tacrolimus is used to reduce the risk of rejection by the body of liver and kidney allogeneic transplants and of bone marrow transplants, usually used with corticosteroids. Recent trials show it to be effective in managing heart, pancreas, pancreatic island cell transplants, and small bowel disease patients. Tacrolimus prevents rejection by impeding T lymphocyte cells, cells that are in the immune system. A lower dose can be used than with cyclosporine because of its potency. Tacrolimus should not be used at the same time as cyclosporine. The current drug should be stopped at least 24 hours before beginning the other one. Tacrolimus can be administered orally, topically, or via intravenous infusion.

J7527

J7527 Everolimus, oral, 0.25 mg

Everolimus inhibits a serine-threonine kinase protein pathway that does not function appropriately in certain human cancers. Everolimus binds to a protein site within the cell preventing the completion of the kinase pathway. It ultimately reduces the expression of vascular endothelial growth factor, which retards cell growth. Everolimus is indicated as a treatment for pancreatic progressive neuroendocrine tumors in patients who cannot be treated with surgery or who have advanced metastatic disease, advanced renal cell carcinoma after failed treatment with sunitinib or sorafenib, and subependymal giant cell astrocytoma (SEGA) associated with tuberous sclerosis who are not candidates for surgical resection. Recommended dose is 2.5 to 10 mg daily based on patient condition and disease process.

J7599

J7599 Immunosuppressive drug, not otherwise classified

Immunosuppressive drugs are chemical compounds that inhibit or prevent the activity of the immune system. These drugs are indicated for the prevention of rejection of a transplanted organ or tissue, to treat autoimmune diseases (e.g., rheumatoid arthritis, ulcerative colitis), and to treat inflammatory diseases not of autoimmune origin (e.g., long-term asthma). This code should be used only for immunosuppressive drugs that are not otherwise classified among the other HCPCS Level II codes.

J7604

J7604 Acetylcysteine, inhalation solution, compounded product, administered through DME, unit dose form, per g

Acetylcysteine is a derivative of the naturally occurring amino acid L-cysteine. The drug is available in inhalation solution, oral, and injectable forms. It is a mucolytic agent when inhaled, used to lower the viscosity (i.e., thin) mucous secretions to allow easier expulsion or easier breathing. The oral and injectable forms are used as an antidote for acetaminophen overdose to prevent life-threatening liver damage. Acetylcysteine reacts with the acetaminophen, rendering some of the acetaminophen harmless. The inhaled form is indicated as an adjunct treatment for patients with acute and chronic bronchopulmonary diseases, cystic fibrosis, tracheostomies, pulmonary complications associated with surgery, post-traumatic chest conditions, and atelectasis due to mucous obstruction. It is also used during anesthesia and in diagnostic bronchial studies. As an antidote for acetaminophen poisoning, acetylcysteine should be administered as soon as possible, but within 24 hours after the overdose. The inhaled form is administered by nebulizer, tent, or as a compressed gas. The injectable form is administered by intravenous infusion over 60 minutes. The oral form should be administered after gastric lavage or emesis. The dosage depends on the indication and drug form.

J7605

J7605 Arformoterol, inhalation solution, FDA-approved final product, noncompounded, administered through DME, unit dose form, 15 mcg

Arformoterol tartrate is a mirror image of the drug formoterol that exhibits slightly different properties. The drug, similar to formoterol, is a long-acting, selective, $beta_2$ -adrenergic receptor agonist. Arformoterol has twice as much potency as formoterol. Inhaled arformoterol acts locally in the lung as a bronchodilator. Arformoterol tartrate inhalation solution is indicated for the long-term maintenance treatment of patients with chronic obstructive pulmonary disease (COPD), including chronic bronchitis and emphysema. The recommended dosage is 15 mcg administered twice a day (morning and evening) by nebulization. The drug is inhaled and should be administered by a standard nebulizer connected to an air compressor.

J7606

J7606 Formoterol fumarate, inhalation solution, FDA-approved final product, noncompounded, administered through DME, unit dose form, 20 mcg

Formoterol fumarate is a long-acting selective $beta_2$-adrenergic receptor agonist 33 ($beta_2$ -agonist). Inhaled formoterol acts locally in the lung as a bronchodilator. This is a long-term medication used to treat chronic obstructive pulmonary disease (COPD), including bronchitis and emphysema. The recommended dose is 20 micrograms twice a day through a nebulizer.

J7607

J7607 Levalbuterol, inhalation solution, compounded product, administered through DME, concentrated form, 0.5 mg

Levalbuterol is a selective beta2-adrenergic receptor agonist that functions as a bronchodilator. The drug blocks the action of enzymes that cause the smooth muscles within the respiratory tract to contract. This relaxation of smooth muscles allows easier breathing. Levalbuterol is indicated for the prevention and relief of bronchospasm in patients with reversible obstructive pulmonary disease and for the prevention of exercise-induced bronchospasm. Effects of the drug may last up to six hours after administration.

J7608

J7608 Acetylcysteine, inhalation solution, FDA-approved final product, noncompounded, administered through DME, unit dose form, per g

Acetylcysteine is a derivative of the naturally occurring amino acid L-cysteine. The drug is available in inhalation solution, oral, and injectable forms. It is a mucolytic agent when inhaled, used to lower the viscosity (i.e., thin) mucous secretions to allow easier expulsion or easier breathing. The oral and injectable forms are used as an antidote for acetaminophen overdose to prevent life-threatening liver damage. Acetylcysteine reacts with the acetaminophen, rendering some of the acetaminophen harmless. The inhaled form is indicated as an adjunct treatment for patients with acute and chronic bronchopulmonary diseases, cystic fibrosis, tracheostomies, pulmonary complications associated with surgery, post-traumatic chest conditions, and atelectasis due to mucous obstruction. It is also used during anesthesia and in diagnostic bronchial studies. As an antidote for acetaminophen poisoning, acetylcysteine should be administered as soon as possible, but within 24 hours after the overdose. The inhaled form is administered by nebulizer, tent, or as a compressed gas. The injectable form is administered by intravenous infusion over 60 minutes. The oral form should be administered after gastric lavage or emesis. The dosage depends on the indication and drug form.

J7609-J7615

J7609 Albuterol, inhalation solution, compounded product, administered through DME, unit dose, 1 mg

J7610 Albuterol, inhalation solution, compounded product, administered through DME, concentrated form, 1 mg

J7611 Albuterol, inhalation solution, FDA-approved final product, noncompounded, administered through DME, concentrated form, 1 mg

J7612 Levalbuterol, inhalation solution, FDA-approved final product, noncompounded, administered through DME, concentrated form, 0.5 mg

J7613 Albuterol, inhalation solution, FDA-approved final product, noncompounded, administered through DME, unit dose, 1 mg

J7614 Levalbuterol, inhalation solution, FDA-approved final product, noncompounded, administered through DME, unit dose, 0.5 mg

J7615 Levalbuterol, inhalation solution, compounded product, administered through DME, unit dose, 0.5 mg

Albuterol and levalbuterol are selective beta2-adrenergic receptor agonists that function as bronchodilators. The drugs block the actions of enzymes that cause the smooth muscles within the respiratory tract to contract. This relaxation of smooth muscles allows easier breathing. Albuterol and levalbuterol are indicated for the prevention and relief of bronchospasm in patients with reversible obstructive pulmonary disease and for the prevention of exercise-induced bronchospasm. Effects of the drug may last up to six hours after administration.

J7620

J7620 Albuterol, up to 2.5 mg and ipratropium bromide, up to 0.5 mg, FDA-approved final product, noncompounded, administered through DME

Albuterol and ipratropium bromide is a combination bronchodilator used in inhalation solutions. Albuterol is a selective beta^{2} -adrenergic receptor agonist that blocks the actions of enzymes that cause the smooth muscles within the respiratory tract to contract. This relaxation of smooth muscles allows easier breathing. Ipratropium bromide is an anticholinergic agent that binds to receptors of vascular smooth muscle and endothelial cells and increases intracellular concentrations of guanosine cyclic monophosphate (cGMP), which creates smooth muscle cell relaxation. Albuterol and ipratropium bromide is indicated as a treatment for bronchospasms associated with chronic obstructive pulmonary disease (COPD). One vial usually contains 2.5 mg or albuterol combined with 0.5 mg of ipratropium bromide. The drug is available as a metered dose inhaler or in a solution for administration via a reusable nebulizer.
Recommended dosage for inhalation is one vial four times a day administered administration via a reusable nebulizer.

J7622

J7622 Beclomethasone, inhalation solution, compounded product, administered through DME, unit dose form, per mg

Beclomethasone is a corticosteroid. Beclomethasone is indicated for the treatment of bronchial asthma when administered as an oral inhalant.
Beclomethasone controls symptoms of asthma and other lung diseases but does not cure them.

J7624

J7624 Betamethasone, inhalation solution, compounded product, administered through DME, unit dose form, per mg

Betamethasone valerate is a corticosteroid with anti-inflammatory and immunosuppressive abilities. The inhalation solution is used to prevent moderate to severe asthma.

J7626-J7627

J7626 Budesonide, inhalation solution, FDA-approved final product, noncompounded, administered through DME, unit dose form, up to 0.5 mg

J7627 Budesonide, inhalation solution, compounded product, administered through DME, unit dose form, up to 0.5 mg

Budesonide is a corticosteroid with anti-inflammatory and immunosuppressive abilities. It is available as an inhalation solution in several formulations including a non-compounded unit dose form, a powder compounded for inhalation, and a concentrated form. The inhalation solution is used to prevent wheezing, shortness of breath, and difficulty breathing caused by severe asthma and other lung diseases. Budesonide controls symptoms of asthma and other lung diseases but does not cure them. Budesonide is usually inhaled once or twice a day.

J7628-J7629

J7628 Bitolterol mesylate, inhalation solution, compounded product, administered through DME, concentrated form, per mg

J7629 Bitolterol mesylate, inhalation solution, compounded product, administered through DME, unit dose form, per mg

Bitolterol mesylate is a bronchodilator used in the treatment of bronchospasm associated with asthma. It may also be helpful in the treatment of emphysema and chronic bronchitis. Asthma is a condition that causes narrowing of the bronchial tubes due to muscle spasm and inflammation within the bronchial tubes. Bitolterol mesylate relaxes the smooth muscles surrounding these airway tubes, thereby increasing the diameter and ease of air flow through the tubes. Bitolterol mesylate is unique in that it is a "prodrug" because the body must first metabolize it before it becomes active. Bitolterol is administered in an aerosol inhaled by mouth. It usually is taken as needed to relieve symptoms or every eight hours to prevent symptoms.

J7631-J7632

J7631 Cromolyn sodium, inhalation solution, FDA-approved final product, noncompounded, administered through DME, unit dose form, per 10 mg

J7632 Cromolyn sodium, inhalation solution, compounded product, administered through DME, unit dose form, per 10 mg

Cromolyn sodium is a nonsteroidal anti-inflammatory that works by preventing the release of substances in the body that cause inflammation. More specifically, cromolyn sodium acts indirectly by blocking calcium ions from entering the mast cell, thereby preventing mediator release. This prevents the release of substances that cause inflammation in the air passages of the lungs. Cromolyn sodium is used to prevent wheezing, shortness of breath, and difficulty breathing caused by asthma. It is also used to prevent breathing difficulties (bronchospasm) during exercise. Cromolyn comes as powder-filled capsules and solution to take by mouth and an aerosol to inhale by mouth. The inhalant form is used to prevent asthma attacks and other conditions involving inflammation of the lung tissues. It is usually inhaled three or four times a day to prevent asthma attacks or within an hour before activities to prevent breathing difficulties caused by exercise.

J7633-J7634

J7633 Budesonide, inhalation solution, FDA-approved final product, noncompounded, administered through DME, concentrated form, per 0.25 mg

J7634 Budesonide, inhalation solution, compounded product, administered through DME, concentrated form, per 0.25 mg

Budesonide is a corticosteroid with anti-inflammatory and immunosuppressive abilities. It is available as an inhalation solution in several formulations, including a non-compounded unit dose form, a powder compounded for inhalation, and a concentrated form. The inhalation solution is used to prevent wheezing, shortness of breath, and difficulty breathing caused by severe asthma and other lung diseases. Budesonide controls symptoms of asthma and other lung diseases but does not cure them. Budesonide is usually inhaled once or twice a day.

J7635-J7636

J7635 Atropine, inhalation solution, compounded product, administered through DME, concentrated form, per mg

J7636 Atropine, inhalation solution, compounded product, administered through DME, unit dose form, per mg

Atropine is an extract of an alkaloid from the plants belladonna, hyoscyamus, or stramonium. It is also made synthetically. Atropine sulfate is a highly toxic compound of atropine and sulfuric acid that has the same uses and effects as atropine. It blocks the neurotransmitter acetylcholine in muscarinic receptors of the parasympathetic system. Muscarinic receptors occur throughout the nervous system including in the heart, smooth muscles of the blood vessels, lungs, salivary glands, gastrointestinal tract, and eye. Atropine sulfate in clinical doses counteracts the peripheral vessel dilatation and abrupt decrease in blood pressure produced by other drugs or biologicals. Atropine is used to reduce secretions in the respiratory tract.

J7637-J7638

J7637 Dexamethasone, inhalation solution, compounded product, administered through DME, concentrated form, per mg

J7638 Dexamethasone, inhalation solution, compounded product, administered through DME, unit dose form, per mg

Dexamethasone is a synthetic corticosteroid that is similar to a natural hormone produced by the adrenal gland. It is 25 times as potent as cortisol. Dexamethasone has anti-inflammatory, antiemetic and immunosuppressant properties. It is used to treat a wide variety of disorders.

J7639

J7639 Dornase alfa, inhalation solution, FDA-approved final product, noncompounded, administered through DME, unit dose form, per mg

Dornase alpha is an inhaled drug indicated for the treatment of cystic fibrosis. Healthy lungs continually secrete fluid into the airways to keep them moist. However, in cystic fibrosis, a reduced amount of water is present in the secretions making them thick and difficult to cough up or spit out. These thickened secretions block the airways, causing labored breathing and promoting the growth of bacteria and infection. These thickened secretions contain high concentrations of deoxyribonucleic acid (DNA) and dornase alpha, a genetically engineered form of the human enzyme deoxyribonuclease or DNAse. Dornase alpha works by breaking down the DNA, thereby reducing the thickness of the fluids. Dornase alpha is supplied in single-use ampules that contain 2.5 ml of a sterile, clear, colorless solution containing 1 mg/ml of dornase alpha.

J7640

J7640 Formoterol, inhalation solution, compounded product, administered through DME, unit dose form, 12 mcg

Formoterol is a long-acting selective beta2 adrenergic receptor agonist 33 (beta2 agonist). Inhaled formoterol acts locally in the lung as a bronchodilator. This is a long-term medication used to treat asthma and to prevent exercise-induced bronchospasm in adults and children older than 12. It can also be used long term to treat chronic obstructive pulmonary disease (COPD), including bronchitis and emphysema. The usual dose is 12 micrograms every 12 hours through an inhaler.

J7641

J7641 Flunisolide, inhalation solution, compounded product, administered through DME, unit dose, per mg

Flunisolide is a corticosteroid used as maintenance treatment for asthma. It is shown to be several hundred times stronger in animal anti-inflammatory assays than the cortisol standard. This may reduce or eliminate the need for oral corticosteroids. Corticosteroids reduce or eliminate inflammation in the lining of the airways. They may also reduce the reaction to inhaled allergen and can be used for the management of the nasal symptoms of seasonal or perennial rhinitis. The recommended dose varies depending on the treatment.

J7642-J7643

J7642 Glycopyrrolate, inhalation solution, compounded product, administered through DME, concentrated form, per mg

J7643 Glycopyrrolate, inhalation solution, compounded product, administered through DME, unit dose form, per mg

Glycopyrrolate is an anticholinergic drug that inhibits the action of acetylcholine on structures innervated by postganglionic cholinergic nerves and on smooth muscles that respond to acetylcholine but lack cholinergic innervation. It reduces the amount of free acidity of gastric secretions and controls excessive pharyngeal, tracheal, and bronchial secretions. Glycopyrrolate inhalation solution is used for maintenance treatment for asthma and chronic obstructive pulmonary disease (COPD). It has been shown to be an effective bronchodilator when used once a day.

J7644-J7645

J7644 Ipratropium bromide, inhalation solution, FDA-approved final product, noncompounded, administered through DME, unit dose form, per mg

J7645 Ipratropium bromide, inhalation solution, compounded product, administered through DME, unit dose form, per mg

Ipratropium bromide is an anticholinergic agent that functions as a bronchodilator when inhaled. The drug binds to receptors of vascular smooth muscle and endothelial cells and increases intracellular concentrations of guanosine cyclic monophosphate (cGMP), which creates smooth muscle cell relaxation. Inhaled ipratropium bromide, singularly or in combination with other bronchodilators, is for the treatment of bronchospasms associated with chronic obstructive pulmonary disease (COPD) including chronic bronchitis and emphysema. Recommended dosage for inhalation is 36 mcg four times a day.

J7647-J7650

J7647 Isoetharine HCl, inhalation solution, compounded product, administered through DME, concentrated form, per mg

J7648 Isoetharine HCl, inhalation solution, FDA-approved final product, noncompounded, administered through DME, concentrated form, per mg

J7649 Isoetharine HCl, inhalation solution, FDA-approved final product, noncompounded, administered through DME, unit dose form, per mg

J7650 Isoetharine HCl, inhalation solution, compounded product, administered through DME, unit dose form, per mg

Isoetharine hydrochloride is a bronchodilator that relaxes the smooth muscles of the lungs that constrict due to inflammation or disease. It is used to treat asthma, emphysema, bronchitis, and chronic obstructive pulmonary disease (COPD). The medication comes in a solution that is used with a nebulizer and in a hand-held aerosol form.

J7657-J7660

J7657 Isoproterenol HCl, inhalation solution, compounded product, administered through DME, concentrated form, per mg

J7658 Isoproterenol HCl, inhalation solution, FDA-approved final product, noncompounded, administered through DME, concentrated form, per mg

J7659 Isoproterenol HCl, inhalation solution, FDA-approved final product, noncompounded, administered through DME, unit dose form, per mg

J7660 Isoproterenol HCl, inhalation solution, compounded product, administered through DME, unit dose form, per mg

Isoproterenol hydrochloride (HCl) is a synthetic sympathomimetic amine that is similar to epinephrine but acts almost entirely on beta-receptors. It lowers peripheral vascular resistance in skeletal muscle, renal, and mesenteric vascular beds. Cardiac output is increased due to the lowered peripheral resistance. The inhalation form is used to treat bronchospasms. Commercial inhalation forms of isoproterenol have been discontinued.

J7665

J7665 Mannitol, administered through an inhaler, 5 mg

Mannitol inhalation substance is used in bronchial challenge tests to help diagnose patients with symptoms of asthma. It is a sugar alcohol substance that constricts the bronchial constriction. Respiratory measurements are taken prior to and after the administration of the mannitol inhaler. The mannitol is administered to the patient in graduated doses until the patient has a positive response or 635 mg of mannitol has been administered.

J7667-J7670

J7667 Metaproterenol sulfate, inhalation solution, compounded product, concentrated form, per 10 mg

J7668 Metaproterenol sulfate, inhalation solution, FDA-approved final product, noncompounded, administered through DME, concentrated form, per 10 mg

J7669 Metaproterenol sulfate, inhalation solution, FDA-approved final product, noncompounded, administered through DME, unit dose form, per 10 mg

J7670 Metaproterenol sulfate, inhalation solution, compounded product, administered through DME, unit dose form, per 10 mg

Metaproterenol sulfate is a bronchodilator used to treat asthma, bronchitis, and emphysema. It acts on the beta receptors in the bronchial smooth muscles to relax bronchospasms that cause difficulty breathing. The medication comes in powder form and in a solution that is used with a nebulizer and in a hand-held aerosol.

J7674

J7674 Methacholine chloride administered as inhalation solution through a nebulizer, per 1 mg

Methacholine chloride is a synthetic choline ester that acts to induce bronchoconstriction. This medication is used in a bronchospasm provocation test to diagnose asthma. This is often done when spirometry alone does not provide a definitive diagnosis. Two different dilution schedules are used in North America to perform the test. Both use 100 mg of methacholine. One is based on a two minute tidal breathing dosing protocol and the other is a five breath dosimeter protocol. Both methods utilize a nebulizer to administer the medication.

J7676

J7676 Pentamidine isethionate, inhalation solution, compounded product, administered through DME, unit dose form, per 300 mg

Pentamidine isethionate is an aromatic diamidine that is an anti-protozoal. Its mechanism of action is not completely known. It is thought the drug interferes with the synthesis of DNA, RNA, and protein, causing cell death. Pentamidine isethionate is indicated as a treatment for *Pneumocystis jirovecii*, trypanosomiasis, and leishmaniasis. The drug may be administered by intramuscular injection, inhalation, or intravenous infusion over one hour. The inhalation solution is inhaled through a special breathing unit that ensures the drug reaches deep into the lungs. The recommended dosage for the inhalation solution is 300 mg once a month, administered via a nebulizer. Treatment usually takes 30 to 45 minutes.

J7677

J7677 Revefenacin inhalation solution, FDA-approved final product, noncompounded, administered through DME, 1 mcg

Revefenacin inhalation solution is an anticholinergic used for the treatment of chronic obstructive pulmonary disease (COPD) in adult patients, ages 18 years and older. Anticholinergics inhibit the cholinergic/acetylcholine M3 receptor of smooth muscle, allowing the muscles around the airway of the lungs to remain relaxed, and preventing common symptoms of COPD, such as chest tightness, cough, shortness of breath, and wheezing. It is a clear, colorless, aqueous solution supplied in 175 mcg unit-dose vials, wrapped in a foil pouch, and administered once daily through a standard nebulizer connected to an air compressor. The vial should not be removed from the foil pouch until immediately prior to use and any remaining solution should be discarded.

J7680-J7681

J7680 Terbutaline sulfate, inhalation solution, compounded product, administered through DME, concentrated form, per mg

J7681 Terbutaline sulfate, inhalation solution, compounded product, administered through DME, unit dose form, per mg

Terbutaline sulfate is a beta$_2$ -adrenergic agonist that functions as a bronchodilator. It works, in part, by stimulating the conversion of adenosine triphosphate (ATP) to cyclic 3',5'-adenosine monophosphate, which relaxes bronchial muscles. Terbutaline sulfate is indicated for the prevention and reversal of bronchospasm in asthma, bronchitis, and emphysema.

J7682

J7682 Tobramycin, inhalation solution, FDA-approved final product, noncompounded, unit dose form, administered through DME, per 300 mg

Tobramycin is an aminoglycoside antibiotic, which is derived from various species of *Streptomyces* bacteria or produced synthetically. Aminoglycosides inhibit bacterial protein synthesis by binding with the 30S ribosomal subunit and are bactericidal. Streptomycin is derived from *Streptomyces tenebrarius* and inhibits protein synthesis, causing cell death. Susceptibility studies should be performed prior to the administration of tobramycin. It is indicated in the treatment of infections caused by gram-negative bacillary bacteria, including *Pseudomonas aeruginosa*, *Staphylococcus aureus*, *Escherichia coli*, *Klebsiella* species, *Enterobacter* species, *Serratia* species, *Proteus* species, *Providencia* species, and *Citrobacter* species. The inhalation form is indicated in the treatment of *Pseudomonas aeruginosa* in patients with cystic fibrosis.

J7683-J7684

J7683 Triamcinolone, inhalation solution, compounded product, administered through DME, concentrated form, per mg

J7684 Triamcinolone, inhalation solution, compounded product, administered through DME, unit dose form, per mg

Triamcinolone is a synthetic corticosteroid, which is analogous to corticosteroids produced by the adrenal cortex. The drug is one to two times more potent than prednisone. Its mechanism of actions is not clearly defined. Triamcinolone does decrease inflammation by stabilizing leukocytes, suppress the chemicals normally released in immune response, and stimulate bone marrow. Inhaled triamcinolone is a local anti-inflammatory delivering the drug directly to the lungs. The drug has no effect on acute bronchospasms, but is indicated for prophylactic and maintenance therapy of asthma.

J7685

J7685 Tobramycin, inhalation solution, compounded product, administered through DME, unit dose form, per 300 mg

Tobramycin is an aminoglycoside antibiotic, which is derived from various species of Streptomyces bacteria or produced synthetically. Aminoglycosides inhibit bacterial protein synthesis by binding with the 30S ribosomal subunit and are bactericidal. Streptomycin is derived from *Streptomyces tenebrarius* and inhibits protein synthesis, causing cell death. Susceptibility studies should be performed prior to the administration of tobramycin. It is indicated in the treatment of infections caused by gram-negative bacillary bacteria, including *Pseudomonas aeruginosa*, *Staphylococcus aureus*, *Escherichia coli*, *Klebsiella* species, *Enterobacter* species, *Serratia* species, *Proteus* species, *Providencia* species, and *Citrobacter* species. The inhalation form is indicated in the treatment of *Pseudomonas aeruginosa* in patients with cystic fibrosis.

J7686

J7686 Treprostinil, inhalation solution, FDA-approved final product, noncompounded, administered through DME, unit dose form, 1.74 mg

Treprostinil inhalation solution is used for the treatment of pulmonary arterial hypertension to improve exercise activities. Treprostinil is a prostacyclin analogue and provides direct vasodilation of pulmonary and systemic arterial vascular beds and inhibition of platelet aggregation. Recommended dose is an initial treatment of three breaths per treatment session, four times daily. The dose is increased by an additional three breaths at approximately one to two week intervals, if tolerated, until nine breaths are reached per treatment session, four times daily. The medication is administered through an ultrasonic, pulsed-delivery nebulizer.

J7699

J7699 NOC drugs, inhalation solution administered through DME

Use this code to represent an inhalation drug that has been administered through DME and is not represented by any other level I or level II HCPCS code.

J7799

J7799 NOC drugs, other than inhalation drugs, administered through DME

Use this code to represent a drug that has been administered through DME, but is not an inhalation drug. Be sure the drug does not have any other specified level I or level II HCPCS code to represent it.

J7999

J7999 Compounded drug, not otherwise classified

This code should be used to report compounded drugs that have been approved by the FDA, but do not have a product-specific HCPCS Level II code assigned.

J8498

J8498 Antiemetic drug, rectal/suppository, not otherwise specified

Antiemetic medication may be used in conjunction with anti-cancer drugs such as chemotherapeutic agents and acts to prevent or relieve nausea and vomiting. Antiemetics are antagonists for a specific serotonin subtype receptor located on the nerve terminals of the vagus in the small intestine.

J8499

J8499 Prescription drug, oral, nonchemotherapeutic, NOS

Use this code to represent an oral prescription drug that is not a form of chemotherapy and is not represented by any other Level I or Level II HCPCS code.

J8501

J8501 Aprepitant, oral, 5 mg

Aprepitant is a chemical complex used as an oral antiemetic drug. It seeks cell receptors of human substance P/neurokinin 1 (NK1). NK1s are peptides found in the central and peripheral nervous systems involved in the transmission of a signal from outside the cell wall into the cell. Aprepitant blocks those transmissions. It is used in combination with a corticosteroid and a 5-HT3 antagonist to prevent acute and delayed nausea and vomiting associated with initial and repeat courses of certain chemotherapies, including high-dose cisplatin.

J8510

J8510 Busulfan, oral, 2 mg

Busulfan is an alkylating agent that is used to reduce tumor growth. It causes breaks in the DNA, which prevent replication, thus interfering with tumor cell reproduction. It is used in the treatment of chronic myelogenous leukemia, and disorders such as severe thrombocytosis and polycythemia vera. Side effects commonly reported from busulfan are brittle or thinned hair, dry skin, diarrhea, weight loss, fatigue, and blistering of the mouth. This code is for the oral administration per 2 mg.

J8515

J8515 Cabergoline, oral, 0.25 mg

Cabergoline is a chemical complex that binds to a dopamine receptor on cells and inhibits the secretion of prolactin. Prolactin is a hormone produced by the anterior pituitary gland that stimulates and sustains lactation. Cabergoline is indicated for the treatment of hyperprolactinemia, whether idiopathic or caused by a pituitary adenoma. The recommended initial dosage is 0.25 mg twice weekly increasing to 1 mg twice weekly depending upon the prolactin levels in the patient's blood. Cabergoline is available only as a self-administrable oral tablet.

J8520-J8521

J8520 Capecitabine, oral, 150 mg
J8521 Capecitabine, oral, 500 mg

Capecitabine is an antineoplastic drug that is broken down in the liver into fluorouracil, also known as 5 FU. Fluorouracil is a fluorinated analogue of uracil. Uracil is a chemical compound found in nucleic acids that interferes with the synthesis of DNA and RNA causing cell death. Capecitabine, singularly or in combination with other chemotherapeutic drugs, is indicated as a treatment for colorectal cancer and metastatic breast cancer. The drug is self-administered orally.

J8530

J8530 Cyclophosphamide, oral, 25 mg

Cyclophosphamide is a synthetic antineoplastic drug chemically related to the nitrogen mustards. The drug itself is inert and functions only after transformation in the liver to active alkylating metabolites. These metabolites interfere with the growth of susceptible rapidly proliferating malignant cells. The mechanism of action is thought to be its interference with the DNA of the tumor cell causing cell death. Cyclophosphamide is indicated singularly or in combination with other chemotherapeutic drugs, to treat a wide variety of cancers including Hodgkin's disease, lymphosarcoma, acute lymphocytic leukemia, Burkitt's lymphoma, carcinoma of the breast, multiple myeloma, chronic lymphocytic leukemia, bronchogenic carcinoma, neuroblastoma, ovarian carcinoma, and carcinoma of the uterine cervix. It is also used as an immunosuppressant to prevent transplant rejection and in the treatment of certain diseases with abnormal immune function, including severe lupus manifestations and vasculitis. Cyclophosphamide may be administered via intravenous injection or infusion, or may be injected intramuscularly, intraperitoneally, or intrapleurally. An oral version is also available. Dosage depends upon body weight and the disease being treated. The lyophilized version of cyclophosphamide is a freeze-dried version of the drug.

J8540

J8540 Dexamethasone, oral, 0.25 mg

Dexamethasone is a synthetic corticosteroid that is similar to a natural hormone produced by the adrenal gland. It is 25 times as potent as cortisol. Dexamethasone has anti-inflammatory, antiemetic and immunosuppressant properties. It is used to treat a wide variety of disorders.

J8560

J8560 Etoposide, oral, 50 mg

Etoposide is a semisynthetic derivative of podophyllotoxin, a toxic compound found in the rhizomes and roots of the mandrake plant. It is believed to inhibit the repair of DNA, causing cell death. Etoposide is an antineoplastic drug used in combination with other chemotherapeutic agents. It is available in injectable or oral versions. Injectable etoposide is indicated for the treatment of small-cell lung cancer and refractory testicular cancer that has been treated previously with surgery, radiation, or other chemotherapy. The oral version is indicated for the treatment of small-cell lung cancer. The recommended dosage of the injectable version ranges from 35 to 100 mg per m^2 of body surface depending on which disease is being treated. The injectable version is administered by intravenous infusion over 30 to 60 minutes. The recommended dosage for the oral version is two times the intravenous version.

J8562

J8562 Fludarabine phosphate, oral, 10 mg

Fludarabine phosphate is an antineoplastic drug that is a fluorinated nucleotide analogue of the antiviral agent vidarabine. It is rapidly broken down into 2-fluoro-ara-A, which inhibits DNA synthesis and causes cell death. Fludarabine phosphate is indicated for the treatment of beta-cell chronic lymphocytic leukemia for patients who have not responded to an alkylating drug treatment. This drug is available in liquid form for IV infusions or in tablet form for oral administration. The recommended dose for oral administration is 40 mg per meter squared of body surface area.

J8565

J8565 Gefitinib, oral, 250 mg

Gefitinib is a chemical complex used as an antineoplastic drug. It inhibits forms of the amino acid tyrosine from binding to epidermal growth factor receptor (EGFR) sites. EGFR is expressed on the cell surface of many normal and cancer cells. Gefitinib is indicated for the treatment of patients with locally advanced or metastatic non-small-cell lung cancer after failure of both platinum-based and docetaxel chemotherapies. It is available only as an oral self-administrable drug. The recommended dosage is 250 mg daily. Gefitinib has limited distribution under a risk management plan called the IRESSATM Access Program, to the following patient populations: patients currently receiving and benefiting from gefitinib; patients who have previously received and benefited from gefitinib; and previously enrolled patients or new patients in non-investigational new drug (IND) clinical trials approved by an institutional review board prior to June 17, 2005. New patients may also be able to obtain gefitinib if the manufacturer decides to make it available under IND and the patients meet the criteria for enrollment under the IND.

J8597

J8597 Antiemetic drug, oral, not otherwise specified

This code reports the supply of oral antiemetic drugs that do not have a more specific HCPCS Level II code. An antiemetic drug is given to prevent or relieve nausea and vomiting. An oral antiemetic may be indicated at the time of chemotherapy treatment to help allay the side effect of nausea and vomiting that often accompanies chemotherapy.

J8600

J8600 Melphalan, oral, 2 mg

Melphalan hydrochloride is a derivative of nitrogen mustard used as an antineoplastic drug. It interferes with RNA synthesis causing cell death. Melphalan is indicated for the treatment of multiple myeloma and advanced epithelial ovarian cancer. The injectable form is used for the treatment of multiple myeloma when the oral form is inappropriate. The recommended oral dosage for ovarian cancer is 0.2 mg pr kg of body weight for five days. The recommended oral dosage for multiple myeloma is 6 mg per day for two to three weeks. Each course can be repeated after four weeks.

J8610

J8610 Methotrexate, oral, 2.5 mg

Methotrexate sodium is a chemical complex that blocks cell metabolism. It works by hindering the production of an enzyme needed for the metabolism of dividing cells, like those involved in inflammation and the immune response. Methotrexate has been found useful in treating diseases linked with abnormally rapid cell growth. It is indicated singularly or in combination as a treatment for gestational choriocarcinoma, chorioadenoma destruens, hydatidiform mole, breast cancer, epidermoid cancers of the head and neck, advanced mycosis fungoides, squamous and small cell lung cancer, advanced non-Hodgkin's lymphoma, acute lymphocytic leukemia, Burkitt's lymphoma, and lymphosarcoma. It is also used to treat rheumatoid and psoriatic arthritis and severe psoriasis that is unresponsive to other treatments.

J8650

J8650 Nabilone, oral, 1 mg

Nabilone is a Schedule II, synthetic cannabinoid that is similar to the active ingredient found in the marijuana plant. Nabilone, like its natural counterpart, produces complex effects on the central nervous system, including alterations in mental status. It is suggested that the antiemetic effect of nabilone is caused by the cannabinoid receptor system in neural tissues. Nabilone is indicated for the treatment of nausea and vomiting associated with cancer chemotherapy in patients who have not adequately responded to conventional antiemetics. Patients should use this drug only when they are under the close supervision of another person. These restrictions are required as many of the patients treated with nabilone experience altered mental states not observed with other antiemetic drugs. Nabilone has the potential for abuse and misuse. This is an oral drug with a recommended dosage of one to two mg twice a day during each cycle of chemotherapy. Maximum recommended dosage is six mg per day. If needed, administration of the drug may continue for 48 hours after the last dose of each chemotherapy cycle.

J8655

J8655 Netupitant 300 mg and palonosetron 0.5 mg, oral

Netupitant/palonosetron is a fixed combination of netupitant (a P/neurokinin 1 receptor antagonist) and palonosetron (a serotonin-3 receptor antagonist) that is used for the prevention of acute and delayed nausea and vomiting associated with cancer chemotherapy treatment. Palonosetron prevents acute onset of nausea and vomiting while netupitant prevents nausea and vomiting during acute and delayed onset following chemotherapy. The fixed combination drug is supplied in capsule form and contains 300 mg netupitant and 0.5 mg palonosetron. Recommended dosage is one capsule administered one hour prior to the start of chemotherapy treatment.

J8670

J8670 Rolapitant, oral, 1 mg

Rolapitant is a chemical complex used as an oral antiemetic drug. It seeks cell receptors of human substance P/neurokinin 1 (NK1). NK1s are peptides found in the central and peripheral nervous systems involved in the transmission of a signal from outside the cell wall into the cell. Rolapitant blocks those transmissions. It is used in combination with a corticosteroid and a 5-HT3 antagonist to prevent acute and delayed nausea and vomiting associated with initial and repeat courses of certain chemotherapies, including high-dose cisplatin. Recommended dosage is 180 mg administered one to two hours prior to chemotherapy.

J8700

J8700 Temozolomide, oral, 5 mg

Temozolomide is a chemical complex that is broken down in the liver into monomethyltriazene, also known as MTIC. MTIC causes breaks in the DNA, which prevents replication, thus interfering with tumor cell reproduction. Temozolomide is indicated for the treatment of adult patients with newly diagnosed glioblastoma multiforme, and for the treatment of adult patients with refractory anaplastic astrocytoma. Temozolomide is available only as a self-administrable oral drug. The recommended dosage is 75 mg per m2 of body surface.

J8705

J8705 Topotecan, oral, 0.25 mg

Topotecan hydrochloride is an antineoplastic drug that is a semisynthetic derivative of camptothecin, an alkaloid extract from plants such as Camptotheca acuminata. The drug works by causing breaks in DNA that the cell cannot repair leading to cell death. Topotecan hydrochloride is indicated as a treatment for metastatic carcinoma of the ovaries after failure of prior chemotherapy. It is also indicated as a treatment for small cell lung cancer that responded to chemotherapy, but subsequently progressed. The recommended dose is 2.3 mg per m2 of body surface once daily for five consecutive days.

J8999

J8999 Prescription drug, oral, chemotherapeutic, NOS

Use this code to represent an oral prescription drug that has been taken as a form of chemotherapy, and is not represented by any other level I or level II HCPCS code.

J9000

J9000 Injection, doxorubicin HCl, 10 mg

Doxorubicin hydrochloride is an anthracycline antibiotic antineoplastic drug isolated from the bacterium *Streptomyces peucetius* var. *caesius*. It binds to DNA and inhibits RNA synthesis, causing cell death. It is utilized to treat many forms of cancer, such as bladder, breast, lung, stomach, and thyroid cancer, as well as Hodgkin's and non-Hodgkin's disease, acute lymphoblastic (ALL) and myeloblastic (AML) leukemia, and Wilms' tumor. The liposome version is the doxorubicin hydrochloride enclosed in a spherical lipid bilayer membrane. Doxorubicin hydrochloride liposome is indicated as a treatment for patients with ovarian cancer whose disease has recurred or progressed after platinum-based chemotherapy, and for patients with AIDS-related Kaposi's sarcoma whose disease has progressed on prior combination chemotherapy or who cannot tolerate such therapy. Both versions are administered via intravenous injection.

J9015

J9015 Injection, aldesleukin, per single use vial

Aldesleukin is an interleukin-2 product produced by recombinant DNA technology using a strain of *Escherichia coli* bacterium. Interleukin-2 is a non-antibody protein produced by T cells in response to an antigen or mitogenic stimulation. It stimulates the production of other T cells, the growth and cytolytic function of NK cells to produce lymphokine-activated killer cells, and is a growth factor for and stimulates antibody synthesis in B cells. It is also thought to promote cell death in antigen-activated T cells. Aldesleukin is indicated for the treatment of adults with metastatic renal cell carcinoma and for the treatment of adults with metastatic melanoma. The recommended dosage is 600,000 IU per kg of body weight administered every eight hours by a 15-minute IV infusion for a maximum of 14 doses. Following nine days of rest, the schedule is repeated for another 14 doses, for a maximum of 28 doses per course.

J9017

J9017 Injection, arsenic trioxide, 1 mg

Arsenic trioxide is a toxic element used as an antineoplastic agent. The actions of the drug are not completely understood. It is known to cause structural cell changes and DNA fragmentation leading to cellular death. Arsenic trioxide is indicated for the induction of remission and consolidation in patients with relapsing or refractory acute promyelocytic leukemia who have undergone retinoid or anthracycline chemotherapy and whose disease has a specific gene expression. The drug must be diluted and administered via an intravenous infusion over one to two hours. The infusion may be extended up to four hours if the patient develops acute vasomotor reactions. Recommended dosage for induction of remission is 0.15 mg per kg of body weight daily until bone marrow remission. The total induction dose should not exceed 60 doses. Recommended dosage for consolidation treatment is 0.15 mg per kg daily for 25 doses over a period up to five weeks. Consolidation treatment should begin three to six weeks after completion of induction therapy.

J9019

J9019 Injection, asparaginase (Erwinaze), 1,000 IU

Asparaginase Erwinia chrysanthemi is an asparaginase derived from the gram negative enterobacterium *Erwinia chrysanthemi*. This is a plant pathogen closely related to *E. coli*. Asparaginase is an enzyme that breaks down the amino acid asparagine into aspartic acid and ammonium. Leukemia cells cannot synthesize their own asparagine and rely on circulating sources to maintain protein survival. This drug deprives the leukemia cells of asparagine and ultimately causes cell death. Asparaginase Erwinia chrysanthemi is indicated as a component of a multi-drug treatment for acute lymphoblastic leukemia in patients who have developed a hypersensitivity to *E. coli* derived asparaginase.

J9020

J9020 Injection, asparaginase, not otherwise specified, 10,000 units

Asparaginase is a synthetic version of the enzyme L-asparaginase produced by recombinant DNA technology using a strain of *Escherichia coli* bacterium. The enzyme catalyzes the breakdown of asparagine, an amino acid. Leukemia cells cannot synthesize asparagine and depend upon exogenous sources. Asparaginase deletes asparagine throughout the body. This depletion kills the leukemia cells. Normal cells can synthesize the asparagine and are unaffected. Asparaginase is indicated in the treatment of acute lymphocytic leukemia for pediatric and adult patients. The dosage depends upon body weight and whether the use is for induction or maintenance therapy. The drug may be administered as an intravenous infusion via an existing IV over 30 minutes. Asparaginase can also be injected intramuscularly with the volume administered at each injection site limited to 2 ml. When used to induce remission, the drug is usually given in combination with other chemotherapeutic agents.

J9021

J9021 Injection, asparaginase, recombinant, (Rylaze), 0.1 mg

Asparaginase recombinant is a synthetic version of the enzyme L-asparaginase produced by recombinant DNA technology produced by fermentation of genetically engineered *Pseudomonas fluorescens* bacterium containing the DNA that encodes for asparaginase *Erwinia chrysanthemi*. The enzyme catalyzes the breakdown of asparagine, an amino acid. Leukemia cells cannot synthesize asparagine and depend upon exogenous sources. Asparaginase deletes asparagine throughout the body. This depletion kills the leukemia cells. Normal cells can synthesize the asparagine and are unaffected. Asparaginase recombinant is indicated in the treatment of acute lymphocytic leukemia for pediatric and adult patients who have developed hypersensitivity to *E. coli*- derived asparaginase. It is intended to be used in combination with other chemotherapeutic agents. The recommended dosage is 25 mg/m^2 administered as an intramuscular (IM) injection every 48 hours.

J9022

J9022 Injection, atezolizumab, 10 mg

Atezolizumab is a programmed death-ligand 1 monoclonal antibody that blocks the interaction of PD-L1 with PD-1 and B7.1 receptors. This releases the PD-L1/PD-1 pathway facilitated inhibition of the immune response, including initiation of the antitumor immune response. It is indicated for the treatment of urothelial carcinoma in patients with disease progression during or following platinum-containing chemotherapy. Recommended dosage is 1,200 mg as an intravenous infusion over 60 minutes. It is administered every three weeks until disease progression or the occurrence of unacceptable toxicity.

J9023

J9023 Injection, avelumab, 10 mg

Avelumab is a programmed cell death-ligand 1 (PD-L1) blocking antibody that binds PD-L1 and blocks interaction of PD-L1 and its PD-1 and B7.1 receptors. This releases inhibitory effects of PD-L1 of the immune response, including the beginning of the antitumor immune response. It is indicated for the treatment of metastatic Merkel cell carcinoma in adult and pediatric patients older than 12 years of age.

Recommended dosage is 10 mg administered as an intravenous infusion over 60 minutes. It is administered every two weeks until disease progression or the occurrence of unacceptable toxicity. Patients should be premedicated with acetaminophen and an antihistamine prior to the first four administrations. For subsequent administrations, premedication should be based upon clinical judgement and the severity of reactions to the previous infusions. Avelumab should not be administered concurrently with other drugs through the same intravenous access line.

J9025

J9025 Injection, azacitidine, 1 mg

Azacitidine is a pyrimidine nucleoside used as an antineoplastic agent. The drug disrupts the chemistry of DNA and causes cellular death in rapidly dividing cells, including cancer cells that no longer respond to normal growth control mechanism. Azacitidine is indicated for the treatment of myelodysplastic syndrome subtypes: refractory anemia or refractory anemia with sideroblasts (if accompanied by neutropenia, thrombocytopenia, or requiring transfusions), refractory anemia with excess blasts, refractory anemia with excess blasts in transformation, and chronic myelomonocytic leukemia. The recommended initial treatment therapy is 75 mg per m^2 of body surface subcutaneously injected daily for seven days, every four weeks. The dosage may be increased to 100 mg per m^2 if no beneficial effect is seen after two treatment cycles and if no side effects other than nausea and vomiting occur. A minimum of four treatment cycles is recommended. However, treatment can continue as long as beneficial effects are evident.

J9027

J9027 Injection, clofarabine, 1 mg

Clofarabine is a purine nucleoside that is an antineoplastic agent. The drug inhibits DNA synthesis and cellular repair leading to cell death. Clofarabine is attracted to rapidly proliferating cells and quiescent cancer cell types. It is indicated for the treatment of pediatric patients, ages 1 to 21 years, with relapsed or refractory acute lymphoblastic leukemia who have undergone at least two prior treatment regimens. Recommended dosage is 52 mg per m^2 of body surface infused intravenously over two hours for five consecutive days. This regimen may be repeated every two to six weeks.

J9030

J9030 BCG live intravesical instillation, 1 mg

BCG live intravesical is a preparation of Bacillus Calmette and Guerin, which is a weakened version of *Mycobacterium bovis. Mycobacterium bovis* is a form of tuberculous originally isolated from cattle. It is indicated for the treatment and prophylaxis of adults with carcinoma in situ of the urinary bladder, and for prophylaxis of primary or recurrent stage Ta and/or stage T1 papillary tumors following transurethral resection. It is supplied as a lyophilized powder, in a single use vial, containing 1 to 8 x 10^8 CFU, equivalent to 50 mg. This product should not be confused with BCG vaccine, which is used for the prevention of tuberculosis. BCG is an infectious agent and should be treated as a biohazard material. BCG should not be administered to patients with current infections or who are being treated with antibiotics, as this may interfere with the effectiveness of BCG. One dose is usually 81 mg of BCG reconstituted by a diluent and further diluted by 50 ml of sterile water. The reconstituted BCG should be refrigerated and administered within two hours. Any unused solution should be discarded after two hours. It causes a local granulomatous reaction of the bladder. The exact antitumor mechanism is unknown. Administration should begin seven to 14 days following bladder biopsy. Patients should be instructed to not drink any fluids for four hours prior to treatment and to empty their bladder prior to administration. BCG is administered intravesically by gravity flow into the urinary bladder, and the patient retains the product in the bladder for two hours and then voids. During retention, patients should be moved from left to right sides, as well as on their abdomen and back, every 15 minutes. This maximizes the surface exposure of the bladder to BCG. Patients should receive one instillation per week for six weeks and the schedule may be repeated once if tumor regression has not been achieved. BCG may then be continued once per month for six to 12 months.

J9032

J9032 Injection, belinostat, 10 mg

Belinostat is a histone (any of a group of small basic proteins present in cell nuclei that organizes DNA strands by forming molecular complexes around which the DNA winds) deacetylase inhibitor indicated for the treatment of patients with relapsed or refractory peripheral T-cell lymphoma. Histone deacetylase are a class of enzymes that remove acetyl groups from an amino acid on a histone, allowing the histone to wrap the DNA more tightly. The accumulation of acetylated histones and other proteins disrupts the cell cycle and causes cell death. Belinostat shows preferred cytotoxicity toward tumor cells compared to normal cells. Recommended dosage is 10,000 mg/m2 over a 30-minute intravenous infusion, once a day on days one to five of a 21-day cycle. Repeat the cycle until the disease progresses or unacceptable toxicity occurs.

J9033

J9033 Injection, bendamustine HCl (Treanda), 1 mg

Bendamustine HCl is an antineoplastic alkylating drug. It is indicated as a treatment for chronic lymphocytic leukemia and indolent B-cell non-Hodgkin's lymphoma when the disease has progressed after being treated with rituximab. The recommended dose is 100 mg per m^2 administered by IV administration on days one and two of a 28-day cycle, for up to six cycles.

J9034

J9034 Injection, bendamustine HCl (Bendeka), 1 mg

Bendamustine HCl is an alkylating drug indicated for treatment of patients with chronic lymphocytic leukemia (CLL) and indolent B-cell non-Hodgkin lymphoma (NHL) that has progressed during or within six months of treatment with rituximab or a rituximab-containing regimen. The exact mechanism of action of bendamustine remains unknown. Recommended dosage for CLL is 100 mg/m2 infused intravenously over 10 minutes on days one and two of a 28-day cycle, for up to six cycles. Efficacy relative to first line therapies other than chlorambucil has not been established. Recommended dosage for NHL is 120 mg/m2 infused intravenously over 10 minutes on days one and two of a 21-day cycle, for up to eight cycles.

J9035

J9035 Injection, bevacizumab, 10 mg

Bevacizumab is a monoclonal antibody produced by recombinant DNA technology in Chinese hamster ovaries. This monoclonal antibody binds to and inhibits the biologic activity of human vascular endothelial growth factor preventing the formation of new blood vessels. Bevacizumab, used in combination with intravenous 5-fluorouracil, is indicated for first-line treatment of patients with metastatic carcinoma of the colon or rectum. The recommended dose is 5 mg per kg of body weight administered once every 14 days disease progression is detected. Bevacizumab is administered by intravenous infusion. The initial dose infusion should be delivered over 90 minutes. If the first infusion is well tolerated, the second infusion may be administered over 60 minutes. If the 60-minute infusion is well tolerated, all subsequent infusions may be administered over 30 minutes.

J9036

J9036 Injection, bendamustine HCl, (Belrapzo/bendamustine), 1 mg

Bendamustine HCl is an alkylating drug indicated for treatment of pediatric and adult patients with chronic lymphocytic leukemia (CLL) and indolent B-cell non-Hodgkin lymphoma (NHL) that has progressed during or within six months of treatment with rituximab or a rituximab-containing regimen. The exact mechanism of action of bendamustine remains unknown. It is supplied in multiple dose vials as a ready-to-dilute solution of 100 mg/4mL. Recommended dosage for CLL is 100 mg/m^2 administered by intravenous infusion over 30 minutes on days one and two of a 28-day cycle, for up to six cycles. Recommended dosage for NHL is 120 mg/m^2 administered by intravenous infusion over 60 minutes on days one and two of a 21-day cycle, for up to eight cycles.

J9037

J9037 Injection, belantamab mafodontin-blmf, 0.5 mg

Belantamab mafodotin-blmf is an injectable B-cell maturation antigen (BCMA)-directed antibody and microtubule inhibitor conjugate. It is indicated for the treatment of adult patients with relapsed or refractory multiple myeloma who have received a minimum of four prior therapies including an anti-CD38 monoclonal antibody, an immunomodulatory agent, and a proteasome inhibitor. The recommended dosage is 2.5 mg/kg of actual body weight given as an intravenous (IV) infusion over approximately 30 minutes once every three weeks until disease progression or unacceptable toxicity.

J9039

J9039 Injection, blinatumomab, 1 mcg

Blinatumomab is a bispecific, CD19-directed, CD3 T-cell engager that activates endogenous T-cells, which in turn releases cytokines and causes a proliferation of T-cells. It is used for the treatment of Philadelphia, chromosome-negative relapsed or refractory B-cell precursor acute lymphoblastic leukemia (ALL), a rare and rapidly developing cancer of blood and bone marrow. Recommended dosage is administered in a cycle of treatment that consists of four weeks of continuous infusion, by infusion pump, followed by a two-week treatment-free period. In the first cycle, the drug is administered by continuous intravenous infusion at 9 mcg per day on days one through seven, 28 mcg per day on days eight through 28, and then a two-week, treatment-free period. In the second and any subsequent cycles, the drug is administered by continuous intravenous infusion at 28 mcg per day on days one through 28. Hospitalization is recommended for the first nine days of the first cycle and for the first two days of the subsequent cycles. A treatment course includes up to two cycles of blinatumomab for induction of treatment, followed by up to three additional cycles (up to a total of five cycles) for treatment consolidation.

J9040

J9040 Injection, bleomycin sulfate, 15 units

Bleomycin sulfate is an antibiotic antineoplastic drug produced from a strain of Streptomyces verticillus. It is thought to cause cell death by the inhibition of DNA synthesis with some inhibition of RNA and protein synthesis. Bleomycin sulfate is indicated as a single agent or in combination with other therapeutic agents for squamous cell carcinoma, Hodgkin's disease, non-Hodgkin's lymphoma, testicular carcinoma, and for treatment of malignant pleural effusion. It can be administered as an intravenous, intramuscular, or subcutaneous injection. Bleomycin sulfate may also be administered into the pleural cavity. The recommended dosage for pleural cavity administration is 60 units. The recommended dosage for other administration is 0.25 to 0.50 units per kg of body weight administered once or twice a week.

J9041

J9041 Injection, bortezomib, 0.1 mg

Bortezomib is a modified form of boronic acid used as an antineoplastic agent. Boron is a nonmetallic element and boric acid is a form of boron. The drug inhibits the activity of a protein complex that regulates the intracellular concentration of specific proteins within a cell. This disruption of cell stability can lead to cell death. Bortezomib is indicated for the treatment of mantle cell lymphoma in adults, ages 18 years and older, who have undergone at least one prior treatment and newly diagnosed or relapsed multiple myeloma in patients who have received at least two prior therapies and who have demonstrated disease progression since the last therapy. It is supplied in single use vials and must be reconstituted with 0.9% sodium chloride. The recommended dosage is 1.3 mg per m^2 (concentration of 1 mg/ml) administered via a three to five second bolus intravenous (IV) injection or via subcutaneous (SC) injections at a concentration of 2.5 mg/ml. Dosage and frequency vary based on the condition treated and toxicities. See full prescribing information for complete administration instructions.

J9042

J9042 Injection, brentuximab vedotin, 1 mg

Brentuximab vedotin is an antibody-drug conjugate (ADC) used to treat patients with Hodgkin lymphoma (HL) after at least two multi-agent chemotherapy treatment courses have failed. It is also used to treat patients with systemic anaplastic large cell lymphoma (sALCL) after at least one prior multi-agent chemotherapy treatment course has been unsuccessful. The antibody binds to CD30-expressing cells and ultimately causes the cell destruction. The recommended dose of brentuximab vedotin is 1.8 mg/kg administered only as an intravenous infusion over 30 minutes every three weeks. The dose for patients weighing greater than 100 kg should be calculated based on a weight of 100 kg.

J9043

J9043 Injection, cabazitaxel, 1 mg

Cabazitaxel is an antineoplastic taxane class agent extracted from yew needles. It is indicated as a treatment for hormone-refractory metastatic prostate cancer previously treated with a docetaxel-containing treatment regimen. The medication binds with the tubulin and disrupts the function and reproduction of the cell. Recommended dose is based on body surface area and is administered by IV infusion over the course of one hour.

J9045

J9045 Injection, carboplatin, 50 mg

Carboplatin is a chemical complex containing the metal platinum used as an antineoplastic drug. It binds to DNA disrupting synthesis and causing cell death. Carboplatin is similar to, but more stable than cisplatin. It is indicated as an initial treatment for advanced ovarian cancer in combination with other chemotherapeutic agents. Carboplatin is also indicated as a secondary treatment of recurrent ovarian carcinoma after prior chemotherapy, including patients who have been previously treated with cisplatin. Dosage depends upon patient body surface, patient reactions to the drug, and whether it is used as a single agent or in combination. Carboplatin is administered by an intravenous infusion lasting 15 minutes or longer. Aluminum reacts with carboplatin causing a loss of potency, therefore, needles or intravenous sets containing aluminum parts that may come in contact with the drug must not be used for its preparation or administration.

J9046

J9046 Injection, bortezomib (Dr. Reddy's), not therapeutically equivalent to J9041, 0.1 mg

Bortezomib is a modified form of boronic acid used as an antineoplastic agent. Boron is a nonmetallic element and boric acid is a form of boron. The drug inhibits the activity of a protein complex that regulates the intracellular concentration of specific proteins within a cell. This disruption of cell stability can lead to cell death. Bortezomib is indicated for the treatment of mantle cell lymphoma in adults, ages 18 years and older, who have undergone at least one prior treatment and for treatment of multiple myeloma. It is supplied in single dose vials of 3.5 mg and must be reconstituted with 0.9% sodium chloride. The recommended dosage is 1.3 mg per m^2 (concentration of 1 mg/ml) administered via a three to five second bolus intravenous (IV) injection. Dosage and frequency vary based on the condition treated and toxicities. See full prescribing information for complete administration instructions. Report J9046 only for bortezomib manufactured by Dr. Reddy's.

J9047

J9047 Injection, carfilzomib, 1 mg

Carfilzomib is a proteasome inhibitor. Proteasomes are protein complexes that assist in the breakdown and elimination of other damaged or unneeded cellular proteins. Proteasome inhibitors block the action of proteasomes allowing debris to build and ultimately causing cellular death. This drug is indicated for the treatment of patients with multiple myeloma who have received at least two prior therapies, including bortezomib and an immunomodulatory agent, and have demonstrated disease progression on or within 60 days of completion of the last therapy. Carfilzomib is administered intravenously over two to 10 minutes, on two consecutive days each week for three weeks (days one, two, eight, nine, 15, and 16), followed by a 12-day rest period (days 17 to 28). The recommended cycle 1 dose is 20 mg/m2/day. If the initial cycle is tolerated, then subsequent cycles can be increased to 27 mg/m2/day.

J

J9048

J9048 Injection, bortezomib (Fresenius Kabi), not therapeutically equivalent to J9041, 0.1 mg

Bortezomib is a modified form of boronic acid used as an antineoplastic agent. Boron is a nonmetallic element and boric acid is a form of boron. The drug inhibits the activity of a protein complex that regulates the intracellular concentration of specific proteins within a cell. This disruption of cell stability can lead to cell death. Bortezomib is indicated for the treatment of mantle cell lymphoma in adults, ages 18 years and older, who have undergone at least one prior treatment and for treatment of multiple myeloma. It is supplied in single dose vials of 3.5 mg and must be reconstituted with 0.9% sodium chloride. The recommended dosage is 1.3 mg per m^2 (concentration of 1 mg/ml) administered via a three to five second bolus intravenous (IV) injection. Dosage and frequency vary based on condition treated and toxicities. See full prescribing information for complete administration instructions. Report J9048 only for bortezomib manufactured by Fresenius Kabi.

J9049

J9049 Injection, bortezomib (Hospira), not therapeutically equivalent to J9041, 0.1 mg

Bortezomib is a modified form of boronic acid used as an antineoplastic agent. Boron is a nonmetallic element and boric acid is a form of boron. The drug inhibits the activity of a protein complex that regulates the intracellular concentration of specific proteins within a cell. This disruption of cell stability can lead to cell death. Bortezomib is indicated for the treatment of mantle cell lymphoma in adults, ages 18 years and older, who have undergone at least one prior treatment and for treatment of multiple myeloma. It is supplied in single dose vials of 3.5 mg and must be reconstituted with 0.9% sodium chloride. The recommended dosage is 1.3 mg per m^2 (concentration of 1 mg/ml) administered via a three to five second bolus intravenous (IV) injection. Dosage and frequency vary based on condition treated and toxicities. See full prescribing information for complete administration instructions. Report J9049 only for bortezomib manufactured by Hospira.

J9050

J9050 Injection, carmustine, 100 mg

Carmustine is one of the nitrosoureas, alkylating agents used as antineoplastic drugs. Nitrosoureas are a group of similar drugs that are highly lipid-soluble and cross the blood-brain barrier. Carmustine inhibits DNA repair causing cell death. It is indicated as a single agent or in combination therapy for the treatment of brain tumors, multiple myeloma, colorectal cancer, Hodgkin's disease, and non-Hodgkin's lymphoma. Dosage depends upon patient body surface, patient reactions to the drug, and whether it is used as a single agent or in combination. Carmustine is administered as an intravenous injection.

J9055

J9055 Injection, cetuximab, 10 mg

Cetuximab is monoclonal antibody produced by recombinant DNA technology in a murine cell culture. This antibody binds specifically to the epidermal growth factor receptor (EGFR, HER1, c-ErbB-1) on both normal and tumor cells resulting in inhibition of cell growth and causing cell death. Cetuximab, used in combination with irinotecan, is indicated for the treatment of EGFR-expressing, metastatic colorectal carcinoma in patients who are refractory to irinotecan-based chemotherapy. Cetuximab, administered as a single agent, is also indicated for the treatment of EGFR-expressing, metastatic colorectal carcinoma in patients who are intolerant to irinotecan-based chemotherapy. The recommended initial dosage for combination or as a single agent is 400 mg per m2 of body surface administered as a 120-minute intravenous infusion. The recommended weekly maintenance dose is 250 mg per m^2 of body surface infused intravenously over 60 minutes.

J9057

J9057 Injection, copanlisib, 1 mg

Copanlisib is a PI3K protein kinase inhibitor indicated for the treatment of relapsed follicular lymphoma (FL) in adult patients, 18 years of age and older, that have received at least two other prior systemic therapies. The mechanism of action of copanlisib is not fully understood. It is thought to target the PI3K-alpha and PI3K-delta protein cells, thus killing cancer cells. Copanlisib is administered by intravenous infusion and is supplied in single dose vials, ready for reconstitution. It should be reconstituted only with a 0.9% sodium chloride (NaCl) solution and should not be mixed with other diluents or drugs. Recommended dose is 60 mg administered by intravenous infusion over one hour on days one, eight, and 15 of a 28-day intermittent cycle consisting of three weeks on and one week off. Treatment should be continued until disease progression or if the patient attains an unacceptable toxicity. When used concomitantly in patients also taking CYP3A inhibitors, the copanlisib dosage should be reduced to 45 mg. Copanlisib should not be used concomitantly in patients also taking CYP3A inducers.

J9060

J9060 Injection, cisplatin, powder or solution, 10 mg

Cisplatin is a chemical complex containing the metal platinum used as an antineoplastic drug. It binds to DNA disrupting synthesis and causing cell death. Cisplatin is indicated in combination therapy for treatment of metastatic testicular and ovarian cancer after surgical and radiation therapy. Cisplatin is indicated as a single agent treatment for advanced transitional cell bladder cancer that can no longer be treated locally, such as with surgery or radiation therapy. As a single agent, it may also be used as a secondary treatment for metastatic ovarian cancer that is refractory to standard chemotherapy where cisplatin has not been previously administered. Cisplatin is administered as an intravenous infusion. Dosage depends upon patient body surface, patient reactions to the drug, and whether it is used as a single agent or in combination. Aluminum reacts with cisplatin causing a loss of potency; therefore, needles or intravenous sets containing aluminum parts that may come in contact with the drug must not be used for its preparation or administration.

J9061

J9061 Injection, amivantamab-vmjw, 2 mg

Amivantamab-vmjw is a bispecific epidermal growth factor receptor (EGFR)-directed and MET receptor-directed antibody that is indicated for the treatment of adults, ages 18 and older, with locally advanced or metastatic non-small cell lung cancer (NSCLC) with EGFR exon 20 insertion mutations, and whose disease has progressed on or following platinum-based chemotherapy. It is supplied in a single dose vial of 350 mg/7 mL (50 mg/mL) that requires either 5% dextrose or 0.9% sodium chloride for dilution (7 mL diluent for each vial of amivantamab-vmjw required). Dosage is based on baseline body weight. Premedication with an antihistamine and an antipyretic are required for all infusions. Premedication with a glucocorticoid is required on week one, days one and two. Glucocorticoid can be administered as needed for subsequent infusions. Amivantamab-vmjw is administered via intravenous (IV) infusion. See full prescribing information for complete administration instructions.

J9065

J9065 Injection, cladribine, per 1 mg

Cladribine is a synthetic version of adenosine used as an antineoplastic drug. Cladribine interferes with DNA repair and causes cell death. Cladribine is indicated as a treatment for active hairy cell leukemia. The recommended initial dosage is 0.9 mg per kg of body weight. It is administered by a continuous intravenous infusion over 24 hours. This continuous infusion is repeated daily for seven consecutive days.

J9070

J9070 Cyclophosphamide, 100 mg

Cyclophosphamide is a synthetic antineoplastic drug chemically related to the nitrogen mustards. The drug itself is inert and functions only after transformation in the liver to active alkylating metabolites. These metabolites interfere with the growth of susceptible rapidly proliferating malignant cells. The mechanism of action is thought to be its interference with the DNA of the tumor cell causing cell death. Cyclophosphamide is indicated singularly or in combination with other chemotherapeutic drugs, to treat a wide variety of cancers including Hodgkin's disease, lymphosarcoma, acute lymphocytic leukemia, Burkitt's lymphoma, carcinoma of the breast, multiple myeloma, chronic lymphocytic leukemia, bronchogenic carcinoma, neuroblastoma, ovarian carcinoma, and carcinoma of the uterine cervix. It is also used as an immunosuppressant to prevent transplant rejection and in the treatment of certain diseases with abnormal immune function, including severe lupus manifestations and vasculitis. Cyclophosphamide may be administered via intravenous injection or infusion, or may be injected intramuscularly, intraperitoneally, or intrapleurally. An oral version is also available. Dosage depends upon body weight and the disease being treated. The lyophilized version of cyclophosphamide is a freeze-dried version of the drug.

J9071

J9071 Injection, cyclophosphamide, (AuroMedics), 5 mg

Cyclophosphamide is a synthetic antineoplastic drug chemically related to the nitrogen mustards. The drug itself is inert and functions only after transformation in the liver to active alkylating metabolites. These metabolites interfere with the growth of susceptible, rapidly proliferating malignant cells. The mechanism of action is thought to be its interference with the DNA of the tumor cell causing cell death. Cyclophosphamide is indicated singularly or in combination with other chemotherapeutic drugs to treat a wide variety of cancers, including adenocarcinoma of the ovary, carcinoma of the breast, leukemias, malignant lymphomas, multiple myeloma, mycosis fungoides, neuroblastoma, and retinoblastoma. Cyclophosphamide may be administered via intravenous injection or infusion, or may be injected intramuscularly, intraperitoneally, or intrapleurally. Dosage and route of administration depends upon body weight and the disease being treated.

J9098-J9100

J9098 Injection, cytarabine liposome, 10 mg
J9100 Injection, cytarabine, 100 mg

Cytarabine is a synthetic nucleoside used as an antineoplastic drug. The drug interferes with DNA synthesis causing cell death. Cytarabine is indicated singularly or in combination with other chemotherapeutic drugs to induce remission in acute nonlymphocytic leukemia in adults and children and to treat acute lymphocytic leukemia and the blast phase of chronic myelocytic leukemia. Intrathecal cytarabine is indicated in the prophylaxis and treatment of meningeal leukemia. Cytarabine may be administered via intravenous injection or infusion, or may be injected intramuscularly, intraperitoneally, intrapleurally, or intrathecally. Dosage depends upon body weight and the disease being treated. The liposome version of cytarabine is a suspension of cytarabine encapsulated with liposomes. The liposome version is administered intrathecally to treat meningitis associated with lymphoma.

J9118

J9118 Injection, calaspargase pegol-mknl, 10 units

Calaspargase pegol-mknl is an asparagine specific enzyme that is indicated as part of a multi-agent chemotherapy regimen for the treatment of acute lymphoblastic leukemia (ALL) in pediatric and adult patients, aged 1 month to 21 years. The mechanism of action is not fully understood, but is thought to be the selective killing of leukemic cells caused by a depletion of plasma L-asparagine. It is supplied in a single dose vial of 3,750 units per 5 mL (750 units/mL) of solution. It requires dilution in 100 mL of 0.9% sodium chloride or 5% dextrose. After dilution, it should be administered intravenously into a running infusion of 0.9% sodium chloride or 5% dextrose over one hour. Other drugs should not be administered through the same line. The recommended dosage is 2,500 to 3,750 units/m^2 administered via intravenous infusion no more frequently than every 21 days.

J9119

J9119 Injection, cemiplimab-rwlc, 1 mg

Cemiplimab-rwlc is a programmed death receptor-1 (PD-1) blocking antibody. It is utilized for the treatment of adult patients with metastatic cutaneous squamous cell carcinoma (CSCC) or locally advanced CSCC patients who are not candidates for curative radiation or surgery. It is supplied in a single dose vial of 350 mg/7 mL (50 mg/mL) that requires dilution with 0.9% sodium chloride or 5% dextrose and should be refrigerated until use. The recommend dosage is 350 mg administered by intravenous infusion over 30 minutes every three weeks.

J9120

J9120 Injection, dactinomycin, 0.5 mg

Dactinomycin, also known as actinomycin D, is an antibiotic produced by a strain of *Streptomyces parvulus* bacterium that is used as an antineoplastic agent. The drug inhibits RNA synthesis, leading to cellular death. Dactinomycin is indicated in combination therapy for the treatment of Wilms' tumor, childhood rhabdomyosarcoma, Ewing's sarcoma, and metastatic nonseminomatous testicular cancer. The drug may be used as a single agent or in combination as a treatment for gestational trophoblastic neoplasia. Dactinomycin is also indicated as a part of a regional perfusion for the palliative and/or adjunctive treatment of locally recurrent or locoregional sarcoma, carcinoma, and adenocarcinoma. Recommended dosages vary by the type of neoplasm being treated and the patient's body surface or weight. The drug is highly toxic even in powdered form and is extremely corrosive to soft tissue. Dactinomycin is administered intravenously.

J9130

J9130 Dacarbazine, 100 mg

Dacarbazine, also known as DTIC, is a chemical complex that is an antineoplastic agent. The drug interferes with DNA synthesis causing cell death. Dacarbazine is indicated in the treatment of metastatic malignant melanoma. It is also used in combination with other chemotherapeutic agents as a treatment for Hodgkin's disease. The drug is administered by intravenous injection or infusion. The recommended dosage depends upon body surface, the disease being treated, and the treatment plan.

J9144

J9144 Injection, daratumumab, 10 mg and hyaluronidase-fihj

Daratumumab, 10 mg and hyaluronidase-fihj (trade name Darzalex Faspro) is a combination of daratumumab, a human CD38-directed cytolytic antibody, and hyaluronidase, an endoglycosidase, that is indicated for the treatment of adults, ages 18 years and older, with multiple myeloma. As a monotherapy, it is used for patients who have received at least three prior therapies, including a proteasome inhibitor (PI) and an immunomodulatory agent, or in patients who are double-refractory to a PI and an immunomodulatory agent; in combination with bortezomib and dexamethasone in patients who have received at least one prior therapy; in combination with bortezomib, melphalan, and prednisone in newly diagnosed patients ineligible for autologous stem cell transplant; and in combination with lenalidomide and dexamethasone in newly diagnosed patients ineligible for autologous stem cell transplants or with relapsed or refractory multiple myeloma who have received at least one prior therapy. The drug is administered by subcutaneous (SC) injection and is supplied in a single dose vial. The recommended dosage is 1,800 mg daratumumab and 30,000 units hyaluronidase administered by SC injection into the abdomen over three to five minutes. When administered as monotherapy, it is given every week for the first eight weeks, every two weeks for weeks nine to 24, then every four weeks until disease progression. Alternate dosing schedules for combination therapies are outlined on the package insert. Patients should be premedicated with corticosteroids, acetaminophen, and an antihistamine. On the first- and second-day post-infusion, the patient should be given corticosteroids to reduce the risk of delayed reactions.

J9145

J9145 Injection, daratumumab, 10 mg

Daratumumab is a human CD38-directed monoclonal antibody used as an antineoplastic agent and is indicated for the treatment of multiple myeloma in patients who have received at least three prior therapies, including a proteasome inhibitor (PI) and an immunomodulatory agent, or in patients who are double-refractory to a PI and an immunomodulatory agent. Patients should be premedicated with corticosteroids, antihistamines, and antipyretics. On the first and second day post-infusion, the patient should be given corticosteroids to reduce the risk of delayed reactions. The drug is administered by intravenous infusion. The recommended dosage is 16 mg/kg body weight weekly for weeks one through eight, every two weeks for weeks nine through 24, and every four weeks from week 25 forward.

J9150-J9151

J9150 Injection, daunorubicin, 10 mg

J9151 Injection, daunorubicin citrate, liposomal formulation, 10 mg

Daunorubicin hydrochloride is an anthracycline antibiotic, produced by a strain of Streptomyces coeruleorubidus bacterium, that is used as an antineoplastic agent. The drug interrupts DNA synthesis creating breaks within the DNA strands leading to cellular death. Daunorubicin hydrochloride is indicated in combination with other chemotherapeutic agents for the remission induction of acute nonlymphocytic leukemia (myelogenous, monocytic, and erythroid) in adults and for acute lymphocytic leukemia in both children and adults. Recommended dosages are 25 to 30 mg per m^2 of body surface infused intravenously. In children younger than 2 years of age, it is recommended that the dose be based on body weight rather than body surface. The drug should never be given by intramuscular or subcutaneous injection. The length of a regimen and the subsequent courses of therapy depend upon the patient and type of leukemia being treated. Daunorubicin citrate liposome is indicted for the treatment of HIV-related advanced Kaposi's sarcoma.

J9153

J9153 Injection, liposomal, 1 mg daunorubicin and 2.27 mg cytarabine

Liposomal, 1 mg daunorubicin and 2.27 mg cytarabine, is a combination of an anthracycline topoisomerase inhibitor (daunorubicin) and a nucleoside metabolic inhibitor (cytarabine) indicated for the treatment of adults with therapy-related acute myeloid leukemia (t-AML) or AML with myelodysplasia-related changes (AML-MRC). The liposomes enter and persist in the patient's bone marrow, are taken up by leukemia cells where the liposomes degrade, and release the drug combination directly inside the intracellular environment. It is supplied in a lyophilized cake that must be reconstituted with sterile water prior to use. The induction dosage is 44 mg/m^2 daunorubicin and 100 mg/m^2 cytarabine liposome by intravenous injection over 90 minutes on days one, three, and five, and on days one and three for subsequent induction cycles, if indicated. The consolidation dosage is 29 mg/m^2 daunorubicin and 65 mg/m^2.

J9155

J9155 Injection, degarelix, 1 mg

Degarelix is a gonadotropin releasing hormone (GnRH) receptor inhibitor used to treat patients with advanced prostate cancer. It inhibits the testosterone, which retards the growth of cancer in the prostate. It's a synthetic mixture that contains seven amino acids. The recommended dose is 240 mg initially administered by two subcutaneous injections of 120 mg each. The recommended maintenance dose is 80 mg given as a single subcutaneous injection every 28 days.

J9160

J9160 Injection, denileukin diftitox, 300 mcg

Denileukin diftitox is a modified form of the diphtheria toxin produced from *E. coli* bacterium using recombinant DNA technology. This biological is used as an antineoplastic agent. It binds to IL-2 receptor sites on certain cells delivering the diphtheria toxin, which inhibits cellular protein synthesis causing the death of the cell. This receptor is usually highly active in activated B and T lymphocytes and macrophages. Denileukin diftitox is indicated for the treatment of persistent or recurrent cutaneous T cell lymphoma where the cells express the CD25 component of the IL-2 receptor. The biological is administered via an intravenous infusion of at least 15 minutes, daily for five consecutive days. This regimen should be administered every 21 days. The recommended dose is 9 or 18 mcg per kg of body weight.

J9165

J9165 Injection, diethylstilbestrol diphosphate, 250 mg

Diethylstilbestrol (DES) diphosphate is a synthetic estrogen used as a hormone treatment for advanced prostate cancer. Estrogen is a hormone produced by the ovaries, adrenal gland, testis, and placenta. While small amounts are present in males, it is generally referred to as the female sex hormone. The high levels of estrogen within the body cause a decrease in testosterone production that can slow the growth of prostatic cancer cells.

J9171

J9171 Injection, docetaxel, 1 mg

Docetaxel is a semisynthetic antineoplastic drug created from the needles of the yew tree. The drug inhibits cell division, which stops the cancer cells from reproducing. Docetaxel is indicated as a single agent for the treatment of locally advanced or metastatic breast cancer after failure of prior chemotherapy and for locally advanced or metastatic non-small-cell lung cancer after failure of prior platinum-based chemotherapy. In combination with other chemotherapeutic agents, it is indicated as induction treatment for patients with inoperable locally advanced squamous cell carcinoma of the head and neck and adjuvant treatment of patients with

J

operable node-positive breast cancer and hormone refractory metastatic prostate cancer; patients with unresectable, locally advanced or metastatic non-small-cell lung cancer who have not previously received chemotherapy for this condition; and those with advanced gastric adenocarcinoma who have not received prior chemotherapy for advanced disease. Docetaxel is infused intravenously over one hour. Dosage depends upon m2 of patient body surface and the disease being treated.

J9173

J9173 Injection, durvalumab, 10 mg

Durvalumab is a human immunoglobulin G1 kappa (IgG1k) monoclonal antibody produced in Chinese hamster ovary cells. This antibody is specifically directed against the interaction of programmed cell death-ligand 1 (PD-L1) with PD-1 and B7.1 molecules. Blocking the interaction between PD-L1/PD-1 or PD-L1/CD80 (B7.1) releases the inhibition of immune responses without inducing antibody dependent cell-mediated cytotoxicity (ADCC). This mechanism increases T-cell activation and decreases tumor size. It is indicated for the treatment of locally advanced or metastatic urothelial carcinoma or unresectable Stage II non-small cell lung cancer in adult patients that have disease progression, have had previous platinum-containing chemotherapy, or have disease progression within 12 months of receiving neoadjuvant or adjuvant platinum-containing chemotherapy. Recommended dosage is 10 mg/kg of weight administered as an intravenous infusion over 60 minutes. It is administered every two weeks until disease progression or the occurrence of unacceptable toxicity. Patients should be premedicated with acetaminophen and an antihistamine prior to the first four administrations. For subsequent administrations, premedication should be based upon clinical judgement and the severity of reactions to the previous infusions.

J9175

J9175 Injection, Elliotts' B solution, 1 ml

Elliotts' B solution is a diluent of buffered electrolytes and dextrose that is comparable in pH, composition, and osmolarity to cerebrospinal fluid. Elliotts' B solution is indicated as a diluent for the intrathecal administration of methotrexate sodium and cytarabine for the prevention or treatment of meningeal leukemia or lymphocytic lymphoma.

J9176

J9176 Injection, elotuzumab, 1 mg

Elotuzumab is a SLAMF-directed immunostimulatory antibody used for the treatment of patients with multiple myeloma who have been treated with one to three prior therapies. Elotuzumab targets the SLAMF7 protein found on Natural Killer Cells (NKC), myeloma cells, and plasma cells. Patients should be premedicated with corticosteroids, antihistamines, an H2 blocker, and antipyretics on the days Elotuzumab is administered. The drug is administered by intravenous infusion. The recommended dosage is 10 mg/kg body weight weekly for the first two cycles and then every two weeks forward concurrently with Lenalidomide on days one to 21 of each dosage cycle. Treatment is continued until full disease progression or patient has unacceptable toxicity.

J9177

J9177 Injection, enfortumab vedotin-ejfv, 0.25 mg

Enfortumab vedotin-ejfv is a Nectin-4-directed antibody and microtubule inhibitor conjugate that is indicated for the treatment of adults, ages 18 years and older, with locally advanced or metastatic urothelial cancer who were previously treated with a programmed death receptor-1 (PD-1) or programmed death-ligand 1 (PD-L1) inhibitor, and a platinum containing chemotherapy in the neoadjuvant/adjuvant, locally advanced, or metastatic setting. The drug is administered via an intravenous (IV) infusion and should not be given as an IV push or bolus and should not be mixed with other medicinal products. It is supplied in 20 and 30 mg single dose vials for reconstitution with sterile water. The 20 mg vial should be reconstituted with 2.3 mL sterile water. The 30 mg vial should be reconstituted with 3.3 mL sterile water. Once reconstituted, the final concentration should be further diluted in an IV bag of either 5% dextrose, 0.9% sodium chloride, or Lactated Ringer's injection. The recommended dosage is 1.25 mg/kg of body weight (up to a maximum of 125 mg) administered via IV infusion over 30 minutes on days one, eight, and 15 of a 28-day cycle until disease progression or unacceptable toxicity.

J9178

J9178 Injection, epirubicin HCl, 2 mg

Epirubicin hydrochloride (HCl) is an anthracycline, antibiotic, antineoplastic drug that is chemically similar to doxorubicin hydrochloride, but has a lower toxicity. It binds to DNA inhibiting RNA and protein synthesis creating cell death. Epirubicin hydrochloride is used as an adjunctive therapy for patients with primary breast cancer who have evidence of axillary node involvement following surgical resection. It is also indicated in the treatment of cancers of the lung, stomach, ovary, colon, and rectum, and for treatment of leukemia, lymphoma, and multiple myeloma. The initial recommended dosage is 100 to 120 mg per m^2 of body surface administered as an intravenous infusion over 15 to 20 minutes. Dosages administered after the initial dose depend upon the patient's reaction and the infusion time for subsequent doses may be significantly decreased.

J9179

J9179 Injection, eribulin mesylate, 0.1 mg

Eribulin mesylate is used to treat patients with metastatic breast cancer who have received at least two other forms of treatment, including taxane-based and anthracycline-based therapy. The drug inhibits the growth phase of microtubules. Recommended dose of eribulin mesylate is 1.4 mg/m2 administered intravenously over two to five minutes on days one and eight of a 21-day cycle. The dose may vary based on renal and hepatic function.

J9181

J9181 Injection, etoposide, 10 mg

Etoposide is a semisynthetic derivative of podophyllotoxin, a toxic compound found in the rhizomes and roots of the mandrake plant. It is believed to inhibit the repair of DNA causing cell death. Etoposide is an antineoplastic drug used in combination with other chemotherapeutic agents. It is available in injectable or oral versions. Injectable etoposide is indicated for the treatment of small cell lung cancer and refractory testicular cancer that has been previously treated with surgery, radiation, or other chemotherapy. The oral version is indicated for the treatment of small cell lung cancer. The recommended dosage of the injectable version ranges from 35 to 100 mg per m2 of body surface depending on which disease is being treated. The injectable version is administered by intravenous infusion over 30 to 60 minutes. The recommended dosage for the oral version is two times the intravenous version.

J9185

J9185 Injection, fludarabine phosphate, 50 mg

Fludarabine phosphate is an antineoplastic drug that is a fluorinated nucleotide analogue of the antiviral agent vidarabine. It is rapidly broken down into 2-fluoro-ara-A which inhibits DNA synthesis and causes cell death. Fludarabine phosphate is indicated for the treatment of beta-cell chronic lymphocytic leukemia for patients who have not responded to an alkylating drug treatment. It is administered through intravenous infusion over 30 minutes for five consecutive days. The recommended dosage is 25 mg per m^2 of body surface.

J9190

J9190 Injection, fluorouracil, 500 mg

Fluorouracil, also known as 5 FU, is an antineoplastic drug that is a fluorinated analogue of uracil. Uracil is a chemical compound found in nucleic acids. Once broken down, it interferes with the synthesis of DNA and RNA causing cell death. Fluorouracil is available in injectable and topical versions. The injectable version is indicated for the treatment of many different cancers, among them cancer of the breast, stomach, pancreas, and colon. The topical version is used to treat actinic or solar keratoses and superficial basal cell carcinomas. Dosage for the injectable version depends upon body weight and is administered by intravenous injection.

J9198

J9198 Injection, gemcitabine HCl, (Infugem), 100 mg

Gemcitabine HCl is a nucleoside metabolic inhibitor indicated in combination with carboplatin for the treatment of advanced ovarian cancer that has relapsed at least six months after completion of platinum-based therapy; in combination with paclitaxel for first-line treatment of metastatic breast cancer after failure of prior anthracycline-containing adjuvant chemotherapy (unless anthracyclines were clinically contraindicated); in combination with cisplatin for the treatment of non-small cell lung cancer; or as a single agent for the treatment of pancreatic cancer. Administered via intravenous (IV) infusion, the dosage is dependent upon the type of cancer and the treatment protocol. It is supplied in single dose, premixed infusion bags containing 10 mg/mL of gemcitabine in 0.9% sodium chloride ranging from 1,200 mg to 2,200 mg. See full prescribing information for recommended dosages by cancer type and protocol.

J9200

J9200 Injection, floxuridine, 500 mg

Floxuridine, also known as FUDR, is an antineoplastic drug that is broken down into the same substance as fluorouracil. It interferes with the synthesis of DNA and RNA causing cell death. Floxuridine is administered by continuous intra-arterial infusion using a pump. It is indicated as a palliative treatment of gastrointestinal adenocarcinoma that has metastasized to the liver in patients who are considered incurable by surgery or other means. The recommended dosage is 0.1 to 0.6 mg per kg of body weight per day.

J9201

J9201 Injection, gemcitabine HCl, not otherwise specified, 200 mg

Gemcitabine hydrochloride is a nucleoside analogue used as an antineoplastic drug. It interferes with the synthesis of DNA and RNA causing cell death. Gemcitabine hydrochloride in combination with paclitaxel is indicated as a treatment for metastatic breast cancer after the failure of prior chemotherapy. It is indicated in combination with cisplatin in the treatment of inoperable locally advanced or metastatic non-small cell lung cancer. As a sole agent, gemcitabine hydrochloride is indicated as a treatment for inoperable, locally advanced, or metastatic pancreatic cancer previously treated with fluorouracil. The recommended initial dosage is from 1,000 to 1,250 mg per m^2 of body surface administered by intravenous infusion over 30 minutes. Report J9201 when the gemcitabine HCl is not otherwise specified by other HCPCS codes.

J9202

J9202 Goserelin acetate implant, per 3.6 mg

Goserelin acetate is a synthetic analogue of the luteinizing hormone-releasing hormone (LHRH) used as an antineoplastic drug. The implant is a biodegradable tube containing 3.6 mg of goserelin acetate that is slowly released over 28 days. This continued administration leads to suppression of pituitary gonadotropins and subsequently to lower levels of estrogen and testosterone. The goserelin acetate implant is indicated as a palliative treatment for advanced breast and prostatic cancer. In combination with flutamide, it is indicated for treatment of locally confined prostate cancer stage T2b-T4 (Stage B2-C). It may also be indicated as a treatment for endometriosis and as an endometrial-thinning agent prior to ablation. The goserelin acetate implant is injected subcutaneously into the upper abdominal wall every 28 days.

J9203

J9203 Injection, gemtuzumab ozogamicin, 0.1 mg

Gemtuzumab ozogamicin is a monoclonal antibody produced by recombinant DNA coupled with an antineoplastic antibiotic, calicheamicin. Calicheamicin is derived from the bacterium *Micromonospora echinospora subsp. calichensis*. The antibody portion of the drug binds specifically to the CD33 antigen, a protein found on the surface of leukemic blasts and immature normal cells of myelomonocytic lineage, but not on normal hematopoietic stem cells. Once bound with the CD33 antigen, the calicheamicin interferes with DNA replication and causes cell death. Gemtuzumab ozogamicin is indicated for the treatment of patients with CD33 positive acute myeloid leukemia (AML) in adults and refractory/relapsed patients 2 years of age and older. For the combination regimen to treat newly diagnosed de novo AML, the recommended induction dosage is 3 mg/m^2 (up to one 4.5 mg vial) on days one, four, and seven, administered in combination with daunorubicin and cytarabine. The recommended consolidation dosage is 3 mg/m^2 (up to one 4.5 mg vial) on day one. For the single agent regiment to treat newly diagnosed AML, the induction dosage is 6 mg/m^2 on day one and 3 mg/m^2 on day eight. Subsequent dosage for patients without disease progression after induction is up to eight courses of 2 mg/m^2 on day one every four weeks. For refractory or relapsed AMG, 3 mg/m^2 on days one, four, and seven. All patients should be premedicated with acetaminophen, an antihistamine, and a corticosteroid one hour prior to the infusion.

J9204

J9204 Injection, mogamulizumab-kpkc, 1 mg

Mogamulizumab-kpkc is a CC chemokine receptor type 4 (CCR4)-directed monoclonal antibody that is indicated for the treatment of adults with refractory or relapsed mycosis fungoides or Sezary syndrome following at least one previous systemic therapy. It is supplied in 20 mg/5 mL (4 mg/mL) single-dose vials that must be transferred into an intravenous bag containing 0.9% sodium chloride. The concentration should be between 0.1 mg/mL to 30 mg/mL and is administered via intravenous infusion over 60 minutes on days one, eight, 15, and 22 of the first 28-day cycle, and then on days one and 15 of each successive cycle. It should not be administered by rapid intravenous infusion or subcutaneously. Acetaminophen and diphenhydramine should be administered before the first infusion.

J9205

J9205 Injection, irinotecan liposome, 1 mg

Irinotecan liposome is a topoisomerase inhibitor for the treatment of patients aged 18 years and older with metastatic pancreatic cancer with progression of the disease, following gemcitabine-based therapy. Irinotecan liposome should not be used as the sole treatment for patients with metastatic pancreatic cancer, but should be used in combination with fluorouracil and leucovorin. The dosage is 70 mg/m^2 administered over a 90-minute intravenous infusion every two weeks. For patients known to be homozygous for the UGT1A1*28 allele, the starting dose should be 50 mg/m^2 with the dose increased in subsequent cycles to 70 mg/m^2, as tolerated.

J9206

J9206 Injection, irinotecan, 20 mg

Irinotecan hydrochloride (HCL) is an antineoplastic drug that is a semisynthetic derivative of camptothecin, an alkaloid extract from plants such as Camptotheca acuminata. The drug works by causing strand breaks in DNA that the cell cannot repair leading to cell death. Irinotecan is indicated as a first line treatment in combination with fluorouracil and leucovorin for metastatic carcinoma of the colon or rectum. Irinotecan is also indicated for patients with metastatic carcinoma of the colon or rectum whose disease has recurred or progressed following initial fluorouracil-based therapy. The recommended dosage varies from 125 to 300 mg depending on the regimen. Irinotecan hydrochloride is administered by intravenous infusion over 90 minutes.

J9207

J9207 Injection, ixabepilone, 1 mg

Ixabepilone is an antineoplastic drug used to treat metastatic or locally advanced breast cancer that is resistant to anthracycline and taxane or if those treatments are contraindicated. It inhibits cell division, which leads to cell death. The recommended dose is 40 mg/m^2 by intravenous infusion over three hours. The treatment is administered every three weeks.

J9208

J9208 Injection, ifosfamide, 1 g

Ifosfamide is an antineoplastic that is a synthetic analogue of cyclophosphamide and is related to the nitrogen mustards. The drug functions only after transformation in the liver to active alkylating metabolites. These metabolites interfere with the DNA causing cell death. Ifosfamide is indicated as a third-line treatment for germ cell testicular cancer. The recommended dosage is 1.2 g per m^2 of body surface administered by slow intravenous infusion over 30 minutes, through five consecutive days. Mesna is often given with ifosfamide as a prophylactic agent against hemorrhagic cystitis.

J9209

J9209 Injection, mesna, 200 mg

Mesna is a synthetic sulfur-hydrogen compound that is used as a detoxifying agent to inhibit the hemorrhagic cystitis caused by ifosfamide. Once broken down in the body, the drug combines with the urotoxic byproducts of ifosfamide rendering them harmless. Mesna is available in injectable and oral versions. The dosage is dependent upon the amount of ifosfamide given calculated at 20 percent the amount of ifosfamide. Mesna is administered as an intravenous injection at the time of ifosfamide administration, and then repeated at four and eight hours following the administration. Alternately, the first does may be by intravenous injection and the subsequent doses may be oral.

J9210

J9210 Injection, emapalumab-lzsg, 1 mg

Emapalumab-lzsg is an interferon gamma blocking antibody that is indicated for the treatment of children and adults with primary hemophagocytic lymphohistiocytosis (HLH) who have refractory, recurrent, or progressive disease, or patients who are intolerant to conventional HLH therapy. It is supplied in single dose vials of 10 mg/2 ml (5mg/ml) or 50 mg/10 ml (5mg/ml) solution and requires dilution with 0.9% sodium chloride for a maximum concentration of 2.5 mg/ml. The number of vials required is determined by the patient's weight and prescribed dose. The recommended starting dosage is 1 mg/kg body weight administered via intravenous infusion over 60 minutes twice per week. Subsequent doses can be increased to 3, 6, or 10 mg/kg body weight based on clinical and laboratory findings. Patients should be premedicated with a prophylaxis for Herpes Zoster, *Pneumocystis jirovecii,* and for fungal infections. Dexamethasone should also be administered.

J9211

J9211 Injection, idarubicin HCl, 5 mg

Idarubicin hydrochloride is an antineoplastic drug that is a semisynthetic analogue of daunorubicin. It interferes with DNA synthesis causing cell death. Idarubicin hydrochloride is indicated in combination with other chemotherapeutic drugs for the treatment of acute myeloid leukemia. The recommended dosage is 12 mg per m^2 of body surface. Idarubicin hydrochloride is administered by intravenous infusion over 10 to 15 minutes.

J9212

J9212 Injection, interferon alfacon-1, recombinant, 1 mcg

Interferon alfacon-1 is a non-natural form of human interferon alpha proteins that are produced by recombinant DNA technology. Interferons are small, naturally occurring proteins that bind to specific cell membranes and initial a series of events that include the inhibition of virus replication and the enhancement of macrophage and lymphocyte destruction of foreign cells. Interferon alfacon-1 is indicated for the treatment of chronic hepatitis C. The recommended dosage is 9 to 15 mcg administered as a subcutaneous injection every 48 hours for 24 weeks.

J9213

J9213 Injection, interferon, alfa-2a, recombinant, 3 million units

Interferon alfa-2a is a purified form of human interferon alpha proteins that are produced by recombinant DNA technology using *Escherichia coli* bacteria. Interferons are small, naturally occurring proteins that bind to specific cell membranes and initial a series of events that include the inhibition of virus replication and the enhancement of macrophage and lymphocyte destruction of foreign cells. Interferon alfa-2a is indicated for the treatment of AIDS-related Kaposi's sarcoma, hairy cell leukemia, chronic hepatitis C, and in Philadelphia chromosome-positive chronic myelogenous leukemia. The recommended dosage is 3 to 9 million IU depending upon the disease being treated. Interferon alfa-2a is administered as an intramuscular or subcutaneous injection daily. Prefilled syringes are intended for subcutaneous injection only.

J9214

J9214 Injection, interferon, alfa-2b, recombinant, 1 million units

Interferon alfa-2b is a purified form of human interferon alpha proteins that are produced by recombinant DNA technology using *Escherichia coli* bacteria. Interferons are small, naturally occurring proteins that bind to specific cell membranes and initial a series of events that include the inhibition of virus replication and the enhancement of macrophage and lymphocyte destruction of foreign cells. Interferon alfa-2b is indicated for the treatment of hairy cell leukemia, malignant melanoma, genital or venereal warts, Kaposi's sarcoma, and chronic hepatitis B and C. It is also indicated in combination with other chemotherapeutic agents as an initial treatment of clinically aggressive follicular non-Hodgkin's lymphoma. The recommended dosage

J

varies from 5 to 25 million IU depending upon the disease being treated. Interferon alfa-2b can be administered as an intramuscular, subcutaneous, or intravenous infusion over 20 minutes or intralesional injection.

J9215

J9215 Injection, interferon, alfa-N3, (human leukocyte derived), 250,000 IU

Interferon alfa-N3 is a purified form of human interferon alpha proteins that is derived from human leukocytes. The human leukocytes are induced by inoculation with a murine virus to produce the interferon alfa proteins. Interferons are small naturally occurring proteins that bind to specific cell membranes and initiate a series of events that include the inhibition of virus replication and the enhancement of macrophage and lymphocyte destruction of foreign cells. Interferon alfa-N3 is indicated for the treatment of condylomata acuminata (genital warts) where it is injected intralesionally. Interferon alfa-N3 has also been used off-label to treat multiple sclerosis, hepatitis C, and some cancers.

J9216

J9216 Injection, interferon, gamma 1-b, 3 million units

Interferon gamma-1b is a purified form of human interferon gamma proteins that are produced by recombinant DNA technology using *Escherichia coli* bacteria. Interferons are small, naturally occurring proteins that bind to specific cell membranes and initial a series of events that include the inhibition of virus replication and the enhancement of macrophage and lymphocyte destruction of foreign cells. Interferon gamma-1b is indicated for the treatment of chronic granulomatous disease and severe malignant osteopetrosis. The recommended dosage varies from 1 to 1.5 million units per m2 of body surface. Interferon gamma-1b is administered as a subcutaneous injection.

J9217-J9219

J9217 Leuprolide acetate (for depot suspension), 7.5 mg

J9218 Leuprolide acetate, per 1 mg

J9219 Leuprolide acetate implant, 65 mg

Leuprolide acetate is a synthetic analogue of the luteinizing hormone-releasing hormone (LHRH) that is used as an antineoplastic drug and a treatment for central precocious puberty, endometriosis, and uterine fibroids. It first stimulates and then suppresses follicle stimulating and luteinizing hormone release, resulting in suppression of testosterone and estrogen. A depot suspension is a drug that remains in the body long-term in storage and is slowly released into the blood. The leuprolide acetate depot suspension in dosages of 3.75 mg monthly and the 12.25 mg every three months are injected intramuscularly to treat endometriosis and uterine fibroids. When used to treat central precocious puberty, the dosage is individualized to the child and can range from 7.5 to 15 mg. Leuprolide acetate in doses of 7.5 mg and greater is injected subcutaneously and is used as a palliative treatment for advanced prostate cancer. The leuprolide acetate implant is a non-biodegradable tube containing 72 mg. The implant delivers the drug over a 12-month period. The implant is inserted subcutaneously in the inner portion of the upper arm. It must be removed or replaced when the drug is depleted. The leuprolide acetate implant is used as a palliative treatment of advanced prostate cancer.

J9223

J9223 Injection, lurbinectedin, 0.1 mg

Lurbinectedin is an alkylating drug indicated for the treatment of adult patients with metastatic small cell lung cancer (SCLC) with disease progression on or after platinum-based chemotherapy. The recommended dose is 3.2 mg/m2 by intravenous (IV) infusion over 60 minutes repeated every 21 days until disease progression or unacceptable toxicity. This code reports a 0.1 mg injection.

J9225-J9226

J9225 Histrelin implant (Vantas), 50 mg

J9226 Histrelin implant (Supprelin LA), 50 mg

A histrelin implant is a thin, flexible tube inserted subcutaneously that contains 50 mg of histrelin acetate, a synthetic version of luteinizing hormone-releasing hormone or gonadotropin-releasing hormone. Luteinizing hormone-releasing hormone is produced by the pituitary gland that stimulates the ovaries (to release an ovum), the release of estrogen, and certain cells in the testis. A histrelin implant is indicated as a palliative treatment for advanced prostate cancer. Histrelin decreases testosterone levels to castrate levels. A histrelin implant is also indicated for the treatment of children with central precocious puberty, who have an early onset of secondary sexual characteristics (earlier than 8 years of age in females and 9 years of age in males). They also show a significantly advanced bone age that can result in diminished adult height attainment. The implant contains 50 mg of histrelin, administered continuously over a 12-month period. When depleted, the implant must be removed and can be replaced with another implant.

J9227

J9227 Injection, isatuximab-irfc, 10 mg

Isatuximab-irfc is a CD38-directed cytolytic antibody used as an antineoplastic agent and is indicated for the treatment of multiple myeloma in adult patients, ages 18 years or older, who have received at least two prior therapies, including lenalidomide and a proteasome inhibitor. Patients should be premedicated with acetaminophen, dexamethasone, diphenhydramine, and H2 antagonists. It is supplied in single dose vials of 100 mg/5 mL (20 mg/mL) and 500 mg/25 mL (20 mg/mL) and is administered by intravenous infusion. The recommended dosage is 10 mg/kg body weight weekly for weeks one through four, then every two weeks until disease progression or toxicity.

J9228

J9228 Injection, ipilimumab, 1 mg

Ipilimumab is a recombinant, human monoclonal antibody used as an antineoplastic agent. The drug is an IgG1 kappa immunoglobulin produced in Chinese hamster ovary cell cultures. Ipilimumab binds and blocks the cytotoxic T-lymphocyte antigen-4 (CTLA-4). This augments T-cell activation and proliferation, which indirectly enhances the T-cell mediated anti-tumor immune response. Ipilimumab is indicated for the treatment of unresectable or metastatic melanoma and cutaneous melanoma with pathologic involvement of regional lymph nodes of more than 1 mm who have undergone complete resection, including total lymphadenectomy. The recommended dosage is 3 mg/kg administered every three weeks for a total of four doses. Ipilimumab is administered as an IV infusion over 90 minutes and should not be administered as IV push or bolus injection.

J9229

J9229 Injection, inotuzumab ozogamicin, 0.1 mg

Inotuzumab ozogamicin is a CD22-directed antibody-drug conjugate (ADC) indicated for the treatment of adult patients with refractory or relapsed B-cell precursor acute lymphoblastic leukemia (ALL). The ADC binds to CD22-expressing tumor cells, ultimately causing breaks in double-stranded DNA, which induces cell-cycle arrest and apoptotic cell death. Patients should be premedicated with an antihistamine, antipyretic, and corticosteroid prior to all infusions. It is administered via intravenous infusion over one hour. The recommended dosage for all patients in cycle one is 0.8 mg/m^2 on day one, 0.5 mg/m^2 on day eight, and 0.5 mg/m^2 on day 15, for each 21-day cycle. For patients on subsequent cycles two through six, that have achieved a complete remission (CR) or complete remission with incomplete hematologic recovery (CRi), the dosage is 0.5 mg/m^2 on days one, eight, and 15 of the 28-day cycle. For patients who have not achieved a CR or CRi, the cycle one regimen is repeated.

J9230

J9230 Injection, mechlorethamine HCl, (nitrogen mustard), 10 mg

Mechlorethamine hydrochloride, also known as nitrogen mustard, is a highly toxic chemical complex used as an antineoplastic drug. In water or body fluids, it is rapidly transformed and acts by interfering with RNA synthesis causing an imbalance of growth, which then leads to cell death. Administered as an intravenous injection, mechlorethamine hydrochloride is indicated for the treatment of Hodgkin's disease, lymphosarcoma, polycythemia vera, chronic lymphocytic and myelocytic leukemias, mycosis fungoides, and bronchogenic cancers. When administered intrapleurally, intraperitoneally, or intrapericardially, it is used to treat malignant effusions. The recommended dosage is 0.4 mg per kg of body weight per day. The dosage may be divided into smaller doses.

J9245

J9245 Injection, melphalan HCl, not otherwise specified, 50 mg

Melphalan hydrochloride is a derivative of nitrogen mustard used as an antineoplastic drug. It interferes with RNA synthesis causing cell death. Melphalan is indicated for the treatment of multiple myeloma and advanced epithelial ovarian cancer. The drug is available in oral and injectable form. The injectable form is used for the treatment of multiple myeloma when the oral form is inappropriate. The recommended oral dosage for ovarian cancer is 0.2 mg per kg of body weight for five days. The recommended intravenous dosage is 16 mg per m^2 of body surface administered as a single infusion over 15 to 20 minutes. The intravenous dosage is administered at two-week intervals for four doses, then at four-week intervals. Report J9245 for melphalan HCl not otherwise specified.

J9246

J9246 Injection, melphalan (Evomela), 1 mg

Melphalan hydrochloride is an alkylating drug indicated for the treatment of adults, ages 18 years and older, for conditioning treatment prior to autologous stem cell transplantation in the treatment of multiple myeloma or for the palliative treatment of patients with multiple myeloma for whom oral therapy is not appropriate. It is supplied as 50 mg lyophilized powder, in a single dose vial, requiring reconstitution with 8.6 mL of 0.9% sodium chloride to make a 50 mg/10 mL (5 mg/mL) concentration. The required volume needed for treatment is added to the appropriate volume of 0.9% sodium chloride to make a final concentration of 0.4 mg/mL. The final concentration should be administered via intravenous (IV) infusion through an injection port or central venous catheter. For conditioning treatment, the recommended dosage is 100 mg/m^2/day administered via IV infusion for two consecutive days (day -3 and day -2) prior to autologous stem cell transplantation. For palliative treatment, the recommended dosage is 16 mg per m^2 of body surface administered as a single IV infusion over 15 to 20 minutes. The intravenous dosage is administered at two-week intervals for four doses, then at four-week intervals. Report J9246 for Evomela (trade name).

J9247

J9247 Injection, melphalan flufenamide, 1 mg

Melphalan flufenamide HCl is an alkylating drug that inhibits proliferation and induces apoptosis of hematopoietic and solid tumor cells. It is indicated for the treatment of adults, ages 18 and older, with relapsed or refractory multiple myeloma who have received a minimum of four prior therapies, including an anti-CD38 monoclonal antibody, an immunomodulatory agent, and a proteasome inhibitor. The recommended dose is 40 mg administered as an intravenous (IV) infusion over 30 minutes on day one of each 28-day cycle until disease progression or until unacceptable toxicity. Additionally, a dose of dexamethasone, 40 mg oral or IV, should be administered on days one, eight, 15, and 22 of each cycle. This dose should be reduced to 20 mg for patients ages 75 and older. A serotonin-3 (5-HT3) receptor antagonist or other antiemetics can be considered prior to and during treatment. See full prescribing information for complete administration instructions.

J9250-J9260

J9250 Methotrexate sodium, 5 mg

J9260 Methotrexate sodium, 50 mg

Methotrexate sodium is a chemical complex that blocks cell metabolism. It works by hindering the production of an enzyme needed for the metabolism of dividing cells, like those involved in inflammation and the immune response. Methotrexate has been found useful in treating diseases linked with abnormally rapid cell growth. It is indicated singularly or in combination as a treatment for gestational choriocarcinoma, chorioadenoma destruens, hydatidiform mole, breast cancer, epidermoid cancers of the head and neck, advanced mycosis fungoides, squamous and small cell lung cancer, advanced non-Hodgkin's lymphoma, acute lymphocytic leukemia, Burkitt's lymphoma, and lymphosarcoma. It is also used to treat rheumatoid and psoriatic arthritis and severe psoriasis that is unresponsive to other treatments.

J9261

J9261 Injection, nelarabine, 50 mg

Nelarabine is an antineoplastic prodrug that is converted in the body into arabinofuranosyl-guanine (ara-G). Ara-G accumulates in leukemic blast cells and is incorporated into cellular DNA. The ara-G inhabits synthesis and causes cell death. Nelarabine is indicated for the treatment of T-cell acute lymphoblastic leukemia and T-cell lymphoblastic lymphoma in patients who have not responded or relapsed following treatment with at least two chemotherapeutic regimens. The drug is administered by intravenous infusion. Recommended adult dosage is 1,500 mg per mc2 of body surface administered over two hours on days one, three, and five. Recommended pediatric dosage is 650 mg per mc^2 of body surface administered over one hour daily for five consecutive days. This chemotherapy cycle is repeated every 21 days until induction of complete response.

J9262

J9262 Injection, omacetaxine mepesuccinate, 0.01 mg

Omacetaxine mepesuccinate is derived from the leaves of the *Cephalotaxus harringtonia* plant (Cowtail Pine or Japanese Plum Yew). The drug functions as a protein synthesis inhibitor. The mechanism of action of omacetaxine mepesuccinate is not fully understood. It binds to the center of a large ribosomal unit and reduces protein levels in cells harboring the BCR-ABL T3151I mutation. Omacetaxine mepesuccinate is indicated for the treatment of chronic or accelerated phase chronic myeloid leukemia that is resistant to tyrosine kinase inhibitors. Omacetaxine mepesuccinate is administered by subcutaneous injection. Recommended induction and maintenance dose is 1.25 mg per m^2 administered twice daily for 14 consecutive days in a 28-day period.

J9263

J9263 Injection, oxaliplatin, 0.5 mg

Oxaliplatin is a chemical complex containing the metal platinum used as an antineoplastic drug. It binds to DNA disrupting synthesis and causing cell death. It is thought to have a greater cytotoxicity than cisplatin and carboplatin, which are other antineoplastic drugs containing platinum. The exact mechanism of action of oxaliplatin is not known. Oxaliplatin forms reactive platinum. Oxaliplatin is indicated with fluorouracil and leucovorin as a treatment for metastatic colon or rectum cancer that has recurred or progressed following irinotecan, fluorouracil, and leucovorin therapy. The recommended dosage is 85 mg per m^2 of body surface. Oxaliplatin is administered by intravenous infusion over two hours. It is administered in a separate bag, but simultaneously with leucovorin.

J9264

J9264 Injection, paclitaxel protein-bound particles, 1 mg

Paclitaxel protein-bound particles are an albumin-bound form of paclitaxel, an antineoplastic agent. Paclitaxel protein-bound particles are indicated for the treatment of breast cancer after the failure of combination chemotherapy for metastatic disease, or relapse within six months of chemotherapy. The recommended therapy is 260 mg per m^2 of body surface infused intravenously over 30 minutes every three weeks. Paclitaxel protein-bound particles are contraindicated in patients with baseline neutrophil counts of less than 1,500.

J9266

J9266 Injection, pegaspargase, per single dose vial

Pegaspargase is a modified version of the enzyme L-asparaginase produced from *E. coli* bacterium and used as an antineoplastic agent. The enzyme catalyzes the breakdown of asparagine, an amino acid.

Leukemia cells cannot synthesize asparagine and depend upon exogenous sources. Pegaspargase depletes asparagine throughout the body. This depletion kills the leukemia cells. Normal cells can synthesize the asparagine and are unaffected. Pegaspargase is indicated as a treatment for acute lymphoblastic leukemia in patients who have developed hypersensitivity to native forms of L-asparaginase. The drug is usually administered in combination with other chemotherapeutic agents and should only be administered as a single therapy when multi-agent therapy is inappropriate. The recommended dose is 2,500 IU per m^2 of body surface via intravenous or intramuscular injection every 14 days. Lower doses of 82.5 IU per kg are recommended for children with a body surface of less than 0.6 m^2.

J9267

J9267 Injection, paclitaxel, 1 mg

Paclitaxel is a chemical compound isolated from the Pacific yew tree used as an antineoplastic drug. It disrupts intercellular functions causing cell death. Paclitaxel, singularly or in combination with other chemotherapeutic drugs, is indicated as a treatment for Kaposi's sarcoma, advanced breast cancer, advanced ovarian cancer, and non-small cell lung cancer. Recommended dosage varies from 100 to 175 mg per m^2 of body surface depending on the disease and treatment regimen. It is administered via intravenous infusion over three hours or over 24 hours depending on the treatment regimen.

J9268

J9268 Injection, pentostatin, 10 mg

Pentostatin is an antibiotic isolated from the soil bacterium Streptomyces antibioticus used as antineoplastic drug. It interferes with enzyme activity preventing cellular reproduction. Pentostatin is indicated as a treatment for hairy cell leukemia refractory to alpha interferon. Pentostatin is given by intravenous injection or diluted in normal saline and infused over approximately 30 minutes. The recommended dosage is 4 mg per m^2 of body surface.

J9269

J9269 Injection, tagraxofusp-erzs, 10 mcg

Tagraxofusp-erzs is a CD123-directed cytotoxin indicated for the treatment of adult and children, 2 years of age and older, with blastic plasmacytoid dendritic cell neoplasm (BPDCN). BPDCN is a rare disease of the bone marrow affecting multiple organs, including the lymph nodes and skin, and often presents as or evolves into leukemia. Tagraxofusp-erzs is made of recombinant human interleukin-3 (IL-3) and truncated diphtheria toxin (DT) fusion protein, which inhibits protein synthesis, causing cell death in CD123-expressing cells. It is supplied as a clear, colorless solution of 1,000 mcg in 1 mL, in a single-dose glass vial. Tagraxofusp-erzs should be administered by intravenous infusion at a rate of 12 mcg/kg over 15 minutes once daily on days one to five of a 21-day cycle. The first cycle of treatment should be administered in an inpatient setting and patients should be observed for at least 24 hours. Subsequent cycles may be administered as an inpatient or in another appropriate outpatient ambulatory care setting, with observation for at least four hours following infusion. Treatment should be continued until disease progression or unacceptable toxicity. Patients should be premedicated with an H1-histamine antagonist, acetaminophen, corticosteroid, and H2-histamine antagonist 60 minutes prior to each infusion.

J9270

J9270 Injection, plicamycin, 2.5 mg

Plicamycin, also known as mithramycin, is an antibiotic with antineoplastic effects. The drug is derived from *Streptomyces plicatus*. It binds to DNA inhibiting RNA synthesis. Plicamycin is indicated for the treatment of testicular cancer in patients for whom surgery or radiotherapy is not an option. Plicamycin may also be considered in the treatment of symptomatic patients with hypercalcemia caused by chemotherapy for whom conventional therapy has failed. The drug may lower serum calcium by blocking the actions of vitamin D and inhibiting the effects of parathyroid hormone. The recommended antineoplastic dose is 25 to 30 mcg per kg of ideal body weight for a period of eight to 10 days. The recommended dose for hypercalcemia treatment is 25 mcg per kg of body weight for a period of three or four days. Plicamycin is administered via an intravenous infusion over four to six hours. The drug may cause severe thrombocytopenia and hemorrhagic syndrome.

J9271

J9271 Injection, pembrolizumab, 1 mg

Pembrolizumab is a humanized monoclonal antibody that blocks the interaction of PD-1 and its ligands PD-L1 and PD-L2. This releases PD-1 pathway mediated inhibition of the immune response, including antitumor immune response. Pembrolizumab is an IgG4 kappa immunoglobulin. It is indicated for the treatment of unresectable or metastatic melanoma with disease progression following ipilimumab and a BRAF inhibitor (when BRAF V6000 mutation is positive). Recommended dosage is 2 mg/kg as an intravenous infusion over 30 minutes. It is administered every three weeks until disease progression or unacceptable toxicity.

J9272

J9272 Injection, dostarlimab-gxly, 10 mg

Dostarlimab-gxly is a programmed death receptor-1 (PD-1) blocking antibody. It is indicated for the treatment of adults, ages 18 and older, with mismatch repair deficient (dMMR) recurrent or advanced endometrial cancer that has progressed while on or following treatment with a platinum-containing regimen or solid tumors that have progressed on or following prior treatment without satisfactory alternative treatment options. It is supplied in a single dose vial of 500 mg/10 mL (50 mg/mL) that requires dilution with 0.9% sodium chloride or 5% dextrose. The recommended initial dosage is 500 mg every three weeks for doses one through four. Subsequent dosing is 1,000 mg every six weeks beginning three weeks following dose four. It should be administered as an intravenous (IV) infusion over 30 minutes. See full prescribing information for complete administration instructions.

J9273

J9273 Injection, tisotumab vedotin-tftv, 1 mg

Tisotumab vedotin-tftv is a tissue factor (TF)-directed antibody drug conjugate (ADC) produced by recombinant DNA technology using Chinese hamster ovaries. It binds to TF expressing cancer cells, leading to cell-cycle arrest and cell death. It is intended for the treatment of adults, ages 18 years and older, with recurrent or metastatic cervical cancer with disease progression on or after chemotherapy. It is supplied as a lyophilized cake for reconstitution in a single dose vial of 40 mg. The recommended dose is 2 mg/kg body weight (maximum of 200 mg for patients weighing 100 kg or more) via intravenous (IV) infusion over 30 minutes every three weeks until disease progression or unacceptable toxicity. See full prescribing information for complete administration instructions.

J9274

J9274 Injection, tebentafusp-tebn, 1 mcg

Tebentafusp-tebn is a bispecific gp100 peptide-HLA-A*02:01 CD3 T-cell receptor (TCR) indicated for the treatment of adult patients, ages 18 years and older, with HLA-A*02:01-positive unresectable or metastatic uveal melanoma. The TCR binds to gp100 peptides on HLA-A*02:01-positive uveal melanoma cells, releasing inflammatory cytokines and cytolytic proteins resulting in direct lysis of tumor cells. It is supplied in single dose vials of 100 mcg/0.5 ml and is administered via intravenous (IV) injection over 15 to 20 minutes following dilution. The recommended dosage is 20 mcg on day one, 30 mcg on day eight, 68 mcg on day 15, and 68 mcg once weekly thereafter. See full prescribing information for complete administration instructions.

J9280

J9280 Injection, mitomycin, 5 mg

Mitomycin is an antibiotic with antineoplastic effects. The drug is derived from Streptomyces caespitosus plicatus. It selectively inhibits DNA synthesis. Mitomycin is not recommended as a single agent primary therapy. Mitomycin is indicated for the treatment of disseminated adenocarcinoma of the stomach or pancreas in combination with other approved chemotherapeutic agents, or as a palliative treatment when other modalities have failed. The drug is not recommended as a replacement for surgery or radiotherapy. Mitomycin is administered intravenously via a catheter with a recommended dosage of 20 mg per m^2 of body surface in six to eight week cycles. The patient must have a full hematological recovery from any previous therapy prior to the administration of mitomycin. The drug has a cumulative effect on bone marrow causing suppression and may cause hemolytic uremic syndrome at doses higher than 60 mg.

J9281

J9281 Mitomycin pyelocalyceal instillation, 1 mg

Mitomycin pyelocalyceal is an alkylating drug that is indicated for the treatment of adults, ages 18 years and older, for the treatment of low-grade upper tract urothelial cancer (LG-UTUC). The drug is derived from *Streptomyces caespitosus* and selectively inhibits DNA synthesis. Mitomycin pyelocalyceal is supplied in a single dose carton that contains two vials of lyophilized mitomycin for pyelocalyceal solution (40 mL each) and one vial of sterile hydrogel (20 mL) for reconstitution. It is administered by instillation via ureteral catheter or nephrostomy tube directly into the kidney. The recommended dosage is 4 mg per mL, with a total volume not to exceed 15 mL (60 mg of mitomycin) instilled once per week for a total of six weeks. The administration should be complete within one minute. For patients who have a complete response after three months of instillation, administer once per month for no more than 11 additional instillations. Patients should receive 1.3 g sodium bicarbonate orally the night prior to, the morning of, and 30 minutes prior to the instillation procedure. Patients should be carefully monitored for signs for ureteric obstruction and bone marrow suppression. It should not be used in patients with a glomerular filtration rate of <30 mL/min.

J9285

J9285 Injection, olaratumab, 10 mg

Olaratumab is a human IgG1 antibody that binds platelet-derived growth factor receptor alpha (PDGFR-Î±). Olaratumab disrupts the PDGFR-Î± signaling pathway in in vivo tumor cells. It is indicated for the treatment of adult patients with soft tissue sarcoma (STS) that is not amenable to radiotherapy or surgery, and should be administered in combination with doxorubicin for the first eight cycles. Doxorubicin, and other medications, should not be administered through the same intravenous line. The recommended dosage is 15 mg per kg, administered through intravenous infusion over 60 minutes, on days one and eight of each 21-day cycle until disease progression or patient has unacceptable toxicity. Prior to infusion on day one, the patient should be premedicated with dexamethasone and diphenhydramine.

J9293

J9293 Injection, mitoxantrone HCl, per 5 mg

Mitoxantrone hydrochloride is a synthetic antineoplastic anthracenedione drug that disrupts the DNA of cells causing cell death. The drug is used in combination with corticosteroids as an initial treatment for pain related to advanced hormone-refractory prostate cancer. Mitoxantrone hydrochloride is also indicated in combination with other approved drugs as the initial treatment for acute nonlymphocytic leukemia, including myelogenous, promyelocytic, monocytic, and erythroid leukemias. Mitoxantrone is also indicated for the treatment of secondary progressive, progressive relapsing, or worsening relapsing-remitting multiple sclerosis. The drug must be diluted and administered via an intravenous infusion.

J9295

J9295 Injection, necitumumab, 1 mg

Necitumumab is an epidermal growth factor receptor (EGFR) for the treatment of patients with metastatic squamous non-small cell lung cancer. It is intended to be used as a first-line treatment, for patients aged 18 years and older, in combination with gemcitabine and cisplatin. Necitumumab is provided in a single dose vial containing 800 mg/50 ml. The dosage is 800 mg administered over 60 minutes of intravenous infusion on days one and eight of each three-week cycle prior to administration of gemcitabine and cisplatin infusion.

J9298

J9298 Injection, nivolumab and relatlimab-rmbw, 3 mg/1 mg

Nivolumab and relatlimab-rmbw is a combination of a programmed death receptor-1 (PD1) blocking antibody (nivolumab) and a lymphocyte activation gene-3 (LAG-3) blocking antibody (relatlimab) that is indicated for the treatment of adults and children, ages 12 years and older, with unresectable or metastatic melanoma. It is supplied in single dose vials of 240 mg nivolumab/80 mg relatlimab per 20 ml and is administered via intravenous (IV) infusion over 30 minutes. The recommended dosage for patients weighing at least 40 kg is 480 mg nivolumab and 160 mg relatlimab every four weeks. See full prescribing information for complete administration instructions.

J9299

J9299 Injection, nivolumab, 1 mg

Nivolumab is a programmed death receptor-1 (PD-1) blocking antibody. It is utilized for the treatment of unresectable or metastatic melanoma, after treatment with ipilimumab and, if the melanoma is BRAF V600 mutation positive, treatment with a BRAF inhibitor. It is also utilized for the treatment of metastatic squamous non-small cell lung cancer with progression following platinum-based chemotherapy. Nivolumab is administered by intravenous infusion, 3 mg/kg over one hour, every two weeks.

J9301

J9301 Injection, obinutuzumab, 10 mg

Obinutuzumab is a humanized monoclonal antibody that is produced using Chinese hamster ovaries. It targets the CD20 antigen found on the surface of pre and mature B-lymphocytes. After binding to these sites, obinutuzumab activates intracellular pathways that lead to the death of the cell. Obinutuzumab, in combination with chlorambucil, is indicated as a treatment for patients with chronic lymphocytic leukemia that have not been previously treated. It is administered as an intravenous infusion. Six cycles are recommended with a dosage of 1,000 mg except for day one and day two of cycle one. Recommended dosage for day one of cycle one is 100 mg with 900 mg recommended for day two of cycle one.

J9302

J9302 Injection, ofatumumab, 10 mg

Ofatumumab is a human monoclonal antibody produced in murine cells. The drug binds specifically to the CD20 molecule contained in B lymphocytes, causing the breakdown of the cell. This drug is indicated for the treatment of patients who have chronic lymphocytic leukemia refractory to fludarabine and alemtuzumab. The drug is administered as a prolonged IV infusion. The recommended dosage is 2,000 mg after an initial 300 mg dose.

J9303

J9303 Injection, panitumumab, 10 mg

Panitumumab is a monoclonal antibody produced by recombinant DNA technology using Chinese hamster ovaries. The drug binds to human epidermal growth factor receptor (EGFR) sites inhibiting its effects. EGFR is a glycoprotein expressed in many normal epithelial cells including skin and hair follicles. Over-expression of EGFR usually accompanies many human epithelial cells including those of the colon and rectum. Panitumumab is indicated for the treatment of EGFR-expressing metastatic colorectal cancer in patients whose disease has progressed after treatment with fluoropyrimidine, oxaliplatin and irinotecan chemotherapy regimens. The drug is administered via an intravenous infusion over 60 minutes. Recommended dosage is 6 mg per kg of patient body weight every 14 days. Total dosages greater than 1000 mg should be administered over 90 minutes.

J9304

J9304 Injection, pemetrexed (Pemfexy), 10 mg

Pemetrexed is a chemical complex used as an antineoplastic drug. It disrupts folate-dependent metabolic processes essential for cell reproduction. Pemetrexed in combination with cisplatin is indicated for the treatment of patients with malignant pleural mesothelioma whose disease is unresectable or who are otherwise not candidates for curative surgery metastatic lung cancer. As a singular agent, pemetrexed is indicated as a treatment for locally advanced or metastatic non-small cell lung cancer after prior chemotherapy. The recommended dosage is 500 mg per m^2 of body surface administered by intravenous injection. The code should be reported for Pemfexy (trade name).

J9305

J9305 Injection, pemetrexed, NOS, 10 mg

Pemetrexed is a chemical complex used as an antineoplastic drug. It disrupts folate-dependent metabolic processes essential for cell reproduction. Pemetrexed in combination with cisplatin is indicated for the treatment of patients with malignant pleural mesothelioma whose disease is unresectable or who are otherwise not candidates for curative surgery metastatic lung cancer. As a singular agent, pemetrexed is indicated as a treatment for locally advanced or metastatic non-small cell lung cancer after prior chemotherapy. The recommended dosage is 500 mg per m^2 of body surface administered by intravenous injection.

J9306

J9306 Injection, pertuzumab, 1 mg

Pertuzumab is a monoclonal antibody produced in Chinese hamster ovaries using recombinant DNA technology. The drug targets the human epidermal growth factor 2 protein (HER2) inhibiting two intracellular signal pathways, which can halt cellular growth and cause cell destruction. Pertuzumab is indicated for use in combination with trastuzumab and docetaxel for the treatment of patients with HER2-positive metastatic breast cancer who have not received prior anti-HER2 therapy or chemotherapy. The initial dose of pertuzumab is 840 mg administered as a 60-minute intravenous infusion. Subsequent recommended dose is 420 mg in an intravenous infusion over 30 to 60 minutes, administered every three weeks.

J9307

J9307 Injection, pralatrexate, 1 mg

Pralatrexate is a folate analogue that is a metabolic inhibitor that prevents the synthesis of thymidine. Thymidine is one of the nucleosides in DNA. This drug is used to treat patients with relapsed or refractory peripheral T-cell lymphoma. The drug is administered via an IV push over three to five minutes. The recommended dose is 30 mg per meter squared of body surface area.

J9308

J9308 Injection, ramucirumab, 5 mg

Ramucirumab is a recombinant human IgG1 monoclonal antibody produced in genetically engineered mammalian cells. It specifically binds to vascular endothelial growth factor (VEGF2) 2 receptor sites. Ramucirumab is indicated for the treatment of advanced or metastatic gastric carcinoma or gastroesophageal junction adenocarcinoma as a single agent after prior fluoropyrimidine or platinum-containing chemotherapy. It is administered as an intravenous infusion over 60 minutes. Recommended dosage is 8 mg per kg every two weeks.

J9309

J9309 Injection, polatuzumab vedotin-piiq, 1 mg

Polatuzumab vedotin-piiq is a CD79b-directed antibody–drug conjugate indicated for the treatment of adult patients with relapsed or refractory diffuse large B-cell lymphoma, not otherwise specified, after at least two prior therapies. The recommended dosage is 1.8 mg/kg as an intravenous infusion over 90 minutes every 21 days for six cycles in combination with bendamustine and a rituximab product. Subsequent infusions may be administered over 30 minutes if the previous infusion is tolerated.

J9311

J9311 Injection, rituximab 10 mg and hyaluronidase

Rituximab and hyaluronidase is a combination of rituximab, which is a CD20 directed cytolytic antibody, and hyaluronidase human, an endoglycosidase. This drug is used to treat adult patients with relapsed or refractory follicular lymphoma as a single agent; non-progressing follicular lymphoma as a single agent after first-line cyclophosphamide, vincristine, and prednisone (CVP) chemotherapy; previously untreated follicular lymphoma combined with first-line chemotherapy and in patients achieving complete or partial response to rituximab combined with chemotherapy, as a single agent maintenance therapy; previously untreated diffuse, large B-cell lymphoma (DLBCL) combined with cyclophosphamide, doxorubicin, vincristine, prednisone (CHOP), or another anthracycline-based chemotherapy; and previously untreated chronic lymphocytic leukemia (CLL) combined with fludarabine and cyclophosphamide (FC). It is supplied in single dose vials. The 1,400 mg rituximab/23,400 units hyaluronidase solution is administered by subcutaneous injection over five minutes, and the 1,600 mg rituximab/26,800 units hyaluronidase solution is administered by subcutaneous injection over seven minutes. Treatment with this drug should only begin after the patient has received at least one full dose of a rituximab product by intravenous infusion. Once rituximab has been administered, rituximab and hyaluronidase is administered as a subcutaneous injection into the abdomen, according to the appropriate schedule for the condition being treated. Patients should be premedicated with acetaminophen and an antihistamine prior to each dose, and use of glucocorticoids should be considered.

J9312

J9312 Injection, rituximab, 10 mg

Rituximab is a monoclonal antibody produced by recombinant DNA in Chinese hamster ovaries used as an antineoplastic drug. It binds to the CD20 antigen on the surface of normal and malignant B-lymphocytes and causes cell death. This drug is used to treat the relapsed or refractory, low-grade, or follicular, CD20-positive, B-cell non-Hodgkin's lymphoma. In combination with other chemotherapeutic drugs, it is indicated as a treatment for diffuse large B-cell, CD20-positive non-Hodgkin's lymphoma, chronic lymphocytic leukemia, and moderate to severe active rheumatoid arthritis that has displayed inadequate response to other therapies. Rituximab is also approved for use in Wegener's granulomatosis and microscopic polyangiitis. The recommended dosage is 375 mg per m^2 of body surface administered by intravenous infusion.

J9313

J9313 Injection, moxetumomab pasudotox-tdfk, 0.01 mg

Moxetumomab pasudotox-tdfk is a CD22-directed cytotoxin that is indicated for the treatment of adults, aged 18 years and older, with relapsed or refractory hairy cell leukemia (HCL) who have received at least two previous systemic therapies, including treatment with a purine nucleoside analog (PNA). It is supplied as a lyophilized cake or powder in a 1 mg single dose vial that requires reconstitution with 1.1 mL of sterile water. One mL of IV solution stabilizer should be added to a 50 mL 0.9% sodium chloride infusion bag prior to the moxetumomab pasudotox-tdfk solution. The recommended dosage is 0.04 mg per kg of weight administered by intravenous infusion over 30 minutes on days one, three, and five of each 28-day cycle, for a maximum of six cycles, disease progression, or unacceptable toxicity. Patients should receive one liter of 5% dextrose and 0.45% or 0.9% sodium chloride via intravenous infusion over two to four hours before and after each moxetumomab pasudotox-tdfk infusion. Patients should be advised to ingest up to three L of oral fluids every 24 hours. Patients less than 50 kg should receive one half liter of 5% dextrose and 0.45% or 0.9% sodium chloride via intravenous infusion over two to four hours before and after each moxetumomab pasudotox-tdfk infusion, and should consume up to three liters of oral fluids every 24 hours on days one through eight of each 28-day cycle. Prior to infusion of moxetumomab pasudotox-tdfk, all patients should be premedicated with an antihistamine, an antipyretic, and a histamine-2 receptor antagonist. Post infusion, patients may be given oral antihistamines and antipyretics for up to 24 hours, an oral corticosteroid to decrease nausea and vomiting, and should be advised to maintain oral hydration.

J9314

J9314 Injection, pemetrexed (Teva) not therapeutically equivalent to J9305, 10 mg

Pemetrexed is a chemical complex used as an antineoplastic drug. It disrupts folate-dependent metabolic processes essential for cell reproduction. Pemetrexed is indicated for the treatment of adults, ages 18 years and older, with recurrent, metastatic non-squamous non-small cell lung cancer (NSCLC) following prior chemotherapy and for the maintenance treatment for locally advanced or metastatic non-squamous NSCLC whose disease has not progressed, following four cycles of a platinum-based first-line chemotherapy. It is supplied in single dose vials of 100 mg/4 ml, 500 mg/20 ml, or 1 g/40 ml and requires dilution with 5% dextrose. The recommended dosage, for patients with a creatinine clearance of 45 ml/min or greater, is 500 mg per m² of body surface administered by intravenous (IV) infusion over 10 minutes on day one of each 21-day cycle until disease progression or unacceptable toxicity. There are no dosage adjustment recommendations for patients with a creatinine clearance less than 45 ml/min. Patients should be premedicated with folic acid, vitamin B12, and dexamethasone. See full prescribing information for complete administration instructions.

J9316

J9316 Injection, pertuzumab, trastuzumab, and hyaluronidase-zzxf, per 10 mg

Pertuzumab, trastuzumab, and hyaluronidase-zzxf is a combination of pertuzumab and trastuzumab (HER2/neu receptor antagonists) and hyaluronidase (an endoglycosidase). Indications include the treatment of patients with HER2-positive breast cancer when it is 1) used in conjunction with chemotherapy as neoadjuvant treatment when the cancer is locally advanced, inflammatory, or early stage, 2) used in conjunction with chemotherapy as adjuvant treatment for early breast cancer that has a high risk of recurrence, or 3) used in combination with docetaxel for treatment of patients with metastatic breast cancer who have not received prior anti-HER2 therapy or chemotherapy for their metastatic disease. The recommended initial dose is 1,200 mg pertuzumab, 600 mg trastuzumab, and 30,000 units hyaluronidase in 15 mL, administered by subcutaneous (SC) injection over approximately eight minutes. Recommended maintenance dose is 600 mg pertuzumab, 600 mg trastuzumab, and 20,000 units hyaluronidase in 10 mL, administered subcutaneously over approximately five minutes every three weeks.

J9317

J9317 Injection, sacituzumab govitecan-hziy, 2.5 mg

Sacituzumab govitecan-hziy is a Trop-2-directed antibody and topoisomerase inhibitor that is indicated for the treatment of adult patients, ages 18 years and older, with metastatic triple-negative breast cancer (mTNBC) who have two prior therapies for metastatic disease. It is supplied in single dose vials of 180 mg lyophilized powder requiring reconstitution with 20 mL 0.9% sodium chloride, for a resulting concentration of 10 mg/mL. The recommended dosage is 10 mg/kg body weight administered via intravenous (IV) infusion over three hours once per week, on days one and eight of a continuous 21-day cycle, until disease progression or toxicity. Subsequent infusions may be administered over one to two hours if prior infusions tolerated. Patients should be premedicated with antipyretics, corticosteroids, and H1 and H2 blockers to prevent infusion reactions and chemotherapy-induced nausea and vomiting (CINV). Sacituzumab govitecan-hziy should not be administered as an IV bolus or push. Do not administer concomitantly with UGT1A1 inhibitors or inducers or with other drugs containing irinotecan or its active metabolite SN-38. This code reports a 2.5 mg injection.

J9318

J9318 Injection, romidepsin, nonlyophilized, 0.1 mg

Romidepsin is a histone (any of a group of small basic proteins present in cell nuclei that organizes DNA strands by forming molecular complexes around which the DNA winds) deacetylase inhibitor indicated for the treatment of adult patients, ages 18 years and older, with cutaneous T-cell lymphoma (CTCL) who have received at least one prior systemic therapy or with peripheral T-cell lymphoma (PTCL) who have received at least one prior therapy. Histone deacetylase are a class of enzymes that remove acetyl groups from an amino acid on a histone, allowing the histone to wrap the DNA more tightly. The accumulation of acetylated histones and other proteins disrupts the cell cycle and causes cell death. It is supplied in single dose vials of 10 mg non-lyophilized liquid and 2 mL of diluent (5 mg/mL) and is administered via intravenous (IV) infusion. The recommended dosage is 14 mg/m^2 administered over four hours via IV infusion, on days one, eight, and 15 of a 28-day cycle. Repeat the cycle every 28 days until the disease progresses or unacceptable toxicity occurs.

J9319

J9319 Injection, romidepsin, lyophilized, 0.1 mg

Romidepsin is a histone (any of a group of small basic proteins present in cell nuclei that organizes DNA strands by forming molecular complexes around which the DNA winds) deacetylase inhibitor indicated for the treatment of adult patients, ages 18 years and older, with cutaneous T-cell lymphoma (CTCL) who have received at least one prior systemic therapy. Histone deacetylase are a class of enzymes that remove acetyl groups from an amino acid on a histone, allowing the histone to wrap the DNA more tightly. The accumulation of acetylated histones and other proteins disrupts the cell cycle and causes cell death. It is supplied in single dose vials of 10 mg lyophilized powder and 2 mL of diluent (5 mg/mL) and is administered via intravenous (IV) infusion. The recommended dosage is 14 mg/m^2 administered over four hours via IV infusion, on days one, eight, and 15 of a 28-day cycle. Repeat the cycle every 28 days until the disease progresses or unacceptable toxicity occurs.

J9320

J9320 Injection, streptozocin, 1 g

Streptozocin is a synthetic antineoplastic drug chemically related to other nitro ureas that inhibits DNA synthesis causing cell death. Streptozocin is indicated for the treatment of metastatic islet cell carcinoma of the pancreas for both functioning and nonfunctioning carcinomas. Due to its renal toxicity, streptozocin should be limited to patients with symptomatic or progressive metastatic disease. The drug is administered intravenously by injection or via infusion.

J9325

J9325 Injection, talimogene laherparepvec, per 1 million plaque forming units

Talimogene laherparepvec is a genetically modified oncolytic viral therapy for the local treatment of unresectable cutaneous, subcutaneous, and nodal lesions in patients aged 18 years and older with recurrent melanoma following initial surgery. It is provided in single-vials in two dose strengths: 10^6 (1 million) plaque-forming units (PFU) per mL for the initial dose only; and 10^8 (100 million) PFU per mL for all subsequent doses. Talimogene laherparepvec is administered by an injection into cutaneous, subcutaneous, or nodal lesions that are visible, palpable, or detectable by ultrasound guidance. The drug should be injected along multiple tracks, via a single insertion point, as far as the radial reach of the needle allows within the lesion to obtain even and complete dispersion. Multiple insertion points can be used if a lesion is larger than the radial reach of the needle. The total volume injected during each treatment should not exceed 4 mL total for the injected lesions combined.

J9328

J9328 Injection, temozolomide, 1 mg

Temozolomide is a chemical complex that is broken down in the liver into monomethyl triazine, also known as MTIC. MTIC causes breaks in the DNA, which prevents replication, thus interfering with tumor cell reproduction. Temozolomide is indicated for the treatment of adult patients with newly diagnosed glioblastoma multiforme and for the treatment of adult patients with refractory anaplastic astrocytoma. Dosage is calculated based on the patient's body surface area. Temozolomide is administered by IV infusion.

J9330

J9330 Injection, temsirolimus, 1 mg

Temsirolimus is an antineoplastic drug used to treat advanced renal cancer. It inhibits mammalian target of rapamycin (mTOR) and binds to the protein that controls cell division. The recommended dose of temsirolimus is 25 mg administered by IV infusion over 30 to 60 minutes. The drug is usually administered once a week.

J9331

J9331 Injection, sirolimus protein-bound particles, 1 mg

Sirolimus is an inhibitor of mechanistic target or rapamycin kinase (mTOR). mTOR controls key cellular processes and is commonly dysregulated in several human cancers. Sirolimus binds to and inhibits mTOR, reducing cell proliferation, angiogenesis, and glucose uptake, resulting in tumor growth inhibition. It is intended for the treatment of adults, ages 18 years and older, with locally advanced, unresectable, or metastatic malignant perivascular epithelioid cell tumor (PEComa). It is supplied as a lyophilized powder requiring reconstitution with 0.9% sodium chloride in a single dose vial. The recommended dose is 100 mg/m^2 administered via intravenous (IV) infusion over 30 minutes on days one and eight of a 21-day cycle, until disease progression or toxicity. See full prescribing information for complete administration instructions.

J9332

J9332 Injection, efgartigimod alfa-fcab, 2 mg

Efgartigimod alfa-fcab is a neonatal Fc receptor blocker indicated for the treatment of adults, ages 18 years and older, with generalized myasthenia gravis (gMG) who are anti-acetylcholine receptor (AChR) antibody positive. Age-appropriate immunizations with live-attenuated or live vaccines is not recommended during treatment. Evaluate need for immunizations prior to initiation of treatment. It is supplied in a single dose vial of 400 mg (20 mg/ml) requiring reconstitution with 0.9% sodium chloride. The recommended dose is 10 mg/kg body weight administered via intravenous (IV) infusion over one hour weekly for four weeks. For patients weighing 120 kg or more, the recommended dose is 1,200 mg per infusion. Subsequent treatment cycles are based on clinical evaluation but should not be initiated sooner than 50 days from the start of the previous cycle. See full prescribing information for complete administration instructions.

J9340

J9340 Injection, thiotepa, 15 mg

Thiotepa is a synthetic antineoplastic compound drug related chemically and pharmacologically to nitrogen mustard. The drug disrupts cell DNA producing cell death. Thiotepa may be administered intravenously, intracavitary, or intravesically. The drug has been tried in the treatment of a wide variety of neoplastic diseases with varying results. It has shown success in treating adenocarcinoma of the breast and ovary, superficial papillary carcinoma of the urinary bladder, and in controlling intracavity effusions secondary to diffuse or localized neoplastic diseases of various serosal cavities. While usually superseded by other treatments, thiotepa has been effective in the treatment of other lymphomas such as lymphosarcoma and Hodgkin's disease.

J9348

J9348 Injection, naxitamab-gqgk, 1 mg

Naxitamab-gqgk is a GD2-binding monoclonal antibody that is indicated for the treatment of adults and children, ages 1 and older, with relapsed or refractory high-risk neuroblastoma in the bone or bone marrow who have demonstrated a partial response, minor response, or have stable disease prior to treatment. The recommended dose is 3 mg per kg of body weight, up to 150 mg/day, administered via intravenous (IV) infusion on days one, three, and five of each treatment cycle. Treatment cycles are repeated every four weeks until complete or partial response, and then repeated by five additional treatment cycles every four weeks. Subsequent cycles may be repeated every eight weeks. Granulocyte-macrophage colony-stimulating factor (GM-CSF) should be administered subcutaneously (SC) prior to and during each treatment cycle as recommended. Pre-infusion medications and supportive treatment should be administered as appropriate during infusion. See full prescribing information for complete administration details.

J9349

J9349 Injection, tafasitamab-cxix, 2 mg

Tafasitamab-cxix, a CD19-directed cytolytic antibody, is indicated in combination with lenalidomide (a thalidomide derivative chemotherapy drug) for the treatment of adult patients, 18 years and older, with relapsed or refractory diffuse large B-cell lymphoma (DLBCL) that is not otherwise specified (including that arising from low grade lymphoma), and who are ineligible for autologous stem cell transplant (ASCT). Administered as an intravenous (IV) infusion, the recommended dosage is 12 mg/kg according to a predetermined dosing schedule. Tafasitamab-cxix is administered in combination with lenalidomide for a maximum of 12 cycles and then continued as monotherapy until disease progresses or there is unacceptable toxicity.

J9351

J9351 Injection, topotecan, 0.1 mg

Topotecan hydrochloride is an antineoplastic drug that is a semisynthetic derivative of camptothecin, an alkaloid extract from plants such as Camptotheca acuminata. The drug works by causing breaks in DNA that the cell cannot repair leading to cell death. Topotecan hydrochloride is indicated as a treatment for metastatic carcinoma of the ovaries after failure of prior chemotherapy. It is also indicated as a treatment for small cell lung cancer that responded to chemotherapy, but subsequently progressed. The recommended dosage is 1.5 mg per m^2 of body surface administered by intravenous infusion over 30 minutes for five consecutive days.

J9352

J9352 Injection, trabectedin, 0.1 mg

Trabectedin is an alkylating drug for the treatment of patients with metastatic or unresectable liposarcoma or leiomyosarcoma who have received prior treatment with an anthracycline-containing regimen. Trabectedin binds to guanine residues in the minor groove of DNA and generates multiple events that ultimately cause the displacement of the oncogenic protein, FUS-CHOP, disrupting the cell cycle, and leading to eventual death of the cells. The recommended dosage is 1.5 mg/m^2 body surface area via intravenous infusion. The infusion is administered through a central line, every three weeks. Patients should be premedicated with corticosteroids 30 minutes prior to each infusion.

J9353

J9353 Injection, margetuximab-cmkb, 5 mg

Margetuximab-cmkb is a chimeric Fc-engineered IgG1 kappa monoclonal antibody (HER2/neu receptor antagonist) indicated for the treatment of adults, ages 18 and older, with metastatic HER2-positive breast cancer who have received two or more prior anti-HER2 therapies, one of which was for metastatic disease. It is supplied in a 250 mg/10 mL single dose vial. The recommended initial dose is 15 mg/kg body weight administered via intravenous (IV) infusion over 120 minutes. Subsequent infusions should be administered for a minimum of 30 minutes every three weeks until disease progression or unacceptable toxicity. When administered on the same day as chemotherapy, margetuximab-cmkb should be administered immediately following chemotherapy completion. Dose modifications may be required for patients with left ventricular dysfunction. See full prescribing information for complete administration information.

J9354

J9354 Injection, ado-trastuzumab emtansine, 1 mg

Ado-trastuzumab emtansine is an HER-2 targeted therapy. It consists of an antibody linked to a drug, called an ADC or antibody-drug conjugate. The antibody links to the target cell. The ADC is then internalized by the cell and the drug is released to perform its function. The trastuzumab is a humanized anti-HER2 IgG1 that is linked to a microtubule inhibitory drug, DM1 with a chemical link called MCC. The emtansine refers to the MCC-DM1 links. Trastuzumab is a monoclonal antibody produced by recombinant technology in Chinese hamster ovaries. After internalization, the DM1 disrupts the microtubule networks of the cell causing cellular death. Ado-trastuzumab emtansine is indicated as a treatment for HER2-positive, metastatic breast cancer in patients who have previously received trastuzumab and a taxane. Ado-trastuzumab emtansine is administered via an IV infusion every three weeks. The recommended dosage is 3.6 mg per kg of patient weight.

J9355

J9355 Injection, trastuzumab, excludes biosimilar, 10 mg

Trastuzumab is a monoclonal antibody produced using recombinant DNA technology from Chinese hamster ovaries. The drug is an antineoplastic agent indicated for treatment of metastatic breast cancer that overexpresses the human epidermal growth factor receptor 2 (HER2) protein. Trastuzumab selectively binds to the HER2 protein site and inhibits the production of cells that overexpress HER2. Trastuzumab is indicated as a treatment for HER2 overexpressing breast cancer in patients who do not have heart failure or cardiomyopathy in the following circumstances: as a single therapy for patients who have undergone one or more chemotherapy regimens for metastatic breast cancer; in combination therapy with doxorubicin, cyclophosphamide, and paclitaxel for node-positive breast cancer that has been surgically treated; and in combination with paclitaxel for patients who have not received chemotherapy for metastatic breast cancer. The drug is administered via an intravenous infusion and should not be given as an IV push or bolus. Recommended dosage for the initial infusion is 4 mg per kg of patient body weight infused over 90 minutes. Subsequent recommended dosage is 2 mg per kg of patient body weight infused over 30 minutes. The infusions are administered every seven days. Code J9355 should not be used to report biosimilar formulations of trastuzumab.

J9356

J9356 Injection, trastuzumab, 10 mg and hyaluronidase-oysk

Trastuzumab and hyaluronidase-oysk is a combination of an IgG1 kappa monoclonal antibody (trastuzumab) and hyaluronidase-oysk, an endoglycosidase that increases the dispersion and absorption of co-administered subcutaneously (SC) injected drugs. Both drugs are produced using recombinant DNA technology from Chinese hamster ovaries and are indicated for the treatment of adults with HER2-overexpressing breast cancer. It is supplied as a colorless to yellowish solution in a single dose vial, providing 600 mg of trastuzumab and 10,000 units of hyaluronidase per 5 mL. The recommended dosage is 600 mg/10,000 units (600 mg trastuzumab and 10,000 unites hyaluronidase) administered by SC injection over two to five minutes, once every three weeks. There is no loading dose or adjustments required for patient body weight or adjuvant chemotherapy regimens. Care should be taken to ensure the proper drug is being administered. This drug is not the same as ado-trastuzumab emtansine.

J9357

J9357 Injection, valrubicin, intravesical, 200 mg

Valrubicin intravesical is a synthetic version of anthracycline doxorubicin that is an antineoplastic agent instilled into the urinary bladder. The drug disrupts cell DNA causing chromosomal damage. Valrubicin is indicated for the intravesical treatment of BCG-refractory carcinoma in situ of the urinary bladder for those patients who cannot undergo an immediate cystectomy.

J9358

J9358 Injection, fam-trastuzumab deruxtecan-nxki, 1 mg

Fam-trastuzumab deruxtecan-nxki is a HER2-directed antibody and topoisomerase inhibitor conjugate comprised of three components: 1) a humanized anti-HER2 IgG1 monoclonal antibody (mAb), covalently linked to 2) a topoisomerase inhibitor, via 3) a tetrapeptide-based cleavable linker. The mAb is produced in Chinese hamster ovary cells through recombinant DNA technology. The topoisomerase inhibitor and tetrapeptide-based linker are produced by chemical synthesis. Fam-trastuzumab deruxtecan-nxki binds to HER2 on tumor cells causing damage and cell death. It is indicated as a treatment for adults, 18 years of age and older, with unresectable or metastatic HER2-positive breast cancer who have received two or more previous anti-HER2-based regimens in the metastatic setting. The drug is administered via an intravenous (IV) infusion and should not be given as an IV push or bolus. It is supplied as 100 mg lyophilized powder in a single dose vial requiring reconstitution with 5 mL sterile water for a concentration of 20 mg/mL. The calculated volume needed for treatment should be further diluted into an IV infusion bag of 100 mL of 5% dextrose solution. Sodium chloride should not be used. The recommended dosage is 5.4 mg/kg body weight administered via IV infusion once every three weeks (21-day cycle) until disease progression or unacceptable toxicity. The first infusion should be administered over 90 minutes. Subsequent infusion may be administered over 30 minutes if patient tolerates.

J9359

J9359 Injection, loncastuximab tesirine-lpyl, 0.075 mg

Loncastiuximab tesirine-lpyl is a CD19-directed antibody and alkylating agent conjugate that is indicated for the treatment of adults, ages 18 and older, with relapsed or refractory diffuse large B-cell lymphoma (DLBCL) that is not otherwise specified, DLBCL that arises from low grade lymphoma, and high-grade B-cell lymphoma. Administered as an intravenous (IV) infusion over 30 minutes on day one of each three-week cycle, the recommended dosages are 0.15 mg/kg body weight every three weeks for two cycles, followed by 0.075 mg/kg body weight every three weeks for subsequent cycles. Patients should be premedicated with 4 mg dexamethasone twice daily for three days starting the day before loncastuximab tesirine-lpyl infusion. See full prescribing information for complete administration instructions.

J9360

J9360 Injection, vinblastine sulfate, 1 mg

Vinblastine sulfate is an antineoplastic drug that is an alkaloid extract from the herb known as Madagascar periwinkle or Vinca rosea Linn. It interferes with the cell metabolism of amino acids and nucleic acid synthesis causing cell death. Vinblastine sulfate, singularly or in combination, is indicated for the treatment of Hodgkin's disease, lymphocytic lymphoma, histiocytic lymphoma, mycosis fungoides, Kaposi's sarcoma, Letterer-Siwe disease, advanced carcinoma of the testis, choriocarcinoma resistant to other chemotherapeutic agents, and breast cancer that is unresponsive to surgery and hormonal therapy. The recommended dosage varies from 2.5 mg to 18.5 mg per m^2 of body surface depending upon the patient's age and response. Vinblastine sulfate is administered by intravenous injection.

J9370-J9371

J9370 Vincristine sulfate, 1 mg

J9371 Injection, vincristine sulfate liposome, 1 mg

Vincristine sulfate is an antineoplastic drug that is an alkaloid extract from the herb known as Madagascar periwinkle or Vinca rosea Linn. It interferes with the cell metabolism of amino acids and nucleic acid synthesis causing cell death. Vincristine sulfate, singularly or in combination, is indicated for the treatment of acute leukemia, non-Hodgkin's lymphoma, Hodgkin's disease, neuroblastoma, rhabdomyosarcoma, and Wilms' tumor. A liposome is an artificially prepared vesicle composed of a lipid bilayer. It is used to deliver nutrients and drugs . The recommended dosage varies from 0.5 to 1.4 mg per m^2 of body surface depending upon the patient's age and response. Vincristine sulfate is administered by intravenous injection.

J9390

J9390 Injection, vinorelbine tartrate, 10 mg

Vinorelbine tartrate is an antineoplastic drug that is a semisynthetic derivative of vinblastine. Vinblastine is an alkaloid extract from the herb known as Madagascar periwinkle or Vinca rosea Linn. It interferes with the cell metabolism of amino acids and nucleic acid synthesis causing cell death. Vinorelbine tartrate, singularly or in combination with cisplatin, is indicated for the treatment of unresectable, advanced non-small cell lung cancer. The recommended dosage is from 25 to 30 mg per m^2 of body surface depending upon the regimen. It is administered by intravenous injection over six to 10 minutes.

J9393

J9393 Injection, fulvestrant (Teva) not therapeutically equivalent to J9395, 25 mg

Fulvestrant is an antineoplastic estrogen receptor antagonist. Many breast cancers have estrogen receptors, and their growth can be stimulated by estrogen. Fulvestrant binds to the estrogen receptor preventing the estrogen from reaching the cells. It is indicated for the treatment of hormone receptor (HR)-positive, human epidermal growth factor receptor 2 (HER2)-negative advanced breast cancer in postmenopausal women not previously treated with or with disease progression following endocrine therapy; HR-positive, HER2-negative advanced or metastatic breast cancer in postmenopausal women in combination with ribociclib, as initial therapy or following disease progression on endocrine-based therapy; HR-positive, HER2-negative advanced or metastatic breast cancer in combination with palbociclib or abemaciclib in women with disease progression after endocrine therapy. It is supplied in a single dose prefilled syringe of 250 mg/5 ml and is administered via intramuscular (IM) injection. The recommended dosage is 500 mg administered into the buttocks slowly as two 5 ml injections, one into each buttock, on days one, 15, 29, and once monthly thereafter. For patients with hepatic impairment, the recommended dosage is 250 mg administered in the buttock as one 5 ml injection on days one, 15, 29, and once monthly thereafter. See full prescribing information for complete administration instructions. Report J9393 only for fulvestrant manufactured by Teva.

J9394

J9394 Injection, fulvestrant (Fresenius Kabi) not therapeutically equivalent to J9395, 25 mg

Fulvestrant is an antineoplastic estrogen receptor antagonist. Many breast cancers have estrogen receptors, and their growth can be stimulated by estrogen. Fulvestrant binds to the estrogen receptor, preventing the estrogen from reaching the cells. It is indicated for the treatment of hormone receptor (HR)-positive, human epidermal growth factor receptor 2 (HER2)-negative advanced breast cancer in postmenopausal women not previously treated or with disease progression following endocrine therapy; HR-positive, HER2-negative advanced or metastatic breast cancer in postmenopausal women in combination with ribociclib, as initial therapy or following disease progression on endocrine-based therapy; HR-positive, HER2-negative advanced or metastatic breast cancer in combination with Palbociclib or abemaciclib in women with disease progression after endocrine therapy. It is supplied in a single dose prefilled syringe of 250 mg/5 ml and is administered via intramuscular (IM) injection. The recommended dosage is 500 mg administered into the buttocks slowly as two 5 ml injections, one into each buttock, on days one, 15, 29, and once monthly thereafter. For patients with hepatic impairment, the recommended dosage is 250 mg administered in the buttock as one 5 ml injection on days one, 15, 29, and once monthly thereafter. See full prescribing information for complete administration instructions. Report J9394 only for fulvestrant manufactured by Fresenius Kabi.

J9395

J9395 Injection, fulvestrant, 25 mg

Fulvestrant is an antineoplastic estrogen receptor antagonist. Many breast cancers have estrogen receptors and their growth can be stimulated by estrogen. Fulvestrant binds to the estrogen receptor preventing the estrogen from reaching the cells. It is indicated for the treatment of estrogen receptor, positive metastatic breast cancer in postmenopausal women who have not responded to other antiestrogen therapy. The recommended dosage is 250 mg. Fulvestrant is administered as a slow intramuscular injection into the buttocks. It may be administered as a single 5 ml injection or as two 2.5 ml injections.

J9400

J9400 Injection, ziv-aflibercept, 1 mg

Ziv-aflibercept is a recombinant fusion protein composed of vascular endothelial growth factor (VEGF)-binding portions from the domains of human VEGF Receptors 1 and 2 then fused to a portion of the human Immunoglobulin G (IgG1). When the drug binds to these receptors, it blocks their activation and can result in the decreased growth of new blood vessels and decreased vascular permeability. Ziv-aflibercept is produced by recombinant DNA technology in a Chinese hamster ovary. Ziv-aflibercept is indicated for patients with metastatic colorectal cancer that is resistant to or has progressed following an oxaliplatin-containing regimen. It is to be used in combination with 5-fluorouracil (5-FU), leucovorin, and irinotecan. The recommended dosage is 4 mg/kg as an intravenous infusion over one hour every two weeks.

J9600

J9600 Injection, porfimer sodium, 75 mg

Porfimer sodium is a mixture of porphyrins that sensitizes cells to light. The drug is injected into neoplastic cells as step one of a two-step photodynamic treatment. Two to three days following injection, the neoplasm is irradiated with a laser light producing a cytotoxic reaction that destroys the cells. As the penetration of the light is limited, the photodynamic therapy is primarily used to treat small thin lesions on accessible surfaces. This type of photodynamic therapy is indicated for the palliative care of patients with completely obstructing esophageal cancer, patients with have partially obstructing esophageal cancer who cannot be satisfactorily treated with laser therapy alone, patients with partially or completely obstructive endobronchial non-small cell lung cancer, or patients who have microinvasive endobronchial non-small cell lung cancer for whom surgery and radiotherapy are not indicated.

J9999

J9999 Not otherwise classified, antineoplastic drugs

Use this code to represent an antineoplastic drug that has been administered and is not represented by any other HCPCS Level I or Level II code.

K

K0001

K0001 Standard wheelchair

A standard wheelchair has a seat width of 16 (narrow) or 18 inches (adult), a seat depth of 16 inches, and 21 inches from seat to floor. It comes with a nonadjustable back height of 16 to 21 inches, a chrome plated frame, 24 inch molded rear wheels, 8 inch molded casters, nylon or vinyl upholstery, and fixed or swing away detachable footrests. The footplate extension is between 16 and 21 inches. The standard wheelchair weighs more than 36 pounds.

K0002

K0002 Standard hemi (low seat) wheelchair

This code reports a standard hemi (low seat) wheelchair. A hemi wheelchair has a seat height of 16 to 18 inches and is made for patients with a short stature or for patients who have an inability to place feet directly on the ground for propulsion. The hemi wheelchair has a weight capacity of 250 pounds and weighs 36 pounds or less. It comes with a chrome plated frame, 24-inch molded rear wheels, 8-inch molded casters, nylon or vinyl upholstery, and fixed or swing away detachable footrests.

K0003

K0003 Lightweight wheelchair

A lightweight wheelchair is indicated for patients requiring a chair for self-propulsion, and when the seat measurements required cannot be accommodated by a standard or hemi standard wheelchair. This device weighs less than 36 pounds, is fully reclining, and has swing away detachable leg rests. The seat width is 14, 16, or 18 inches, has a seat depth of 16 inches, and seat height between 17 and 21 inches. It has a nonadjustable back height of 16 to 17 inches, 24 inch molded rear wheels; 8 inch molded casters, nylon or vinyl upholstery, fixed-height detachable arms, and fixed or swing away detachable footrests. The footplate extension is between 14 and 17 inches.

K0004

K0004 High strength, lightweight wheelchair

A high strength, lightweight wheelchair is indicated for patients requiring a chair for self propulsion that is extra strong in frame construction, and when the seat measurements required cannot be accommodated by a standard or hemi standard wheelchair. This device weighs less than 34 pounds, with cross braces. The seat width is 14, 16, or 18 inches, has a seat depth of 14 (child) or 16 inches (adult), and a seat height between 17 and 21 inches. It has a sectional or adjustable back height of 15 to 19 inches. It has 24 inch molded rear wheels, 8 inch molded casters, nylon upholstery, fixed-height detachable arms, and fixed or swing away detachable footrests. The footplate extension is 16 to 21 inches.

K0005

K0005 Ultralightweight wheelchair

An ultra-lightweight wheelchair weighs less than 30 pounds, with cross braces, has a seat width of 14, 16, or 18 inches, a seat depth of 14 (child) or 16 inches (adult), and a seat height between 17 and 21 inches. It has an adjustable rear axle position, nylon upholstery, fixed or detachable arms, and fixed or swing away detachable footrests. The footplate extension is 16 to 21 inches.

K0006-K0007

K0006 Heavy-duty wheelchair

K0007 Extra heavy-duty wheelchair

Wide, heavy-duty, and extra heavy-duty wheelchairs are indicated for obese patients when the seat measurements required cannot be accommodated by a standard wheelchair. The seat width is 18 inches, has a seat depth of 16 to 17 inches, and a seat height between 19 and 21 inches. It has a nonadjustable back height of 16 to 17 inches. It has reinforced back and seat upholstery, fixed-height detachable arms, and fixed or swing away detachable footrests. The footplate extension is 16 to 21 inches.

K0008

K0008 Custom manual wheelchair/base

A custom manual wheelchair or base is a uniquely constructed or substantially modified wheelchair or base adapted to a specific patient according to the physician's description and orders. Customized items are rarely necessary and are rarely furnished. It is expected to be a one-of-a-kind item fabricated to meet specific needs.

K0009

K0009 Other manual wheelchair/base

Use this code to report manual wheelchair bases that are not described by any other HCPCS Level II code.

K0010-K0014

K0010 Standard-weight frame motorized/power wheelchair

K0011 Standard-weight frame motorized/power wheelchair with programmable control parameters for speed adjustment, tremor dampening, acceleration control and braking

K0012 Lightweight portable motorized/power wheelchair

K0013 Custom motorized/power wheelchair base

K0014 Other motorized/power wheelchair base

Motorized (powered) wheelchairs are those not included in the manual wheelchair categories. They can be standard, lightweight, and customized, and can be fitted with a variety of accessories. These wheelchairs are generally slow-speed and fairly good at maneuvering and negotiating corners and certain inclines. They usually work from a battery power source. Motorized wheelchairs are not suited to patients who cannot operate the controls, such as stroke patients. Wheelchairs, in general, assist the patient in the activities of daily living (ADL), both in and out of the home. They enable the patient to move about in confined and open spaces. While some patients and/or their caretakers may prefer motorized wheelchairs, depending on the patient's clinical needs and ADL restrictions, payers' policies can differ widely in coverage. The patient's medical condition may dictate whether or not the patient can operate (maneuver and control) a motorized wheelchair alone or with limited assistance and/or observation. A custom manual wheelchair or base is a uniquely constructed or substantially modified wheelchair or base adapted to a specific patient according to the physician's description and orders. It is expected to be a one-of-a-kind item fabricated to meet specific needs.

K0015-K0020

K0015 Detachable, nonadjustable height armrest, each

K0017 Detachable, adjustable height armrest, base, replacement only, each

K0018 Detachable, adjustable height armrest, upper portion, replacement only, each

K0019 Arm pad, replacement only, each

K0020 Fixed, adjustable height armrest, pair

Armrests are used with wheelchairs to provide comfort to the patient. They help with the patient position, allowing for better posture. There are several different types of armrests. Fixed armrests are bolted to the chair and cannot be removed. Detachable armrests can be removed to make moving the patient easier and to allow the patient better access to tables and desks. The armrests may also be adjustable to different heights for comfort and function. Armrest pads are attached to the armrest; they may be upholstered, hard plastic, or covered with soft material.

K0037

K0037 High mount flip-up footrest, each

The flip up footrest forms the support surface on which the patient's foot is supported and may be flipped up out of the way when the patient is transferred in or out of the wheelchair. Use this code to report a flip up footrest that is mounted high up on the wheelchair.

K0038-K0039

K0038 Leg strap, each

K0039 Leg strap, H style, each

Use these codes to report the fabric strap that is placed over the legs to secure the lower leg to the legrest. The H-style leg strap covers more of the leg and provides greater stability for the patient with severely impaired legs. Typically, the H-strap is used for quadriplegics, hemiplegics, paraplegics, and patients with palsy.

K0040-K0042

K0040 Adjustable angle footplate, each

K0041 Large size footplate, each

K0042 Standard size footplate, replacement only, each

Footplates are flat surfaces designed to support the feet while in a wheelchair. They may be aluminum (usually found in heavy duty wheelchairs) or made of a plastic composite material, which is lightweight and easy to keep clean. Footplates come in various sizes but usually support the individual's foot from the back of his/her heel to around the ball of the foot. An adjustable angle footplate is usually aluminum and has two or three adjustment features, depending on the model of the wheelchair. Adjustable angle footplates are generally longer since they support more of the foot than the standard footplates and may be adjusted with the toes pointing down or up. Use these codes to report each wheelchair footplate.

K0043-K0045

K0043 Footrest, lower extension tube, replacement only, each

K0044 Footrest, upper hanger bracket, replacement only, each

K0045 Footrest, complete assembly, replacement only, each

Footrests are available in two or three angles, depending on the individual's needs, and may be removed. The lower extension tube attaches to the footplate. The upper hanger bracket attaches the footrest to the wheelchair. The complete assembly includes all three components.

K

K0046-K0047

K0046 Elevating legrest, lower extension tube, replacement only, each

K0047 Elevating legrest, upper hanger bracket, replacement only, each

Elevating legrests attach to the lower front of the chair and are used to support the legs. The elevating legrest can be positioned to maintain the leg in an extended position or at varying angles. These codes represent pieces of a footrest.

K0050

K0050 Ratchet assembly, replacement only

A wheelchair ratchet assembly is a device that allows continuous linear or rotary movement in one direction while preventing motion in the opposite direction. A ratchet may allow the wheels to roll forward, but prevent any backward motion.

K0051

K0051 Cam release assembly, footrest or legrest, replacement only, each

A cam release assembly device allows quick and easy release and removal of the legrest or footrest of a wheelchair. The legrest or footrest can be removed for access to the patient and transporting the wheelchair.

K0052

K0052 Swingaway, detachable footrests, replacement only, each

Swing away footrests form a platform on which the foot is supported. The hinged connection enables the footrest to rotate out of the way when the patient is transferred into or out of the wheelchair. Use this code to report removable swing away footrests.

K0053

K0053 Elevating footrests, articulating (telescoping), each

Elevating footrests can be raised up to elevate and support the patient's legs. The telescopic feature allows the legrest to be lengthened as a support for patients with longer limbs. Use this code to report each elevating, articulating footrest.

K0056

K0056 Seat height less than 17 in or equal to or greater than 21 in for a high-strength, lightweight, or ultralightweight wheelchair

A standard wheelchair has a nonadjustable back height of 16 to 21 inches. The standard wheelchair weighs more than 36 pounds. This code reports a seat height less than 17 inches or equal to or greater than 21 inches that is designed for use in a high-strength, lightweight, or ultra lightweight wheelchair.

K0065

K0065 Spoke protectors, each

Wheelchair spoke protectors, or spoke guards, are lightweight discs designed to cover the back wheels of wheelchairs. These protectors prevent fingers from going into the spokes of the wheelchairs.

K0069-K0070

K0069 Rear wheel assembly, complete, with solid tire, spokes or molded, replacement only, each

K0070 Rear wheel assembly, complete, with pneumatic tire, spokes or molded, replacement only, each

The rear wheels are the large wheels on the back of a wheelchair often used for propulsion. The wheel assembly is comprised of the rear wheel, spokes, and hub. The wheels may come with solid or pneumatic tires. Use these codes to report the rear wheel assembly (based on type of tire).

K0071-K0077

K0071 Front caster assembly, complete, with pneumatic tire, replacement only, each

K0072 Front caster assembly, complete, with semipneumatic tire, replacement only, each

K0073 Caster pin lock, each

K0077 Front caster assembly, complete, with solid tire, replacement only, each

Casters are the front wheels of a wheelchair and are designed to pivot and allow the patient to steer the chair. The caster assembly is composed of the front wheel and the castor fork assembly. Casters may come with pneumatic, semi pneumatic, or solid tires. Use these codes to report the complete front caster assembly (based on type of tire) or to report the pin that locks the caster in place.

K0098

K0098 Drive belt for power wheelchair, replacement only

A drive belt is used with the belt-drive power wheelchair to connect the motor to the drive wheels.

K0105

K0105 IV hanger, each

The IV hanger is a pole that attaches to a wheelchair to allow the patient to receive an infusion.

K0108

K0108 Wheelchair component or accessory, not otherwise specified

A wheelchair component or accessory is an addition or a part of a wheelchair. Report this code for a wheelchair component or accessory that is not identified by a more specific HCPCS Level II code.

K0195

K0195 Elevating legrests, pair (for use with capped rental wheelchair base)

An elevating legrest is a wheelchair accessory required by patients who have musculoskeletal conditions, casts, or braces that prevent 90-degree flexion at the knee. It may also be required for patients with significant edema of the lower extremities requiring elevation of the legs and for patients who require a reclining back on the wheelchair. This code reports a single elevating legrest and all hardware required for complete assembly. Report this code twice for patients who require elevating legrests for both legs.

K0455

K0455 Infusion pump used for uninterrupted parenteral administration of medication, (e.g., epoprostenol or treprostinol)

Epoprostenol (Flolan) is a medication used primarily to treat pulmonary hypertension. Its brief half-life typically requires continuous parenteral infusion. The infusion pump is usually delivered through the subclavian or jugular veins, sometimes through a tunneled catheter that exits in an area maintainable by the patient. The pump is typically portable, worn on a harness or belt, and powered by 9-volt or AA alkaline batteries. Often a second unit is worn, or immediately available, and alternated every 24 hours to ensure uninterrupted delivery.

K0462

K0462 Temporary replacement for patient-owned equipment being repaired, any type

This code reports temporary replacement of patient equipment that is being repaired.

K0552

K0552 Supplies for external noninsulin drug infusion pump, syringe type cartridge, sterile, each

This code reports the sterile supplies required for the syringe type cartridge external drug infusion pump. The pump runs on electrical current.

K0601-K0605

K0601 Replacement battery for external infusion pump owned by patient, silver oxide, 1.5 volt, each

K0602 Replacement battery for external infusion pump owned by patient, silver oxide, 3 volt, each

K0603 Replacement battery for external infusion pump owned by patient, alkaline, 1.5 volt, each

K0604 Replacement battery for external infusion pump owned by patient, lithium, 3.6 volt, each

K0605 Replacement battery for external infusion pump owned by patient, lithium, 4.5 volt, each

The external infusion pump (EIP) is a small portable device that provides a continuous infusion therapy over an extended time period. The EIP requires batteries for operation. Use these codes to report the batteries required by an EIP that is owned by the patient.

K0606-K0609

K0606 Automatic external defibrillator, with integrated electrocardiogram analysis, garment type

K0607 Replacement battery for automated external defibrillator, garment type only, each

K0608 Replacement garment for use with automated external defibrillator, each

K0609 Replacement electrodes for use with automated external defibrillator, garment type only, each

Automatic external defibrillators are compact and portable devices that deliver an electrical shock to a person who has a sudden cardiac arrest. Automatic external defibrillator units use a microprocessor inside of a portable defibrillator to interpret a person's heart rhythm through electrodes. The computer recognizes ventricular fibrillation or ventricular tachycardia. Once recognized, the computer advises the operator/user that electrical defibrillation is needed or it will automatically deliver a countershock. The patient wears the external defibrillator in a vest.

K0669

K0669 Wheelchair accessory, wheelchair seat or back cushion, does not meet specific code criteria or no written coding verification from DME PDAC

Wheelchair seat cushions can provide leg positioning, pelvic stability, and pressure management for patients with postural asymmetry. A cushion may provide support and pressure relief for individuals sitting in a wheelchair. The cushions can be made out of various material and filling. The Pricing, Data Analysis and Coding (PDAC) contractor maintains the Durable Medical Equipment Coding System.

K0672

K0672 Addition to lower extremity orthotic, removable soft interface, all components, replacement only, each

A soft interface is worn under an orthosis to provide skin cushioning and protection. It also lessens the pressure and irritation that the orthosis can cause. The interface can be made of different kinds of fibers and are usually seam free.

K0730

K0730 Controlled dose inhalation drug delivery system

A controlled dose inhalation drug delivery system provides a precise, monitored dose of inhaled medication. The dose provided in nebulizers may vary somewhat from patient to patient based on breathing patterns. The medications through a nebulizer are administered in a continuous flow. Some medications require precise dosing that cannot be obtained with other nebulizers. The controlled dose inhaler monitors the patient's breathing pattern and adjusts the drug delivery. Medication is only administered during inhalation and not during exhalation.

K0733

K0733 Power wheelchair accessory, 12 to 24 amp hour sealed lead acid battery, each (e.g., gel cell, absorbed glassmat)

A 12 to 24 amp hour lead-acid battery is a valve-regulated type that may be referred to as sealed or maintenance-free. This type of battery fixes the acid electrolyte in a gel or in an absorptive fiberglass mat. A gel cell suspends the electrolyte in a silica-based gel producing a thick pasty material. An absorbed glassmat (AGM) suspends the electrolyte in fiberglass matt separators that act as absorbent sponges. The battery needs no added water and can be safely operated in any position.

K0738

K0738 Portable gaseous oxygen system, rental; home compressor used to fill portable oxygen cylinders; includes portable containers, regulator, flowmeter, humidifier, cannula or mask, and tubing

A rented portable gaseous oxygen system is equipment that includes a home compressor used to fill portable oxygen cylinders. This type of system allows individuals to fill their own oxygen cylinders in their homes. This is accomplished by attaching the home compressor to an oxygen concentrator that provides the oxygen for the cylinders. The home compressor takes the oxygen and compresses it into the portable cylinders, which the patient uses when away from home. The home compressor can be used simultaneously to receive stationary oxygen while at the same time filling portable cylinders. This code includes all delivery hardware associated with use of the portable gaseous oxygen system, including portable containers, regulator, flowmeter, humidifier, cannula/mask, and tubing.

K0739-K0740

K0739 Repair or nonroutine service for durable medical equipment other than oxygen equipment requiring the skill of a technician, labor component, per 15 minutes

K0740 Repair or nonroutine service for oxygen equipment requiring the skill of a technician, labor component, per 15 minutes

These codes report the repair or non-routine service of durable medical equipment, such as wheelchair repair or oxygen equipment, that requires the skill of a technician. The labor involved in the repair or service is reported in 15-minute increments.

K0743

K0743 Suction pump, home model, portable, for use on wounds

Home wound suction is achieved with a system of components. The wound suction pump provides a controlled atmospheric pressure without the use of a collection canister. The pump is used with separately reportable special dressings that absorb the drainage. Use this code to report use of a home suction pump.

K0744-K0746

K0744 Absorptive wound dressing for use with suction pump, home model, portable, pad size 16 sq in or less

K0745 Absorptive wound dressing for use with suction pump, home model, portable, pad size more than 16 sq in but less than or equal to 48 sq in

K0746 Absorptive wound dressing for use with suction pump, home model, portable, pad size greater than 48 sq in

These codes report the dressing sets used with the portable suction pump that does not require a collection canister. These codes include all of the necessary components of a complete dressing change, such as the drainage tubing, the porous non-adherent dressing, and an occlusive dressing that creates the seal around the wound site.

K0800-K0812

K0800 Power operated vehicle, group 1 standard, patient weight capacity up to and including 300 pounds

K0801 Power operated vehicle, group 1 heavy-duty, patient weight capacity 301 to 450 pounds

K0802 Power operated vehicle, group 1 very heavy-duty, patient weight capacity 451 to 600 pounds

K0806 Power operated vehicle, group 2 standard, patient weight capacity up to and including 300 pounds

K0807 Power operated vehicle, group 2 heavy-duty, patient weight capacity 301 to 450 pounds

K0808 Power operated vehicle, group 2 very heavy-duty, patient weight capacity 451 to 600 pounds

K0812 Power operated vehicle, not otherwise classified

A power operated vehicle (POV) is a battery powered mobility device with tiller operated steering and three or four wheels. POVs may also be referred to as scooters. POVs are designed for a combination of indoor use with moderate outdoor capabilities on flat terrain and hard surfaces with minimal to moderate surface irregularity. A POV assists patients for whom a wheelchair is unsuitable in the activities of daily living, but POVs are not suited to all types of patients such as stroke victims or some quadriplegic and/or hemiplegic patients who cannot operate the controls nor be left alone while the vehicle is in operation. POVs are divided into two groups. Group 1 POVs have the following specifications: length 48 inches, width 28 inches, obstacle height 20 mm, minimum top end speed-flat 3 MPH, range 5 miles, and dynamic stability incline 6 degrees. Group 2 POVs have the following specifications: length 48 inches, width 28 inches, obstacle height 50 mm, minimum top end speed-flat 4 MPH, range 10 miles, and dynamic stability incline 7.5 degrees. POVs are further classified by weight capacity. Standard refers to a weight capacity up to and including 300 pounds. Heavy duty refers to a weight capacity of between 301 and 450 pounds. Very heavy duty refers to a weight capacity of between 451 and 600 pounds.

K0813-K0816

K0813 Power wheelchair, group 1 standard, portable, sling/solid seat and back, patient weight capacity up to and including 300 pounds

K0814 Power wheelchair, group 1 standard, portable, captain's chair, patient weight capacity up to and including 300 pounds

K0815 Power wheelchair, group 1 standard, sling/solid seat and back, patient weight capacity up to and including 300 pounds

K0816 Power wheelchair, group 1 standard, captain's chair, patient weight capacity up to and including 300 pounds

These codes describe Group 1 standard power wheelchairs. Group 1 power wheelchairs have the following specifications: length 40 inches, width 24 inches, obstacle height 20 mm, minimum top end speed-flat 3 MPH, range 5 miles, dynamic stability incline 6 degrees, fatigue test on a level 200,000 cycles with 0.5 inch slats under all wheels, and 6,666 drop cycles. Standard wheelchairs have a maximum weight capacity of 300 pounds. Chairs represented by these four codes have been further subdivided by portability. Portable chairs are defined as being easily disassembled without the use of tools for transport in a vehicle whereas nonportable chairs cannot be easily disassembled. Each of these subcategories has been further defined by the type of chair.

K0820-K0823

K0820 Power wheelchair, group 2 standard, portable, sling/solid seat/back, patient weight capacity up to and including 300 pounds

K0821 Power wheelchair, group 2 standard, portable, captain's chair, patient weight capacity up to and including 300 pounds

K0822 Power wheelchair, group 2 standard, sling/solid seat/back, patient weight capacity up to and including 300 pounds

K0823 Power wheelchair, group 2 standard, captain's chair, patient weight capacity up to and including 300 pounds

These codes describe Group 2 standard power wheelchairs. Group 2 power wheelchairs have the following specifications: length 48 inches, width 34 inches, obstacle height 40 mm, minimum top speed-flat 3 MPH, range 7 miles, dynamic stability incline 6 degrees, fatigue test on a level 200,000 cycles with 0.5 inch slats under all wheels, and 6,666 drop cycles. Standard wheelchairs have a maximum weight capacity of 300 pounds. Chairs represented by these four codes have been further subdivided by portability. Portable chairs are defined as being easily disassembled without use of tools for transport in a vehicle whereas nonportable chairs cannot be easily disassembled. Each of these subcategories has been further defined by the type of chair.

K0824-K0825

K0824 Power wheelchair, group 2 heavy-duty, sling/solid seat/back, patient weight capacity 301 to 450 pounds

K0825 Power wheelchair, group 2 heavy-duty, captain's chair, patient weight capacity 301 to 450 pounds

These codes describe Group 2 heavy duty power wheelchairs. Group 2 power wheelchairs have the following specifications: length 48 inches, width 34 inches, obstacle height 40 mm, minimum top speed-flat 3 MPH, range 7 miles, dynamic stability incline 6 degrees, fatigue test on a level 200,000 cycles with 0.5 inch slats under all wheels, and 6,666 drop cycles. Heavy duty wheelchairs have a weight capacity of between 301 to 450 pounds. Chairs represented by these two codes have been further subdivided by type of chair.

K0826-K0827

K0826 Power wheelchair, group 2 very heavy-duty, sling/solid seat/back, patient weight capacity 451 to 600 pounds

K0827 Power wheelchair, group 2 very heavy-duty, captain's chair, patient weight capacity 451 to 600 pounds

These codes describe Group 2 very heavy duty power wheelchairs. Group 2 power wheelchairs have the following specifications: length 48 inches, width 34 inches, obstacle height 40 mm, minimum top speed-flat 3 MPH, range 7 miles, dynamic stability incline 6 degrees, fatigue test on a level 200,000 cycles with 0.5 inch slats under all wheels, and 6,666 drop cycles. Very heavy duty wheelchairs have a weight capacity of 451 to 600 pounds. Chairs represented by these two codes have been further subdivided by type of chair.

K0828-K0829

K0828 Power wheelchair, group 2 extra heavy-duty, sling/solid seat/back, patient weight capacity 601 pounds or more

K0829 Power wheelchair, group 2 extra heavy-duty, captain's chair, patient weight 601 pounds or more

These codes describe Group 2 extra heavy duty power wheelchairs. Group 2 power wheelchairs have the following specifications: length 48 inches, width 34 inches, obstacle height 40 mm, minimum top speed-flat 3 MPH, range 7 miles, dynamic stability incline 6 degrees, fatigue test on a level 200,000 cycles with 0.5 inch slats under all wheels, and 6,666 drop cycles. Extra heavy duty wheelchairs have a weight capacity of 601 pounds or more. Chairs represented by these two codes have been further subdivided by type of chair: sling/solid seat/back and a captain's chair.

K0830-K0831

K0830 Power wheelchair, group 2 standard, seat elevator, sling/solid seat/back, patient weight capacity up to and including 300 pounds

K0831 Power wheelchair, group 2 standard, seat elevator, captain's chair, patient weight capacity up to and including 300 pounds

These codes describe Group 2 standard power wheelchairs with the added feature of a seat elevator. Seat elevators are used to assist with transfers and to reach items that would be out of reach from a standard wheelchair height. Group 2 power wheelchairs have the following specifications: length 48 inches, width 34 inches, obstacle height 40 mm, minimum top speed-flat 3 MPH, range 7 miles, dynamic stability incline 6 degrees, fatigue test on a level 200,000 cycles with 0.5 inch slats under all wheels, and 6,666 drop cycles. Standard wheelchairs have a maximum weight capacity of 300 pounds. Chairs represented by these two codes have been further subdivided by type of chair.

K0835-K0840

K0835 Power wheelchair, group 2 standard, single power option, sling/solid seat/back, patient weight capacity up to and including 300 pounds

K0836 Power wheelchair, group 2 standard, single power option, captain's chair, patient weight capacity up to and including 300 pounds

K0837 Power wheelchair, group 2 heavy-duty, single power option, sling/solid seat/back, patient weight capacity 301 to 450 pounds

K0838 Power wheelchair, group 2 heavy-duty, single power option, captain's chair, patient weight capacity 301 to 450 pounds

K0839 Power wheelchair, group 2 very heavy-duty, single power option sling/solid seat/back, patient weight capacity 451 to 600 pounds

K0840 Power wheelchair, group 2 extra heavy-duty, single power option, sling/solid seat/back, patient weight capacity 601 pounds or more

These codes describe Group 2 power wheelchairs with the added feature of a single power option. Group 2 power wheelchairs have the following specifications: length 48 inches, width 34 inches, obstacle height 40 mm, minimum top speed-flat 3 MPH, range 7 miles, dynamic stability incline 6 degrees, fatigue test on a level 200,000 cycles with 0.5 inch slats under all wheels, and 6,666 drop cycles. The single power option is available in all weight capacities, including standard (weight capacity up to and including 300 pounds), heavy duty (weight capacity 301 to 450 pounds), very heavy duty (weight capacity 451 to 600 pounds), and extra heavy duty (weight capacity 601 pounds or more). Standard and heavy duty weight capacity chairs with single power option are further classified by type of chair.

K0841-K0843

K0841 Power wheelchair, group 2 standard, multiple power option, sling/solid seat/back, patient weight capacity up to and including 300 pounds

K0842 Power wheelchair, group 2 standard, multiple power option, captain's chair, patient weight capacity up to and including 300 pounds

K0843 Power wheelchair, group 2 heavy-duty, multiple power option, sling/solid seat/back, patient weight capacity 301 to 450 pounds

These codes describe Group 2 power wheelchairs with the added feature of a multiple power option. Group 2 power wheelchairs have the following specifications: length 48 inches, width 34 inches, obstacle height 40 mm, minimum top speed-flat 3 MPH, range 7 miles, dynamic stability incline 6 degrees, fatigue test on a level 200,000 cycles with 0.5 inch slats under all wheels, and 6,666 drop cycles. The multiple power option is available in only standard and heavy duty weight capacities. Standard weight capacity is defined as up to and including 300 pounds and heavy duty weight capacity is 301 to 450 pounds. Standard weight capacity chairs with single power option are further classified by type of chair.

K0848-K0851

K0848 Power wheelchair, group 3 standard, sling/solid seat/back, patient weight capacity up to and including 300 pounds

K0849 Power wheelchair, group 3 standard, captain's chair, patient weight capacity up to and including 300 pounds

K0850 Power wheelchair, group 3 heavy-duty, sling/solid seat/back, patient weight capacity 301 to 450 pounds

K0851 Power wheelchair, group 3 heavy-duty, captain's chair, patient weight capacity 301 to 450 pounds

These codes describe standard and heavy duty Group 3 power wheelchairs. Group 3 power wheelchairs have the following specifications: length 48 inches, width 34 inches, obstacle height 60 mm, minimum top speed-flat 4.5 MPH, range 12 miles, dynamic stability incline 7.5 degrees, fatigue test on a level 200,000 cycles with 0.5 inch slats under all wheels, and 6,666 drop cycles. Standard weight capacity is defined as up to and including 300 pounds and heavy duty weight capacity is 301 to 450 pounds. Standard and heavy duty weight capacity chairs are further classified by type of chair.

K0852-K0855

K0852 Power wheelchair, group 3 very heavy-duty, sling/solid seat/back, patient weight capacity 451 to 600 pounds

K0853 Power wheelchair, group 3 very heavy-duty, captain's chair, patient weight capacity 451 to 600 pounds

K0854 Power wheelchair, group 3 extra heavy-duty, sling/solid seat/back, patient weight capacity 601 pounds or more

K0855 Power wheelchair, group 3 extra heavy-duty, captain's chair, patient weight capacity 601 pounds or more

These codes describe very heavy duty and extra heavy duty Group 3 power wheelchairs. Group 3 power wheelchairs have the following specifications: length 48 inches, width 34 inches, obstacle height 60 mm, minimum top speed-flat 4.5 MPH, range 12 miles, dynamic stability incline 7.5 degrees, fatigue test on a level 200,000 cycles with 0.5 inch slats under all wheels, and 6,666 drop cycles. Very heavy duty weight capacity is 451 to 600 pounds and extra heavy duty is 601 pounds or more. Very heavy duty and extra heavy duty weight capacity chairs are further classified by type of chair.

K0856-K0860

K0856 Power wheelchair, group 3 standard, single power option, sling/solid seat/back, patient weight capacity up to and including 300 pounds

K0857 Power wheelchair, group 3 standard, single power option, captain's chair, patient weight capacity up to and including 300 pounds

K0858 Power wheelchair, group 3 heavy-duty, single power option, sling/solid seat/back, patient weight 301 to 450 pounds

K0859 Power wheelchair, group 3 heavy-duty, single power option, captain's chair, patient weight capacity 301 to 450 pounds

K0860 Power wheelchair, group 3 very heavy-duty, single power option, sling/solid seat/back, patient weight capacity 451 to 600 pounds

These codes describe Group 3 power wheelchairs with the added feature of a single power option. Group 3 power wheelchairs have the following specifications: length 48 inches, width 34 inches, obstacle height 60 mm, minimum top speed-flat 4.5 MPH, range 12 miles, dynamic stability incline 7.5 degrees, fatigue test on a level 200,000 cycles with 0.5 inch slats under all wheels, and 6,666 drop cycles. The single power option is available in standard (weight capacity up to and including 300 pounds), heavy duty (weight capacity 301 to 450 pounds), and very heavy duty (weight capacity 451 to 600 pounds). Standard and

K

heavy duty weight capacity chairs are further classified by type of chair.

K0861-K0864

K0861 Power wheelchair, group 3 standard, multiple power option, sling/solid seat/back, patient weight capacity up to and including 300 pounds

K0862 Power wheelchair, group 3 heavy-duty, multiple power option, sling/solid seat/back, patient weight capacity 301 to 450 pounds

K0863 Power wheelchair, group 3 very heavy-duty, multiple power option, sling/solid seat/back, patient weight capacity 451 to 600 pounds

K0864 Power wheelchair, group 3 extra heavy-duty, multiple power option, sling/solid seat/back, patient weight capacity 601 pounds or more

These codes describe Group 3 power wheelchairs with the added feature of a multiple power option. Group 3 power wheelchairs have the following specifications: length 48 inches, width 34 inches, obstacle height 60 mm, minimum top speed-flat 4.5 MPH, range 12 miles, dynamic stability incline 7.5 degrees, fatigue test on a level 200,000 cycles with 0.5 inch slats under all wheels, and 6,666 drop cycles. The multiple power option is available with sling/solid seat/back in all weight capacities.

K0868-K0871

K0868 Power wheelchair, group 4 standard, sling/solid seat/back, patient weight capacity up to and including 300 pounds

K0869 Power wheelchair, group 4 standard, captain's chair, patient weight capacity up to and including 300 pounds

K0870 Power wheelchair, group 4 heavy-duty, sling/solid seat/back, patient weight capacity 301 to 450 pounds

K0871 Power wheelchair, group 4 very heavy-duty, sling/solid seat/back, patient weight capacity 451 to 600 pounds

These codes describe Group 4 power wheelchairs. Group 4 power wheelchairs have the following specifications: length 48 inches, width 34 inches, obstacle height 75 mm, minimum top speed-flat 6 MPH, range 16 miles, dynamic stability incline 9 degrees, fatigue test on a level 200,000 cycles with 0.5 inch slats under all wheels, and 6,666 drop cycles. Group 4 power wheelchairs are available in three weight capacities, including standard (up to and including 300 pounds), heavy duty (301 to 450 pounds), and very heavy duty (450 to 600 pounds). Standard weight capacity chairs are further classified by type of chair. Heavy duty and very heavy duty chairs are available only as sling/solid seat/back.

K0877-K0880

K0877 Power wheelchair, group 4 standard, single power option, sling/solid seat/back, patient weight capacity up to and including 300 pounds

K0878 Power wheelchair, group 4 standard, single power option, captain's chair, patient weight capacity up to and including 300 pounds

K0879 Power wheelchair, group 4 heavy-duty, single power option, sling/solid seat/back, patient weight capacity 301 to 450 pounds

K0880 Power wheelchair, group 4 very heavy-duty, single power option, sling/solid seat/back, patient weight 451 to 600 pounds

These codes describe Group 4 power wheelchairs with the added feature of a single power option. Group 4 power wheelchairs have the following specifications: length 48 inches, width 34 inches, obstacle height 75 mm, minimum top speed-flat 6 MPH, range 16 miles, dynamic stability incline 9 degrees, fatigue test on a level 200,000 cycles with 0.5 inch slats under all wheels, and 6,666 drop cycles. The single power option is available in three weight capacities, including standard (up to and including 300 pounds), heavy duty (301 to 450 pounds), and very heavy duty (450 to 600 pounds). Standard weight capacity chairs with a single power option are further classified by type of chair. Heavy duty and very heavy duty chairs are available only as sling/solid seat/back.

K0884-K0886

K0884 Power wheelchair, group 4 standard, multiple power option, sling/solid seat/back, patient weight capacity up to and including 300 pounds

K0885 Power wheelchair, group 4 standard, multiple power option, captain's chair, patient weight capacity up to and including 300 pounds

K0886 Power wheelchair, group 4 heavy-duty, multiple power option, sling/solid seat/back, patient weight capacity 301 to 450 pounds

These codes describe Group 4 power wheelchairs with the added feature of a multiple power option. Group 4 power wheelchairs have the following specifications: length 48 inches, width 34 inches, obstacle height 75 mm, minimum top speed-flat 6 MPH, range 16 miles, dynamic stability incline 9 degrees, fatigue test on a level 200,000 cycles with 0.5 inch slats under all wheels, and 6,666 drop cycles. Group 4 power wheelchairs with a multiple power option are available in standard (up to and including 300 pounds) and heavy duty (301 to 450 pounds) weight capacities. Standard weight capacity chairs are further classified by type of chair. Heavy duty chairs are available only as sling/solid seat/back.

K0890-K0891

K0890 Power wheelchair, group 5 pediatric, single power option, sling/solid seat/back, patient weight capacity up to and including 125 pounds

K0891 Power wheelchair, group 5 pediatric, multiple power option, sling/solid seat/back, patient weight capacity up to and including 125 pounds

These codes describe Group 5 power wheelchairs, which are pediatric wheelchairs with a patient weight capacity up to and including 125 pounds. Group 5 power wheelchairs have the following specifications: length 48 inches, width 28 inches, obstacle height 60 mm, minimum top speed-flat 4.5 MPH, range 12 miles, dynamic stability incline 7.5 degrees, fatigue test on a level 200,000 cycles with 0.5 inch slats under all wheels, and 6,666 drop cycles. Group 5 power wheelchairs are available with single and multiple power options in a sling/solid seat/back chair.

K0898-K0899

K0898 Power wheelchair, not otherwise classified

K0899 Power mobility device, not coded by DME PDAC or does not meet criteria

Power wheelchairs and power mobility device codes are assigned based on specific criteria related to length, width, obstacle height, minimum top end speed on a flat surface, range, dynamic stability on incline, fatigue tests on a level with 0.5-inch slats, and drop cycles. Criteria were defined by the Pricing, Data Analysis and Coding (PDAC) contractor, a national entity that provides services under contract to CMS related to DMEPOS HCPCS coding and pricing.

K0900

K0900 Customized durable medical equipment, other than wheelchair

Customized durable medical equipment is uniquely constructed or substantially modified wheelchair or base adapted to a specific patient according to the physician's description and orders. Customized items are rarely necessary and are rarely furnished. It is expected to be a one-of-a-kind item fabricated to meet specific needs. Use this code for durable medical equipment, other than wheelchairs, that meet the customized requirements explained above.

K1001

K1001 Electronic positional obstructive sleep apnea treatment, with sensor, includes all components and accessories, any type

This mask-free device for positional obstructive sleep apnea (POSA) is intended for patients whose sleep apnea most commonly occurs when they are sleeping on their back (supine position). The device consists of a palm-sized electronic sensor with adjustable vibration feedback. It allows the person to fall asleep in any position and delivers gentle vibrations intended to cause the person to avoid the supine position. This code includes all accessories and components.

K1002

K1002 Cranial electrotherapy stimulation (CES) system, any type

A cranial electrotherapy stimulation (CES) device delivers electronic microcurrent that is supposedly at a natural level. The current is delivered via small clips worn on the earlobes, and travels through the brain to stimulate specific groups of nerve cells. It is reportedly able to provide significant anxiety relief, mood normalization, pain relief, and better sleep. The device is controlled via two handheld probes. Report K1002 for the CES device. Report A4596 monthly for system supplies and accessories.

K1003

K1003 Whirlpool tub, walk in, portable

This device is a therapeutic water device that uses circulating water and water jets to stimulate circulation, relieve pain, and massage the body. Whirlpools may have a single pump that circulates the water or multiple pumps—one to circulate the water and the others to drive the hydrotherapy jets. This version is portable and walk-in.

K1004

K1004 Low frequency ultrasonic diathermy treatment device for home use, includes all components and accessories

This treatment uses an ultrasound device to apply heat to the tissues in the body with a transducer/applicator that is incorporated into a patch, similar to a bandage, that adheres to the skin. It generates continuous surface acoustic waves ultrasound at 90KHZ through a reusable applicator/transducer that covers an area of about 6 sq cm. The small applicator allows treatment of less accessible body parts such as the heel and wrist. The device includes a transducer/applicator, rechargeable battery powered driver unit, and a cable that connects the driver to the transducer. It is indicated for the treatment of specific medical conditions such as pain relief, muscle spasm, and joint contractures.

K1005

K1005 Disposable collection and storage bag for breast milk, any size, any type, each

Disposable milk bags are intended for use with a wearable breast pump. This single-use, four-ounce milk collection and storage bag is contained within the breast pump housing and flange during pumping and has a one-way valve that ensures the milk goes into the bag and remains spill-proof. The milk bag can be used for refrigerator or freezer storage.

K1006

K1006 Suction pump, home model, portable or stationary, electric, any type, for use with external urine management system

An external urine management system is a urine collection system that is indicated for non-invasive treatment of female patients with permanent urinary incontinence. It should not be used for patients with urinary retention. The system consists of a female external catheter and a urine collection system: collection canister, connector port and tubing, base, pump tubing, power cord, and privacy cover. The system is portable and may be used with batteries or the supplied power cord. The system should remain stationary during use. The external catheter is connected to the pump tubing. Once connected, the gauze side of the external catheter should be placed against the separated labia, which should fit snugly against the body. The external catheter should be removed and replaced when soiled, or at least once every eight to 12 hours. This code represents the suction pump. Report A5102 for the collection canister. Report A4331 for tubing. Report A4328 for the female external catheter.

K1007

K1007 Bilateral hip, knee, ankle, foot (HKAFO) device, powered, includes pelvic component, single or double upright(s), knee joints any type, with or without ankle joints any type, includes all components and accessories, motors, microprocessors, sensors

A bilateral hip, knee, ankle, foot (HKAFO) device is a wearable robotic exoskeleton system that is intended for use by patients with lower body paralysis due to spinal cord injury (SCI) to restore function of motor movement and return to activities of daily living. It enables patients with SCI to stand upright and walk. Users independently control initiation, speed, and direction through controller commands and a shift in body weight. This code represents a customizable exoskeleton system consisting of a bilateral pelvic component, single or double uprights, knee joints, ankle joints, along with all required accessories and components, microprocessors, motors, and sensors.

K1009

K1009 Speech volume modulation system, any type, including all components and accessories

A speech volume modulation system is a prosthetic, in-ear device that plays noise (multi-talker babble) only when the wearer speaks. The system is used to treat patients with Parkinson's who have been diagnosed with dysarthria and anarthria. The noise produces the Lombard effect, an involuntary vocal response, that automatically increases the patient's vocal intensity resulting in a slower speech rate, increasing the clarity of the patient's speech. The effect is similar to speaking louder in a loud environment. The system includes an ear worn device, charging station, and charging cord.

K1013

K1013 Enema tube, with or without adapter, any type, replacement only, each

This code reports a percutaneous antegrade continence enema device indicated for patients who have nonfunctioning colons and who have been unresponsive to conservative treatments such as laxatives, high-fiber diets, or rectal enemas. The device may be inserted into the cecum via a cecostomy or a Malone/appendicostomy procedure and is held in place by an external silicone bolster and an internal silicone balloon. An irrigation port and balloon inflation port are contained by the external bolster, which allows the user to administer an enema and inflate/deflate the balloon. Using the same replacement method as a low-profile gastrostomy tube, the device can be replaced in the hospital, clinic, or at home. This code may also be reported for a specialized adapter with connecting tube for use in patients who have been implanted with a proprietary cecostomy catheter. This single-patient, reusable connecting tube is a replaceable accessory that allows connection between the catheter and the delivery tubing of an enema bag/irrigation system, permitting the enema solution to flow into the cecum through the catheter. Report this code for each replacement tube.

K1014

K1014 Addition, endoskeletal knee-shin system, 4 bar linkage or multiaxial, fluid swing and stance phase control

A proprietary microprocessor-controlled knee is indicated for use by amputees who are missing the leg through the knee joint or higher. It uses a four-bar knee geometry in conjunction with a microprocessor-controlled hydraulic unit that affords various levels of resistance depending on the patient's stance or swing phase of gait. Range of motion (ROM) and toe clearance are improved, and an enhanced safety feature automatically locks knee flexion when a load is supported on a flexed, stationary knee. The lock feature releases upon knee extension, returning the knee to normal function. This code reports the addition to an endoskeletal knee-shin system that provides increased functionality and stability on slopes, uneven terrain, or in crouched positions.

K1015

K1015 Foot, adductus positioning device, adjustable

This proprietary, adjustable orthopedic device is an alternative to serial casting and functions by stabilizing the heel in the heel cage and the remainder of the foot in the brace. Corrective pressure is applied to the midfoot, resulting in realignment of the deformed foot. Indicated for the treatment of metatarsus adductus/varus (also known as pigeon toe), in which the front half of the foot turns inward, this short foot orthopedic device is worn below the ankle. Components include a rigid plastic insert and an adjustable strap.

K1016-K1017

K1016 Transcutaneous electrical nerve stimulator for electrical stimulation of the trigeminal nerve

K1017 Monthly supplies for use of device coded at K1016

A proprietary external trigeminal nerve stimulation (eTNS) system treats pediatric attention deficit hyperactivity disorder (ADHD). This nonimplantable device is indicated as a monotherapy, available by prescription only, for patients ages 7 through 12 years, who do not currently take prescription ADHD meds. Intended to be utilized in the home environment during periods of sleep and under caregiver supervision, the system functions by providing therapeutic electrical stimulation of the V1 branch of the trigeminal nerve in the forehead, where it increases metabolic activity in the areas of the brain associated with attention, executive function, and mood. In this therapy, which is initiated just prior to sleep and ends upon wakening in the morning, a customized disposable electrical patch is placed in the center of the patient's forehead just over the eyebrows. A hand-held pulse generator is connected to the patch, where it produces and transmits a proprietary signal to the patch. Report K1016 for the eTNS system and K1017 for associated monthly supplies, including disposable refill electric patches.

K1018-K1019

K1018 External upper limb tremor stimulator of the peripheral nerves of the wrist

K1019 Replacement supplies and accessories for external upper limb tremor stimulator of the peripheral nerves of the wrist

A proprietary, peripherally worn nerve stimulating device treats essential tremor, a chronic, progressive movement disorder. The noninvasive stimulation device, which is physician prescribed for a patient's home use, is worn on the wrist and ensures that the electrical impulses are appropriately targeted to the individual patient's nerves. An initial calibration is performed in which sensors measure the patient's tremor frequency to individualize the amount of stimulation delivered. The wrist device is attached to the rechargeable stimulator that generates electrical impulses during periods of active therapy; a base station recharges the stimulator. Electrical impulses are delivered to the nerves in the wrist to stimulate the central tremor network through the peripheral nervous system. Report K1018 for the stimulation device and initial components and K1019 for associated monthly supplies, which includes the replacement component of the wrist-worn connector.

K1020

K1020 Noninvasive vagus nerve stimulator

A proprietary, noninvasive vagus nerve stimulator is indicated in the prevention and treatment of cluster headaches. By externally stimulating the cervical branch of the vagus nerve, the hand-held device can decrease the severity of acute cluster attacks; preventive use can also reduce the number of cluster headaches that occur.

K1021

K1021 Exsufflation belt, includes all supplies and accessories

Exsufflation belt is a stand-alone, intermittent abdominal daytime pressure ventilator device. It is a body wearable, noninvasive method of forcing diaphragmatic exhalation for support of pulmonary restrictive or pulmonary obstructive breathing. It consists of a fabric corset containing an air sac/bladder by a patient-supplied positive pressure ventilator. The pressure supplied from the ventilator compresses the abdomen, raising the diaphragm and causing active exhalation. When the sac/bladder deflates, passive inhalation occurs. This code reports the supply of the fabric corset.

K1022

K1022 Addition to lower extremity prosthesis, endoskeletal, knee disarticulation, above knee, hip disarticulation, positional rotation unit, any type

This code reports the addition of a rotation adaptor to a hip or knee joint of an endoskeletal system for above-the-knee amputation or hip disarticulation. The adapter provides medically necessary rotation of the prosthetic limb, allowing the patient to adjust to surroundings without additional torsional loads or strains on the prosthetic socket or residual limb.

K1023

K1023 Distal transcutaneous electrical nerve stimulator, stimulates peripheral nerves of the upper arm

A distal transcutaneous electrical nerve stimulator is a neuromodulation device that uses electrical current delivered through electrodes placed on the surface of the skin for the acute treatment of episodic and chronic migraines. The mechanism of action, conditioned pain modulation, is an endogenous, descending, analgesic mechanism triggered by the remote stimulation of nociceptive nerve fibers. It is applied on the upper arm, remote from the trigeminal nerve, and employs a smartphone application to control intensity and to track efficacity.

K1024-K1025

K1024 Nonpneumatic compression controller with sequential calibrated gradient pressure

K1025 Nonpneumatic sequential compression garment, full arm

A segmental compression device is a sequential gradient, non-pneumatic system used to treat and manage lymphedema, venous insufficiency, and to promote wound healing. It consists of a non-pneumatic segmental compressor controller, a liner, and a full-arm compression garment. The system connects to a separately supplied pneumatic pump. The compressor creates calibrated, gradient pressure that moves excess fluid, from distal to proximal, in a rhythmic manner. The wearable compression garment allows the patient to remain mobile during treatment. Report K1024 for the non-pneumatic compression controller. Report K1025 for the full-arm, non-pneumatic sequential compression garment.

K1026

K1026 Mechanical allergen particle barrier/inhalation filter, cream, nasal, topical

Alzair (trade name) inhalation powder is a drug-free inhaled powder indicated for the treatment of hay fever and other allergies by relieving mild allergic symptoms (i.e., itchy, runny, or congested nasal passages) that may be triggered by various airborne allergens. It is comprised of pharmaceutical grade hydroxypropyl methylcellulose (HPMC) and high-quality peppermint that are formulated into a micronized powder. It is supplied in a bottle designed to deliver the appropriate dose. The fine powder provides a protective barrier covering the nasal membranes that blocks inhaled allergens. It can be used in combination with oral antihistamines and following use of any other inhaled medications or nasal sprays.

K1027

K1027 Oral device/appliance used to reduce upper airway collapsibility, without fixed mechanical hinge, custom fabricated, includes fitting and adjustment

An intra-oral device or appliance is designed to treat snoring and mild to moderate obstructive sleep apnea syndrome (OSAS). The device consists of two custom fitted trays, worn on the mandible and maxilla, which reposition the mandible and increase the pharyngeal space, reducing airway obstructions during sleep. The custom 3D printed trays include integrally formed molar extensions and forward leaning ramps to keep open the anterior pharyngeal gap and allow more space for the tongue.

K1028-K1029

K1028 Power source and control electronics unit for oral device/appliance for neuromuscular electrical stimulation of the tongue muscle for the reduction of snoring and obstructive sleep apnea, controlled by phone application

K1029 Oral device/appliance for neuromuscular electrical stimulation of the tongue muscle, used in conjunction with the power source and control electronics unit, controlled by phone application, 90-day supply

Neuromuscular stimulators are used to stimulate muscles into activity through an electrical impulse. An oral device/appliance for neuromuscular electrical stimulation (NMES) of the tongue muscle is a daytime therapy for the reduction of snoring and obstructive sleep apnea (OSA). The system consists of a control unit, a disposable one-size fits all silicone mouthpiece, and USB-C charger. In addition, a smartphone application with an adherence coach can be downloaded. The mouthpiece is inserted into the control unit, connects the device to the Bluetooth-enabled smartphone application, and places the mouthpiece on the tongue. Through electrical stimulation, the device trains the tongue and upper airway muscles to remain in proper position during sleep, reducing snoring and OSA. Report K1028 for the power source and control electronics. Report K1029 for the oral device/appliance.

K1030

K1030 External recharging system for battery (internal) for use with implanted cardiac contractility modulation generator, replacement only

A cardiac contractility modulation (CCM) generator is a small implantable pulse generator (IPG), similar to a pacemaker, intended for the treatment of chronic heart failure in patients who are symptomatic despite appropriate medical treatment. In contrast to a pacemaker or a defibrillator, the system is designed to modulate the strength of contraction of the heart muscle rather than the rhythm. The CCM delivers electrical signals to the ventricles during the ventricular absolute refractory period. The expected result is improvement in six-minute hall walking distance, quality of life, functional status, and exercise tolerance. Typically implanted in the right pectoral region, the IPG is connected to two standard leads (electrodes) that are used to sense ventricular activity. Two electrodes in the right ventricular septum ensure the precise timing of the cardiac contractility modulation (CCM) signals, delivering them just after the heart contracts (the absolute refractory period). The expected result is improvement in six-minute hall walking distance, quality of life, functional status, and exercise tolerance. In addition, the system contains an external charging device. The IPG unit should be recharged weekly for optimal device and battery performance. This code reports replacement of the external battery recharging system only.

K1031-K1033

K1031 Nonpneumatic compression controller without calibrated gradient pressure

K1032 Nonpneumatic sequential compression garment, full leg

K1033 Nonpneumatic sequential compression garment, half leg

A segmental compression device is a sequential, nonpneumatic system used to treat and manage lymphedema, venous insufficiency, and to promote wound healing. It consists of a nonpneumatic segmental compressor controller, a liner, and a compression garment. The compressor creates calibrated pressure that moves excess fluid, from distal to proximal, in a rhythmic manner. The wearable compression garment allows the patient to remain mobile during treatment. Report K1031 for a nonpneumatic compression controller. Report K1032 for a full-leg, and K1033 for a half-leg, nonpneumatic sequential compression garment.

K1034

K1034 Provision of COVID-19 test, nonprescription self-administered and self-collected use, FDA approved, authorized or cleared, one test count

For self-administered tests, CMS has created a code that may be reported to identify and cover over the counter (OTC) COVID-19 tests at no cost, including deductible and copays, for Medicare Part B and Medicare Advantage (MA) beneficiaries. Eligible beneficiaries can receive up to eight tests per calendar month from an eligible provider until the Public Health Emergency (PHE) ends. This code may be reported for single-test and multiple-test packages. One test equals one unit. Claims must be submitted by the provider, not the patient. All payer types, including Medicaid and private insurance, may report K1034.

L

L0112

L0112 Cranial cervical orthosis, congenital torticollis type, with or without soft interface material, adjustable range of motion joint, custom fabricated

A custom fabricated cranial cervical orthosis for congenital muscular torticollis (CMT) is used to treat infants with CMT complicated by plagiocephaly. CMT is a postural deformity that results primarily from unilateral shortening and fibrosis of the sternocleidomastoid muscle. This causes the head to tilt to one side. Plagiocephaly, manifested as deformities of the skull base, cranium, or face, may occur in infants with CMT. These deformities may be the result of intrauterine compression or may occur after birth due to consistent positioning of the head to one side during sleep. A cranial cervical orthosis is designed to treat both the torticollis and any resulting plagiocephaly. The cranial orthosis consists of a custom fabricated helmet that may be lined with a soft interface material. The helmet remolds the skull to a more normal shape. The helmet is attached to an adjustable cervical orthosis that supports the neck and relieves the tilting of the head. The cervical component can be adjusted as the sternocleidomastoid muscle lengthens and the head tilt becomes less severe.

L0113

L0113 Cranial cervical orthosis, torticollis type, with or without joint, with or without soft interface material, prefabricated, includes fitting and adjustment

A prefabricated cranial cervical orthosis for muscular torticollis is used to treat patients with torticollis. Torticollis is a postural deformity that results primarily from unilateral shortening and fibrosis of the sternocleidomastoid muscle. This causes the head to tilt to one side. The cranial orthosis consists of a prefabricated helmet that may be lined with a soft interface material. The helmet is attached to an adjustable cervical orthosis that supports the neck and relieves the tilting of the head. The cervical component can be adjusted as the sternocleidomastoid muscle lengthens and the head tilt becomes less severe.

L0120-L0130

L0120 Cervical, flexible, nonadjustable, prefabricated, off-the-shelf (foam collar)

L0130 Cervical, flexible, thermoplastic collar, molded to patient

Cervical collars are used to limit the range of motion in the head and neck. By having the jaws and chin supported, the angle between the chin and the chest is maintained, which alleviates stress on the posterior neck/nuchal and suboccipital areas. This reduces the potential for cervical root irritation and adds an extra measure of head/neck immobilization. There is still a minute degree of mobilization capability while the patient is in the cervical collar. These codes report flexible cervical collars. Cervical foam collars are nonadjustable in terms of collar width but can be easily adjusted to the circumference of the patient's neck by simply pulling the collar closed and securing it in an overlapping fashion using the Velcro anchor at the back of the collar. Some collars can be obtained in low, medium, or high contour styles, depending on the collar width and degree of head and/or neck immobilization desired.

L0140-L0160

L0140 Cervical, semi-rigid, adjustable (plastic collar)

L0150 Cervical, semi-rigid, adjustable molded chin cup (plastic collar with mandibular/occipital piece)

L0160 Cervical, semi-rigid, wire frame occipital/mandibular support, prefabricated, off-the-shelf

Cervical collars are used to limit the range of motion in the head and neck. By having the jaws and chin supported, the angle between the chin and the chest is maintained, which alleviates stress on the posterior neck/nuchal and suboccipital areas. This reduces the potential for cervical root irritation and adds an extra measure of head/neck immobilization. There is still a minute degree of mobilization capability while the patient is in the cervical collar. These codes report semi-rigid cervical collars. Semi-rigid collars are typically constructed from plastic or like materials, with padded inner surfaces and may have an added jaw/chin support.

L0170

L0170 Cervical, collar, molded to patient model

Cervical collars are used to limit the range of motion in the head and neck. By having the jaws and chin supported, the angle between the chin and the chest is maintained, which alleviates stress on the posterior neck/nuchal and suboccipital areas. This reduces the potential for cervical root irritation and adds an extra measure of head/neck immobilization. There is still a minute degree of mobilization capability while the patient is in the cervical collar.

L0172

L0172 Cervical, collar, semi-rigid thermoplastic foam, two piece, prefabricated, off-the-shelf

Cervical collars are used to limit the range of motion in the head and neck. By having the jaws and chin supported, the angle between the chin and the chest is maintained, which alleviates stress on the posterior neck/nuchal and suboccipital areas. This reduces the potential for cervical root irritation and adds an extra measure of head/neck immobilization. There is still a minute degree of mobilization capability while the patient is in the cervical collar. This collar has two pieces, is semi-rigid, usually light in weight though constructed from sturdy plastics, and also has padded or lined surfaces so as not to chafe the patient's skin. Sizes vary according to source.

L0174

L0174 Cervical, collar, semi-rigid, thermoplastic foam, two piece with thoracic extension, prefabricated, off-the-shelf

This code reports the supply of a specific type of two-piece cervical collar. Cervical orthoses are used to restrict motion to prevent pain, to protect spinal instability before or after surgery, and as emergency protection from the effects of trauma. The cervical spine (neck) offers the ability for a wide range of motion. The head normally rotates almost 180 degrees; about 145 degrees of flexion and extension is considered a clinical base as is about 90 degrees of lateral flexion. This type of orthosis restricts these movements by immobilizing the head. The design reported by this code has two semi-rigid pieces. One piece may be a chin support component that drops into the support collar. Other models may feature front and back components. Velcro closures are used to close and adjust the two pieces. The design reported by this code also features an extension to the thoracic region to further stabilize the cervical spine. This may be an upper waistband connected by rigid bars (front and back) to the cervical collar. The thoracic component essentially converts the device to a cervical thoracic orthosis.

L0180-L0200

L0180 Cervical, multiple post collar, occipital/mandibular supports, adjustable

L0190 Cervical, multiple post collar, occipital/mandibular supports, adjustable cervical bars (SOMI, Guilford, Taylor types)

L0200 Cervical, multiple post collar, occipital/mandibular supports, adjustable cervical bars, and thoracic extension

These codes report the supply of multiple post cervical collars. Cervical orthoses are used to restrict motion to prevent pain or to address spinal instability before or after surgery. The healthy cervical spine (neck) offers a wide range of motion. The head normally rotates almost 180 degrees; about 145 degrees of flexion and extension is considered a clinical base as is about 90 degrees of lateral flexion. These types of orthoses restrict these movements by immobilizing the head. All collars will have more than one bar or post to support and immobilize the cervical spine. The SOMI brace is named as an acronym for sternal occipital mandibular immobilizer. The SOMI brace features three adjustable vertical bars on the front of the device that connects a rigid upper sternal band to the cervical and head support. The head and neck component supports against the mandible (lower jaw) and occiput (back of head). The Guilford brace is an eponym for the designer and features two adjustable posts (front and back) that extend from a shoulder harness to a ring that supports the head. Some designs may also feature an extension to the thoracic region to further stabilize the cervical spine. This may be a rigid extension to the thoracic region. The thoracic component essentially converts the device to a cervical thoracic orthosis.

L0220

L0220 Thoracic, rib belt, custom fabricated

A thoracic rib belt is an elastic belt used to support the thoracic area and rib cage. This code represents a belt crafted specifically for the patient.

L0450-L0490

L0450 Thoracic-lumbar-sacral orthosis (TLSO), flexible, provides trunk support, upper thoracic region, produces intracavitary pressure to reduce load on the intervertebral disks with rigid stays or panel(s), includes shoulder straps and closures, prefabricated, off-the-shelf

L0452 Thoracic-lumbar-sacral orthosis (TLSO), flexible, provides trunk support, upper thoracic region, produces intracavitary pressure to reduce load on the intervertebral disks with rigid stays or panel(s), includes shoulder straps and closures, custom fabricated

L0454 Thoracic-lumbar-sacral orthosis (TLSO), flexible, provides trunk support, extends from sacrococcygeal junction to above T-9 vertebra, restricts gross trunk motion in the sagittal plane, produces intracavitary pressure to reduce load on the intervertebral disks with rigid stays or panel(s), includes shoulder straps and closures, prefabricated item that has been trimmed, bent, molded, assembled, or otherwise customized to fit a specific patient by an individual with expertise

L0455 Thoracic-lumbar-sacral orthosis (TLSO), flexible, provides trunk support, extends from sacrococcygeal junction to above T-9 vertebra, restricts gross trunk motion in the sagittal plane, produces intracavitary pressure to reduce load on the intervertebral disks with rigid stays or panel(s), includes shoulder straps and closures, prefabricated, off-the-shelf

L0456 Thoracic-lumbar-sacral orthosis (TLSO), flexible, provides trunk support, thoracic region, rigid posterior panel and soft anterior apron, extends from the sacrococcygeal junction and terminates just inferior to the scapular spine, restricts gross trunk motion in the sagittal plane, produces intracavitary pressure to reduce load on the intervertebral disks, includes straps and closures, prefabricated item that has been trimmed, bent, molded, assembled, or otherwise customized to fit a specific patient by an individual with expertise

L0457 Thoracic-lumbar-sacral orthosis (TLSO), flexible, provides trunk support, thoracic region, rigid posterior panel and soft anterior apron, extends from the sacrococcygeal junction and terminates just inferior to the scapular spine, restricts gross trunk motion in the sagittal plane, produces intracavitary pressure to reduce load on the intervertebral disks, includes straps and closures, prefabricated, off-the-shelf

L0458 Thoracic-lumbar-sacral orthosis (TLSO), triplanar control, modular segmented spinal system, two rigid plastic shells, posterior extends from the sacrococcygeal junction and terminates just inferior to the scapular spine, anterior extends from the symphysis pubis to the xiphoid, soft liner, restricts gross trunk motion in the sagittal, coronal, and transverse planes, lateral strength is provided by overlapping plastic and stabilizing closures, includes straps and closures, prefabricated, includes fitting and adjustment

L0460 Thoracic-lumbar-sacral orthosis (TLSO), triplanar control, modular segmented spinal system, two rigid plastic shells, posterior extends from the sacrococcygeal junction and terminates just inferior to the scapular spine, anterior extends from the symphysis pubis to the sternal notch, soft liner, restricts gross trunk motion in the sagittal, coronal, and transverse planes, lateral strength is provided by overlapping plastic and stabilizing closures, includes straps and closures, prefabricated item that has been trimmed, bent, molded, assembled, or otherwise customized to fit a specific patient by an individual with expertise

L0462 Thoracic-lumbar-sacral orthosis (TLSO), triplanar control, modular segmented spinal system, three rigid plastic shells, posterior extends from the sacrococcygeal junction and terminates just inferior to the scapular spine, anterior extends from the symphysis pubis to the sternal notch, soft liner, restricts gross trunk motion in the sagittal, coronal, and transverse planes, lateral strength is provided by overlapping plastic and stabilizing closures, includes straps and closures, prefabricated, includes fitting and adjustment

L0464 **Thoracic-lumbar-sacral orthosis (TLSO), triplanar control, modular segmented spinal system, four rigid plastic shells, posterior extends from sacrococcygeal junction and terminates just inferior to scapular spine, anterior extends from symphysis pubis to the sternal notch, soft liner, restricts gross trunk motion in sagittal, coronal, and transverse planes, lateral strength is provided by overlapping plastic and stabilizing closures, includes straps and closures, prefabricated, includes fitting and adjustment**

L0466 **Thoracic-lumbar-sacral orthosis (TLSO), sagittal control, rigid posterior frame and flexible soft anterior apron with straps, closures and padding, restricts gross trunk motion in sagittal plane, produces intracavitary pressure to reduce load on intervertebral disks, prefabricated item that has been trimmed, bent, molded, assembled, or otherwise customized to fit a specific patient by an individual with expertise**

L0467 **Thoracic-lumbar-sacral orthosis (TLSO), sagittal control, rigid posterior frame and flexible soft anterior apron with straps, closures and padding, restricts gross trunk motion in sagittal plane, produces intracavitary pressure to reduce load on intervertebral disks, prefabricated, off-the-shelf**

L0468 **Thoracic-lumbar-sacral orthosis (TLSO), sagittal-coronal control, rigid posterior frame and flexible soft anterior apron with straps, closures and padding, extends from sacrococcygeal junction over scapulae, lateral strength provided by pelvic, thoracic, and lateral frame pieces, restricts gross trunk motion in sagittal, and coronal planes, produces intracavitary pressure to reduce load on intervertebral disks, prefabricated item that has been trimmed, bent, molded, assembled, or otherwise customized to fit a specific patient by an individual with expertise**

L0469 **Thoracic-lumbar-sacral orthosis (TLSO), sagittal-coronal control, rigid posterior frame and flexible soft anterior apron with straps, closures and padding, extends from sacrococcygeal junction over scapulae, lateral strength provided by pelvic, thoracic, and lateral frame pieces, restricts gross trunk motion in sagittal and coronal planes, produces intracavitary pressure to reduce load on intervertebral disks, prefabricated, off-the-shelf**

L0470 **Thoracic-lumbar-sacral orthosis (TLSO), triplanar control, rigid posterior frame and flexible soft anterior apron with straps, closures and padding extends from sacrococcygeal junction to scapula, lateral strength provided by pelvic, thoracic, and lateral frame pieces, rotational strength provided by subclavicular extensions, restricts gross trunk motion in sagittal, coronal, and transverse planes, provides intracavitary pressure to reduce load on the intervertebral disks, includes fitting and shaping the frame, prefabricated, includes fitting and adjustment**

L0472 **Thoracic-lumbar-sacral orthosis (TLSO), triplanar control, hyperextension, rigid anterior and lateral frame extends from symphysis pubis to sternal notch with two anterior components (one pubic and one sternal), posterior and lateral pads with straps and closures, limits spinal flexion, restricts gross trunk motion in sagittal, coronal, and transverse planes, includes fitting and shaping the frame, prefabricated, includes fitting and adjustment**

L0480 **Thoracic-lumbar-sacral orthosis (TLSO), triplanar control, one-piece rigid plastic shell without interface liner, with multiple straps and closures, posterior extends from sacrococcygeal junction and terminates just inferior to scapular spine, anterior extends from symphysis pubis to sternal notch, anterior or posterior opening, restricts gross trunk motion in sagittal, coronal, and transverse planes, includes a carved plaster or CAD-CAM model, custom fabricated**

L0482 **Thoracic-lumbar-sacral orthosis (TLSO), triplanar control, one-piece rigid plastic shell with interface liner, multiple straps and closures, posterior extends from sacrococcygeal junction and terminates just inferior to scapular spine, anterior extends from symphysis pubis to sternal notch, anterior or posterior opening, restricts gross trunk motion in sagittal, coronal, and transverse planes, includes a carved plaster or CAD-CAM model, custom fabricated**

L0484 Thoracic-lumbar-sacral orthosis (TLSO), triplanar control, two-piece rigid plastic shell without interface liner, with multiple straps and closures, posterior extends from sacrococcygeal junction and terminates just inferior to scapular spine, anterior extends from symphysis pubis to sternal notch, lateral strength is enhanced by overlapping plastic, restricts gross trunk motion in the sagittal, coronal, and transverse planes, includes a carved plaster or CAD-CAM model, custom fabricated

L0486 Thoracic-lumbar-sacral orthosis (TLSO), triplanar control, two-piece rigid plastic shell with interface liner, multiple straps and closures, posterior extends from sacrococcygeal junction and terminates just inferior to scapular spine, anterior extends from symphysis pubis to sternal notch, lateral strength is enhanced by overlapping plastic, restricts gross trunk motion in the sagittal, coronal, and transverse planes, includes a carved plaster or CAD-CAM model, custom fabricated

L0488 Thoracic-lumbar-sacral orthosis (TLSO), triplanar control, one-piece rigid plastic shell with interface liner, multiple straps and closures, posterior extends from sacrococcygeal junction and terminates just inferior to scapular spine, anterior extends from symphysis pubis to sternal notch, anterior or posterior opening, restricts gross trunk motion in sagittal, coronal, and transverse planes, prefabricated, includes fitting and adjustment

L0490 Thoracic-lumbar-sacral orthosis (TLSO), sagittal-coronal control, one-piece rigid plastic shell, with overlapping reinforced anterior, with multiple straps and closures, posterior extends from sacrococcygeal junction and terminates at or before the T-9 vertebra, anterior extends from symphysis pubis to xiphoid, anterior opening, restricts gross trunk motion in sagittal and coronal planes, prefabricated, includes fitting and adjustment

A thoracic-lumbar-sacral orthosis (TLSO) is a rigid or semirigid brace used to support weak or deformed areas of the spine or to restrict or eliminate motion (immobilization) in diseased or injured areas of the spine. An orthosis can be either prefabricated (custom fitted) or custom fabricated. These particular orthoses can have various features and can be constructed or have component parts of different types of materials. The benefits from orthotics use, specifically during convalescence from an injury or illness (useful to the weak or deformed body area) or as a postoperative treatment measure, can include the following: restricted range of motion of the affected area (immobilization); support of the affected area; and/or protection from injury, reinjury, suture tearing, and/or wound dehiscence. A prefabricated or custom-fitted orthosis is one that the manufacturer has produced in quantity, without a specific patient in mind. A prefabricated orthosis may be trimmed, bent, molded (with or without heat), or otherwise modified for use by a specific patient (i.e., custom fitted). An orthosis that is assembled from prefabricated components is considered prefabricated. Any orthosis that does not meet the definition of a custom-fabricated orthosis is considered prefabricated. A custom-fabricated orthosis is individually made for a specific patient, starting with basic materials, including but not limited to plastic, metal, leather, or cloth in the form of sheets, bars, and so forth. This type of orthosis must involve substantial work, such as cutting, bending, molding, sewing, and so forth. Although it may involve the incorporation of some prefabricated components, the device involves more than trimming, bending, or making other modifications to a substantially prefabricated item. A molded-to-patient-model orthosis is a particular type of custom-fabricated orthosis in which an impression of the specific body part is made (by means of a plaster cast, CAD-CAM technology, etc.). This impression is then used to make a positive model (of plaster or other material) of the body part to be braced. The orthosis is then molded on this positive model to be fit exactly to the patient's body part.

L0491-L0492

L0491 Thoracic-lumbar-sacral orthosis (TLSO), sagittal-coronal control, modular segmented spinal system, two rigid plastic shells, posterior extends from the sacrococcygeal junction and terminates just inferior to the scapular spine, anterior extends from the symphysis pubis to the xiphoid, soft liner, restricts gross trunk motion in the sagittal and coronal planes, lateral strength is provided by overlapping plastic and stabilizing closures, includes straps and closures, prefabricated, includes fitting and adjustment

L0492 Thoracic-lumbar-sacral orthosis (TLSO), sagittal-coronal control, modular segmented spinal system, three rigid plastic shells, posterior extends from the sacrococcygeal junction and terminates just inferior to the scapular spine, anterior extends from the symphysis pubis to the xiphoid, soft liner, restricts gross trunk motion in the sagittal and coronal planes, lateral strength is provided by overlapping plastic and stabilizing closures, includes straps and closures, prefabricated, includes fitting and adjustment

A thoracic-lumbar-sacral orthosis (TLSO) is a brace that is a rigid or semirigid device used for the purpose of supporting weak or deformed areas of the spine, or for restricting or eliminating motion (immobilization) in diseased or injured areas of the spine. An orthosis can be prefabricated (custom fitted) or custom fabricated. These particular orthoses can have various features and can be constructed or have component parts of different types of materials. The benefits from orthotics use, specifically during convalescence from an injury or illness or as a postoperative treatment measure, can include the following: restricted range of motion of the affected area (immobilization), support of the affected area (useful to the weak or deformed body area), and/or protection from injury, reinjury, suture tearing, and/or wound dehiscence. A prefabricated (also known as custom-fitted) orthosis is one that the manufacturer has produced in quantity, without a specific patient in mind. A prefabricated orthosis may be trimmed, bent, molded (with or without heat), or otherwise modified for use by a specific patient (i.e., custom fitted). An orthosis that is assembled from prefabricated components is considered prefabricated. Any orthosis that does not meet the definition of a custom-fabricated orthosis is considered prefabricated. In contrast to a prefabricated orthosis, a custom-fabricated orthosis is individually made for a specific patient, starting with basic materials including, but not limited to, plastic, metal, leather, or cloth in the form of sheets, bars, and so forth. It involves substantial work, such as cutting, bending, molding, sewing, and so forth. Although it may involve the incorporation of some prefabricated components, it involves more than trimming, bending, or making other modifications to a prefabricated item. A molded-to-patient-model orthosis is a particular type of custom-fabricated orthosis in which an impression of the specific body part is made (by means of a plaster cast, CAD-CAM technology, etc.). This impression is then used to make a positive model (of plaster or other material) of the body part to be braced. The orthosis is then molded on this positive model to be fit exactly to the patient's body part.

L0621-L0624

L0621 Sacroiliac orthosis (SO), flexible, provides pelvic-sacral support, reduces motion about the sacroiliac joint, includes straps, closures, may include pendulous abdomen design, prefabricated, off-the-shelf

L0622 Sacroiliac orthosis (SO), flexible, provides pelvic-sacral support, reduces motion about the sacroiliac joint, includes straps, closures, may include pendulous abdomen design, custom fabricated

L0623 Sacroiliac orthosis (SO), provides pelvic-sacral support, with rigid or semi-rigid panels over the sacrum and abdomen, reduces motion about the sacroiliac joint, includes straps, closures, may include pendulous abdomen design, prefabricated, off-the-shelf

L0624 Sacroiliac orthosis (SO), provides pelvic-sacral support, with rigid or semi-rigid panels placed over the sacrum and abdomen, reduces motion about the sacroiliac joint, includes straps, closures, may include pendulous abdomen design, custom fabricated

Sacroiliac orthoses may be flexible, rigid, or semi-rigid. These orthoses provide support for the lower portion of the torso, including the pelvic region, and reduce motion about the sacroiliac joint. Because of the narrow width of these types of orthoses, they are commonly referred to as belts or corsets. An orthosis can be prefabricated or custom fabricated. A prefabricated (also known as custom fitted) orthosis is one that the manufacturer has produced in quantity, without a specific patient in mind. A prefabricated orthosis may be trimmed, bent, molded (with or without heat), or otherwise modified for use by a specific patient (i.e., custom fitted). An orthosis that is assembled from prefabricated components is considered prefabricated. In contrast, a custom-fabricated orthosis is one that is individually made for a specific patient, starting with basic materials, including plastic, metal, leather, or cloth in the form of sheets, bars, and so forth. It involves substantial work, such as cutting, bending, molding, sewing, and so forth. It may involve the incorporation of some prefabricated components. It involves more than

L

trimming, bending, or making other modifications to a prefabricated item. Sacroiliac orthoses are usually prescribed to reduce sacroiliac diastasis or to reduce pelvic symphysis separation, and can even be given on a prophylactic basis to workers whose day-to-day tasks involve heavy lifting.

L0625-L0627

L0625 Lumbar orthosis (LO), flexible, provides lumbar support, posterior extends from L-1 to below L-5 vertebra, produces intracavitary pressure to reduce load on the intervertebral discs, includes straps, closures, may include pendulous abdomen design, shoulder straps, stays, prefabricated, off-the-shelf

L0626 Lumbar orthosis (LO), sagittal control, with rigid posterior panel(s), posterior extends from L-1 to below L-5 vertebra, produces intracavitary pressure to reduce load on the intervertebral discs, includes straps, closures, may include padding, stays, shoulder straps, pendulous abdomen design, prefabricated item that has been trimmed, bent, molded, assembled, or otherwise customized to fit a specific patient by an individual with expertise

L0627 Lumbar orthosis (LO), sagittal control, with rigid anterior and posterior panels, posterior extends from L-1 to below L-5 vertebra, produces intracavitary pressure to reduce load on the intervertebral discs, includes straps, closures, may include padding, shoulder straps, pendulous abdomen design, prefabricated item that has been trimmed, bent, molded, assembled, or otherwise customized to fit a specific patient by an individual with expertise

Lumbar orthoses may be flexible, rigid, or semi-rigid. These orthoses provide support to the lumbar (L1-L5) spinal area. They function by producing pressure within the abdominal and body cavities, creating space between the vertebrae, and allowing the intervertebral disk enough space to comfortably fit between the vertebrae. An orthosis can be prefabricated (custom fitted) or custom fabricated. A prefabricated (also known as custom fitted) orthosis is one that the manufacturer has produced in quantity, without a specific patient in mind. A prefabricated orthosis may be trimmed, bent, molded (with or without heat), or otherwise modified for use by a specific patient (i.e., custom fitted). An orthosis that is assembled from prefabricated components is considered prefabricated. In contrast to a prefabricated orthosis, a custom fabricated orthosis is one that is individually made for a specific patient, starting with basic materials including, but not limited to, plastic, metal, leather, or cloth in the form of sheets, bars, and so forth. It involves substantial work, such as cutting, bending, molding, sewing, and so forth. It may involve the incorporation of some prefabricated components. Flexible lumbar orthoses are used to treat mild spinal instability, painful arthritis, vertebral fractures of the lumbar and lower thoracic spine, and may be used immediately after lumbar surgery (e.g., discectomy, fusion) to provide back support. The rigid lumbar orthoses are used postfracture to reduce risk of further injury, or postoperatively for complex spinal surgeries when increased support is required. Rigid devices are also recommended for the treatment of scoliosis.

L0628-L0651

L0628 Lumbar-sacral orthosis (LSO), flexible, provides lumbo-sacral support, posterior extends from sacrococcygeal junction to T-9 vertebra, produces intracavitary pressure to reduce load on the intervertebral discs, includes straps, closures, may include stays, shoulder straps, pendulous abdomen design, prefabricated, off-the-shelf

L0629 Lumbar-sacral orthosis (LSO), flexible, provides lumbo-sacral support, posterior extends from sacrococcygeal junction to T-9 vertebra, produces intracavitary pressure to reduce load on the intervertebral discs, includes straps, closures, may include stays, shoulder straps, pendulous abdomen design, custom fabricated

L0630 Lumbar-sacral orthosis (LSO), sagittal control, with rigid posterior panel(s), posterior extends from sacrococcygeal junction to T-9 vertebra, produces intracavitary pressure to reduce load on the intervertebral discs, includes straps, closures, may include padding, stays, shoulder straps, pendulous abdomen design, prefabricated item that has been trimmed, bent, molded, assembled, or otherwise customized to fit a specific patient by an individual with expertise

L0631 Lumbar-sacral orthosis (LSO), sagittal control, with rigid anterior and posterior panels, posterior extends from sacrococcygeal junction to T-9 vertebra, produces intracavitary pressure to reduce load on the intervertebral discs, includes straps, closures, may include padding, shoulder straps, pendulous abdomen design, prefabricated item that has been trimmed, bent, molded, assembled, or otherwise customized to fit a specific patient by an individual with expertise

L0632 **Lumbar-sacral orthosis (LSO), sagittal control, with rigid anterior and posterior panels, posterior extends from sacrococcygeal junction to T-9 vertebra, produces intracavitary pressure to reduce load on the intervertebral discs, includes straps, closures, may include padding, shoulder straps, pendulous abdomen design, custom fabricated**

L0633 **Lumbar-sacral orthosis (LSO), sagittal-coronal control, with rigid posterior frame/panel(s), posterior extends from sacrococcygeal junction to T-9 vertebra, lateral strength provided by rigid lateral frame/panels, produces intracavitary pressure to reduce load on intervertebral discs, includes straps, closures, may include padding, stays, shoulder straps, pendulous abdomen design, prefabricated item that has been trimmed, bent, molded, assembled, or otherwise customized to fit a specific patient by an individual with expertise**

L0634 **Lumbar-sacral orthosis (LSO), sagittal-coronal control, with rigid posterior frame/panel(s), posterior extends from sacrococcygeal junction to T-9 vertebra, lateral strength provided by rigid lateral frame/panel(s), produces intracavitary pressure to reduce load on intervertebral discs, includes straps, closures, may include padding, stays, shoulder straps, pendulous abdomen design, custom fabricated**

L0635 **Lumbar-sacral orthosis (LSO), sagittal-coronal control, lumbar flexion, rigid posterior frame/panel(s), lateral articulating design to flex the lumbar spine, posterior extends from sacrococcygeal junction to T-9 vertebra, lateral strength provided by rigid lateral frame/panel(s), produces intracavitary pressure to reduce load on intervertebral discs, includes straps, closures, may include padding, anterior panel, pendulous abdomen design, prefabricated, includes fitting and adjustment**

L0636 **Lumbar-sacral orthosis (LSO), sagittal-coronal control, lumbar flexion, rigid posterior frame/panels, lateral articulating design to flex the lumbar spine, posterior extends from sacrococcygeal junction to T-9 vertebra, lateral strength provided by rigid lateral frame/panels, produces intracavitary pressure to reduce load on intervertebral discs, includes straps, closures, may include padding, anterior panel, pendulous abdomen design, custom fabricated**

L0637 **Lumbar-sacral orthosis (LSO), sagittal-coronal control, with rigid anterior and posterior frame/panels, posterior extends from sacrococcygeal junction to T-9 vertebra, lateral strength provided by rigid lateral frame/panels, produces intracavitary pressure to reduce load on intervertebral discs, includes straps, closures, may include padding, shoulder straps, pendulous abdomen design, prefabricated item that has been trimmed, bent, molded, assembled, or otherwise customized to fit a specific patient by an individual with expertise**

L0638 **Lumbar-sacral orthosis (LSO), sagittal-coronal control, with rigid anterior and posterior frame/panels, posterior extends from sacrococcygeal junction to T-9 vertebra, lateral strength provided by rigid lateral frame/panels, produces intracavitary pressure to reduce load on intervertebral discs, includes straps, closures, may include padding, shoulder straps, pendulous abdomen design, custom fabricated**

L0639 **Lumbar-sacral orthosis (LSO), sagittal-coronal control, rigid shell(s)/panel(s), posterior extends from sacrococcygeal junction to T-9 vertebra, anterior extends from symphysis pubis to xyphoid, produces intracavitary pressure to reduce load on the intervertebral discs, overall strength is provided by overlapping rigid material and stabilizing closures, includes straps, closures, may include soft interface, pendulous abdomen design, prefabricated item that has been trimmed, bent, molded, assembled, or otherwise customized to fit a specific patient by an individual with expertise**

L0640 **Lumbar-sacral orthosis (LSO), sagittal-coronal control, rigid shell(s)/panel(s), posterior extends from sacrococcygeal junction to T-9 vertebra, anterior extends from symphysis pubis to xyphoid, produces intracavitary pressure to reduce load on the intervertebral discs, overall strength is provided by overlapping rigid material and stabilizing closures, includes straps, closures, may include soft interface, pendulous abdomen design, custom fabricated**

L0641 **Lumbar orthosis (LO), sagittal control, with rigid posterior panel(s), posterior extends from L-1 to below L-5 vertebra, produces intracavitary pressure to reduce load on the intervertebral discs, includes straps, closures, may include padding, stays, shoulder straps, pendulous abdomen design, prefabricated, off-the-shelf**

L0642 Lumbar orthosis (LO), sagittal control, with rigid anterior and posterior panels, posterior extends from L-1 to below L-5 vertebra, produces intracavitary pressure to reduce load on the intervertebral discs, includes straps, closures, may include padding, shoulder straps, pendulous abdomen design, prefabricated, off-the-shelf

L0643 Lumbar-sacral orthosis (LSO), sagittal control, with rigid posterior panel(s), posterior extends from sacrococcygeal junction to T-9 vertebra, produces intracavitary pressure to reduce load on the intervertebral discs, includes straps, closures, may include padding, stays, shoulder straps, pendulous abdomen design, prefabricated, off-the-shelf

L0648 Lumbar-sacral orthosis (LSO), sagittal control, with rigid anterior and posterior panels, posterior extends from sacrococcygeal junction to T-9 vertebra, produces intracavitary pressure to reduce load on the intervertebral discs, includes straps, closures, may include padding, shoulder straps, pendulous abdomen design, prefabricated, off-the-shelf

L0649 Lumbar-sacral orthosis (LSO), sagittal-coronal control, with rigid posterior frame/panel(s), posterior extends from sacrococcygeal junction to T-9 vertebra, lateral strength provided by rigid lateral frame/panels, produces intracavitary pressure to reduce load on intervertebral discs, includes straps, closures, may include padding, stays, shoulder straps, pendulous abdomen design, prefabricated, off-the-shelf

L0650 Lumbar-sacral orthosis (LSO), sagittal-coronal control, with rigid anterior and posterior frame/panel(s), posterior extends from sacrococcygeal junction to T-9 vertebra, lateral strength provided by rigid lateral frame/panel(s), produces intracavitary pressure to reduce load on intervertebral discs, includes straps, closures, may include padding, shoulder straps, pendulous abdomen design, prefabricated, off-the-shelf

L0651 Lumbar-sacral orthosis (LSO), sagittal-coronal control, rigid shell(s)/panel(s), posterior extends from sacrococcygeal junction to T-9 vertebra, anterior extends from symphysis pubis to xyphoid, produces intracavitary pressure to reduce load on the intervertebral discs, overall strength is provided by overlapping rigid material and stabilizing closures, includes straps, closures, may include soft interface, pendulous abdomen design, prefabricated, off-the-shelf

A lumbosacral orthotic (LSO) can be flexible, rigid, or semi-rigid. An LSO provides lumbosacral support from the sacrococcygeal junction to the T-9 vertebrae. It is a device that is used for the purpose of supporting weak or deformed areas of the spine, or for restricting or eliminating motion (immobilization) in diseased or injured areas of the spine. An orthosis can be prefabricated or custom fabricated. A prefabricated (also known as off-the-shelf) orthosis is one that the manufacturer has produced in quantity, without a specific patient in mind. A prefabricated orthosis may be trimmed, bent, molded (with or without heat), or otherwise modified for use by a specific patient (i.e., custom fitted). In contrast, a custom-fabricated orthosis is one that is individually made for a specific patient, starting with basic materials including plastic, metal, leather, or cloth in the form of sheets, bars, and so forth. It involves substantial work, such as cutting, bending, molding, sewing, and/or other modifications. It may involve the incorporation of some minor prefabricated components, but involves more than the minor modifications to a fully prefabricated item. The benefits of orthotics use, specifically during convalescence from an injury or illness (useful to the weak or deformed body area) or as a postoperative treatment measure, can include the following: restricted range of motion of the affected area (immobilization); support of the affected area; protection from injury or reinjury, suture tearing, and/or wound dehiscence. An LSO can be designed to control movement of the trunk and between the segments of the vertebrae in one or more planes of motion. The most common planes are coronal/frontal, sagittal, and transverse.

L0700-L0710

L0700 Cervical-thoracic-lumbar-sacral orthosis (CTLSO), anterior-posterior-lateral control, molded to patient model, (Minerva type)

L0710 Cervical-thoracic-lumbar-sacral orthosis (CTLSO), anterior-posterior-lateral control, molded to patient model, with interface material, (Minerva type)

These codes report a specific type of cervical thoracic lumbar sacral orthosis (CTLSO). These orthoses control all spinal movement, lateral as well as anterior and posterior. Since the unit has a cervical component, the patient's head and neck are also immobilized. In addition to immobilization, the orthosis reduces compression load on the affected area of the spine. These devices are usually prepared ahead of a planned surgery. Measurements, scans, and moldings are taken by an orthotist. The orthosis is fashioned out of plastic polymers based on the patient data. The orthosis is bivalved, or cut into front and back pieces for donning and adjustment. Ventilation holes may be cut into the body of the orthosis, since they are typically worn over the course of the day. The Minerva component is an extension from the body of the orthosis that supports the mandible and occiput and stabilizes the cervical spine.

L0810-L0861

L0810 Halo procedure, cervical halo incorporated into jacket vest

L0820 Halo procedure, cervical halo incorporated into plaster body jacket

L0830 Halo procedure, cervical halo incorporated into Milwaukee type orthotic

L0859 Addition to halo procedure, magnetic resonance image compatible systems, rings and pins, any material

L0861 Addition to halo procedure, replacement liner/interface material

This system represents the non-conductive halo traction ring and skull pins. These component parts represent pieces of what is commonly called the halo system. The halo system consists of a metal ring that is secured to the upper part of the skull (mid-forehead area) with pins. A cervical halo is used to immobilize the cervical spine usually due to an odontoid fracture (fracture of the second cervical vertebrae). Two metal rods extend from the halo along the sides of the head to the shoulder area and are attached to a well-fitted plastic vest, jacket, or other type of orthotic. While the patient is wearing the halo system, the patient may be required to have diagnostic imaging such as MRI or CT procedures. These additions to the halo system ensure patient safety by eliminating the risk of scalp burns, while also allowing for a clearer, higher-quality image.

L0970-L0976

L0970 Thoracic-lumbar-sacral orthosis (TLSO), corset front

L0972 Lumbar-sacral orthosis (LSO), corset front

L0974 Thoracic-lumbar-sacral orthosis (TLSO), full corset

L0976 Lumbar-sacral orthosis (LSO), full corset

This range of codes reports specific corset additions to spinal orthoses. Some spinal orthoses, such as the "chair back" designs, require a closure addition for the anterior of the device. The corset front is attached to this type of posterior orthosis and provides a means to close and adjust tension of the device. The corset closure is a lace-and-eyelet configuration. Some designs feature a full corset design. These devices will have a stiff fabric body, sometimes with semi-rigid ribbing, and a corset closure, usually on the front.

L0978

L0978 Axillary crutch extension

This code reports the supply of an axillary crutch extension. The axillary crutch is the most common type of crutch in use today. A pad under the armpit, or axilla, bears most of the user's weight over the length of double uprights that extend to the floor. An extra upright piece makes the crutch adjustable (extension crutch). A handle bridges the double uprights about one-third the length down the crutch.

L0980

L0980 Peroneal straps, prefabricated, off-the-shelf, pair

This code reports the supply of each pair of perineal straps. These straps, or belts, are used occasionally with spinal orthoses that tend to migrate upward as the wearer engages in activities. The belt connects to the lower aspect of the orthosis, front to rear, by passing in a crisscross fashion under the groin, or perineum. Certain ankle straps used to provide traction during endoscopic surgery may be referred to as peroneal straps, but are not reported by this spinal orthosis code.

L0982

L0982 Stocking supporter grips, prefabricated, off-the-shelf, set of four (4)

Compression and support stocking are frequently singular stockings not permanently attached to a panty or other support garment. Stocking supporter grips are devices that attach to the top of the stocking and the bottom of the support garment, such as a garter belt. The grips help to hold the stockings in place.

L0984

L0984 Protective body sock, prefabricated, off-the-shelf, each

A protective body sock is a garment made up of soft, cushiony fabric that is used under spinal orthotics and body jackets. This item does not meet the definition of a brace and is considered more as a convenience item for the patient.

L0999

L0999 Addition to spinal orthosis, not otherwise specified

A spinal orthotic is a flexible, rigid, or semi-rigid device that provides support to the spinal area. It functions by producing pressure within the abdominal and body cavities, creating space between the vertebrae, and allowing the intervertebral disk enough space to comfortably fit between the vertebrae. Use this code to report an addition to a spinal orthotic that is not identified by a more specific code.

L1000

L1000 Cervical-thoracic-lumbar-sacral orthosis (CTLSO) (Milwaukee), inclusive of furnishing initial orthotic, including model

This code reports the supply of a Milwaukee-style cervical thoracic lumbar sacral orthosis (CTLSO). This is among the oldest designs of spinal braces still in use today, most commonly as treatment for idiopathic scoliosis, a lateral curvature of the spine that usually presents around puberty. A variety of brace configurations is seen, but all reported by this code will have a component that supports the head, limiting movement of the cervical spine (neck). Traditional braces were made of rigid leather, although most modern versions are constructed of thermoplastic and natural and artificial padding. The classic model features rigid waist and upper torso components. Metal rods, front and back, connect these components and the cervical support. Various padding may be placed to further manipulate the spine. Computer models based on detailed patient measurements and radiographs are used to calculate spinal geometries and loading. Several initial orthoses may be generated before a long-term brace is fabricated.

L1001

L1001 Cervical-thoracic-lumbar-sacral orthosis (CTLSO), immobilizer, infant size, prefabricated, includes fitting and adjustment

This is a cervical thoracic lumbar sacral orthosis (CTLSO) that is intended for use on infants with suspected or diagnosed spinal injury resulting from trauma or delivery complications or a tumor impinging on the spine, or it can be used for temporary immobilization for IV placement. This orthotic stabilizes the child's head and spine, and its unique shape keeps the child's spine aligned with the airway to promote an optimal healing process.

L1005

L1005 Tension based scoliosis orthosis and accessory pads, includes fitting and adjustment

This code reports the supply of a tension based scoliosis orthosis. Idiopathic scoliosis is a lateral curvature of the spine that usually presents by adolescence. Girls are affected at a ratio of five to one over boys. The classic nonsurgical approach is to stabilize the spine and manipulate development toward normal anatomy through the use of cervical thoracic lumbar sacral orthoses (CTLSO) or TLSOs. Tension based orthoses address scoliosis by exerting correctional forces on the spine through use of elastic fabrics and bands. Fabrics with elastic properties, pads, and elastic bands are fitted on the patient, often in configurations that change as development occurs. The orthosis is worn over the trunk, without a cervical component.

L1010

L1010 Addition to cervical-thoracic-lumbar-sacral orthosis (CTLSO) or scoliosis orthosis, axilla sling

This code reports the addition of an axilla sling to a scoliosis orthosis. Idiopathic scoliosis is a lateral curvature of the spine that usually presents by adolescence. Girls are affected at a ratio of five to one over boys. The classic nonsurgical approach is to stabilize the spine and manipulate development toward normal anatomy through the use of cervical thoracic lumbar sacral orthoses (CTLSO) or TLSOs. An axilla sling may be added to an orthosis to provide corrective leverage on the upper spine, usually in combination with fabric pads elsewhere on the apparatus. As the name implies, the sling runs under the armpit and connects the anterior and posterior components of the orthosis. It may be added to either a CTLSO or TLSO.

L1020-L1025

L1020 Addition to cervical-thoracic-lumbar-sacral orthosis (CTLSO) or scoliosis orthosis, kyphosis pad

L1025 Addition to cervical-thoracic-lumbar-sacral orthosis (CTLSO) or scoliosis orthosis, kyphosis pad, floating

These codes report the addition of pads to a scoliosis orthosis. Idiopathic scoliosis is a lateral curvature of the spine that usually presents by adolescence. Girls are affected at a ratio of five to one over boys. The classic non-surgical approach is to stabilize the spine and manipulate development toward normal anatomy through the use of cervical thoracic lumbar sacral orthoses (CTLSO) or TLSOs. Fabric pads are often added to an orthosis, often at the area of greatest thoracic curve (kyphosis) and usually in combination with a thoracic strap or axilla sling. When a pad is suspended from the apparatus on a movable strap, it is known as a "floating" pad, as opposed to one that is mounted onto the rigid shell. Maximum pad adjustment is ideal to adjust the amount of pressure and angle of applied force.

L1030-L1040

L1030 Addition to cervical-thoracic-lumbar-sacral orthosis (CTLSO) or scoliosis orthosis, lumbar bolster pad

L1040 Addition to cervical-thoracic-lumbar-sacral orthosis (CTLSO) or scoliosis orthosis, lumbar or lumbar rib pad

These codes report addition of specific types of pads to a scoliosis orthosis. Idiopathic scoliosis is a lateral curvature of the spine that usually presents by adolescence. Girls are affected at a ratio of five to one over boys. The classic non-surgical approach is to stabilize the spine and manipulate development toward normal anatomy through the use of cervical thoracic lumbar sacral orthoses (CTLSO). Fabric or foam pads are often added to an orthosis, often at the area of lumbar curve. The pads are considered accessories to flexible corset-style orthoses and occasionally to rigid models. The pads are typically rectangular shaped and may be referred to informally as a "shingle." The actual pad may be fabric-based, urethane, closed cell foam, or other material. Lumbar pads may be available as inflatable units. The addition may be made to a CTLSO or other type of scoliosis orthosis.

L1050

L1050 Addition to cervical-thoracic-lumbar-sacral orthosis (CTLSO) or scoliosis orthosis, sternal pad

This code reports the addition of a sternal pad to a scoliosis orthosis. Idiopathic scoliosis is a lateral curvature of the spine that usually presents by adolescence. Girls are affected at a ratio of five to one over boys. The classic non-surgical approach is to stabilize the spine and manipulate development toward normal anatomy through the use of cervical thoracic lumbar sacral orthoses (CTLSO). Other forms of scoliosis may be treated with orthoses as well. The padded sternal component reported by this code may be added to a scoliosis orthosis to provide a pressure point against the sternal bone. Some may be applied and held in place by straps. But most models feature an integrated pad and rigid outer shell, sometimes including a tension hinge on an armature to adjust pressure on the sternum. The actual pad may be fabric-based, urethane, closed cell foam, or other material. The addition may be made to a CTLSO or other type of scoliosis orthosis.

L1060

L1060 Addition to cervical-thoracic-lumbar-sacral orthosis (CTLSO) or scoliosis orthosis, thoracic pad

This code reports the addition of a thoracic pad to a scoliosis orthosis. Idiopathic scoliosis is a lateral curvature of the spine that usually presents by adolescence. Girls are affected at a ratio of five to one over boys. The classic non-surgical approach is to stabilize the spine and manipulate development toward normal anatomy through the use of cervical thoracic lumbar sacral orthoses (CTLSO). These devices rely on pressure points to manipulate spinal development and strategically placed padding provides this pressure. Other forms of scoliosis may be treated with orthoses as well. Thoracic pads may be applied and held in place by straps. Others are integrated into the rigid shell that comprises the thoracic component of the orthosis.

L1070

L1070 Addition to cervical-thoracic-lumbar-sacral orthosis (CTLSO) or scoliosis orthosis, trapezius sling

This code reports the addition of a trapezius sling to a scoliosis orthosis. Idiopathic scoliosis is a lateral curvature of the spine that usually presents by adolescence. Girls are affected at a ratio of five to one over boys. The classic non-surgical approach is to stabilize the spine and manipulate development toward normal anatomy through the use of cervical thoracic lumbar sacral orthoses (CTLSO). These devices rely on pressure points to manipulate spinal development and strategically placed padding provides this pressure. Other forms of scoliosis may be treated with orthoses as well. The trapezius muscle is on the upper back and works to move the shoulder blade. A trapezius sling is an addition to the anterior and posterior thoracic components that cross high on the shoulder near the neck. Padding on the sling provides a pressure point, usually to address the upper thoracic and lower cervical vertebra.

L1080-L1085

L1080 Addition to cervical-thoracic-lumbar-sacral orthosis (CTLSO) or scoliosis orthosis, outrigger

L1085 Addition to cervical-thoracic-lumbar-sacral orthosis (CTLSO) or scoliosis orthosis, outrigger, bilateral with vertical extensions

These codes report outrigger additions to scoliosis orthoses. Idiopathic scoliosis is a lateral curvature of the spine that usually presents by adolescence. Girls are affected at a ratio of five to one over boys. The classic non-surgical approach is to stabilize the spine and manipulate development toward normal anatomy through the use of cervical thoracic lumbar sacral orthoses (CTLSO). These devices rely on pressure points to manipulate spinal development. Other forms of scoliosis may be treated with orthoses as well. Outriggers are components added to the rigid portion of the orthosis. They are most often associated with Milwaukee-style orthoses. Outriggers themselves are often stainless steel bars and attachment may be to a vertical bar of the orthosis. The outrigger usually contributes leverage for pressure points.

L1090

L1090 Addition to cervical-thoracic-lumbar-sacral orthosis (CTLSO) or scoliosis orthosis, lumbar sling

A lumbar sling is an addition to a scoliosis orthotic device. Scoliosis is an abnormal curvature of the spine from side to side, giving the spine an "S" shape. The sling addition is a padded strap or sling used to hold or put pressure on the lumbar spine.

L1100-L1110

L1100 Addition to cervical-thoracic-lumbar-sacral orthosis (CTLSO) or scoliosis orthosis, ring flange, plastic or leather

L1110 Addition to cervical-thoracic-lumbar-sacral orthosis (CTLSO) or scoliosis orthosis, ring flange, plastic or leather, molded to patient model

These codes report the addition of a custom molded ring flange to a scoliosis orthosis. This device supports the mandible and occiput of a cervical thoracic lumbar sacral orthoses (CTLSO). Idiopathic scoliosis is a lateral curvature of the spine that usually presents by adolescence. Girls are affected at a ratio of five to one over boys. The classic nonsurgical approach is to stabilize the spine and manipulate development toward normal anatomy through the use of CTLSO. Certain CTLSO models employ a plastic ring to immobilize the cervical spine and head, which is less visible than the larger supports seen on some models.

L1120

L1120 Addition to cervical-thoracic-lumbar-sacral orthosis (CTLSO), scoliosis orthosis, cover for upright, each

A CTLSO is an orthosis used for the treatment of scoliosis and/or kyphosis, and consists of pelvic interface molded to the patient. Metal anterior and posterior uprights attach to the pelvic interface and terminate in the occipital mandibular area. The cover for the uprights protects the skin and prevents skin breakdown.

L1200

L1200 Thoracic-lumbar-sacral orthosis (TLSO), inclusive of furnishing initial orthosis only

This code reports the supply of a thoracic lumbar sacral orthosis (TLSO). These devices are sometimes referred to as "low profile" because they lack the "high profile" of a cervical component and many designs fit unobtrusively under clothing. These braces are not specifically limited to correction of scoliosis. Some may be prescribed following certain surgeries or to treat symptoms of trauma. Numerous fittings may be required, as idiopathic scoliosis requires adjustments as the patient's spine develops. Report this code for an initial TLSO only.

L1210

L1210 Addition to thoracic-lumbar-sacral orthosis (TLSO), (low profile), lateral thoracic extension

A TLSO is an orthotic designed for scoliosis and/or kyphosis. It is a heat moldable plastic insert for rigid support of the lower areas of the spine. This orthotic is used on the lateral aspect of a patient.

L1220

L1220 Addition to thoracic-lumbar-sacral orthosis (TLSO), (low profile), anterior thoracic extension

A TLSO is an orthotic designed for scoliosis and/or kyphosis. It is a heat moldable plastic insert for rigid support of the lower areas of the spine. This orthotic is used on the anterior aspect of a patient in a low profile scoliosis TLSO.

L1230

L1230 Addition to thoracic-lumbar-sacral orthosis (TLSO), (low profile), Milwaukee type superstructure

This code reports the addition of a Milwaukee type superstructure to a thoracic lumbar sacral orthosis (TLSO). The Milwaukee brace is among the oldest designs of spinal braces still in use today, most commonly as treatment for idiopathic scoliosis, a lateral curvature of the spine that usually presents around puberty. A variety of Milwaukee brace configurations are seen, but the classic model features rigid waist and upper torso components. Vertical metal rods, front and back, connect these components. Various padding arrangements and slings may be placed to further manipulate the spine.

L1240

L1240 Addition to thoracic-lumbar-sacral orthosis (TLSO), (low profile), lumbar derotation pad

A TLSO is an orthotic made from molded plastic designed for scoliosis and/or kyphosis in the lower areas of the spine. TLSOs have built-in pads (derotation) in the lumbar area that exert pressure on the spinal column at three points to apply the corrective force to improve the malposition of the spinal column. These three point corsets are fitted with derotation pressure pads along the lumbar spine, around the outer pelvis, and along the rib cage. Correction of the existing spinal malposition is achieved through derotation pad pressure in a low profile scoliosis TLSO.

L1250

L1250 Addition to thoracic-lumbar-sacral orthosis (TLSO), (low profile), anterior ASIS pad

This code reports the addition of an anterior ASIS pad to a thoracic lumbar sacral orthosis (TLSO). The acronym ASIS stands for anterior sacroiliac spine, which is the prominence of the hipbone at the front of the waist. This type of pad typically is used to provide a pressure point across the lower abdomen. Pressure here raises intraabdominal pressure, which in turn supports the lumbosacral spine.

L1260

L1260 Addition to thoracic-lumbar-sacral orthosis (TLSO), (low profile), anterior thoracic derotation pad

A TLSO is a molded plastic orthotic designed for scoliosis and/or kyphosis in the lower areas of the spine. TLSOs have built-in pads (derotation) in the anterior thoracic area that exert pressure on the spinal column at three points to apply the corrective force to improve the malposition of the spinal column. These three point corsets are fitted with derotation pressure pads along the anterior thoracic spine, around the outer pelvis, and along the rib cage. Correction of the existing spinal malposition is achieved through derotation pad pressure in a low profile scoliosis TLSO.

L1270

L1270 Addition to thoracic-lumbar-sacral orthosis (TLSO), (low profile), abdominal pad

A pad is attached to or incorporated into the abdominal area of a low profile scoliosis TLSO to counteract rotation of the thoracic spine.

L1280

L1280 Addition to thoracic-lumbar-sacral orthosis (TLSO), (low profile), rib gusset (elastic), each

A rib gusset is an addition to a spinal orthotic. It is an elastic support used to provide structural integrity and to lower the pressure on the ribs.

L1290

L1290 Addition to thoracic-lumbar-sacral orthosis (TLSO), (low profile), lateral trochanteric pad

A pad is installed in the trochanter area to control the lumbar curve.

L1300-L1310

L1300 Other scoliosis procedure, body jacket molded to patient model

L1310 Other scoliosis procedure, postoperative body jacket

These codes report the supply of a body jacket to treat scoliosis. Idiopathic scoliosis is a lateral curvature of the spine that usually presents by adolescence. Girls are affected at a ratio of five to one over boys. The non-surgical approach to idiopathic scoliosis is to stabilize the spine and manipulate development toward normal anatomy, and may include use of a body jacket. Body jackets may also be used for other cases of scoliosis. Preparation of a body jacket entails taking a plaster mold of the patient's body. Radiography, body scans, and computer modeling may also be employed. A plastic shell is prepared from the modeling and manipulated for optional therapy. The jacket may be bi-valved, or split into front and back halves for entry. The shell is vented and lined with cushion material. In some instances, a body jacket is required for recovery from surgery. In these cases, the casting and measurements are usually, but not always, taken prior to surgery.

L1499

L1499 Spinal orthosis, not otherwise specified

A spinal orthotic is an external apparatus that is applied to the body to limit the motion of, correct a deformity in, reduce the axial load on, or improve the function of a particular segment of the spine. Report this code for any spinal orthotic device not described in more specific HCPCS Level II codes.

L1600-L1650

L1600 Hip orthosis (HO), abduction control of hip joints, flexible, Frejka type with cover, prefabricated item that has been trimmed, bent, molded, assembled, or otherwise customized to fit a specific patient by an individual with expertise

L1610 Hip orthosis (HO), abduction control of hip joints, flexible, (Frejka cover only), prefabricated item that has been trimmed, bent, molded, assembled, or otherwise customized to fit a specific patient by an individual with expertise

L1620 Hip orthosis (HO), abduction control of hip joints, flexible, (Pavlik harness), prefabricated item that has been trimmed, bent, molded, assembled, or otherwise customized to fit a specific patient by an individual with expertise

L1630 Hip orthosis (HO), abduction control of hip joints, semi-flexible (Von Rosen type), custom fabricated

L1640 Hip orthosis (HO), abduction control of hip joints, static, pelvic band or spreader bar, thigh cuffs, custom fabricated

L1650 Hip orthosis (HO), abduction control of hip joints, static, adjustable, (Ilfled type), prefabricated, includes fitting and adjustment

This range of codes reports the supply of flexible hip orthoses designed to control hip abduction (spreading the legs). Many of these designs address congenital anomalies, such as hip dysplasia in infants and pre-toddlers. The Frejka orthosis is a pillow-like device that separates and immobilizes the legs. The Pavlik harness features cuffs that fit to the femurs; front and back harness arrangement fits over the shoulders and chest and may be adjusted to maintain the desired leg position. Like the Frejka device, this design also immobilizes the upper legs in a flexed and abducted position. The Von Rosen orthosis is a cross-shaped, semi-rigid pad that is custom fitted to the baby and then fixed into the desired position. The Ilfeld-style device uses a spreader bar fitted to cuffs on the baby's thighs and is prefabricated or custom fabricated. Either is adjustable and the degree of abduction is controlled by adjusting the length of the cross bar. A waistband is generally used to hold the splint in place more securely. None of the above devices completely immobilize the legs and hips. All prefabricated devices include fitting and adjustment.

L1652-L1686

L1652 Hip orthosis (HO), bilateral thigh cuffs with adjustable abductor spreader bar, adult size, prefabricated, includes fitting and adjustment, any type

L1660 Hip orthosis (HO), abduction control of hip joints, static, plastic, prefabricated, includes fitting and adjustment

L1680 Hip orthosis (HO), abduction control of hip joints, dynamic, pelvic control, adjustable hip motion control, thigh cuffs (Rancho hip action type), custom fabricated

L1685 Hip orthosis (HO), abduction control of hip joint, postoperative hip abduction type, custom fabricated

L1686 Hip orthosis (HO), abduction control of hip joint, postoperative hip abduction type, prefabricated, includes fitting and adjustment

These codes report supply of prefabricated hip orthoses designed to control hip abduction (spreading the legs) in adults. Such devices may be for any number of disorders, following certain surgeries, or to treat symptoms of trauma.

L1690

L1690 Combination, bilateral, lumbo-sacral, hip, femur orthosis providing adduction and internal rotation control, prefabricated, includes fitting and adjustment

This code represents a type of assistive technology often referred to as SWASH (standing, walking, and sitting hip orthosis). A SWASH is most commonly used on children with cerebral palsy, who often have difficulties with dystonia, hip migration, and a scissoring gait that interferes with ambulation and limits independent sitting. When properly fitted, the SWASH stabilizes the hip and prevents excessive adduction and internal rotation. This ultimately helps the child with stability while standing and gait during walking. When the child sits, the orthosis dictates continuous abduction, resulting in a wider base. This allows for a balanced posture and keeps the child from having to use their hands for support. Because of the technical nature of the SWASH orthosis, providers interested in using the device are required to attend a specialized training course.

L

L1700-L1755

L1700 Legg Perthes orthosis, (Toronto type), custom fabricated

L1710 Legg Perthes orthosis, (Newington type), custom fabricated

L1720 Legg Perthes orthosis, trilateral, (Tachdijan type), custom fabricated

L1730 Legg Perthes orthosis, (Scottish Rite type), custom fabricated

L1755 Legg Perthes orthosis, (Patten bottom type), custom fabricated

These codes report supply of a specific type of custom fabricated orthosis used to treat Legg Calve Perthes disease (LCPD or, more commonly, Legg Perthes). Legg Perthes disease is an osteonecrosis of the femoral head and hip socket found only in children, usually boys between the ages of 2 and 12. Bone death occurs in the ball of the hip due to interruption in blood flow. The disease is of unknown etiology. The Toronto type orthosis addresses the disorder with an unusual splint design. Each leg is secured by cuffs high on the thigh. A single vertical tube is connected to these thigh cuffs near the crotch. The lower end is connected to horizontal spreader bars fixed to special shoes. A ball joint between the vertical tube and the spreader bar allows knee flexibility. Shoe blocks are attached to the shoes to maintain alignment.

L1810-L1833

L1810 Knee orthosis (KO), elastic with joints, prefabricated item that has been trimmed, bent, molded, assembled, or otherwise customized to fit a specific patient by an individual with expertise

L1812 Knee orthosis (KO), elastic with joints, prefabricated, off-the-shelf

L1820 Knee orthosis (KO), elastic with condylar pads and joints, with or without patellar control, prefabricated, includes fitting and adjustment

L1830 Knee orthosis (KO), immobilizer, canvas longitudinal, prefabricated, off-the-shelf

L1831 Knee orthosis (KO), locking knee joint(s), positional orthosis, prefabricated, includes fitting and adjustment

L1832 Knee orthosis (KO), adjustable knee joints (unicentric or polycentric), positional orthosis, rigid support, prefabricated item that has been trimmed, bent, molded, assembled, or otherwise customized to fit a specific patient by an individual with expertise

L1833 Knee orthosis (KO), adjustable knee joints (unicentric or polycentric), positional orthosis, rigid support, prefabricated, off-the shelf

Knee orthotics (braces) come in a variety of sizes and shapes, and are made differently depending on their intended use. A prophylactic brace is used to prevent or reduce the severity of knee ligament injuries. A rehabilitative brace allows protected movement of the injured knee, and usually has hinges that allow the knee to be locked into certain positions. A functional brace is used to support an unsteady knee during daily activities or is used during a sporting activity. A derotation brace is used after an injury to a ligament and typically has bars, straps, and hinges; it is used during sporting activities and is most often made up of lightweight materials so that it allows significant motion and speed. An unloader brace is specifically designed for patients suffering from pain and disability due to osteoarthritis. This brace works by keeping the knee in the valgus position, which allows unloading of the compressive forces on the medial compartment.

L1834

L1834 Knee orthosis (KO), without knee joint, rigid, custom fabricated

This code reports the supply of a rigid knee orthotic, without knee joint, custom fabricated. Certain knee orthoses are designed to immobilize the knee completely and therefore do not feature a joint system. These devices may be applied to a knee injury to facilitate healing or to protect the joint following surgery.

L1836

L1836 Knee orthosis (KO), rigid, without joint(s), includes soft interface material, prefabricated, off-the-shelf

This code reports the supply of a prefabricated rigid knee orthosis. Certain knee orthoses (KO) are designed to immobilize the knee completely and therefore do not feature a joint system. Such devices may be applied to a knee injury to facilitate healing, or to protect the joint following surgery. The orthosis holds the knee in a fixed position, usually slightly flexed. Cushion material to interface between the rigid orthosis and the patient's skin is included in the code description as are fitting sessions.

L1840

L1840 Knee orthosis (KO), derotation, medial-lateral, anterior cruciate ligament, custom fabricated

This code reports supply of a custom made knee orthosis that limits medial and lateral rotation of the knee for patients with compromised anterior cruciate ligament function. This is a dynamic rigid body orthosis, meaning that muscle actions against the orthosis work to stabilize the joint. The anterior cruciate ligament (ACL) is the most often injured ligament in the knee, often without external contact. The ACL limits forward motion and rotation of the tibia. Patients with compromised ACL exhibit muscle movement abnormalities in activities as simple as walking on level surfaces. Stopping, landing from a jump, running downhill, or making rapid lateral maneuvers causes a sense of instability. Most knee orthoses that address ACL instability exert pressures to prevent the knee from coming into full extension. Devices such as the Lenox-Hill orthosis also work to control torque, or twisting, actions of the tibia.

L1843-L1846

L1843 Knee orthosis (KO), single upright, thigh and calf, with adjustable flexion and extension joint (unicentric or polycentric), medial-lateral and rotation control, with or without varus/valgus adjustment, prefabricated item that has been trimmed, bent, molded, assembled, or otherwise customized to fit a specific patient by an individual with expertise

L1844 Knee orthosis (KO), single upright, thigh and calf, with adjustable flexion and extension joint (unicentric or polycentric), medial-lateral and rotation control, with or without varus/valgus adjustment, custom fabricated

L1845 Knee orthosis (KO), double upright, thigh and calf, with adjustable flexion and extension joint (unicentric or polycentric), medial-lateral and rotation control, with or without varus/valgus adjustment, prefabricated item that has been trimmed, bent, molded, assembled, or otherwise customized to fit a specific patient by an individual with expertise

L1846 Knee orthosis (KO), double upright, thigh and calf, with adjustable flexion and extension joint (unicentric or polycentric), medial-lateral and rotation control, with or without varus/valgus adjustment, custom fabricated

Knee orthotic devices (braces) come in a variety of sizes and shapes, and are made differently depending on their intended use. A prophylactic brace is used to prevent or reduce the severity of knee ligament injuries. A rehabilitative brace allows protected movement of the injured knee, and usually has hinges that allow the knee to be locked into certain positions. A functional brace is used to support an unsteady knee during daily activities or is used during a sporting activity. A derotation brace is used after an injury to a ligament and typically has bars, straps, and hinges; it is used during sporting activities and is most often made up of lightweight materials so that it allows significant motion and speed. An unloader brace is specifically designed for patients suffering from pain and disability due to osteoarthritis. This brace works by keeping the knee in the valgus position, which allows unloading of the compressive forces on the medial compartment.

L1847-L1848

L1847 Knee orthosis (KO), double upright with adjustable joint, with inflatable air support chamber(s), prefabricated item that has been trimmed, bent, molded, assembled, or otherwise customized to fit a specific patient by an individual with expertise

L1848 Knee orthosis (KO), double upright with adjustable joint, with inflatable air support chamber(s), prefabricated, off-the-shelf

This code reports the supply of a specific type of prefabricated knee orthosis that uses air-support chambers. Many varieties of knee brace orthoses are available, and many feature a lateral and medial upright and an adjustable joint. The type reported by this code, however, also supports the knee with air-filled chambers rather than cushion material alone. This type of orthosis may be used to initially stabilize the joint following trauma.

L1850

L1850 Knee orthosis (KO), Swedish type, prefabricated, off-the-shelf

This code reports the supply of a particular design of knee orthosis (KO) known as the Swedish cage, or Swedish type. Great varieties of knee brace orthoses are available, and many feature a lateral and medial upright and an adjustable joint. The Swedish cage design also features a posterior support piece to further stabilize the joint and prevent hyperextension. The Swedish style brace is further distinguished by its longer length. The thigh and calf cuffs are generally positioned at a further extreme than similar hinged KOs. This type of orthosis is "off-the-shelf," or prefabricated.

L1851-L1852

L1851 Knee orthosis (KO), single upright, thigh and calf, with adjustable flexion and extension joint (unicentric or polycentric), medial-lateral and rotation control, with or without varus/valgus adjustment, prefabricated, off-the-shelf

L1852 Knee orthosis (KO), double upright, thigh and calf, with adjustable flexion and extension joint (unicentric or polycentric), medial-lateral and rotation control, with or without varus/valgus adjustment, prefabricated, off-the-shelf

Prefabricated knee orthoses (KO) are ready-made knee braces that are purchased off-the-shelf with no custom fitting or adjustment. Report L1851 for a single upright hinge and L1852 for a double upright hinge. Both are secured to the leg at the thigh and calf, have adjustable flexion and extension joint (unicentric or polycentric), and medial-lateral and rotation control, with or without varus/valgus adjustment.

L1860

L1860 Knee orthosis (KO), modification of supracondylar prosthetic socket, custom fabricated (SK)

This code reports a custom fabricated modification to a knee orthosis (KO) that is fitted in combination with a specific type of prosthetic socket. A prosthetic socket is the device that secures to the residual limb. The prosthetic leg attaches to the socket. In this instance, the socket is a variety that fits above the bony protuberance, or condyles, that constitute the distal end of the femur and the proximal end of the tibia (supracondylar). A KO may be required in patients with lower limb prosthetics to stabilize the joint, particularly during training in the use of an artificial limb.

L1900

L1900 Ankle-foot orthosis (AFO), spring wire, dorsiflexion assist calf band, custom fabricated

This code reports the supply of a custom made, specialty ankle foot orthosis (AFO). Most AFOs employ medial and lateral upright bars attached from a calf band to an orthotic shoe or footplate. This device uses heavy gauge stainless steel spring wire rather than upright bars. The coiled spring action is at the attachment to the shoe or footplate and assists in dorsiflexion of the ankle joint (raising the foot at the ankle). These devices hold an advantage in being lightweight while offering good dorsiflexion assistance.

L1902-L1906

L1902 Ankle orthosis (AO), ankle gauntlet or similar, with or without joints, prefabricated, off-the-shelf

L1904 Ankle orthosis (AO), ankle gauntlet or similar, with or without joints, custom fabricated

L1906 Ankle foot orthosis (AFO), multiligamentous ankle support, prefabricated, off-the-shelf

Ankle orthotics, gauntlets, and supports are generalized under the heading ankle-foot orthosis (AFO). (An exception within this range is the simple, prefabricated neoprene sock-type device.) AFOs within this range are prescribed for a variety of conditions for ambulatory patients, including congenital anomalies, pronation of the ankle, tendon problems, arthritis, and amputation. These devices generally extend well above the ankle, often to the upper calf, and may accommodate multiple planes of ankle movement. Some devices also limit ankle movement. The units may be built from standardized molds or custom fabricated from a plaster impression taken of the patient's foot and ankle. The units themselves may be made of metal, plastic polymers, or leather, sometimes in combination, and usually with various fabrics, cushions, and closure systems. A custom-fabricated orthosis involves substantial work, such as cutting, bending, molding, or sewing. It may involve the incorporation of some prefabricated components. It involves more than trimming, bending, or making other modifications to a substantially prefabricated item. Polypropylene models are close fitting and are often worn inside the shoe. Gauntlets usually feature lateral and medial stabilizers to address eversion and inversion, arch support, heel lock, padded tongue to facilitate application, and side panels for additional reinforcement. Fitting and adjustment is included in the supply of the product. Some gauntlets use natural heat therapy to gently warm troubled areas on the ankle and foot. They consist of stabilizers (usually plastic) on either side to help resist inversion and eversion. Other features usually offered are arch support and complete heel lock, elastic back section to eliminate blistering, padded tongue to facilitate application, and side panels for more reinforcement. A molded-to-patient-model orthosis is a particular type of custom fabricated orthosis in which an impression of the foot is taken, by means of a plaster cast, CAD-CAM technology, etc. This impression is then used to make a positive model (of plaster or other material) of the body part to be braced. The orthosis is then molded on this positive model to be fit exactly to the patient's foot. It may require several castings and fittings by an orthotist/MD.

L1907

L1907 Ankle orthosis (AO), supramalleolar with straps, with or without interface/pads, custom fabricated

Ankle foot orthotics (AFO) are orthoses or braces made of plastic or other material encompassing the ankle joint and all (or part) of the foot. AFOs are externally applied and intended to control position and motion of the ankle, compensate for weakness, or correct deformities. A variety of straps are available, including standard Velcro turn-back straps or custom designed leather and Dacron straps with padding.

L1910

L1910 Ankle-foot orthosis (AFO), posterior, single bar, clasp attachment to shoe counter, prefabricated, includes fitting and adjustment

This code reports the supply of a prefabricated single bar ankle foot orthosis (AFO). This type of AFO involves a single upright bar that attaches to a cuff near the top of the back of the calf and spans to an attachment that fits at the heel of the foot with a clasp attachment. The bar is shaped to the curve of the back of the calf and ankle. The AFO is available "off-the-shelf," and fitting and adjustment to a specific patient is required.

L1920

L1920 Ankle-foot orthosis (AFO), single upright with static or adjustable stop (Phelps or Perlstein type), custom fabricated

The type of ankle-foot orthosis (AFO) represented by this code involves a single upright bar that attaches to a band near the top of the calf and spans to an attachment that fits at the ankle-foot. The bar is usually on the lateral side of the orthotic and its length may be adjustable. The AFO is custom fabricated to address a specific disorder and to fit a specific patient.

L1930-L1940

L1930 Ankle-foot orthosis (AFO), plastic or other material, prefabricated, includes fitting and adjustment

L1932 Ankle-foot orthosis (AFO), rigid anterior tibial section, total carbon fiber or equal material, prefabricated, includes fitting and adjustment

L1940 Ankle-foot orthosis (AFO), plastic or other material, custom fabricated

Ankle-foot orthoses extend well above the ankle (usually to near the top of the calf) and are fastened around the lower leg above the ankle. A prefabricated ankle-foot orthosis (AFO) involves producing many generic AFOs from a single mold. This device is constructed for many patients and is generic in design, made of plastic or other material. A custom fabricated (molded to patient model) AFO involves taking a mold of the patient first and fabricating an AFO from that mold. This device is constructed for only one patient and is not generic in design. It is made of plastic or other material.

L1945

L1945 Ankle-foot orthosis (AFO), plastic, rigid anterior tibial section (floor reaction), custom fabricated

This code reports the supply of a specific type of custom-made ankle foot orthosis (AFO). Typically a plaster mold is made of the patient's calf, ankle, and foot, although scans and computer modeling may also be used. A thermoplastic orthosis is created based on the patient's image. The device reported by this code features an anterior plastic upright piece, known as floor reaction. This upright is integrated into a solid footplate. A floor reaction AFO is often used for patients with lower limb weaknesses, since it prevents dorsiflexion collapse at the ankle. It is ordinarily prescribed bilaterally. The orthosis is rear-entry with Velcro or strap closures.

L1950

L1950 Ankle-foot orthosis (AFO), spiral, (Institute of Rehabilitative Medicine type), plastic, custom fabricated

This code reports supply of a specific type of custom-made ankle foot orthosis (AFO). The IRM is typically a single-piece AFO. The calf cuff is integrated into a single upright that spirals around the lower calf to join a footplate. Some designs are hemi-spiral others make a full spiral. This thermoplastic component is based on patient specific measurements or moldings.

L1951

L1951 Ankle-foot orthosis (AFO), spiral, (Institute of rehabilitative Medicine type), plastic or other material, prefabricated, includes fitting and adjustment

Ankle foot orthotics (AFO) are orthoses or braces made of plastic or other material encompassing the ankle joint and all (or part) of the foot. AFOs are externally applied and intended to control position and motion of the ankle, compensate for weakness, or correct deformities. The spiral AFO helps patients control medial-lateral movement. This code includes the fitting and adjustment of the AFO.

L1960

L1960 Ankle-foot orthosis (AFO), posterior solid ankle, plastic, custom fabricated

A custom fabricated (molded to patient model) ankle-foot orthosis (AFO) involves taking a mold of a patient first and fabricating an AFO from that mold. This device is constructed of plastic for only one patient and has a posterior solid ankle.

L1970

L1970 Ankle-foot orthosis (AFO), plastic with ankle joint, custom fabricated

A custom-fabricated orthosis is one that is individually made for a specific patient starting with basic materials including, but not limited to, plastic, metal, leather, or cloth in the form of sheets, bars, and so forth. It involves substantial work, such as cutting, bending, molding, sewing, and so forth. It may involve the incorporation of some prefabricated components. It involves more than trimming, bending, or making other modifications to a substantially prefabricated item. A molded-to-patient-model orthosis is a particular type of custom fabricated orthosis in which an impression of the ankle joint is made by means of a plaster cast, CAD-CAM technology, etc. This impression is then used to make a model of plastic of the ankle joint to be braced. The orthosis is then molded on this model to be fit exactly to the ankle. This provides for free limited motion or assists in dorsiflexion and plantar flexion while limiting inversion and eversion of the ankle. The plastic design is lightweight and allows the patient to interchange shoes. It may provide critical foot and arch support. Neutral arch position promotes healing of injured ligaments. Side supports help position the brace correctly and tightly to move in harmony with the foot and ankle and assure full time protection and support.

L1971

L1971 Ankle-foot orthosis (AFO), plastic or other material with ankle joint, prefabricated, includes fitting and adjustment

Ankle foot orthotics (AFO) are orthoses or braces made of plastic or other material encompassing the ankle joint and all (or part) of the foot. AFOs are externally applied and intended to control position and motion of the ankle, compensate for weakness, or correct deformities.

L1980-L1990

L1980 Ankle-foot orthosis (AFO), single upright free plantar dorsiflexion, solid stirrup, calf band/cuff (single bar 'BK' orthosis), custom fabricated

L1990 Ankle-foot orthosis (AFO), double upright free plantar dorsiflexion, solid stirrup, calf band/cuff (double bar 'BK' orthosis), custom fabricated

This type of ankle-foot orthosis (AFO) involves use of upright bars that attach to a band near the top of the calf and spans to a stirrup attachment that fits at the ankle-foot. A single bar is usually on the lateral side of the orthotic. The double bar model has upright supports on the medial and lateral sides of the AFO. Both models allow for free plantarflexion and dorsiflexion (movement to raise and lower the foot) at the hinged stirrup. The AFO is custom fabricated to address a specific disorder and to fit a specific patient.

L2000-L2034

L2000 Knee-ankle-foot orthosis (KAFO), single upright, free knee, free ankle, solid stirrup, thigh and calf bands/cuffs (single bar 'AK' orthosis), custom fabricated

L2005 Knee-ankle-foot orthosis (KAFO), any material, single or double upright, stance control, automatic lock and swing phase release, any type activation, includes ankle joint, any type, custom fabricated

L2006 Knee ankle foot device, any material, single or double upright, swing and stance phase microprocessor control with adjustability, includes all components (e.g., sensors, batteries, charger), any type activation, with or without ankle joint(s), custom fabricated

L2010 Knee-ankle-foot orthosis (KAFO), single upright, free ankle, solid stirrup, thigh and calf bands/cuffs (single bar 'AK' orthosis), without knee joint, custom fabricated

L2020 Knee-ankle-foot orthosis (KAFO), double upright, free ankle, solid stirrup, thigh and calf bands/cuffs (double bar 'AK' orthosis), custom fabricated

L2030 Knee-ankle-foot orthosis (KAFO), double upright, free ankle, solid stirrup, thigh and calf bands/cuffs, (double bar 'AK' orthosis), without knee joint, custom fabricated

L2034 Knee-ankle-foot orthosis (KAFO), full plastic, single upright, with or without free motion knee, medial-lateral rotation control, with or without free motion ankle, custom fabricated

These codes report the supply of specific, custom-fabricated knee-ankle-foot orthotics (KAFO). Designs for KAFO devices are similar to ankle-foot devices. Similar materials are employed. Some units may be built from standardized molds, but most are custom fabricated for a specific patient based on plaster molds and measurements. In addition to the solid stirrup ankle-foot features reported by this range of codes, a KAFO has an upper thigh band or plastic shell and a hinged apparatus to eliminate (static) or limit knee movement. Code L2006 includes microprocessor sensor technology.

L2035

L2035 Knee-ankle-foot orthosis (KAFO), full plastic, static (pediatric size), without free motion ankle, prefabricated, includes fitting and adjustment

A knee-ankle-foot orthotic (KAFO) is a device that extends from the thigh to the foot and is generally used to control instabilities in the lower limb by maintaining alignment and controlling motion. In L2035, a prefabricated plastic KAFO is designed to hold a child's ankle and knee in a fixed position. It is non-adjustable and is sometimes used to treat infantile club foot disorders. Fitting and adjustment is included in this code.

L2036-L2038

L2036 Knee-ankle-foot orthosis (KAFO), full plastic, double upright, with or without free motion knee, with or without free motion ankle, custom fabricated

L2037 Knee-ankle-foot orthosis (KAFO), full plastic, single upright, with or without free motion knee, with or without free motion ankle, custom fabricated

L2038 Knee-ankle-foot orthosis (KAFO), full plastic, with or without free motion knee, multi-axis ankle, custom fabricated

A knee-ankle-foot orthotic (KAFO) is a device that extends from the thigh to the foot and is generally used to control instabilities in the lower limb by maintaining alignment and controlling motion. These codes describe a custom-fabricated KAFO that is used to control the knee and ankle, with free motion joints or rigid control at the ankle, with or without bilateral unicentric free motion joints at the knee, and molded plastic thigh and calf/ankle/foot sections. A single or double upright metal KAFO is an AFO with one or two metal uprights extending proximally to the thigh to control knee motion and alignment. This orthosis consists of a mechanical knee joint and two thigh bands between one or two uprights. Free motion knee joint refers to a joint that has unrestricted knee flexion and extension with a stop to prevent hyperextension. The free motion knee joint is used for patients with recurvatum but good strength of the quadriceps to control knee motion. A multi-axis ankle allows movement along multiple planes.

L2040

L2040 Hip-knee-ankle-foot orthosis (HKAFO), torsion control, bilateral rotation straps, pelvic band/belt, custom fabricated

This custom fabricated hip-knee-ankle-foot orthotic (HKAFO) is used to assist in controlling rotation at the hips. It consists of a pelvic band and belt with elastic or webbing straps that twist around the legs and attach to shoes.

L2050

L2050 Hip-knee-ankle-foot orthosis (HKAFO), torsion control, bilateral torsion cables, hip joint, pelvic band/belt, custom fabricated

This custom fabricated hip-knee-ankle-foot orthotic (HKAFO) is used to control the internal or external rotation of the hips and consists of a pelvic band and belt, unicentric free motion hip joints, bilateral torsion cables, and calf straps attached to shoes.

L2060

L2060 Hip-knee-ankle-foot orthosis (HKAFO), torsion control, bilateral torsion cables, ball bearing hip joint, pelvic band/ belt, custom fabricated

This custom fabricated hip-knee-ankle-foot orthotic (HKAFO) is used to control the internal or external rotation of the hips and consists of a pelvic band and belt, unicentric free motion ball bearing hip joints, bilateral torsion cables, and calf straps attached to shoes.

L2070-L2090

L2070 Hip-knee-ankle-foot orthosis (HKAFO), torsion control, unilateral rotation straps, pelvic band/belt, custom fabricated

L2080 Hip-knee-ankle-foot orthosis (HKAFO), torsion control, unilateral torsion cable, hip joint, pelvic band/belt, custom fabricated

L2090 Hip-knee-ankle-foot orthosis (HKAFO), torsion control, unilateral torsion cable, ball bearing hip joint, pelvic band/ belt, custom fabricated

These custom fabricated hip-knee-ankle-foot orthotics (HKAFO) are used to assist in controlling rotation of one hip. In L2070, the orthotic includes a pelvic band and belt with an elastic or a webbing rotation strap that twists around the leg and attaches to a shoe. In L2080 and L2090, the orthotic includes a unicentric free motion hip joint (L2080) or a unicentric ball bearing free motion hip joint (L2090) in conjunction with a unilateral torsion cable, calf strap, pelvic band, and belt to control the internal or external rotation of one hip. The orthosis attaches to a shoe and is custom fabricated.

L2106-L2116

L2106 Ankle-foot orthosis (AFO), fracture orthosis, tibial fracture cast orthosis, thermoplastic type casting material, custom fabricated

L2108 Ankle-foot orthosis (AFO), fracture orthosis, tibial fracture cast orthosis, custom fabricated

L2112 Ankle-foot orthosis (AFO), fracture orthosis, tibial fracture orthosis, soft, prefabricated, includes fitting and adjustment

L2114 Ankle-foot orthosis (AFO), fracture orthosis, tibial fracture orthosis, semi-rigid, prefabricated, includes fitting and adjustment

L2116 Ankle-foot orthosis (AFO), fracture orthosis, tibial fracture orthosis, rigid, prefabricated, includes fitting and adjustment

Certain tibial fractures may be treated with ankle-foot orthoses (AFO). These devices generally extend well above the ankle, often to the upper calf. Ankle movement may be locked or limited, or multiple planes of ankle movement allowed. The units may be built from standardized prefabricated molds or custom fabricated from a plaster impression taken of the patient's foot, ankle, and lower leg. The units themselves may be made of metal, plastic polymers, or leather, sometimes in combination, and usually with various fabrics, cushions, and closure systems. Some models are "thermoplastic," which means shape can be adjusted by application of heat. Fracture AFOs may also be custom built from rigid materials such as plaster or synthetic polymers, as well as from prefabricated and easily manipulated semi-rigid (polypropylene) and soft materials (rubber, plastic foam). Fitting and adjustment is included in the supply of the product.

L2126-L2136

L2126 Knee-ankle-foot orthosis (KAFO), fracture orthosis, femoral fracture cast orthosis, thermoplastic type casting material, custom fabricated

L2128 Knee-ankle-foot orthosis (KAFO), fracture orthosis, femoral fracture cast orthosis, custom fabricated

L2132 Knee-ankle-foot orthosis (KAFO), fracture orthosis, femoral fracture cast orthosis, soft, prefabricated, includes fitting and adjustment

L2134 Knee-ankle-foot orthosis (KAFO), fracture orthosis, femoral fracture cast orthosis, semi-rigid, prefabricated, includes fitting and adjustment

L2136 Knee-ankle-foot orthosis (KAFO), fracture orthosis, femoral fracture cast orthosis, rigid, prefabricated, includes fitting and adjustment

These codes report the supply of specific femoral fracture cast orthoses. Codes are differentiated by casting material and rigidity and whether the device is custom made or prefabricated. Custom fabricated orthoses are generally manufactured for a specific patient based on measurements, castings, and sometimes computer modeling. Prefabricated orthoses are generally produced in volume, with variations only for size, and are intended for use by any patient in need of such a device. Prefabricated devices require fitting and adjustment sessions. Knee ankle foot orthotics (KAFO) typically extend well above the knee and in these instances address fractures of the femur. Thermoplastic is shaped and contoured by heat application.

L2180-L2192

L2180 Addition to lower extremity fracture orthosis, plastic shoe insert with ankle joints

L2182 Addition to lower extremity fracture orthosis, drop lock knee joint

L2184 Addition to lower extremity fracture orthosis, limited motion knee joint

L2186 Addition to lower extremity fracture orthosis, adjustable motion knee joint, Lerman type

L2188 Addition to lower extremity fracture orthosis, quadrilateral brim

L2190 Addition to lower extremity fracture orthosis, waist belt

L2192 Addition to lower extremity fracture orthosis, hip joint, pelvic band, thigh flange, and pelvic belt

Fracture orthoses stabilize the fracture site and promote callus formation, while allowing weight bearing and joint movement after initial subsiding pain and edema. The bony motion at the fracture site is prevented through circumferential compression of the soft tissue. Fracture orthoses include the tibial fracture orthosis and femoral fracture orthosis. Fracture orthoses are commonly referred to as "removable casts." These codes report additions to lower extremity fracture orthotics.

L2200

L2200 Addition to lower extremity, limited ankle motion, each joint

This code reports an addition to a previously provided orthosis. This code represents the supply of a device or service to limit ankle motion on an ankle-foot orthosis. The ankle joint moves the foot in flexion (plantarflexion is the dropping of the foot downward and dorsiflexion moves the foot upward), as well as inversion and eversion. A previously supplied orthosis is adjusted to limit ankle motion. This may entail molding a block to the interface of the ankle/foot parts of the orthosis, or otherwise manipulating the orthosis to limit movement.

L2210-L2265

L2210 Addition to lower extremity, dorsiflexion assist (plantar flexion resist), each joint

L2220 Addition to lower extremity, dorsiflexion and plantar flexion assist/resist, each joint

L2230 Addition to lower extremity, split flat caliper stirrups and plate attachment

L2232 Addition to lower extremity orthosis, rocker bottom for total contact ankle-foot orthosis (AFO), for custom fabricated orthosis only

L2240 Addition to lower extremity, round caliper and plate attachment

L2250 Addition to lower extremity, foot plate, molded to patient model, stirrup attachment

L2260 Addition to lower extremity, reinforced solid stirrup (Scott-Craig type)

L2265 Addition to lower extremity, long tongue stirrup

This range of codes reports additions to previously provided orthoses. Dorsiflexion assist (as well as plantarflexion assist/resist) devices involve the application of a small spring-loaded cylinder on the ankle portion of the orthosis that works against a piston rod on the foot section. The spring tension assists or resists the flexing action of the foot as prescribed. (Plantarflexion is the dropping of the foot downward; dorsiflexion moves the foot upward.) Certain devices, such as caliper plates, stirrup plates, and stirrups can be mounted to an existing orthosis. Others may be molded directly to a plastic polymer orthosis. These additions are used to manipulate the flexion mobility of the ankle joint.

L2270-L2275

L2270 Addition to lower extremity, varus/valgus correction (T) strap, padded/lined or malleolus pad

L2275 Addition to lower extremity, varus/valgus correction, plastic modification, padded/lined

Varus/valgus is usually a congenital condition (or pathological condition, such as in poliomyelitis). Varus is the condition where the joint is bent outward; valgus is the condition where the joint is bent inward, or medially. Treatment may entail an ankle-foot orthosis (AFO). Valgus of the ankle, or inversion, might be treated by an AFO with a bar on the medial side and a t-strap on the lateral side. Varus, or eversion, might be treated by an AFO with a bar on the lateral side and a t-strap on the medial side.

L2280

L2280 Addition to lower extremity, molded inner boot

A molded inner boot is a rigid protective covering for the ankle and foot. It is usually composed of polypropylene or a similar material and is vacuum formed to a plaster mold of the patient's foot and ankle.

L2300-L2310

L2300 Addition to lower extremity, abduction bar (bilateral hip involvement), jointed, adjustable

L2310 Addition to lower extremity, abduction bar, straight

These codes report the supply of abduction bars added to a fracture orthosis. The fracture bar added to the orthosis maintains abduction (legs spread) during healing. The bar is jointed and adjustable.

L2320-L2340

L2320 Addition to lower extremity, nonmolded lacer, for custom fabricated orthosis only

L2330 Addition to lower extremity, lacer molded to patient model, for custom fabricated orthosis only

L2335 Addition to lower extremity, anterior swing band

L2340 Addition to lower extremity, pretibial shell, molded to patient model

A leather, or similar material, lacer is a cuff-like support that fits around the calf area. It may be custom to measurement or molded from a model of the patient. An anterior swing band is a rigid anterior (front) articulating metal band for attachment to a lower extremity orthosis. An anterior (front) pretibial shell is a lower limb orthoses that is custom molded to a model of the patient's leg.

L2350

L2350 Addition to lower extremity, prosthetic type, (BK) socket, molded to patient model, (used for PTB, AFO orthoses)

This code reports a custom-fabricated plastic prosthetic type socket, molded from a model of the patient's knee section, used on ankle-foot orthotics (AFO). It includes casting and cast preparation.

L2360

L2360 Addition to lower extremity, extended steel shank

This orthotic is a steel shank inserted between the inner and outer sole of a shoe to provide more rigidity to the shoe.

L2370

L2370 Addition to lower extremity, Patten bottom

This code reports the addition to a lower extremity orthosis of a Patten bottom. A Patten bottom is a type of strike boot added to the bottom of a knee ankle foot orthosis (KAFO). The Patten bottom is connected to the rigid outer shell of the orthotic so that with the limb slightly flexed, weight is transferred to the orthosis and upper leg rather than on the foot and ankle.

L2375

L2375 Addition to lower extremity, torsion control, ankle joint and half solid stirrup

This orthosis is a half stirrup attached to a shoe and a free motion ankle joint for torsion control.

L2380

L2380 Addition to lower extremity, torsion control, straight knee joint, each joint

This code reports a lower extremity addition and refers to a free motion knee joint used only for torsion control.

L2385

L2385 Addition to lower extremity, straight knee joint, heavy-duty, each joint

This code reports a free motion knee joint used only for torsion control. It is a heavy duty, 180-degree stop unicentric knee joint for a knee orthotic (KO) or a knee-ankle-foot orthotic (KAFO).

L2387

L2387 Addition to lower extremity, polycentric knee joint, for custom fabricated knee-ankle-foot orthosis (KAFO), each joint

This code reports a polycentric knee joint for a custom knee-ankle-foot orthotic (KAFO) only. It provides stability at full extension and easy movement during swing phase.

L2390-L2395

L2390 Addition to lower extremity, offset knee joint, each joint

L2395 Addition to lower extremity, offset knee joint, heavy-duty, each joint

These codes refer to an orthosis that has a design of a 180-degree stop unicentric knee joint or heavy-duty knee joint for a knee orthotic (KO) or knee-ankle-foot orthotic (KAFO). This addition puts the joint center posterior to the weight line providing more knee stability.

L2397

L2397 Addition to lower extremity orthosis, suspension sleeve

Orthoses of the lower extremities are sometimes attached by a suspension sleeve. These interface devices often feature a soft silicone or neoprene liner that makes a non-slip suction-type contact to the skin.

L2405-L2492

L2405 Addition to knee joint, drop lock, each

L2415 Addition to knee lock with integrated release mechanism (bail, cable, or equal), any material, each joint

L2425 Addition to knee joint, disc or dial lock for adjustable knee flexion, each joint

L2430 Addition to knee joint, ratchet lock for active and progressive knee extension, each joint

L2492 Addition to knee joint, lift loop for drop lock ring

This range of codes addresses additions to external knee joint orthoses used to treat knee dysfunctions. The codes report additions or adaptations to the joint mechanism of a base orthosis. Many of these types of orthoses minimally feature a manual adjustment that locks the joint for walking and another to release the knee for comfortable sitting. The traditional manual drop lock system requires the patient to lift a locking mechanism to release the fixed walking position. More advanced adaptations automatically lock and unlock the joint as the patient goes through gait motions (swing-phase or pendulum lock systems). Some adaptations add a release mechanism, such as a bail or cable, or a dial lock. A polycentric joint works like a cam, offering more rigidity as the joint is extended and less during flexion. A ratchet joint features a series of locking positions that can be selected or skipped over by the wearer, either for active use or as a means to progressively increase range of motion. A lift loop is a gripping device for the wearer to raise the locking ring of a drop lock mechanism.

L2500

L2500 Addition to lower extremity, thigh/weight bearing, gluteal/ischial weight bearing, ring

This code reports an addition to the upper part of a knee-ankle-foot orthotic (KAFO) designed to assist with weight bearing at the ischium during walking and standing.

L2510

L2510 Addition to lower extremity, thigh/weight bearing, quadri-lateral brim, molded to patient model

A molded plastic model of a patient's thigh is constructed. It is then used at the upper portion of a knee-ankle-foot orthotic (KAFO) to reduce the weight off the extremity during walking and standing. This custom fabricated quadrilateral socket design includes casting and cast preparation.

L2520

L2520 Addition to lower extremity, thigh/weight bearing, quadri-lateral brim, custom fitted

This code reports a prefabricated, adjustable plastic brim that is used at the upper portion of a knee-ankle-foot orthotic (KAFO). It is designed to reduce the weight on the extremity during walking and standing. It is custom fitted.

L2525-L2526

L2525 Addition to lower extremity, thigh/weight bearing, ischial containment/narrow M-L brim molded to patient model

L2526 Addition to lower extremity, thigh/weight bearing, ischial containment/narrow M-L brim, custom fitted

These codes report a thigh/weight bearing orthosis that has a foam cast brim that may be custom fitted or custom molded. These models have a tighter medial-lateral (M-L) design and greater weight bearing ability from the standard quadrilateral model.

L2530-L2540

L2530 Addition to lower extremity, thigh/weight bearing, lacer, nonmolded

L2540 Addition to lower extremity, thigh/weight bearing, lacer, molded to patient model

These codes report a thigh/weight bearing lacer, which is a corset-like device wrapped around a thigh, and used at the top portion of a knee-ankle-foot orthotic (KAFO) to reduce the weight on the extremity during walking and standing. It may be molded to a patient model or nonmolded.

L2550

L2550 Addition to lower extremity, thigh/weight bearing, high roll cuff

This code reports a high roll cuff used for thigh/weight bearing. A high roll cuff is a padded and rolled special top edge of a lacer, which is a corset-like device wrapped around a thigh to give greater support and comfort.

L2570

L2570 Addition to lower extremity, pelvic control, hip joint, Clevis type two-position joint, each

This code reports a specially designed hip joint that can be locked in 90- and 180-degree positions.

L2580

L2580 Addition to lower extremity, pelvic control, pelvic sling

This code reports a narrow band of leather or other flexible material that is attached to an orthotic hip joint to apply pressure to the gluteal area to stabilize the pelvic area.

L2600

L2600 Addition to lower extremity, pelvic control, hip joint, Clevis type, or thrust bearing, free, each

This code reports a free motion unicentric hip joint for a knee-ankle-foot orthotic (KAFO). This device controls motion at the hip, knee, and ankle.

L2610

L2610 Addition to lower extremity, pelvic control, hip joint, Clevis or thrust bearing, lock, each

This refers to a free motion unicentric hip joint. This KAFO device controls motion at hip, knee, and ankle and has a drop lock.

L2620

L2620 Addition to lower extremity, pelvic control, hip joint, heavy-duty, each

This is a free motion, unicentric hip joint KAFO that is heavy duty. This device controls motion at hip, knee, and ankle.

L2622

L2622 Addition to lower extremity, pelvic control, hip joint, adjustable flexion, each

This is an adjustable flexion, free motion unicentric hip joint for a KAFO. This device controls motion at hip, knee, and ankle. The adjustable flexion control range of motion of the affected limb.

L2624

L2624 Addition to lower extremity, pelvic control, hip joint, adjustable flexion, extension, abduction control, each

This code reports an adjustable extension, flexion, and abduction free, motion unicentric hip joint on a knee-ankle-foot orthotic (KAFO). These hip joints control flexion/extension and abduction/adduction and control range of motion of the affected area.

L2627

L2627 Addition to lower extremity, pelvic control, plastic, molded to patient model, reciprocating hip joint and cables

This refers to a hip/pelvic control system that provides a reciprocating gait action. The way RGA works is with every step a patient takes, as one leg flexes, the other leg must extend and thereby stretch out the hip contracting structures. This orthoses is custom fabricated, a molded plastic pelvic section, molded from a model of the patient, special hip joints, vertical lateral uprights, and a thoracic belt.

L2628

L2628 Addition to lower extremity, pelvic control, metal frame, reciprocating hip joint and cables

This refers to a hip/pelvic control system that provides a reciprocating gait action. The way RGA works is with every step a patient takes, as one leg flexes, the other leg must extend and thereby stretch out the hip contracting structures. This KAFO orthoses includes a metal pelvic band, special hip joints, vertical lateral uprights, and a thoracic belt. It is custom fabricated.

L2630

L2630 Addition to lower extremity, pelvic control, band and belt, unilateral

This refers to a pelvic band and belt for use with a unilateral KAFO that is secured to the hip joint for control and is custom fabricated

L2640

L2640 Addition to lower extremity, pelvic control, band and belt, bilateral

This refers to a pelvic band and belt for use with bilateral orthosis and is secured to both hip joints for control and is custom fabricated.

L2650

L2650 Addition to lower extremity, pelvic and thoracic control, gluteal pad, each

This code reports a specially designed pad that provides gluteal pressure. This aids in support and balance and is custom fabricated.

L2660

L2660 Addition to lower extremity, thoracic control, thoracic band

This code reports a thoracic band that is added to a bilateral hip-knee-ankle-foot orthotic (HKAFO). A pelvic band and paraspinal uprights are also used to provide greater torso control and spinal alignment.

L2670-L2680

L2670 Addition to lower extremity, thoracic control, paraspinal uprights

L2680 Addition to lower extremity, thoracic control, lateral support uprights

These codes report thoracic bands that are added to a bilateral hip-knee-ankle-foot orthotic (HKAFO). One has paraspinal uprights (L2670) between the pelvic and thoracic bands to provide greater control of the torso and spinal alignment. The other has lateral uprights (L2680) between the pelvic and thoracic bands to provide greater control of the torso and spinal alignment.

L2750

L2750 Addition to lower extremity orthosis, plating chrome or nickel, per bar

This refers to a process of adding a durable, protective finish to steel components on any orthoses.

L2755

L2755 Addition to lower extremity orthosis, high strength, lightweight material, all hybrid lamination/prepreg composite, per segment, for custom fabricated orthosis only

This code reports supply of a segmental addition to a lower extremity orthosis of high strength, lightweight material, such as carbon graphite laminates. These high-end materials are extremely lightweight yet possess good torsional and structural properties. This additional segment is for custom fabricated orthosis only.

L2760-L2780

L2760 Addition to lower extremity orthosis, extension, per extension, per bar (for lineal adjustment for growth)

L2768 Orthotic side bar disconnect device, per bar

L2780 Addition to lower extremity orthosis, noncorrosive finish, per bar

This range of codes reports supply of additions to lower extremity orthoses support bars and associated devices. These bars are usually paired medially and laterally on the orthosis, although single-bar units are also used. Growth in children necessitates regular changing of bars and disconnect devices may be added to facilitate bar change and adjustment.

L2785

L2785 Addition to lower extremity orthosis, drop lock retainer, each

This refers to a clip or a spring and a steel ball inserted into a metal upright on an orthoses. It is designed to hold a drop lock in a locked or unlocked position.

L2795-L2810

L2795 Addition to lower extremity orthosis, knee control, full kneecap

L2800 Addition to lower extremity orthosis, knee control, knee cap, medial or lateral pull, for use with custom fabricated orthosis only

L2810 Addition to lower extremity orthosis, knee control, condylar pad

This range of codes reports supply of additions to lower extremity orthoses designed to improve knee stability and control through manipulative padding and coverings. These additions may allow for greater loading or unloading of a side of the joint, possibly relieving pressure on an arthritic or injured site.

L2820-L2830

L2820 Addition to lower extremity orthosis, soft interface for molded plastic, below knee section

L2830 Addition to lower extremity orthosis, soft interface for molded plastic, above knee section

These codes report supply of soft interface additions to lower extremity orthoses. This is padding against the skin for molded plastic pieces. A great deal of orthosis design engineering focuses on above-the-joint and below-the-joint supports. These supports must work through the skin surface to stabilize skeletal bone as well as softer-tissue structures such as ligaments, cartilage, and musculature.

L2840-L2850

L2840 Addition to lower extremity orthosis, tibial length sock, fracture or equal, each

L2850 Addition to lower extremity orthosis, femoral length sock, fracture or equal, each

These codes report supply of fracture socks, or the equivalent. These are highly elastic stockings, often with a natural fabric liner on the skin contact side. The stockings are often made of a closed mesh that can be trimmed for length. Fracture socks may be applied for certain types of closed fractures of the lower extremity, usually in combination with a rigid orthosis. The sock/orthosis combination holds certain advantages over traditional plaster casting in that patients often experience less muscle shrinkage.

L2861

L2861 Addition to lower extremity joint, knee or ankle, concentric adjustable torsion style mechanism for custom fabricated orthotics only, each

This code describes concentric adjustable torsion style mechanisms used for the lower extremity joint, knee or ankle, for custom fabricated orthotics only. These components incorporate adjustable and removable dynamic power assist. The power assist add-on component is mounted to a conventionally functioning knee or ankle component within a custom orthotic and adds the prescribed function to dynamic assist/resist as required. These additions are used to improve stability and walking functions.

L2999

L2999 Lower extremity orthoses, not otherwise specified

This code reports the supply of an orthosis of the lower extremity that is not defined elsewhere in the HCPCS listing. Certain wraps, splints, shoes, or other supplies may be reported by the code. Generally speaking, a Medicare claim for L2999 must include "a narrative description of the item, the brand name and model name/number of the item, and a statement defining the medical necessity of the item for the particular patient."

L3000-L3030

L3000 Foot insert, removable, molded to patient model, UCB type, Berkeley shell, each

L3001 Foot, insert, removable, molded to patient model, Spenco, each

L3002 Foot insert, removable, molded to patient model, Plastazote or equal, each

L3003 Foot insert, removable, molded to patient model, silicone gel, each

L3010 Foot insert, removable, molded to patient model, longitudinal arch support, each

L3020 Foot insert, removable, molded to patient model, longitudinal/metatarsal support, each

L3030 Foot insert, removable, formed to patient foot, each

This range of codes reports supply of a variety of prescription orthosis shoe inserts, differentiated largely by product type, construction material, and method of preparation and fitting. These devices fit inside the shoe. Most are molded to a plaster or foam replica of the patient's foot, but some are modeled to electronic images of the foot. Inserts molded to the patient's foot directly are often made of thermo-formable materials that can be heat softened, custom applied, and trimmed in a single session. The UCB (also known as UCBL or "Berkeley shell") is named for the University of California Biomechanics Laboratories, the developer of several types of rigid inserts. Materials for this range of codes include high and low heat plastic, leather, and various synthetics. Plastazote is a type of closed cell polyethylene foam and Spenco is manufactured from closed cell neoprene. Most inserts address a variety of foot corrections.

L3031

L3031 Foot, insert/plate, removable, addition to lower extremity orthosis, high strength, lightweight material, all hybrid lamination/prepreg composite, each

This code refers to a lower extremity orthosis of high strength, lightweight material, such as carbon graphite laminates. These high-end materials are extremely lightweight and have good structural properties. This device fits inside the shoe.

L3040-L3060

L3040 Foot, arch support, removable, premolded, longitudinal, each

L3050 Foot, arch support, removable, premolded, metatarsal, each

L3060 Foot, arch support, removable, premolded, longitudinal/metatarsal, each

This range of codes reports the supply of arch support products that are available premolded and not modeled to a replica of the patient's foot. These prefabricated "stock" devices may still require a custom fitting, however. Materials are usually various synthetics.

L3070-L3090

L3070 Foot, arch support, nonremovable, attached to shoe, longitudinal, each

L3080 Foot, arch support, nonremovable, attached to shoe, metatarsal, each

L3090 Foot, arch support, nonremovable, attached to shoe, longitudinal/metatarsal, each

These codes report the supply of nonremovable arch support products that are attached to the patient's shoe. Materials are usually various synthetics.

L3100

L3100 Hallus-valgus night dynamic splint, prefabricated, off-the-shelf

This type of night splint addresses poor alignment of the base joint of the great toe (hallux-valgus) through strapping, padding, and rigid splinting. A slip-on type splint is applied to the great toe and straps are applied to correctly align the toe while the patient sleeps.

L3140-L3150

L3140 Foot, abduction rotation bar, including shoes

L3150 Foot, abduction rotation bar, without shoes

These codes report the supply of abduction rotation bars. Abduction is the movement away from the median plane, in this case of the foot outward. These bars maintain the position of the feet and, consequently, the femoral head in a fixed position. The abduction bar is often prescribed to treat cases of talipes (clubfoot) and genu varus (pigeon toe-in) and certain types of hip dysplasia in toddlers. The prototypical orthosis is the Denis-Browne splint, which is an abduction rotation bar that attaches to the footplate of a baby shoe or is wrapped to the foot. The variety that attaches to a shoe may be adjusted with a special wrench.

L3160

L3160 Foot, adjustable shoe-styled positioning device

This is a pediatric two piece shoe that enables the forefoot and hind foot can be positioned independently for the forefoot adduction or abduction. The two pieces have separate closures for control.

L3170

L3170 Foot, plastic, silicone or equal, heel stabilizer, prefabricated, off-the-shelf, each

Report this code for supply of prefabricated plastic silicone or equivalent heel stabilizer bars to control abduction and rotation. Ordinarily, this is an insert or modification to a shoe that is part of a lower extremity orthosis system.

L3201-L3203

L3201 Orthopedic shoe, Oxford with supinator or pronator, infant

L3202 Orthopedic shoe, Oxford with supinator or pronator, child

L3203 Orthopedic shoe, Oxford with supinator or pronator, junior

These codes report supply of specific orthopedic footwear. The codes are differentiated by whether the footwear is modeled for infants, children, or juniors. The shoes reported by this range of codes are oxford style. The shoes are fitted with adjustment for supination or pronation. Supination is bowing out of the foot and adjustment is usually to raise the lateral edge of the shoe or to lower the medial edge. Pronation is a "flat foot" or bowing in of the foot. Adjustment is usually to raise the medial edge or lower the lateral edge of the shoe.

L3204-L3207

L3204 Orthopedic shoe, hightop with supinator or pronator, infant

L3206 Orthopedic shoe, hightop with supinator or pronator, child

L3207 Orthopedic shoe, hightop with supinator or pronator, junior

These codes report supply of specific orthopedic footwear. The codes are differentiated by whether the footwear is modeled for infants, children, or juniors. The shoes reported by this range of codes are high-top style. The shoes are fitted with adjustment for supination or pronation. Supination is bowing out of the foot and adjustment is usually to raise the lateral edge of the shoe or to lower the medial edge. Pronation is a "flat foot" or bowing in of the foot. Adjustment is usually to raise the medial edge or lower the lateral edge of the shoe.

L3208-L3211

L3208 Surgical boot, each, infant

L3209 Surgical boot, each, child

L3211 Surgical boot, each, junior

A surgical boot or shoe is a special type of footwear, usually high-top style, designed to accommodate post-surgical wrappings and dressings and to allow the patient a degree of mobility. Ordinarily these boots are manufactured without left-foot or right-foot design considerations and are sold as single units.

L3212-L3214

L3212 Benesch boot, pair, infant

L3213 Benesch boot, pair, child

L3214 Benesch boot, pair, junior

Benesch boots are shoes that have a clear plastic window in the back that permit a view of the heel while in the shoe. It is used to ensure that the heel is held in the correct position within the shoe.

L3215-L3230

L3215 Orthopedic footwear, ladies shoe, Oxford, each

L3216 Orthopedic footwear, ladies shoe, depth inlay, each

L3217 Orthopedic footwear, ladies shoe, hightop, depth inlay, each

L3219 Orthopedic footwear, mens shoe, Oxford, each

L3221 Orthopedic footwear, mens shoe, depth inlay, each

L3222 Orthopedic footwear, mens shoe, hightop, depth inlay, each

L3224 Orthopedic footwear, woman's shoe, Oxford, used as an integral part of a brace (orthosis)

L3225 Orthopedic footwear, man's shoe, Oxford, used as an integral part of a brace (orthosis)

L3230 Orthopedic footwear, custom shoe, depth inlay, each

This range of codes reports supply of orthopaedic footwear. The codes are differentiated by whether the footwear is modeled for men or women, whether the shoe is an integral part of a lower-extremity orthosis, and the style of the shoe. Depth inlay is a design feature to accommodate an in-the-shoe component of a lower-extremity orthosis. The inlay may be removable for use of the shoe with or without the brace component. Shoes that are an integral part of a lower-extremity orthosis generally feature a stirrup or caliper and plate attachment system to an external brace. Custom shoes are made for a specific patient. Generally, a code reports supply of a single shoe when sold as a single unit.

L3250

L3250 Orthopedic footwear, custom molded shoe, removable inner mold, prosthetic shoe, each

Report this code for each prosthetic shoe that is custom molded for a patient and has a removable inner mold and a custom fabricated insert designed for toe or distal partial foot amputation.

L3251

L3251 Foot, shoe molded to patient model, silicone shoe, each

This code reports a custom-fabricated shoe molded from a model of the patient that is lined with a silicone material. It is designed for sensitive feet and accommodates pressure areas. Casting and cast preparation is included.

L3252

L3252 Foot, shoe molded to patient model, Plastazote (or similar), custom fabricated, each

This is a custom fabricated shoe. It is molded from a model of the patient. The upper portion of the shoe is made of foam plastic or a similar material. It is designed to accommodate pressure areas. This code includes the casting and cast preparation.

L3253

L3253 Foot, molded shoe, Plastazote (or similar), custom fitted, each

This code is used to report a molded foam plastic (or like material) shoe, designed for temporary use. It is custom fitted and designed for sensitive feet and pressure areas.

L3254-L3255

L3254 Nonstandard size or width

L3255 Nonstandard size or length

These codes report a shoe or shoes that are not a normal size or width or a shoe or shoes that are not a normal size or length.

L3257

L3257 Orthopedic footwear, additional charge for split size

This code reports an additional charge when the two orthopedic shoes for a patient are of different sizes (split shoes).

L3260

L3260 Surgical boot/shoe, each

A surgical boot or shoe is a special type of footwear, usually high-top style, designed to accommodate post-surgical wrappings and dressings and to allow the patient a degree of mobility. Ordinarily these boots are manufactured without left-foot or right-foot design considerations and are sold as single units.

L3265

L3265 Plastazote sandal, each

Plastazote is a type of closed cell polyethylene foam and this code reports supply of each Plastazote sandal. This type of footwear is often prescribed for patients who have undergone surgery of the toes or metatarsal area or who have problems in the forefoot zone. The sole of the sandal is manufactured from polyethylene foam to protect and cushion the plantar surface. Closures are usually Velcro strapping.

L3300-L3334

L3300 Lift, elevation, heel, tapered to metatarsals, per in

L3310 Lift, elevation, heel and sole, neoprene, per in

L3320 Lift, elevation, heel and sole, cork, per in

L3330 Lift, elevation, metal extension (skate)

L3332 Lift, elevation, inside shoe, tapered, up to one-half in

L3334 Lift, elevation, heel, per in

This range of codes reports lift modification to shoes. The codes are differentiated largely by type of material, style, and application in the shoe.

L3340-L3350

L3340 Heel wedge, SACH

L3350 Heel wedge

Heel wedges are modifications to shoes to lift medial or lateral aspects of the foot (pronation or supination) or otherwise address foot or posture problems. SACH is an acronym for solid ankle, cushioned heel.

L3360-L3370

L3360 Sole wedge, outside sole

L3370 Sole wedge, between sole

Heel wedges are modifications to shoes to lift medial or lateral aspects of the foot (pronation or supination) or otherwise address foot or posture problems.

L3380

L3380 Clubfoot wedge

This code reports a shoe modification wedge to address clubfoot. Talipes equinovarus is the Latin-based medical term for clubfoot. Equino is a reference to horse and varus means to "toe-in." Babies born with clubfoot exhibit extreme plantarflexion, which, as in horses, means weight is born on the extreme forefoot and toes. The feet are also characteristically turned inward. Talipes refers to the talus bone of the foot, which is not fully developed in clubfoot. Optimally, cases of clubfoot are aggressively addressed early in life. Shoe wedges may be of some benefit to those patients who still exhibit characteristics as children, teens, and adults. The wedge is usually fitted to fill the extreme arch of the foot seen in these patients.

L3390

L3390 Outflare wedge

An outflare wedge refers to a heel or sole that is extended and flared out from the shoe to provide greater efficiency in controlling pronation and supination of the ankle.

L3400

L3400 Metatarsal bar wedge, rocker

Bar wedges and rockers are used to transfer and alleviate pressure and improve the gait. Rocker soles assist in the burring of energy that forces the body forward after the center of gravity goes over the peak of the rocker. The rockers also assist in cases of limited range of motion with regards to the ankle or metatarsophalangeal joints. Rockers are created by adding extra crepe to the midsole portion of the shoe and then beveling it away just proximal to the point of pressure. There are different types of rockers, but they should all have a stable flat area at mid-stance. There are also many styles of rockers. There are also metatarsophalangeal bars that refer to specific shoe modifications. All metatarsophalangeal bars are to help metatarsalgia and relieve plantar pressure by adding a wedge of firm material across the sole of the shoe. By placing the bar to the metatarsophalangeal heads it unloads the pressure from the metatarsophalangeal heads, which allows transfer from the shafts of the metatarsals to the distal end of the toes.

L3410

L3410 Metatarsal bar wedge, between sole

This code reports a style of metatarsal bar that is placed between the sole layers.

L3420

L3420 Full sole and heel wedge, between sole

This refers to a wedge that is placed between sole layers over the full length of the shoe.

L3430-L3440

L3430 Heel, counter, plastic reinforced

L3440 Heel, counter, leather reinforced

These codes report a firm plastic liner or a firm leather liner that reinforces the heel section of a shoe. These are permanently attached to a shoe.

L3450

L3450 Heel, SACH cushion type

This code reports a solid ankle cushion heel, also known as a SACH cushion heel. It is made of a softer durometer material that replaces a portion of the posterior heel base. SACH heels reduce shock at heel strike and compensate for the absence of ankle motion.

L3455-L3460

L3455 Heel, new leather, standard

L3460 Heel, new rubber, standard

These codes report a conventional leather heel or a conventional rubber heel for shoes.

L3465-L3470

L3465 Heel, Thomas with wedge

L3470 Heel, Thomas extended to ball

These codes report modifications to a shoe heel known as the Thomas wedge. This is a bar applied to the exterior of the sole of the shoe posterior to the metatarsal heads. The bar is shaved at either end. The wedge provides pressure relief off the metatarsal heads, or ball of the foot.

L3480-L3485

L3480 Heel, pad and depression for spur

L3485 Heel, pad, removable for spur

Bone spurs often form on the bones of the feet, particularly on the calcaneus or heel bone. These spurs can be extremely painful, particularly as pressure is placed against them.

L3500

L3500 Orthopedic shoe addition, insole, leather

This code reports a full leather insole to an orthopedic shoe.

L3510

L3510 Orthopedic shoe addition, insole, rubber

This code reports a full rubber or similar material insole for an orthopedic shoe.

L3520

L3520 Orthopedic shoe addition, insole, felt covered with leather

This code reports a full-length lining made of felt and leather that is placed inside an orthopedic shoe.

L3530-L3540

L3530 Orthopedic shoe addition, sole, half

L3540 Orthopedic shoe addition, sole, full

These codes report an addition, repair, and/or modification to half of the sole or the complete sole of an orthopedic shoe.

L3550-L3560

L3550 Orthopedic shoe addition, toe tap, standard

L3560 Orthopedic shoe addition, toe tap, horseshoe

These codes report a small metal insert, sometimes shaped like a horseshoe (L3560), secured to the sole (near the toe) of an orthopedic shoe to reduce wear.

L3570

L3570 Orthopedic shoe addition, special extension to instep (leather with eyelets)

This code reports an extension piece added to an existing lace area of an orthopedic shoe that allows a patient with an extremely high instep or deformity to tie his or her own shoes.

L3580

L3580 Orthopedic shoe addition, convert instep to Velcro closure

This code reports an addition to an orthopedic shoe that converts an instep of a shoe that has laces to an instep that has straps with Velcro, which is a hook/loop tape fastener. This is easier for donning and removing shoes.

L3590

L3590 Orthopedic shoe addition, convert firm shoe counter to soft counter

This code reports the conversion of a firm counter (the cup the heel fits into) of an orthopedic shoe to a soft counter.

L3595

L3595 Orthopedic shoe addition, March bar

This code reports an external sole buildup to an orthopedic shoe that has an elevation placed behind the metatarsal heads to relieve pressure.

L3600-L3610

L3600 Transfer of an orthosis from one shoe to another, caliper plate, existing

L3610 Transfer of an orthosis from one shoe to another, caliper plate, new

These codes report the transfer or replacement of caliper plates from one shoe to another. The caliper plate is the footplate of an ankle foot orthosis (AFO) or knee ankle foot orthosis (KAFO). The plate features short, integrated medial and lateral uprights that connect to the upper portion of the AFO. The caliper plate is usually incorporated into a shoe, typically by cutting or splitting the sole. These plates are subject to some wear and occasionally need to be replaced. More commonly, though, the shoe becomes worn and the caliper plate is switched to a new shoe.

L3620-L3630

L3620 Transfer of an orthosis from one shoe to another, solid stirrup, existing

L3630 Transfer of an orthosis from one shoe to another, solid stirrup, new

These codes report the transfer or replacement of solid stirrups from one shoe to another. The solid stirrup is a particular design component of many ankle foot orthoses (AFO) or knee ankle foot orthoses (KAFO). Stirrups usually are attached directly to the shoe between the sole and heel, although the footplate inside the shoe occasionally is used. A solid stirrup reported by these codes integrates the upright with the footplate portion. A medial and lateral upright connects to the upper portion of the AFO. The stirrup may be subject to some wear and occasionally needs to be replaced. More commonly, though, the shoe becomes worn and the stirrup is switched to a new shoe.

L3640

L3640 Transfer of an orthosis from one shoe to another, Dennis Browne splint (Riveton), both shoes

This code reports the transfer of a specific type of orthosis from one shoe to another. The Denis Browne splint is named for the British pediatric surgeon who invented the device early in the last century. It is a static orthotic device used to treat babies and young children with congenital disorders such as hip dysplasia and congenital genu varus (toe-in). An abduction bar is attached to a special footplate of the patient's baby shoes. The bar and footplates fix the patient's feet and, therefore, the femoral heads into a therapeutic position. Adjustment on the footplate allows for positioning of the feet. In infancy, the splint may be left on for long periods. In toddlers, the splint may be used only at night and during nap times. As the patient grows, new shoes must be fitted. The Denis Browne splint can be detached from the old pair of shoes and mounted to the new pair.

L3649

L3649 Orthopedic shoe, modification, addition or transfer, not otherwise specified

This code reports any orthopedic shoe modification or addition that has not been individually listed in previous HCPCS Level II codes.

L3650-L3660

L3650 Shoulder orthosis (SO), figure of eight design abduction restrainer, prefabricated, off-the-shelf

L3660 Shoulder orthosis (SO), figure of eight design abduction restrainer, canvas and webbing, prefabricated, off-the-shelf

A shoulder orthosis (SO) or shoulder immobilizer is a support device (usually not rigid or semirigid) used for sustaining injured, postsurgical, and/or weak or deformed areas of the shoulder girdle and for restricting or eliminating motion (immobilization). The benefits from orthotic and immobilizer use, specifically during convalescence from an injury (strain, chip fracture with strain, fracture) or illness or as a postoperative treatment measure can include the following: restricted range of motion of the affected area (immobilization), support of the affected area, and/or protection from injury, reinjury, suture tearing, and/or wound dehiscence. Some of the devices support the shoulder while limiting most ranges of motion, particularly abduction, which is the movement that raises the arm. All of these items usually require the assistance of a person other than the patient for appropriate application. Most of these items can be adjusted to fit the patient and come in a variety of sizes.

L3670-L3678

L3670 Shoulder orthosis (SO), acromio/clavicular (canvas and webbing type), prefabricated, off-the-shelf

L3671 Shoulder orthosis (SO), shoulder joint design, without joints, may include soft interface, straps, custom fabricated, includes fitting and adjustment

L3674 Shoulder orthosis (SO), abduction positioning (airplane design), thoracic component and support bar, with or without nontorsion joint/turnbuckle, may include soft interface, straps, custom fabricated, includes fitting and adjustment

L3675 Shoulder orthosis (SO), vest type abduction restrainer, canvas webbing type or equal, prefabricated, off-the-shelf

L3677 Shoulder orthosis (SO), shoulder joint design, without joints, may include soft interface, straps, prefabricated item that has been trimmed, bent, molded, assembled, or otherwise customized to fit a specific patient by an individual with expertise

L3678 Shoulder orthosis (SO), shoulder joint design, without joints, may include soft interface, straps, prefabricated, off-the-shelf

A shoulder orthosis (SO) or shoulder immobilizer is a support device (usually not rigid or semirigid) used for sustaining injured, postsurgical, and/or weak or deformed areas of the shoulder girdle and for restricting or eliminating motion (immobilization). The benefits from orthotic and immobilizer use, specifically during convalescence from an injury (strain, chip fracture with strain, fracture) or illness or as a postoperative treatment measure, can include the following: restriction of the range of motion of the affected area (immobilization); support of the affected area; and/or protection from injury, reinjury, suture tearing, and/or wound dehiscence. Some of the devices support the shoulder while limiting most ranges of motion, particularly abduction, which is the movement that raises the arm. All of these items usually require the assistance of a person other than the patient for appropriate application. Most of these items can be adjusted to fit the patient and come in a variety of sizes.

L

L3702

L3702 Elbow orthosis (EO), without joints, may include soft interface, straps, custom fabricated, includes fitting and adjustment

This code reports a static/rigid elbow orthotic that is custom fabricated and may have a soft interface. It is used particularly for elbow immobilization in patients who have had recent elbow surgery and/or inflammation.

L3710

L3710 Elbow orthosis (EO), elastic with metal joints, prefabricated, off-the-shelf

This code reports supply of a simple, prefabricated elastic elbow orthotic with metal joints. The device is prefabricated, which means the orthotist selects from mass produced products based on the size of the patient and fits the device accordingly. These devices may be neoprene or Lycra sleeves pulled over the elbow or wrapped around the elbow and closed with Velcro straps. Incorporated into the fabric of the orthosis are rigid, jointed bars, typically on the medial and lateral sides.

L3720

L3720 Elbow orthosis (EO), double upright with forearm/arm cuffs, free motion, custom fabricated

This code reports a custom fitted elbow orthotic designed to provide control of the elbow joint. It consists of upper and lower arm sections made of plastic or leather and bilateral unicentric free motion joints.

L3730

L3730 Elbow orthosis (EO), double upright with forearm/arm cuffs, extension/ flexion assist, custom fabricated

This code reports a custom fabricated elbow orthotic that provides control of the elbow and flexion or extension support. It consists of upper and lower arm sections made of plastic or leather, bilateral unicentric free motion joints, and a unilateral spring device at a joint.

L3740

L3740 Elbow orthosis (EO), double upright with forearm/arm cuffs, adjustable position lock with active control, custom fabricated

This code reports a custom fabricated elbow orthotic designed to provide control and function to a weak elbow. It consists of upper and lower arm sections made of plastic or leather, bilateral unicentric joints (one of which is lockable at various levels of flexion), and a shoulder harness assembly with a cable used to operate the elbow lock.

L3760

L3760 Elbow orthosis (EO), with adjustable position locking joint(s), prefabricated, item that has been trimmed, bent, molded, assembled, or otherwise customized to fit a specific patient by an individual with expertise

This code reports a custom fitted elbow orthosis that is designed to control the elbow. It consists of upper and lower arm sections and has adjustable locking joints.

L3761

L3761 Elbow orthosis (EO), with adjustable position locking joint(s), prefabricated, off-the-shelf

This code reports the supply of an elbow orthosis that is designed to control the elbow. It consists of upper and lower arm sections and has adjustable locking joints. The device is prefabricated and off-the-shelf, which means the orthotist selects from mass produced products based on the size of the patient and fits the device accordingly.

L3762

L3762 Elbow orthosis (EO), rigid, without joints, includes soft interface material, prefabricated, off-the-shelf

This code reports the supply of a prefabricated, rigid elbow orthosis. In certain instances the elbow must be immobilized as completely as possible, such as following trauma or during recovery from a surgery of the joint capsule. This type of orthosis acts much like a cast in that the joint is locked in position, usually in several degrees of flexion. The brace is rigid and includes cushion material between the hard structure and the patient's skin. The device is prefabricated, which means the orthotist selects from mass produced products based on the size of the patient and fits the device accordingly.

L3763-L3766

L3763 Elbow-wrist-hand orthosis (EWHO), rigid, without joints, may include soft interface, straps, custom fabricated, includes fitting and adjustment

L3764 Elbow-wrist-hand orthosis (EWHO), includes one or more nontorsion joints, elastic bands, turnbuckles, may include soft interface, straps, custom fabricated, includes fitting and adjustment

L3765 Elbow-wrist-hand-finger orthosis (EWHFO), rigid, without joints, may include soft interface, straps, custom fabricated, includes fitting and adjustment

L3766 Elbow-wrist-hand-finger orthosis (EWHFO), includes one or more nontorsion joints, elastic bands, turnbuckles, may include soft interface, straps, custom fabricated, includes fitting and adjustment

Fracture orthoses may be similar in design, depending on the manufacturer and the intended application. These are bracing devices, typically containing hardware such as aluminum or other lightweight arm supports for the desired degree of abduction, as well as plastic, polyethylene, or foam. These devices may use the patient torso or neck as an anchor, as well as the phalanges. There may be hinges at certain points in the device to allow for a certain degree of elbow or wrist motion. The treating provider must initially apply these items, but a person other than the patient can be instructed in the proper application when/if the patient removes the device during specified intervals. Sizes can vary according to the manufacturer (there may be pediatric sizes as well). The items are generally manufactured in right and left models. Shoulder braces with arm, elbow, and wrist immobilization support and control the range of motion of the upper extremity, including the upper arm, scapula, clavicle, elbow, forearm, and/or wrist. They also support most muscles and ligamentous tissues related to the movement of the upper extremity. They maintain a degree of abduction between the patient's torso and the affected upper limb, at the degree desired (usually 45-90 degrees). Each of these devices typically leaves the fingers free, but grasping heavy items is usually unable to be accomplished and is not advised. They are used posttraumatically for severe fractures.

L3806-L3809

L3806 Wrist-hand-finger orthosis (WHFO), includes one or more nontorsion joint(s), turnbuckles, elastic bands/springs, may include soft interface material, straps, custom fabricated, includes fitting and adjustment

L3807 Wrist-hand-finger orthosis (WHFO), without joint(s), prefabricated item that has been trimmed, bent, molded, assembled, or otherwise customized to fit a specific patient by an individual with expertise

L3808 Wrist-hand-finger orthosis (WHFO), rigid without joints, may include soft interface material; straps, custom fabricated, includes fitting and adjustment

L3809 Wrist-hand-finger orthosis (WHFO), without joint(s), prefabricated, off-the-shelf, any type

A wrist-hand-finger orthosis (WHFO) is typically a rigid or semirigid device used for the purpose of supporting injured, post-surgical, and/or weak or deformed areas of the wrist, hand, and metacarpal regions (phalanges are usually freely mobile with these types of devices) and for restricting or eliminating motion (immobilization) of the affected structure. While orthoses are usually prefabricated (custom fitted) or custom fabricated, these types of orthoses are generally not customized. Many of these items appear as sleeves or stockinette types of items. The benefits from WHFO use, specifically during convalescence from an injury or illness or as a postoperative treatment measure, can include the following: restricted range of motion of the affected area (immobilization); support of the affected area; and/or protection from injury, reinjury, suture tearing, and/or wound dehiscence.

L3891

L3891 Addition to upper extremity joint, wrist or elbow, concentric adjustable torsion style mechanism for custom fabricated orthotics only, each

This code describes concentric adjustable torsion style mechanisms used for the upper extremity joint, wrist or elbow, for custom fabricated orthotics only. Each component is used to describe the removable components used with custom orthotics. These components incorporate adjustable and removable dynamic power assist. The power assist add-on component is mounted to a conventionally functioning wrist or elbow within a custom orthotic and they add the prescribed function to dynamic assist/resist as required. These additions are used to improve reach, grasp, and pinching functions.

L

L3900-L3935

L3900 Wrist-hand-finger orthosis (WHFO), dynamic flexor hinge, reciprocal wrist extension/ flexion, finger flexion/extension, wrist or finger driven, custom fabricated

L3901 Wrist-hand-finger orthosis (WHFO), dynamic flexor hinge, reciprocal wrist extension/ flexion, finger flexion/extension, cable driven, custom fabricated

L3904 Wrist-hand-finger orthosis (WHFO), external powered, electric, custom fabricated

L3905 Wrist-hand orthosis (WHO), includes one or more nontorsion joints, elastic bands, turnbuckles, may include soft interface, straps, custom fabricated, includes fitting and adjustment

L3906 Wrist-hand orthosis (WHO), without joints, may include soft interface, straps, custom fabricated, includes fitting and adjustment

L3908 Wrist-hand orthosis (WHO), wrist extension control cock-up, nonmolded, prefabricated, off-the-shelf

L3912 Hand-finger orthosis (HFO), flexion glove with elastic finger control, prefabricated, off-the-shelf

L3913 Hand-finger orthosis (HFO), without joints, may include soft interface, straps, custom fabricated, includes fitting and adjustment

L3915 Wrist-hand orthosis (WHO), includes one or more nontorsion joint(s), elastic bands, turnbuckles, may include soft interface, straps, prefabricated item that has been trimmed, bent, molded, assembled, or otherwise customized to fit a specific patient by an individual with expertise

L3916 Wrist-hand orthosis (WHO), includes one or more nontorsion joint(s), elastic bands, turnbuckles, may include soft interface, straps, prefabricated, off-the-shelf

L3917 Hand orthosis (HO), metacarpal fracture orthosis, prefabricated item that has been trimmed, bent, molded, assembled, or otherwise customized to fit a specific patient by an individual with expertise

L3918 Hand orthosis (HO), metacarpal fracture orthosis, prefabricated, off-the-shelf

L3919 Hand orthosis (HO), without joints, may include soft interface, straps, custom fabricated, includes fitting and adjustment

L3921 Hand-finger orthosis (HFO), includes one or more nontorsion joints, elastic bands, turnbuckles, may include soft interface, straps, custom fabricated, includes fitting and adjustment

L3923 Hand-finger orthosis (HFO), without joints, may include soft interface, straps, prefabricated item that has been trimmed, bent, molded, assembled, or otherwise customized to fit a specific patient by an individual with expertise

L3924 Hand-finger orthosis (HFO), without joints, may include soft interface, straps, prefabricated, off-the-shelf

L3925 Finger orthosis (FO), proximal interphalangeal (PIP)/distal interphalangeal (DIP), nontorsion joint/spring, extension/flexion, may include soft interface material, prefabricated, off-the-shelf

L3927 Finger orthosis (FO), proximal interphalangeal (PIP)/distal interphalangeal (DIP), without joint/spring, extension/flexion (e.g., static or ring type), may include soft interface material, prefabricated, off-the-shelf

L3929 Hand-finger orthosis (HFO), includes one or more nontorsion joint(s), turnbuckles, elastic bands/springs, may include soft interface material, straps, prefabricated item that has been trimmed, bent, molded, assembled, or otherwise customized to fit a specific patient by an individual with expertise

L3930 Hand-finger orthosis (HFO), includes one or more nontorsion joint(s), turnbuckles, elastic bands/springs, may include soft interface material, straps, prefabricated, off-the-shelf

L3931 Wrist-hand-finger orthosis (WHFO), includes one or more nontorsion joint(s), turnbuckles, elastic bands/springs, may include soft interface material, straps, prefabricated, includes fitting and adjustment

L3933 Finger orthosis (FO), without joints, may include soft interface, custom fabricated, includes fitting and adjustment

L3935 Finger orthosis (FO), nontorsion joint, may include soft interface, custom fabricated, includes fitting and adjustment

A wrist-hand-finger orthosis (WHFO) is typically a rigid or semirigid device used for the purpose of supporting injured, post-surgical, and/or weak or deformed areas of the wrist, hand, and metacarpal regions (phalanges are usually freely mobile with these types of devices) and for restricting or eliminating motion (immobilization) of the affected structure. While orthoses are usually prefabricated (custom fitted) or custom fabricated, these types of orthoses are generally not customized. Many of these items appear as sleeves or stockinette types of items. The benefits from WHFO use, specifically during convalescence from an injury or illness or as a postoperative treatment measure, can include the following:

L

restricted range of motion of the affected area (immobilization); support of the affected area; and/or protection from injury, reinjury, suture tearing, and/or wound dehiscence.

L3956

L3956 Addition of joint to upper extremity orthosis, any material; per joint

This code reports the incorporation of a joint into an upper extremity orthosis in which the base code does not include an articulation.

L3960-L3962

L3960 Shoulder-elbow-wrist-hand orthosis (SEWHO), abduction positioning, airplane design, prefabricated, includes fitting and adjustment

L3961 Shoulder-elbow-wrist-hand orthosis (SEWHO), shoulder cap design, without joints, may include soft interface, straps, custom fabricated, includes fitting and adjustment

L3962 Shoulder-elbow-wrist-hand orthosis (SEWHO), abduction positioning, Erb's palsy design, prefabricated, includes fitting and adjustment

A shoulder-elbow-wrist-hand orthosis (SEWHO) is used for the purpose of supporting injured, post-surgical, and/or weak or deformed areas of the shoulder, elbow, wrist, or hand. These codes may be similar in design, depending on the manufacturer and the intended application. These are bracing devices used on wheelchairs, typically containing hardware such as aluminum or other lightweight arm supports for the desired degree of abduction, as well as plastic, polyethylene, or foam. These devices may use the patient torso or neck as an anchor as well as the phalanges. There may be hinges at certain points in the device to allow for a certain degree of elbow or wrist motion. The treating provider must initially apply these items, but a person other than the patient can be instructed in the proper application when/if the patient removes the device during specified intervals. Sizes can vary according to the manufacturer (there may be pediatric sizes as well). The items are generally manufactured in right and left models. Shoulder braces, with arm, elbow, and wrist immobilization, support and control the range of motion of the upper extremity, including the upper arm, scapula, clavicle, elbow, forearm, and/or wrist. They also support most muscles and ligamentous tissues related to the movement of the upper extremity. They maintain a degree of abduction between the patient's torso and the affected upper limb, at the degree desired (usually 45-90 degrees). Each of these devices will typically leave the fingers free, but grasping heavy items is usually unable to be accomplished and is not advised. They are used post-traumatically for severe fractures and for certain types of surgical procedures, such as partial or total shoulder replacement. A prefabricated or custom fitted orthosis is one that the manufacturer has produced in quantity, without a specific patient in mind. A prefabricated orthosis may be trimmed, bent, molded (with or without heat), or otherwise modified for use by a specific patient (i.e., custom fitted). An orthosis that is assembled from prefabricated components is considered prefabricated. Any orthosis that does not meet the definition of a custom fabricated orthosis is considered prefabricated. A custom fabricated orthosis is one that is individually made for a specific patient, starting with basic materials including, but not limited to, plastic, metal, leather, or cloth in the form of sheets, bars, and so forth. It involves substantial work, such as cutting, bending, molding, sewing, and so forth. It may involve the incorporation of some prefabricated components. It involves more than trimming, bending, or making other modifications to a substantially prefabricated item. A molded-to-patient-model orthosis is a particular type of custom fabricated orthosis in which an impression of the specific body part is made (by means of a plaster cast, CAD-CAM technology, etc.).

L3967-L3978

L3967 Shoulder-elbow-wrist-hand orthosis (SEWHO), abduction positioning (airplane design), thoracic component and support bar, without joints, may include soft interface, straps, custom fabricated, includes fitting and adjustment

L3971 Shoulder-elbow-wrist-hand orthotic (SEWHO), shoulder cap design, includes one or more nontorsion joints, elastic bands, turnbuckles, may include soft interface, straps, custom fabricated, includes fitting and adjustment

L3973 Shoulder-elbow-wrist-hand orthosis (SEWHO), abduction positioning (airplane design), thoracic component and support bar, includes one or more nontorsion joints, elastic bands, turnbuckles, may include soft interface, straps, custom fabricated, includes fitting and adjustment

L3975 Shoulder-elbow-wrist-hand-finger orthosis (SEWHO), shoulder cap design, without joints, may include soft interface, straps, custom fabricated, includes fitting and adjustment

L3976 Shoulder-elbow-wrist-hand-finger orthosis (SEWHO), abduction positioning (airplane design), thoracic component and support bar, without joints, may include soft interface, straps, custom fabricated, includes fitting and adjustment

L3977 Shoulder-elbow-wrist-hand-finger orthosis (SEWHO), shoulder cap design, includes one or more nontorsion joints, elastic bands, turnbuckles, may include soft interface, straps, custom fabricated, includes fitting and adjustment

L3978 Shoulder-elbow-wrist-hand-finger orthosis (SEWHO), abduction positioning (airplane design), thoracic component and support bar, includes one or more nontorsion joints, elastic bands, turnbuckles, may include soft interface, straps, custom fabricated, includes fitting and adjustment

A shoulder-elbow-wrist-hand orthosis (SEWHO) is used for the purpose of supporting injured, post-surgical, and/or weak or deformed areas of the shoulder, elbow, wrist, or hand. These codes may be similar in design, depending on the manufacturer and the intended application. These are bracing devices attached to wheelchairs, typically containing hardware such as aluminum or other lightweight arm supports for the desired degree of abduction, as well as plastic, polyethylene, or foam. These devices may use the patient torso or neck as an anchor, as well as the phalanges. There may be hinges at certain points in the device to allow for a certain degree of elbow or wrist motion. The treating provider must initially apply these items, but a person other than the patient can be instructed in the proper application when/if the patient removes the device during specified intervals. Sizes can vary according to the manufacturer (there may be pediatric sizes as well). The items are generally manufactured in right and left models. Shoulder braces with arm, elbow, and wrist immobilization support and control the range of motion of the upper extremity, including the upper arm, scapula, clavicle, elbow, forearm, and/or wrist. They also support most muscles and ligamentous tissues related to the movement of the upper extremity. They maintain a degree of abduction between the patient's torso and the affected upper limb, at the degree desired (usually 45-90 degrees). Each of these devices typically leaves the fingers free, but grasping heavy items is usually unable to be accomplished and is not advised. They are used posttraumatically for severe fractures and for certain types of surgical procedures, such as partial or total shoulder replacement. A prefabricated or custom fitted orthosis is one that the manufacturer has produced in quantity, without a specific patient in mind. A prefabricated orthosis may be trimmed, bent, molded (with or without heat), or otherwise modified for use by a specific patient (i.e., custom fitted). An orthosis that is assembled from prefabricated components is considered prefabricated. Any orthosis that does not meet the definition of a custom fabricated orthosis is considered prefabricated. A custom fabricated orthosis is one that is individually made for a specific patient, starting with basic materials including, but not limited to, plastic, metal, leather, or cloth in the form of sheets, bars, and so forth. It involves substantial work, such as cutting, bending, molding, sewing, and so forth. It may involve the incorporation of some prefabricated components. It involves more than trimming, bending, or making other modifications to a substantially prefabricated item. A molded-to-patient-model orthosis is a particular type of custom fabricated orthosis in which an impression of the specific body part is made (by means of a plaster cast, CAD-CAM technology, etc.). These codes describe shoulder-elbow-wrist-hand orthoses that are supports attached to a wheelchair.

L3980-L3984

L3980 Upper extremity fracture orthosis, humeral, prefabricated, includes fitting and adjustment

L3981 Upper extremity fracture orthosis, humeral, prefabricated, includes shoulder cap design, with or without joints, forearm section, may include soft interface, straps, includes fitting and adjustments

L3982 Upper extremity fracture orthosis, radius/ulnar, prefabricated, includes fitting and adjustment

L3984 Upper extremity fracture orthosis, wrist, prefabricated, includes fitting and adjustment

Fracture orthoses may be similar in design, depending on the manufacturer and the intended application. These are bracing devices, typically containing hardware such as aluminum or other lightweight arm supports for the desired degree of abduction, as well as plastic, polyethylene, or foam. These devices may use the patient torso or neck as an anchor, as well as the phalanges. There may be hinges at certain points in the device to allow for a certain degree of elbow or wrist motion. The treating provider must initially apply these items, but a person other than the patient can be instructed in the proper application when/if the patient removes the device during specified intervals. Sizes can vary according to the manufacturer (there may be pediatric sizes as well). The items are generally manufactured in right and left models. Shoulder braces, with arm, elbow, and wrist immobilization, support and control the range of motion of the upper extremity, including the upper arm, scapula, clavicle, elbow, forearm, and/or wrist. They also support most muscles and ligamentous tissues related to the movement of the upper extremity. They maintain a degree of abduction between the patient's torso and the affected upper limb, at the degree desired (usually 45 to 90 degrees). Each of these devices typically leave the fingers free, but grasping heavy items is usually unable to be accomplished and is not advised. They are used posttraumatically for severe fractures. A prefabricated or custom-fitted orthosis is one that the manufacturer has produced in quantity, without a specific patient in mind. A prefabricated orthosis may be trimmed, bent, molded (with or without heat), or otherwise modified for use by a specific patient (e.g., custom fitted). An orthosis that is assembled from prefabricated components is considered prefabricated. Any orthosis that does not meet the definition of a custom-fabricated orthosis is considered prefabricated. A custom-fabricated orthosis is one that is individually made for a specific patient, starting with basic materials including, but not limited to, plastic, metal, leather, or cloth in the form of sheets, bars, and so forth. It involves substantial work, such as cutting, bending, molding, sewing, and so forth. It may involve the incorporation of some prefabricated components. It involves more than trimming, bending, or making other modifications to a substantially prefabricated item. A molded-to-patient-model orthosis is a particular type of custom fabricated orthosis in which an impression of the specific body part is made (by means of a plaster cast, CAD-CAM technology, etc.).

L3995

L3995 Addition to upper extremity orthosis, sock, fracture or equal, each

This code reports an addition to an upper extremity fracture orthosis. It consists of a special sock that is used as an interface between the arm and the orthosis.

L3999

L3999 Upper limb orthosis, not otherwise specified

This code reports an upper limb orthosis not specified in previous HCPCS Level II codes. Upper extremity orthoses are devices applied externally to restore or improve functional and structural characteristics of the musculoskeletal and nervous systems.

L4000

L4000 Replace girdle for spinal orthosis (cervical-thoracic-lumbar-sacral orthosis (CTLSO) or spinal orthosis SO)

This code reports replacement of a molded plastic or leather pelvic girdle for a spinal orthosis. It is custom fabricated from a model of the patient and includes casting and cast preparation.

L4002

L4002 Replacement strap, any orthosis, includes all components, any length, any type

This code reports replacement of a dysfunctional strap on an orthosis and includes all attachment components.

L4010-L4030

L4010 Replace trilateral socket brim

L4020 Replace quadrilateral socket brim, molded to patient model

L4030 Replace quadrilateral socket brim, custom fitted

These codes report replacement of a molded plastic ischial weight bearing socket of trilateral (L4010) or quadrilateral design for a knee-ankle-foot orthotic (KAFO). The quadrilateral design can be custom fabricated from a model of a patient (L4020) and/or custom fitted (L4030). Casting and cast preparation are included.

L4040-L4055

L4040 Replace molded thigh lacer, for custom fabricated orthosis only

L4045 Replace nonmolded thigh lacer, for custom fabricated orthosis only

L4050 Replace molded calf lacer, for custom fabricated orthosis only

L4055 Replace nonmolded calf lacer, for custom fabricated orthosis only

These codes report the replacement of molded lacers. Lacers are cuff-like devices that fit around a portion of a limb. They have a slit opening on one side to don the device and a lace-string corset-style closure of gussets and eyelets. Often they are of thermoplastic material with cushion liners built from patient molds, but many are still manufactured of leather, or have leather incorporated into the design. An orthotic device may attach to this device. Many are used for suspension of a prosthetic attachment.

L4060-L4130

L4060 Replace high roll cuff

L4070 Replace proximal and distal upright for KAFO

L4080 Replace metal bands KAFO, proximal thigh

L4090 Replace metal bands KAFO-AFO, calf or distal thigh

L4100 Replace leather cuff KAFO, proximal thigh

L4110 Replace leather cuff KAFO-AFO, calf or distal thigh

L4130 Replace pretibial shell

These codes report replacements/repairs of any dysfunctional pieces to various parts of a knee-ankle-foot orthotic (KAFO) and/or ankle-foot orthotic (AFO).

L4205

L4205 Repair of orthotic device, labor component, per 15 minutes

This code reports the labor component of repair of a previously provided orthosis except for any labor involved in the replacement of an orthotic component that has a specific L code. Report the time in 15-minute increments.

L

L4210

L4210 Repair of orthotic device, repair or replace minor parts

This code reports the replacement or repair of any minor parts on any type of orthosis.

L4350

L4350 Ankle control orthosis, stirrup style, rigid, includes any type interface (e.g., pneumatic, gel), prefabricated, off-the-shelf

This code reports a prefabricated ankle brace support comprised of a stirrup that goes under the foot with pads on both sides, which are wrapped around the ankle. Rigid brace shells fit the ankle comfortably and provide the needed medial/lateral stabilization.

L4360-L4361

L4360 Walking boot, pneumatic and/or vacuum, with or without joints, with or without interface material, prefabricated item that has been trimmed, bent, molded, assembled, or otherwise customized to fit a specific patient by an individual with expertise

L4361 Walking boot, pneumatic and/or vacuum, with or without joints, with or without interface material, prefabricated, off-the-shelf

This code reports a boot-shaped brace for an injured foot. It is a lightweight, rigid knee-length boot with a reinforced sole and other supporting devices embedded in the plaster to facilitate walking. This device has compressing air in chambers between the rigid outer shell and the patient's leg.

L4370

L4370 Pneumatic full leg splint, prefabricated, off-the-shelf

This code reports the supply of pneumatic splints or air splints. These devices immobilize the limb by compressing air in chambers between the rigid outer shell and the patient's leg. These orthoses are used commonly in first response situations to trauma, although some models may be prescribed for more extended use to support the knee joint. The devices reported by these codes are prefabricated and may require fitting and adjustment sessions to suit individual patient needs. Typically, the chambers are inflated by a hand pump or electric pump until the desired level of pressure against the limb is attained.

L4386-L4387

L4386 Walking boot, nonpneumatic, with or without joints, with or without interface material, prefabricated item that has been trimmed, bent, molded, assembled, or otherwise customized to fit a specific patient by an individual with expertise

L4387 Walking boot, nonpneumatic, with or without joints, with or without interface material, prefabricated, off-the-shelf

This code reports a boot-shaped brace for an injured foot. It is a lightweight, rigid knee-length boot with a reinforced sole and other supporting devices embedded in the plaster to facilitate walking. It is prefabricated and includes fitting and adjustment.

L4392-L4394

L4392 Replacement, soft interface material, static AFO

L4394 Replace soft interface material, foot drop splint

These codes represent replacements of softer interface materials for static ankle foot orthotics and foot drop splints. Ankle flexion contracture is a condition in which there is shortening of the muscles and/or tendons that plantarflex the ankle with the resulting inability to bring the ankle to 0 degrees by passive range of motion (0 degrees ankle position is when the foot is perpendicular to the lower leg). "Foot drop" is a condition in which there is weakness and/or lack of use of the muscles that dorsiflex the ankle, but there is the ability to bring the ankle to 0 degrees by passive range of motion. A foot drop splint/recumbent positioning device is a prefabricated ankle-foot orthosis, with a soft interface, that has all of the following characteristics: designed to maintain the foot at a fixed position of 0 degrees (i.e., perpendicular to the lower leg), not designed to accommodate an ankle with a plantar flexion contracture, and used by a patient who is nonambulatory.

L4396-L4397

L4396 Static or dynamic ankle foot orthosis, including soft interface material, adjustable for fit, for positioning, may be used for minimal ambulation, prefabricated item that has been trimmed, bent, molded, assembled, or otherwise customized to fit a specific patient by an individual with expertise

L4397 Static or dynamic ankle foot orthosis, including soft interface material, adjustable for fit, for positioning, may be used for minimal ambulation, prefabricated, off-the-shelf

A static ankle foot orthosis (AFO) is a prefabricated AFO that may be adjustable for fit and positioning and is designed to accommodate an ankle with a plantar flexion contracture up to 45 degrees. It applies a dorsiflexion force to the ankle, allows pressure

L

reduction, is used by a patient who is minimally ambulatory or nonambulatory, and has a soft interface. AFOs extend well above the ankle (usually to near the top of the calf) and are fastened around the lower leg above the ankle. A dynamic AFO allows a more gradual stretch, and allows the patient to progress as tolerance is increased. The low-load stretching also allows the patient to maintain gains in range of motion. The dynamic AFO has an adjustable cord and articulating dorsal shell that assists in controlling the degree of stretch, while at the same time allowing for an adjustment of the cord's tension. This code includes the fitting, adjustment, and supply of a static or dynamic ankle foot orthosis.

L4398

L4398 Foot drop splint, recumbent positioning device, prefabricated, off-the-shelf

A foot drop splint/recumbent positioning device is a prefabricated ankle-foot orthosis that is designed to maintain the foot at a fixed position of 0 degrees (i.e., perpendicular to the lower leg), but not designed to accommodate an ankle with a plantar flexion contracture. The foot drop splint is used by a patient who is nonambulatory and has a soft interface. This code includes the fitting and adjustment as well as the supply of the static ankle foot orthosis.

L4631

L4631 Ankle-foot orthosis (AFO), walking boot type, varus/valgus correction, rocker bottom, anterior tibial shell, soft interface, custom arch support, plastic or other material, includes straps and closures, custom fabricated

This code reports an ankle-foot orthotic (AFO) intended to protect the affected ankle/foot from further damage by replacing the shoe with a device suitable for ambulation. This AFO includes a metal "rocker" to the sole of the plastic form to reduce plantar pressures during gait and a varus/valgus correction wedging lift. It is custom fabricated and includes straps and closures.

L5000-L5020

L5000 Partial foot, shoe insert with longitudinal arch, toe filler

L5010 Partial foot, molded socket, ankle height, with toe filler

L5020 Partial foot, molded socket, tibial tubercle height, with toe filler

These codes report the supply of partial foot orthoses. Partial amputations of the foot often entail disarticulation of the forefoot (phalanges and metatarsals), leaving the heel (calcaneus) intact. Prosthesis preparation for partial foot amputations is complicated by several factors, including socket fitting to the foot remnant and filler material for the amputation. Typically, a toe filler is prepared from artificial materials to resemble the size and shape of the missing toes and metatarsal pad. This is designed to fit into a conventional shoe. Based on moldings or castings taken before amputation, a flexible sleeve is custom fabricated from rubber or other material with elastic properties. The fore end is designed to attach to the toe filler. The proximal end may be fitted with a zipper that closes up the back of the ankle in the general area over the Achilles tendon. This design is usually fitted up to the tibial tubercle, the bony prominence at the ankle. Other designs simply fit over the residual foot/ankle by elastic compression. A molded socket is the interface between the residual foot/ankle and the toe filler. The prosthesis is designed to fit into a conventional or orthotic shoe.

L5050-L5060

L5050 Ankle, Symes, molded socket, SACH foot

L5060 Ankle, Symes, metal frame, molded leather socket, articulated ankle/foot (SACH)

These codes report the supply of specific prostheses for Symes-type amputations. The Symes amputation is a disarticulation at the ankle joint with preservation of the fatty heel pad, which is rotated over the distal closure. The heel pad becomes the most distal part of the residual limb and an interface for a prosthesis. Based on moldings or castings taken before or after amputation, a flexible sleeve is custom fabricated from rubber or other material with elastic properties. This constitutes the molded socket that interfaces between the residual ankle and the prosthetic foot. A solid ankle, cushioned heel (SACH) foot prosthesis is a basic passive device.

L5100-L5105

L5100 Below knee (BK), molded socket, shin, SACH foot

L5105 Below knee (BK), plastic socket, joints and thigh lacer, SACH foot

These codes report the supply of specific prostheses for below-the-knee amputations. Based on moldings or castings taken before or after amputation, a flexible sleeve is custom fabricated from rubber or other material with elastic properties. This constitutes the molded socket that interfaces between the residual limb and the prosthesis that attaches to it. Plastic sockets are typically custom fabricated, sometimes from thermoplastic materials that are molded and shaped as heat is applied. A thigh lacer is a cuff-like device that fits around that portion of the residual limb. It has a slit opening on the front side to don the device and a lace-string corset-style closure of gussets and eyelets. Often lacers are of thermoplastic material with cushion liners built from patient molds, but many are still manufactured of leather, or have leather incorporated into the design. The thigh lacer supports and suspends the below-the-knee prosthesis from above. A solid ankle, cushioned heel (SACH) foot prosthesis is a basic passive device.

L5150-L5160

L5150 Knee disarticulation (or through knee), molded socket, external knee joints, shin, SACH foot

L5160 Knee disarticulation (or through knee), molded socket, bent knee configuration, external knee joints, shin, SACH foot

These codes report the supply of specific prostheses for knee disarticulation (or through knee) amputations. A flexible sleeve is custom fabricated from rubber or other material with elastic properties based on moldings or castings taken before or after amputation. This constitutes the molded socket that interfaces between the residual limb and the prosthesis that attaches to it. Plastic sockets are typically custom fabricated, sometimes from thermoplastic materials that are molded and shaped as heat is applied. Knee disarticulation results in an excellent weight-bearing stump.

L5200-L5230

L5200 Above knee (AK), molded socket, single axis constant friction knee, shin, SACH foot

L5210 Above knee (AK), short prosthesis, no knee joint (stubbies), with foot blocks, no ankle joints, each

L5220 Above knee (AK), short prosthesis, no knee joint (stubbies), with articulated ankle/foot, dynamically aligned, each

L5230 Above knee (AK), for proximal femoral focal deficiency, constant friction knee, shin, SACH foot

These codes report the supply of a specific above-the-knee prosthetic system. Based on moldings or castings taken before or after amputation, a flexible sleeve is custom fabricated from rubber or other material with elastic properties. This constitutes the molded socket that interfaces between the residual limb and the prosthetic system that attaches to it. Plastic sockets may be custom fabricated from moldings as well, sometimes from thermoplastic materials that are molded and shaped as heat is applied. A single-axis friction knee is a prosthetic component to replace the knee joint. This type of joint is among the oldest designs and consists of a simple axle connecting the thigh and shank segments. The joint is capable of flexion and extension, but cannot bear the user's weight unless locked in an extended position. Constant friction is applied to the joint hinge to keep it from swinging too freely, particularly in gait. A solid ankle, cushioned heel (SACH) foot prosthesis is a basic passive device. These prostheses are considered inexpensive and simple to manufacture.

L5250-L5270

L5250 Hip disarticulation, Canadian type; molded socket, hip joint, single axis constant friction knee, shin, SACH foot

L5270 Hip disarticulation, tilt table type; molded socket, locking hip joint, single axis constant friction knee, shin, SACH foot

These codes report the supply of prostheses for patients who have had hip disarticulation amputations (removal of the entire leg at the juncture of the hip socket and femoral head). The Canadian type prosthesis consists of a plastic waistband at the trunk line of the iliac crests. Any residual stump may also be utilized for prosthesis attachment and a molded plastic socket encloses the ischial tuberosity to bear weight. The artificial hip joint is toward the anterior of the prosthesis and is unlocked, as is the knee joint. The "tilt table" type prosthesis refers to a specific device that takes the patient's weight off the fresh incisions during early rehabilitation following disarticulation. Based on moldings or castings taken before or after amputation, a flexible sleeve is custom fabricated from rubber or other material with elastic properties. This constitutes the molded socket that interfaces between the residual limb and the prosthetic system that attaches to it. Plastic sockets may be custom fabricated from moldings as well, sometimes from thermoplastic materials that are molded and shaped as heat is applied. A single-axis friction knee is a prosthetic component to replace the knee joint. This type of joint is among the oldest designs and consists of a simple axle connecting the thigh and shank segments. The joint is capable of flexion and extension, but cannot bear the user's weight unless locked in an extended position. Constant friction is applied to the joint hinge to keep it from swinging too freely, particularly in gait. A solid ankle, cushioned heel (SACH) foot prosthesis is a basic passive device. The knee and foot components are considered inexpensive and simple to manufacture.

L5280

L5280 Hemipelvectomy, Canadian type; molded socket, hip joint, single axis constant friction knee, shin, SACH foot

This code reports a Canadian type prosthesis that consists of a plastic waistband at the trunk line of the iliac crests. Any residual stump may also be utilized for prosthesis attachment and a molded plastic socket encloses the ischial tuberosity to bear weight. The artificial hip joint is toward the anterior of the prosthesis and is unlocked, as is the knee joint. A single-axis friction knee is a prosthetic component to replace the knee joint and consists of a simple axle connecting the thigh and shank segments. The joint is capable of flexion and extension, but cannot bear the user's weight unless locked in an extended position. Constant friction is applied to the joint hinge to keep it from swinging too freely, particularly in gait. A solid

L

ankle, cushioned heel (SACH) foot prosthesis is a basic passive device.

L5301

L5301 Below knee (BK), molded socket, shin, SACH foot, endoskeletal system

This code reports a below knee prosthesis. Based on moldings or castings taken before or after amputation, a flexible sleeve is custom fabricated from rubber or other material with elastic properties. This constitutes the molded socket that interfaces between the residual limb and the prosthetic system that attaches to it. Plastic sockets may be custom fabricated from moldings as well, sometimes from thermoplastic materials that are molded and shaped as heat is applied. A solid ankle, cushioned heel (SACH) foot prosthesis is a basic passive device.

L5312

L5312 Knee disarticulation (or through knee), molded socket, single axis knee, pylon, SACH foot, endoskeletal system

This code reports a through the knee prosthesis. Based on moldings or castings taken before or after amputation, a flexible sleeve is custom fabricated from rubber or other material with elastic properties. This constitutes the molded socket that interfaces between the residual limb and the prosthetic system that attaches to it. Plastic sockets may be custom fabricated from moldings as well, sometimes from thermoplastic materials that are molded and shaped as heat is applied. A pylon is a post-like structure fitted to the plaster socket on one end and the prosthetic foot component on the other. It is a feature of many lower limb prosthetic designs. The pylon may be a tube made of aluminum, titanium, steel, or carbon fiber reinforced plastic and in early fittings is usually adjustable for length. The artificial knee component is a single axis, which means the joint is capable of simple flexion and extension actions only. A solid ankle, cushioned heel (SACH) foot prosthesis is a basic passive device.

L5321

L5321 Above knee (AK), molded socket, open end, SACH foot, endoskeletal system, single axis knee

This code reports an above-the-knee prosthesis. Based on moldings or castings taken before or after amputation, a flexible sleeve is custom fabricated from rubber or other material with elastic properties. This constitutes the molded socket that interfaces between the residual limb and the prosthetic system that attaches to it. Plastic sockets may be custom fabricated from moldings as well, sometimes from thermoplastic materials that are molded and shaped as heat is applied. The artificial knee component is single axis, which means the joint is capable of simple flexion and extension actions only. Rather than internal rigid supports, this type of prosthesis uses the external hard shell to transfer the patient's weight from the thigh and knee to the foot component. A solid ankle, cushioned heel (SACH) foot prosthesis is a basic passive device.

L5331-L5341

L5331 Hip disarticulation, Canadian type, molded socket, endoskeletal system, hip joint, single axis knee, SACH foot

L5341 Hemipelvectomy, Canadian type, molded socket, endoskeletal system, hip joint, single axis knee, SACH foot

These codes report a prosthetic system for patients who have undergone a hemipelvectomy (removal of half of the pelvic girdle and an entire leg). This type of amputation presents numerous problems for the prosthetist, since there is no residual limb with which to anchor a device. The socket is based on moldings and castings taken before or after amputation and may extend well up the torso. The Canadian type prosthesis features a molded plastic socket to enclose the remaining ischial tuberosity to bear weight. An artificial hip joint is toward the anterior of the prosthesis and is unlocked, as is the knee joint, which is single axis. This means the joint is capable of simple flexion and extension actions only. Rather than internal rigid supports, this type of leg prosthesis uses the external hard shell to transfer the patient's weight from the thigh and knee to the foot component (endoskeletal). A solid ankle, cushioned heel (SACH) foot prosthesis is a basic passive device.

L5400-L5430

L5400 Immediate postsurgical or early fitting, application of initial rigid dressing, including fitting, alignment, suspension, and one cast change, below knee (BK)

L5410 Immediate postsurgical or early fitting, application of initial rigid dressing, including fitting, alignment and suspension, below knee (BK), each additional cast change and realignment

L5420 Immediate postsurgical or early fitting, application of initial rigid dressing, including fitting, alignment and suspension and one cast change above knee (AK) or knee disarticulation

L5430 Immediate postsurgical or early fitting, application of initial rigid dressing, including fitting, alignment and suspension, above knee (AK) or knee disarticulation, each additional cast change and realignment

These codes report supply of early fittings and dressings following below-the-knee amputation or disarticulation at the knee joint. A major consideration for prosthetists is the constantly changing size and shape of the residual limb, or stump, which is the attachment site for a prosthesis. Following amputation of the limb, post-surgical or "early" dressings are applied to the surgical stump, sometimes during the same operative session. These early applications are designed to compress and prepare the distal tissues in anticipation of fitting a test socket and later a permanent socket. Early applications may be known as immediate post-surgical fittings (IPSF). The accepted plan for most lower limb amputations is to transition the patient as quickly as possible to use of a prosthesis. This minimizes muscle atrophy and limb weakness seen in longer convalescences. In some instances, a plaster cast or other rigid dressing is hand molded to the residual limb as the amputation session is completed. In other instances, the initial dressing is applied up to several days following surgery. As swelling diminishes and also to access the surgical closure, the dressing must be periodically changed out. These early dressings may be fitted to interface with test prosthetic devices.

L5450-L5460

L5450 Immediate postsurgical or early fitting, application of nonweight bearing rigid dressing, below knee (BK)

L5460 Immediate postsurgical or early fitting, application of nonweight bearing rigid dressing, above knee (AK)

These codes report supply of early non-weight bearing fittings and dressings following amputation of a lower limb. Following amputation of the limb, post-surgical or "early" dressings are applied to the surgical stump, sometimes during the same operative session. These early applications are designed to compress and prepare the distal tissues in anticipation of fitting a test socket and later a permanent socket. In some instances, a plaster cast or other rigid dressing is hand molded to the residual limb as the amputation session is completed. In other instances, the initial dressing is applied up to several days following surgery. As swelling diminishes and also to access the surgical closure, the dressing must be periodically changed out. For plaster and rigid dressings, this entails cutting off the cast and reapplying the dressing. In some cases, removable casts or caps are devised. These devices may be removed and reapplied several times. The dressings reported by these codes are never fitted to interface with test prostheses.

L5500-L5505

L5500 Initial, below knee (BK) PTB type socket, nonalignable system, pylon, no cover, SACH foot, plaster socket, direct formed

L5505 Initial, above knee (AK), knee disarticulation, ischial level socket, nonalignable system, pylon, no cover, SACH foot, plaster socket, direct formed

These codes report the supply of initial hand molded plaster socket systems for amputation of a lower limb. These are initial sockets that are the transition between the initial rigid dressings applied post-surgery and the test socket systems that prepare the patient for a long-term prosthesis. A patella tendon bearing (PTB) type socket generally features an adjustable cuff worn just above the knee joint. This cuff suspends the lower components, comprised in this instance of the direct-formed plaster socket over the stump, the pylon, and foot components. Plaster sockets may be directly formed from bandages saturated with plaster of paris. Once fitted, the plaster socket cannot be aligned. A pylon is a post-like structure fitted to the plaster socket on one end and the prosthetic foot component on the other. It is a feature of most lower limb prosthetic designs. The pylon may be a tube made of aluminum, titanium, steel, or carbon fiber reinforced plastic and in early fittings is usually adjustable for length. Unlike many long-term prostheses, this unit does not feature a cosmetic covering. A solid ankle, cushioned heel (SACH) foot prosthesis is a basic passive device. A high, above-the-knee amputation or disarticulation at the femoral head presents numerous challenges for the prosthetist, since there is very little residual limb to attach the prosthesis. An ischial level socket in this instance is a direct-formed plaster encasement of the ischial tuberosity, to bear the patient's weight. Once fitted, it cannot be aligned. A pylon is fitted to the plaster socket on one end and the prosthetic foot component on the other.

L5510-L5540

L5510 Preparatory, below knee (BK) PTB type socket, nonalignable system, pylon, no cover, SACH foot, plaster socket, molded to model

L5520 Preparatory, below knee (BK) PTB type socket, nonalignable system, pylon, no cover, SACH foot, thermoplastic or equal, direct formed

L5530 Preparatory, below knee (BK) PTB type socket, nonalignable system, pylon, no cover, SACH foot, thermoplastic or equal, molded to model

L5535 Preparatory, below knee (BK) PTB type socket, nonalignable system, no cover, SACH foot, prefabricated, adjustable open end socket

L5540 Preparatory, below knee (BK) PTB type socket, nonalignable system, pylon, no cover, SACH foot, laminated socket, molded to model

These codes report a variety of non-alignable preparatory prostheses for below-the-knee amputations. Preparatory prostheses are transition devices between the initial rigid dressings and pylons applied post-surgery and the finished long-term prosthetic system. The codes are differentiated by the style of socket and the material used in its fabrication. As is typical with preparatory sockets, none can be aligned once fitted. A patella tendon bearing (PTB) type socket generally features an adjustable cuff worn just above the knee joint. This cuff suspends the socket, which can be made of any of a variety of materials. A plaster socket, in this instance, is formed from bandages saturated with plaster of paris applied over a previously cast model of the stump. A thermoplastic socket may be formed by applying heat to the rough-formed socket and modeling it to the patient's stump directly or to a previously cast model of the stump. Another style of preparatory socket involves laminating together two or more resin-saturated materials over a previously cast model of the stump. Other preparatory sockets are prefabricated or selected from mass produced components based only on patient size. This type of preparatory socket is adjustable. A pylon is a post-like structure fitted to the plaster socket on one end and the prosthetic foot component on the other. It is a feature of most lower limb prosthetic designs. The pylon may be a tube made of aluminum, titanium, steel, or carbon fiber reinforced plastic and in early fittings is usually adjustable for length. Unlike many long-term prostheses, none of these units feature cosmetic coverings. A solid ankle, cushioned heel (SACH) foot prosthesis is a basic passive device.

L5560-L5590

L5560 Preparatory, above knee (AK), knee disarticulation, ischial level socket, nonalignable system, pylon, no cover, SACH foot, plaster socket, molded to model

L5570 Preparatory, above knee (AK), knee disarticulation, ischial level socket, nonalignable system, pylon, no cover, SACH foot, thermoplastic or equal, direct formed

L5580 Preparatory, above knee (AK), knee disarticulation, ischial level socket, nonalignable system, pylon, no cover, SACH foot, thermoplastic or equal, molded to model

L5585 Preparatory, above knee (AK), knee disarticulation, ischial level socket, nonalignable system, pylon, no cover, SACH foot, prefabricated adjustable open end socket

L5590 Preparatory, above knee (AK), knee disarticulation, ischial level socket, nonalignable system, pylon, no cover, SACH foot, laminated socket, molded to model

These codes report preparatory prostheses for knee disarticulations with ischial level sockets. Preparatory prostheses are transition devices between the initial rigid dressings and pylons applied post-surgery and the finished long-term prosthetic system. The codes are differentiated by the style of socket and the material used in its fabrication. Ischial level sockets embrace the thigh to the level of the ischial tuberosity, or so-called "sit bones." Preparatory sockets extending to this level are for transition and are unsuitable for aggressive ambulation. Permanent sockets for knee disarticulations are usually three-quarter-thigh length. As is typical with preparatory sockets, none can be aligned once fitted. A plaster socket, in this instance, is formed from bandages saturated with plaster of Paris applied over a previous cast model of the stump and ischium. A thermoplastic socket may be formed by applying heat to the rough-formed socket and modeling it to either the patient's stump and ischium directly or to a previously cast model of the stump. Another style of preparatory socket involves laminating together two or more resin-saturated materials over a previously cast model of the stump. Other preparatory sockets are prefabricated selected from mass-produced components based only on patient size and are adjustable. A pylon is a post-like structure fitted to the socket on one end and the prosthetic foot component on the other. It is a feature of most lower limb prosthetic designs. The pylon may be a tube made of aluminum, titanium, steel, or carbon fiber reinforced plastic and in early fittings is usually adjustable for length. Unlike many long-term prostheses, none of these units features cosmetic coverings, and none of the units reported by this range of codes features knee joints. A solid ankle, cushioned heel (SACH) foot prosthesis is a basic passive device.

L5595-L5600

L5595 Preparatory, hip disarticulation/hemipelvectomy, pylon, no cover, SACH foot, thermoplastic or equal, molded to patient model

L5600 Preparatory, hip disarticulation/hemipelvectomy, pylon, no cover, SACH foot, laminated socket, molded to patient model

These codes report preparatory prostheses for hip disarticulation/hemipelvectomy. Preparatory prostheses are a cosmetically unfinished functional replacement for an amputated extremity, fitted and aligned in accordance with sound biomechanical principles, which is worn for a limited period of time to expedite prosthetic wear and use and to aid in the evaluation of amputee adjustment. This transition device is used between the initial rigid dressings and pylons applied postsurgery and the finished long-term prosthetic system. Preparatory sockets extending to this level are for transition and are unsuitable for aggressive ambulation. As is typical with preparatory sockets, none can be aligned once fitted. A thermoplastic socket may be formed by applying heat to the rough-formed socket and modeling it to the patient's stump directly or to a previously cast model of the stump. Another style of preparatory socket involves laminating together two or more resin-saturated materials over a previously cast model of the stump. A pylon is a post-like structure fitted to the socket on one end and the prosthetic foot component on the other. It is a feature of most lower limb prosthetic designs. The pylon may be a tube made of aluminum, titanium, steel, or carbon fiber reinforced plastic and in early fittings is usually adjustable for length. Unlike many long-term prostheses, none of these units feature cosmetic coverings. None of the units reported by this range of codes feature knee joints. A solid ankle, cushioned heel (SACH) foot prosthesis is a basic passive device.

L5610

L5610 Addition to lower extremity, endoskeletal system, above knee (AK), hydracadence system

This code reports the addition of above knee devices to knee joints fitted to patients who have undergone above-the-knee amputation or disarticulation at the knee joint. This code reports the hydracadence system. Hydracadence knee is a single axis hydraulic knee whose specific feature is a unique functional coupling between the knee and the ankle joint during flexion and extension movements. It incorporates some ankle control, as well as swing-phase control. This system is available only in a metal frame, with a specially designed foot-ankle assembly. The swing-phase unit is a relatively simple piston type. In addition to control of the shank during swing phase, resistance to plantar flexion is controlled hydraulically, and motion between the ankle and knee are coordinated so that dorsiflexion of the ankle takes place after the knee has been flexed 20 degrees.

L5611-L5614

L5611 Addition to lower extremity, endoskeletal system, above knee (AK), knee disarticulation, four-bar linkage, with friction swing phase control

L5613 Addition to lower extremity, endoskeletal system, above knee (AK), knee disarticulation, four-bar linkage, with hydraulic swing phase control

L5614 Addition to lower extremity, exoskeletal system, above knee (AK), knee disarticulation, four-bar linkage, with pneumatic swing phase control

These codes report the addition of specific types of swing control devices to knee joints fitted to patients who have undergone above-the-knee amputation or disarticulation at the knee joint. The codes report supply of polycentric-type knee joints. Single-axis knee joints are capable of simple flexion and extension only. The polycentric joint offers greater range of motion. The center of rotation for a polycentric knee joint varies as the flexion angle changes. This feature offers the patient better toe clearance during the swing phase of gait. A common type of polycentric knee is known as the four-bar linkage. This device has four axes of rotation connected by four rigid linkages, and all codes in this range describe this type of knee component. Friction control over the knee joint means that the joint adjustments are tightened down to prevent unwanted movement during gait. Hydraulic swing phase control means the joint is fitted with a fluid-filled piston to dampen unwanted movement during gait, whereas pneumatic swing phase control involves an air-filled piston. All codes in the range report an endoskeletal prosthesis. In this type of design, a pylon, or pole, bears most of the weight load from the thigh to the prosthetic foot, rather than the exterior prosthetic shell in exoskeletal systems.

L5616

L5616 Addition to lower extremity, endoskeletal system, above knee (AK), universal multiplex system, friction swing phase control

This code reports an addition to an endoskeletal above-the-knee prosthesis of a specific design of knee joint. There are two major design differences for the shank component of a leg prosthesis. Endoskeletal shank designs transfer most of the weight from the residual limb to the prosthetic foot through a pylon, a post-like structure fitted to the socket on one end and the prosthetic foot component on the other. The pylon may be a tube made of aluminum, titanium, steel, or carbon fiber reinforced plastic. The pylon may be adjustable and may feature shock absorption characteristics. Most endoskeletal systems are modular and components can be fairly easily upgraded. The endoskeletal pylon system may be covered with an entirely cosmetic outer shell that resembles an actual leg. Exoskeletal designs feature a rigid and structural outer shell that transfers most of the weight from the residual limb to the prosthetic foot. Exoskeletal designs also usually have a pylon, but most of the weight is distributed by the shell. Exoskeletal systems are usually covered and painted to resemble an actual leg. In general, exoskeletal systems are considered durable and easy to maintain. Both systems offer special versions for active and athletic amputees. The universal multiplex is a particular design suited for moderately active use. This code reports friction swing phase control, which means the joint may be adjusted more tightly to control unwanted movement during gait. Report L5616 for addition of a universal multiplex system with friction swing phase control to an existing endoskeletal above-the-knee prosthesis.

L5617

L5617 Addition to lower extremity, quick change self-aligning unit, above knee (AK) or below knee (BK), each

This code reports a device that allows the distal section of the prosthetic to be quickly disconnected and reconnected whenever desired without loss of alignment.

L5618-L5628

L5618 Addition to lower extremity, test socket, Symes

L5620 Addition to lower extremity, test socket, below knee (BK)

L5622 Addition to lower extremity, test socket, knee disarticulation

L5624 Addition to lower extremity, test socket, above knee (AK)

L5626 Addition to lower extremity, test socket, hip disarticulation

L5628 Addition to lower extremity, test socket, hemipelvectomy

A socket is the portion of a prosthesis that fits around the residual limb (or stump) and to which prosthetic components are attached. Test sockets are typically soft and often have transparent fittings that allow the prosthetist to visualize the fit. A test socket tests the interface between the prosthesis and the residual limb. The use of a test/temporary socket allows a refinement in the fit and allows repeated modifications for increased comfort.

L5629

L5629 Addition to lower extremity, below knee, acrylic socket

This code reports an acrylic resin used to laminate the socket.

L5630

L5630 Addition to lower extremity, Symes type, expandable wall socket

This code reports the addition of a Symes-type expandable wall socket to a test socket. A socket is the portion of a prosthesis that fits around the residual limb (or stump) and to which prosthetic components are attached. Test sockets are typically soft and often have transparent fittings that allow the prosthetist to visualize the fit. A test socket tests the interface between the prosthesis and the residual limb. The eponym Symes derives from the Scottish surgeon James Syme, who introduced many orthopaedic procedures in the early 19th century. The Symes disarticulation at the ankle joint remains in common use.

L5631

L5631 Addition to lower extremity, above knee (AK) or knee disarticulation, acrylic socket

This code reports the addition of a specific variation to a test socket for knee disarticulations or above-the-knee amputations. A socket is the portion of a prosthesis that fits around the residual limb (or stump) and to which prosthetic components are attached. A test socket, also known as a "check" socket, tests the interface between the prosthesis and the residual limb. The type of socket reported by this code is of acrylic material that is often clear. A clear socket allows the prosthetist to visualize the fit and see points of contact and potential problem areas.

L5632-L5636

L5632 Addition to lower extremity, Symes type, PTB brim design socket

L5634 Addition to lower extremity, Symes type, posterior opening (Canadian) socket

L5636 Addition to lower extremity, Symes type, medial opening socket

These codes report the addition of specific alterations to test sockets. A socket is the portion of a prosthesis that fits around the residual limb (or stump) and to which prosthetic components are attached. Test sockets are typically soft and often have transparent fittings that allow the prosthetist to visualize the fit. A test socket tests the interface between the prosthesis and the residual limb. The eponym Symes derives from the Scottish surgeon James Syme, who introduced many orthopaedic procedures in the early 19th century. The Symes disarticulation at the ankle joint remains in common use. Among prostheses, however, Symes refers to a particular design in which a door is cut into the prosthetic device or, in this instance, the test socket. A patella tendon bearing (PTB) brim design is a socket that extends up to the area above the knee joint; the stump is held in place by the brim shape of the socket.

L5637-L5639

L5637 Addition to lower extremity, below knee (BK), total contact

L5638 Addition to lower extremity, below knee (BK), leather socket

L5639 Addition to lower extremity, below knee (BK), wood socket

These codes address socket variations for below-the-knee prostheses. A socket is the portion of a prosthesis that fits around the residual limb and to which prosthetic components are attached. Several test sockets may be required as the dimensions of the residual limb stabilize following amputation and as the musculature changes over time. A total contact socket, also known as a total surface bearing, is one that fully interfaces with the entire residual limb (or stump). Traditionally, there is a bit of space between the stump and the contact area of the test socket. This space is accessed and injected with a substance that dries to a gel-like consistency, conforming exactly to the shape of the stump and the socket. A total contact interface allows more surface area to bear weight against the prosthesis.

L5640

L5640 Addition to lower extremity, knee disarticulation, leather socket

A knee-disarticulation prosthesis is very similar to an above-knee prosthesis, except for the lower part of the socket and the knee mechanism. Before the introduction of the present day polycentric knee units, sockets for the prosthesis were usually made of leather and metal hinges were used to attach the

L

socket to the shin. Leather sockets are held on by a lacing.

L5642

L5642 Addition to lower extremity, above knee (AK), leather socket

This code reports an above knee leather socket. A leather socket has several advantages, including widespread availability, increased comfort in hot weather, and ease of adjustment to the stump as it becomes smaller. Also, leather is soft and easily takes the shape of the stump, and therefore self-corrects molding mistakes.

L5643

L5643 Addition to lower extremity, hip disarticulation, flexible inner socket, external frame

This code reports a hip disarticulation socket that utilizes a semi flexible, molded plastic inner socket that is supported by a rigid structural frame. Plastic sockets usually have a foam liner in the lower part for the bulbous end of the stump to slip by so as to keep the socket in place.

L5644

L5644 Addition to lower extremity, above knee (AK), wood socket

The oldest, traditional way of making artificial limbs is to make the socket out of wood. Wood always has a preponderant place in the fabrication of above knee sockets. Wood is easier to work on the actual object (the socket) rather than on its negative image (positive plaster). In the first fitting, corrections of depth, volume, and form are easy to make while maintaining an acceptable aspect for a definitive socket. When it comes to performing the final adjustments to a finished socket, the thickness of the medial border enables modifications to be effected that are difficult to make on a plastic socket, just as are modifications of volume.

L5645-L5653

L5645 Addition to lower extremity, below knee (BK), flexible inner socket, external frame

L5646 Addition to lower extremity, below knee (BK), air, fluid, gel or equal, cushion socket

L5647 Addition to lower extremity, below knee (BK), suction socket

L5648 Addition to lower extremity, above knee (AK), air, fluid, gel or equal, cushion socket

L5649 Addition to lower extremity, ischial containment/narrow M-L socket

L5650 Additions to lower extremity, total contact, above knee (AK) or knee disarticulation socket

L5651 Addition to lower extremity, above knee (AK), flexible inner socket, external frame

L5652 Addition to lower extremity, suction suspension, above knee (AK) or knee disarticulation socket

L5653 Addition to lower extremity, knee disarticulation, expandable wall socket

This range of codes addresses additions to lower extremity prostheses of test sockets. Above and below the knee amputations are addressed. A socket is the portion of a prosthesis that fits around the residual limb and to which prosthetic components are attached. Amputees consistently report that the comfort and fit of the socket is crucial to the success of the prosthesis. Test sockets are used to determine optimal interface between the patient's skin at the residual limb and the artificial material of the prosthesis. Several test sockets may be required as the dimensions of the residual limb stabilize following amputation and as the musculature changes over time. Some socket designs feature a flexible inner socket combined with an external frame and/or strapping. Air cushion sockets were developed for aggressive ambulation and running. Suction sockets usually employ a silicone interface. The vacuum is created by the natural properties of the silicone as the socket is donned and weight placed against the interface. Some systems feature a release button to aid in removal. An ischial containment socket is a traditional above-the-knee design by which the ischial tuberosity is contained within the walls of the socket (also known as "plug fit" or anatomical fit). The M-L socket is another variety of anatomical fit, above-the-knee designs. The M-L (medial-lateral) socket is tight fitting with most of the squeezing taking place on the lateral side followed by the medial side.

L5654-L5658

L5654 Addition to lower extremity, socket insert, Symes, (Kemblo, Pelite, Aliplast, Plastazote or equal)

L5655 Addition to lower extremity, socket insert, below knee (BK) (Kemblo, Pelite, Aliplast, Plastazote or equal)

L5656 Addition to lower extremity, socket insert, knee disarticulation (Kemblo, Pelite, Aliplast, Plastazote or equal)

L5658 Addition to lower extremity, socket insert, above knee (AK) (Kemblo, Pelite, Aliplast, Plastazote or equal)

Socket inserts help to protect the fragile skin of the residual limb while compensating for daily changes in limb volume. Some manufacturers of prostheses require socket inserts. Other designs can be comfortably fit without use of an insert. Irregular or bony residual limbs present complications that can be addressed by inserts. The codes in this range are differentiated by type of amputation and length of residual limb. Symes-type disarticulation occurs at the ankle joint with the fat pad of the heel preserved and rotated over the closure. The specific insert materials mentioned in the code descriptions are trade names for foams or other synthetic materials that are generally lightweight and can be molded and shaped when heat is applied.

L5661-L5665

L5661 Addition to lower extremity, socket insert, multidurometer Symes

L5665 Addition to lower extremity, socket insert, multidurometer, below knee (BK)

These codes report the supply of multidurometer socket inserts for either a Symes-type disarticulation at the ankle or a below-the-knee amputation. Some manufacturers of prostheses require socket inserts. Other designs can be comfortably fit without use of an insert. A durometer is a device to measure surface resiliency of material, and a firmness scale is used by fabricators of prosthetic devices. Multidurometer, in this context, is used to define an insert material made up of three or more materials, each with a different firmness rating. Combinations may include laminates of Plastazote, Poron, or other materials.

L5666

L5666 Addition to lower extremity, below knee (BK), cuff suspension

This code reports supply of a specific type of suspension socket for patients who have had below-the-knee amputation. A cuff is a gripping device that fits, in this instance, around the residual limb below the knee. A cuff is smaller than a corset or "lacer" but works similarly. It is made of rigid or semi-rigid material lined on the inside with cushioning material. The cuff may be closed snugly around the limb by straps, Velcro, or eyelet and gusset lacing. The socket and prosthesis may make full contact with the residual limb, particularly when weight is brought to bear, but the attachment integrity of the system is the suspension from the cuff.

L5668

L5668 Addition to lower extremity, below knee (BK), molded distal cushion

This code reports supply of a molded distal cushion addition to a prosthesis liner. These types of cushions are now made of viscoelastic materials; gel-like substances that may be molded or provided off-the-shelf. In this instance, the cushion is molded to a positive image of the residual distal stump for precise fit.

L5670-L5672

L5670 Addition to lower extremity, below knee (BK), molded supracondylar suspension (PTS or similar)

L5671 Addition to lower extremity, below knee (BK)/above knee (AK) suspension locking mechanism (shuttle, lanyard, or equal), excludes socket insert

L5672 Addition to lower extremity, below knee (BK), removable medial brim suspension

These codes report suspension style additions to lower extremity prostheses. A patella tendon bearing (PTB) type of prosthesis may have already been fitted to a below-the-knee amputation. Above-the-knee amputations may require the addition of a suspension-locking device to hold the prosthesis. The supracondylar suspension (PTS) is a prosthesis that suspends from the prominence of the condyles of the tibial plateau just distal to the knee joint. The prosthesis is allowed to hang from just below the knee joint until weight is placed upon it. A shuttle system incorporates a pin and lock at the bottom of the socket to suspend the prosthesis and may be used for amputations above or below the knee.

L5673

L5673 Addition to lower extremity, below knee (BK)/above knee (AK), custom fabricated from existing mold or prefabricated, socket insert, silicone gel, elastomeric or equal, for use with locking mechanism

This socket insert has an interface that surrounds the residual limb in a layer of skin friendly, mineral-oil based gel. Made from thermoplastic elastomer, the gel gently adheres to the skin to protect against abrasion and breakdown. The gel is covered in a layer of durable fabric that helps to extend the life of the liners and allows the amputees to easily slide into the sockets. These locking liners are designed for use with a shuttle lock and 10mm pin.

L

L5676

L5676 Additions to lower extremity, below knee (BK), knee joints, single axis, pair

This basic lower-extremity prosthesis includes a single-axis, constant friction knee. This device is a basic knee that acts as a door-and-hinge device, is free swinging and does not allow stance control. It allows one-speed ambulation and is often used in children.

L5677

L5677 Additions to lower extremity, below knee (BK), knee joints, polycentric, pair

The polycentric knee is a device that has multiple rotational axes and is sometimes referred to as the "four bar" knee. It has four points of rotation connected by a linkage bar. The device is very stable in early stance and easy to flex in swing phase.

L5678

L5678 Additions to lower extremity, below knee (BK), joint covers, pair

This is an accessory that aids in the effective use of a lower-limb prosthetic.

L5679

L5679 Addition to lower extremity, below knee (BK)/above knee (AK), custom fabricated from existing mold or prefabricated, socket insert, silicone gel, elastomeric or equal, not for use with locking mechanism

This socket insert has an interface that surrounds the residual limb in a layer of skin-friendly, mineral-oil based gel. Made from thermoplastic elastomer, the gel gently adheres to the skin to protect against abrasion and breakdown. The gel is covered in a layer of durable fabric that helps to extend the life of the liners and allows the amputees to easily slide into the sockets.

L5680

L5680 Addition to lower extremity, below knee (BK), thigh lacer, nonmolded

This code reports the supply of so-called thigh lacers, or corsets, for patients who have undergone below-the-knee amputations. These corset-like cuffs are often made of leather or composites and may be custom manufactured or off-the-shelf. Custom-made devices are usually molded to a positive image of the leg. The devices are typically closed using lacing through eyelets and gussets along the anterior face. A lower leg prosthesis is attached to the corset, usually by two vertical metal sidebars, thus forming a type of suspension system. At one time thigh lacers were a common form of suspension for transtibial prostheses. With the rise of total contact sockets, however, thigh lacer suspension has seen diminishing use. Thigh lacers still offer an advantage in that much of the weight is distributed from the thigh to the lower leg over the vertical sidebars and may be prescribed for patients who do not tolerate full contact pressure on the residual limb.

L5681

L5681 Addition to lower extremity, below knee (BK)/above knee (AK), custom fabricated socket insert for congenital or atypical traumatic amputee, silicone gel, elastomeric or equal, for use with or without locking mechanism, initial only (for other than initial, use code L5673 or L5679)

This is a polyurethane liner that sits directly against the skin. The suspension sleeve creates a seal between the prosthesis and the residual limb. One code is for an initial liner for a congenital or atypical traumatic amputee and the other for other than a congenital or atypical traumatic amputee.

L5682

L5682 Addition to lower extremity, below knee (BK), thigh lacer, gluteal/ischial, molded

This code reports the supply of so-called thigh lacers, or corsets, for patients who have undergone below-the-knee amputations. These corset-like cuffs are often made of leather or composites and may be custom manufactured or off-the-shelf. Custom-made devices are usually molded to a positive image of the leg. The devices are typically closed using lacing through eyelets and gussets along the anterior face. A lower leg prosthesis is attached to the corset, usually by two vertical metal sidebars, thus forming a type of suspension system. At one time thigh lacers were a common form of suspension for transtibial prostheses. With the rise of total contact sockets, however, thigh lacer suspension has seen diminishing use. Thigh lacers still offer an advantage in that much of the weight is distributed from the thigh to the lower leg over the vertical sidebars and may be prescribed for patients who do not tolerate full contact pressure on the residual limb.

L5683

L5683 Addition to lower extremity, below knee (BK)/above knee (AK), custom fabricated socket insert for other than congenital or atypical traumatic amputee, silicone gel, elastomeric or equal, for use with or without locking mechanism, initial only (for other than initial, use code L5673 or L5679)

This is a polyurethane liner that sits directly against the skin. The suspension sleeve creates a seal between the prosthesis and the residual limb. This code is for an initial liner for other than a congenital or atypical traumatic amputee.

L5684

L5684 Addition to lower extremity, below knee, fork strap

This type of suspension incorporates a fork strap, with or without a waist belt. A fork strap has two diagonal straps attached to a third strap. The advantages of straps are that they are patient adjustable and provide auxiliary suspension for participation in activities such as sports, hunting, or hiking.

L5685

L5685 Addition to lower extremity prosthesis, below knee, suspension/sealing sleeve, with or without valve, any material, each

This is a suspension component consisting of a sleeve that fits over the socket and onto the thigh of the wearer. A valve may or may not be incorporated into the sleeve.

L5686

L5686 Addition to lower extremity, below knee (BK), back check (extension control)

This code reports the supply of a device that, when added to a lower prosthesis, prevents the knee joint from hyperextension, or bending backward. This device may be a strap, blocking, or locking mechanism that prevents the artificial knee from moving beyond the position needed for normal standing.

L5688-L5690

L5688 Addition to lower extremity, below knee (BK), waist belt, webbing

L5690 Addition to lower extremity, below knee (BK), waist belt, padded and lined

Waist belt suspension is designed to work with transtibial prostheses. This belt is made of leather, cotton webbing, or nylon webbing and is worn around the patient's waist. Padding and/or a leather liner may be included to minimize the discomfort caused by the edges of the belt digging into the skin of the waist. An elastic strap extends from the belt to a leather strap attached to the medial and lateral (side) surfaces of the prosthetic socket. The design helps with extension of the residual limb and is indicated for patients with weak musculature. Waist belt suspension is primarily used for patients who have experienced difficulty with, or cannot tolerate, other forms of suspension.

L5692-L5695

L5692 Addition to lower extremity, above knee (AK), pelvic control belt, light

L5694 Addition to lower extremity, above knee (AK), pelvic control belt, padded and lined

L5695 Addition to lower extremity, above knee (AK), pelvic control, sleeve suspension, neoprene or equal, each

These codes report additions of pelvic control systems to above-the-knee amputation prosthetics. These are often belt systems worn around the lower waist. A light belt is a simple fabric belt worn around the lower waist. The Silesian belt consists of a broad and often padded belt that fits around the lower back and halfway around the hips. A thinner cinch belt fits over the broad portion and closes and adjusts the system. The belt systems partially suspend the prosthesis, usually from a single location on the lateral side. A sleeve suspension is pulled over the residual limb and in this instance extends over the ischium and pelvis. Neoprene is specifically cited in the code description, but gel-like materials made from silicon are probably used most often today.

L5696

L5696 Addition to lower extremity, above knee (AK) or knee disarticulation, pelvic joint

This code reports the addition of a pelvic joint to an above-the-knee amputation or pelvic joint disarticulation. The pelvic joint may be single or multiple axes and typically is mounted at the anterior of the prosthesis. Various designs and features are available. The joint allows for flexibility at the hip and may allow ambulation.

L5697-L5698

L5697 Addition to lower extremity, above knee (AK) or knee disarticulation, pelvic band

L5698 Addition to lower extremity, above knee (AK) or knee disarticulation, Silesian bandage

These codes report the supply of additional supports to an above-the-knee amputation or pelvic joint disarticulation prosthetic system. Most modern femoral amputation prostheses are designed to attach and hold firmly to the residual limb without use of hip belts or additional supports. In some instances, however, patients may require additional support or suspension in the form of pelvic bands or bandages. These are typically broad, padded bands or wrappings worn around the lower waist and from which the prosthesis can be attached. The site of attachment is usually at a lateral and/or anterior location on the prosthesis.

L5699

L5699 All lower extremity prostheses, shoulder harness

This code reports the supply of a shoulder harness support to an above-the-knee amputation or a pelvic joint disarticulation prosthetic system. Most modern femoral amputation prostheses are designed to attach and hold firmly to the residual limb without use of hip belts or additional supports at the shoulder. In some instances, however, patients may require additional support or suspension in the form of a shoulder harness. This type of device may involve both shoulders or be a simpler single-shoulder harness sling. The site of attachment is usually at a lateral and/or anterior location on the prosthesis.

L5700-L5703

L5700 Replacement, socket, below knee (BK), molded to patient model

L5701 Replacement, socket, above knee (AK)/knee disarticulation, including attachment plate, molded to patient model

L5702 Replacement, socket, hip disarticulation, including hip joint, molded to patient model

L5703 Ankle, Symes, molded to patient model, socket without solid ankle cushion heel (SACH) foot, replacement only

These codes report replacement for molded sockets for lower limb prosthetic systems. The codes are differentiated by the level of amputation. Amputation patients routinely see significant daily changes in the volume and physical dimensions of the residual limb, or stump. This challenge is addressed as best as possible by fitting test or "check" sockets during the early phase of adjustment to a prosthetic limb. Liners and stockings of varying thickness also compensate for volume changes in the stump. Terminal sockets designed for extended use have limited life spans and must be changed out for various reasons, including changes in stump volume. These codes report supply of a replacement socket molded to a plaster positive model taken of the residual limb. Changes in the limb may require that a new model be prepared, or an earlier model may still be workable. Increasingly, computer models and scans are used. The socket material may be heat molded or otherwise shaped to conform precisely to the patient model.

L5704-L5707

L5704 Custom shaped protective cover, below knee (BK)

L5705 Custom shaped protective cover, above knee (AK)

L5706 Custom shaped protective cover, knee disarticulation

L5707 Custom shaped protective cover, hip disarticulation

A custom-shaped protective covering for a prosthesis is one of two general varieties. Prostheses with internal supports (endoskeletal) usually feature an outer protective cover made of closed cell foam and a skin-color finish. Externally supported prostheses (exoskeletal) usually feature a hard, synthetic shell, also usually finished to resemble human skin. Both varieties may start out from an off-the-shelf blank but are carefully customized to match the size and length, thickness, and coloring of an opposing or lost limb. This range of codes reports the replacement of these protective outer surface cover systems (POSCS).

L5710

L5710 Addition, exoskeletal knee-shin system, single axis, manual lock

This code refers to an addition of a manual lock to a single-axis knee/shin system. A manual locking knee incorporates an automatic lock that can be unlocked voluntarily. The manual locking knee is appropriate for weak or unstable patients as well as more active individuals who frequently walk on unstable terrain.

L5711

L5711 Additions exoskeletal knee-shin system, single axis, manual lock, ultra-light material

This code refers to an addition of a manual lock to a single-axis knee/shin system made of ultra-light material. A manual locking knee incorporates an automatic lock that can be unlocked voluntarily. The manual locking knee is appropriate for weak or unstable patients as well as more active individuals who frequently walk on unstable terrain.

L5712

L5712 Addition, exoskeletal knee-shin system, single axis, friction swing and stance phase control (safety knee)

This is a transfemoral or hip disarticulation knee/shin unit that is unicentric and locks when weight is placed on it (otherwise known as stance locking).

L5714

L5714 Addition, exoskeletal knee-shin system, single axis, variable friction swing phase control

This code refers to a mechanical variable friction knee unit that utilizes two brakes to terminate the flexion and extension portions of swing phase, simulating the functions of the quadriceps and hamstring muscles. The deceleration and braking function is performed by two bumpers attached to a tubular knee bolt, which provide continuous friction throughout the gait cycle.

L5716

L5716 Addition, exoskeletal knee-shin system, polycentric, mechanical stance phase lock

The geometric lock feature, also referred to as a mechanical stance phase lock, locks the knee on full extension (initial contact) and does not release it until the weight line passes over the forefoot and the knee unit is hyperextended. Mechanical-knee users must exert muscular and mechanical control to alter speed and step length. This provides stability in the weight-bearing phase of gait.

L5718

L5718 Addition, exoskeletal knee-shin system, polycentric, friction swing and stance phase control

Friction is used in the knee to control the knee joint during walking. Friction controls how far and how fast the knee bends and straightens during gait. A manual locking knee incorporates an automatic lock that can be unlocked voluntarily. The manual locking knee is appropriate for weak or unstable patients as well as more active individuals who frequently walk on unstable terrain.

L5722

L5722 Addition, exoskeletal knee-shin system, single axis, pneumatic swing, friction stance phase control

This code refers to a hydraulic unit that includes piston cylinders and contains air (pneumatic) added to the knee device to allow swing control as the amputee speeds up or slows down. Swing control may allow the amputee to walk at variable speeds. The limitation of the lack of stance control can be addressed by locking knee or safety knee features.

L5724

L5724 Addition, exoskeletal knee-shin system, single axis, fluid swing phase control

This is a hydraulic knee control unit that includes a knee/shin set-up that is unicentric and controls swing phase only.

L5726

L5726 Addition, exoskeletal knee-shin system, single axis, external joints, fluid swing phase control

This is a hydraulic knee control unit that consists of a knee/shin set-up that is unicentric with external uprights above the knee center and that controls swing phase only.

L5728

L5728 Addition, exoskeletal knee-shin system, single axis, fluid swing and stance phase control

This is a hydraulic knee control unit that includes the knee/shin set-up that is unicentric and controls both swing and stance.

L5780

L5780 Addition, exoskeletal knee-shin system, single axis, pneumatic/hydra pneumatic swing phase control

This is a hydra-pneumatic knee unit that is unicentric and is for swing phase control and provides smooth, coordinated hip and knee motion.

L5781-L5782

L5781 Addition to lower limb prosthesis, vacuum pump, residual limb volume management and moisture evacuation system

L5782 Addition to lower limb prosthesis, vacuum pump, residual limb volume management and moisture evacuation system, heavy-duty

These codes report a specialized vacuum system for the socket. Amputation patients routinely see significant daily changes in the volume and physical dimensions of the residual limb, or stump. This volume can change significantly in the course of a day and some suction socket systems are believed to exacerbate short-term volume loss. The vacuum system reported by these codes is designed to create a greater vacuum between the liner and the wall of the socket than is found in standard suction socket systems. Moisture trapped between the liner and socket is also removed. The system purportedly stabilizes volume fluctuation in the residual limb.

L5785-L5795

L5785 Addition, exoskeletal system, below knee (BK), ultra-light material (titanium, carbon fiber or equal)

L5790 Addition, exoskeletal system, above knee (AK), ultra-light material (titanium, carbon fiber or equal)

L5795 Addition, exoskeletal system, hip disarticulation, ultra-light material (titanium, carbon fiber or equal)

These codes report the addition of ultra-light weight material components to an exoskeletal lower limb prosthesis. The codes are differentiated by level of amputation. Two major types of lower limb prostheses are currently offered. Endoskeletal shank designs transfer most of the weight from the residual limb to the prosthetic foot through a pylon, a post-like structure fitted to the socket on one end and the prosthetic foot component on the other. The pylon may be a tube made of aluminum, titanium, steel, or carbon fiber-reinforced plastic. Most endoskeletal systems are modular and components can be fairly easily upgraded. The endoskeletal pylon system may be covered with an entirely cosmetic outer shell that resembles an actual leg. Exoskeletal designs feature a rigid and structural outer shell that transfers most of the weight from the residual limb to the prosthetic foot. Exoskeletal designs also often have a pylon, but most of the weight is distributed by the shell. Exoskeletal systems are usually covered and painted to resemble an actual leg. In general, exoskeletal systems are considered durable and easy to maintain. Both systems offer special versions for active and athletic amputees. These codes report modification to an exoskeletal system by the addition of carbon fiber, titanium, or other lightweight materials, either to the pylon component, the exoskeletal shell, or both.

L5810-L5812

L5810 Addition, endoskeletal knee-shin system, single axis, manual lock

L5811 Addition, endoskeletal knee-shin system, single axis, manual lock, ultra-light material

L5812 Addition, endoskeletal knee-shin system, single axis, friction swing and stance phase control (safety knee)

These codes report additions to endoskeletal prosthetic systems of single axis knees. Endoskeletal shank designs transfer most of the weight from the residual limb to the prosthetic foot through a pylon, a post-like structure fitted to the socket on one end and the prosthetic foot component on the other. The pylon may be a tube made of aluminum, titanium, steel, or carbon fiber-reinforced plastic. Most endoskeletal systems are modular and components can be easily upgraded. The endoskeletal pylon system may be covered with a cosmetic outer shell that resembles an actual leg. Addition of a single axis knee joint to an endoskeletal system entails proper interface with the upper component and the pylon (shin) component. A single axis joint is capable of straight-on flexion and extension only. The type reported by L5810 features a locking pin that maintains the standing position. The device must be manually released for the patient to flex the joint and to sit down. Friction control over the knee joint means that the adjustments can be tightened down to prevent unwanted joint movement, especially during gait. The joint also features a braking or locking mechanism to maintain proper standing position and to prevent overextension of the joint.

L5814-L5818

L5814 Addition, endoskeletal knee-shin system, polycentric, hydraulic swing phase control, mechanical stance phase lock

L5816 Addition, endoskeletal knee-shin system, polycentric, mechanical stance phase lock

L5818 Addition, endoskeletal knee-shin system, polycentric, friction swing and stance phase control

These codes report additions to endoskeletal prosthetic systems of multiple axis, or polycentric knee joints. These knees flex and extend like single axis joints, but also offer limited lateral movement and twisting action. Endoskeletal shank designs transfer most of the weight from the residual limb to the prosthetic foot through a pylon, a post-like structure fitted to the socket on one end and the prosthetic foot component on the other. The pylon may be a tube made of aluminum, titanium, steel, or carbon fiber-reinforced plastic. Most endoskeletal systems are modular and components can be easily upgraded. The endoskeletal pylon system may be covered with a cosmetic outer shell that resembles an actual leg. Addition of a single axis knee joint to an endoskeletal system entails proper interface with the upper component and the pylon (shin) component. A hydraulic cylinder may be used to assist joint movement, especially during the swing phase of gait. A locking mechanism or a friction brake may be added to support the system as the patient stands.

L5822-L5830

L5822 Addition, endoskeletal knee-shin system, single axis, pneumatic swing, friction stance phase control

L5824 Addition, endoskeletal knee-shin system, single axis, fluid swing phase control

L5826 Addition, endoskeletal knee-shin system, single axis, hydraulic swing phase control, with miniature high activity frame

L5828 Addition, endoskeletal knee-shin system, single axis, fluid swing and stance phase control

L5830 Addition, endoskeletal knee-shin system, single axis, pneumatic/swing phase control

These codes report additions to endoskeletal prosthetic systems of single axis knee joints. Specific devices are added to the joints to assist the swing phase of gait and sometimes to control stance, or standing. Single axis knee joints are capable of simple flexion and extension only. Endoskeletal shank designs transfer most of the weight from the residual limb to the prosthetic foot through a pylon, a post-like structure fitted to the socket on one end and the prosthetic foot component on the other. The pylon may be a tube made of aluminum, titanium, steel, or carbon fiber-reinforced plastic. Most endoskeletal systems are modular and components can be easily upgraded. The endoskeletal pylon system may be covered with a cosmetic outer shell that resembles an actual leg. Friction control over the knee joint means that adjustments can be tightened down to slow down joint movement, especially during gait. Consequently, friction control joints may be fitted with assistance devices to help extend the joint during the swing phase of gait. These devices may employ a cylinder filled with air or gas (pneumatic) or fluids such as oil (hydraulic). Pressure in the cylinder forces a piston to assist movement of the joint while dampening impact during heel strike. The pressure may also be employed to act as a brake to control joint movement while standing. A high activity frame is a supportive structure around the knee joint and is designed for high levels of activity and uneven terrain. The framework may assist in special functions such as shortening the shin component for better heel and toe clearance over uneven terrain.

L5840

L5840 Addition, endoskeletal knee-shin system, four-bar linkage or multiaxial, pneumatic swing phase control

This code refers to an addition of a specific endoskeletal knee-shin system known for its multiaxial features. Endoskeletal shank designs

L

transfer most of the weight from the residual limb to the prosthetic foot through a pylon, a post-like structure fitted to the socket on one end with the prosthetic foot component on the other. The pylon may be a tube made of aluminum, titanium, steel, or carbon fiber-reinforced plastic. Most endoskeletal systems are modular, and components can be easily upgraded. The endoskeletal pylon system may be covered with a cosmetic outer shell that resembles an actual leg. As the name denotes, a four-bar joint system features four vertical bars paired anteriorly and posteriorly, and superior and inferior hinges are linked together to pivot the joint. The additional bars affect the center of gravity and provide for a stable joint. Other multiaxial joints may feature bearings or other innovations to provide additional movement. Certain joints may be fitted with assistance devices to help extend and/or flex the joint during the swing phase of gait. These devices may employ a cylinder filled with air or gas (pneumatic). Pressure in the cylinder forces a piston to assist movement of the joint while dampening impact during heel strike.

L5845

L5845 Addition, endoskeletal knee-shin system, stance flexion feature, adjustable

This code refers to an addition to an endoskeletal knee-shin system of an adjustable stance flexion feature. Endoskeletal shank designs transfer most of the weight from the residual limb to the prosthetic foot through a pylon, a post-like structure fitted to the socket on one end and the prosthetic foot component on the other. The pylon may be a tube made of aluminum, titanium, steel, or carbon fiber-reinforced plastic. Most endoskeletal systems are modular, and components can be easily upgraded. The endoskeletal pylon system may be covered with a cosmetic outer shell that resembles an actual leg. This code reports the addition of an adjustable device that limits movement of the knee joint while standing, while still assisting the bending, or flexion, of the joint during gait. This type of device may be piston-driven, either pneumatic or hydraulic. Some models activate stance control as the patient "bounces" weight on the knee, which locks and unlocks the device for prolonged standing.

L5848

L5848 Addition to endoskeletal knee-shin system, fluid stance extension, dampening feature, with or without adjustability

This code reports the addition to a knee-shin endoskeletal system of an adjustable fluid stance extension with dampening feature, with or without adjustability addition. Endoskeletal shank designs transfer most of the weight from the residual limb to the prosthetic foot through a pylon, a post-like structure fitted to the socket on one end and the prosthetic foot component on the other. The pylon may be a tube made of aluminum, titanium, steel, or carbon fiber-reinforced plastic. Most endoskeletal systems are modular and components can be easily upgraded. The endoskeletal pylon system may be covered with a cosmetic outer shell that resembles an actual leg. This type of addition is to a knee joint prosthesis and involves the use of a hydraulic driven device. Fluid such as oil is compressed in a chamber. As the joint moves, the oil is further compressed or relaxed, which governs the stance phase of the prosthesis. The compression chamber further works to dampen shock as weight is placed on the fully extended joint to engage the stance phase. Most of these designs are integrated into the joint interior. Adjustments allow the patient to open and close valves to control fluid movement through the chambers.

L5850-L5855

L5850 Addition, endoskeletal system, above knee (AK) or hip disarticulation, knee extension assist

L5855 Addition, endoskeletal system, hip disarticulation, mechanical hip extension assist

These codes refer to the addition of mechanical joint assists to prosthetic joints of the knee or hip. Various prosthetic joint designs are available, particularly for endoskeletal systems with knee components. Almost all feature some type of control to temper joint movement when not needed. Constant friction control involves adjusting tension against the joint pivot, essentially making it more difficult to move throughout its range. Other designs may involve external brakes that slow or stop joint action, particularly in the full extension stance phase. Mechanical assist devices are often added to prosthetic joints to make them move more easily in one direction, particularly during the swing phase of gait. These devices may feature an air-filled or fluid-filled cylinder and piston design that helps to push the knee joint into extension. Others may entail spring action to operate the mechanical assistance. Prosthetic hip joints are usually on the anterior side near the top of the femoral pylon somewhat removed from the natural anatomic location. Disarticulation of the hip constitutes only about 2 percent of lower-limb amputations. Several types of mechanical assistance designs are used for hip joints. Some employ cords with elastic properties to assist flexion. More modern designs entail spring-driven assistance devices with components integrated into the joint.

L5856

L5856 Addition to lower extremity prosthesis, endoskeletal knee-shin system, microprocessor control feature, swing and stance phase, includes electronic sensor(s), any type

This is a computerized limb prosthesis that is a nonstandard, external prosthetic device that incorporates a microprocessor for movement control.

This use of a microprocessor control in both the swing and stance phases of gait improves stance control and may provide increased safety, stability, and function; for example, the sensors are designed to recognize a stumble and stiffen the knee, thus avoiding a fall. Other potential benefits of microprocessor-controlled knee prostheses are improved ability to navigate stairs, slopes, and uneven terrain, and reduction in energy expenditure and concentration required for ambulation.

L5857

L5857 Addition to lower extremity prosthesis, endoskeletal knee-shin system, microprocessor control feature, swing phase only, includes electronic sensor(s), any type

This is a computerized limb prosthesis that is a nonstandard, external prosthetic device incorporating a microprocessor for movement control. These devices are equipped with a sensor that detects when the knee is in full extension and adjusts the swing phase automatically, permitting a more natural walking pattern of varying speeds.

L5858

L5858 Addition to lower extremity prosthesis, endoskeletal knee-shin system, microprocessor control feature, stance phase only, includes electronic sensor(s), any type

This is a computerized limb prosthesis that is a nonstandard, external prosthetic device incorporating a microprocessor for movement control. This device improves stance control and may provide increased safety, stability, and function; for example, the sensors are designed to recognize a stumble and stiffen the knee, thus avoiding a fall.

L5859

L5859 Addition to lower extremity prosthesis, endoskeletal knee-shin system, powered and programmable flexion/extension assist control, includes any type motor(s)

A motorized prosthetic knee is provided as an addition to a lower extremity prosthetic. The knee contains an electromechanical actuator that actively initiates and controls all aspects of the user's gait. It also provides powered knee flexion and extension for the patient. The knee functions based on data collected through accelerometers, gyroscopes, a torque sensor, and a load sensor. When the patient walks, the addition samples knee position and loads at a high rate of speed. It is able to help replace hip, leg, and foot muscle function to allow a more natural gait and stance. It also provides stability and support and reduces impact to the patient. The motor in the knee is battery operated.

L5910-L5920

L5910 Addition, endoskeletal system, below knee (BK), alignable system

L5920 Addition, endoskeletal system, above knee (AK) or hip disarticulation, alignable system

These codes report the addition of an alignable system for lower extremity endoskeletal prostheses. Alignment of the prosthesis usually occurs during the latter phases of the manufacturing process. Endoskeletal systems feature internal supports. Preliminary alignment of an above-the-knee prosthesis may occur at a fitting session before the protective covering is applied. Ordinarily, however, alignment is performed at the time of final fitting. Below-the-knee systems sometimes feature alignment settings for the foot/ankle component that can be adjusted by the person who wears the prosthesis.

L5925

L5925 Addition, endoskeletal system, above knee (AK), knee disarticulation or hip disarticulation, manual lock

This code reports the addition of a manual lock to a hip or knee joint of an endoskeletal system for above-the-knee amputation or hip disarticulation. A manual lock to a joint prosthesis is usually designed to be easily engaged and disengaged by the wearer. Some may feature a ring or lever that pulls a cable triggering locking mechanism. The lock itself may be a simple drop-pin design that engages the two main components of the joint, usually in full extension. This allows the patient to confidently stand without worry that the joint will collapse into flexion or hyperextend backward. The wearer must actively disengage the lock to allow the joint to flex for sitting. For some prostheses, the lock is engaged for walking as well as standing. Some manual locks can be engaged while the joint is in any variety of positions as needed by the user.

L5930

L5930 Addition, endoskeletal system, high activity knee control frame

This code refers to the addition of a high-activity knee control frame to an endoskeletal prosthesis. Lower-limb prosthesis users are usually classified in some manner according to their physical abilities. Those with good prospects for high activity levels and athletes may be fitted with special adaptations to accommodate additional stresses on the knee prosthesis. A knee control frame is usually employed in more advanced prostheses and is most often used to support high-end joint components to accommodate extreme use. These typically include a polycentric knee joint with hydraulic features and possibly microprocessor controls.

L

L5940

L5940 Addition, endoskeletal system, below knee (BK), ultra-light material (titanium, carbon fiber or equal)

This is a global code that includes ultra-light materials and encompasses all areas of a below-knee prosthesis.

L5950

L5950 Addition, endoskeletal system, above knee (AK), ultra-light material (titanium, carbon fiber or equal)

This is a global code that includes ultra-light materials and encompasses all areas of an above knee prosthesis.

L5960

L5960 Addition, endoskeletal system, hip disarticulation, ultra-light material (titanium, carbon fiber or equal)

An endoskeletal system is an internal support composed of natural skeletal parts or artificial parts that replace missing natural parts. This system is used to replace an entire lower limb that was removed at the hip joint. Ultralight materials allow greater ease in movement.

L5961

L5961 Addition, endoskeletal system, polycentric hip joint, pneumatic or hydraulic control, rotation control, with or without flexion and/or extension control

An endoskeletal system is an internal support composed of natural skeletal parts or artificial parts that replace missing natural parts. A polycentric hip joint with pneumatic or hydraulic control is a three-dimensional joint system using mechanical means to mimic natural hip movement.

L5962-L5966

L5962 Addition, endoskeletal system, below knee (BK), flexible protective outer surface covering system

L5964 Addition, endoskeletal system, above knee (AK), flexible protective outer surface covering system

L5966 Addition, endoskeletal system, hip disarticulation, flexible protective outer surface covering system

These codes refer to a skin-like material that is either brushed or sprayed over the soft foam covering that is attached to the outside of a definitive prosthesis that forms a water- and tear-resistant flexible surface.

L5968

L5968 Addition to lower limb prosthesis, multiaxial ankle with swing phase active dorsiflexion feature

This code reports the addition of a specific design of multiaxial ankle to a lower limb prosthesis. A multiaxial ankle prosthesis is capable of dorsiflexion and plantarflexion (the single axis movement of the foot up and down), as well as limited twisting motion and medial and lateral movement. This offers stability and allows the user to better negotiate uneven terrain. In addition, this prosthesis automatically moves the foot into dorsiflexion (foot up) during the swing phase of gait to prepare for heel strike. This feature may be accomplished several ways. A spring-loaded cylinder acting on a piston rod is one approach. Spring tension pushes the heel down and raises the forefoot into dorsiflexion. Other designs may be activated by energy storing capabilities as weight is released from the foot.

L5969

L5969 Addition, endoskeletal ankle-foot or ankle system, power assist, includes any type motor(s)

An endoskeletal system is an internal support composed of natural skeletal parts or artificial parts that replace missing natural parts. A polycentric hip joint with pneumatic or hydraulic control is a three-dimensional joint system using mechanical means to mimic natural hip movement. The power assist add-on component is mounted to a conventionally functioning ankle-foot component within a custom orthotic and adds the prescribed function to dynamic assist/resist as required. This addition is used to improve stability and walking functions.

L5970-L5972

L5970 All lower extremity prostheses, foot, external keel, SACH foot

L5971 All lower extremity prostheses, solid ankle cushion heel (SACH) foot, replacement only

L5972 All lower extremity prostheses, foot, flexible keel

These codes report the supply of a variety of prosthetic foot types. The keel of a prosthetic foot is the rigid (or spring-like) section that generally runs from heel to toe near the footplate. It may serve merely as a structural piece, as in designs using wooden or rigid keels. In other designs, the keel absorbs impact and transfers energy as weight rolls from heel strike to "toe-off," the moment when weight is released from the forefoot. The keel may be made of wood, plastic, carbon-reinforced fibers, or metal. An external keel, as the name implies, is exposed and the prosthesis may be hollow, or exoskeletal. A solid ankle, cushion heel type foot is known by the acronym SACH and a variety of models are available. In some, the external keel is part of the shell. Flexible keels are integral components of many energy storing prosthetic feet. A stationary ankle, flexible exoskeleton type of foot is known by the acronym SAFE. These types of prosthetic feet have flexible keels, either internally or as external components of the shell. The SAFE foot is known for its ability to slightly invert and evert and to absorb shock. Some designs of SACH and SAFE feet have a pylon-type bolt that penetrates through the prosthesis and connects to the ankle component and pylon. The STEN foot is named for "STored ENergy," which is largely accomplished through use of a flexible keel and other resilient materials.

L5973

L5973 Endoskeletal ankle foot system, microprocessor controlled feature, dorsiflexion and/or plantar flexion control, includes power source

Endoskeletal ankle foot system, microprocessor controlled feature, dorsiflexion and/or plantar flexion control, includes power source is an electronic, microprocessor controlled prosthetic ankle-foot system. This system was designed to assist lower extremity amputees with walking on level ground or on uneven terrain, up and down inclines and declines, up and down stairs, and standing up from a sitting position. The system permits a more dynamic, real-time adjustment of the prosthetic as the patient takes a step.

L5974-L5975

L5974 All lower extremity prostheses, foot, single axis ankle/foot

L5975 All lower extremity prostheses, combination single axis ankle and flexible keel foot

These codes report the supply of specific types of prosthetic feet. A single axis ankle is capable of dorsiflexion and plantarflexion only (the movement of the foot up and down). This is among the more fundamental designs of prosthetic feet. The keel is the component of a prosthetic foot that generally runs from heel to toe near the footplate. A flexible keel may be made of carbon reinforced fibers, metal, or resilient materials. The flexible keel absorbs impact and transfers energy as weight rolls from heel strike to "toe-off," the moment when weight is released from the forefoot. Flexible keels are integral components of many energy storing prosthetic feet.

L5976

L5976 All lower extremity prostheses, energy storing foot (Seattle Carbon Copy II or equal)

This code refers to the supply of a specific level of energy-storing prosthetic foot, whereby some type of material deforms with weight pressure but then resumes its original shape as pressure is removed with a consequent release of energy. The keel is the component of a prosthetic foot that generally runs from heel to toe near the footplate. A flexible keel, which may be made of carbon-reinforced fibers, metal, or resilient materials, absorbs impact and transfers energy as weight rolls from heel strike to "toe-off" the moment when weight is released from the forefoot. Flexible keels are integral components of many energy-storing prosthetic feet.

L5978-L5979

L5978 All lower extremity prostheses, foot, multiaxial ankle/foot

L5979 All lower extremity prostheses, multiaxial ankle, dynamic response foot, one-piece system

These codes report the supply of a specific type of foot prosthesis. A multi-axial ankle is capable of dorsiflexion and plantarflexion (the movement of the foot up and down), as well as limited twisting motion, medial and lateral movement, and internal and external rotation. This offers stability and allows the user to better negotiate uneven terrain. The dynamic response foot is a type of energy storing prosthetic foot. It falls well within the range of active use, but somewhat short of the high-end athletic prostheses. The keel in this type of foot is energy absorbing with good transfer upon "toe-off." Sure-Flex, Genesis II, and Seattle Lite are considered in this category.

L5980-L5981

L5980 All lower extremity prostheses, flex-foot system

L5981 All lower extremity prostheses, flex-walk system or equal

These codes report the supply of a specific type of foot prosthesis. The original flex-foot system was a unique design to accommodate active users. The foot was developed in the early 1980s using a single L-shaped strip of carbon fiber, which at the time was a material new to prosthesis fabrication. The lower horizontal portion was fitted to sole material, and the upper vertical part was attached to the pylon. A separate strip was attached to the rear of the footplate like a leaf spring to act as the heel. The design provides springlike compression action, as well as some torque and flexibility properties. The foot is known for high flexibility and good energy-storing capabilities and remains in widespread use. The flex-walk system is a second generation of the flex-foot design and addresses the needs of amputees with longer residual limbs with moderate activity levels, as well as pediatric applications. Both versions adapt well to both endoskeletal and exoskeletal shank designs.

L5982-L5984

L5982 All exoskeletal lower extremity prostheses, axial rotation unit

L5984 All endoskeletal lower extremity prostheses, axial rotation unit, with or without adjustability

When the prosthesis incorporates an axial rotation device, this net torque acting about the long axis of the socket is able to rotate the socket externally, the only resistance to such rotation being the relatively weak return spring in the axial rotation device. The axial rotation tends to relieve the contact pressures that caused the torque and thus reduces pressures in the critical anteromedial region of the brim. With an axial rotation device, the socket is free to respond to the demands of the stump and relieve the pressures and torque caused by cyclic action of the musculature.

L5985

L5985 All endoskeletal lower extremity prostheses, dynamic prosthetic pylon

This code reports the supply of a dynamic pylon for a lower-extremity prosthesis system. A pylon is a post-like structure fitted to the residual limb socket on one end and the prosthetic foot component on the other. The pylon may be a tube made of aluminum, titanium, steel, or carbon fiber-reinforced plastic. A dynamic pylon has energy-storing properties, typically provided by an internal spring or series of springs. Some models, such as the Endolite telescopic torsion pylon, also allow for some twisting movement. The energy-return feature absorbs shock and in some users provides gait efficiency with less energy outlay.

L5986

L5986 All lower extremity prostheses, multiaxial rotation unit (MCP or equal)

This code reports the supply of a multiaxial system for artificial ankles that incorporate rubber compression springs bonded to reversible adapters. This allows the adapters to be bolted to the ankle plate and function with the maximum efficiency in all the planes of motion.

L5987

L5987 All lower extremity prostheses, shank foot system with vertical loading pylon

This code refers to a pylon foot system that deflects vertically on weight bearing and reflexes to its original posture as it is unloaded.

L5988

L5988 Addition to lower limb prosthesis, vertical shock reducing pylon feature

This code reports the supply of a vertical shock-reducing pylon for a lower-extremity prosthesis system. A pylon is a post-like structure fitted to the residual limb socket on one end and the prosthetic foot component on the other. The pylon may be a tube made of aluminum, titanium, steel, or carbon fiber-reinforced plastic. A pylon may be fitted with a device to absorb vertical shock, as occurs during heel strike. These additions have energy-storing properties, typically provided by an internal spring or series of springs. This feature absorbs shock and in some users provides gait efficiency with less energy outlay.

L5990

L5990 Addition to lower extremity prosthesis, user adjustable heel height

The adjustable heel height prosthetic foot is an anatomical gliding ankle that maintains appropriate foot alignment to provide knee stability and consistent performance at all heel heights. A person can adjust the heel to accommodate wearing a sandal to wearing a two-inch heel on a dress shoe.

L5999

L5999 Lower extremity prosthesis, not otherwise specified

A lower extremity prosthetic is used to replace function for a patient who is missing all or part of a leg or foot. Use this code to report a lower extremity prosthetic when there is not a more specific HCPCS Level II code available.

L6000-L6020

L6000 Partial hand, thumb remaining

L6010 Partial hand, little and/or ring finger remaining

L6020 Partial hand, no finger remaining

This range of codes reports the supply of a traditional type of shoulder-powered hand prosthesis. They are designed for patients with partial hand amputation. The prosthesis is functional through use of a simple mechanical shoulder harness with a cable extending to the prosthesis. The length of socket depends on the amputation and the types of tasks demanded of the prosthesis. Heavy-duty use typically requires a deeper socket. A cosmetic glove-like covering may finish the prosthesis. A two-position prosthetic thumb is used when that digit is missing. Other digits may feature single or multiple joints.

L6026

L6026 Transcarpal/metacarpal or partial hand disarticulation prosthesis, external power, self-suspended, inner socket with removable forearm section, electrodes and cables, two batteries, charger, myoelectric control of terminal device, excludes terminal device(s)

A myoelectric prosthesis of the hand is an electronic device used as a replacement for an amputation at the transcarpal or metacarpal area. This type of prosthesis uses an external battery pack to supply power to electric motors and microprocessors that control the movement of the device in different directions. The myoelectric prosthetic has a more realistic appearance and provides the patient with increased function. Control of the device is through skin electrodes inside the socket of the prosthetic. The electrodes can detect and amplify the electrical activity of muscle groups left in the hand. These impulses are cycled through the microprocessor units and result in movement of the hand through electric motors.

L6050-L6055

L6050 Wrist disarticulation, molded socket, flexible elbow hinges, triceps pad

L6055 Wrist disarticulation, molded socket with expandable interface, flexible elbow hinges, triceps pad

These codes report the supply of hand prostheses for disarticulations at the wrist. As is typical of traditional below-the-elbow prostheses, an upper-arm harness assists the mechanical operation. Movement is transferred by cable from the harness to the prosthesis. A cuff or half-cuff is situated over the triceps muscle. Paired medial and lateral elbow hinges act as leverage points to assist movement. The socket is the interface between the residual limb and the prosthesis. Traditionally, a plaster mold is taken of the residual stump and a positive replica is made. The socket is then vacuum fitted to the replica. A socket may be made from any variety of materials, although modern ones are increasingly fabricated from thermoplastic resins or elastic sleeves. Many are designed for use with gel liners. Patients with wrist disarticulation amputations can retain a high level of pronation and supination movement. An expandable interface at the socket end may be fashioned to accommodate limb growth in children or for interchangeable prostheses.

L6100-L6110

L6100 Below elbow, molded socket, flexible elbow hinge, triceps pad

L6110 Below elbow, molded socket (Muenster or Northwestern suspension types)

These codes report two types of sockets for below-the-elbow or transradial amputations. A cuff or half-cuff is situated over the triceps muscle. Paired medial and lateral elbow hinges act as leverage points to assist movement. The socket is the interface between the residual limb and the prosthesis. Traditionally, a plaster mold is taken of the residual stump, and a positive replica is made. The socket is then vacuum fitted to the replica. A socket may be made from any variety of materials, although modern ones are increasingly fabricated from thermoplastic resins or elastic sleeves. Many are designed for use with gel liners. The Muenster and Northwestern-style sockets traditionally extend proximally to the elbow condyles. The Muenster fits snugly on the anterior and posterior aspects; the Northwestern on the medial and lateral sides. Modified versions of both are available, often with the upper posterior side cut away for movement and breathability. Both styles are suspension sockets, which hold snugly to the residual limb and suspend the prosthetic components.

L6120

L6120 Below elbow, molded double wall split socket, step-up hinges, half cuff

This code refers to an exoskeletal prosthesis for a short, transradial amputation. It includes a custom-fitted socket fabricated from a model of a patient, custom-fabricated forearm using step-up hinges to increase range of motion, a triceps cuff, and a friction wrist unit.

L6130

L6130 Below elbow, molded double wall split socket, stump activated locking hinge, half cuff

This code refers to an exoskeletal prosthesis for a short, transradial amputation. It includes a custom-fitted socket fabricated from a model of a patient, custom-fabricated forearm using stump-activated locking hinges, a triceps cuff, and a friction wrist unit.

L6200-L6205

L6200 Elbow disarticulation, molded socket, outside locking hinge, forearm

L6205 Elbow disarticulation, molded socket with expandable interface, outside locking hinges, forearm

These codes report an exoskeletal prosthesis for an elbow disarticulation or long, transhumeral amputation. It includes a custom-fitted socket fabricated from a model of a patient and a custom-fabricated forearm using an outside locking hinge and a friction wrist unit. An expandable interface allows for differences in residual limb size.

L6250

L6250 Above elbow, molded double wall socket, internal locking elbow, forearm

A transhumeral prothesis is an artificial limb that replaces an arm missing above the elbow. This code refers to a transhumeral amputation that includes a custom-fitted double wall socket fabricated from a model of the patient, a custom-fabricated forearm using an internal locking elbow, and a friction wrist unit.

L6300

L6300 Shoulder disarticulation, molded socket, shoulder bulkhead, humeral section, internal locking elbow, forearm

This code refers to an exosketetal prosthesis for a shoulder disarticulation amputation. It includes a custom-fitted socket fabricated from a model of a patient, a custom-fabricated humeral section, and a forearm using a shoulder bulkhead, an internal locking elbow, and friction wrist unit. Exoskeletal prostheses have a hard outer shell, which can usually withstand considerable force. Exoskeletal designs are usually preferred for prostheses designed to perform work.

L6310

L6310 Shoulder disarticulation, passive restoration (complete prosthesis)

This code refers to an exoskeletal passive prosthesis for a shoulder disarticulation amputation. It includes a custom-fitted socket fabricated from a model of the patient, a custom-fabricated humeral section and forearm using a passive elbow, a passive terminal device (the most distal part of a prosthesis that substitutes for the hand; it may be a prosthetic hand, a hook, or another device), and a friction wrist unit and suspension. Exoskeletal prostheses have a hard outer shell, which can usually withstand considerable force. Exoskeletal designs are usually preferred for prostheses designed to perform work. A passive functional prosthesis offers very realistic cosmetics and can perform limited function.

L6320

L6320 Shoulder disarticulation, passive restoration (shoulder cap only)

The code refers to an upper extremity restoration (cap) prosthesis for the shoulder of a shoulder disarticulation amputation. It includes a custom-fitted socket fabricated from a model of the patient with special modifications to restore shoulder shape and protect the amputation area. A passive system is primarily cosmetic but also functions as a stabilizer. A passive system is fabricated if the patient does not have enough strength or movement to control a prosthesis or wears a prosthesis only because of cosmetic concerns.

L6350

L6350 Interscapular thoracic, molded socket, shoulder bulkhead, humeral section, internal locking elbow, forearm

An interscapular-thoracic amputation is the surgical separation of the humerus (upper arm bone), scapula (shoulder blade), and a portion of the clavicle (collar bone) from the body. In this procedure the entire shoulder and arm are removed. This code refers to an exoskeletal prosthesis for an interscapular thoracic amputation. It includes a custom-fitted socket fabricated from a model of the patient, a custom-fabricated humeral section, forearm utilizing a shoulder bulkhead, an internal locking elbow, and a friction wrist unit.

L6360

L6360 Interscapular thoracic, passive restoration (complete prosthesis)

An interscapular-thoracic amputation is the surgical separation of the humerus (upper arm bone), scapula (shoulder blade), and a portion of the clavicle (collar bone) from the body. In this procedure, the entire shoulder and arm are removed. This code refers to the complete passive restoration. A passive system is primarily cosmetic but also functions as a stabilizer. A passive system is fabricated if the patient does not have enough strength or movement to control a prosthesis or wears a prosthesis only because of cosmetic concerns.

L6370

L6370 Interscapular thoracic, passive restoration (shoulder cap only)

An interscapular-thoracic amputation is the surgical separation of the humerus (upper arm bone), scapula (shoulder blade), and a portion of the clavicle (collar bone) from the body. In this procedure the entire shoulder and arm are removed. This code refers to an upper-extremity restoration (shoulder cap) prosthesis for the shoulder of an interscapular thoracic amputation. It includes a custom-fitted socket fabricated from a model of the patient with special modification to restore shoulder shape and to provide protection to the amputation area.

L6380-L6384

L6380 Immediate postsurgical or early fitting, application of initial rigid dressing, including fitting alignment and suspension of components, and one cast change, wrist disarticulation or below elbow

L6382 Immediate postsurgical or early fitting, application of initial rigid dressing including fitting alignment and suspension of components, and one cast change, elbow disarticulation or above elbow

L6384 Immediate postsurgical or early fitting, application of initial rigid dressing including fitting alignment and suspension of components, and one cast change, shoulder disarticulation or interscapular thoracic

These codes report supply of early fittings and dressings following an upper limb amputation or disarticulation at the shoulder joint. A major consideration for prosthetists is the constantly changing size and shape of the residual limb, or stump, which is the attachment site for the prosthesis. Following amputation of the limb, post-surgical or "early" dressings are applied to the surgical stump, sometimes during the same operative session. These early applications are designed to compress and prepare the distal tissues in anticipation of fitting a test socket and later a permanent socket. Early applications may be known as immediate post-surgical fittings (IPSF). The accepted plan for most limb amputations is to transition the patient as quickly as possible to the use of prosthesis. This minimizes muscle atrophy and limb weakness seen in longer convalescences. In some instances, a plaster cast or other rigid dressing is hand molded to the residual limb as the amputation session is completed. In other instances, the initial dressing is applied up to several days following surgery. As swelling diminishes and also to access the surgical closure, the dressing must be periodically changed out. These early dressings may be fitted to interface with test prosthetic devices.

L6386

L6386 Immediate postsurgical or early fitting, each additional cast change and realignment

This code refers to the removal and reapplication of the direct formed socket (codes L6380, L6382, and L6384) and includes alignment and any adjustments.

L6388

L6388 Immediate postsurgical or early fitting, application of rigid dressing only

This code refers to an application of a dressing immediately post-op or soon after surgery, consisting of a socket fabricated directly to the amputee's residual limb at any level.

L6400

L6400 Below elbow, molded socket, endoskeletal system, including soft prosthetic tissue shaping

A transradial prosthesis is an artificial limb that replaces an arm missing below the elbow. This code refers to an endoskeletal prosthesis for a transradial amputation. It includes a custom-fitted socket fabricated from a patient model, a forearm (always made of similar material as the arm section), friction wrist unit, custom-shaped cover, and a nonprotective covering. An endoskeletal system is covered with a cosmetic foam that is shaped to match the sound side limb (the noninvolved limb).

L6450

L6450 Elbow disarticulation, molded socket, endoskeletal system, including soft prosthetic tissue shaping

This code refers to an endoskeletal prosthesis for an elbow disarticulation or long transradial amputation. It includes a custom-fitted socket fabricated from a patient model, a nonalignable forearm, friction wrist unit, custom-shaped cover, and a nonprotective covering.

L6500

L6500 Above elbow, molded socket, endoskeletal system, including soft prosthetic tissue shaping

This code refers to an endoskeletal prosthesis for a transradial amputation. It includes a custom-fitted socket fabricated from a patient model, nonalignable humeral section, nonalignable forearm section, friction wrist unit, custom-shaped cover, and nonprotective covering.

L6550

L6550 Shoulder disarticulation, molded socket, endoskeletal system, including soft prosthetic tissue shaping

This code refers to an upper-extremity, endoskeletal prosthesis for a shoulder disarticulation amputation. It includes a custom-fitted socket fabricated from a patient model, nonalignable humeral section, nonalignable forearm section, friction wrist unit, custom-shaped cover, and nonprotective covering.

L6570

L6570 Interscapular thoracic, molded socket, endoskeletal system, including soft prosthetic tissue shaping

This code refers to an upper-extremity, endoskeletal prosthesis for an interscapular thoracic amputation. It includes a custom-fitted socket fabricated from a patient model, nonalignable humeral section, nonalignable forearm section, friction wrist unit, custom-shaped cover, and nonprotective covering.

L6580

L6580 Preparatory, wrist disarticulation or below elbow, single wall plastic socket, friction wrist, flexible elbow hinges, figure of eight harness, humeral cuff, Bowden cable control, USMC or equal pylon, no cover, molded to patient model

This code refers to an upper-extremity, preparatory prosthesis for a wrist disarticulation or transradial amputation. It includes a custom-fitted socket fabricated from a patient model, single-wall construction, nonalignable pylon, triceps cuff flexible hinges, friction wrist unit, Bowden control cable, and figure-eight harness. No cover is allowed with this code.

L6582

L6582 Preparatory, wrist disarticulation or below elbow, single wall socket, friction wrist, flexible elbow hinges, figure of eight harness, humeral cuff, Bowden cable control, USMC or equal pylon, no cover, direct formed

This code refers to an upper-extremity, preparatory prosthesis for a wrist disarticulation or transradial amputation. It includes a direct formed socket, single-wall construction, nonalignable pylon, triceps cuff, flexible hinges, Bowden control cable, figure-eight harness, and friction wrist unit. No cover is allowed for this code.

L6584

L6584 Preparatory, elbow disarticulation or above elbow, single wall plastic socket, friction wrist, locking elbow, figure of eight harness, fair lead cable control, USMC or equal pylon, no cover, molded to patient model

This code refers to an upper-extremity, preparatory prosthesis for a wrist disarticulation or transradial amputation. It includes a custom-fitted socket fabricated from a patient, single-wall construction, locking elbow, nonalignable pylon, fair lead control cable, figure-eight harness, and friction wrist unit. No cover is allowed for this code.

L

L6586

L6586 Preparatory, elbow disarticulation or above elbow, single wall socket, friction wrist, locking elbow, figure of eight harness, fair lead cable control, USMC or equal pylon, no cover, direct formed

This code refers to an upper-extremity, preparatory prosthesis for a wrist disarticulation or transradial amputation. It includes a direct formed socket, single-wall construction, locking elbow, nonalignable pylon, fair lead control cable, figure-eight harness, and friction wrist unit. No cover is allowed for this code.

L6588

L6588 Preparatory, shoulder disarticulation or interscapular thoracic, single wall plastic socket, shoulder joint, locking elbow, friction wrist, chest strap, fair lead cable control, USMC or equal pylon, no cover, molded to patient model

This code refers to an upper-extremity, preparatory prosthesis for a shoulder disarticulation or an interscapular thoracic amputation. It includes a custom-fitted socket fabricated from a patient model, single-wall fabrication using a plastic shoulder joint, locking elbow, friction wrist joint, nonalignable pylon, fair lead control cable, and chest harness. No cover is allowed for this code.

L6590

L6590 Preparatory, shoulder disarticulation or interscapular thoracic, single wall socket, shoulder joint, locking elbow, friction wrist, chest strap, fair lead cable control, USMC or equal pylon, no cover, direct formed

This code refers to an upper-extremity, preparatory prosthesis for a shoulder disarticulation or an interscapular thoracic amputation. It includes a direct formed socket, single-wall fabrication using a plastic shoulder joint, locking elbow, friction wrist unit, nonalignable pylon, fair lead control cable, and chest harness. No cover is allowed for this code.

L6600-L6611

L6600 Upper extremity additions, polycentric hinge, pair

L6605 Upper extremity additions, single pivot hinge, pair

L6610 Upper extremity additions, flexible metal hinge, pair

L6611 Addition to upper extremity prosthesis, external powered, additional switch, any type

In the prosthetics armamentarium (all of the equipment necessary for prosthetic fitting or use), a patient or doctor needs a complete range of components to be available to provide a proper fitting prosthesis for all sites of amputations. These codes refer to the array of components necessary for the prescription fitting of prostheses in relation to the site of upper-extremity amputation.

L6615-L6616

L6615 Upper extremity addition, disconnect locking wrist unit

L6616 Upper extremity addition, additional disconnect insert for locking wrist unit, each

The disconnect locking wrist unit refers to a quick disconnect wrist unit that allows interchanging of terminal device (supination and pronation of a device) in locked positions. The disconnect locking wrist unit includes one wrist unit insert. An additional insert to be utilized with the quick disconnect wrist unit is also available.

L6620

L6620 Upper extremity addition, flexion/extension wrist unit, with or without friction

This code refers to a wrist unit that allows flexion of the terminal device into a locked position. The wrist unit flexes in only one plane.

L6621

L6621 Upper extremity prosthesis addition, flexion/extension wrist with or without friction, for use with external powered terminal device

This code refers to a wrist unit that allows flexion of the terminal device into locked positions. The wrist unit flexes in only one plane. This is for use with external powered devices.

L6623

L6623 Upper extremity addition, spring assisted rotational wrist unit with latch release

This code refers to a wrist unit that utilizes a spring to assist supination and pronation. A locking mechanism locks the terminal in a fixed position.

L6624

L6624 Upper extremity addition, flexion/extension and rotation wrist unit

Flexion and extension, along with rotation, give the prosthesis two additional degrees of freedom, and rotational wrist units are cable-controlled, positive-locking mechanisms. Flexion and extension in a prosthetic wrist make it easier for users to grip and see objects.

L6625

L6625 Upper extremity addition, rotation wrist unit with cable lock

This code refers to a wrist unit that utilizes a cable to unlock the terminal device to allow supination and pronation.

L

L6628

L6628 Upper extremity addition, quick disconnect hook adapter, Otto Bock or equal

The code refers to a wrist unit for an external powered prosthesis that allows for the interchange of an external powered or body powered terminal device. This device allows supination or pronation and allows the wearer to release the hand quickly in an emergency or reposition objects without having to go through the open/close cycle.

L6629

L6629 Upper extremity addition, quick disconnect lamination collar with coupling piece, Otto Bock or equal

This code refers to a lamination collar and a coupling piece to accept a terminal device for an external powered prosthesis. It is used in the fabrication of the forearm.

L6630

L6630 Upper extremity addition, stainless steel, any wrist

This code refers to any wrist unit made of stainless steel.

L6632

L6632 Upper extremity addition, latex suspension sleeve, each

This code refers to a suspension sleeve (which suspends the prosthesis) made of latex. These sleeves provide optimal distribution of weight between the upper arm and forearm. It is also formulated with a medical grade mineral oil that soothes and protects the skin from shearing, abrasion, and friction between the residual limb and the prosthesis.

L6635

L6635 Upper extremity addition, lift assist for elbow

Lift assists are used to counterbalance the weight of the forearm, making elbow flexion easier. It is a spring mechanism that somewhat compensates for gravity forces.

L6637

L6637 Upper extremity addition, nudge control elbow lock

This code refers to a device used by high-level amputees to lock and unlock the prosthetic elbow when shoulder excursion (linear displacement) is limited.

L6638

L6638 Upper extremity addition to prosthesis, electric locking feature, only for use with manually powered elbow

An electric locking feature is attached to a prosthetic elbow to allow locking in various positions. The locking mechanism is activated electronically rather than manually using a myoelectrode, touch pad, or switch.

L6640

L6640 Upper extremity additions, shoulder abduction joint, pair

This code reports shoulder joints that provide passive abduction for the humeral section of a high-level prosthesis.

L6641-L6642

L6641 Upper extremity addition, excursion amplifier, pulley type

L6642 Upper extremity addition, excursion amplifier, lever type

A cable-operated prosthesis uses body movements to supply power for its operation. An excursion amplifier is used to amplify the patient's motion that is necessary to operate the cables in upper extremity prosthesis. It consists of a small pulley attached near the posterior end of the chest strap of the harness or an actuation lever that can be moved to different places on the device. The pulley amplifier reduces the required body motion in half (and doubles the required body force). The lever amplifier can be varied by placement of the control strap cable on the lever.

L6645

L6645 Upper extremity addition, shoulder flexion-abduction joint, each

A shoulder flexion-abduction joint is a two-way joint that is attached to residual limb of the shoulder. This addition allows the patient to flex and abduct the prosthetic arm.

L6646

L6646 Upper extremity addition, shoulder joint, multipositional locking, flexion, adjustable abduction friction control, for use with body powered or external powered system

This code reports an addition to an upper extremity prosthesis. It is a shoulder joint that can swing in a natural arc and can also be locked in 36 positions, every 10 degrees. The user can free the joint manually or by using a nudge control. Abduction (pushing away) and adduction (pulling in) is achieved through a second hinge with adjustable friction. This joint can be used with body powered or external powered systems.

L6647-L6648

L6647 Upper extremity addition, shoulder lock mechanism, body powered actuator

L6648 Upper extremity addition, shoulder lock mechanism, external powered actuator

A locking feature is attached to a prosthetic shoulder to allow locking in various positions. The mechanism can be powered by cables that use body movements for control or it can be an externally powered locking device that is powered by electric motors and an external battery pack.

L6650

L6650 Upper extremity addition, shoulder universal joint, each

This code reports a universal shoulder joint that provides passive abduction, flexion, rotation, and circumduction.

L6655-L6660

L6655 Upper extremity addition, standard control cable, extra

L6660 Upper extremity addition, heavy-duty control cable

These codes report a standard or heavy duty control cable and housing for a body-powered prosthesis.

L6665

L6665 Upper extremity addition, Teflon, or equal, cable lining

Control cables are attached to the prosthesis and are used to link the patient's movements to control movement of the prosthesis. These cables run through lined housings. The housing can be lined to reduce the friction generated as the cable moves.

L6670

L6670 Upper extremity addition, hook to hand, cable adapter

This code reports a cable adapter utilized to allow a hook and hand to be interchanged on a body-powered prosthesis.

L6672-L6677

L6672 Upper extremity addition, harness, chest or shoulder, saddle type

L6675 Upper extremity addition, harness, (e.g., figure of eight type), single cable design

L6676 Upper extremity addition, harness, (e.g., figure of eight type), dual cable design

L6677 Upper extremity addition, harness, triple control, simultaneous operation of terminal device and elbow

A harness system holds the prosthetic device securely to the residual limb, distributes the weight and lifting load, and positions the prosthesis for greatest ease of use. For the figure-8 strap, a harness wraps around the axilla on the intact side of the body. This holds the harness and provides the counterforce for suspension and control-cable forces. On the residual limb side, the front strap provides most of the suspending forces to the prosthesis by attaching directly to the socket in transhumeral prosthesis or indirectly to a transradial socket through an intermediate Y-strap and triceps cuff. The back strap on the side with the prosthesis attaches to the control cable. A saddle type harness provides the ability for the patient to lift heavier loads and is an alternative to the figure-8 harness. A shoulder saddle is a fairly wide leather piece that rests on the shoulder of the amputated arm. Straps are attached to the saddle and the prosthesis and the saddle is secured with a strap around the chest. This provides less pressure on the axilla than the figure-8 harness.

L6680-L6684

L6680 Upper extremity addition, test socket, wrist disarticulation or below elbow

L6682 Upper extremity addition, test socket, elbow disarticulation or above elbow

L6684 Upper extremity addition, test socket, shoulder disarticulation or interscapular thoracic

A socket is the portion of a prosthesis that fits around the residual limb (or stump) and to which prosthetic components are attached. Test sockets are typically soft and often have transparent fittings that allow the prosthetist to visualize the fit. A test socket tests the interface between the prosthesis and the residual limb. The use of a test/temporary socket allows a refinement in the fit and allows repeated modifications for increased comfort.

L6686

L6686 Upper extremity addition, suction socket

A suction socket uses a vacuum action to attach the prosthesis to the socket. The residual limb is put into the socket. It is fit with a one-way air valve to remove air and create the suction force to keep the socket in place until air is reintroduced to remove the socket. Suction sockets require total contact with the residual limb to maintain the vacuum.

L6687-L6690

L6687 Upper extremity addition, frame type socket, below elbow or wrist disarticulation

L6688 Upper extremity addition, frame type socket, above elbow or elbow disarticulation

L6689 Upper extremity addition, frame type socket, shoulder disarticulation

L6690 Upper extremity addition, frame type socket, interscapular-thoracic

A socket is the piece of the prosthetic that fits the residual limb of a patient who has experienced an amputation. A frame type of socket has a flexible plastic inner piece for contact and fit. This is surrounded by a flexible liner and a rigid frame for support and to which the necessary cables and joints are attached as needed. Windows are created in the outer sock to allow movement and reduce pressure and pain over bony prominences.

L6691-L6692

L6691 Upper extremity addition, removable insert, each

L6692 Upper extremity addition, silicone gel insert or equal, each

A prosthetic socket insert surrounds the residual limb in a layer of skin friendly material. A gel insert gently adheres to the skin to protect against abrasion and breakdown. The gel is covered in a layer of durable fabric that helps extend the life of liners and allows amputees to easily slide into the sockets.

L6693

L6693 Upper extremity addition, locking elbow, forearm counterbalance

A locking elbow is an addition to an upper extremity prosthesis. It allows the elbow joint to flex and can be locked into various positions. Elbow spring-lift devices are used to counterbalance the weight of the forearm to make flexion easier for the patient.

L6694-L6697

L6694 Addition to upper extremity prosthesis, below elbow/above elbow, custom fabricated from existing mold or prefabricated, socket insert, silicone gel, elastomeric or equal, for use with locking mechanism

L6695 Addition to upper extremity prosthesis, below elbow/above elbow, custom fabricated from existing mold or prefabricated, socket insert, silicone gel, elastomeric or equal, not for use with locking mechanism

L6696 Addition to upper extremity prosthesis, below elbow/above elbow, custom fabricated socket insert for congenital or atypical traumatic amputee, silicone gel, elastomeric or equal, for use with or without locking mechanism, initial only (for other than initial, use code L6694 or L6695)

L6697 Addition to upper extremity prosthesis, below elbow/above elbow, custom fabricated socket insert for other than congenital or atypical traumatic amputee, silicone gel, elastomeric or equal, for use with or without locking mechanism, initial only (for other than initial, use code L6694 or L6695)

A socket insert is a soft device designed to fit around a residual limb and inside the socket to provide increased padding and comfort. This code reports socket inserts for prosthetic arms. The inserts may be composed of silicone gel and elastic polymers (elastomers), and can be custom-made from an existing mold or prefabricated (ready-made). Locking mechanics hold the arm or a portion thereof in a set position until the lock is released. The designation of "initial only" represents the first creation of a mold of the residual arm and the socket insert for a specific patient.

L6698

L6698 Addition to upper extremity prosthesis, below elbow/above elbow, lock mechanism, excludes socket insert

A prosthetic locking mechanism is a device using suction, pins, or similar means to hold the prosthesis to the residual limb.

L6703-L6704

L6703 Terminal device, passive hand/mitt, any material, any size

L6704 Terminal device, sport/recreational/work attachment, any material, any size

A terminal device is an addition to an upper extremity prosthesis that replaces a missing hand in function, appearance, or both. The device attaches to a base wrist unit. Terminal devices are interchangeable, and a patient may use different versions at different times. Terminal devices may be passive or active. Passive devices more cosmetically resemble a hand and are usually less functional.

L6706-L6722

L6706 Terminal device, hook, mechanical, voluntary opening, any material, any size, lined or unlined

L6707 Terminal device, hook, mechanical, voluntary closing, any material, any size, lined or unlined

L6708 Terminal device, hand, mechanical, voluntary opening, any material, any size

L6709 Terminal device, hand, mechanical, voluntary closing, any material, any size

L6711 Terminal device, hook, mechanical, voluntary opening, any material, any size, lined or unlined, pediatric

L6712 Terminal device, hook, mechanical, voluntary closing, any material, any size, lined or unlined, pediatric

L6713 Terminal device, hand, mechanical, voluntary opening, any material, any size, pediatric

L6714 Terminal device, hand, mechanical, voluntary closing, any material, any size, pediatric

L6715 Terminal device, multiple articulating digit, includes motor(s), initial issue or replacement

L6721 Terminal device, hook or hand, heavy-duty, mechanical, voluntary opening, any material, any size, lined or unlined

L6722 Terminal device, hook or hand, heavy-duty, mechanical, voluntary closing, any material, any size, lined or unlined

A terminal device is an addition to an upper extremity prosthesis that replaces a missing hand in function, appearance, or both. The device attaches to a base wrist unit. Terminal devices are interchangeable, and a patient may use different versions at different times. Terminal devices may be passive or active. Passive devices more cosmetically resemble a hand and are usually less functional. Active devices provide some of the normal hand functions. These active terminal devices may be in the form of a hook or a hand. A hook is a metal device with two fingers that can be opened or closed and is usually made of aluminum or steel. Hands are more esthetically pleasing and allow finger position control. Body-powered or manual prostheses use cables and gross limb movement to control the device. They are usually of moderate weight and cost. Active devices may have voluntary opening or closing mechanisms. Multiple articulating digits allow individual, multiple movements in the fingers and/or thumb. Each digit has a separate motor to control the movement. Voluntary opening mechanisms are closed at relaxation and open when the patient exerts control. Control may be mechanical or electric using patient muscle contractions. Relaxation of the muscles allows the device to close around the object. Voluntary closing mechanisms are open at rest. Residual forearm flexors control the grasp of the desired object.

L6805

L6805 Addition to terminal device, modifier wrist unit

A terminal device is the distal potion of an upper extremity prosthesis that replaces a missing hand in function, appearance, or both. Terminal devices are interchangeable and a patient may use different versions at different times. This device attaches to a modified wrist unit. Wrist units may be modified for use with designated sports or occupational equipment.

L6810

L6810 Addition to terminal device, precision pinch device

A precision grip is designed to perform more refined thumb and index finger movement. It allows the user to pinch or pick up small objects.

L6880

L6880 Electric hand, switch or myoelectric controlled, independently articulating digits, any grasp pattern or combination of grasp patterns, includes motor(s)

A terminal device is an addition to an upper extremity prosthesis that replaces a missing hand in function, appearance, or both. The device attaches to a base wrist unit. Terminal devices are interchangeable and a patient may use different versions at different times. Hands are more esthetic and allow finger position control. Myoelectric prostheses transmit electrical impulses from electrodes on the surface of the residual muscles to an electric motor that operates the terminal device. Myoelectric devices are heavier and more expensive than manual prostheses. Myoelectric devices use electrodes to generate muscle contraction strength controlling the function. Multi-articulating digits allow various finger and grip positions.

L6881

L6881 Automatic grasp feature, addition to upper limb electric prosthetic terminal device

A terminal device is an addition to an upper extremity prosthesis that replaces a missing hand in function, appearance, or both. The device attaches to a base wrist unit. Terminal devices are interchangeable and a patient may use different versions at different times. Electric prosthesis uses a small electric motor to provide movement. An automatic grasp feature in an electric hand monitors the shear force and the grip force and automatically adjusts the grip strength so that an object can be securely held within the hand even if its center of gravity changes.

L6882

L6882 Microprocessor control feature, addition to upper limb prosthetic terminal device

A microprocessor is a single integrated circuit that contains all the functions of a computer's central processing. In this instance, the microprocessor controls the terminal device attached to a prosthetic arm. Sensors determine the current parameters (weight load, position, etc.) of the prosthesis and send a message to the prosthesis that guides its subsequent motion. Greater control allows a more natural motion.

L6883-L6885

L6883 Replacement socket, below elbow/wrist disarticulation, molded to patient model, for use with or without external power

L6884 Replacement socket, above elbow/elbow disarticulation, molded to patient model, for use with or without external power

L6885 Replacement socket, shoulder disarticulation/interscapular thoracic, molded to patient model, for use with or without external power

A socket is the portion of a prosthesis that fits around the residual limb (or stump) and to which prosthetic components are attached. When the initial socket is created, a mold of the extremity is taken along with measurements and notations on cosmetic features. These codes report replacement sockets created using patient models. The differentiation between these sockets is through which joint the amputation (disarticulation) occurred.

L6890-L6895

L6890 Addition to upper extremity prosthesis, glove for terminal device, any material, prefabricated, includes fitting and adjustment

L6895 Addition to upper extremity prosthesis, glove for terminal device, any material, custom fabricated

A terminal device is an addition to an upper extremity prosthesis that replaces a missing hand in function, appearance, or both. The device attaches to a base wrist unit. Terminal devices are interchangeable, allowing the patient to use different versions for different functions. A glove is put over the terminal device to enhance the appearance and protect the device from water and dirt. The gloves can be made from various materials, such as silicone or polyvinyl chloride (PVC). The gloves range from prefabricated gloves that may come in different skin shades to custom painted covers that closely match the patient's own skin, applying acrylic nails and even tattoos and hair to further customize the glove.

L6900-L6915

L6900 Hand restoration (casts, shading and measurements included), partial hand, with glove, thumb or one finger remaining

L6905 Hand restoration (casts, shading and measurements included), partial hand, with glove, multiple fingers remaining

L6910 Hand restoration (casts, shading and measurements included), partial hand, with glove, no fingers remaining

L6915 Hand restoration (shading and measurements included), replacement glove for above

Partial hand restoration replaces part of a hand. A mold is made of the affected hand and a glove is made with holes for any remaining fingers. Realistic looking custom fingers are created to replace the missing digits. The glove adheres to the hand by suction. The glove can be customized to closely match the patient's own skin, applying acrylic nails and jewelry on the prosthetic fingers to create a natural appearance.

L6920-L6925

L6920 Wrist disarticulation, external power, self-suspended inner socket, removable forearm shell, Otto Bock or equal switch, cables, two batteries and one charger, switch control of terminal device

L6925 Wrist disarticulation, external power, self-suspended inner socket, removable forearm shell, Otto Bock or equal electrodes, cables, two batteries and one charger, myoelectronic control of terminal device

These prostheses are replacement devices for an amputation at the wrist. This type of prosthesis uses a self-suspended inner socket to which a terminal device is attached. The socket and terminal device interface are covered by a removable forearm shell. The myoelectric prosthetic uses an external battery pack to supply power to electric motors and microprocessors that control the movement of the device in different directions. The myoelectric prosthetic has a more realistic appearance and provides the patient with increased function. Control of the device is through skin electrodes inside the socket of the prosthetic. They are able to detect and amplify the electrical activity of muscle groups left in the limb. These impulses are cycled through the microprocessor units and result in movement through electric motors. Switch control of the terminal device requires the user to toggle, nudge, or otherwise operate a switch to create movement in the terminal device.

L6930-L6935

L6930 Below elbow, external power, self-suspended inner socket, removable forearm shell, Otto Bock or equal switch, cables, two batteries and one charger, switch control of terminal device

L6935 Below elbow, external power, self-suspended inner socket, removable forearm shell, Otto Bock or equal electrodes, cables, two batteries and one charger, myoelectronic control of terminal device

These prostheses are replacement devices for a below-elbow amputation. This type of prosthesis uses a self-suspended inner socket to which a terminal device is attached. The socket and terminal device interface is covered by a removable forearm shell. A myoelectric prosthesis uses an external battery pack to supply power to electric motors and microprocessors that control the movement of the device in different directions. The myoelectric prosthetic has a more realistic appearance and provides the patient with increased function. The device is controlled through skin electrodes inside the socket of the prosthetic that can detect and amplify the electrical activity of muscle groups left in the limb. These impulses are cycled through the microprocessor units and result in movement through electric motors. Switch control of the terminal device requires the user to toggle, nudge, or otherwise operate a switch to create movement in the terminal device.

L6940-L6945

L6940 Elbow disarticulation, external power, molded inner socket, removable humeral shell, outside locking hinges, forearm, Otto Bock or equal switch, cables, two batteries and one charger, switch control of terminal device

L6945 Elbow disarticulation, external power, molded inner socket, removable humeral shell, outside locking hinges, forearm, Otto Bock or equal electrodes, cables, two batteries and one charger, myoelectronic control of terminal device

These prostheses are replacement devices for an amputation at the elbow. The myoelectric prosthetic uses an external battery pack to supply power to electric motors and microprocessors that control the movement of the device in different directions. The myoelectric prosthetic has a more realistic appearance and provides the patient with increased function. This type of prosthesis uses a self-suspended inner socket to which a terminal device is attached. The socket and terminal device interface are covered by a removable forearm shell. The device is controlled through skin electrodes inside the socket of the prosthetic that can detect and amplify the electrical activity of muscle groups left in the limb. These impulses are cycled through the microprocessor units and result in movement through electric motors. Switch control of the terminal device requires the user to toggle, nudge, or otherwise operate a switch to create movement in the terminal device.

L6950-L6955

L6950 Above elbow, external power, molded inner socket, removable humeral shell, internal locking elbow, forearm, Otto Bock or equal switch, cables, two batteries and one charger, switch control of terminal device

L6955 Above elbow, external power, molded inner socket, removable humeral shell, internal locking elbow, forearm, Otto Bock or equal electrodes, cables, two batteries and one charger, myoelectronic control of terminal device

These prostheses are replacement devices for an amputation above the elbow. The myoelectric prosthetic uses an external battery pack to supply power to electric motors and microprocessors that control the movement of the device in different directions. The myoelectric prosthetic has a more realistic appearance and provides the patient with increased function. This type of prosthesis uses a self-suspended inner socket to which a terminal device is attached. The socket and terminal device interface are covered by a removable forearm shell. The device is controlled through skin electrodes inside the socket of the prosthetic that can detect and amplify the electrical activity of muscle groups left in the limb. These impulses are cycled through the microprocessor units and result in movement through electric motors. Switch control of the terminal device requires the user to toggle, nudge, or otherwise operate a switch to create movement in the terminal device.

L6960

L6960 Shoulder disarticulation, external power, molded inner socket, removable shoulder shell, shoulder bulkhead, humeral section, mechanical elbow, forearm, Otto Bock or equal switch, cables, two batteries and one charger, switch control of terminal device

A switch controlled prosthesis device is an electronic device used as a replacement for an amputation through the shoulder joint. This type of prosthesis uses switches instead of muscle tightening to control the prosthesis. The switches are located inside the socket or harness and can be activated by pulling a harness or triggered by movement of a bony protrusion against the switch. An external battery pack is used to supply power to electric motors that control the movement of the device.

L

L6965

L6965 Shoulder disarticulation, external power, molded inner socket, removable shoulder shell, shoulder bulkhead, humeral section, mechanical elbow, forearm, Otto Bock or equal electrodes, cables, two batteries and one charger, myoelectronic control of terminal device

A myoelectric prosthesis is an electronic device used as a replacement for an amputation through the shoulder joint. This type of prosthesis uses an external battery pack to supply power to electric motors and microprocessors that control the movement of the device in different directions. The myoelectric prosthetic has a more realistic appearance and provides the patient with increased function. Control of the device is through skin electrodes inside the socket of the prosthetic. They are able to detect and amplify the electrical activity of muscle groups. These impulses are cycled through the microprocessor units and result in movement through electric motors.

L6970

L6970 Interscapular-thoracic, external power, molded inner socket, removable shoulder shell, shoulder bulkhead, humeral section, mechanical elbow, forearm, Otto Bock or equal switch, cables, two batteries and one charger, switch control of terminal device

A switch controlled prosthesis device is an electronic device used as a replacement for an amputation at the interscapulothoracic region, also referred to as a forequarter amputation. This type of prosthesis uses switches instead of muscle tightening to control the prosthesis. The switches are located inside the socket or harness and can be activated by pulling a harness or triggered by movement of a bony protrusion against the switch. An external battery pack is used to supply power to electric motors that control the movement of the device.

L6975

L6975 Interscapular-thoracic, external power, molded inner socket, removable shoulder shell, shoulder bulkhead, humeral section, mechanical elbow, forearm, Otto Bock or equal electrodes, cables, two batteries and one charger, myoelectronic control of terminal device

A myoelectric prosthesis is an electronic device used as a replacement for an amputation at the interscapulothoracic region, also referred to as a forequarter amputation. This type of prosthesis uses an external battery pack to supply power to electric motors and microprocessors that control the movement of the device in different directions. The myoelectric prosthetic has a more realistic appearance and provides the patient with increased function. Control of the device is through skin electrodes inside the socket of the prosthetic. They are able to detect and amplify the electrical activity of muscle groups. These impulses are cycled through the microprocessor units and result in movement through electric motors.

L7007-L7009

L7007 Electric hand, switch or myoelectric controlled, adult

L7008 Electric hand, switch or myoelectric, controlled, pediatric

L7009 Electric hook, switch or myoelectric controlled, adult

A terminal device is an addition to an upper extremity prosthesis that replaces a missing hand in function, appearance, or both. The device attaches to a base wrist unit. Terminal devices are interchangeable and a patient may use different versions at different times. Terminal devices may be passive or active. Passive devices more cosmetically resemble a hand and are usually less functional. Active devices provide some of the normal hand functions. These active terminal devices may be in the form of a hook or a hand. A hook is a metal device with two fingers that can be opened or closed and are usually made of aluminum or steel. Hands are more esthetic and allow finger position control. Body powered or manual prostheses use cables and gross limb movement to control the device. They are usually of moderate weight and cost. Electric hands may be switch activated or myoelectric. Myoelectric prostheses transmit electrical impulses from electrodes on the surface of the residual muscles to an electric motor that operates the terminal device. Myoelectric devices are heavier and more expensive than manual prostheses. Myoelectric devices can have one or two electrodes. The two electrode version has separate electrodes for flexion and extension. The one electrode version uses only one electrode for both flexion and extension with differing muscle contraction strength controlling each function.

L7040

L7040 Prehensile actuator, switch controlled

An actuator is a small mechanical device that converts energy into motion. In this case it controls the grasping action of a terminal device. It uses a switch rather than muscle signals to activate the device. The switches can be activated by movement of a residual digit or movement of a bony prominence against the switch. Another method to active the switch is by pulling on the suspension harness.

L7045

L7045 Electric hook, switch or myoelectric controlled, pediatric

A terminal device is an addition to an upper extremity prosthesis that replaces a missing hand in function, appearance, or both. The device attaches to a base wrist unit. Terminal devices are interchangeable and a patient may use different versions at different times. Terminal devices may be passive or active. Passive devices more cosmetically resemble a hand and are usually less functional. Active devices provide some of the normal hand functions. These active terminal devices may be in the form of a hook or a hand. A hook is a metal device with two fingers that can be opened or closed and are usually made of aluminum or steel. Hands are more esthetic and allow finger position control. Body powered or manual prostheses use cables and gross limb movement to control the device. They are usually of moderate weight and cost. Electric hands may be switch activated or myoelectric. Myoelectric prostheses transmit electrical impulses from electrodes on the surface of the residual muscles to an electric motor that operates the terminal device. Myoelectric devices are heavier and more expensive than manual prostheses. Myoelectric devices can have one or two electrodes. The two electrode version has separate electrodes for flexion and extension. The one electrode version uses only one electrode for both flexion and extension with differing muscle contraction strength controlling each function. This code represents the pediatric version of an electric hook, switch or myoelectric control.

L7170-L7191

L7170 Electronic elbow, Hosmer or equal, switch controlled

L7180 Electronic elbow, microprocessor sequential control of elbow and terminal device

L7181 Electronic elbow, microprocessor simultaneous control of elbow and terminal device

L7185 Electronic elbow, adolescent, Variety Village or equal, switch controlled

L7186 Electronic elbow, child, Variety Village or equal, switch controlled

L7190 Electronic elbow, adolescent, Variety Village or equal, myoelectronically controlled

L7191 Electronic elbow, child, Variety Village or equal, myoelectronically controlled

Electronic elbows are additions to arm prostheses that use an external power source, electric motor, and/or a microprocessing unit to enable the movement of the elbow in several different planes. Some allow the sequential or simultaneous movement of both the elbow and terminal device. Myoelectrically controlled devices use surface electrodes embedded in the socket to detect and amplify the electrical activity of muscle groups in the residual limb. The myoelectric impulses are then translated through microprocessors and electric motors into limb functions. Switch controlled motors allow a patient to move the prosthetic device using toggle switches or buttons. The switches can be toggled using the remaining muscles in a residual limb or by using the opposite shoulder.

L7259

L7259 Electronic wrist rotator, any type

Electric wrist rotator devices attach to an arm prosthesis and provide movement of the terminal device. Rotators provide pronation and supination of the terminal device and can sometimes allow for the opening and closing of the device. These devices are intended for use with the specific type of prosthetic device listed in the description.

L7360-L7368

L7360 Six volt battery, each

L7362 Battery charger, six volt, each

L7364 Twelve volt battery, each

L7366 Battery charger, 12 volt, each

L7367 Lithium ion battery, rechargeable, replacement

L7368 Lithium ion battery charger, replacement only

These codes report the supply of batteries and chargers for prosthetic devices. These battery systems fall into two major categories: primary or single-use batteries, which are cells containing lithium-metal anodes, and secondary or rechargeable batteries, which are systems utilizing lithium-ion chemistry. Nickel cadmium (NiCad) batteries are usually acceptable for air travel and have other advantages, but they tend to lose charge over time while not in use. All of these cells share the characteristics of high safety, reliability, energy density, and predictability of performance.

L7400-L7405

L7400 Addition to upper extremity prosthesis, below elbow/wrist disarticulation, ultra-light material (titanium, carbon fiber or equal)

L7401 Addition to upper extremity prosthesis, above elbow disarticulation, ultra-light material (titanium, carbon fiber or equal)

L7402 Addition to upper extremity prosthesis, shoulder disarticulation/interscapular thoracic, ultra-light material (titanium, carbon fiber or equal)

L7403 Addition to upper extremity prosthesis, below elbow/wrist disarticulation, acrylic material

L7404 Addition to upper extremity prosthesis, above elbow disarticulation, acrylic material

L7405 Addition to upper extremity prosthesis, shoulder disarticulation/interscapular thoracic, acrylic material

These codes report additions to upper arm prosthetics for amputations at various levels. Code selection is based on the material used for the addition. These codes should only be reported if a more specific HCPCS Level II code is not available.

L7499

L7499 Upper extremity prosthesis, not otherwise specified

An upper extremity prosthetic is used to replace function for a patient who is missing all or part of an arm or hand. This code reports an upper extremity prosthetic if there is not a more specific HCPCS Level II code available.

L7510

L7510 Repair of prosthetic device, repair or replace minor parts

Report this code for any minor materials (those without specific HCPCS codes) used as replacement parts or used to adjust and/or repair a prosthetic device.

L7520

L7520 Repair prosthetic device, labor component, per 15 minutes

Adjustments and repairs made to prostheses are billed as a labor charge using this code with one unit of service representing 15 minutes of labor time. The time reported must be only for laboratory repair time and associated prosthetic evaluation.

L7600

L7600 Prosthetic donning sleeve, any material, each

A donning sleeve is a cone-shaped sleeve that is used to help the patient place the residual limb into the prosthesis. It reduces the friction to allow the patient to more easily pull on the prosthetic liner or prosthetic. This code should be reported for a sleeve made out of any material.

L7700

L7700 Gasket or seal, for use with prosthetic socket insert, any type, each

This code represents a gasket or seal for use with a prosthetic socket insert of any type. The gasket or seal secures the residual limb to the prosthesis. It provides a secure attachment, locking the limb to the socket wall, and improves user comfort.

L7900-L7902

L7900 Male vacuum erection system

L7902 Tension ring, for vacuum erection device, any type, replacement only, each

Vacuum erection systems are used to treat erectile dysfunction in men. In normal circumstances, sexual arousal in men causes blood to flow into the corpus cavernosum, the blood storage columns of the penis, which creates an erection for sexual activity. Erectile dysfunction occurs when blood flow is inadequate, sometimes in combination with defects in the natural blood trapping mechanism that allows an erection to be sustained. A vacuum device is usually a clear silastic cylinder that fits externally over the penis. A vacuum is created, manually or by an electronic pump, causing blood to be drawn into the penis. Typically a release valve on the device prevents too much vacuum pressure from building. A special elastic, metal, or leather ring is slipped around the base of the member, holding the blood within the erect penis. The vacuum pump is then removed. The ring is left on during intercourse and removed immediately afterward.

L8000-L8002

L8000 Breast prosthesis, mastectomy bra, without integrated breast prosthesis form, any size, any type

L8001 Breast prosthesis, mastectomy bra, with integrated breast prosthesis form, unilateral, any size, any type

L8002 Breast prosthesis, mastectomy bra, with integrated breast prosthesis form, bilateral, any size, any type

Mastectomy bras come in various materials and sizes to fit patients who have undergone a mastectomy. The bras provide support and shape, usually so that the patient looks the same as she did prior to the mastectomy.

L8010-L8031

L8010 Breast prosthesis, mastectomy sleeve

L8015 External breast prosthesis garment, with mastectomy form, post mastectomy

L8020 Breast prosthesis, mastectomy form

L8030 Breast prosthesis, silicone or equal, without integral adhesive

L8031 Breast prosthesis, silicone or equal, with integral adhesive

This range of codes reports the supply of specific breast prosthetics. A mastectomy sleeve is a full-length elastic support sleeve for the upper arm and axilla. Removal of lymph nodes during mastectomy surgery can cause lymphedema, fluid retention and swelling, in this instance in the axilla and upper arm region. Mastectomy sleeves address this condition. Some may feature a shoulder cap and support straps around the upper torso; others just fit the arm and are held in place by the tensor properties of the fabric. Forms are external cosmetic breast devices that fit on the skin or onto garments following a patient's mastectomy surgery. Certain lightweight models may be made of silicone or other synthetics. Many designs adhere to the skin while others feature tabs to attach to bras or other garments.

L8032-L8033

L8032 Nipple prosthesis, prefabricated, reusable, any type, each

L8033 Nipple prosthesis, custom fabricated, reusable, any material, any type, each

An areola/nipple prosthesis is a reusable, washable, self-sticking adhesive device formed in the shape of a human nipple. It can be used daily over several months and assists patients who are status post nipple/breast reconstructive surgery in achieving a natural looking breast. Indicated for patients undergoing mastectomies and breast reconstruction, the prosthesis may be utilized prior to or as an alternative to nipple reconstruction. Code L8032 reports a prefabricated prosthesis, while L8033 reports an individualized, custom fabricated device formed by creating a rubber impression of the nipple-areolar complex prior to a mastectomy. Made from biocompatible silicone, the individualized prosthesis is colored to match the specific patient's skin.

L8035-L8039

L8035 Custom breast prosthesis, post mastectomy, molded to patient model

L8039 Breast prosthesis, not otherwise specified

A custom fabricated breast prosthesis is individually made for a patient who is post-mastectomy status, starting with basic materials. This particular type of custom fabricated prosthesis involves using an initial impression of the chest wall to make a positive model of the chest wall. The breast prosthesis is molded on this positive model. Report the other code for a breast prosthesis that is not otherwise specified by other HCPCS codes.

L8040

L8040 Nasal prosthesis, provided by a nonphysician

A nasal prosthesis is a removable superficial prosthesis that restores all or part of the nose. It may include the nasal septum. Report this code when a nonphysician provides the prosthesis.

L8041

L8041 Midfacial prosthesis, provided by a nonphysician

A midfacial prosthesis is a removable superficial prosthesis that restores part or all of the nose plus significant adjacent facial tissue/structures but does not include the orbit or any intraoral maxillary component. Adjacent facial tissue or structures include one or more of the following: soft tissue of the cheek, upper lip, or forehead.

L

L8042

L8042 Orbital prosthesis, provided by a nonphysician

An orbital prosthesis is a removable superficial prosthesis that restores the eyelids and the hard and soft tissue of the orbit. It may also include the eyebrow. This code does not include the ocular prosthesis component.

L8043

L8043 Upper facial prosthesis, provided by a nonphysician

An upper facial prosthesis is a removable superficial prosthesis that restores the orbit plus significant adjacent facial tissue/structures but does not include the nose or any intraoral maxillary component. Adjacent facial tissue and structures include one or more of the following: soft tissue of the cheek or forehead. This code does not include the ocular prosthesis component.

L8044

L8044 Hemi-facial prosthesis, provided by a nonphysician

A hemifacial prosthesis is a removable superficial prosthesis that restores part or all of the nose plus the orbit and significant adjacent facial tissue/structures but does not include any intraoral maxillary component. This code does not include the ocular prosthesis component.

L8045

L8045 Auricular prosthesis, provided by a nonphysician

An auricular prosthesis is a removable superficial prosthesis that restores all or part of the ear.

L8046

L8046 Partial facial prosthesis, provided by a nonphysician

A partial facial prosthesis is a removable superficial prosthesis that restores a portion of the face but does not specifically involve the nose, orbit, or ear.

L8047

L8047 Nasal septal prosthesis, provided by a nonphysician

A nasal septal prosthesis is a removable prosthesis that occludes a hole in the nasal septum but does not include superficial nasal tissue.

L8048

L8048 Unspecified maxillofacial prosthesis, by report, provided by a nonphysician

Report this code for any materials used for repair or modification of a maxillofacial prosthesis provided by a nonphysician. This code is also used for a facial prosthesis that is not described by a specific code.

L8049

L8049 Repair or modification of maxillofacial prosthesis, labor component, 15 minute increments, provided by a nonphysician

Modifications or repairs of a maxillofacial prosthesis are reported using this code for the labor component by a nonphysician provider. Report the time in 15-minute increments. Time reported should be only for laboratory modification/repair time and associated prosthetic evaluation used only for services after 90 days from the date of delivery of the prosthesis.

L8300-L8330

L8300 Truss, single with standard pad

L8310 Truss, double with standard pads

L8320 Truss, addition to standard pad, water pad

L8330 Truss, addition to standard pad, scrotal pad

A truss is a supportive device mainly used for hernias. It can be a belt or a brief type garment that provides extra support where needed. A double truss would be used for a bilateral hernia. The pads that can add extra support and comfort can be added or replaced within the truss.

L8400-L8417

L8400 Prosthetic sheath, below knee, each

L8410 Prosthetic sheath, above knee, each

L8415 Prosthetic sheath, upper limb, each

L8417 Prosthetic sheath/sock, including a gel cushion layer, below knee (BK) or above knee (AK), each

This range of codes reports supply of prosthetic sheaths. Many wearers of prostheses use nylon (or other artificial or natural fabric) sleeves over the residual limb to interface between skin and the socket material. The sheath may be a stocking in the case of ankle/foot prostheses, although the term prosthetic sock refers to a sleeve that is closed on one end and may be used on either upper or lower extremity amputations. A special gel cushion layer may be used to improve the attachment capabilities of the socket. Sheaths and socks play an important role in adjusting for volume changes in the residual limb, and many products provide thickness padding against the socket.

L8420-L8435

L8420 Prosthetic sock, multiple ply, below knee (BK), each

L8430 Prosthetic sock, multiple ply, above knee (AK), each

L8435 Prosthetic sock, multiple ply, upper limb, each

The term prosthetic sock refers to a sleeve that is closed on one end and may be used on either upper or lower extremity amputations. The sock may be nylon, wool, or other artificial or natural fabric or blends. The sock plays an important role in adjusting for volume changes in the residual limb, and many products provide thickness padding against the socket. This thickness is expressed as a ply rating; generally one- to six-ply socks are most commonly available. By selecting a ply rating, usually in combination with liners, the wearer can adjust for changes in the size of the residual limb.

L8440-L8465

L8440 Prosthetic shrinker, below knee (BK), each

L8460 Prosthetic shrinker, above knee (AK), each

L8465 Prosthetic shrinker, upper limb, each

This range of codes reports the supply of prosthetic shrinkers, or stump shrinkers. These elastic stockings are usually applied shortly after amputation to control swelling of the residual limb and to prepare the site for a temporary prosthesis. Most shrinkers are made of elastic material, and the devices may be strapped on or simply held in place by the tensor properties of the fabric. Most devices are designed to mold and shape the site in preparation for eventual fitting of a prosthesis.

L8470-L8485

L8470 Prosthetic sock, single ply, fitting, below knee (BK), each

L8480 Prosthetic sock, single ply, fitting, above knee (AK), each

L8485 Prosthetic sock, single ply, fitting, upper limb, each

This range of codes reports the fitting of single ply prosthetic socks. The term prosthetic sock refers to a sleeve that is closed on one end and may be used on either upper or lower extremity amputations. The sock may be nylon, wool, or other artificial or natural fabric or blends. The sock plays an important role in adjusting for volume changes in the residual limb, and many products provide thickness padding against the socket. This thickness is expressed as a ply rating. This range of codes reports only single-ply thickness fittings.

L8499

L8499 Unlisted procedure for miscellaneous prosthetic services

This code reports miscellaneous prosthetic services that are not described by more specific HCPCS Level II codes.

L8500

L8500 Artificial larynx, any type

An artificial larynx is a prosthetic speech device intended to assume some of the function of the natural larynx in the absence of the human organ. A natural larynx generates sound waves that become speech. It also controls the pitch and volume of the sounds. Air expelled from the lungs adds to the volume. The sound waves move from the larynx up the throat to the oral cavity where movement of the lips, teeth, palate, and tongue contribute to the final sound that emerges as speech. The artificial larynx may be electronically-controlled or pneumatically-controlled. It is held against the throat or cheek and creates sound that the user could then form into words. An electronically controlled larynx generates the sound by creating a battery driven vibration.

L8501

L8501 Tracheostomy speaking valve

A tracheostomy speaking valve is used for patients who have had a tracheostomy which is an incision in the anterior portion of the neck that opens a direct path to the trachea. A tube is usually placed in this pathway to maintain the opening. Following this procedure, patients are not able to speak normally because air is diverted through the tracheostomy tube and it doesn't pass through the vocal folds. Speaking valves can be attached to the tracheostomy tube to allow air to move through the tracheostomy tube but not out through it. This forces air around the tracheostomy tube, through the vocal cords and out the mouth upon expiration allowing the patient to speak. The vocalization may not sound like the patient's normal speech but allows a patient with a tracheostomy to be able communicate more effectively.

L8505

L8505 Artificial larynx replacement battery/accessory, any type

An artificial larynx is a prosthetic speech device intended to assume some of the function of the natural larynx in the absence of the human organ. A natural larynx generates sound waves that become speech. It also controls the pitch and volume of the sounds. Air expelled from the lungs adds to the volume. The sound waves move from the larynx up the throat to the oral cavity where movement of the lips, teeth, palate, and tongue contribute to the final sound that emerges as speech. The artificial larynx may be electronically-controlled or pneumatically-controlled. It is held against the throat or cheek and creates sound that the user could then form into words. An electronically controlled larynx generates the sound by creating a battery driven vibration.

L8507-L8509

L8507 Tracheo-esophageal voice prosthesis, patient inserted, any type, each

L8509 Tracheo-esophageal voice prosthesis, inserted by a licensed health care provider, any type

A tracheo-esophageal voice prosthesis shunts air from the lungs into the esophagus and vibrates the esophageal tissue to produce speech sounds. These may be indwelling devices and are considered semi-permanent. The device is inserted into a tracheostoma and secured using flanges on the device. There is a one-way valve at the end of the prosthesis that is inserted into the esophagus that allows air to flow into the esophagus. The life span of a tracheo-esophageal voice prosthesis is three to six months after which it is replaced with a new device.

L8510

L8510 Voice amplifier

A voice amplifier is an external device worn or carried in a pocket, on a waistband, or in a similar manner that makes speech stronger and louder. This can be used by a person who has a weakened voice due to conditions such as vocal nodules, Parkinson's disease, Lou Gehrig's disease, multiple sclerosis, Guillain Barre, impairment of throat or chest muscles, damaged or partially paralyzed vocal cords, diminished lung capacity, artificial larynx users, and esophageal and TEP speakers. The device makes the voice louder and reduces the strain on the patient's voice.

L8511-L8515

L8511 Insert for indwelling tracheo-esophageal prosthesis, with or without valve, replacement only, each

L8512 Gelatin capsules or equivalent, for use with tracheo-esophageal voice prosthesis, replacement only, per 10

L8513 Cleaning device used with tracheoesophageal voice prosthesis, pipet, brush, or equal, replacement only, each

L8514 Tracheo-esophageal puncture dilator, replacement only, each

L8515 Gelatin capsule, application device for use with tracheo-esophageal voice prosthesis, each

An indwelling tracheo-esophageal voice prosthesis must be cleaned several times a day and replaced every three to six months. The tract that holds the prosthesis may need to be dilated periodically to maintain the diameter necessary for the prosthesis. Gelatin capsules aid in insertion as they dissolve within seconds and allow the prosthesis to expand and adhere to the anterior esophageal wall.

L8600

L8600 Implantable breast prosthesis, silicone or equal

A breast implant is a prosthesis used to modify the size, form, and feel of a woman's breast in a post-mastectomy reconstruction, improve chest wall congenital deformities, augment the breast, or perform gender transition (male to female). Breast implants are surgically placed in anatomical relation to the pectoralis major muscle.

L8603

L8603 Injectable bulking agent, collagen implant, urinary tract, 2.5 ml syringe, includes shipping and necessary supplies

Collagen is a protein based substance of strength and flexibility that is the major component of connective tissue, found in cartilage, bone, tendons, and skin. Collagen can be used as an implanted bulking agent to treat urinary incontinence due to intrinsic sphincter deficiency. A cystoscope is inserted into the urethra and the collagen is injected into and around the urethral sphincter to plump up the tissue and inhibit the urine leakage.

L8604

L8604 Injectable bulking agent, dextranomer/hyaluronic acid copolymer implant, urinary tract, 1 ml, includes shipping and necessary supplies

Dextranomer/hyaluronic acid is a bulking agent used to treat vesicoureteral reflux (VUR) in children. VUR occurs when there is a defect in the area where the ureters connect to the bladder.
Dextranomer/hyaluronic acid is a biocompatible, biodegradable gel that is injected in the bladder near the opening of each ureter to prevent the flow of urine back into the ureter and kidneys. It is injected with the aid of a cystoscope.

L8605

L8605 Injectable bulking agent, dextranomer/hyaluronic acid copolymer implant, anal canal, 1 ml, includes shipping and necessary supplies

Dextranomer/hyaluronic acid is a bulking agent used to treat fecal incontinence in patients 18 years of age or older who have failed conservative therapy. Although the exact mechanism of action isn't known, it is theorized that it works by causing a chemical reaction within the body that may narrow the anal canal and expand the submucosal tissue, which in turn, allows better sphincter control. Using an anoscope, the physician injects 1 mL of the agent into the submucosal layer of the anal canal in four different sites.

L8606

L8606 Injectable bulking agent, synthetic implant, urinary tract, 1 ml syringe, includes shipping and necessary supplies

Synthetic material such as copolymer can be used as a bulking agent to treat urinary incontinence due to intrinsic sphincter deficiency. A cystoscope is inserted into the urethra and the substance is injected into and around the urethral sphincter to plump up the tissue and inhibit the urine leakage.

L8607

L8607 Injectable bulking agent for vocal cord medialization, 0.1 ml, includes shipping and necessary supplies

Injection for vocal cord medialization is considered medically necessary for vocal cord paralysis. It has been established to improve the vocal quality and assist in the prevention of aspiration pneumonia that often affects patients with this paralysis.

L8608

L8608 Miscellaneous external component, supply or accessory for use with the Argus II Retinal Prosthesis System

A retinal prosthesis, also known as a bionic eye or retinal implant, is an implantable medical device intended to provide electrical stimulation of the retina to induce visual perception in patients who are profoundly blind due to retinitis pigmentosa (RP). The system employs electrical signals to bypass dead photoreceptor cells and stimulate the overlying neurons. There are three primary components: an implanted epiretinal prosthesis that is fully implanted on and in the eye (there are no percutaneous leads); external components, such as an externally worn video camera, contained in glasses, that wirelessly transmits a real-time video signal; and a "fitting" system for the clinician that is periodically used to perform diagnostic tests with the system and to custom program the external unit. This code represents an external component, supply, or accessory for the prosthetic system.

L8609

L8609 Artificial cornea

An artificial cornea is used to treat patients who are not candidates for human donor corneas because of rejection or eye diseases that would interfere with a human cornea transplant. The cornea is made from a clear hydrogel center and surrounded by a mesh that allows the patient's tissue to secure the implant.

L8610

L8610 Ocular implant

An ocular implant is a spherical shaped device that can be implanted at the time of an eye removal or during a subsequent surgery. It is surgically implanted into the orbit to replace the lost volume and maintain the shape of the missing eye. It is inserted and the eye muscles are usually attached to it to allow it to move in conjunction with the other eye. This implant stays in place permanently. An artificial eye can be attached to the implant to restore a natural appearance.

L8612

L8612 Aqueous shunt

Aqueous shunts are small tubes used in surgery to treat glaucoma. Glaucoma is an eye disease that causes increased pressure in the eye. The increased pressure in the eye is caused by the inability of the aqueous fluid to drain normally. An aqueous shunt is surgically inserted into the anterior chamber of the eye. The shunt maintains an opening to allow drainage of the eye fluid. The fluid is absorbed into the body through the lymph nodes and blood system.

L8613

L8613 Ossicula implant

Ossicular implants are small surgically implanted components used to replace one or more of the ear ossicles. They can be made from various materials such as stainless steel, ceramic material, or Gelfoam.

L8614-L8629

L8614 Cochlear device, includes all internal and external components

L8615 Headset/headpiece for use with cochlear implant device, replacement

L8616 Microphone for use with cochlear implant device, replacement

L8617 Transmitting coil for use with cochlear implant device, replacement

L8618 Transmitter cable for use with cochlear implant device or auditory osseointegrated device, replacement

L8619 Cochlear implant, external speech processor and controller, integrated system, replacement

L8621 Zinc air battery for use with cochlear implant device and auditory osseointegrated sound processors, replacement, each

L8622 Alkaline battery for use with cochlear implant device, any size, replacement, each

L8623 Lithium ion battery for use with cochlear implant device speech processor, other than ear level, replacement, each

L8624 Lithium ion battery for use with cochlear implant or auditory osseointegrated device speech processor, ear level, replacement, each

L8625 External recharging system for battery for use with cochlear implant or auditory osseointegrated device, replacement only, each

L8627 Cochlear implant, external speech processor, component, replacement

L8628 Cochlear implant, external controller component, replacement

L8629 Transmitting coil and cable, integrated, for use with cochlear implant device, replacement

A cochlear implant is a surgically implanted electronic device that provides a sense of sound to a person who is profoundly deaf or severely hard-of-hearing. A cochlear implant consists of one or more external microphones that pick up sound from the environment; an external speech processor that filters sound, splits it into channels, and sends the sound signals through a thin cable to a transmitter; and a transmitter, which may be a coil held in place by a magnet placed behind the external ear. The transmitter sends the power and sound to the internal receiver and stimulator that is surgically implanted in bone. The receiver and stimulator convert the signals into electric impulses and send them through an internal cable to an electrode array that winds through the cochlea. The cochlea transmits the impulses through the auditory nerve system to the brain. The external system may be worn entirely behind the ear or its parts may be worn in a pocket, belt pouch, or harness. These codes report replacement pieces for the different components of a cochlear implant.

L8630-L8659

L8630 Metacarpophalangeal joint implant

L8631 Metacarpal phalangeal joint replacement, two or more pieces, metal (e.g., stainless steel or cobalt chrome), ceramic-like material (e.g., pyrocarbon), for surgical implantation (all sizes, includes entire system)

L8641 Metatarsal joint implant

L8642 Hallux implant

L8658 Interphalangeal joint spacer, silicone or equal, each

L8659 Interphalangeal finger joint replacement, two or more pieces, metal (e.g., stainless steel or cobalt chrome), ceramic-like material (e.g., pyrocarbon) for surgical implantation, any size

These codes report implants in the hands or feet to restore function or relieve pain in those joints. Total joint replacements are usually comprised of two components that fit together to mimic joint function. They are made of various materials such a silicone or titanium or a combination of materials to best mimic joint function. A joint spacer does not replace the total joint. It is implanted into the interphalangeal joint for an interpositional arthroplasty.

L8670

L8670 Vascular graft material, synthetic, implant

A vascular graft consists of material used to patch a damaged, diseased, or injured area of an artery or for replacement of whole segments of vessels. Synthetic grafts are usually made from Dacron or polytetrafluoroethylene (PTFE).

L

L8679-L8689

L8679 Implantable neurostimulator, pulse generator, any type

L8680 Implantable neurostimulator electrode, each

L8681 Patient programmer (external) for use with implantable programmable neurostimulator pulse generator, replacement only

L8682 Implantable neurostimulator radiofrequency receiver

L8683 Radiofrequency transmitter (external) for use with implantable neurostimulator radiofrequency receiver

L8684 Radiofrequency transmitter (external) for use with implantable sacral root neurostimulator receiver for bowel and bladder management, replacement

L8685 Implantable neurostimulator pulse generator, single array, rechargeable, includes extension

L8686 Implantable neurostimulator pulse generator, single array, nonrechargeable, includes extension

L8687 Implantable neurostimulator pulse generator, dual array, rechargeable, includes extension

L8688 Implantable neurostimulator pulse generator, dual array, nonrechargeable, includes extension

L8689 External recharging system for battery (internal) for use with implantable neurostimulator, replacement only

An implantable neurostimulator generator is a device that creates small electrical impulses that are transmitted to electrodes implanted near the spinal cord or a peripheral nerve. The small electrical impulses interrupt pain signals sent to the brain. The neurostimulator has either an external power source worn outside the body or batteries that can be implanted. A programmer allows signals to be sent to an internal receiver to adjust the neurostimulator impulses.

L8690-L8694

L8690 Auditory osseointegrated device, includes all internal and external components

L8691 Auditory osseointegrated device, external sound processor, excludes transducer/actuator, replacement only, each

L8692 Auditory osseointegrated device, external sound processor, used without osseointegration, body worn, includes headband or other means of external attachment

L8693 Auditory osseointegrated device abutment, any length, replacement only

L8694 Auditory osseointegrated device, transducer/actuator, replacement only, each

An auditory osseointegrated implant is a device that is implanted behind the patient's ear to provide hearing function for patients with a missing or diseased middle ear. It consists of an internal titanium implant that attaches to the temporal bone, an external abutment, and an external sound processor. The initial code for the osseointegrated implant includes all of the components. Occasionally components may need to be replaced. Specific codes are used to report the replacement devices. Code L8692 represents a device used for patients who are not candidates for implanted auditory osseointegrated systems. It consists of an adjustable headband to which the amplification disk is attached. The headband positions the device appropriately behind the ear.

L8695

L8695 External recharging system for battery (external) for use with implantable neurostimulator, replacement only

An implantable neurostimulator generator is a device that creates small electrical impulses that are transmitted to electrodes implanted near the spinal cord or a peripheral nerve. The small electrical impulses interrupt pain signals sent to the brain. The neurostimulator has either an external power source worn outside the body or batteries that can be implanted. A programmer allows signals to be sent to an internal receiver to adjust the neurostimulator impulses. This code reports an external recharging system for the external battery used with an implantable neurostimulator.

L8696

L8696 Antenna (external) for use with implantable diaphragmatic/phrenic nerve stimulation device, replacement, each

Implantable diaphragmatic/phrenic nerve stimulation devices are pacemakers used to stimulate the diaphragm/phrenic nerve in adult and pediatric patients who have chronic respiratory insufficiency and would otherwise be dependent upon a ventilator. These devices are often used for the treatment of patients who have sustained C1-C3 brainstem injuries, central hypoventilation syndromes, or paralysis of the diaphragm. The patient must retain residual function of the diaphragm, lungs, and phrenic nerves to be considered. A receiver and electrode are surgically implanted and connected to an external radio transmitter, which is then connected to an external antenna. The stimulated pulses allow the patient to inhale air into the lungs under negative pressure, rather than air being forced into the chest through positive pressure of a ventilator. This code reports the replacement of the external antenna.

L8698

L8698 Miscellaneous component, supply or accessory for use with total artificial heart system

A total artificial heart system, or artificial heart, is a temporary measure until transplantation or to prolong life for patients not eligible for transplant. One type of artificial heart system, described here, is a self-contained, electrohydraulic action heart, charged from a battery source through the skin. Once attached, the natural atria pumps blood into the artificial ventricles of the replacement heart and the hydraulic pump moves the blood into circulation. Internal components include the implanted rechargeable battery, which is continually charged by external battery packs, the internal transcutaneous coil for receiving the battery charge across the skin, and the control unit, which monitors and controls the pumping speed of the artificial heart. This code represents an external component, supply, or accessory for use with the total artificial heart system, such as onboard batteries, portable driver, power supply system, and other miscellaneous items.

L8699

L8699 Prosthetic implant, not otherwise specified

This code reports prosthetic implants that are not otherwise described in more specific HCPCS Level II codes.

L8701-L8702

L8701 Powered upper extremity range of motion assist device, elbow, wrist, hand with single or double upright(s), includes microprocessor, sensors, all components and accessories, custom fabricated

L8702 Powered upper extremity range of motion assist device, elbow, wrist, hand, finger, single or double upright(s), includes microprocessor, sensors, all components and accessories, custom fabricated

A powered upper extremity range of motion assist device is intended to restore function to arms and hands of patients who have sustained an injury, or who suffer from cerebral palsy, neuromuscular disease, or stroke. It is a custom fabricated upper arm orthosis that has noninvasive sensors on the surface of the skin. The sensors read the nerve signals and activate small motors in the orthosis, allowing the patient to move their arm or hand. It consists of the custom fabricated orthosis; noninvasive sensors, motors, and electronics that amplify and process the nerve signals; and batteries. Code L8701 represents an orthosis that includes the elbow, hand, and wrist. Code L8702 represents an orthosis that includes the elbow, hand, wrist, and fingers.

L9900

L9900 Orthotic and prosthetic supply, accessory, and/or service component of another HCPCS L code

This code is to be used for an orthotic or prosthetic supply, accessory, and/or service that is a component of another HCPCS Level II code.

M

M0075

M0075 Cellular therapy

Cellular therapy is the practice of injecting humans with foreign proteins, such as those derived from the placenta or lungs of unborn lambs. Cellular therapy is currently without scientific or statistical evidence to document its therapeutic efficacy and, in fact, is considered a potentially dangerous practice.

M0076

M0076 Prolotherapy

Prolotherapy is also known as proliferative injection therapy or sclerotherapy. The practice of prolotherapy is used by physicians to treat a number of different types of chronic pain. Prolotherapy consists of a series of trigger point injections of "proliferative" solutions into ligaments and tendons near the pained area to induce the proliferation of new cells. Proponents of this treatment suggest that looseness in the supporting ligaments and tendons around the joints causes the pain, inducing the muscles to contract against the ligament and irritate the nerve endings. Three types of solutions are used to initiate inflammation: chemical irritants (e.g., phenol), osmotic shock agents (e.g., hypertonic dextrose and glycerin), and chemotactic agents (e.g., morrhuate sodium, a fatty acid derivative of cod liver oil). These injections irritate or inflame the area where they are injected and are intended to mimic the natural healing process by causing an influx of fibroblasts that synthesize collagen at the injection site, leading to the formation of new ligament and tendon tissue. The newly produced collagen is intended to support the injured or loosened ligaments, creating a more stable and strong muscle base, in the process, alleviating pain.

M0100

M0100 Intragastric hypothermia using gastric freezing

Intragastric hypothermia using gastric freezing is an obsolete treatment for chronic peptic ulcer disease. The treatment is a non-surgical procedure designed to reduce or eliminate the production of gastric acid by freezing the secretory cells with a supercooled fluid introduced into a balloon positioned in the stomach. The treatment was popular about 20 years ago but now is seldom performed. Gastric freezing provided provides only temporary improvement to most patients. It has been largely abandoned due to a high complication rate and its lack of effectiveness in double-blind, controlled clinical trials.

M0201

M0201 COVID-19 vaccine administration inside a patient's home; reported only once per individual home, per date of service, when only COVID-19 vaccine administration is performed at the patient's home

This code is reported for the administration of a COVID-19 vaccine, when administered in a patient's home.

M0220-M0221

M0220 Injection, tixagevimab and cilgavimab, for the pre-exposure prophylaxis only, for certain adults and pediatric individuals (12 years of age and older weighing at least 40kg) with no known SARS-CoV-2 exposure, who either have moderate to severely compromised immune systems or for whom vaccination with any available COVID-19 vaccine is not recommended due to a history of severe adverse reaction to a COVID-19 vaccine(s) and/or COVID-19 vaccine component(s), includes injection and post administration monitoring

M0221 Injection, tixagevimab and cilgavimab, for the pre-exposure prophylaxis only, for certain adults and pediatric individuals (12 years of age and older weighing at least 40kg) with no known SARS-CoV-2 exposure, who either have moderate to severely compromised immune systems or for whom vaccination with any available COVID-19 vaccine is not recommended due to a history of severe adverse reaction to a COVID-19 vaccine(s) and/or COVID-19 vaccine component(s), includes injection and post administration monitoring in the home or residence; this includes a beneficiary's home that has been made provider-based to the hospital during the COVID-19 public health emergency

Tixagevimab and cilgavimab are recombinant human IgG1^{K} monoclonal antibodies that bind to the receptor-binding domain of the spike protein of severe acute respiratory syndrome coronavirus 2 (SARS-CoV-2/coronavirus disease/COVID-19). The combination is indicated for pre-exposure prophylaxis of COVID-19 in adult and pediatric patients, ages 12 and older, weighing at least 40 kg, who are not currently infected with SARS-CoV-2, have not had known recent exposure to SARS-CoV-2, and who have moderate to severe immune compromise due to a medical condition or medications or have a history of severe allergic reaction to COVID-19 vaccines or vaccine components. It should not be used for treatment or for post-exposure prophylaxis. This investigational monoclonal antibody therapy was issued an emergency use authorization (EUA) by the FDA in December 2021. Effective February 24, 2022, the authorized dosage is 600 mg (300 mg tixagevimab and 300 mg cilgavimab) administered as two separate consecutive intramuscular (IM) injections in separate injection sites, preferably one in each gluteal muscle. Patients should be monitored for at least one hour following administration. For patients who received an initial dose of 150 mg tixagevimab and 150 mg cilgavimab, a second dose of 150 mg tixagevimab and 150 mg cilgavimab should be administered as soon as possible. For patients who have received a COVID-19 vaccine, it should be administered at least two weeks following vaccination. There are no current recommendations for repeat dosing. Report M0220 for administration in a health care setting and M0221 for administration in the patient's home or residence.

M0222-M0223

M0222 Intravenous injection, bebtelovimab, includes injection and post administration monitoring

M0223 Intravenous injection, bebtelovimab, includes injection and post administration monitoring in the home or residence; this includes a beneficiary's home that has been made provider-based to the hospital during the COVID-19 public health emergency

Bebtelovimab is a recombinant human IgG1^{K} monoclonal antibody that binds to the receptor-binding domain of the spike protein of severe acute respiratory syndrome coronavirus 2 (SARS-CoV-2/coronavirus disease/COVID-19). It is indicated for pre-exposure prophylaxis of COVID-19 in adult and pediatric patients, ages 12 and older, weighing at least 40 kg, with mild-to-moderate coronavirus disease 2019 (COVID-19) with positive results to SARS-CoV-2 viral testing, are at high risk for illness progression or hospitalization, and for whom alternative FDA-approved treatment options are not clinically appropriate or accessible. This investigational monoclonal antibody therapy was issued an emergency use authorization (EUA) by the FDA in February 2022. The authorized dosage is 175 mg administered via intravenous (IV) injection over at least 30 seconds. It should be administered within seven days of the onset of symptoms. Patients should be monitored for at least one hour following administration. Report M0222 for administration in a health care setting and M0223 for administration in the patient's home or residence.

M0240-M0241

M0240 Intravenous infusion or subcutaneous injection, casirivimab and imdevimab, includes infusion or injection and post administration monitoring, subsequent repeat doses

M0241 Intravenous infusion or subcutaneous injection, casirivimab and imdevimab, includes infusion or injection, and post administration monitoring in the home or residence. This includes a beneficiary's home that has been made provider-based to the hospital during the covid-19 public health emergency, subsequent repeat doses

Casirivimab and imdevimab are monoclonal antibodies that bind to the receptor-binding domain of the spike protein of severe acute respiratory syndrome coronavirus 2 (SARS-CoV-2/coronavirus disease/COVID-19). Indicated for the postexposure prophylaxis of COVID-19 in adult and pediatric patients 12 years of age and older, weighing at least 40 kg, who are at high risk for progression to severe COVID-19 and/or hospitalization, are not fully vaccinated or not expected to mount an adequate immune response to complete vaccination, and have been or are at high risk of exposure to an infected individual. This postexposure prophylaxis therapy was issued an emergency use authorization (EUA) by the FDA in July 2021. The recommended dosage is 600 mg of casirivimab and 600 mg of imdevimab administered together as a single subcutaneous (SC) injection or an intravenous (IV) infusion as soon as possible following exposure. For individuals with ongoing exposure, a subsequent repeat dose of 300 mg of casirivimab and 300 mg of imdevimab may be administered once every four weeks for duration of exposure. See full prescribing information for complete administration instructions. These codes report only the administration by IV infusion or SC injection and include post-administration monitoring. Report M0240 for administration in a healthcare setting or M0241 for administration in the patient's home or residence.

M0243

M0243 Intravenous infusion or subcutaneous injection, casirivimab and imdevimab, includes infusion or injection, and post administration monitoring

Casirivimab and imdevimab are monoclonal antibodies that bind to the receptor-binding domain of the spike protein of severe acute respiratory syndrome coronavirus 2 (SARS-CoV-2/Coronavirus disease/COVID-19). Indicated for the treatment of mild to moderate COVID-19 in adult and pediatric patients 12 years of age and older, weighing at least 40 kg, whose test results are positive for COVID-19 and who are at high risk for progression to severe COVID-19 and/or hospitalization, this investigational monoclonal antibody combination therapy was issued an emergency use authorization (EUA) by the FDA in November 2020. The dosage is 1,200 mg of casirivimab and 1,200 mg of imdevimab administered together as a single intravenous (IV) infusion over at least 60 minutes. The solutions must be diluted prior to administration and should be given together as soon as possible after a positive result of direct SARS-CoV-2 viral testing and within 10 days of symptom onset. Administration is allowed only in settings where healthcare providers have immediate access to medications that can treat anaphylaxis or other severe infusion reactions and can activate the emergency medical system (EMS) when necessary. This code reports only the administration by IV infusion and includes post-administration monitoring.

M0244

M0244 Intravenous infusion or subcutaneous injection, casirivimab and imdevimab, includes infusion or injection and post administration monitoring in the home or residence; this includes a beneficiary's home that has been made provider-based to the hospital during the COVID-19 public health emergency

Casirivimab and imdevimab are monoclonal antibodies that bind to the receptor-binding domain of the spike protein of severe acute respiratory syndrome coronavirus 2 (SARS-CoV-2/Coronavirus disease/COVID-19). Indicated for the treatment of mild to moderate COVID-19 in adult and pediatric patients, age 12 and older, weighing at least 40 kg, whose test results are positive for COVID-19 and who are at high risk for progression to severe COVID-19 and/or hospitalization, this investigational monoclonal antibody combination therapy was issued an emergency use authorization (EUA) by the FDA in November 2020. The dosage is 1,200 mg of casirivimab and 1,200 mg of imdevimab administered together as a single intravenous (IV) infusion over at least 60 minutes. The solutions must be diluted prior to administration and should be given together as soon as possible after a positive result of direct SARS-CoV-2 viral testing and within 10 days of symptom onset. This code reports only the administration by IV infusion in the patient's home or residence and includes post-administration monitoring. Health care providers must have immediate access to medications that can treat anaphylaxis or other severe infusion reactions, as well as the ability to activate the emergency medical system (EMS) when necessary.

M0245

M0245 Intravenous infusion, bamlanivimab and etesevimab, includes infusion and post administration monitoring

Bamlanivimab is a neutralizing IgG1 monoclonal antibody that binds to the receptor-binding domain of the spike protein of severe acute respiratory syndrome coronavirus 2 (SARS-CoV-2/Coronavirus disease/COVID-19). Etesevimab is a monoclonal antibody against the surface spike protein of SARS-CoV-2. Indicated for the treatment of mild to moderate COVID-19 in adult and pediatric patients ages 12 years and older, weighing at least 40 kg, whose test results are positive for COVID-19, and who are at high risk for progression to severe COVID-19 and/or hospitalization, this investigational monoclonal antibody therapy was issued an emergency use authorization (EUA) by the FDA in February 2021. The authorized dosage is a single intravenous (IV) infusion of 700 mg bamlanivimab and 1400 mg etesevimab over at least 60 minutes via pump or gravity. It should be administered as soon as possible after a positive viral test for SARS-CoV-2 and within 10 days of symptom onset. Administration is allowed only in settings where healthcare providers have immediate access to medications that can treat anaphylaxis or other severe infusion reactions and can activate the emergency medical system (EMS) when necessary. This code reports only the administration by IV infusion and includes post-administration monitoring.

M0246

M0246 Intravenous infusion, bamlanivimab and etesevimab, includes infusion and post administration monitoring in the home or residence; this includes a beneficiary's home that has been made provider-based to the hospital during the COVID-19 public health emergency

Bamlanivimab is a neutralizing IgG1 monoclonal antibody that binds to the receptor-binding domain of the spike protein of severe acute respiratory syndrome coronavirus 2 (SARS-CoV-2/Coronavirus disease/COVID-19). Etesevimab is a monoclonal antibody against the surface spike protein of SARS-CoV-2. Indicated for the treatment of mild to moderate COVID-19 in adult and pediatric patients, ages 12 and older, weighing at least 40 kg, whose test results are positive for COVID-19, and who are at high risk for progression to severe COVID-19 and/or hospitalization, this investigational monoclonal antibody therapy was issued an emergency use authorization (EUA) by the FDA in February 2021. The authorized dosage is a single intravenous (IV) infusion of 700 mg bamlanivimab and 1,400 mg etesevimab over at least 60 minutes via pump or gravity. It should be administered as soon as possible after a positive viral test for SARS-CoV-2 and within 10 days of symptom onset. This code reports only the administration by IV infusion in the patient's home or residence and includes post-administration monitoring. Health care providers must have immediate access to medications that can treat anaphylaxis or other severe infusion reactions, as well as the ability to activate the emergency medical system (EMS) when necessary.

M0247-M0248

M0247 Intravenous infusion, sotrovimab, includes infusion and post administration monitoring

M0248 Intravenous infusion, sotrovimab, includes infusion and post administration monitoring in the home or residence; this includes a beneficiary's home that has been made provider-based to the hospital during the COVID-19 public health emergency

Sotrovimab is a neutralizing IgG1 monoclonal antibody that binds to the receptor-binding domain of the spike protein of severe acute respiratory syndrome coronavirus 2 (SARS-CoV-2/coronavirus disease/COVID-19). Sotrovimab is a monoclonal antibody against the surface spike protein of SARS-CoV-2. Indicated for the treatment of mild to moderate COVID-19 in adult and pediatric patients, ages 12 and older, weighing at least 40 kg, whose test results are positive for COVID-19, and who are at high risk for progression to severe COVID-19 and/or hospitalization, this investigational monoclonal antibody therapy was issued an emergency use authorization (EUA) by the FDA in February 2021. The authorized dosage is a single intravenous (IV) infusion of 500 mg of sotrovimab over 30 minutes via pump or gravity. It should be administered as soon as possible after a positive viral test for SARS-CoV-2 and within 10 days of symptom onset. Report M0247 for administration by IV infusion only, including post-administration monitoring. Report M0248 for the administration by IV infusion in the patient's home or residence, including post-administration monitoring. Healthcare providers must have immediate access to medications that can treat anaphylaxis or other severe infusion reactions, as well as the ability to activate the emergency medical system (EMS) when necessary.

M0249-M0250

M0249 Intravenous infusion, tocilizumab, for hospitalized adults and pediatric patients (2 years of age and older) with COVID-19 who are receiving systemic corticosteroids and require supplemental oxygen, non-invasive or invasive mechanical ventilation, or extracorporeal membrane oxygenation (ECMO) only, includes infusion and post administration monitoring, first dose

M0250 Intravenous infusion, tocilizumab, for hospitalized adults and pediatric patients (2 years of age and older) with COVID-19 who are receiving systemic corticosteroids and require supplemental oxygen, non-invasive or invasive mechanical ventilation, or extracorporeal membrane oxygenation (ECMO) only, includes infusion and post administration monitoring, second dose

Tocilizumab is a recombinant humanized anti-human interleukin 6 (IL-6) monoclonal antibody, subclass IgG1k (gamma 1, kappa), that binds to IL-6 receptors and inhibits IL-6 mediated signaling. It is indicated for the treatment of severe acute respiratory syndrome coronavirus 2 (SARS-CoV-2/coronavirus disease/COVID-19) in hospitalized adult and pediatric patients, ages 2 and older, weighing at least 30 kg, who are receiving systemic corticosteroids and require supplemental oxygen, invasive or noninvasive mechanical ventilation, or extracorporeal membrane oxygenation (ECMO). This investigational monoclonal antibody therapy was issued an emergency use authorization (EUA) by the FDA in June 2021. The authorized dosage for patients weighing less than 30 kg is 12 mg/kg diluted to 50 mL in 0.9% or 0.45% sodium chloride. For patients weighing 30 kg or more, the authorized dosage is 8 mg/kg diluted to 100 mL in 0.9% or 0.45% sodium chloride. The maximum dosage is 800 mg per infusion. It is administered as a single intravenous (IV) infusion over 60 minutes. It should not be administered via a bolus, push, or subcutaneous (SC) injection. If signs or symptoms do not improve or worsen after the first dose, an additional infusion may be given eight hours following the first dose. Report M0249 for administration of the first dose. Report M0250 for administration of the second dose.

M0300

M0300 IV chelation therapy (chemical endarterectomy)

Intravenous chelation therapy is infusion of a solution, traditionally a synthetic amino acid called ethylene diamine tetraacetic acid (EDTA). The EDTA binds with metals and minerals, which are then excreted from the body with the EDTA. This therapy, which removes unwanted metal ions from the body purportedly has therapeutic and preventative effects. Chelation therapy, when used as a treatment for atherosclerosis, is sometimes referred to as a chemical endarterectomy. The application of chelation therapy using EDTA for the treatment and prevention of atherosclerosis is controversial. There is no widely accepted rationale to explain the beneficial effects attributed to this therapy. Its safety is questioned and its clinical effectiveness has never been established by well-designed, controlled clinical trials.

M0301

M0301 Fabric wrapping of abdominal aneurysm

Fabric wrapping of an abdominal aneurysm is a treatment where the aneurysm is wrapped with cellophane or fascia lata. No other procedure is performed on the aneurysm or its surrounding tissue. The procedure has not been shown to prevent eventual rupture. In extremely rare instances, external wall reinforcement may be indicated when the current accepted treatment (excision of the aneurysm and reconstruction with synthetic materials) is not a viable alternative, but external wall reinforcement is not fabric wrapping. CMS believes that this treatment is ineffective and it is not covered by Medicare and many other payers.

P

P2028

P2028 Cephalin floculation, blood

Cephalin flocculation is a test performed on serum using cephalin or a cephalin-cholesterol emulation. The flocculation or dispersion of the blood into discrete visible particles may indicate the presence of liver cell disease. This test is considered obsolete.

P2029

P2029 Congo red, blood

Congo red is an odorless dark red or brown powder that decomposes upon exposure to acid fumes. It is used as a diagnostic aid in amyloidosis. The Congo red dye is injected intravenously. If after one hour more than 60 percent of the dye has disappeared, amyloidosis is indicated. This test is considered obsolete.

P2031

P2031 Hair analysis (excluding arsenic)

Laboratory analysis of hair may be used to detect the presence of drugs, chemicals, and other substances. Note that many insurance payers only cover hair analysis for the detection of arsenic. This code reports hair analysis, excluding arsenic.

P2033

P2033 Thymol turbidity, blood

Thymol turbidity is a test performed on serum using the chemical thymol. The serum precipitates into albumin and globulin, which can then be measured to look for indications of liver disease. Although popular in the past, it has been superseded by quantitative determination of specific proteins and direct measurement of liver enzymes. This test is considered obsolete.

P2038

P2038 Mucoprotein, blood (seromucoid) (medical necessity procedure)

Mucoprotein is a general term for a protein-polysaccharide complex, wherein the protein component is the major part of the complex. The compound is present in all connective and supporting tissues. It is sometimes called glycoprotein, although this term usually refers to those mucoproteins that contain less than four percent carbohydrate. This code represents an assay of the mucoproteins contained in a sample of blood. Most testing performed currently are for a more specific component of the complex.

P3000-P3001

P3000 Screening Papanicolaou smear, cervical or vaginal, up to three smears, by technician under physician supervision

P3001 Screening Papanicolaou smear, cervical or vaginal, up to three smears, requiring interpretation by physician

A screening Papanicolaou (commonly referred to as Pap) smear, cervical or vaginal, is a microscopic examination of cells scraped from the cervix or vaginal wall. The smears are examined for any cells that appear to be abnormal. It is a screening procedure when no known disease process exists.

P7001

P7001 Culture, bacterial, urine; quantitative, sensitivity study

A culture is the inoculation and incubation of a growth medium. In this case, urine is inoculated onto a growth medium with the intention of determining the types and amounts of bacteria that grow. A sensitivity test follows. The bacteria that have been grown are tested against antibiotics to determine which antibiotic has the greatest efficacy against the bacteria. This code should be used only for urine cultures when both a culture and sensitivity are performed consecutively on the same specimen.

P9010-P9011

P9010 Blood (whole), for transfusion, per unit

P9011 Blood, split unit

Whole blood is blood without any component removed. Whole blood is the liquid medium containing the microscopic elements of erythrocytes (red blood cell), leukocytes (white blood cells), and thrombocytes (blood platelets). Whole blood is drawn from a selected donor under strict aseptic conditions. The blood is usually mixed with a citrate ion or heparin to prevent coagulation. It may be banked and used as a replacement when blood is lost. Blood is classified into four phenotypes based upon the characteristics present: A, B, AB, and O. Additionally, an Rh factor of negative or positive is assigned, denoting the absence or presence of an Rh antigen. Before any blood, with the exception of type O negative, can be transfused into a patient, tests must be run to determine the compatibility of the donor blood with the patient's own blood. Type O negative is said to be the universal donor as this type of blood contains no factors that may adversely interact with the blood of the recipient. Due to the variety and number of incompatibilities that may exist, whole blood is used only when absolutely necessary and blood components are more routinely transfused.

P9012

P9012 Cryoprecipitate, each unit

Cryoprecipitate is the cold insoluble portion of plasma that precipitates (settles into solid particles) when fresh frozen plasma is thawed at 1-6 degrees C. The supernatant (or liquid plasma) is removed and the residual cryoprecipitate (approximately 15 ml) is refrozen and stored at -18 degrees C. A single unit of cryoprecipitate contains an average of 80-100 units of factor VIII and von Willebrand factor, 150-250 mg of fibrinogen and some factor XIII and fibronectin. No compatibility testing is required and typing is not necessary. When cryoprecipitate is ordered, units are thawed, suspended in sterile, normal saline (20ml/bag) and pooled. Cryoprecipitate is the only fibrinogen concentrate available for intravenous use. In the past, cryoprecipitate had been used as a treatment for von Willebrand's disease and hemophilia A. However, newer products are the treatment of choice now. Cryoprecipitate may also be used in the preparation of fibrin glue. This glue is used in neurosurgery, orthopedic, and other surgeries. Although widespread, such use is not FDA-approved. Autologous (the patient's own blood) units can be collected prior to surgery and processed into fibrin glue. This code represents one unit of cryoprecipitate.

P9016

P9016 Red blood cells, leukocytes reduced, each unit

Red blood cells (RBCs) are a singular component of whole blood. RBCs are prepared from whole blood by the removal of most of the plasma, or by apheresis collection. RBCs are stored in one of several saline-based anticoagulant/preservative solutions, yielding a hematocrit (Hct) between 55 to 80 percent. Leukocytes (or WBCs) are reduced or removed from the unit as the leukocytes may provoke an adverse reaction or antibody formation when they interact with the patient's own blood. RBC transfusions increase the oxygen-carrying capacity of blood. Transfusions may also treat chronic anemia when pharmacologic therapy is not effective or available, active bleeding, sickle cell disease, or other conditions. RBCs require compatibility testing. Transfusions should be completed within four hours per unit. A unit may be divided by the blood bank in advance and administered in two or more aliquots. This code represents one unit of RBCs.

P9017

P9017 Fresh frozen plasma (single donor), frozen within 8 hours of collection, each unit

Plasma is the liquid portion of whole blood. Plasma is prepared by separating it from whole blood using a centrifuge, or by hemapheresis using centrifugation or filtration. The volume of plasma varies and appears on the label. One unit of fresh frozen plasma contains the plasma from one unit of whole blood, approximately 250 ml, separated and frozen within eight hours of collection. While plasma may be pooled (multiple units of whole blood are separated and combined), this code represents plasma obtained from a single donor. Plasma contains all soluble clotting factors, though some may be substantially reduced, such as Factors V and VIII. Units of plasma transfused should be ABO compatible with the recipient, but crossmatching and Rh compatibility are not required. Plasma may be indicated in the treatment of thrombotic thrombocytopenic purpura and related syndromes, congenital or acquired coagulation factor deficiency when no concentrate is available, and for specific plasma protein deficiencies such as an anti-thrombin III or C-1 esterase deficiency. Plasma may also be indicated for bleeding, preoperative, or massively transfused patients with a deficiency of multiple coagulation factors, or for patients on warfarin therapy who are bleeding and/or who are facing urgent invasive procedures. Report this code for one unit of fresh frozen plasma that was frozen within eight hours of its collection from a single donor.

P9019-P9020

P9019 Platelets, each unit

P9020 Platelet rich plasma, each unit

Platelets are thrombocyte cells removed from whole blood. Platelets may be separated from the whole blood of many different donors by the use of a centrifuge or may be harvested from a single donor by hemapheresis. Pooled random donor platelets are typically prepared from four to six units of random donor platelets. Platelet-rich plasma contains pooled amounts of platelets. Platelets may be suspended in donor plasma. Volume is specified on the label. Compatibility testing is not required, but units of platelets transfused should be ABO compatible when possible. Transfusion of large quantities of ABO-incompatible plasma may lead to a positive direct antiglobulin test and, rarely, clinically significant red cell destruction. Rh compatibility is important but not always possible. Platelets may be indicated for the prevention and treatment of nonsurgical bleeding due to thrombocytopenia and for patients with accelerated platelet destruction with significant bleeding (such as autoimmune or drug-induced thrombocytopenia), those with documented low-level platelet counts who are bleeding or who face major invasive procedures, and for patients with diffuse microvascular bleeding following cardiopulmonary bypass or massive transfusions.

P9021

P9021 Red blood cells, each unit

This code reports each unit of red blood cells. Whole blood is run through centrifugation where plasma (liquid portion of the whole blood) and red blood cells are separated. Red blood cells contain hemoglobin. Hemoglobin is a complex iron-containing protein that carries oxygen through the body and gives blood its red coloring. There are approximately 1 billion red blood cells in two to three drops of blood. Red blood cells are manufactured in the bone marrow.

P9022

P9022 Red blood cells, washed, each unit

Whole blood is run through centrifugation where the plasma (liquid portion of the whole blood) and the red blood cells are separated. Red blood cells contain hemoglobin. Hemoglobin is a complex iron containing protein that carries oxygen through the body and gives blood its red coloring. There are approximately one billion red blood cells in two to three drops of blood. Red blood cells are manufactured in the bone marrow. These red blood cells are washed with normal saline.

P9023

P9023 Plasma, pooled multiple donor, solvent/detergent treated, frozen, each unit

Plasma is the liquid portion of whole blood. Plasma is prepared by separating it from whole blood using a centrifuge, or by hemapheresis using centrifugation or filtration. The volume of plasma varies and appears on the label. One unit of fresh frozen plasma contains the plasma from one unit of whole blood, approximately 250 ml, separated and frozen within eight hours of collection. While plasma may be obtained from a single donor, this code represents plasma that has been pooled (multiple units of whole blood separated and combined). Plasma contains all soluble clotting factors, though some may be substantially reduced, such as Factors V and VIII. Plasma may be "washed" or treated with a solvent or detergent to destroy any lipid bound viruses, including HIV1 and 2, hepatitis B and C, and HTLVI and II. The process does not destroy non-enveloped viruses or prion particles. Units of plasma transfused should be ABO compatible, but crossmatching and Rh compatibility are not required. Plasma may be indicated in the treatment of thrombotic thrombocytopenic purpura and related syndromes, congenital or acquired coagulation factor deficiency when no concentrate is available, and specific plasma protein deficiencies such as an anti-thrombin III or C-1 esterase deficiency. Plasma may also be indicated for bleeding, preoperative, or massively transfused patients with a deficiency of multiple coagulation factors, or for patients on warfarin therapy who are bleeding and/or who are facing urgent invasive procedures. This code should be used for one unit of plasma that has been pooled from multiple donors, solvent or detergent treated, and frozen.

P9025

P9025 Plasma, cryoprecipitate reduced, pathogen reduced, each unit

Plasma that is cryoprecipitate reduced and plasma reduced is the solution remaining once the cold insoluble portion has been removed. Cryoprecipitate settles into solid particles when fresh frozen plasma is thawed at 1-6 degrees C. The liquid plasma removed is the cryoprecipitate-reduced plasma. Amotosalen, a photoactive compound to target DNA and RNA, is activated by ultraviolet A (UVA), permanently cross linking the nucleic acids and creating plasma, cryoprecipitate reduced, pathogen reduced (PCRPR). PCRPR blocks replication of bacteria, parasites, and viruses. It is indicated for the treatment of thrombotic thrombocytopenic purpura (TTP) and to provide coagulation factors except for fibrinogen, factor VIII, factor XIII, and vWF. This code represents one unit.

P9026

P9026 Cryoprecipitated fibrinogen complex, pathogen reduced, each unit

Cryoprecipitated fibrinogen complex, plasma reduced (CFCPR) is the solution remaining once the cold insoluble portion has been removed. Cryoprecipitate settles into solid particles when fresh frozen plasma is thawed at 1-6 degrees C. The liquid plasma removed is the cryoprecipitate-reduced plasma. Amotosalen, a photoactive compound to target DNA and RNA, is activated by ultraviolet A (UVA), permanently cross linking the nucleic acids and creating cryoprecipitated fibrinogen complex, plasma reduced. CFCPR blocks replication of bacteria, parasites, and viruses. It is indicated for the treatment and control of bleeding associated with fibrinogen deficiency, control of bleeding when recombinant or other specific virally inactivated factor XIII or von Willebrand disease (vWF) are not available, as a second-line treatment for vWF, and control of uremic bleeding when other treatment has failed. This code represents one unit.

P9031-P9037

P9031 Platelets, leukocytes reduced, each unit
P9032 Platelets, irradiated, each unit
P9033 Platelets, leukocytes reduced, irradiated, each unit
P9034 Platelets, pheresis, each unit
P9035 Platelets, pheresis, leukocytes reduced, each unit
P9036 Platelets, pheresis, irradiated, each unit
P9037 Platelets, pheresis, leukocytes reduced, irradiated, each unit

Platelets are the thrombocyte cells removed from whole blood. Platelets may be separated from the whole blood of many different donors by the use of a centrifuge, or may be harvested from a single donor by hemapheresis. Pooled random donor platelets are typically prepared from four to six units of random donor platelets. Platelet rich plasma contains pooled amounts of platelets. Platelets may be suspended in donor plasma. Volume is specified on the label. Compatibility testing is not required, but units of platelets transfused should be ABO compatible when possible. Rh compatibility is important but not always possible. Platelets may be leukocyte (white blood cell) reduced, which is the filtered removal of contaminating leukocytes. Platelets may be irradiated using gamma radiation to destroy the ability of lymphocytes (a type of leukocyte) to respond to foreign antigens, such as those in the recipient's blood. Leukocytes may provoke an adverse reaction or antibody formation in the patient's blood. They may also transmit certain viruses, including cytomegalovirus (CMV) and human T-cell lymphotropic virus (HTLV-I/II). Pheresis (apheresis) is a targeted removal of blood component from whole blood with the return of the remaining blood components to the donor. Pheresis uses a centrifuge device to separate blood components. Plasma, platelet, and leukocytes are the components that may be removed using pheresis. The designated component (in this case platelets) is removed and the remaining blood components are retransfused into the donor. Platelets are indicated for the prevention and treatment of non-surgical bleeding due to thrombocytopenia, for patients with accelerated platelet destruction with significant bleeding (such as autoimmune or drug-induced thrombocytopenia), for patients with documented low level platelet counts who are bleeding or who face major invasive procedures, and for patients with diffuse microvascular bleeding following cardiopulmonary bypass or massive transfusions.

P9038-P9040

P9038 Red blood cells, irradiated, each unit
P9039 Red blood cells, deglycerolized, each unit
P9040 Red blood cells, leukocytes reduced, irradiated, each unit

Red blood cells (RBC) are a singular component of whole blood. RBCs are prepared from whole blood by the removal of most of the plasma or by apheresis collection. RBCs are stored in one of several saline-based anticoagulant/preservative solutions, yielding a hematocrit (Hct) between 55 to 80 percent. RBCs may be leukocyte (or white blood cell) reduced, which is the filter removal of contaminating leukocytes. RBCs may be irradiated using gamma radiation to destroy the ability of lymphocytes (a type of leukocyte) to respond to foreign antigens in the recipient's blood. Leukocytes may provoke an adverse reaction or antibody formation when they interact with the patient's own blood. They may also transmit certain viruses, including cytomegalovirus (CMV) and human T-cell lymphotropic virus (HTLV-I/II). Prior to freezing, glycerol may be added to the RBCs. When this glycerol is removed upon thawing, the RBCs are termed "deglycerolized." A major indication for RBC transfusions is prevention or treatment of symptoms of tissue hypoxia by increasing the oxygen-carrying capacity of blood. RBCs may also be indicated in the treatment of symptomatic chronic anemia when pharmacologic therapy is not effective or available, active bleeding with signs and symptoms of hypovolemia, preoperative anemia with impending major blood loss, sickle cell disease, and anemia due to renal failure/hemodialysis. RBCs require compatibility testing and should be ABO and Rh compatible. The initial transfusion period may be carefully monitored with a slow transfusion rate to allow early detection of a reaction. Transfusions should be completed within four hours per unit. Alternatively, the unit may be divided by the blood bank in advance and administered in two or more aliquots.

P9041

P9041 Infusion, albumin (human), 5%, 50 ml

Albumin is a protein manufactured by the liver and carried throughout the body by plasma and is the most prevalent protein found in blood plasma. Plasma is collected and pooled, then fractionated to separate the albumin. Unlike other plasma proteins, albumin has several essential physiologic functions in the human body and is an important therapeutic agent. Albumin maintains the osmotic pressure that causes fluid to remain within the blood stream instead of leaking out into the tissues. It also transports thyroid hormone, drugs, and bilirubin. It increases total blood volume by drawing fluid from body tissues. Albumin may be indicated as a treatment for shock, hypovolemia, acute liver failure, burns and other thermal injuries, hypoproteinemia, adult respiratory distress syndrome, cardiopulmonary bypass, neonatal hemolytic disease, renal dialysis, acute nephrosis, erythrocyte, acute peritonitis, pancreatitis, and cellulitis. Albumin is available with varying concentrations of protein: 5 percent, 20 percent, and 25 percent. The recommended concentration and dosage depends upon the patient and reason for administration. It is administered by intravenous infusion.

P9043

P9043 Infusion, plasma protein fraction (human), 5%, 50 ml

Plasma protein fraction is a sterile solution of selected proteins derived from the blood plasma of adult human donors. It typically contains 4.5 to 5.5 grams of protein per 100 ml. This protein consists of 83 to 90 percent albumin, with the remainder alpha- and beta-globulins. Plasma protein fraction is the solution remaining once cryoprecipitate, fibrinogen, and immunoglobulins have been removed. Plasma protein faction is usually heat treated to destroy viruses. Indications for its use are similar to those for albumin. Administered intravenously, it increases total blood volume by drawing fluid from body tissues. Other indications include shock, hypovolemia, acute liver failure, burns and other thermal injuries, hypoproteinemia, adult respiratory distress syndrome, cardiopulmonary bypass, neonatal hemolytic disease, renal dialysis, acute nephrosis, erythrocyte resuspension, acute peritonitis, pancreatitis, mediastinitis, and cellulitis. This code represents 50 ml of a 5 percent concentration of plasma protein fraction.

P9044

P9044 Plasma, cryoprecipitate reduced, each unit

Cryoprecipitate reduced plasma is the solution remaining once the cold insoluble portion has been removed. Cryoprecipitate settles into solid particles when fresh frozen plasma is thawed at 1-6 degrees C. The liquid plasma removed is the cryoprecipitate-reduced plasma. Cryoprecipitate reduced plasma is deficient in Von Willebrand factor, Factor VIII, Factor XIII, fibrinogen, and fibronectin. It may be indicated for the treatment of thrombotic thrombocytopenic purpura. This code represents one unit.

P9045-P9047

P9045 Infusion, albumin (human), 5%, 250 ml

P9046 Infusion, albumin (human), 25%, 20 ml

P9047 Infusion, albumin (human), 25%, 50 ml

Albumin is a protein manufactured by the liver and carried throughout the body by plasma and is the most prevalent protein found in blood plasma. Plasma is collected and pooled, then fractionated to separate the albumin. Unlike other plasma proteins, albumin has several essential physiologic functions in the human body and is an important therapeutic agent. Albumin maintains the osmotic pressure that causes fluid to remain within the blood stream instead of leaking out into the tissues. It also transports thyroid hormone, drugs, and bilirubin. It increases total blood volume by drawing fluid from body tissues. Albumin may be indicated as a treatment for shock, hypovolemia, acute liver failure, burns and other thermal injuries, hypoproteinemia, adult respiratory distress syndrome, cardiopulmonary bypass, neonatal hemolytic disease, renal dialysis, acute nephrosis, erythrocyte, acute peritonitis, pancreatitis, and cellulitis. Albumin is available with varying concentrations of protein: 5 percent, 20 percent, and 25 percent. The recommended concentration and dosage depends upon the patient and reason for administration. It is administered by intravenous infusion.

P9048

P9048 Infusion, plasma protein fraction (human), 5%, 250 ml

Plasma protein fraction is a sterile solution of selected proteins derived from the blood plasma of adult human donors. It contains 4.5 to 5.5 grams of protein per 100 ml. This protein consists of 83 to 90 percent albumin with the remainder alpha-and beta-globulins. Plasma Protein Fraction is the solution remaining once cryoprecipitate, fibrinogen, and immunoglobulins have been removed from plasma. Plasma protein faction is usually heat treated to destroy HIV, hepatitis viruses, and CMV. Indications for its use are similar to those for albumin. Administered intravenously, it increases total blood volume by drawing fluid from body tissues. Other indications include shock, hypovolemia, acute liver failure, burns and other thermal injuries, hypoproteinemia, adult respiratory distress syndrome, cardiopulmonary bypass, neonatal hemolytic disease, renal dialysis, acute nephrosis, erythrocyte resuspension, acute peritonitis, pancreatitis, mediastinitis, and cellulitis. This code represents 250 ml of a 5 percent concentration of plasma protein fraction.

P9050

P9050 Granulocytes, pheresis, each unit

Granulocytes are types of leukocytes (white blood cells) consisting of neutrophils, basophils, or eosinophils. They are distinguished by the granules (insoluble nonmembranous particles) found within their cytoplasm. Granulocytes surround and destroy microorganisms. These granules within each cell are filled with chemicals, which upon their release, help to degrade the microorganism that the granulocyte surrounds. The cells are named for the way they stain in the laboratory. For example, eosinophils absorb acidic dyes such as eosin. Pheresis (apheresis) is a targeted removal of blood component from whole blood with the return of the remaining blood components to the donor. Pheresis uses a centrifuge to separate blood components. Plasma, platelet, and leukocytes are the components that may be removed using pheresis. The designated component (in this case granulocytes) is removed and the remaining blood components are retransfused into the donor. A standard adult concentrate contains approximately 20-50x109 granulocytes, 20-50 ml red blood cells, and 200-400 ml plasma. Granulocyte concentrates for neonates contain approximately 5x109 granulocytes in 30 µl plasma. Prior to the collection of granulocytes, donors are given G-CSF to stimulate their production. Granulocytes must be ABO and RH compatible with the recipient as there are large numbers of red cells in granulocyte concentrates. Granulocyte concentrates are always irradiated using gamma radiation to destroy the ability of lymphocytes to respond to foreign antigens, such as those in the recipient's blood. Granulocytes may be indicated as a treatment for infections that are unresponsive to antibiotic therapy.

P9051

P9051 Whole blood or red blood cells, leukocytes reduced, CMV-negative, each unit

Whole blood is blood without any component removed. Blood consists of plasma, or the liquid medium containing the microscopic elements of erythrocytes (red blood cells), leukocytes (white blood cells), and thrombocytes (blood platelets). Red blood cells (RBCs) are a singular component of whole blood. RBCs are prepared from whole blood by the removal of most of the plasma or by apheresis collection. RBCs are stored in one of several saline-based anticoagulant/preservative solutions, yielding a hematocrit (Hct) between 55 to 80 percent. Both whole blood and RBCs require compatibility testing and should be ABO and Rh compatible. Leukocytes (or white blood cells) are reduced or removed from the unit as the leukocytes may provoke an adverse reaction or antibody formation when they interact with the patient's own blood. Cytomegalovirus (CMV) is a herpes type virus that is found universally throughout all geographic locations and socioeconomic groups and infects between 50 to 85percent of adults in the United States by 40 years of age. For most healthy persons who acquire CMV, there are few symptoms and no long-term health consequences. For the vast majority of people, CMV infection is not a serious problem. However, CMV infection is important to certain high-risk groups. These groups include pregnant women, people who work with children, and immunocompromised people, such as organ transplant recipients and persons infected with human immunodeficiency virus (HIV). Blood products intended for people in a high-risk group are usually tested for CMV. The major indication for RBC transfusions is prevention or treatment of symptoms of tissue hypoxia by increasing the oxygen-carrying capacity of blood. RBCs may also be indicated in the treatment of symptomatic chronic anemia when pharmacologic therapy is not effective or available, active bleeding, with signs and symptoms of hypovolemia, preoperative anemia with impending major blood loss, sickle cell disease, and anemia due to renal failure/hemodialysis refractory to erythropoietin therapy. Due to the variety and number of incompatibilities that may exist, whole blood is used only when necessary and blood components are more routinely transfused. This code represents one unit of either whole body or RBCs that has been leukocyte reduced and has tested negative for the presence of the CMV virus.

P9052-P9053

P9052 Platelets, HLA-matched leukocytes reduced, apheresis/pheresis, each unit

P9053 Platelets, pheresis, leukocytes reduced, CMV-negative, irradiated, each unit

Platelets are the thrombocyte cells removed from whole blood. They may be separated from the whole blood of many different donors by the use of a centrifuge or may be harvested from a single donor by hemapheresis. Platelets may be suspended in donor plasma. Volume is specified on the label. Human leukocyte antigens (HLAs) are proteins located on the surface of white blood cells (WBCs) and certain tissues within the body. HLAs are inherited. There are three groups of HLA: HLA-A, HLA-B and HLA-DR. Each group contains many specific proteins, each labeled with a number (e.g., HLA-A1). Not every person possesses every type of protein (e.g., one person may be HLA-A1 and another HLA-A2). HLA testing determines the compatibility between the donor and recipient blood at the level of the A and B antigens. HLA-matched blood products are then crossmatched. HLA platelets are irradiated. Leukocytes (or WBCs) are reduced or removed from the unit, as the leukocytes may provoke an adverse reaction or antibody formation when they interact with the patient's own blood. Leukocytes may also transmit certain viruses, including cytomegalovirus (CMV) and human T-cell lymphotropic virus (HTLV-I/II). Pheresis (apheresis) is a targeted removal of blood component from whole blood with the return of the remaining blood components to the donor. Essentially, the blood is centrifuged to separate components, in this case the platelets. The remaining blood components are retransfused into the donor. Cytomegalovirus (CMV) is a herpes-type virus that is found universally throughout all geographic locations and socioeconomic groups, and infects between 50 and 85 percent of adults in the United States by 40 years of age. Most healthy persons who acquire CMV exhibit few symptoms and no long-term health consequences. Some persons may experience a mononucleosis-like syndrome with prolonged fever, and mild hepatitis. Once a person is infected, the virus remains alive, but usually dormant within that person's body for life. Recurrent disease rarely occurs unless the person's immune system is suppressed due to therapeutic drugs or disease. Blood products intended for people in high-risk groups are usually tested for CMV. HLA-matched platelets may be indicated for patients who have become refractory to random donor platelets. Report P9052 for one unit of HLA-matched, leukocyte reduced platelets obtained via pheresis (apheresis). Report P9053 for one unit of leukocyte reduced platelets that has been irradiated, has tested negative for CMV, and has been obtained via pheresis (apheresis).

P9054

P9054 Whole blood or red blood cells, leukocytes reduced, frozen, deglycerol, washed, each unit

Whole blood is blood without any component removed. Whole blood contains the microscopic elements of erythrocytes (red blood cells), leukocytes (white blood cells), and thrombocytes (blood platelets). Red blood cells (RBCs) are a singular component of whole blood. RBCs are prepared from whole blood by the removal of most of the plasma or by apheresis collection. RBCs are stored in one of several saline-based anticoagulant/preservative solutions, yielding a hematocrit (Hct) between 55 to 80 percent. Both whole blood and RBCs require compatibility testing. Leukocytes (or WBCs) are reduced or removed from the unit as the leukocytes may provoke an adverse reaction or antibody formation when they interact with the recipient blood. Glycerol may be added to the RBCs prior to freezing. When this glycerol is removed after thawing, the RBCs are termed "deglycerolized." Both whole blood and RBCs may be "washed" or treated with solvent to destroy any lipid bound viruses including HIV and hepatitis B and C. RBC transfusions increase the oxygen-carrying capacity of blood. Transfusions may also treat chronic anemia when pharmacologic therapy is not effective or available, active bleeding, sickle cell disease, and other conditions. Due to the variety and number of incompatibilities that may exist, whole blood is used only when necessary and blood components are more routinely transfused. This code represents a unit of either whole body or RBCs that has been leukocyte reduced, frozen, deglycerolized, and washed.

P9055

P9055 Platelets, leukocytes reduced, CMV-negative, apheresis/pheresis, each unit

Platelets are the thrombocyte cells removed from whole blood. Platelets may be separated from the whole blood of many different donors by a centrifuge or may be harvested from a single donor by hemapheresis. Pooled random donor platelets are typically prepared from four to six units of random donor platelets. Platelet-rich plasma is plasma containing pooled amounts of platelets. Platelets may be suspended in donor plasma; volume is specified on the label. Compatibility type testing is not generally required. Rh compatibility is important but not always possible. Platelets may be leukocyte (or white blood cell) reduced, which is the filter removal of contaminating leukocytes. Leukocytes may provoke an adverse reaction or antibody formation when they interact with the patient's own blood. They may also transmit certain viruses, including cytomegalovirus (CMV) and human T-cell lymphotropic virus (HTLV-I/II). Blood products intended for people in a high-risk group are usually tested for CMV. Pheresis (apheresis) is a targeted removal of blood component from whole blood with the return of the remaining blood components to the donor. Essentially, the blood is centrifuged to separate components. Plasma, platelets, and leukocytes are components that may be removed by pheresis. The designated component, in this case platelets, is removed, and the remaining blood components are retransfused into the donor.

P9056

P9056 Whole blood, leukocytes reduced, irradiated, each unit

Whole blood is blood without any component removed. Blood consists of plasma or the liquid medium containing the microscopic elements of erythrocytes (red blood cell), leukocytes (white blood cells) and thrombocytes (blood platelets). Whole blood is drawn from a selected donor under strict aseptic conditions. The whole blood is usually mixed with a citrate ion or heparin to prevent coagulation. It is typically used as a replacement for blood loss. Blood is classified into four phenotypes based upon the characteristics present: A, B, AB, and O. Additionally, an Rh factor of negative or positive is assigned denoting the absence or presence of an Rh antigen. Tests are run to determine compatibility of the donor blood with the patient's own blood. Type O negative is said to be the universal donor, as this blood type contains no factors that may adversely affect or interact with the blood of the recipient. Whole blood may be leukocyte (white blood cell) reduced using a filter. Whole blood may be gamma irradiated to destroy the ability of lymphocytes (a type of leukocyte) to respond to foreign antigens, such as those in the recipient's blood. Leukocytes may provoke an adverse reaction or antibody formation when they interact with the patient's own blood. Due to the variety and number of incompatibilities that may exist, whole blood is used only when absolutely necessary and blood components are more routinely transfused.

P9057-P9058

P9057 Red blood cells, frozen/deglycerolized/washed, leukocytes reduced, irradiated, each unit

P9058 Red blood cells, leukocytes reduced, CMV-negative, irradiated, each unit

Red blood cells (RBCs) are a singular component of whole blood. RBCs are prepared from whole blood by the removal of most of the plasma, or by apheresis collection. RBCs are stored in one of several saline-based anticoagulant/preservative solutions, yielding a hematocrit (Hct) between 55 and 80 percent. RBCs require ABO and Rh compatibility testing. Leukocytes (white blood cells) are reduced or removed from the unit, as the leukocytes may provoke an adverse reaction or antibody formation when they interact with the patient's own blood. RBCs may also be gamma irradiated to destroy the ability of lymphocytes (a type of leukocyte) to respond to foreign antigens, such as those in the recipient's blood. Glycerol may be added to the RBCs prior to freezing. When this glycerol is removed after thawing, the RBCs are termed "deglycerolized." RBCs may be "washed," or treated with solvent, to destroy any lipid-bound viruses. Blood products intended for people in a high-risk group are usually tested for cytomegalovirus (CMV). RBC transfusions increase the oxygen-carrying capacity of blood. RBC transfusion may be indicated for symptomatic chronic anemia when pharmacologic therapy is not effective or available, active bleeding, preoperative anemia with impending major blood loss, and sickle cell disease, among other conditions. Due to the variety and number of incompatibilities that may exist, whole blood is used only when absolutely necessary and blood components are more routinely transfused.

P9059-P9060

P9059 Fresh frozen plasma between 8-24 hours of collection, each unit

P9060 Fresh frozen plasma, donor retested, each unit

Plasma is the liquid portion of whole blood. Plasma is prepared by separating it from whole blood by centrifuge, or by hemapheresis using centrifugation or filtration. The volume of plasma varies and appears on the label. One unit of fresh frozen plasma contains the plasma from one unit of whole blood, approximately 250 ml, separated and frozen. Plasma may be pooled (multiple units of whole blood separated and combined). Plasma contains all soluble clotting factors, though some may be substantially reduced, such as Factors V and VIII. Units of plasma transfused should be ABO compatible with the recipient, but crossmatching and Rh compatibility are not typically required. Donors may be tested and retested for communicable diseases. Plasma may be indicated for a number of conditions and syndromes, including for preoperative or massively transfused patients with a deficiency of multiple coagulation factors.

P9070-P9071

P9070 Plasma, pooled multiple donor, pathogen reduced, frozen, each unit

P9071 Plasma (single donor), pathogen reduced, frozen, each unit

The FDA approved a plasma pathogen reduction system for use in reducing the risk of transfusion transmitted infections often present in plasma from whole blood and/or apheresis. This system exposes the specimen to ultraviolet light and a chemical called amotosalen. The specimen is purified to remove the chemical and any remaining byproducts. It can then be utilized for transfusion purposes.

P9073

P9073 Platelets, pheresis, pathogen-reduced, each unit

The FDA approved a pathogen reduction system for use in reducing the risk of transfusion transmitted infections often present in platelets from whole blood and/or apheresis. This system exposes the specimen to ultraviolet light and a chemical called amotosalen. The specimen is purified to remove the chemical and any remaining byproducts. The process is effective against multiple infectious agents, including bacteria, parasites, protozoa, and viruses. It also reduces T-cell levels to lower the risk of transfusion-associated graft-versus-host disease (TA-GVHD). It can then be utilized for transfusion purposes. Report P9073 for the administration of platelets that have been tested for pathogen contamination. Report P9100 for the testing of platelets for pathogen contamination.

P9099

P9099 Blood component or product not otherwise classified

This code reports any blood component not otherwise identified by a more specific HCPCS code.

P9100

P9100 Pathogen(s) test for platelets

The FDA approved a pathogen reduction system for use in reducing the risk of transfusion transmitted infections often present in platelets from whole blood and/or apheresis. This system exposes the specimen to ultraviolet light and a chemical called amotosalen. The specimen is purified to remove the chemical and any remaining byproducts. The process is effective against multiple infectious agents, including bacteria, parasites, protozoa, and viruses. It also reduces T-cell levels to lower the risk of transfusion-associated graft-versus-host disease (TA-GVHD). It can then be utilized for transfusion purposes. Report P9073 for the administration of platelets that have been tested for pathogen contamination. Report P9100 for the testing of platelets for pathogen contamination.

P9603-P9604

P9603 Travel allowance, one way in connection with medically necessary laboratory specimen collection drawn from homebound or nursing homebound patient; prorated miles actually travelled

P9604 Travel allowance, one way in connection with medically necessary laboratory specimen collection drawn from homebound or nursing homebound patient; prorated trip charge

When a patient is unable to travel to the laboratory, some laboratories send technicians to a person's home or to a nursing home to collect the specimens necessary to perform a physician-ordered test. The laboratory may have a set travel fee that is charged for such collections, or it may charge by the number of miles traveled. HCPCS Level II code P9603 is used to report the actual number of one-way miles traveled. This mileage must be prorated or divided between all the patients that had specimen collection performed during one specific trip. Report P9604 when the laboratory has a set fee charged for each trip. This fee must also be prorated among the patients that had specimen collection performed during the trip.

P9612-P9615

P9612 Catheterization for collection of specimen, single patient, all places of service

P9615 Catheterization for collection of specimen(s) (multiple patients)

Patients who cannot produce a urine specimen when required for physician-ordered testing may need to be catheterized. Catheterization is the insertion of a small tube through the urethra to the bladder. Urine ordinarily flows freely through the tube, allowing for collection and testing. Catheterizations may be performed in hospitals, physician offices, nursing homes, or the patient's home.

Q

Q0035

Q0035 Cardiokymography

Cardiokymography involves the use of a noninvasive device to record the anterior left ventricle segmental wall motion. The device typically consists of a 5 cm diameter capacitive plate transducer as part of a high-frequency, low-power oscillator with recording probe. Changes in wall motion affect the magnetic field and thus the oscillatory frequency, which is then recorded on a multichannel analog waveform polygraph. Medicare and most payers cover this type of test only as an adjunct to electrocardiographic stress testing to evaluate coronary artery disease and only when specific clinical indications are present. For male patients there must be atypical angina pectoris or nonischemic chest pain. For female patients, there must be angina, either typical or atypical.

Q0081

Q0081 Infusion therapy, using other than chemotherapeutic drugs, per visit

Intravenous infusion is the administration of a liquid through the patient's veins for therapeutic or diagnostic purposes. This code should not be used for the infusion of any chemotherapeutic drug. This code should be reported only once per visit.

Q0083

Q0083 Chemotherapy administration by other than infusion technique only (e.g., subcutaneous, intramuscular, push), per visit

This code reports the administration of chemotherapy by any technique other than infusion. Chemotherapy administration may include intramuscular or subcutaneous injection or a "push." A push is the direct intravenous injection of a drug slowly over one to two minutes. Typically drugs that are pushed are not diluted with any type of intravenous solution (e.g., D5W, saline). Chemotherapy is the treatment of any disease with chemical agents, but commonly refers to the administration of anti-neoplastic drugs. This code should be reported only once per visit.

Q0084

Q0084 Chemotherapy administration by infusion technique only, per visit

This code reports the administration of chemotherapy through the patient's vascular system for therapeutic purposes. Chemotherapy is the treatment of any disease with chemical agents, but commonly refers to the administration of anti-neoplastic drugs. This code should be reported only once per visit.

Q0085

Q0085 Chemotherapy administration by both infusion technique and other technique(s) (e.g. subcutaneous, intramuscular, push), per visit

This code reports the administration of chemotherapy by both infusion and other techniques. Chemotherapy is the treatment of any disease with chemical agents, but commonly refers to the administration of anti-neoplastic drugs. This code should be reported only once per visit.

Q0091

Q0091 Screening Papanicolaou smear; obtaining, preparing and conveyance of cervical or vaginal smear to laboratory

A screening Papanicolaou (commonly referred to as Pap) smear, cervical or vaginal, is a microscopic examination of cells scraped from the cervix or vaginal wall. The smears are examined for any abnormal appearing cells. It is a screening procedure when no known disease process currently exists and the test is looking for any possible abnormalities. This code reports the collection and preparation of a screening vaginal or cervical Pap smear and includes the conveyance or transportation of the smear to the laboratory.

Q0092

Q0092 Set-up portable x-ray equipment

The set-up of portable x-ray equipment is the procedure of unpacking and readying portable radiologic devices for use. This code should only be used by portable x-ray suppliers when the equipment is transported and set-up in a place of residence used as the patient's home (such as a nursing home) or in a nonparticipating institution. Portable x-ray services and their set-up must be performed under the general supervision of a physician and certain health and safety conditions must be met. Portable studies should be performed only when there is true medical necessity and when the patient cannot access or otherwise be examined on fixed conventional x-ray equipment. These studies should not be performed for "routine" purposes or for reasons of minor convenience. A set-up component can be paid for each radiological procedure (other than retakes of the same procedure) during single patient and multiple patient trips. This code should not be used when the portable x-ray supplier performs an EKG.

Q0111

Q0111 Wet mounts, including preparations of vaginal, cervical or skin specimens

A wet mount is the placement of a specimen on a microscope slide with the addition of a liquid. The liquid helps support the specimen and fills space between the cover slip and slide, which allows more light to pass and better visualization of the specimen. Wet mounts may be used for cervical, vaginal, and prostate smears, and examination of skin or feces specimens.

Q0112

Q0112 All potassium hydroxide (KOH) preparations

Potassium hydroxide (KOH) preparations are wet mounted slides where the added liquid is potassium hydroxide. The KOH dissolves cellular elements, such as skin cells, leaving only fungus and yeast visible.

Q0113

Q0113 Pinworm examinations

Pinworms are nematodes or round worms that live in the perianal area and migrate from the bowel to the skin to lay eggs. The eggs are very resistant to dehydration and can easily be dispersed into the air. Pinworm examinations involve the application of a special tape or swab at different times. The tape or swab is then examined for the presence of the pinworm or its eggs.

Q0114

Q0114 Fern test

A fern test is named for the pattern that the fluid takes when viewed under a microscope. The liquid crystallizes into a fern pattern. Cervical fluids may be analyzed in this manner to detect estrogen activity. As ovulation approaches, the pattern features more ferning. The test may also be used to detect amniotic fluid leakage in a pregnant uterus. A slide of vaginal fluid is allowed to dry. Amniotic fluid crystallizes to form a fern-like pattern due to its concentrations of sodium chloride, proteins, and carbohydrates.

Q0115

Q0115 Postcoital direct, qualitative examinations of vaginal or cervical mucous

The microscopic analysis of cervical mucus may be performed within hours of timed intercourse in order to observe and evaluate the interaction of sperm, semen, and cervical mucus. A small sample is obtained and examined under a microscope to determine the quality of sperm and its interaction with the cervical mucosa.

Q0138-Q0139

Q0138 Injection, ferumoxytol, for treatment of iron deficiency anemia, 1 mg (non-ESRD use)

Q0139 Injection, ferumoxytol, for treatment of iron deficiency anemia, 1 mg (for ESRD on dialysis)

Ferumoxytol is an iron oxide used to treat low iron in patients with chronic kidney disease. It is coated with a carbohydrate layer that helps surround the iron from the plasma until it can be used for hemoglobin. The recommended dose starts with 510 mg with a follow-up injection three to eight days later. Ferumoxytol is administered as an IV injection.

Q0144

Q0144 Azithromycin dihydrate, oral, capsules/powder, 1 g

Azithromycin dehydrate is an antibiotic indicated for use in patients with mild to moderate infections caused by susceptible strains of various microorganisms. Indications include pneumonia, pharyngitis and tonsillitis, staph and strep skin infections, cervicitis and urethritis due to gonorrhea and chlamydia, and genital ulcers. This code represents one gram of the oral tablets or powder.

Q0161

Q0161 Chlorpromazine HCl, 5 mg, oral, FDA-approved prescription antiemetic, for use as a complete therapeutic substitute for an IV antiemetic at the time of chemotherapy treatment, not to exceed a 48-hour dosage regimen

Chlorpromazine hydrochloride (HCl) is used in the treatment of manic psychosis, preoperative sedation, acute intermittent porphyria, an adjunct treatment for tetanus, intractable hiccups, some behavior problems in children, and nausea and vomiting. The main pharmacological actions are psychotropic. The mechanism of action is not known. It has a sedative and antiemetic effect.

Q0162

Q0162 Ondansetron 1 mg, oral, FDA-approved prescription antiemetic, for use as a complete therapeutic substitute for an IV antiemetic at the time of chemotherapy treatment, not to exceed a 48-hour dosage regimen

Ondansetron hydrochloride is a chemical compound that is a selective blocker of serotonin 5-HT3 receptors. It is an antiemetic drug available in oral and injectable forms. Serotonin 5-HT3 receptors are present on the vagal nerve and at sensory nerve endings. Cytotoxic chemotherapy appears to trigger the release of serotonin in the small intestine, which may trigger the 5-HT3 receptors and initiate the vomiting reflex. Ondansetron hydrochloride is indicated for the prevention of nausea and vomiting associated with surgery and antineoplastic drugs. The oral version is also indicated for the prevention of nausea and vomiting associated with radiation therapy. The drug is available in oral and injectable versions. The recommended dose is 4 mg or 0.1 mg/kg of body weight administered by intravenous or intramuscular injection. Dosages for the oral version vary from 8 to 24 mg depending on the indication and patient. This code should be used to report ondansetron hydrochloride for use as a complete therapeutic substitute for an IV antiemetic at the time of chemotherapy treatment, not to exceed a 48 hour dosage regimen.

Q0163

Q0163 Diphenhydramine HCl, 50 mg, oral, FDA-approved prescription antiemetic, for use as a complete therapeutic substitute for an IV antiemetic at time of chemotherapy treatment not to exceed a 48-hour dosage regimen

Diphenhydramine hydrochloride is an antihistamine, a histamine receptor antagonist that has anticholinergic, antitussive, antiemetic, antivertigo, antipruritic, antidyskinetic, and sedative effects. It blocks the effects of histamine on the smooth muscle of the bronchial tubes, GI tract, uterus, and blood vessels. It also acts as a local anesthetic by preventing transmission of nerve impulses. Diphenhydramine hydrochloride is indicated for the treatment of anaphylaxis, Parkinsonism when the patient cannot tolerate other medications, drug-induced extrapyramidal disorders, motion sickness, allergies, vertigo, and insomnia, and to suppress nausea and prevent vomiting. Its antiemetic effects allow it to be prescribed to treat nausea and vomiting associated with chemotherapy. Diphenhydramine hydrochloride is available in self-administrable oral forms and in an injectable form. The injectable form is administered by intramuscular or intravenous injection.

Q0164

Q0164 Prochlorperazine maleate, 5 mg, oral, FDA-approved prescription antiemetic, for use as a complete therapeutic substitute for an IV antiemetic at the time of chemotherapy treatment, not to exceed a 48-hour dosage regimen

Prochlorperazine/prochlorperazine maleate is an antiemetic used for severe nausea and vomiting, such as that associated with the administration of chemotherapy and prior to induction of anesthesia to control nausea and vomiting during and after surgery. The drug inhibits nausea and vomiting by acting on the chemoreceptor trigger zone and partially depresses the vomiting center. Prochlorperazine is also indicated for treating adult psychiatric illnesses including schizophrenia, non-psychotic anxiety, and mild psychotic disorders. Prochlorperazine is available in injection form for intramuscular (IM) and intravenous (IV) use, in tablets, extended release capsules and syrup for oral administration, and in suppository form. The dosage, route of administration, and frequency of administration depends on the patient's diagnosis, the severity of symptoms, and, in the injectable form, by the patient's weight. Parenteral adult doses range from 2.5 to 10 mg at no more than 5 mg/minute IV for adults or 5 to 20 mg IM. The maximum parenteral adult dose is 40 mg a day. The drug should be injected or infused slowly. For children, 0.132 mg/kg may be administered IM. Oral doses range from 5 to 10 mg three or four times a day for tablets, or for extended-release capsules, 15 mg daily or 10 mg every 12 hours.

Q0166

Q0166 Granisetron HCl, 1 mg, oral, FDA-approved prescription antiemetic, for use as a complete therapeutic substitute for an IV antiemetic at the time of chemotherapy treatment, not to exceed a 24-hour dosage regimen

An antiemetic is a drug given to suppress nausea and prevent vomiting. Patients receiving chemotherapy treatment have to contend with a great deal of nausea and vomiting as a side-effect and are given an antiemetic at the time of treatment. These codes all report FDA-approved prescription antiemetics to be taken orally, for use as a complete therapeutic substitute for an antiemetic given by IV injection at the time of therapy, not to exceed a 48-hour dosage regimen.

Q0167

Q0167 Dronabinol, 2.5 mg, oral, FDA-approved prescription antiemetic, for use as a complete therapeutic substitute for an IV antiemetic at the time of chemotherapy treatment, not to exceed a 48-hour dosage regimen

Dronabinol is a cannabinoid with an active ingredient that is found in marijuana. It is used to treat anorexia associated with weight loss in patients with AIDS and nausea and vomiting for patients on chemotherapy. Dronabinol may be used as a complete therapeutic substitute for intravenous antiemetic therapy at the time of a chemotherapy treatment. When used to treat anorexia associated with AIDS or as a prolonged treatment for nausea and vomiting for patients on chemotherapy, an initial dose of 2.5 mg of dronabinol is administered before lunch and dinner. This can be gradually increased to 20 mg per day. Dronabinol is administered orally.

Q0169

Q0169 Promethazine HCl, 12.5 mg, oral, FDA-approved prescription antiemetic, for use as a complete therapeutic substitute for an IV antiemetic at the time of chemotherapy treatment, not to exceed a 48-hour dosage regimen

Promethazine hydrochloride is a phenothiazine derivative with antihistamine, sedative, antiemetic, and anticholinergic properties. The drug binds to histamine receptors preventing the histamine from dilating capillaries, constricting the bronchial smooth muscles, and increasing gastric secretions. Promethazine hydrochloride is indicated as an antiemetic, a sedative in anesthesia, as a treatment for motion sickness, and for allergic reactions, including rhinitis and pruritic skin reactions. The drug may be combined with other drugs in cough and cold preparations. Promethazine hydrochloride is available in injectable, oral, and rectal suppository forms. The injectable form is administered by intramuscular or intravenous injection. Dosage varies from 25 to 50 mg.

Q0173

Q0173 Trimethobenzamide HCl, 250 mg, oral, FDA-approved prescription antiemetic, for use as a complete therapeutic substitute for an IV antiemetic at the time of chemotherapy treatment, not to exceed a 48-hour dosage regimen

Trimethobenzamide hydrochloride (HCl) is an antiemetic used to alleviate nausea and vomiting. The mechanism of action is not known but it appears to act on the chemoreceptor trigger zone (CTZ) in the brain where vomiting impulses are transmitted. It can be administered via intramuscular injection. Trimethobenzamide HCl also comes in capsule and suppository forms.

Q0174

Q0174 Thiethylperazine maleate, 10 mg, oral, FDA-approved prescription antiemetic, for use as a complete therapeutic substitute for an IV antiemetic at the time of chemotherapy treatment, not to exceed a 48-hour dosage regimen

Thiethylperazine maleate is indicated for the relief of nausea and vomiting. The exact mechanism of action is not known. However, it appears to have an effect on the vomiting center and the chemoreceptor trigger zone (CTZ) of the brain. Recommended oral dose is 10 to 30 mg a day. Thiethylperazine maleate can be administered orally or by intramuscular injection. Recommended intramuscular injection dose is 10 mg one to three times a day.

Q0175

Q0175 Perphenazine, 4 mg, oral, FDA-approved prescription antiemetic, for use as a complete therapeutic substitute for an IV antiemetic at the time of chemotherapy treatment, not to exceed a 48-hour dosage regimen

Perphenazine is used in treating psychosis and severe nausea and vomiting. The mechanism of action is not known. However, it does have an effect on the entire central nervous system particularly the hypothalamus. Dose is based on the condition and response of the patient. Perphenazine is administered orally.

Q0177

Q0177 Hydroxyzine pamoate, 25 mg, oral, FDA-approved prescription antiemetic, for use as a complete therapeutic substitute for an IV antiemetic at the time of chemotherapy treatment, not to exceed a 48-hour dosage regimen

Hydroxyzine is a piperazine derivative that has central nervous system depressant, antispasmodic, antihistamine, and antifibrillatory properties. It is used to treat a variety of conditions such as anxiety, pruritus from allergies, psychiatric and emotional emergencies, and nausea and vomiting. Hydroxyzine may be used as a complete therapeutic substitute for intravenous antiemetic therapy at the time of a chemotherapy treatment. It is often used as a preoperative medication. It tends to increase the effect of meperidine and barbiturates. It can be administered via intravenous push, intramuscular injection, or orally. Hydroxyzine hydrochloride is used to treat anxiety, manifestations of allergic dermatoses, as an antiemetic, and as a preoperative medication. It is administered by intramuscular injection or orally. Hydroxyzine pamoate has uses similar to the hydrochloride version. The pamoate version is administered orally.

Q0180

Q0180 Dolasetron mesylate, 100 mg, oral, FDA-approved prescription antiemetic, for use as a complete therapeutic substitute for an IV antiemetic at the time of chemotherapy treatment, not to exceed a 24-hour dosage regimen

Dolasetron mesylate is an antiemetic drug with a chemical compound that is a selective blocker of serotonin 5-HT3 receptors. Serotonin 5-HT3 receptors are present on the vagal nerve and at sensory nerve endings. Cytotoxic chemotherapy appears to trigger the release of serotonin in the small intestine, which may trigger the 5-HT3 receptors and initiate the vomiting reflex. It is indicated to prevent and treat nausea and vomiting associated with chemotherapy or surgery.

Q0181

Q0181 Unspecified oral dosage form, FDA-approved prescription antiemetic, for use as a complete therapeutic substitute for an IV antiemetic at the time of chemotherapy treatment, not to exceed a 48-hour dosage regimen

Oral antiemetic drugs are a therapeutic substitute for intravenous antiemetic drugs. Oral antiemetic drugs help patients better tolerate the effects of chemotherapy. Report this code for an unspecified oral dosage of an antiemetic drug used as a complete therapeutic substitute for an IV antiemetic at the time of chemotherapy treatment.

Q0220

Q0220 Injection, tixagevimab and cilgavimab, for the pre-exposure prophylaxis only, for certain adults and pediatric individuals (12 years of age and older weighing at least 40kg) with no known SARS-CoV-2 exposure, who either have moderate to severely compromised immune systems or for whom vaccination with any available COVID-19 vaccine is not recommended due to a history of severe adverse reaction to a COVID-19 vaccine(s) and/or COVID-19 vaccine component(s), 300 mg

Tixagevimab and cilgavimab are recombinant human IgG1^{K} monoclonal antibodies that bind to the receptor-binding domain of the spike protein of severe acute respiratory syndrome coronavirus 2 (SARS-CoV-2/coronavirus disease/COVID-19). The combination is indicated for pre-exposure prophylaxis of COVID-19 in adult and pediatric patients, ages 12 and older, weighing at least 40 kg, who are not currently infected with SARS-CoV-2, have not had known recent exposure to SARS-CoV-2, and who have moderate to severe immune compromise due to a medical condition or medications or have a history of severe allergic reaction to COVID-19 vaccines or vaccine components. It should not be used for treatment or for post-exposure prophylaxis. This investigational monoclonal antibody therapy was issued an emergency use authorization (EUA) by the FDA in December 2021. Effective February 24, 2022, the authorized dosage is 600 mg (300 mg tixagevimab and 300 mg cilgavimab) administered as two separate consecutive intramuscular (IM) injections in separate injection sites, preferably one in each gluteal muscle. Patients should be monitored for at least one hour following administration. For patients who received an initial dose of 150 mg tixagevimab and 150 mg cilgavimab, a second dose of 150 mg tixagevimab and 150 mg cilgavimab should be administered as soon as possible. For patients who have received a COVID-19 vaccine, it should be administered at least two weeks following vaccination. There are no current recommendations for repeat dosing.

Q0221

Q0221 Injection, tixagevimab and cilgavimab, for the pre-exposure prophylaxis only, for certain adults and pediatric individuals (12 years of age and older weighing at least 40kg) with no known SARS-CoV-2 exposure, who either have moderate to severely compromised immune systems or for whom vaccination with any available COVID-19 vaccine is not recommended due to a history of severe adverse reaction to a COVID-19 vaccine(s) and/or COVID-19 vaccine component(s), 600 mg

Tixagevimab and cilgavimab are recombinant human IgG1K monoclonal antibodies that bind to the receptor-binding domain of the spike protein of severe acute respiratory syndrome coronavirus 2 (SARS-CoV-2/coronavirus disease/COVID-19). The combination is indicated for pre-exposure prophylaxis of COVID-19 in adult and pediatric patients, ages 12 and older, weighing at least 40 kg, who are not currently infected with SARS-CoV-2, have not had known recent exposure to SARS-CoV-2, and who have moderate to severe immune compromise due to a medical condition or medications or have a history of severe allergic reaction to COVID-19 vaccines or vaccine components. It should not be used for treatment or for post-exposure prophylaxis. This investigational monoclonal antibody therapy was issued an emergency use authorization (EUA) by the FDA in December 2021. Effective February 24, 2022, the authorized dosage is 600 mg (300 mg tixagevimab and 300 mg cilgavimab) administered as two separate consecutive intramuscular (IM) injections in separate injection sites, preferably one in each gluteal muscle. Patients should be monitored for at least one hour following administration. For patients who received an initial dose of 150 mg tixagevimab and 150 mg cilgavimab, a second dose of 150 mg tixagevimab and 150 mg cilgavimab should be administered as soon as possible. For patients who have received a COVID-19 vaccine, it should be administered at least two weeks following vaccination. There are no current recommendations for repeat dosing.

Q0222

Q0222 Injection, bebtelovimab, 175 mg

Bebtelovimab is a recombinant human IgG1K monoclonal antibody that binds to the receptor-binding domain of the spike protein of severe acute respiratory syndrome coronavirus 2 (SARS-CoV-2/coronavirus disease/COVID-19). It is indicated for pre-exposure prophylaxis of COVID-19 in adult and pediatric patients, ages 12 and older, weighing at least 40 kg, with mild-to-moderate coronavirus disease 2019 (COVID-19) with positive results to SARS-CoV-2 viral testing, are at high risk for illness progression or hospitalization, and for whom alternative FDA-approved treatment options are not clinically appropriate or accessible. This investigational monoclonal antibody therapy was issued an emergency use authorization (EUA) by the FDA in February 2022. The authorized dosage is 175 mg administered via intravenous (IV) injection over at least 30 seconds. It should be administered within seven days of the onset of symptoms. Patients should be monitored for at least one hour following administration.

Q0240

Q0240 Injection, casirivimab and imdevimab, 600 mg

Casirivimab and imdevimab are monoclonal antibodies that bind to the receptor-binding domain of the spike protein of severe acute respiratory syndrome coronavirus 2 (SARS-CoV-2/coronavirus disease/COVID-19). Indicated for the postexposure prophylaxis of COVID-19 in adult and pediatric patients 12 years of age and older, weighing at least 40 kg, who are at high risk for progression to severe COVID-19 and/or hospitalization, are not fully vaccinated or not expected to mount an adequate immune response to complete vaccination, and have been or are at high risk of exposure to an infected individual. This postexposure prophylaxis therapy was issued an emergency use authorization (EUA) by the FDA in July 2021. The recommended dosage is 600 mg of casirivimab and 600 mg of imdevimab administered together as a single subcutaneous (SC) injection or an intravenous (IV) infusion as soon as possible following exposure. For individuals with ongoing exposure, a subsequent repeat dose of 300 mg of casirivimab and 300 mg of imdevimab may be administered once every four weeks for duration of exposure. See full prescribing information for complete administration instructions. This code reports only the updated dosing for postexposure prophylaxis.

Q0243-Q0244

Q0243 Injection, casirivimab and imdevimab, 2400 mg

Q0244 Injection, casirivimab and imdevimab, 1200 mg

Casirivimab and imdevimab are monoclonal antibodies that bind to the receptor-binding domain of the spike protein of severe acute respiratory syndrome coronavirus 2 (SARS-CoV-2/coronavirus disease/COVID-19). Indicated for the treatment of mild to moderate COVID-19 in adult and pediatric patients, ages 12 and older, weighing at least 40 kg, whose test results are positive for COVID-19 and who are at high risk for progression to severe COVID-19 and/or hospitalization or death, this investigational monoclonal antibody combination therapy was issued an emergency use authorization (EUA) by the FDA in November 2020. The dosage is 600 mg of casirivimab and 600 mg of imdevimab administered together as a single subcutaneous (SC) injection or an intravenous (IV) infusion over at least 60 minutes. Patients should be monitored for at least one hour following

Q

administration. The solutions must be diluted prior to administration and should be given together as soon as possible after a positive result of direct SARS-CoV-2 viral testing and within 10 days of symptom onset. Administration by SC injection should only be considered when IV infusion is either not feasible or would delay treatment. Healthcare providers must have immediate access to medications that can treat anaphylaxis or other severe infusion reactions, as well as the ability to activate the emergency medical system (EMS) when necessary. Code Q0243 represents the original dosing information of 1,200 mg of casirivimab and 1,200 mg of imdevimab under the EUA in November 2020. Code Q0244 represents the updated dosing information effective June 3, 2021.

Q0245

Q0245 Injection, bamlanivimab and etesevimab, 2100 mg

Bamlanivimab is a neutralizing IgG1 monoclonal antibody that binds to the receptor-binding domain of the spike protein of severe acute respiratory syndrome coronavirus 2 (SARS-CoV-2/coronavirus disease/COVID-19). Etesevimab is a monoclonal antibody against the surface spike protein of SARS-CoV-2. Indicated for the treatment of mild to moderate COVID-19 in adult and pediatric patients ages 12 years and older, weighing at least 40 kg, whose test results are positive for COVID-19, and who are at high risk for progression to severe COVID-19 and/or hospitalization, this investigational monoclonal antibody therapy was issued an emergency use authorization (EUA) by the FDA in February 2021. The authorized dosage is a single intravenous (IV) infusion of 700 mg bamlanivimab and 1400 mg etesevimab over at least 60 minutes via pump or gravity. It should be administered as soon as possible after a positive viral test for SARS-CoV-2 and within 10 days of symptom onset. Administration is allowed only in settings where healthcare providers have immediate access to medications that can treat anaphylaxis or other severe infusion reactions and can activate the emergency medical system (EMS) when necessary. This code reports a 700 mg bamlanivimab and 1400 mg etesevimab combination injection and applies to the monoclonal antibody product only.

Q0247

Q0247 Injection, sotrovimab, 500 mg

Sotrovimab is a neutralizing IgG1 monoclonal antibody that binds to the receptor-binding domain of the spike protein of severe acute respiratory syndrome coronavirus 2 (SARS-CoV-2/coronavirus disease/COVID-19). Sotrovimab is a monoclonal antibody against the surface spike protein of SARS-CoV-2. Indicated for the treatment of mild to moderate COVID-19 in adult and pediatric patients, ages 12 and older, weighing at least 40 kg, whose test results are positive for COVID-19, and who are at high risk for progression to severe COVID-19 and/or hospitalization, this investigational monoclonal antibody therapy was issued an emergency use authorization (EUA) by the FDA in February 2021. The authorized dosage is a single intravenous (IV) infusion of 500 mg of sotrovimab over 30 minutes via pump or gravity. It should be administered as soon as possible after a positive viral test for SARS-CoV-2 and within 10 days of symptom onset.

Q0249

Q0249 Injection, tocilizumab, for hospitalized adults and pediatric patients (2 years of age and older) with COVID-19 who are receiving systemic corticosteroids and require supplemental oxygen, non-invasive or invasive mechanical ventilation, or extracorporeal membrane oxygenation (ECMO) only, 1 mg

Tocilizumab is a recombinant humanized anti-human interleukin 6 (IL-6) monoclonal antibody, subclass IgG1k (gamma 1, kappa), that binds to IL-6 receptors and inhibits IL-6 mediated signaling. It is indicated for the treatment of severe acute respiratory syndrome coronavirus 2 (SARS-CoV-2/coronavirus disease/COVID-19) in hospitalized adult and pediatric patients, ages 2 and older, weighing at least 30 kg, who are receiving systemic corticosteroids and require supplemental oxygen, invasive or noninvasive mechanical ventilation, or extracorporeal membrane oxygenation (ECMO). This investigational monoclonal antibody therapy was issued an emergency use authorization (EUA) by the FDA in June 2021. The authorized dosage for patients weighing less than 30 kg is 12 mg/kg diluted to 50 mL in 0.9% or 0.45% sodium chloride. For patients weighing 30 kg or more, the authorized dosage is 8 mg/kg diluted to 100 mL in 0.9% or 0.45% sodium chloride. The maximum dosage is 800 mg per infusion. It is administered as a single intravenous (IV) infusion over 60 minutes. It should not be administered via a bolus, push, or subcutaneous (SC) injection. If signs or symptoms do not improve or worsen after the first dose, an additional infusion may be given eight hours following the first dose.

Q0477-Q0509

Q0477 Power module patient cable for use with electric or electric/pneumatic ventricular assist device, replacement only

Q0478 Power adapter for use with electric or electric/pneumatic ventricular assist device, vehicle type

Q0479 Power module for use with electric or electric/pneumatic ventricular assist device, replacement only

Q0480 Driver for use with pneumatic ventricular assist device, replacement only

Q0481 Microprocessor control unit for use with electric ventricular assist device, replacement only

Q0482 Microprocessor control unit for use with electric/pneumatic combination ventricular assist device, replacement only

Q0483 Monitor/display module for use with electric ventricular assist device, replacement only

Q0484 Monitor/display module for use with electric or electric/pneumatic ventricular assist device, replacement only

Q0485 Monitor control cable for use with electric ventricular assist device, replacement only

Q0486 Monitor control cable for use with electric/pneumatic ventricular assist device, replacement only

Q0487 Leads (pneumatic/electrical) for use with any type electric/pneumatic ventricular assist device, replacement only

Q0488 Power pack base for use with electric ventricular assist device, replacement only

Q0489 Power pack base for use with electric/pneumatic ventricular assist device, replacement only

Q0490 Emergency power source for use with electric ventricular assist device, replacement only

Q0491 Emergency power source for use with electric/pneumatic ventricular assist device, replacement only

Q0492 Emergency power supply cable for use with electric ventricular assist device, replacement only

Q0493 Emergency power supply cable for use with electric/pneumatic ventricular assist device, replacement only

Q0494 Emergency hand pump for use with electric or electric/pneumatic ventricular assist device, replacement only

Q0495 Battery/power pack charger for use with electric or electric/pneumatic ventricular assist device, replacement only

Q0496 Battery, other than lithium-ion, for use with electric or electric/pneumatic ventricular assist device, replacement only

Q0497 Battery clips for use with electric or electric/pneumatic ventricular assist device, replacement only

Q0498 Holster for use with electric or electric/pneumatic ventricular assist device, replacement only

Q0499 Belt/vest/bag for use to carry external peripheral components of any type ventricular assist device, replacement only

Q0500 Filters for use with electric or electric/pneumatic ventricular assist device, replacement only

Q0501 Shower cover for use with electric or electric/pneumatic ventricular assist device, replacement only

Q0502 Mobility cart for pneumatic ventricular assist device, replacement only

Q0503 Battery for pneumatic ventricular assist device, replacement only, each

Q0504 Power adapter for pneumatic ventricular assist device, replacement only, vehicle type

Q0506 Battery, lithium-ion, for use with electric or electric/pneumatic ventricular assist device, replacement only

Q0507 Miscellaneous supply or accessory for use with an external ventricular assist device

Q0508 Miscellaneous supply or accessory for use with an implanted ventricular assist device

Q0509 Miscellaneous supply or accessory for use with any implanted ventricular assist device for which payment was not made under Medicare Part A

A ventricular assist device (VAD) is a mechanical device that compresses the heart to aid pumping function in patients with heart failure. The device is implanted into the chest and connects to an external controlling mechanism. The codes listed above are used to report the replacement of various components of the VAD.

Q

Q

Q0510-Q0512

Q0510 Pharmacy supply fee for initial immunosuppressive drug(s), first month following transplant

Q0511 Pharmacy supply fee for oral anticancer, oral antiemetic, or immunosuppressive drug(s); for the first prescription in a 30-day period

Q0512 Pharmacy supply fee for oral anticancer, oral antiemetic, or immunosuppressive drug(s); for a subsequent prescription in a 30-day period

Medicare pays a dispensing or supplying fee for immunosuppressive drugs, oral anti-cancer chemotherapeutic drugs, and oral anti-emetic drugs used as part of an anti-cancer chemotherapeutic regimen. These fees are payable to a pharmacy, dialysis facility, or any hospital outpatient department not subject to the OPPS for each supplied prescription of the above-mentioned drugs. Medicare also pays a separately billable supplying fee for the initial supplied prescription of immunosuppressive drugs during the first month following a patient's transplant. When multiple prescriptions are supplied in a 30-day period, Medicare will pay a specified amount for the first prescription of the above-mentioned drugs as well as each subsequent prescription. A pharmacy will be limited to one predetermined fee per 30-day period even if the pharmacy supplies drugs from more than one of the above-mentioned categories to a beneficiary (e.g., an oral-anticancer drug and an oral anti-emetic drug). Supply fees and dispensing fees must be billed on the same claim as the drug.

Q0513-Q0514

Q0513 Pharmacy dispensing fee for inhalation drug(s); per 30 days

Q0514 Pharmacy dispensing fee for inhalation drug(s); per 90 days

Medicare pays a dispensing or supplying fee for inhalation drugs furnished through durable medical equipment. Medicare will pay a specified dispensing fee to a pharmacy for the initial 30-day period of inhalation drugs furnished through DME, regardless of the number of shipments or drugs dispensed or the number of pharmacies used by a beneficiary during that time. This is a one-time fee applicable only to someone who is using inhalation drugs for the first time as a Medicare beneficiary. Subsequently, Medicare will also pay a dispensing fee to a pharmacy/supplier for each 30-day supply of inhalation drugs furnished through DME, regardless of the number of shipments or drugs dispensed during the 30-day period. Medicare will pay a dispensing fee to a pharmacy/supplier for each 90-day period of inhalation drugs furnished through DME, regardless of the number of shipments or drugs dispensed during the 90 days. Only one 30-day dispensing fee will be payable per 30-day period, and only one 90-day dispensing fee will be payable per 90-day period, regardless of the number of suppliers used. A 30-day and 90-day supplying fee cannot be applied to drugs supplied for the same month. Medicare will not pay separately for compounding drugs; this cost is in the dispensing fees. Supply fees and dispensing fees must be billed on the same claim as the drug.

Q0515

Q0515 Injection, sermorelin acetate, 1 mcg

Sermorelin acetate is a synthetic peptide that contains a portion of the 191 amino acids that compromise natural human growth hormone (HGH). The drug stimulates the pituitary gland to produce HGH. HGH has a direct effect on the metabolism of protein, carbohydrates, and fat and controls skeletal and visceral growth. Sermorelin acetate is used in the diagnosis of HGH deficiencies and is indicated for the treatment of idiopathic HGH deficiency in children with growth failure. Treatment with sermorelin acetate should begin at a bone age of younger than 7.5 years for females and younger than 8 years for males and should be discontinued when the epiphyses are fused. The drug is administered subcutaneously daily at a dosage of 30 mcg per kg body weight and may be self-administered.

Q1004-Q1005

Q1004 New technology, intraocular lens, category 4 as defined in Federal Register notice

Q1005 New technology, intraocular lens, category 5 as defined in Federal Register notice

Cataracts are the clouding of the crystalline lens of the eye, which obstructs vision. An intraocular lens (IOL) is usually placed during or subsequent to cataract extraction. New-technology intraocular lenses (NTIOL) are FDA-approved prosthetic implants that demonstrate clinical advantages and superiority over existing intraocular lenses. The FDA, based upon published clinical data, determines if a lens has clinical advantages and superiority over existing IOLs with regard to reduced risk of intraoperative or postoperative complication or trauma, accelerated postoperative recovery, reduced induced astigmatism, improved postoperative visual acuity, more stable postoperative vision, or other comparable clinical advantages. Each subset or category of NTIOLs is separated into groups that meet the criteria for being treated as NTIOLs and share a common feature that distinguishes them from other IOLs. For example, all new-technology IOLs that are made of a particular bioengineered material could make up one subset, while all that rely on a particular optical innovation would encompass another. Any assignment and definition of the categories of four and five will be announced in the *Federal Register* notice prior to their use.

Q2004

Q2004 Irrigation solution for treatment of bladder calculi, for example renacidin, per 500 ml

Irrigation solution for treatment of bladder calculi is a liquid containing various minerals and weak acids that is used to irrigate or wash calculi from the bladder. The solution acts upon the stones by dissolving portions or all of the calculi.

Q2009

Q2009 Injection, fosphenytoin, 50 mg phenytoin equivalent

Fosphenytoin is a prodrug that is converted within the body to the anticonvulsant phenytoin. It is indicated for the control of status epilepticus, the prevention or control of seizures during neurosurgery, and for short-term parenteral administration when other means of phenytoin administration are unavailable, inappropriate, or less advantageous. It is thought to alter the sodium channels and block the calcium flow across the neuronal membranes, modulate the voltage-dependent calcium channels of neurons, and enhance the sodium-potassium ATPase activity of neurons and glial cells. Fosphenytoin may be administered by intravenous injection, intravenous infusion, or intramuscular.

Q2017

Q2017 Injection, teniposide, 50 mg

Teniposide is a semisynthetic derivative of podophyllotoxin, a toxic compound found in the rhizomes and roots of the mandrake plant. Teniposide is closely related to etoposide. It is an antineoplastic drug used in combination with other approved antineoplastic agents for induction therapy in patients with refractory childhood acute lymphoblastic leukemia. It acts on cells by preventing them from entering mitosis. Teniposide is administered via intravenous infusion over 30 to 60 minutes.

Q2026

Q2026 Injection, Radiesse, 0.1 ml

Radiesse is an injectable implant placed under the skin for treatment of defects such as moderate to severe wrinkles and folds such as nasolabial folds and facial lipoatrophy in patients with human immunodeficiency virus (HIV). It is also used to treat certain dental defects, as a tissue marker, and for treatment of vocal fold insufficiency. Radiesse contains a synthetic calcium hydroxylapatite in an injectable gel. It provides temporary filling and helps stimulate the body's collagen formation. The treatment can last up to one year or more. The recommended dose varies based on location and severity of the defect.

Q2028

Q2028 Injection, sculptra, 0.5 mg

Sculptra is an injectable implant placed under the skin for treatment of facial lipoatrophy in patients with human immunodeficiency virus (HIV). Sculptra contains microparticles of poly-L-lactic acid, a biodegradable, biocompatible synthetic polymer from the alpha-hydroxy-acid family. It provides temporary fullness to improve the sunken appearance from the fat loss that may accompany HIV therapy. Sculptra treatments can last up to two years. The recommended dose varies based on location and size of the treatment area.

Q2034-Q2039

Q2034 Influenza virus vaccine, split virus, for intramuscular use (Agriflu)

Q2035 Influenza virus vaccine, split virus, when administered to individuals 3 years of age and older, for intramuscular use (AFLURIA)

Q2036 Influenza virus vaccine, split virus, when administered to individuals 3 years of age and older, for intramuscular use (FLULAVAL)

Q2037 Influenza virus vaccine, split virus, when administered to individuals 3 years of age and older, for intramuscular use (FLUVIRIN)

Q2038 Influenza virus vaccine, split virus, when administered to individuals 3 years of age and older, for intramuscular use (Fluzone)

Q2039 Influenza virus vaccine, not otherwise specified

These codes report the supply of the vaccine only. A vaccine produces active immunization by inducing the immune system to build its own antibodies against specific microorganisms/viruses. The body retains memory of the antibody production pattern for long-term protection. A split virus suspension of the expected strains of influenza is prepared for intramuscular use. The vaccine induces active immunity to the highly contagious infection of the respiratory tract caused by a myxovirus and transmitted by airborne droplet infection. Vaccines are administered by IM injection. Report these codes with the appropriate administration code.

Q2041

Q2041 Axicabtagene ciloleucel, up to 200 million autologous anti-CD19 CAR positive T cells, including leukapheresis and dose preparation procedures, per therapeutic dose

Axicabtagene ciloleucel is a CD19-directed, genetically modified autologous T cell immunotherapy indicated to treat refractory B-cell lymphoma, including diffuse large B-cell lymphoma (DLBCL) not otherwise specified, DLBCL arising from follicular lymphoma, high grade B-cell lymphoma, and

Q

primary mediastinal large B-cell lymphoma in adult patients who have completed two or more lines of systemic therapy. It should not be used for the treatment of primary central nervous system lymphoma. The therapy is designed to reprogram a patient's own T cells with a chimeric antigen receptor (CAR) to eliminate CD10-expressing cells. Axicabtagene ciloleucel is derived from the patient's own white blood cells (WBC). After leukapheresis, the WBCs are sent to the manufacturer and axicabtagene ciloleucel is returned in approximately three to four weeks. Axicabtagene ciloleucel is supplied in a frozen, single dose unit that contains CAR-positive viable T cells based on patient weight at the time of treatment, and must be thawed prior to use. The thawed product should be infused within three hours. A treatment course includes lymphodepleting chemotherapy on the fifth, fourth, and third day before infusion, followed by administration of axicabtagene ciloleucel. Tocilizumab and emergency equipment should be available during infusion and recovery. The patient should be premedicated with acetaminophen and an antihistamine one hour prior to infusion. No corticosteroids should be administered unless required for life-saving measures. Axicabtagene ciloleucel should be administered by intravenous infusion. Patients must be monitored for seven days after infusion, and are not permitted to drive or operate heavy machinery for eight weeks following infusion.

Q2042

Q2042 Tisagenlecleucel, up to 600 million CAR-positive viable T cells, including leukapheresis and dose preparation procedures, per therapeutic dose

Tisagenlecleucel is a CD19-directed, genetically modified, autologous T cell immunotherapy indicated to treat refractory B-cell precursor acute lymphoblastic leukemia (ALL), or ALL in a second or later relapse, for patients up to 25 years of age. The therapy is designed to reprogram a patient's own T cells with a chimeric antigen receptor (CAR) to eliminate CD10-expressing cells. Tisagenlecleucel is derived from the patient's own white blood cells (WBC). After leukapheresis, the WBCs are sent to the manufacturer and tisagenlecleucel is returned in approximately three to four weeks. A treatment course includes lymphodepleting chemotherapy followed by administration of tisagenlecleucel, two to 14 days after the chemotherapy. Tisagenlecleucel is supplied in a frozen, single dose unit that contains CAR-positive viable T cells based on patient weight at the time of treatment, and must be thawed prior to use. The thawed product should be infused within 30 minutes. Tocilizumab and emergency equipment should be available during infusion and recovery. The patient should be premedicated with acetaminophen and an antihistamine 30 to 60 minutes prior to infusion. No corticosteroids should be administered unless required for life saving measures. Tisagenlecleucel should be administered by intravenous infusion at a rate of 10 mL to 20 mL per minute, and the rate should be adjusted for smaller children who need smaller volumes. For patients weighing 50 kg or less, administer 0.2 to 5.0 x 10^6 CAR-positive viable T cells per kg of body weight. For patients weighing more than 50 kg, administer 0.1 to 2.5 x 10^8 CAR-positive T cells.

Q2043

Q2043 Sipuleucel-T, minimum of 50 million autologous CD54+ cells activated with PAP-GM-CSF, including leukapheresis and all other preparatory procedures, per infusion

Sipuleucel T is an autologous cellular immunotherapy used in the treatment of asymptomatic or minimally symptomatic metastatic castrate resistant (hormone refractory) prostate cancer. Sipuleucel T consists of autologous peripheral blood mononuclear cells (PBMC) obtained by leukapheresis and cultured or activated using a recombinant human protein (PAP GM CSF) that consists of prostatic acid phosphatase linked to granulocyte macrophage colony stimulating factor. Sipuleucel T is administered by intravenous infusion over a period of approximately 60 minutes.

Q2049

Q2049 Injection, doxorubicin HCl, liposomal, imported Lipodox, 10 mg

Doxorubicin hydrochloride is an anthracycline antibiotic antineoplastic drug isolated from the bacterium *Streptomyces peucetius var. caesius*. It binds to DNA and inhibits RNA synthesis, causing cell death. It is utilized to treat many forms of cancer, such as bladder, breast, lung, stomach, and thyroid cancer, as well as Hodgkin's and non-Hodgkin's disease, acute lymphoblastic (ALL) and myeloblastic (AML) leukemia, and Wilms' tumor. The liposome version is the doxorubicin hydrochloride enclosed in a spherical lipid bilayer membrane. Doxorubicin hydrochloride liposome is indicated as a treatment for patients with ovarian cancer whose disease has recurred or progressed after platinum-based chemotherapy and for patients with AIDS-related Kaposi's sarcoma whose disease has progressed on prior combination chemotherapy or who cannot tolerate such therapy. Both versions are administered via intravenous (IV) injection.

Q2050

Q2050 Injection, doxorubicin HCl, liposomal, not otherwise specified, 10 mg

Doxorubicin hydrochloride is an anthracycline antibiotic antineoplastic drug isolated from the bacterium *Streptomyces peucetius* var. *caesius*. It binds to DNA and inhibits RNA synthesis, causing cell death. It is utilized to treat many forms of cancer, such as bladder, breast, lung, stomach, and thyroid cancer, as well as Hodgkin's and non-Hodgkin's disease, acute lymphoblastic (ALL) and myeloblastic (AML) leukemia, and Wilms' tumor. The liposome version is the doxorubicin hydrochloride enclosed in a spherical lipid bilayer membrane. Doxorubicin hydrochloride liposome is indicated as a treatment for patients with ovarian cancer whose disease has recurred or progressed after platinum-based chemotherapy, and for patients with AIDS-related Kaposi's sarcoma whose disease has progressed on prior combination chemotherapy or who cannot tolerate such therapy. Both versions are administered via intravenous injection.

Q2052

Q2052 Services, supplies and accessories used in the home under the Medicare intravenous immune globulin (IVIG) demonstration

The Medicare IVIG Access and Strengthening Medicare and Repaying Taxpayers Act of 2012 established a three year demonstration to evaluate the benefits of providing payment for items and services needed for the in-home administration of intravenous immune globulin (IVIG) for the treatment of primary immune deficiency disease (PIDD). This is a not a regular or a new Medicare benefit. It is a special demonstration limited to 4,000 beneficiaries diagnosed with PIDD who voluntarily apply to participate. Medicare currently pays for IVIG medications for beneficiaries who have primary immune deficiency who wish to receive the drug at home. However, the traditional Medicare fee for service benefit does not currently cover any services to administer the drug to a beneficiary at home, such as nursing services and certain supplies. Under the demonstration, Medicare will pay a bundled payment for the administration and supplies related to the administration of IVIG for beneficiaries who are otherwise eligible to receive IVIG in the home.

Q2053

Q2053 Brexucabtagene autoleucel, up to 200 million autologous anti-CD19 CAR positive viable T cells, including leukapheresis and dose preparation procedures, per therapeutic dose

Brexucabtagene autoleucel, a CD19-directed genetically modified autologous T-cell immunotherapy, is also known as chimeric antigen receptor (CAR) T-cell therapy. It is indicated for the treatment of adult patients with relapsed or refractory mantle cell lymphoma (MCL). In MCL, a rare form of non-Hodgkin's lymphoma typically occurring in middle-aged or older adults, the B-cells mutate into cancer cells that form tumors in the lymph nodes that rapidly metastasize to other areas of the body. This engineered cell-based antitumor immunotherapy utilizes gene transfer of tumor antigen-specific T cell receptors (TCR) or synthetic chimeric antigen receptors. The cells are prepared from the patient's peripheral blood mononuclear cells, obtained through a standard leukapheresis procedure. After the blood is sent to the manufacturer, the cells are enriched for T-cells, which are expanded in cell culture, washed, made into a suspension, and cryopreserved. This product is then infused back into the patient, where the modified CAR T-cells help the body's immune system better target and treat the tumor cells.

Q2054

Q2054 Lisocabtagene maraleucel, up to 110 million autologous anti-CD19 CAR-positive viable T cells, including leukapheresis and dose preparation procedures, per therapeutic dose

Lisocabtagene maraleucel, a CD19-directed genetically modified autologous T-cell immunotherapy, is also known as chimeric antigen receptor (CAR) T-cell therapy. It is indicated for the treatment of adult patients with relapsed or refractory large B-cell lymphoma following treatment with two or more systemic therapies, including diffuse large B-cell lymphoma (DLBCL) not otherwise specified, high-grade B-cell lymphoma, primary mediastinal large B-cell lymphoma, and follicular lymphoma grade 3B. It should not be used for the treatment of patients with primary central nervous system lymphoma. This engineered cell-based antitumor immunotherapy utilizes gene transfer of tumor antigen-specific T cell receptors (TCR) or synthetic chimeric antigen receptors. The cells are prepared from the patient's peripheral blood mononuclear cells, obtained through a standard leukapheresis procedure. After the blood is sent to the manufacturer, the cells are enriched for T-cells, which are expanded in cell culture, washed, made into a suspension, and cryopreserved. This product is infused back into the patient, where the modified CAR T-cells help the body's immune system better target and treat the tumor cells. The patient should be premedicated with acetaminophen and an antihistamine prior to treatment. It must be administered in a certified healthcare facility and availability of tocilizumab must be confirmed prior to infusion. See full prescribing information for complete administration instructions.

Q2055

Q2055 Idecabtagene vicleucel, up to 460 million autologous B-cell maturation antigen (BCMA) directed CAR-positive T cells, including leukapheresis and dose preparation procedures, per therapeutic dose

Idecabtagene vicleucel is a B-cell maturation antigen (BCMA)-directed genetically modified autologous T-cell immunotherapy. It is indicated for the treatment of adults, ages 18 and older, with refractory or relapsed multiple myeloma following treatment with four or more prior lines of therapy, including an anti-CD38 monoclonal antibody, an immunomodulatory agent, and a proteasome inhibitor. This engineered cell-based antitumor immunotherapy utilizes gene transfer of tumor antigen-specific T cell receptors or synthetic chimeric antigen receptors. The cells are prepared from the patient's peripheral blood mononuclear cells and obtained through a standard leukapheresis procedure. After the blood is sent to the manufacturer, the cells are enriched for T-cells, which are expanded in cell culture, washed, made into a suspension, and cryopreserved. This product is infused back into the patient, where CAR T-cell proliferation, cytokine secretion, and cytolytic killing of BCMA-expressing cells help the body's immune system better target and treat the tumor cells. The patient should be premedicated with acetaminophen and an antihistamine prior to treatment. See full prescribing information for complete administration instructions.

Q2056

Q2056 Ciltacabtagene autoleucel, up to 100 million autologous B-cell maturation antigen (BCMA) directed CAR-positive T cells, including leukapheresis and dose preparation procedures, per therapeutic dose

Ciltacabtagene autoleucel, a BCMA-directed genetically modified autologous T-cell immunotherapy, is also known as chimeric antigen receptor (CAR) T-cell therapy. T-cell immunotherapy involves reprogramming a patient's own T cells with a transgene encoding a chimeric antigen receptor (CAR) that identifies and eliminates cells that express BCMA. The cells are prepared from the patient's peripheral blood mononuclear cells, obtained through a standard leukapheresis procedure. After the blood is sent to the manufacturer, the cells are enriched for T-cells, which are expanded in cell culture, washed, made into a suspension, and cryopreserved. This product is infused back into the patient, where the modified CAR T-cells help the body's immune system better target and treat the tumor cells. It is indicated for the treatment of adult patients with relapsed or refractory multiple myeloma following four or more previous lines of therapy, including a proteasome inhibitor, an immunomodulatory agent, and an anti-CD38 monoclonal antibody. See full prescribing information for complete administration instructions.

Q3001

Q3001 Radioelements for brachytherapy, any type, each

Brachytherapy is a form of radiotherapy in which physicians place the source of irradiation close to the tumor or within a body cavity. Brachytherapy includes placing radioactive sources inside a body cavity (intracavitary brachytherapy) or putting radioactive material directly into body tissue using hollow needles (interstitial brachytherapy). Brachytherapy may be given in addition to external beam radiation or it may be used as the only form of radiotherapy. In some cases, the radioactive sources may be permanently left in place; in other cases, they are removed after a specified time. Placement of radioactive sources may be repeated several times. Use this code to report the radioelement used in brachytherapy.

Q3014

Q3014 Telehealth originating site facility fee

Telehealth is the delivery of health-related services via telecommunications equipment. The term encompasses technology that includes e-mail, video conferencing, and the transmission of medical images or medical data. The telecommunications most often involve a primary care practitioner with a patient at a remote site and a consulting medical specialist at an urban or referral facility. As applicable to Medicare, an originating site is the location of the patient at the time the service is being furnished via a telecommunications system. Originating sites authorized by law include the following: Physician or practitioner's office; Hospital; Critical access hospital; Rural health clinic; Federally qualified health center; Community mental health center; Skilled nursing facility; Hospital-based or CAH-based renal dialysis center. A fee that is set annually is paid to the originating site. A separate payment is made for the professional fee(s) of the physician or practitioner at the distant site.

Q3027-Q3028

Q3027 Injection, interferon beta-1a, 1 mcg for intramuscular use

Q3028 Injection, interferon beta-1a, 1 mcg for subcutaneous use

Interferon beta-1a is a synthetic version of natural interferon beta-1a produced by recombinant DNA technology from Chinese hamster ovaries. Interferons are small, naturally occurring proteins that bind to specific cell membranes and initiate a series of events that include the inhibition of virus replication and the enhancement of macrophage and lymphocyte destruction of foreign cells. There are several types of interferons. Interferon beta-1a has been shown to control symptoms of muscular sclerosis, but its exact mechanism of action is unknown. Interferon beta-1a is indicated for the treatment of patients with relapsing forms of multiple sclerosis to decrease the frequency of clinical exacerbations and delay the onset of the physical disabilities associated with the disease. The drug may be self-administered as a subcutaneous injection. Interferon beta-1a is also available as an intramuscular injection.

Q3031

Q3031 Collagen skin test

This code reports the kit supplied for performing a collagen skin test. A collagen skin test is done to test for delayed hypersensitivity before any collagen procedure is carried out. The test is given as a small injection into and just under the skin, where a small lump is formed and watched for redness or irritation in the days following.

Q4001-Q4051

Q4001 Casting supplies, body cast adult, with or without head, plaster

Q4002 Cast supplies, body cast adult, with or without head, fiberglass

Q4003 Cast supplies, shoulder cast, adult (11 years +), plaster

Q4004 Cast supplies, shoulder cast, adult (11 years +), fiberglass

Q4005 Cast supplies, long arm cast, adult (11 years +), plaster

Q4006 Cast supplies, long arm cast, adult (11 years +), fiberglass

Q4007 Cast supplies, long arm cast, pediatric (0-10 years), plaster

Q4008 Cast supplies, long arm cast, pediatric (0-10 years), fiberglass

Q4009 Cast supplies, short arm cast, adult (11 years +), plaster

Q4010 Cast supplies, short arm cast, adult (11 years +), fiberglass

Q4011 Cast supplies, short arm cast, pediatric (0-10 years), plaster

Q4012 Cast supplies, short arm cast, pediatric (0-10 years), fiberglass

Q4013 Cast supplies, gauntlet cast (includes lower forearm and hand), adult (11 years +), plaster

Q4014 Cast supplies, gauntlet cast (includes lower forearm and hand), adult (11 years +), fiberglass

Q4015 Cast supplies, gauntlet cast (includes lower forearm and hand), pediatric (0-10 years), plaster

Q4016 Cast supplies, gauntlet cast (includes lower forearm and hand), pediatric (0-10 years), fiberglass

Q4017 Cast supplies, long arm splint, adult (11 years +), plaster

Q4018 Cast supplies, long arm splint, adult (11 years +), fiberglass

Q4019 Cast supplies, long arm splint, pediatric (0-10 years), plaster

Q4020 Cast supplies, long arm splint, pediatric (0-10 years), fiberglass

Q4021 Cast supplies, short arm splint, adult (11 years +), plaster

Q4022 Cast supplies, short arm splint, adult (11 years +), fiberglass

Q4023 Cast supplies, short arm splint, pediatric (0-10 years), plaster

Q4024 Cast supplies, short arm splint, pediatric (0-10 years), fiberglass

Q4025 Cast supplies, hip spica (one or both legs), adult (11 years +), plaster

Q4026 Cast supplies, hip spica (one or both legs), adult (11 years +), fiberglass

Q4027 Cast supplies, hip spica (one or both legs), pediatric (0-10 years), plaster

Q4028 Cast supplies, hip spica (one or both legs), pediatric (0-10 years), fiberglass

Q4029 Cast supplies, long leg cast, adult (11 years +), plaster

Q4030 Cast supplies, long leg cast, adult (11 years +), fiberglass

Q4031 Cast supplies, long leg cast, pediatric (0-10 years), plaster

Q4032 Cast supplies, long leg cast, pediatric (0-10 years), fiberglass

Q4033 Cast supplies, long leg cylinder cast, adult (11 years +), plaster

Q4034 Cast supplies, long leg cylinder cast, adult (11 years +), fiberglass

Q4035 Cast supplies, long leg cylinder cast, pediatric (0-10 years), plaster

Q4036 Cast supplies, long leg cylinder cast, pediatric (0-10 years), fiberglass

Q4037 Cast supplies, short leg cast, adult (11 years +), plaster

Q4038 Cast supplies, short leg cast, adult (11 years +), fiberglass

Q4039 Cast supplies, short leg cast, pediatric (0-10 years), plaster

Q4040 Cast supplies, short leg cast, pediatric (0-10 years), fiberglass

Q4041 Cast supplies, long leg splint, adult (11 years +), plaster

Q4042 Cast supplies, long leg splint, adult (11 years +), fiberglass

Q4043 Cast supplies, long leg splint, pediatric (0-10 years), plaster

Q4044 Cast supplies, long leg splint, pediatric (0-10 years), fiberglass

Q4045 Cast supplies, short leg splint, adult (11 years +), plaster

Q4046 Cast supplies, short leg splint, adult (11 years +), fiberglass

Q4047 Cast supplies, short leg splint, pediatric (0-10 years), plaster

Q4048 Cast supplies, short leg splint, pediatric (0-10 years), fiberglass

Q4049 Finger splint, static

Q4050 Cast supplies, for unlisted types and materials of casts

Q4051 Splint supplies, miscellaneous (includes thermoplastics, strapping, fasteners, padding and other supplies)

Casting materials are made of plaster-imbedded strips or bandages or fiberglass wraps or strips, available in varieties pertinent to the type of fracture or post-surgical state requiring the support and protection of a cast. Some of these materials are initially dry and are water-activated, while others come premoistened for immediate application. Plaster varieties can be imbedded with strength-adding chemical compounds such as polyurethane. Splints are used when a cast is

Q

not necessary but the injury or condition requires immobilization. Casts and casting materials support and protect fractured or strained extremities or other body areas. They hold manipulated (set) fractures in place or can assist other devices (pins, wires, screws) in doing so and protect against reinjury. These codes identify the different casting materials (e.g., fiberglass or plaster), the type of immobilization provided such splint or cast for adult or pediatric patients, and the length or shape of casts for the different types of injuries or conditions (e.g., shoulder or body cast, long or short leg or arm).

Q4074

Q4074 Iloprost, inhalation solution, FDA-approved final product, noncompounded, administered through DME, unit dose form, up to 20 mcg

Iloprost is an inhaled form of prostacyclin, an analogue of prostaglandin. Prostaglandin is a naturally occurring, long-chain fatty acid that regulates smooth muscle contractions, is a vasodilator, lowers blood, and affects other hormones. It is an orphan drug indicated for use in pulmonary arterial hypertension (WHO group I) patients who have New York Heart Association (NYHA) Class III or IV symptoms. The NYHA classification system identifies Class II patients as those patients with marked limitation of activity, who are comfortable only at rest. NYHA Class IV patients are those patients who should be at complete rest, for whom any physical activity brings on discomfort. The drug is administered via a pulmonary drug delivery device with an initial inhaled dose of 2.5 mcg increasing to 5.0 mcg if tolerated. Iloprost should be inhaled six to nine times a day during waking hours, no more than once every two hours.

Q4081

Q4081 Injection, epoetin alfa, 100 units (for ESRD on dialysis)

Epoetin alfa (EPO) is a biologically engineered protein that stimulates the bone marrow to make new red blood cells. EPO is administered to treat anemia in patients with end-stage renal disease (ESRD) on a regular course of dialysis, as well as patients with other primary and secondary anemias. EPO is administered by subcutaneous or intravenous injection. This code is specific to patients with ESRD on dialysis and reports 100 units of EPO.

Q4082

Q4082 Drug or biological, not otherwise classified, Part B drug competitive acquisition program (CAP)

This code reports drugs or biologicals (not otherwise classified) that are administered as part of the Medicare Part B drug competitive acquisition program.

Q4100

Q4100 Skin substitute, not otherwise specified

This code represents skin substitutes that are not specifically identified by other HCPCS Level II codes. Skin substitutes may or may not contain bioactive tissue, cells, or matrices from human or animal sources. The skin substitutes are used to protect large or non-healing wounds or burns. Some products promote cellular growth and wound repair. Most substitutes are used in place of grafts.

Q4101

Q4101 Apligraf, per sq cm

Apligraf® is a skin substitute created from biological ingredients found in healthy human skin. It contains an outer layer of protective skin cells and an inner layer to aid in wound healing. It looks like a round piece of skin but does not include hair follicles, sweat glands, or blood vessels. When healthy skin cells get damaged, proteins and growth factors in the skin trigger the body to regenerate new skin. In certain conditions, such as diabetes or circulatory problems, the triggers are missing and wounds do not heal. Apligraf® contains fresh cells, nutrients, and proteins that are applied directly to the wound and initiate the healing process. It is used to heal sores such as diabetic foot and venous leg ulcers that are not healing after three to four weeks, despite treatment with conventional therapies. After debriding the wound of necrotic, damaged, or infected tissue, the physician applies the Apligraf and covers it with a nonadhering dressing and an outer wrap.

Q4102-Q4103

Q4102 Oasis wound matrix, per sq cm

Q4103 Oasis burn matrix, per sq cm

Oasis® is a skin substitute created from a biomaterial found in porcine small intestine. The material is processed to remove all cells and then dehydrated. This leaves a matrix or scaffold material that the body uses to surround cells, binding it to tissue and replacing extracellular matrix (ECM). ECM is a necessary component in wound healing. Oasis® is used to treat nonhealing wounds such as diabetic, venous, and pressure ulcers, as well as second-degree burns. After debriding the wound of necrotic, damaged, or infected tissue, the physician applies Oasis® to the wound and a small area of surrounding tissue. The dehydrated sheet is fixed into place using Steri-strips, sutures, or staples and rehydrated with sterile saline. The wound is covered with a nonadherent dressing, an absorptive dressing for wet wounds, or a moist dressing for dry wounds, and covered with a secure dressing. Oasis® is absorbed and forms a gel leaving ECM material. Oasis® may be reapplied every seven days over the top of the ECM gel.

Q4104

Q4104 Integra bilayer matrix wound dressing (BMWD), per sq cm

Integra® bilayer wound matrix is a biologic matrix that provides coverage for partial- and full-thickness wounds. It is used to treat chronic and traumatic wounds, including pressure ulcers, venous ulcers, diabetic ulcers, chronic and vascular ulcers, surgical wounds, traumatic wound abrasions, lacerations, and draining wounds. It is a two-layer material created from three-dimensional porous material made from the fibers of a cross-linked bovine tendon collagen and a glycosaminoglycan. This provides the framework for dermal tissue and capillary growth. As the tissue is repaired, the matrix dissolves. For large wounds, an epidermal autograft may also be used. The outer layer is made of silicone and provides moisture control and a bacteria barrier. When the Integra® bilayer wound matrix is applied, fluid is quickly adhered to the wound and conforms to the shape of the wound. It can also be adhered with sutures, staples, or other materials. About 21 days after application, the outer silicone layer is removed, which allows further healing of the epidermis. The bilayer wound matrix may be used in conjunction with Integra® matrix wound dressing.

Q4105

Q4105 Integra dermal regeneration template (DRT) or Integra Omnigraft dermal regeneration matrix, per sq cm

Integra® dermal regeneration template is a bilayer matrix or scaffold for dermal regeneration. It is a two-layer material created from the fibers of a cross-linked bovine tendon collagen and a glycosaminoglycan. The outer layer is made of silicone and provides moisture control and bacteria barrier of the wound. The dermal layer is a collagen that provides a scaffold for dermal tissue and blood vessels. This provides a viable surface for autografting. This product is used for the immediate treatment of partial or full-thickness burns. It can also be used to treat scar contractures when there are not adequate donor sites or the patient's condition prohibits immediate grafting. As skin cells grow into the matrix, the collagen is slowly absorbed into the body and replaced with protein that the skin naturally produces. In about 14 to 21 days, new dermal skin is produced and the outer layer can be removed. The physician can then perform an autograft of the patient's epidermis.

Q4106

Q4106 Dermagraft, per sq cm

Dermagraft® is a human dermal substitute manufactured from newborn foreskin tissue. It is made of fibroblasts, extracellular matrix, and a bioabsorbable scaffold. The fibroblasts reproduce and infiltrate the scaffold and secrete human dermal collagen, matrix proteins, growth factors, and cytokines to create a three-dimensional human skin substitute. Dermagraft® does not contain macrophages, lymphocytes, blood vessels, or hair follicles. Dermagraft® is approved for use in the treatment of full-thickness diabetic foot ulcers lasting longer than six weeks but without exposure of the tendon, muscle, joint capsule, or bone. The physician prepares the wound bed, thaws and rinses the Dermagraft®, and applies it to the site. The wound is dressed and left undisturbed for 72 hours.

Q4107

Q4107 GRAFTJACKET, per sq cm

Graftjacket™ is a three-dimensional, freeze dried biologic tissue matrix that forms a tissue scaffold used for diabetic foot ulcers. The material is derived from donated human skin. The epidermal and dermal cells are removed. The result is a matrix of preserved human dermal tissue, including its native protein, collagen structure, blood vessel channels, and essential biochemical composition to allow repair and revascularization. There are two distinct sides to the Graftjacket™. The dermal or vascular side is placed down, closest to the wound bed. The basement membrane side is exposed to the secondary dressing. The wound is prepared to receive the graft, and the graft is cut to size and rehydrated. Two or more sheets can be sewn together for larger wounds. The matrix is applied and fixed into place with sutures or staples and a moist dressing is applied.

Q4108

Q4108 Integra matrix, per sq cm

Integra® matrix is a biologic matrix that provides coverage for partial- and full-thickness wounds. It is used to treat chronic and traumatic wounds, including pressure ulcers, venous ulcers, diabetic ulcers, chronic and vascular ulcers, tunneled or undermined wounds, surgical wounds, traumatic wounds abrasions, lacerations, and draining wounds. It is a single layer material created of three-dimensional porous material made from the fibers of a cross-linked bovine tendon collagen. This provides the framework for tissue and capillary growth. Within seven to 14 days, the tissues and blood vessels invade the scaffold and the matrix is absorbed. For deeper wounds, Integra® matrix can be used in conjunction with Integra bilayer wound dressing. An epidermal autograft can be performed 21 to 56 days later if necessary.

Q4110

Q4110 PriMatrix, per sq cm

PriMatrix® is an acellular collagen matrix that provides the framework for tissue and vascular growth. It is used to treat partial- and full-thickness wounds, pressure ulcers, diabetic ulcers, venous ulcers, second-degree burns, surgical wounds, skin tears, and tunneled or undermined wounds. It is derived from fetal bovine dermal tissue and consists of type I and type III collagen. It delivers collagen to the wound, which stimulates tissue growth and collagen production. The physician debrides the wound as appropriate. The PriMatrix® is cut to size, rehydrated, and applied to the wound. It is affixed with a surgical closure and covered with a nonadherent dressing. Hydrogel is applied and the wound is dressed.

Q4111

Q4111 GammaGraft, per sq cm

GammaGraft™ is a skin substitute derived from human cadaver tissue. It contains a dermal and epidermal layer of human skin that is irradiated. GammaGraft™ is used as a temporary covering when the patient's own skin is not available and provides a protection from bacteria and reduces fluid loss. It is used to treat burns, chronic wounds, and partial- and full-thickness wounds. The physician debrides the wound of infected or necrotic tissue. The GammaGraft™ is applied and affixed with sutures or other means. The wound is covered by a nonadherent dressing and covered with gauze.

Q4112

Q4112 Cymetra, injectable, 1 cc

Cymetra™ is a small, particulate substance derived from donated human tissue. It contains collagens, elastin, proteins, and proteoglycans. It provides a structure for cell regrowth and helps the body produce tissue growth and vascularization. It is used as a substitute for the patient's own tissue to correct soft tissue defects and laryngoplasty.

Q4113

Q4113 GRAFTJACKET XPRESS, injectable, 1 cc

GRAFTJACKET® XPRESS is a micronized substance derived from human dermis. This substance contains biologic components and structure of the dermal matrix. It forms a tissue scaffold and is used for damaged or inadequate integumentary tissue, such as deep dermal wounds. The freeze-dried powder is rehydrated and injected as appropriate.

Q4114

Q4114 Integra flowable wound matrix, injectable, 1 cc

Integra® flowable wound matrix is a biologic gel that provides coverage for partial- and full-thickness wounds. It is used to treat chronic and traumatic wounds including pressure ulcers, venous ulcers, diabetic ulcers, chronic and vascular ulcers, tunneled or undermined wounds, surgical wounds, traumatic wound abrasions, lacerations, and draining wounds. This product is not used for third-degree burns. Since the wound matrix needs to be in contact with the wound bed, the flowable matrix is used for tunneled or irregular shaped defects. It is a single layer material created of three-dimensional porous material made from the fibers of a cross-linked bovine tendon collagen and mixed with sterile saline to form a gel. This provides the framework for tissue and capillary growth. The wound is debrided and probed for depth and tracking. The powdered product is mixed with sterile saline and injected into the site. A dressing is applied to ensure adherence and protect the wound.

Q4115

Q4115 AlloSkin, per sq cm

AlloSkin™ is an allograft made from donated human skin that is used for partial- and full-thickness wounds. It has two layers, epidermal and dermal, and provides protection from infection by covering exposed tissue and allowing time for the wound to heal.

Q4116

Q4116 AlloDerm, per sq cm

AlloDerm® is a regenerative tissue matrix used to repair hernias and in postmastectomy reconstruction. The matrix is derived from donated human skin in which all the dermal and epidermal cells are removed. This provides a scaffold of acellular biological components that encourages revascularization, cell migration, and regeneration.

Q4117

Q4117 HYALOMATRIX, per sq cm

Hyalomatrix® is a temporary dermal substitute composed of an esterified hyaluronan (or hyaluronic acid) scaffold covered by a silicone membrane. The hyaluronan scaffold provides a biodegradable, three-dimensional surface that promotes cellular growth. Hyalomatrix® is indicated for the management of wounds or burns.

Q4118

Q4118 MatriStem micromatrix, 1 mg

MatriStem® is extracellular matrices derived from porcine urinary bladder (also called UBM) used to promote wound healing and tissue growth. The product is noncrosslinked acellular material that is resorbable. This product contains bioactive collagens, elastins, and glycoproteins that trigger new blood vessel formation and attract numerous cell types to the wound area. It is indicated for the management of partial- and full-thickness wounds, ulcers, and burns.

Q4121

Q4121 TheraSkin, per sq cm

TheraSkin® is a cryopreserved human skin allograft. It contains a dermal and epidermal layer with bioactive cells, including collagens, elastins, and glycoproteins that promote wound healing. TheraSkin® is indicated as a wound covering for diabetic, pressure, or venous stasis ulcers; burns; dehisced surgical wounds; or any wound for which a graft is considered.

Q4122

Q4122 DermACELL, DermACELL AWM or DermACELL AWM Porous, per sq cm

DermACELL®, DermACELL AWM®, or DermACELL AWM Porous® are skin substitutes used to treat second- and third-degree burns, breast reconstruction, chronic nonhealing wounds, dehisced wound sites, and cosmetic reconstruction after traumatic burn injuries. The products are derived from human tissue with most of the DNA removed. They provide a mechanical barrier and an allograft collagen scaffold regeneration mesh to protect the wound and promote healing. They are available in various sizes and are sutured to the wound.

Q4123

Q4123 AlloSkin RT, per sq cm

AlloSkin™ RT is a skin replacement used to treat wounds caused by burns or trauma or chronic wounds such as venous and arterial ulcers, neuropathic diabetic ulcers, and pressure ulcers. The tissue is derived from human cadaver skin that is specially treated by low-dose, e-beam irradiation. The AlloSkin™ RT provides protection and promotes healing of the tissue. It is applied surgically and secured into place by sutures, staples, glue, or other methods the physician deems appropriate.

Q4124

Q4124 OASIS ultra tri-layer wound matrix, per sq cm

Oasis® Ultra Tri-layer Matrix is an acellular matrix derived from three layers of porcine small intestinal mucosa. It is indicated for the treatment of partial- and full-thickness wounds that are surgical or traumatic; burns; venous, vascular, diabetic, or pressure ulcers; and draining wounds. It is not for use on third-degree burns.

Q4125

Q4125 ArthroFlex, per sq cm

ArthroFlex® is an allograft used to treat chronic wounds such as diabetic foot ulcers and large surgical wounds. It is comprised of decellularized human skin and contains collagen, cytokines, and elastin. Collagen and elastin provide structure and growth factors to aid tissue growth and wound healing. Cytokines help with epithelializations and adjust the differentiation and growth of epithelium. ArthroFlex® also provides a matrix to provide a scaffold for tissue growth and stimulates cell growth. This biological also creates protection from contamination and helps decrease the rate of water, electrolyte, protein, and heat loss from the wound. It is applied to the wound and anchored using sutures, staples, or adhesive strips.

Q4126

Q4126 MemoDerm, DermaSpan, TranZgraft or InteguPly, per sq cm

MemoDerm® is a thin meshed acellular dermal matrix derived from human cadaver allograft tissue. The epidermal layer and cellular elements have been removed making the matrix acellular. MemoDerm® is sterilized using gamma radiation leaving intact the collagen, proteoglycans, and elastin scaffold. The matrix assists in revascularization and in the repopulation of cells. It is indicated for use as an onlay graft for diabetic foot ulcers and other soft tissue repair.

Q4127

Q4127 Talymed, per sq cm

Talymed® is a bioactive wound matrix used to cover wounds such as diabetic ulcers, venous ulcers, pressure wounds, ulcers caused by mixed vascular etiologies, full-thickness and partial-thickness wounds, second-degree burns, surgical wounds, chronic vascular ulcers, and dehisced surgical wounds and bleeding surface wounds, abrasions, and lacerations. The active ingredient in Talymed® is poly-N-acetylglucosamine (p-GlcNAc). It stimulates tissue growth and aids in wound closure and healing. The dressing is cut to the appropriate size and applied to the wound. It can be replaced as necessary.

Q4128

Q4128 FlexHD, or AllopatchHD, per sq cm

FlexHD® and AllopatchHD® are human allograft tissue processed to remove epidermal and dermal cells. It is processed using a proprietary process that preserves and maintains the natural biochemical, biomechanical, and matrix properties of the dermal graft. It assists in revascularization and in the repopulation of cells at surgical sites. It is indicated for use as a graft to replace damaged or inadequate integumentary tissue or for the repair, reinforcement, or supplemental support of soft tissue defects.

Q4130

Q4130 Strattice TM, per sq cm

Strattice™ is a surgical mesh for soft tissue repair that acts as a scaffold. It is derived from porcine skin and promotes healing and revascularization of the wound. Strattice™ is surgically implanted and used to treat partial and full thickness wounds, pressure ulcers, venous ulcers, diabetic ulcers, chronic vascular ulcers, tunneled/undermined wounds, surgical wounds, trauma wounds, draining wounds, or other bleeding surface wounds. It can also be used as reinforcement tissue. It comes in pliable or firm forms and in assorted sizes.

Q4132-Q4133

Q4132 Grafix Core and GrafixPL Core, per sq cm

Q4133 Grafix PRIME, GrafixPL PRIME, Stravix and StravixPL, per sq cm

Grafix® Core, GrafixPL® Core, Grafix® Prime, GrafixPL® Prime, Stravix®, and StravixPL® are wound matrixes derived from human placental tissue. The matrix in each product includes viable endogenous cells, including mesenchymal stem cells (MSC), fibroblasts of the native tissue, and regenerative growth factors. The matrix provides a scaffold of cellular support and growth factors, encouraging cell regeneration. They are indicated for the treatment of wounds that have exposed bone, muscle, and/or tendon, such as deep diabetic foot ulcers, venous stasis ulcers, and pressure ulcers that have not responded to other wound care. The product is supplied frozen and must be thawed prior to application. Once thawed, it is applied to the wound, without fixation, and covered with a nonadherent dressing. The matrix is applied weekly, as needed, for up to 12 weeks.

Q4134

Q4134 HMatrix, per sq cm

hMatrix® is an acellular dermal scaffold derived from human skin. The epidermal and dermal cells are removed leaving the collagen and elastin matrix. This biological is intended to replace damaged or inadequate integumental tissue, including as a wound cover or for breast reconstruction or abdominal wall repair.

Q4135

Q4135 Mediskin, per sq cm

Mediskin™ is a frozen, irradiated porcine xenograft used to treat burns, abrasions, donor sites, decubitus, and chronic vascular ulcers. It provides protection from fluid loss and external contamination. It also provides a favorable environment for wound healing. Mediskin™ may also be used as a temporary wound cover. As the wound heals, Mediskin™ eventually sloughs off on its own.

Q4136

Q4136 E-Z Derm, per sq cm

EZ-Derm™ is a porcine dermis xenograft that is used as temporary skin coverage for treatment of burns, abrasions, donor sites, and decubitus and chronic vascular ulcers. It provides protection from fluid loss and external contamination. It also provides a favorable environment for wound healing. EZ-Derm™ eventually sloughs off on its own and can be trimmed to avoid shearing.

Q4137

Q4137 AmnioExcel, AmnioExcel Plus or BioDExcel, per sq cm

AmnioExcel®, AmnioExcel® Plus, and BioDExCel™ are sterile, non-crosslinked, resorbable, extracellular amniotic membranes that act as a natural scaffold for cellular attachment creating tissue repair and regeneration. It is indicated for use in traumatic injuries; burns; surgical wounds; complex, chronic, and acute wounds; and other soft tissue defects.

Q4138

Q4138 BioDFence DryFlex, per sq cm

BioDfence™ is an amniotic tissue based allograft derived from human placenta. It is composed of collagens and extracellular substrates that include growth factors, connective proteins, and cytokines. BioDfence™ provides an adhesion barrier reducing fibroblast infiltration. It is procured from live, healthy donors during childbirth and dehydrated to provide optimum handling characteristics. While this product was initially used in the acute care inpatient setting in connection with neurosurgical, orthopedic, and spine surgical procedures, it is now producing positive outcomes in individual wound care cases. The dehydrated (and the hydrated) human amnion allografts are intended for the repair or replacement of lost or damaged dermal tissue. Indications include traumatic injuries, burns, Mohs procedures, or surgical wounds; complex chronic and acute wounds, such as diabetic ulcers, venous and arterial leg ulcers, pressure ulcers, or cutaneous ulcers; wounds with exposed vital structures, such as tendon, bone, and blood vessels; and other soft tissue defects. BioDfence DryFlex™ is dehydrated, making it less sticky and a better choice for use with instrumentation.

Q4139

Q4139 AmnioMatrix or BioDMatrix, injectable, 1 cc

AmnioMatrix™ and BioDMatrix™ are viable human placental allografts composed of morselized amniotic membrane and amniotic fluid components recovered from the same human donor. The amniotic membrane is separated from the placenta and morselized into particulate form, then combined with amniotic fluid components to form the allograft. The processing method is intended to preserve the structural properties of the collagen, growth factors, cellular materials, and matrix present in the tissue to create a micro-scaffold to be used to aid in the wound healing process. AmnioMatrix™ (also to be marketed under the trade name BioDMatrix™) is intended for the treatment of wounds, including surgical wounds, burns, traumatic injury; chronic and acute wound conditions; and supportive treatment of wound-associated bone defects. The product may be mixed with normal saline for application to surgical sites and open, complex or chronic wounds or mixed with the recipient's blood to fill soft tissue defects and wound-associated bone defects. AmnioMatrix™ is cryopreserved and supplied in injectable form in sterile vials.

Q4140

Q4140 BioDFence, per sq cm

BioDfence™ is an amniotic tissue-based allograft derived from human placenta. It is composed of collagens and extracellular substrates that include growth factors, connective proteins, and cytokines. BioDfence™ provides an adhesion barrier reducing fibroblast infiltration. It is procured from live, healthy donors during childbirth and dehydrated to provide optimum handling characteristics. While this product was initially used in the acute care inpatient setting in connection with neurosurgical, orthopedic, and spine surgical procedures, it is now producing positive outcomes in individual wound care cases. The dehydrated (and the hydrated) human amnion allografts are intended for the repair or replacement of lost or damaged dermal tissue. Indications include traumatic injuries, burns, Mohs procedures, or surgical wounds; complex chronic and acute wounds, such as diabetic ulcers, venous and arterial leg ulcers, pressure ulcers, or cutaneous ulcers; wounds with exposed vital structures, such as tendon, bone, and blood vessels; and other soft tissue defects. BioDfence™ is hydrated, which makes it a bit sticky and glue may not be needed, which may make it easier to use for procedures such as on corneal defects.

Q4141

Q4141 AlloSkin AC, per sq cm

Alloskin™ is meshed, biological cadaver dermis that is decellularized and further processed to provide an acellular tissue allograft. Alloskin™ AC allograft is a natural skin replacement that can be used as a scaffold for regeneration of tissue through revascularization and remodeling into the host tissue to achieve wound closure of partial- or full-thickness wounds due to tissue loss from burns, trauma, and chronic wounds, such as venous and arterial ulcers, diabetic foot ulcers, and pressure ulcers. After the epidermal layer is removed, the resulting dermal product is low-dose, e-beam irradiated to preserve the graft in a shelf-stable format. The tissue allograft is surgically applied and secured to the skin by the anchoring method chosen by the surgeon (sutures, staples, adhesive glue, etc.).

Q4142

Q4142 XCM biologic tissue matrix, per sq cm

XCM Biologic Tissue Matrix™ is a sterile, non-cross-linked matrix derived from porcine dermis. It provides a support structure for cellular migration and is incorporated into the surrounding tissue. It is indicated for use in general surgical procedures for the reinforcement and repair of soft tissue where weakness exists including defects of the thoracic wall, suture line reinforcement, and muscle flap reinforcement; urogynecological surgical reinforcement, such as rectal and vaginal prolapse, reconstruction of the pelvic floor, or hernia repair; soft tissue reconstructive procedures including plastic and reconstructive surgical application; and for reinforcement of the soft tissues, which are repaired by suture or suture anchors, such as rotator cuff, patellar, Achilles, biceps, quadriceps, and other tendons. XCM Biologic Tissue Matrix™ is supplied sterile and hydrated in a foil liner pouch. It does not require refrigeration or any preparation before use.

Q4143

Q4143 Repriza, per sq cm

Repriza® is an acellular dermal matrix. It is sterile, hydrated, ready to use upon opening, and it may be stored at ambient temperature. It has no orientation, so either side may be approximated to tissues of the wound or burn. Repriza® is indicated as a skin substitute in the treatment of various types of wounds, including burns, chronic ulcers, and surgical wounds. Repriza® may also be used as an implant during plastic and reconstructive surgeries wherever an acellular dermal matrix may be used. For example, it may be used to support implants in a defined pocket such as in breast reconstruction and abdominal wall reconstruction procedures. It is available in standard sizes with custom sizes and thicknesses available upon request.

Q4145

Q4145 EpiFix, injectable, 1 mg

EpiFix® Injectable is a processed, dehydrated, sterilized cellular amniotic membrane allograft used for wound treatment when it is necessary to replace or repair lost or damaged human collagen tissue. It delivers multiple extracellular matrix proteins, growth factors, cytokines, and other specialty proteins present in amniotic tissue to help regenerate soft tissue. EpiFix® Injectable is indicated for the treatment and management of chronic wounds including neuropathic ulcers, venous stasis ulcers, post traumatic ulcers, post-surgical ulcers, and pressure ulcers. It is particularly suited to deeply creviced, irregularly shaped, or tunneling wounds. The size of the dosing used is based upon the size of the wound defect.

Q4146

Q4146 Tensix, per sq cm

TenSIX™ is an acellular dermal matrix derived from aseptically processed sterile cadaver human skin. It is made from human donor skin, which undergoes a process that removes the epidermis and dermal cells, thereby creating an acellular dermis. TenSIX™ acts as a scaffold to facilitate vessel growth and the migration of growth factors that stimulate cell migration. Once rehydrated, the allograft can be applied topically to the wound and secured by the physician in his manner of choice. It is indicated for the repair or replacement of damaged or inadequate integumental tissue, particularly for wounds resulting from chronic diabetic foot ulcers.

Q4147

Q4147 Architect, Architect PX, or Architect FX, extracellular matrix, per sq cm

Architect™ ECM is type I collagen that has been stabilized and sterilized for ease of use and enhanced durability as a wound dressing. It is made from equine pericardium and utilizes a patented collagen stabilizing technology. It purportedly supports rapid healing by not promoting an inflammatory response; serves as a temporary matrix that provides a platform for cell migration; helps to optimize the wound-healing environment; and facilitates cellular activity.

Q4148

Q4148 Neox Cord 1K, Neox Cord RT, or Clarix Cord 1K, per sq cm

Clarix™ Cord 1K, NEOX™ Cord 1K, and NEOX™ Cord RT are ultra-thick human amniotic membrane products. They are nonimplantable biological skin graft substitutes comprised of human amniotic membrane retrieved from electively donated umbilical cords. Clarix Cord 1K is indicated as surgical wound barrier, cover, or wrap. NEOX™ Cord1K and NEOX™ Cord RT are indicated as wound coverings in chronic nonhealing dermal wounds, such as diabetic ulcers. They are administered by placing the appropriately sized product to completely cover the wound bed after debridement, and is secured to the wound edges using sutures or surgical staples, at the discretion of the physician.

Q4149

Q4149 Excellagen, 0.1 cc

Excellagen® is a highly refined fibrillar Type I bovine collagen gel for wound care management. The collagen is purified using a specialized process that removes impurities (including endotoxins), denatured molecules, and collagen fragments. Excellagen® promotes cellular adhesion, migration, and proliferation to stimulate granulation tissue formation. The flowable, ready to use gel is ideal for use in wounds of varying shapes and surface contours as well as tunneled/undermined wounds. Excellagen® is indicated for non-healing lower extremity ulcers in diabetic patients and other dermal wounds and is intended for physician use during debridement procedures. It is supplied in ready-to-use, prefilled, single-use sterile syringes.

Q4150

Q4150 AlloWrap DS or dry, per sq cm

AlloWrap DS® is a biological barrier composed of human amniotic membrane that is applied to a postsurgical repaired site. The double-sided membrane has two layers of epithelial tissue with the epithelial tissue oriented outward.

Q4151

Q4151 AmnioBand or Guardian, per sq cm

AmnioBand® and Guardian are human tissue allografts made of donated placental membranes. The allograft is composed of native human amnion and chorion, which together create a membrane in which the amnion serves as a covering epithelium. AmnioBand® and Guardian are identical products. They are intended for interior and exterior wounds. They may be used as coverings for surgical sites, wounds, ulcers, and soft tissue defects.

Q4152

Q4152 DermaPure, per sq cm

DermaPure® is derived from split-thickness grafts harvested from human cadaver tissue donors. The tissue is a single layer of decellularized dermal allograft. It is indicated as a treatment for acute and chronic wounds, such as diabetic foot ulcers, venous stasis ulcers, and other wounds that are refractory to more conservative care.

Q4153

Q4153 Dermavest and Plurivest, per sq cm

Dermavest® is a human placental connective tissue matrix. It is intended to replace or supplement damaged or inadequate integumental tissue and to stabilize a debrided wound.

Q4154

Q4154 Biovance, per sq cm

Biovance® is a dehydrated, decellularized, human amniotic membrane. It is derived from the placental amnion and includes epithelial and stromal components in a collagen-rich extracellular matrix. Biovance® also contains extracellular proteins, such as elastin, glycosaminoglycans, and laminins, which are important in extracellular matrix strength, cell attraction, and migration. It is indicated for the treatment of damaged or lost soft tissue.

Q4155

Q4155 Neox Flo or Clarix Flo 1 mg

Neox® Flo and Clarix® Flo are human amniotic membrane and umbilical cord products in particulate form. They are obtained from donated placentas and are indicated as wound coverings for dermal ulcers and defects, such as diabetic ulcers. The particulate form is useful in treating irregularly shaped or tunneled wounds.

Q4156

Q4156 Neox 100 or Clarix 100, per sq cm

Clarix™ 100 and Neox™ 100 are cryopreserved skin graft substitutes composed of human amniotic membrane and umbilical cord tissue. Clarix™ 100 is indicated for use as a surgical covering or wrap. Neox™ 100 is indicated for the treatment of minor, superficial skin wounds and ulcers. Clarix™ 100 and Neox™ 100 modulate inflammation and encourage healing. Both grafts are available in multiple sizes up to 7 x 7 cm. The graft is placed over the wound and secured with staples or sutures, per physician preference.

Q4157

Q4157 Revitalon, per sq cm

Revitalon™ is a human allograft made from donated amniotic membrane derived from the inner lining of the placenta. It is composed of native human amnion and chorion consisting of collagen, laminin, fibronectin, nidogen, and proteoglycans. It is indicated as a covering for full-thickness wounds, damaged membranes, and as a dressing for burns.

Q4158

Q4158 Kerecis Omega3, per sq cm

Kerecis™ Omega3 is an acellular dermal matrix comprised of collagen matrix of cod fish skin. Kerecis™ manufactures four separate products (Omega3 Burn, Omega3 Dura, Omega3 Surgical, and Omega3 Wound) that are indicated as a wound covering for breast and dura reconstruction, burns, chronic wounds, surgical repairs, and traumatic wounds. The matrix provides a strong repair hold and is replaced by the patient's own tissue over time. The products are supplied in sheets of sizes up to 7 x 10 cm.

Q4159

Q4159 Affinity, per sq cm

Affinity® is a minimally processed, amniotic fluid membrane allograft. It is comprised of the amniotic epithelial layer, the amniotic basement membrane, and the amniotic stroma. It is indicated as an onlay graft for acute and chronic wounds, including, but not limited to, neuropathic ulcers, venous stasis ulcers, pressure ulcers, burns, posttraumatic wounds, and postsurgical wounds.

Q4160

Q4160 Nushield, per sq cm

NuShield® is produced from human placental membrane. It includes the amniotic epithelial layer, the amniotic basement membrane, the amniotic stroma, the chorionic basement membrane, and the chorionic stroma. It is intended as a lay-on graft for acute and chronic wounds, including, but not limited to, neuropathic ulcers, venous stasis ulcers, pressure ulcers, burns, posttraumatic wounds, and postsurgical wounds. This product comes in a meshed, expandable form.

Q4161

Q4161 bio-ConneKt wound matrix, per sq cm

bio-ConneKt® wound matrix is a wound dressing made of reconstituted collagen obtained from equine tendon that works to stabilize and help prevent early degradation of a wound. The dressing aids in tissue regrowth while providing moisture to the wound. The product can be used to treat wounds such as diabetic, venous, and pressure ulcers, as well as second-degree burns and other traumatic wounds.

Q4162

Q4162 WoundEx Flow, BioSkin Flow, 0.5 cc

BioSkin® Flow and WoundEx® Flow are fluid wound dressings made of human placental connective tissue. The dressings provide assistance in tissue regrowth and help reduce the risk of scarring. The products are in a concentrated liquid form and are applied by pouring the matrix over the wound in a sterile field. The coverage area may be extended with the addition of saline.

Q4163

Q4163 WoundEx, BioSkin, per sq cm

BioSkin® and WoundEx® are membrane allografts made of dehydrated and decellularized human amniotic membrane and are used as wound coverings. They are indicated for the treatment of acute and chronic wounds, including surgical and traumatic wounds and ulcers. The products contain a zeolite-iodine complex, which also works to stop bleeding and prevent infection. The products can be applied in any direction and adhere to the wound bed. Fixation is not required, and the products are held in place with gauze compression. Replacement may be needed in 24 to 48 hours, as medically necessary.

Q4164

Q4164 Helicoll, per sq cm

Helicoll™ is an acellular dermal matrix made from bovine collagen. It is indicated for the treatment of surgical and traumatic wounds, as well as various types of ulcers. The product provides an environment that promotes the formation of granulation tissue and regeneration of blood vessels. The dermal matrix is applied after soaking for five to 10 minutes in sterile saline, and the edge may be secured with staples, sutures, or tape, depending on physician preference. Removal is not required, except for cases of infection or slowly healing chronic ulcers.

Q4165

Q4165 Keramatrix or Kerasorb, per sq cm

Keramatrix® is a wound matrix made from acellular, animal-derived keratin protein. Kerasorb® is a wound matrix foam that provides keratin to the wound surface and is backed with an absorbent polyurethane foam, which is designed to manage wound exudate. Both products are indicated for the treatment of surgical and traumatic wounds, as well as burns and various types of ulcers. The matrixes provide a scaffolding for the growth of new tissue, degrading into a gel, and is reabsorbed into the wound. Once degradation has occurred, a new matrix should be applied, removing the degraded matrix every two to three dressing changes, as indicated.

Q4166

Q4166 Cytal, per sq cm

Cytal® is a wound matrix composed of an animal-derived extracellular matrix, also known as urinary bladder matrix (UBM). It is intended for the management of second-degree burns, surgical and traumatic wounds, and various types of ulcers. The primary advantage of Cytal® products is that they maintain their natural collagen structure and components that are gradually incorporated within the patients' body, while replacing the product with site-appropriate tissue. The result is constructively remodeled, site-specific tissue. Cytal® is supplied in a sheet configuration composed of one, two, three, or six layers, and in dimensions up to 10 cm x 15 cm.

Q4167

Q4167 Truskin, per sq cm

TruSkin® is a split-thickness cryopreserved human skin allograft. It is intended for the replacement or reconstruction of inadequate or damaged integumental tissue. An advanced skin substitute, it is an off-the-shelf alternative to fresh skin allograft. The product addresses biological deficiencies in the wound, assists in epithelialization, and aids in preserving surrounding tissue. TruSkin® is made using the proprietary processing, which retains all components of fresh skin in their native state, including collagen-rich skin extracellular matrix (ECM), endogenous bioactive factors, and endogenous living skin cells. This product is indicated for patients with acute and chronic wounds who have limited treatment options and are at great risk for wound-related morbidities and mortality. TruSkin® offers patients an alternative to invasive procedures, including autologous skin grafting or limb amputation.

Q4168

Q4168 AmnioBand, 1 mg

AmnioBand® is a placental matrix derived from human donated amnion membranes originating from the inner lining of the placenta. It is intended for internal and external tissue defects, including acute, chronic, and surgically-created wounds. The product is used as a natural wound scaffold to support the body's inherent ability to restore and remodel tissue. AmnioBand® contains biological extracellular matrix proteins, cytokines, growth factors, and viable endogenous cells that work to support host tissue remodeling. This provides a barrier to infections and helps to maintain a moist wound environment for healing. The product is supplied in 2 cm x 2 cm and 5 cm x 5 cm sizes.

Q4169

Q4169 Artacent wound, per sq cm

Artacent® Wound is a dual-layer human amniotic membrane graft used for acute and chronic wound applications. It is derived from the submucosa of donated human placenta. It consists of collagen layers, including basement membrane and stromal matrix. Its dual layer and bilateral application improves handling, while its unique design permits easy manipulation and placement onto the wound bed. Artacent wound is supplied in the following sizes: 2 cm x 2 cm, 2 cm x 3 cm, 3 cm x 3 cm, 3 cm x 4 cm, 4 cm x 4 cm, 4 cm x 6 cm, 4 cm x 8 cm, as well as 9 mm, 12 mm, 15 mm, and 18 mm disks.

Q4170

Q4170 Cygnus, per sq cm

Cygnus® is an amniotic tissue allograft with innate regenerative capability to support healing without adhesion or scar formation. It is used most often to treat acute wounds, chronic wounds, and burns, and it can serve as an adhesion barrier to keep potentially adherent surfaces apart. The product is a dried human amnion membrane allograft composed of a single layer of epithelial cells, a basement membrane, and an avascular connective tissue matrix. It is a minimally manipulated, dried nonviable cellular amniotic membrane allograft that preserves and delivers multiple extracellular matrix proteins, growth factors, cytokines, and other specialty proteins present in amniotic tissue to help regenerate soft tissue. The product is supplied in a variety of sizes, ranging from 1 cm x 2 cm to 7 cm x 7 cm.

Q4171

Q4171 Interfyl, 1 mg

Interfyl is a decellularized and dehydrated placental disc (chorionic plate) derived extracellular matrix (ECM). Its connective-tissue matrix (CTM) serves as a scaffold for recipient cells in the wound to regenerate soft tissue. It is not cross-linked and does not contain cells, and therefore reduces the likelihood of immunogenic and inflammatory responses. Interfyl is intended for use as the replacement or supplementation of damaged or inadequate integumental tissue by providing support for the body's normal healing processes. Indications include treatment of deep dermal wounds, irregularly-shaped and tunneling wounds, augmentation of deficient/inadequate soft tissue, and the repair of small surgical defects. Interfyl is supplied as single-dose flowable product syringes containing 250 mg in 1.5 mL, and as particulate product in vials containing 50 mg and 100 mg.

Q4173

Q4173 PalinGen or PalinGen XPlus, per sq cm

PalinGen® XPlus Membrane and PalinGen® XPlus Hydromembrane are human allografts comprised of amniotic membrane. They provide a wound covering and support for native tissues. They are used to repair or replace soft tissue defects, soft trauma defects, tendinitis, tendinosis, chronic wound repair, and localized inflammation. The product is intended for older patients with diabetes for the treatment of chronic wounds. These products have also been used in the repair and reconstruction of a recipient's cells or tissues. Indications include venous leg ulcers, diabetic ulcers, pressure ulcers, and in orthopedic, cardiac, and ophthalmologic conditions. PalinGen® XPlus Membrane and PalinGen® XPlus Hydromembrane are supplied in 10 different sizes, ranging from 1 sq cm to 64 sq cm.

Q4174

Q4174 PalinGen or ProMatrX, 0.36 mg per 0.25 cc

ProMatrX ACF® is a cryopreserved human allograft comprised of amnion and amniotic fluid, providing a liquid allograft to aid in the healing and repair of chronic wounds. It contains key growth factors, cytokines, amino acids, carbohydrates, hyaluronic acid, extracellular matrix proteins, and cellular components recognized as intrinsic to the complex wound healing process. The product is commonly used in the treatment of chronic wounds that are most prevalent in older populations, particularly in patients with Type I diabetes. The product is applied directly on or in the wound with a 20 to 23 gauge needle. The prescribed dosage varies by the size of the wound. Typical doses range from 0.25 cc to 4.0 cc, depending on the size, depth, and type of wound. ProMatrX® ACF is supplied in liquid form in vials containing 0.25 cc, 0.5 cc, 1 cc, 2 cc, and 4 cc.

Q4175

Q4175 Miroderm, per sq cm

MiroDerm® is a non-crosslinked acellular wound matrix that is derived from porcine liver and is processed and stored in a phosphate buffered aqueous solution. It is clinically indicated for the management of wounds. The product provides a scaffold for chronic wounds to maintain and support a healing environment through constructive remodeling. It is used to cover the entire surface of the wound bed and extend slightly beyond all wound margins. MiroDerm® is available in fenestrated and non-fenestrated form, in seven sizes ranging from 9 cm^2 to 120 cm^2.

Q4176

Q4176 Neopatch or therion, per square centimeter

NeoPatch® and Therion are wound coverings derived from terminally sterilized, dehydrated human placental membrane tissue consisting of amnion and chorionic membrane. They are used as a wound covering for the treatment of acute wounds or chronic lower extremity ulcers. The collagen-rich extracellular matrix (ECM) provides a protective covering to the wound. It is available in 14 mm round, 18 mm round, 24 mm round, 2 cm x 3 cm, 3 cm x 5 cm, 4 cm x 4 cm, and 5 cm x 6 cm sizes.

Q4177-Q4178

Q4177 FlowerAmnioFlo, 0.1 cc

Q4178 FlowerAmnioPatch, per sq cm

FlowerAmnioPatch™ is a dehydrated amniotic membrane allograft that is used as a wound covering for postsurgical wound care. FlowerAmnioPatch is available in various sizes up to 4 x 8 cm for optimal coverage. FlowerAmnioFlo™ is a premixed, placental tissue matrix allograft that is used to replace or supplement damaged or integumental tissue for postsurgical wound care. FlowerAmnioFlo™ is supplied in liquid form, from 0.5 cc to 2.0 cc, and can be extended from 1.0 cc to 4.0 cc. Both products contain extracellular matrix (ECM), including collagens, fibronectin, growth factors, hyaluronan, integrins, and laminins, that promote the body's own regenerative process, and help reduce fibrous tissue growth, graft rejection, inflammation, infection, and scar development.

Q4179

Q4179 FlowerDerm, per sq cm

FlowerDerm™ is an acellular dermal allograft intended to be used as a skin substitute for wound covering. It provides growth factors and proteins to help facilitate healing, as well as a scaffold for cellular production and vascular in-growth. It is also used as a supplemental support for and reinforcement of tendons. FlowerDerm™ is supplied in two forms, standard and meshed sheets, which allow for a variety of applications. The standard form is available in three thicknesses (0.5 mm, 1.0 mm, and 2.2 mm) and various sizes. The meshed form is available in 0.5 mm and 1.0 mm thicknesses, and in sizes from 2 x 4 cm up to 4 x 8 cm. Both forms are prehydrated and stored at room temperature.

Q4180

Q4180 Revita, per sq cm

Revita® is a terminally sterilized, dehydrated allograft used as a wound covering for acute and chronic wounds and for postsurgical wound management. It is derived from donated, intact human placental tissue consisting of amniotic and chorionic membrane. The intact membrane maintains the 3D architecture as well as extracellular matrix (ECM), including collagen, cytokines, extracellular components, and growth factors, which help promote tissue growth and healing. It is available in sheets in sizes from 2 x 2 cm to 6 x 8 cm.

Q4181

Q4181 Amnio Wound, per sq cm

Amnio Wound is a lyophilized human amniotic membrane allograft consisting of an epithelial layer and two fibrous connective tissue layers specifically processed to be used for the repair and replacement of lost or damaged dermal tissue. Amnio Wound is used for the treatment of burns, surgical and traumatic wounds, and various types of ulcers. The graft is administered by applying the stromal side to the external wound area and fixation of the wound, per the physician's preference.

Q4182

Q4182 Transcyte, per sq cm

TransCyte® (formerly Dermagraft-TC™) is a human dermal substitute derived from human tissue and consists of fibroblasts, extracellular matrix (ECM), and a bioabsorbable mesh scaffold. The fibroblasts reproduce and infiltrate the scaffold and secrete human dermal collagen, matrix proteins, growth factors, and cytokines to create a three-dimensional human skin substitute. Over time, the scaffold is absorbed by the body. TransCyte does not contain macrophages, lymphocytes, blood vessels, or hair follicles. TransCyte is approved for use in the treatment of full-thickness diabetic foot ulcers lasting longer than six weeks but without exposure of the tendon, muscle, joint capsule, or bone. The physician prepares the wound bed, thaws and rinses the TransCyte, and applies it to the site. The wound is dressed and left undisturbed for 72 hours. Serial applications can be made without the need for removal of the previously placed application.

Q4183

Q4183 Surgigraft, per sq cm

SurgiGraft™ is an amniotic tissue-based allograft derived from human placenta. It is composed of collagens and extracellular substrates that include growth factors, connective proteins, and cytokines. SurgiGraft™ provides an adhesion barrier reducing fibroblast infiltration. It is procured from live, healthy donors during cesarean childbirth and dehydrated to provide optimum handling characteristics. While this product was initially used in the acute care inpatient setting in connection with neurosurgical, orthopedic, and spine surgical procedures, it is now producing positive outcomes in individual wound care cases. The dehydrated (and the hydrated) human amnion allografts are intended for the repair or replacement of lost or damaged dermal tissue. Indications include traumatic injuries, burns, Mohs procedures, or surgical wounds; complex chronic and acute wounds, such as diabetic ulcers, venous and arterial leg ulcers, pressure ulcers, or cutaneous ulcers; wounds with exposed vital structures, such as tendon, bone, and blood vessels; and other soft tissue defects.

Q4184-Q4185

Q4184 Cellesta or Cellesta Duo, per sq cm

Q4185 Cellesta Flowable Amnion (25 mg per cc); per 0.5 cc

Cellesta™, Cellesta™ Duo, and Cellesta™ Flowable are amniotic tissue-based allografts derived from human placenta. They are composed of collagens and extracellular substrates that include growth factors, connective proteins, and cytokines. Cellesta™ provides an adhesion barrier reducing fibroblast infiltration. It is procured from live, healthy donors during cesarean childbirth and dehydrated to provide optimum handling characteristics. While this product was initially used in the acute care inpatient setting in connection with neurosurgical, orthopedic, and spine surgical procedures, it is now producing positive outcomes in individual wound care cases. The dehydrated (and the hydrated) human amnion allografts are intended for the repair or replacement of lost or damaged dermal tissue. Indications include traumatic injuries, burns, Mohs procedures, or surgical wounds; complex chronic and acute wounds, such as diabetic ulcers, venous and arterial leg ulcers, pressure ulcers, or cutaneous ulcers; wounds with exposed vital structures, such as tendon, bone, and blood vessels; and other soft tissue defects.

Q4186-Q4187

Q4186 Epifix, per sq cm

Q4187 Epicord, per sq cm

EpiFix® is a biologic human tissue allograft used to treat viable, noninfected, full- and partial-thickness wounds, such as venous, diabetic, pressure, and chronic vascular ulcers; traumatic and surgical wounds; and burns. The amniotic tissue lines the inside layer of the placenta. The fibrous layer of the amnion contains collagen IV, V, and VII. The collagen provides an attachment for cell growth. It is a natural barrier and stimulates cell growth and wound healing. The graft is cut to the appropriate size, placed on the wound surface, and secured with sterile strips and a dressing. EpiCord® is a unique, thick membrane derived from umbilical cord. It is a minimally manipulated, dehydrated, nonviable cellular umbilical cord allograft for homologous use. EpiCord® provides a protective environment for the healing process and a connective tissue matrix to replace or supplement damaged or inadequate integumental tissue.

Q4188

Q4188 AmnioArmor, per sq cm

AmnioArmor™ is an amniotic tissue-based allograft derived from human placenta. It is composed of collagens and extracellular substrates that include growth factors, connective proteins, and cytokines. AmnioArmor™ provides an adhesion barrier reducing fibroblast infiltration. It is procured from live, healthy donors during cesarean childbirth and dehydrated to provide optimum handling characteristics. While this product was initially used in the acute care inpatient setting in connection with neurosurgical, orthopedic, and spine surgical procedures, it is now producing positive outcomes in individual wound care cases. The dehydrated human amnion allografts are intended for the repair or replacement of lost or damaged dermal tissue. Indications include traumatic injuries, burns, Mohs procedures, or surgical wounds; complex chronic and acute wounds, such as diabetic ulcers, venous and arterial leg ulcers, pressure ulcers, or cutaneous ulcers; wounds with exposed vital structures, such as tendon, bone, and blood vessels; and other soft tissue defects.

Q4189-Q4190

Q4189 Artacent AC, 1 mg

Q4190 Artacent AC, per sq cm

Artacent® AC is an amniotic tissue-based allograft derived from human placenta. It is composed of collagens and extracellular substrates that include growth factors, connective proteins, and cytokines. Artacent® AC provides an adhesion barrier reducing fibroblast infiltration. It is procured from live, healthy donors during cesarean childbirth and dehydrated to provide optimum handling characteristics. While this product was initially used in the acute care inpatient setting in connection with neurosurgical, orthopedic, and spine surgical procedures, it is now producing positive outcomes in individual wound care cases. The dehydrated human amnion allografts are intended for the repair or replacement of lost or damaged dermal tissue. Indications include traumatic injuries, burns, Mohs procedures, or surgical wounds; complex chronic and acute wounds, such as diabetic ulcers, venous and arterial leg ulcers, pressure ulcers, or cutaneous ulcers; wounds with exposed vital structures, such as tendon, bone, and blood vessels; and other soft tissue defects.

Q4191-Q4192

Q4191 Restorigin, per sq cm

Q4192 Restorigin, 1 cc

Restorigin™ is an extracellular matrix (ECM) allograft procured from live, healthy donors during cesarean childbirth and dehydrated to provide optimum handling characteristics. It is composed of collagens and extracellular substrates that include amino acids, collagen, growth factors, connective proteins, and cytokines. Restorigin™ inhibits fibrogenesis and promotes formation of healthy tissue without adhesion or scar formation. It is indicated for multiple types of applications, such as acute and chronic wounds; burn care; wounds with exposed vital structures, such as tendon, bone, and blood vessels; soft tissue defects; and posttraumatic and postsurgical wounds. Code Q4191 represents the Restorigin™ Amnion Patch that is derived from placental or umbilical cord tissue. It is available in three thicknesses and multiple sizes. Code Q4192 represents Restorigin™, a frozen liquid allograft derived from amniotic fluid, and is available in four sizes: .25 ml, .5 ml, 1 ml, and 2 ml. It requires no dilation and is applied directly to the injury or wound.

Q4193

Q4193 Coll-e-Derm, per sq cm

Coll-e-Derm™ is a non-crosslinked, dermal allograft derived from decellularized human dermal tissue. Human donors lower the risk of an inflammatory response. It is composed of collagen, elastin, and proteoglycans that allow cellular regeneration upon application and provides natural scaffolding that encourages the healing process. It can be utilized for wounds that have not healed with other conventional treatment. It is available in three thicknesses (0.5 mm to 1 mm, 1 mm to 2 mm, >= 2 mm) and can be sutured in place, if necessary. Coll-e-Derm™ is intended for use in the following applications: abdominal wall repair, breast reconstruction, repair of soft tissue defects, replacement of damaged or inadequate homologous tissue, tendon augmentation, and tendon lengthening.

Q4194

Q4194 Novachor, per sq cm

Novachor is a sterile, single-use sheet dressing made from the chorion layer of human placental membranes. The placental membrane contains collagen types I, III, V, VI laminin, fibronectin, and proteoglycans; growth factors; pluripotential cells; tissue inhibitors of matrix metalloproteinases (TIMPs); and trophic proteins. It is intended for the management of acute and chronic wounds. It is supplied dry in sheet form, measuring 2.5 x 2.5 cm. It is surgically applied and fixed to a wound using sutures or other fixation methods based on the size of the wound being treated.

Q4195-Q4197

Q4195 PuraPly, per sq cm

Q4196 PuraPly AM, per sq cm

Q4197 PuraPly XT, per sq cm

PuraPly®, PuraPly® AM, and PuraPly® XT are sterile, single-use sheet dressings made of two layers of porcine intestinal collagen matrix coated with polyhexamethylene biguanide hydrochloride (PHMB). They are intended for the management of wounds and as an effective barrier to resist microbial colonization within the dressings and to reduce microbes penetrating through the dressing. Antimicrobial PHMB wound dressing is supplied dry in sheet form, in sizes ranging from 4 cm x 4 cm to 12 cm x 36 cm. It is intended as a skin substitute for use on acute and chronic partial- and full-thickness wounds. It is surgically applied and fixed to a wound using sutures or other fixation methods based on the size of the wound being treated.

Q4198

Q4198 Genesis Amniotic Membrane, per sq cm

Genesis Amniotic Membrane is a human allograft made from donated amniotic membrane derived from the inner lining of the placenta. It is composed of dehydrated human amnion consisting of collagen, fibronectin, integrin, laminin, and hyaluronan. It is indicated as a wound covering for diabetic patients who have issues with wound healing. The product is applied directly over the wound and does not require any sutures or other fixation. It is available in sizes ranging from 1 x cm^2 to 7 x 15 cm^2.

Q4199

Q4199 Cygnus matrix, per sq cm

Cygnus® matrix is a flexible, multilayer amniotic tissue allograft with innate regenerative capability to support healing without adhesion or scar formation. It is used most often to treat acute wounds, chronic wounds, and burns, and it can serve as an adhesion barrier to keep potentially adherent surfaces apart. The product is a dried human amnion membrane allograft composed of a single layer of epithelial cells, a basement membrane, and an avascular connective tissue matrix. It is a minimally manipulated, dried nonviable cellular amniotic membrane allograft that preserves and delivers multiple extracellular matrix (ECM) proteins, growth factors, cytokines, and other specialty proteins present in amniotic tissue to help regenerate soft tissue. The product is supplied in a variety of sizes, with square/rectangular shapes ranging from 1 cm x 2 cm to 7 cm x 7 cm, and disks ranging from 15 mm to 65 mm.

Q4200

Q4200 SkinTE, per sq cm

SkinTE™ is a human cellular and tissue-based autologous, homologous product for skin reconstruction, regeneration, repair, replacement, and supplementation. It is harvested from a patient's own

Q

skin and can be used for the treatment of acute and chronic wounds, burns, replacement of failed grafts or flaps, scar revision, surgical reconstruction, and traumatic injuries. The SkinTE™ product is obtained with the use of a Harvest Box, which allows the provider to obtain a full-thickness skin sample from the patient. The sample is returned to the manufacturer. SkinTE™ is contained within a syringe and returned to the provider in a Deployment Box, usually within 48 to 72 hours. The provider applies SkinTE™ to the defect or wound, covers it with a dressing, and follows standard wound care protocol.

Q4201

Q4201 Matrion, per sq cm

Matrion™ is a regenerative allograft derived from human placenta. It is a matrix scaffold made from the amniotic and chorionic layers of the placenta. The decellularized membrane is freeze-dried and available in injectable, membrane, and sponge forms and is intended for repair of wounds, tendons, and nerves. It is supplied in 2x2 cm, 2x3 cm, 2x4 cm, 4x4 cm, and 4x6 sizes, and can be fixated if needed.

Q4202

Q4202 Keroxx (2.5 g/cc), 1 cc

Keroxx® is an advanced wound matrix made from acellular, biologically active keratin protein. The protein is derived from sheep wool and is available in an injectable flowable gel format. The gel is injected in the wound bed and the keratin protein is absorbed, providing a scaffold for new tissue growth. The active keratin protein stimulates cells to enter the hyperproliferative phase needed for wound healing.

Q4203

Q4203 Derma-Gide, per sq cm

Derma-Gide® is a wound dressing made from purified porcine collagen and is intended for use as a covering and for healing of soft tissue defects and wounds. It provides protection from infection by covering exposed tissue and promotes wound healing and tissue growth.

Q4204

Q4204 XWRAP, per sq cm

XWRAP® is a chorion-free, extracellular matrix (ECM) derived from human donated amnion membranes originating from the inner lining of the placenta. It is intended for internal and external tissue defects, including acute, chronic, and surgically-created wounds. The product is used as a natural wound scaffold to support the body's inherent ability to restore and remodel tissue. XWRAP® contains collagen, fibronectin, laminin, cytokines, growth factors, and modulates that work to support host tissue remodeling. This provides a barrier to infections and helps to maintain a moist wound environment for healing. The product is supplied in multiple sizes for a broad range of wounds.

Q4205

Q4205 Membrane Graft or Membrane Wrap, per sq cm

Membrane Graft and Membrane Wrap™ are membrane allografts made of dehydrated and decellularized human amniotic membrane and are used as wound coverings. They are indicated for the treatment of acute and chronic wounds, including surgical and traumatic wounds and ulcers, as well as burns. It is available in a variety of sizes, ranging from 1 cm x 1 cm to 4 cm x 8 cm.

Q4206

Q4206 Fluid Flow or Fluid GF, 1 cc

Fluid Flow™ and Fluid GF are amniotic liquid allografts derived from human amniotic tissue. The amniotic membrane is separated from the placenta and morselized into particulate form, then combined with amniotic fluid components to form the allograft. The processing method is intended to preserve the structural properties of the collagen, growth factors, cellular materials, and matrix present in the tissue to create a micro-scaffold to be used to aid in the wound healing process. The wound coverings reduce inflammation and healing time, as well as encourage repair and reconstruction of soft tissue injuries such as bursitis, degenerative joint disorders, fasciitis, ligament and tendon sprains, meniscal and muscle tears, and tendonitis. They are available in 0.5 cc, 1 cc, and 2 cc sizes.

Q4208

Q4208 Novafix, per sq cm

Novafix™ is a dehydrated amniotic membrane allograft that is used as a wound covering for the treatment of acute and chronic wounds, burns, postsurgical wounds, traumatic injuries, various types of ulcers, and wound dehiscence. It contains extracellular matrix (ECM), including collagens, fibronectin, growth factors, hyaluronan, integrins, and laminins, that promote the body's own regenerative process, and help reduce fibrous tissue growth, graft rejection, inflammation, infection, and scar development. Novafix™ should be applied to the wound bed and positioned to completely cover the wound and extend slightly outside of the wound margins. If needed, it can be fixed to the wound site with sutures. It is supplied in a variety of sizes, including 2 cm x 2 cm, 4 cm x 4 cm, 5 cm x 5 cm, as well as a 15 mm disc.

Q4209

Q4209 SurGraft, per sq cm

SurGraft® is a dehydrated amniotic membrane sheet derived from extracellular matrix (ECM), including collagens, fibronectin, growth factors, hyaluronan, integrins, and laminins. It promotes the body's own regenerative process, and helps reduce fibrous tissue growth, graft rejection, inflammation, infection, and scar development. It serves as a scaffold for recipient cells in the wound to regenerate soft tissue. It is not crosslinked and does not contain cells, and therefore reduces the likelihood of immunogenic and inflammatory responses. SurGraft® is intended for the treatment of acute and chronic wounds, burns, noninfected ulcers, and surgical wounds that have not responded to other therapy. It is supplied in five sizes: 2 cm x 2 cm, 2 cm x 3 cm, 2 cm x 4 cm, 4 cm x 4 cm, and 4 cm x 8 cm.

Q4210

Q4210 Axolotl Graft or Axolotl DualGraft, per sq cm

Axolotl Graft™ and Axolotl DualGraft™ are dehydrated amniotic membrane allografts that are used as wound barriers, nerve wraps, and wound coverings for the repair or regeneration of injured or diseased tissues. They contain extracellular matrix (ECM), including collagens, fibronectin, growth factors, hyaluronan, integrins, and laminins, that promote the body's own regenerative process, and help reduce fibrous tissue growth, graft rejection, inflammation, infection, and scar development. Axolotl DualGraft™ is a thicker, bi-layered version of the membrane allograft that provides more protection for wounds vulnerable to damage. Axolotl Graft™ is available in three sizes: 1 cm x 2 cm, 2 cm x 3 cm, and 4 cm x 4 cm. Axolotl DualGraft™ is available in four sizes: 1 cm x 2 cm, 2 cm x 3 cm, 4 cm x 4 cm, and 4 cm x 6 cm.

Q4211

Q4211 Amnion Bio or AxoBioMembrane, per sq cm

AxoBioMembrane™ is a dehydrated human amnion membrane (dHAM) allograft. It contains key growth factors, cytokines, amino acids, carbohydrates, hyaluronic acid, extracellular matrix proteins, and cellular components recognized as intrinsic to the complex wound healing process. It is intended for use as a wound covering, providing a natural wound barrier, for the treatment of acute and chronic wounds. It is available in three sizes: 1 cm x 2 cm, 2 cm x 3 cm, and 4 cm x 4 cm.

Q4212

Q4212 AlloGen, per cc

AlloGen® is a cryopreserved human allograft comprised of amnion and amniotic fluid, providing a liquid allograft designed to cushion within the joint capsule. The product is applied directly into the administration site with a 30 gauge, or larger, needle. The prescribed dosage varies depending on the joint treated. It is supplied in liquid form, both in frozen and ambient temperature format, in single use vials, ranging from 0.25 ml to 2.0 ml.

Q4213

Q4213 Ascent, 0.5 mg

Ascent™ is a dehydrated cell and protein concentrate (dCPC) injectable derived from human amniotic fluid. It provides a liquid allograft designed to cushion, lubricate, and reduce inflammation in osteoarthritic joints and to treat tendinopathies. It contains key growth factors, cytokines, amino acids, carbohydrates, hyaluronic acid, extracellular matrix proteins, and cellular components recognized as intrinsic to the complex wound healing process. The product is injected directly into the joint or injury site. Local or topical anesthetic, as well as ultrasound imaging guidance, may be utilized. A bandage is applied following injection. It is supplied in powdered weights of 7.5 mg, 15 mg, and 30 mg, which require reconstitution with sterile saline volumes of 0.5 cc, 1 cc, and 2 cc, respectively. The prescribed dosage varies depending on the joint or size, depth, and type of wound.

Q4214

Q4214 Cellesta Cord, per sq cm

Cellesta™ Cord is a regenerative wound covering derived from human umbilical cord tissue. It is a minimally manipulated, dehydrated, nonviable cellular allograft that is used to treat acute, chronic, and postsurgical wounds. Once placed over the wound surface, it can be secured with suture material or glue, if needed. It is available in a variety of sizes, ranging from 1.5 cm x 1.5 cm, 3 cm x 2 cm, 3 cm x 4 cm, 3 cm x 6 cm, and 3 cm x 8 cm, as well as 12 mm, 15 mm, and 18 mm disks.

Q4215

Q4215 Axolotl Ambient or Axolotl Cryo, 0.1 mg

Axolotl Ambient™ and Axolotl Cryo™ are human allograft comprised of amnion and amniotic fluid, providing a liquid allograft designed to cushion within the joint capsule. It contains key growth factors, cytokines, amino acids, carbohydrates, hyaluronic acid, extracellular matrix proteins, and cellular components recognized as intrinsic to the complex wound healing process. Axolotl Ambient™ is supplied at ambient temperature. Axolotl Cryo™ is supplied in frozen format. Both products are available in 0.5 ml, 1 ml, and 2 ml vials.

Q4216

Q4216 Artacent Cord, per sq cm

Artacent® Cord is an allograft membrane derived from human umbilical cord tissue. It is a minimally manipulated, dehydrated, nonviable cellular allograft that is used to treat burns and acute and chronic wounds, such as diabetic and venous stasis ulcers. The graft is cut to the appropriate size, placed on the wound surface, and secured with suture material, if needed. The allograft may be hydrated with sterile saline, if required, once it has been applied to the wound site.

Q4217

Q4217 WoundFix, BioWound, WoundFix Plus, BioWound Plus, WoundFix Xplus or BioWound Xplus, per sq cm

WoundFix™, BioWound™, WoundFix™ Plus, BioWound™ Plus, WoundFix™ XPlus, BioWound™ XPlus, WoundFix™ XPlus Membrane, and BioWound™ XPlus Membrane are membrane allografts made of dehydrated and decellularized human amniotic membrane and are used as wound coverings. They are indicated for the treatment of burns, acute and chronic wounds, including postsurgical and traumatic wounds, and ulcers, including those with exposed tendon, muscle, or bone. WoundFix™, BioWound™, WoundFix™ Plus, and BioWound™ Plus are supplied in single use packages, in a variety of sizes, ranging from .786 sq cm to 486 sq cm. WoundFix™ XPlus and BioWound™ XPlus are supplied in single use packages, in a variety of sizes, ranging from .786 sq cm to 192 sq cm. WoundFix™ XPlus Membrane, and BioWound™ XPlus Membrane are supplied in single use packages in 6 sq cm and 12 sq cm sizes.

Q

Q4218

Q4218 SurgiCORD, per sq cm

SurgiCORD is a human umbilical tissue membrane. It is a nonimplantable biological skin graft substitute comprised of human amniotic membrane retrieved from electively donated umbilical cords, containing collagen types IV, V, and VII. It is indicated as a wound covering in chronic, nonhealing dermal wounds. It is applied topically and is available in four sizes: 1.5 cm x 1.5 cm, 3 cm x 2 cm, 3 cm x 4 cm, and 3 cm x 6 cm.

Q4219

Q4219 SurgiGRAFT-DUAL, per sq cm

SurgiGRAFT-DUAL™ is a dehydrated amniotic membrane allograft that is used as a wound barrier and wound covering for the repair or regeneration of injured or diseased tissues. It contains extracellular matrix (ECM), including collagens, fibronectin, growth factors, hyaluronan, integrins, and laminins, that promote the body's own regenerative process, and help reduce fibrous tissue growth, graft rejection, inflammation, infection, and scar development. SurgiGRAFT-DUAL™ is a bi-layered graft and provides more protection for wounds vulnerable to damage. SurgiGRAFT-DUAL™ is available in a variety of sizes, including 2 cm x 2 cm, 2 cm x 3 cm, 2 cm x 4 cm, 2 cm x 8 cm, 4 cm x 4 cm, as well as 12 mm, 15 mm, and 18 mm disks.

Q4220

Q4220 BellaCell HD or Surederm, per sq cm

BellaCell HD and SureDerm® are regenerative tissue matrixes intended for use in skin reconstruction to repair burn injuries, congenital diseases or other malformations, abdominal wall repairs, hiatal hernia repair, periodontal diseases, postmastectomy reconstruction, traumatic injuries, ulcers, and urinary incontinence. The matrix is derived from donated human skin in which all the dermal and epidermal cells are removed. This provides a scaffold of acellular biological components that encourages revascularization, cell migration, and regeneration. BellaCell HD is supplied in a variety of sizes, ranging from 1.0 mm to 3.49 mm. SureDerm® is supplied in a variety of sizes, ranging from 0.25 mm to over 1.8 mm.

Q4221

Q4221 Amnio Wrap2, per sq cm

AmnbioWrap2™ is produced from human placental membrane. It includes the amniotic epithelial layer, the amniotic basement membrane, the amniotic stroma, the chorionic basement membrane, and the chorionic stroma. It is intended for the treatment of chronic wounds, including diabetic ulcers. It is available in a variety of sizes, ranging from 1 cm x 1 cm to 10 cm x 12 cm.

Q4222

Q4222 ProgenaMatrix, per sq cm

ProgenaMatrix™ is a graft matrix derived from keratin proteins extracted from human hair. ProgenaMatrix™ is intended for use on burns, chronic wounds, donor sites and grafts, dry and exuding partial- and full-thickness wounds, postsurgical wounds, and various types of ulcers. It is available in five sizes: 2 cm x 2 cm, 4 cm x 4 cm, 6 cm x 6 cm, 10 cm x 10 cm, and 12 cm x 12 cm.

Q4224

Q4224 Human Health Factor 10 Amniotic Patch (HHF10-P), per sq cm

Human Health Factor 10 Patch™ (HHF10-P™) is a minimally processed sterilized cellular amniotic membrane allograft used for wound treatment when it is necessary to replace or repair lost or damaged human collagen tissue. It delivers multiple extracellular matrix proteins, growth factors, cytokines, and other specialty proteins present in amniotic tissue to help regenerate soft tissue. It is intended for homologous use to act as a barrier or covering for protection from the surrounding environment. It is supplied in sheets measuring 2 cm x 2 cm or 4 cm x 4 cm.

Q4225

Q4225 AmnioBind, per sq cm

AmnioBind™ is a wound covering derived from terminally sterilized, dehydrated human placental membrane tissue consisting of amnion and chorionic membrane. The collagen-rich extracellular matrix (ECM) provides a protective covering to the wound. It is used as a wound covering for the treatment of acute and chronic wounds following debridement and is intended to remain in place for five to seven days.

Q4226

Q4226 MyOwn Skin, includes harvesting and preparation procedures, per sq cm

MyOwn Skin™ is a nonsurgical procedure that utilizes a small sample of the patient's own skin and a blood sample to produce up to three 4 in x 4 in skin grafts in five to seven days. The skin sample is obtained from a partial-thickness skin sample from a healthy donor site and is comprised of viable skin cells and extracellular matrix. These autologous-based patches, which reduce possible tissue rejection, are used as wound coverings to promote the healing of burns, chronic wounds, diabetic foot ulcers, postsurgical wounds, and other hard to heal wounds.

Q4227

Q4227 AmnioCore TM, per sq cm

AmnioCore™ is dehydrated amniotic membrane derived from extracellular matrix (ECM), including proteins, growth factors, cytokines, and other specialty proteins. It serves as a scaffold for recipient cells in the wound to regenerate soft tissue. It is not crosslinked and does not contain cells, and therefore reduces the likelihood of immunogenic and inflammatory responses. AmnioCore™ is intended for the treatment of acute and chronic wounds, to reduce inflammation and scar formation, as well as enhance healing. It has a five-year shelf life but must be used within six hours once the package seal is broken. It is supplied in sheet and particulate forms. Sheets are available in multiple sizes ranging from 16 mm to 9 x 20 cm. The particulate is available in volumes ranging from 20 mg to 160 mg.

Q4229-Q4230

Q4229 Cogenex Amniotic Membrane, per sq cm

Q4230 Cogenex Flowable Amnion, per 0.5 cc

Cogenex Amniotic Membrane and Cogenex Flowable Amnion are amniotic tissue-based allografts derived from human placenta. They are composed of collagens and extracellular substrates that include growth factors, connective proteins, and cytokines procured from live, healthy donors during cesarean childbirth. They provide an adhesion barrier protecting the wound from the surrounding environment in both reparative and reconstructive procedures. While this product was initially used in the acute care inpatient setting in connection with neurosurgical, orthopedic, and spine surgical procedures, it is now producing positive outcomes in individual wound care cases. Cogenex Amniotic Membrane is indicated for, but not limited to, use in chronic wound repair, gynecological and urologic surgeries, and burn wounds. It is available in wet or dry format in eight sizes: 2 cm x 2 cm, 3 cm x 3 cm, 2 cm x 4 cm, 2 cm x 6 cm, 4 cm x 4 cm, 4 cm x 6 cm, 4 cm x 8 cm, and 2 cm x 12 cm. Cogenex Flowable Amnion is a particular powder suspended in a saline solution and is intended for the treatment of deep dermal wounds, augmentation of deficient or inadequate soft tissue, irregularly-shaped, crevassing and tunneling wounds, and other complex wound where a patch may not provide adequate wound coverage. It is available in three volumes: 0.5 cc, 1.0 cc, and 3.0 cc, and is supplied in a prefilled syringe for direct application into the wound.

Q4231-Q4232

Q4231 Corplex P, per cc

Q4232 Corplex, per sq cm

Corplex™ and Corplex™ P are extracellular matrix (ECM) allograft derived from human umbilical cord tissue, including the epithelial layer and the Wharton's Jelly. It is composed of collagens and extracellular substrates that include amino acids, collagen, growth factors, connective proteins, and cytokines. Corplex™ is intended for repair, reconstruction, replacement, or supplementation of tissue, specifically as a wound covering or barrier over deep and challenging acute and chronic wounds. It is supplied in four sizes: 15 mm, 2 cm x 2 cm, 2 cm x 3 cm, and 3 cm x 5 cm sheets. Corplex™ P is intended for use in open wound environments to cushion and protect the surrounding tissue. It should be packed into the wound and covered with a dressing. It is freeze dried and supplied in sterile vials that require rehydration at time of application. It is available in three volumes: 1 cc, 2 cc, and 4 cc.

Q4233

Q4233 SurFactor or NuDyn, per 0.5 cc

SurFactor® and NuDyn™ are decellularized, human amniotic membranes derived from the placental amnion and includes epithelial and stromal components in a collagen-rich extracellular matrix. They also contain hyaluronic acid and extracellular proteins, such as elastin, glycosaminoglycans, and laminins, which are important in extracellular matrix strength, cell attraction, and migration. SurFactor® and NuDyn™ are indicated for the treatment of acute, chronic, surgical, or nonhealing wounds, burns, and for soft tissue conditions and injuries such as ankle capsulitis, bursitis, ligament and tendon sprains, nerve entrapment, plantar fasciitis, and tendonitis. They are supplied in ready to use vials in three sizes: 0.5 cc, 1 cc, and 2 cc, and are injected directly into the lesion, surrounding tissue, or wound margins.

Q4234

Q4234 XCellerate, per sq cm

XCellerate™ is a lyophilized amniotic membrane allograft containing extracellular matrix (ECM), including collagens, fibronectin, growth factors, hyaluronan, integrins, and laminins, that promote the body's own regenerative process, and help reduce fibrous tissue growth, graft rejection, inflammation, infection, and scar development. It is intended for use as a wound covering for nonhealing wounds and burn injuries. It should be applied to the wound bed after proper wound preparation. It is supplied in a variety of sizes: 2 cm x 2 cm, 2 cm x 4 cm, 4 cm x 4 cm, 4 cm x 7 cm, as well as 6 mm, 9 mm, and 12 mm discs.

Q4235

Q4235 AMNIOREPAIR or AltiPly, per sq cm

AMNIOREPAIR® and AltiPly® are lyophilized placental membrane allograft containing extracellular matrix (ECM), including collagens, fibronectin, growth factors, hyaluronan, integrins, and laminins, that promote the body's own regenerative process and help reduce fibrous tissue growth, graft rejection, inflammation, infection, and scar development. They are intended for use as biological barriers or wound covers for acute and chronic wounds. The dry graft absorbs moisture directly from the wound, but a few drops of sterile saline may be applied if not all areas are rehydrated. The wound should be covered with a non-adherent dressing and saline moistened gauze to fill, but not pack, the wound. They are supplied in a variety of sizes: 2 cm x 2 cm, 4 cm x 4 cm, 4 cm x 7 cm, and 6 cm x 9 cm sheets.

Q4236

Q4236 carePATCH, per square centimeter

carePATCH is a dehydrated amniotic membrane allograft containing extracellular matrix (ECM), including collagens, fibronectin, growth factors, hyaluronan, integrins, and laminins, that promote the body's own regenerative process and help reduce fibrous tissue growth, graft rejection, inflammation, infection, and scar development. It is intended for the treatment of nonhealing wounds and burn injuries. Sutures or tissue adhesive may be utilized if necessary. It is supplied in a variety of sizes.

Q4237

Q4237 Cryo-Cord, per sq cm

Cryo-Cord™ is an extracellular matrix (ECM) allograft derived from human placental umbilical cord tissue, including the epithelial layer and the Wharton's Jelly. It is composed of collagens and extracellular substrates that include amino acids, collagen, growth factors, connective proteins, and cytokines. Cryo-Cord™ is intended for use as a wound covering for chronic nonhealing wounds. It is supplied in three sizes: 2 cm x 2 cm, 2 cm x 4 cm, and 3 cm x 6 cm sheets.

Q4238

Q4238 Derm-Maxx, per sq cm

Derm-Maxx™ is a freeze dried decellularized dermal matrix allograft derived from consenting donors that contains extracellular matrix (ECM) composed of collagens and extracellular substrates that include amino acids, collagen, growth factors, connective proteins, and cytokines. It is intended for use as integumentary augmentation and as a covering for wounds and skin defects. It is supplied in multiple sizes and is applied directly to the wound.

Q4239

Q4239 Amnio-Maxx or Amnio-Maxx Lite, per sq cm

Amnio-Maxx™ and Amnio-Maxx™ Lite are amniotic tissue membrane grafts derived from human amniotic tissue during cesarean deliveries. They are composed of collagens and extracellular substrates that include growth factors, connective proteins, and cytokines. Amnio-Maxx™ is dual layer; Amnio-Maxx™ Lite is a single layer. Both products are intended for the treatment of wounds, including surgical wounds, burns, traumatic injury, chronic and acute wound conditions, and supportive treatment of wound-associated bone defects. Amnio-Maxx™ is available in four sizes: 2 cm x 3 cm, 4 cm x 4 cm, 4 cm x 6 cm, and 4 cm x 8 cm sheets. Amnio-Maxx™ Lite is available in two sizes: 3 cm x 6 cm and 3 cm x 8 cm sheets.

Q4240-Q4241

Q4240 CoreCyte, for topical use only, per 0.5 cc

Q4241 PolyCyte, for topical use only, per 0.5 cc

CoreCyte™ and PolyCyte™ are extracellular matrix (ECM) allograft derived from human umbilical cord tissue, including the epithelial layer and the Wharton's Jelly. They are composed of collagens and extracellular substrates that include amino acids, collagen, growth factors, connective proteins, and cytokines. Both products are intended for use in repair, reconstruction, replacement, or supplementation of a patient's cells or tissues. CoreCyte™ and PolyCyte™ are shipped and stored frozen and available in three volumes: 0.5 mL, 1.0 mL, and 2.0 mL. After thawing, the products are drawn up into a syringe and applied directly on or in the wound.

Q4242

Q4242 AmnioCyte Plus, per 0.5 cc

AmnioCyte™ Plus is an amniotic membrane allograft containing extracellular matrix (ECM), including collagens, fibronectin, growth factors, hyaluronan, integrins, and laminins that promote the body's own regenerative process, and help reduce fibrous tissue growth, graft rejection, inflammation, infection, and scar development. It is intended for use in repairing, reconstruction, replacement, or supplementation of a patient's cells or tissues. It is shipped and stored frozen and available in three volumes: 0.5 mL, 1.0 mL, and 2.0 mL. After thawing, the product is drawn up into a syringe and applied directly on or in the wound.

Q4244

Q4244 Procenta, per 200 mg

Procenta® is an extracellular matrix (ECM) placental derived allograft procured from live, healthy donors during cesarean childbirth and dehydrated to provide optimum handling characteristics. It is composed of collagens and extracellular substrates that include amino acids, collagen, growth factors, connective proteins, and cytokines. It is indicated for chronic nonhealing ulcers and wounds. It is available in three sizes: 100 mg, 200 mg, and 300 mg and is applied to the wound intraoperatively.

Q4245

Q4245 AmnioText, per cc

AmnioText™ is an amniotic membrane allograft containing extracellular matrix (ECM), including collagens, fibronectin, growth factors, hyaluronan, integrins, and laminins needed for the repair of damaged tissue. It provides a barrier to help with the healing of a defect. The amount is determined by the size of the defect and is administered directly to the defect through a syringe. It is packaged in a protective pouch in a cryogenic container.

Q4246

Q4246 CoreText or ProText, per cc

CoreText™ and ProText™ are extracellular matrix (ECM) allografts derived from human umbilical cord tissue, including the epithelial layer and the Wharton's Jelly. It is composed of collagens and extracellular substrates that include amino acids, collagen, growth factors, connective proteins, and cytokines. CoreText™ is intended for use for muscle and cartilage tears, as well as wound and tissue defects. ProText™ is intended for use as replacement tissue that is injected or inserted into a joint or other area. Both products are supplied in a cryogenic primary tissue container. The product is drawn into a syringe and applied or injected into the wound or defect.

Q4247

Q4247 Amniotext patch, per sq cm

AmnioText™ patches are amniotic membrane allografts containing extracellular matrix (ECM), including collagens, fibronectin, growth factors, hyaluronan, integrins, and laminins needed for the repair of damaged tissue. It serves as a wound covering for chronic non-healing wounds. The amount is determined by the size of the wound and is applied directly to the wound bed. It is available in various sizes to match the size of wound defects. It is packaged in a protective pouch in a dual package container.

Q4248

Q4248 Dermacyte Amniotic Membrane Allograft, per sq cm

Dermacyte® Amniotic Membrane Allograft is a dehydrated amniotic membrane allograft that is used as a wound covering for the treatment of acute and chronic wounds, burns, postsurgical wounds, traumatic injuries, various types of ulcers, and wound dehiscence. It contains extracellular matrix (ECM), including collagens, fibronectin, growth factors, hyaluronan, integrins, and laminins, that promote the body's own regenerative process and help reduce fibrous tissue growth, graft rejection, inflammation, infection, and scar development. It should be applied to cover the wound, followed by a compression wrap to secure the product.

Q4249

Q4249 AMNIPLY, for topical use only, per sq cm

AMNIPLY® is a human amniotic membrane graft derived from the submucosa of the placenta. It is used for acute and chronic wound applications, and for surgical procedures such as spinal fusions and tendon repairs. The graft should be placed into the affected area or wound bed. It is supplied in single- and dual-layer options that are individually packaged and stored at room temperature. Both options are available in multiple sizes. The size that most closely matches the defect or wound should be selected.

Q4250

Q4250 AmnioAmp-MP, per sq cm

AmnioAMP-MP™ is an allograft made of dehydrated and decellularized human amniotic membrane derived from placental amnion, including epithelial and stromal components, that provides a collagen-rich extracellular matrix, cytokines, and growth factors. The matrix provides a scaffold for cell attachment and proliferation that is required for granulation tissue development, vascularization, and epithelization. The matrix is indicated for the treatment of partial and full-thickness acute and chronic wounds, including those with exposed bone, muscle, and tendon. It is provided in a ready to use dry sheet, available in multiple sizes, and is stored at room temperature. The size that most closely matches the defect or wound should be selected.

Q4251

Q4251 Vim, per sq cm

Vim is a dehydrated, decellularized, human amniotic membrane. It is derived from the placental amnion and includes epithelial and stromal components in a collagen-rich extracellular matrix. Vim contains extracellular proteins, such as collagen, glycoproteins, proteoglycans, cytokines, and growth factors that are important in extracellular matrix strength, cell attraction, and migration. It is indicated for use as a wound cover or barrier in ophthalmic, orthopedic, surgical, and other wound applications. It is available in two sizes, 2 cm x 2 cm and 4 cm x 4 cm, and may be cut to fit the wound. The graft is placed over the wound and secured with staples or sutures, per physician preference.

Q4252

Q4252 Vendaje, per sq cm

Vendaje is a dehydrated, sterilized cellular amniotic membrane allograft used for wound treatment when it is necessary to replace or repair lost or damaged skin. It delivers multiple extracellular matrix proteins, growth factors, cytokines, and other specialty proteins present in amniotic tissue to help regenerate soft tissue. It is indicated for the treatment and management of chronic wounds including chronic ulcers, ulcers due to disease process, partial thickness burns, draining wound, postsurgical wounds, and traumatic wounds. It is available in multiple sizes and the dosage is based on wound size. It is applied over or within the wound and secured by hydrostatic tension.

Q4253

Q4253 Zenith Amniotic Membrane, per sq cm

Zenith Amniotic Membrane is a dehydrated, sterilized cellular amniotic membrane allograft used as a barrier and covering for wounds. It delivers multiple extracellular matrix proteins, growth factors, cytokines, and other specialty proteins present in amniotic tissue to help regenerate soft tissue. It is indicated for the treatment and management of acute and chronic nonhealing wounds such as burns, diabetic foot ulcers, venous leg ulcers, pressure ulcers, and surgical wounds. It is available in multiple sizes and the dosage is based on wound size. It is applied over the burn or wound site following wound preparation.

Q4254

Q4254 Novafix DL, per sq cm

Novafix® DL is a dehydrated human amnion chorion membrane allograft derived from placental extracellular matrix (ECM). The matrix fully absorbs into the wound and provides proteins, cytokines, growth factors, and viable endogenous cells that work to support cellular infiltration and vascularization. It is intended for the treatment of acute and chronic wounds, surgical wounds, traumatic wounds, and wounds that are draining. It is supplied in dry sheets in 2 cm x 2 cm, 4 cm x 4 cm, 4 cm x 6 cm, and 4 cm x 8 cm sizes and is stored at room temperature.

Q4255

Q4255 REGUaRD, for topical use only, per sq cm

REGUaRD is a hydrated acellular human dermal allograft matrix derived from placental extracellular matrix (ECM) that provides a scaffold for cell attachment and proliferation that is required for granulation tissue development, vascularization, and epithelization. The matrix is indicated for the treatment of non-healing wounds and burn injuries, and for a variety of dental and surgical wounds. It is available in 2 cm x 2 cm, 2 cm x 4 cm, 4 cm x 4 cm, 4 cm x 6 cm, and 4 cm x 8 cm sizes and is stored at room temperature.

Q4256

Q4256 MLG-Complete, per sq cm

MLG-Complete™ is a wound covering derived from terminally sterilized, dehydrated human placental membrane tissue consisting of amnion and chorionic membrane. It delivers multiple extracellular matrix proteins, growth factors, cytokines, and other specialty proteins present in amniotic tissue to help regenerate soft tissue. It is intended for the management of acute and chronic wounds such as pressure sores/ulcers, tunneled or undermined wounds, as well as other surgical and traumatic wounds. It is applied directly to the wound, requires no fixation, and is fully resorbable. It is supplied in a single use package in a variety of sizes.

Q4257

Q4257 Relese, per sq cm

Relese™ is a human allograft comprised of amniotic membrane. It provides a wound covering and support for native tissues. It is intended for use as a selective barrier and for protection from the environment for acute and chronic wounds including ulcers and other defects. It can be applied wet or dry. It is supplied in single-use sheets ranging from 2 cm x 2 cm to 6 cm x 8 cm.

Q4258

Q4258 Enverse, per sq cm

Enverse™ is a human allograft comprised of amniotic membrane. It provides a wound covering and support for native tissues. It is intended for use as a selective barrier and for protection from the environment for acute and chronic wounds including ulcers and other defects. It can be applied wet or dry. It is supplied in single-use sheets ranging from 2 cm x 2 cm to 9 cm x 15 cm.

Q4259

Q4259 Celera Dual Layer or Celera Dual Membrane, per sq cm

Celera Dual Layer and Celera Dual Membrane are wound coverings derived from terminally sterilized, dehydrated human placental membrane tissue consisting of amnion and chorionic membrane. The collagen-rich extracellular matrix (ECM) provides a protective covering to the wound. They are available in multiple sizes, ranging from 2 cm x 3 cm through 7 cm x 7 cm.

Q4260

Q4260 Signature APatch, per sq cm

Signature APatch is a cryopreserved amniotic membrane for homologous use as a wound barrier or covering. It is intended for the treatment of acute and chronic wounds, including burns, surgical and traumatic wounds, and ulcers. It is applied directly to the wound weekly for up to 12 weeks or until the wound is closed. The product is thawed in a sterile gloved hand for five minutes, then applied to the wound site with forceps, following wound preparation. It is available in a single, hexagonal size of 16.24 cm^2, which allows for multidirectional expansion to cover various sizes of wounds. It may be used with tissue adhesives or semi-wet dressings if necessary.

Q4261

Q4261 TAG, per sq cm

TAG is a processed, dehydrated, sterilized cellular amniotic membrane allograft obtained from donated human placental tissue, intended for use as a wound barrier and to provide coverage for acute and chronic wounds. It delivers multiple extracellular matrix proteins, growth factors, cytokines, and other specialty proteins present in amniotic tissue to help regenerate soft tissue. Following standard wound preparation, the product is applied directly to the wound. It may be rehydrated with sterile water and secured in place with a secondary dressing. It is available in 2.56 cm x 2.56 cm and 10 cm x 13 cm sizes.

Q4262

Q4262 Dual Layer Impax Membrane, per sq cm

Dual Layer Impax Membrane is a dual-layered, dehydrated human amniotic membrane allograft consisting of an epithelial layer and two fibrous connective tissue layers specifically processed to be used for the repair and replacement of lost or damaged dermal tissue. Dual Layer Impax Membrane is used for the treatment of acute and chronic and as a wound barrier or cover to protect the wounds. The graft is administered by applying directly over the wound. It is available in multiple sizes.

Q4263

Q4263 SurGraft TL, per sq cm

SurGraft® TL is a triple-layer, dehydrated amniotic membrane sheet derived from extracellular matrix (ECM), including collagens, fibronectin, growth factors, hyaluronan, integrins, and laminins. It promotes the body's own regenerative process, and helps reduce fibrous tissue growth, graft rejection, inflammation, infection, and scar development. It serves as a scaffold for recipient cells in the wound to regenerate soft tissue. SurGraft® is intended for the treatment of acute and chronic wounds, burns, noninfected ulcers, and surgical wounds and it adheres directly to the wound bed without fixation. It is supplied in a variety of sizes.

Q4264

Q4264 Cocoon Membrane, per sq cm

Cocoon Membrane is produced from human placental membrane. It includes the amniotic epithelial layer, the amniotic basement membrane, the amniotic stroma, the chorionic basement membrane, and the chorionic stroma. It is intended to use as a barrier and cover for full and partial thickness, acute, and chronic wounds. It is applied directly over the wound and the provider secures it in place using their choice of fixation.

Q5001-Q5010

Q5001 Hospice or home health care provided in patient's home/residence

Q5002 Hospice or home health care provided in assisted living facility

Q5003 Hospice care provided in nursing long-term care facility (LTC) or nonskilled nursing facility (NF)

Q5004 Hospice care provided in skilled nursing facility (SNF)

Q5005 Hospice care provided in inpatient hospital

Q5006 Hospice care provided in inpatient hospice facility

Q5007 Hospice care provided in long-term care facility

Q5008 Hospice care provided in inpatient psychiatric facility

Q5009 Hospice or home health care provided in place not otherwise specified (NOS)

Q5010 Hospice home care provided in a hospice facility

These codes report the location where hospice or home health care services are rendered. Hospice care services are designed to address the physical, mental, emotional, and spiritual needs of terminally ill patients and their families. Hospice care is a palliative service that is provided when a cure is not possible. Services focus on keeping the patient comfortable by relieving pain and other symptoms and supporting the family during the terminal phase of the patient's illness. Hospice services also include bereavement counseling following the patient's death. Hospice care is typically delivered by an interdisciplinary health care team of physicians, nurses, social workers, counselors, home health aides, clergy, therapists, and trained volunteers. Hospice care is most often provided in a home-care setting, but may be provided in other settings if the patient's condition is such that more intensive professional services are required. Hospitals often have inpatient hospice programs. These programs may consist of a separate hospice unit or of a hospice team that provides care to terminally ill patients throughout the hospital. There are also freestanding inpatient hospice facilities that specialize in the care of the terminally ill patient. Other facilities, such as long-term acute care facilities and inpatient psychiatric facilities, may also provide hospice services.

Q5101

Q5101 Injection, filgrastim-sndz, biosimilar, (Zarxio), 1 mcg

Filgrastim-sndz is a synthetic, human granulocyte colony stimulating factor (G-CSF). It is produced by recombinant DNA technology using *E. coli* bacteria. The drug binds to surface receptors on hematopoietic progenitor cells and stimulates neutrophil production, differentiation, maturation, and function. It is indicated as a treatment for neutropenia in patients receiving myelosuppressive therapy for nonmyeloid malignancies. Filgrastim is also used to mobilize hematopoietic progenitor cells for leukapheresis to be used for bone marrow transplants. The drug is administered by subcutaneous or intravenous injection and intravenous infusion. Recommended dosage varies from 5 to 10 mcg/kg of body weight per day depending on the indication. The drug is supplied in prefilled syringes intended for subcutaneous and intravenous injection.

Q5103

Q5103 Injection, infliximab-dyyb, biosimilar, (Inflectra), 10 mg

Infliximab-dyyb is an injectable antibody that blocks the effects of tumor necrosis factor (TNF), a substance made by cells of the body that has an important role in promoting inflammation. Specifically, infliximab is used for treating the inflammation of Crohn's disease, ulcerative colitis, rheumatoid arthritis, psoriatic arthritis, plaque psoriasis, and ankylosing spondylitis. Infliximab is administered by intravenous infusion, and dosage varies depending on body weight (kg) and the condition being treated. It is supplied as a sterile, white, lyophilized powder in a 20 mL single use vial and is administered by intravenous infusion after reconstitution with 10 mL sterile water. The recommended dosage for the treatment of adults with Crohn's disease, pediatric (6 to 17 years old) Crohn's disease, ulcerative colitis, psoriatic arthritis, and plaque psoriasis is an induction of 5 mg/kg at zero, two, and six weeks, followed by a maintenance dose of 5 mg/kg every eight weeks. The recommended dosage for the treatment of adults with rheumatoid arthritis (RA), in conjunction with methotrexate, is an induction of 3 mg/kg at zero, two, and six weeks, followed by a maintenance dose of 3 mg/kg every eight weeks. Some RA patients may be treated with 10 mg/kg every four weeks. The recommended dosage for the treatment of ankylosing spondylitis is 5 mg/kg at zero, two, and six weeks, followed by a maintenance dose of 5 mg/kg every six weeks.

Q5104

Q5104 Injection, infliximab-abda, biosimilar, (Renflexis), 10 mg

Infliximab-abda is an injectable antibody that blocks the effects of tumor necrosis factor (TNF), a substance made by cells of the body that have an important role in promoting inflammation. Specifically, infliximab is used for treating the inflammation of Crohn's disease, ulcerative colitis, rheumatoid arthritis, psoriatic arthritis, plaque psoriasis, and ankylosing spondylitis. Infliximab is supplied as a lyophilized solution and is administered by intravenous infusion. Dosage varies depending on body weight (kg) and the condition being treated. It is supplied as a sterile, white, lyophilized powder in a 20 mL single use vial and is administered by intravenous infusion after reconstitution with 10 mL sterile water. The recommended dosage for the treatment of adults with Crohn's disease, pediatric (6 to 17 years old) Crohn's disease, ulcerative colitis, psoriatic arthritis, and plaque psoriasis is an induction of 5 mg/kg at zero, two, and six weeks, followed by a maintenance dose of 5 mg/kg every eight weeks. The recommended dosage for the treatment of adults with rheumatoid arthritis (RA) is an induction of 3 mg/kg at zero, two, and six weeks, followed by a maintenance dose of 3 mg/kg every eight weeks. Some RA patients may be treated with 10 mg/kg every four weeks. The recommended dosage for the treatment of ankylosing spondylitis is 5 mg/kg at zero, two, and six weeks, followed by a maintenance dose of 5 mg/kg every six weeks.

Q5105-Q5106

Q5105 Injection, epoetin alfa-epbx, biosimilar, (Retacrit) (for ESRD on dialysis), 100 units

Q5106 Injection, epoetin alfa-epbx, biosimilar, (Retacrit) (for non-ESRD use), 1000 units

Epoetin alfa-epbx (EPO) is a biologically engineered protein that stimulates the bone marrow to make new red blood cells. It acts in the body similarly to erythropoietin, which is produced by the kidneys. Erythropoietin is a hormone the kidneys release into the blood system to prompt the production of red blood cells when low levels of oxygen are detected in the blood. Patients with chronic renal failure are not able to produce adequate levels of erythropoietin in the kidneys. Epoetin alfa is used to treat patients with anemia due to chronic kidney disease, for chronic renal failure due to chemotherapy in patients with nonmyeloid cancer, or anemia for HIV patients being treated with zidovudine. Epoetin alfa is also indicated in the preoperative treatment of anemic patients scheduled to undergo surgery with significant, anticipated blood loss who cannot donate autologous blood. The dose is based on the patient's condition and indication. EPO is supplied in 2,000 units/mL, 3,000 units/mL, 4,000 units/mL, 10,000 units/mL, and 40,000 units/mL in single-dose vials. It is administered by subcutaneous or intravenous injection. Retacrit is a biosimilar product.

Q5107

Q5107 Injection, bevacizumab-awwb, biosimilar, (Mvasi), 10 mg

Bevacizumab-awwb is a vascular endothelial growth factor-specific (VEGF) angiogenesis inhibitor. Bevacizumab-awwb binds to and inhibits the biologic activity of VEGF preventing the formation of new blood vessels. It is indicated for first-line treatment of patients with metastatic colorectal cancer, in combination with intravenous 5-fluorouracil; second-line treatment of patients with metastatic colorectal cancer, in combination with fluoropyrimidine-irinotecan- or fluoropyrimidine-oxaliplatin-based chemotherapy who have disease progression on a first-line bevacizumab product–containing regimen; first-line treatment of unresectable, locally advanced, recurrent, or metastatic non-squamous non-small cell lung cancer; treatment of glioblastoma in patients with progressive disease after other therapy; treatment of metastatic renal cell carcinoma with interferon alfa; and for the treatment of persistent, recurrent, or metastatic cervical cancer, in combination with paclitaxel/cisplatin or paclitaxel/topotecan. The recommended dose is 5 mg per kg of body weight administered once every 14 days disease progression is detected. Bevacizumab-awwb is administered via intravenous infusion and should not be administered via intravenous bolus or push. The initial dose infusion should be delivered over 90 minutes. If the first infusion is well tolerated, the second infusion may be administered over 60 minutes. If the 60-minute infusion is well tolerated, all subsequent infusions may be administered over 30 minutes.

Q5108

Q5108 Injection, pegfilgrastim-jmdb, biosimilar, (Fulphila), 0.5 mg

Pegfilgrastim-jmdb is a leukocyte growth factor indicated as a treatment of adult and pediatric patients for febrile neutropenia, who are receiving myelosuppressive therapy for nonmyeloid malignancies. Filgrastim is a synthetic human granulocyte colony-stimulating factor (G-CSF). Pegfilgrastim is produced by recombinant DNA technology using *E. coli* bacteria. Pegfilgrastim-jmdb is a covalent conjugate of recombinant methionyl human G-CSF and monomethoxypolyethylene glycol. Pegfilgrastim-jmdb binds to surface receptors on hematopoietic cells and stimulates neutrophil production, differentiation, maturation, and function. Pegfilgrastim-jmdb is supplied in a 6 mg/0.6 mL single dose prefilled syringe and is administered by subcutaneous injection. The recommended dosage is 6 mg once each chemotherapy cycle. Dosage adjustments are required for pediatric patients weighing less than 45 kg.

Q5109

Q5109 Injection, infliximab-qbtx, biosimilar, (Ixifi), 10 mg

Infliximab-qbtx is an injectable antibody that blocks the effects of tumor necrosis factor (TNF), a substance made by cells of the body that has an important role in promoting inflammation. Specifically, infliximab is used for treating adults and pediatric patients 6 years of age and older with Crohn's disease, ulcerative colitis, rheumatoid arthritis (RA), psoriatic arthritis, plaque psoriasis, and ankylosing spondylitis. Infliximab-qbtx is administered by intravenous infusion, over a minimum of two hours, and the dosage varies depending on body weight (kg) and the condition being treated. The recommended dosage for the treatment of adults with Crohn's disease, pediatric (6 to 17 years old) Crohn's disease, ulcerative colitis, psoriatic arthritis, and plaque psoriasis is an induction of 5 mg/kg at zero, two, and six weeks, followed by a maintenance dose of 5 mg/kg every eight weeks. The recommended dosage for the treatment of adults with RA is an induction of 3 mg/kg at zero, two, and six weeks, followed by a maintenance dose of 3 mg/kg every eight weeks. The recommended dosage for the treatment of ankylosing spondylitis is 5 mg/kg at zero, two, and six weeks, followed by a maintenance dose of 5 mg/kg every six weeks.

Q5110

Q5110 Injection, filgrastim-aafi, biosimilar, (Nivestym), 1 mcg

Filgrastim-aafi is a leukocyte growth factor indicated as a treatment of adult and pediatric patients for febrile neutropenia and to prevent or treat neutropenia in patients undergoing chemotherapy or radiation. It is also used to mobilize hematopoietic progenitor cells for leukapheresis to be used for bone marrow transplants. The drug binds to surface receptors on hematopoietic cells and stimulates neutrophil production, differentiation, maturation, and function. Filgrastim-aafi is supplied in single dose vials and prefilled syringes and can be administered via intravenous or subcutaneous injection. Recommended dosage varies from 5 to 10 mcg/kg of body weight per day depending on the indication.

Q5111

Q5111 Injection, pegfilgrastim-cbqv, biosimilar, (Udenyca), 0.5 mg

Pegfilgrastim-cbqv is a leukocyte growth factor indicated as a treatment of adult and pediatric patients for febrile neutropenia, who are receiving myelosuppressive therapy for nonmyeloid malignancies. Filgrastim is a synthetic human granulocyte colony-stimulating factor (G-CSF). Pegfilgrastim is produced by recombinant DNA technology using *E. coli* bacteria. Pegfilgrastim-cbqv is a covalent conjugate of recombinant methionyl human G-CSF and monomethoxypolyethylene glycol. Pegfilgrastim-cbqv binds to surface receptors on hematopoietic cells and stimulates neutrophil production, differentiation, maturation, and function. Pegfilgrastim-cbqv is supplied in a 6 mg/0.6 mL single dose prefilled syringe and is administered by subcutaneous injection. The recommended dosage is 6 mg once each chemotherapy cycle. Dosage adjustments are required for pediatric patients weighing less than 45 kg.

Q5112

Q5112 Injection, trastuzumab-dttb, biosimilar, (Ontruzant), 10 mg

Trastuzumab-dttb (trade name Ontruzant) is an IgG1 kappa monoclonal antibody produced using recombinant DNA technology from Chinese hamster ovaries. It is indicated for the treatment of adults with HER2-overexpressing breast cancer as well as HER2-overexpressing metastatic gastric or gastroesophageal junction adenocarcinoma. For adjuvant treatment of HER2-overexpressing breast cancer, it is part of a chemotherapy regimen that includes cyclophosphamide, doxorubicin, and either docetaxel or paclitaxel, or along with carboplatin and docetaxel. For the treatment of metastatic HER2-overexpressing breast cancer, it may be used as a first line treatment or as a single agent for patients who previously received one or more chemotherapies for metastatic disease. It is supplied as a white to pale yellow, lyophilized powder, in a 150 mg single dose vial that requires reconstitution with 7.15 mL of diluent yielding 21 mg/mL. For adjuvant treatment of HER2-overexpressing breast cancer, the recommended initial dosage is 4 mg/kg administered over 90 minutes by intravenous (IV) infusion, then 2 mg/kg over 30 minutes by IV infusion each week for a duration of 12 weeks (along with docetaxel or paclitaxel) or for a duration of 18 weeks (along with carboplatin and docetaxel). One week following the final weekly dose, 6 mg/kg over 30 to 90 minutes should be administered by IV infusion every three weeks, for a total of 52 weeks of therapy. The regimen may also be altered to an initial dosage of 8 mg/kg administered over 90 minutes by IV infusion and then 6 mg/kg administered over 30 to 90 minutes by IV infusion every three weeks, for a total of 52 weeks of therapy. For the treatment of metastatic HER2-overexpressing breast cancer, the recommended initial dosage is 4 mg/kg administered over 90 minutes by IV infusion and then 2 mg/kg administered over 30 minutes by IV infusion weekly until disease progression. For the treatment of metastatic HER2-overexpressing gastric cancer, the recommended initial dosage is 8 mg/kg administered over 90 minutes by IV infusion and then 6 mg/kg administered over 30 to 90 minutes by IV infusion every three weeks. Care should be taken to ensure the proper drug is being administered. This drug is not the same as ado-trastuzumab emtansine.

Q5113

Q5113 Injection, trastuzumab-pkrb, biosimilar, (Herzuma), 10 mg

Trastuzumab-pkrb (trade name Herzuma®) is an IgG1 kappa monoclonal antibody produced using recombinant DNA technology from Chinese hamster ovaries. It is indicated for the treatment of adults with HER2-overexpressing node positive or node negative breast cancer. For adjuvant treatment of HER2-overexpressing breast cancer, it is part of a chemotherapy regimen that includes cyclophosphamide, doxorubicin, and docetaxel or paclitaxel, or along with carboplatin and docetaxel. For the treatment of metastatic HER2-overexpressing breast cancer, it may be used as a first line treatment or as a single agent for patients who previously received one or more chemotherapies for metastatic disease. It is supplied as a white to pale yellow, lyophilized powder that requires reconstitution with 20 mL of diluent yielding 21 mg/mL of the drug or approximately 420 mg. For adjuvant treatment of HER2-overexpressing breast cancer, the recommended initial dosage is 4 mg/kg administered over 90 minutes by intravenous (IV) infusion and then 2 mg/kg over 30 minutes by IV infusion each week for a duration of 12 weeks (along with docetaxel or paclitaxel) or for a duration of 18 weeks (along with carboplatin and docetaxel). One week following the final weekly dose, 6 mg/kg over 30 to 90 minutes should be administered by IV infusion every three weeks, for a total of 52 weeks of therapy. For the treatment of metastatic HER2-overexpressing breast cancer, the recommended initial dosage is 4 mg/kg administered over 90 minutes by IV infusion and then 2 mg/kg administered over 30 minutes by IV infusion weekly until disease progression. Care should be taken to ensure the proper drug is being administered. This drug is not the same as ado-trastuzumab emtansine.

Q5114

Q5114 Injection, Trastuzumab-dkst, biosimilar, (Ogivri), 10 mg

Trastuzumab-dkst (trade name Ogivri) is an IgG1 kappa monoclonal antibody produced using recombinant DNA technology from Chinese hamster ovaries. It is indicated for the treatment of adults with HER2-overexpressing breast cancer as well as HER2-overexpressing metastatic gastric or gastroesophageal junction adenocarcinoma. For adjuvant treatment of HER2-overexpressing breast cancer, it is part of a chemotherapy regimen that includes cyclophosphamide, doxorubicin, and docetaxel or paclitaxel, or along with carboplatin and docetaxel. For the treatment of metastatic HER2-overexpressing breast cancer, it may be used as a first line treatment or as a single agent for patients who previously received one or more chemotherapies for metastatic disease. It is supplied as a white to pale yellow, lyophilized powder, in a 420 mg multiple dose vial that requires reconstitution with 20 mL of diluent yielding 21 mg/mL. For adjuvant treatment of HER2-overexpressing breast cancer, the recommended initial dosage is 4 mg/kg administered over 90 minutes by intravenous (IV) infusion and then 2 mg/kg over 30 minutes by IV infusion each week for a duration of 12 weeks (along with docetaxel or paclitaxel) or for a duration of 18 weeks (along with carboplatin and docetaxel). One week following the final weekly dose, 6 mg/kg over 30 to 90 minutes should be administered by IV infusion every three weeks, for a total of 52 weeks of therapy. The regimen may also be altered to an initial dosage of 8 mg/kg administered over 90 minutes by IV infusion and then 6 mg/kg administered over 30 to 90 minutes by IV infusion every three weeks, for a total of 52 weeks of therapy. For the treatment of metastatic HER2-overexpressing breast cancer, the recommended initial dosage is 4 mg/kg administered over 90 minutes by IV infusion and then 2 mg/kg administered over 30 minutes by IV infusion weekly until disease progression. For the treatment of metastatic HER2-overexpressing gastric cancer, the recommended initial dosage is 8 mg/kg administered over 90 minutes by IV infusion and then 6 mg/kg administered over 30 to 90 minutes by IV infusion every three weeks. Care should be taken to ensure the proper drug is being administered. This drug is not the same as ado-trastuzumab emtansine.

Q5115

Q5115 Injection, rituximab-abbs, biosimilar, (Truxima), 10 mg

Rituximab-abbs is a monoclonal antibody produced by recombinant DNA in Chinese hamster ovaries used as an antineoplastic drug. It binds to the CD20 antigen on the surface of normal and malignant B-lymphocytes and causes cell death. This drug is used to treat the relapsed or refractory, low-grade, or follicular, CD20-positive, B-cell non-Hodgkin's lymphoma (NHL) and for previously untreated follicular NHL. In combination with other first-line chemotherapeutic drugs, it is indicated as a treatment for CD20-positive B-cell NHL, and as a single-agent maintenance therapy of patients who have achieved complete or partial response to a rituximab product in combination with chemotherapy. It is also indicated for the treatment of non-progressing, low-grade, CD20-positive B-cell NHL as a single agent following first-line treatment with cyclophosphamide, vincristine, and prednisone (CVP) chemotherapy. The recommended dosage is 375 mg per m^2 of body surface administered by intravenous infusion. The initial infusion should be administered beginning at a rate of 50 mg/hr and if no toxicity is present, can be increased by 50 mg/hr increments every 30 minutes up to a maximum of 400 mg/hr. Subsequent infusions should be administered beginning at a rate of 100 mg/hr and if no toxicity is present, can be increased by 100 mg/hr increments every 30 minutes up to a maximum of 400 mg/hr. For previously untreated NHL, if the patient has no adverse events during the first cycle, rituximab-abbs can be administered over a 90-minute period during the second cycle, along with a glucocorticoid chemotherapy regimen. Patients who have significant cardiovascular disease should not receive the 90-minute infusion.

Q5116

Q5116 Injection, trastuzumab-qyyp, biosimilar, (Trazimera), 10 mg

Trastuzumab-qyyp is an IgG1 monoclonal antibody (HER2/neu receptor antagonist) produced using recombinant DNA technology from Chinese hamster ovaries. The drug is an antineoplastic agent indicated for adjuvant treatment of HER2-overexpressing breast cancer, or primary treatment of HER2-overexpressing metastatic gastric or gastroesophageal junction adenocarcinoma. It selectively binds to the HER2 protein site and inhibits the production of cells that overexpress HER2. Trastuzumab-qyyp is indicated as a treatment for adult patients, 18 years of age and older, who do not have heart failure or cardiomyopathy. The drug is administered via an intravenous (IV) infusion and should not be given as an IV push or bolus. The recommended dosage for adjuvant treatment of patients with HER2-overexpressing breast cancer is an initial dose of 4 mg/kg body weight administered over 90 minutes by IV infusion, then 2 mg/kg body weight over 30 minutes IV infusion each week for a total of 12 weeks when administered with paclitaxel or docetaxel, or for a total of 18 weeks when administered with docetaxel and carboplatin. One week following the last dose of trastuzumab-qyyp, administer 6 mg/kg body weight over 30 to 90 minute IV infusion every three weeks for a total of 52 weeks of treatment. The recommended dosage for primary treatment of patients with HER2-overexpessing breast cancer is an initial dose of 4 mg/kg body weight over 90 minute IV infusion followed by subsequent weekly doses of 2 mg/kg body weight over 30 minute IV infusion. The recommended dosage for primary treatment of patients with HER2-overexpressing gastric cancer is an initial dose of 8 mg/kg body weight followed by subsequent weekly doses of 6 mg/kg body weight over 30 to 90 minute IV infusion every three weeks. Trastuzumab-qyyp should not be substituted for or administered with ado-trastuzumab emtansine.

Q5117

Q5117 Injection, trastuzumab-anns, biosimilar, (Kanjinti), 10 mg

Trastuzumab-anns is an IgG1 monoclonal antibody (HER2/neu receptor antagonist) produced using recombinant DNA technology from Chinese hamster ovaries. The drug is an antineoplastic agent indicated for adjuvant treatment of HER2-overexpressing breast cancer, or primary treatment of HER2-overexpressing metastatic gastric or gastroesophageal junction adenocarcinoma. It selectively binds to the HER2 protein site and inhibits the production of cells that overexpress HER2. Trastuzumab-anns is indicated as a treatment for adult patients, 18 years of age and older, who do not have heart failure or cardiomyopathy. The drug is administered via an intravenous (IV) infusion and should not be given as an IV push or bolus. The recommended dosage for adjuvant treatment of patients with HER2-overexpressing breast cancer is an initial dose of 4 mg/kg body weight administered over 90 minutes by IV infusion, then 2 mg/kg body weight over 30 minutes IV infusion each week for a total of 12 weeks when administered with paclitaxel or docetaxel, or for a total of 18 weeks when administered with docetaxel and carboplatin. One week following the last dose of trastuzumab-qyyp, administer 6 mg/kg body weight over 30 to 90 minute IV infusion every three weeks for a total of 52 weeks of treatment. The recommended dosage for primary treatment of patients with HER2-overexpessing breast cancer is an initial dose of 4 mg/kg body weight over 90 minute IV infusion followed by subsequent weekly doses of 2 mg/kg body weight over 30 minute IV infusion. The recommended dosage for primary treatment of patients with HER2-overexpressing gastric cancer is an initial dose of 8 mg/kg body weight followed by subsequent weekly doses of 6 mg/kg body weight over 30 to 90 minute IV infusion every three weeks. Trastuzumab-anns should not be substituted for or administered with ado-trastuzumab emtansine.

Q5118

Q5118 Injection, bevacizumab-bvzr, biosimilar, (Zirabev), 10 mg

Bevacizumab-bvzr is a vascular endothelial growth factor-specific (VEGF) angiogenesis inhibitor. Bevacizumab-bvzr binds to and inhibits the biologic activity of VEGF preventing the formation of new blood vessels. It is indicated for first- or second-line treatment of patients with metastatic colorectal cancer, in combination with intravenous 5-fluorouracil; second-line treatment of patients with metastatic colorectal cancer, in combination with fluoropyrimidine-irinotecan- or fluoropyrimidine-oxaliplatin-based chemotherapy who have disease progression on a first-line bevacizumab product-containing regimen; first-line treatment of unresectable, locally advanced, recurrent, or metastatic nonsquamous non-small cell lung cancer; treatment of glioblastoma in patients with progressive disease after other therapy; treatment of metastatic renal cell carcinoma with interferon alfa; and for the treatment of persistent, recurrent, or metastatic cervical cancer, in combination with paclitaxel/cisplatin or paclitaxel/topotecan. Bevacizumab-bvzr is not indicated for the adjuvant treatment of colon cancer. It is supplied in single dose vials of 100 mg/4 ml (25 mg/ml) or 400 mg/16 ml (25 mg/ml) and requires dilution for a total volume of 100 ml of 0.9% sodium chloride. Bevacizumab-bvzr is administered via intravenous infusion and should not be administered via intravenous bolus or push. The initial dose infusion should be delivered over 90 minutes. If the first infusion is well tolerated, the second infusion may be administered over 60 minutes. If the 60-minute infusion is well tolerated, all subsequent infusions may be administered over 30 minutes. The recommended dose for the treatment of metastatic colorectal cancer is 5 mg/kg body weight administered every two weeks with bolus-IFL (irinotecan, 5-fluorouracil bolus, and leucovorin); 10 mg/kg body weight every two weeks administered with FOLFOX4 (5-fluomumcil/leucovorin combined and oxaliplatin); 5 mg/kg body weight or 7.5 mg/kg body weight administered every three weeks with fluoropyrimidine-irinotecan- or fluoropyrimidine-oxaliplatin-based chemotherapy who have disease progression on a first-line bevacizumab product–containing regimen. The recommended dose for the first-line treatment nonsquamous, non-small cell lung cancer is 15 mg/kg body weight every three weeks with carboplatin and paclitaxel. The recommended dose for the treatment of recurrent glioblastoma is 10 mg/kg body weight every two weeks. The recommended dose for the treatment of metastatic renal cell carcinoma is 10 mg/kg body weight every two weeks administered with interferon alfa. The recommend dose for the treatment of persistent, recurrent, or metastatic cervical cancer is 15 mg/kg body weight every three weeks administered with paclitaxel and cisplatin or paclitaxel and topotecan.

Q5119

Q5119 Injection, rituximab-pvvr, biosimilar, (RUXIENCE), 10 mg

Rituximab-pvvr is a monoclonal antibody produced by recombinant DNA in Chinese hamster ovaries used as an antineoplastic drug. It binds to the CD20 antigen on the surface of normal and malignant B-lymphocytes and causes cell death. This drug is indicated for the treatment of adults, 18 years of age and older, with the following: relapsed or refractory, low-grade, or follicular, CD20-positive, B-cell non-Hodgkin's lymphoma (NHL) and for previously untreated follicular NHL; in combination with other first-line chemotherapeutic drugs, it is indicated as a treatment for CD20-positive B-cell NHL, and as a single-agent maintenance therapy of patients who have achieved complete or partial response to a rituximab product in combination with chemotherapy; non-progressing, low-grade, CD20-positive B-cell NHL as a single agent following first-line treatment with cyclophosphamide, vincristine, and prednisone (CVP) chemotherapy; previously untreated diffuse large B-cell (DLBCL), CD20-positive NHL in combination with cyclophosphamide, doxorubicin, vincristine, and prednisone (CHOP) or other anthracycline-based chemotherapy regimens; previously untreated CD20-positive chronic lymphocytic leukemia (CLL) in combination with fludarabine and cyclophosphamide (FC); granulomatosis with polyangiitis (GPA) (Wegener's Granulomatosis) and microscopic polyangiitis (MPA) in combination with glucocorticoids. The drug is administered via an intravenous (IV) infusion and should not be given as an IV push or bolus. The recommended dosage for NHL is 375 mg per m^2 of body surface. The recommended dosage for CLL 375 mg per m^2 of body surface in the first cycle and 500 mg/m^2 in cycles two through six, in combination with FC, administered every 29 days. The recommended induction dosage for patients with active GPA and MPA in combination with glucocorticoids is 375 mg per m^2 of body surface once weekly for four weeks. Subsequent dosages for patients with GPA and MPA who have achieved disease control under induction treatment, in combination with glucocorticoids, is two 50 mg IV infusions separated by two weeks, followed by 500 mg IV infusion every six months. The recommended dosage as a component of Zevalin® (ibritumomab tiuxetan) Therapeutic Regiment is 250 mg/m^2 of body surface. The initial infusion should be administered beginning at a rate of 50 mg/hr and if no toxicity is present, can be increased by 50 mg/hr increments every 30 minutes up to a maximum of 400 mg/hr. Subsequent infusions should be administered beginning at a rate of 100 mg/hr and if no toxicity is present, can be increased by 100 mg/hr increments every 30 minutes up to a maximum of 400 mg/hr. For previously untreated Follicular NHL and DLBCL patients, if the patient has no adverse events during the first cycle, rituximab-abbs can be administered over a 90-minute period during the second cycle, along with a glucocorticoid chemotherapy regimen. Patients who have significant cardiovascular disease should not receive the 90-minute infusion.

Q5120

Q5120 Injection, pegfilgrastim-bmez, biosimilar, (ZIEXTENZO), 0.5 mg

Pegfilgrastim-bmez is a leukocyte growth factor indicated as a treatment of adult and pediatric patients for febrile neutropenia receiving myelosuppressive therapy for nonmyeloid malignancies. Filgrastim is a synthetic human granulocyte colony-stimulating factor (G-CSF). Pegfilgrastim is produced by recombinant DNA technology using *E. coli* bacteria. Pegfilgrastim-bmez is a covalent conjugate of recombinant methionyl human G-CSF and monomethoxypolyethylene glycol. It binds to surface receptors on hematopoietic cells and stimulates neutrophil production, differentiation, maturation, and function. It is supplied in a 6 mg/0.6 mL single dose prefilled syringe and is administered by subcutaneous injection. The recommended dosage is 6 mg once each chemotherapy cycle. Dosage adjustments are required for pediatric patients weighing less than 45 kg. See full prescribing information for additional dosage adjustments.

Q5121

Q5121 Injection, infliximab-axxq, biosimilar, (AVSOLA), 10 mg

Infliximab-axxq is an injectable antibody that blocks the effects of tumor necrosis factor (TNF), a substance made by cells of the body that has an important role in promoting inflammation. Specifically, infliximab is used for treating the inflammation of Crohn's disease, ulcerative colitis, rheumatoid arthritis, psoriatic arthritis, plaque psoriasis, and ankylosing spondylitis. Infliximab is administered by intravenous infusion, and dosage varies depending on body weight (kg) and the condition being treated. It is supplied as a sterile, white, lyophilized powder in a 20 mL single use vial and is administered via intravenous (IV) infusion after reconstitution with 10 mL sterile water. The recommended dosage for the treatment of adults with Crohn's disease, pediatric (6 to 17 years old) Crohn's disease, ulcerative colitis, psoriatic arthritis, and plaque psoriasis is an induction of 5 mg/kg at zero, two, and six weeks, followed by a maintenance dose of 5 mg/kg every eight weeks. The recommended dosage for the treatment of adults with rheumatoid arthritis (RA), in conjunction with methotrexate, is an induction of 3 mg/kg at zero, two, and six weeks, followed by a maintenance dose of 3 mg/kg every eight weeks. Some RA patients may be treated with 10 mg/kg every four weeks. The recommended dosage for the treatment of ankylosing spondylitis is 5 mg/kg at zero, two, and six weeks, followed by a maintenance dose of 5 mg/kg every six weeks.

Q5122

Q5122 Injection, pegfilgrastim-apgf, biosimilar, (Nyvepria), 0.5 mg

Pegfilgrastim-apgf is a leukocyte growth factor and a biosimilar to pegfilgrastim. It is indicated to decrease the incidence of infection in patients with nonmyeloid malignancies who receive myelosuppressive anticancer drugs that are associated with significant febrile neutropenia. The recommended dosage is a single subcutaneous (SC) injection of 6 mg administered once per chemotherapy cycle. This code reports a 0.5 mg injection.

Q5123

Q5123 Injection, rituximab-arrx, biosimilar, (Riabni), 10 mg

Rituximab is a genetically engineered chimeric murine/human monoclonal IgG1 kappa (CD20-directed) antibody, produced by recombinant DNA in Chinese hamster ovaries, used as an antineoplastic drug. It binds to the CD20 antigen on the surface of normal and malignant B-lymphocytes, causing cell death. It is used to treat patients with the following diseases: relapsed or refractory, low-grade or follicular, CD20-positive, B-cell non-Hodgkin's lymphoma (NHL) as a single agent; previously untreated follicular CD20-positive B-cell NHL in combination with other first line chemotherapeutic drugs and as a single-agent maintenance therapy; non-progressing or stable low-grade, CD20-positive B-cell NHL as a single agent following first line cyclophosphamide, vincristine, and prednisone (CVP) chemotherapy; previously untreated diffuse large B-cell, CD20-positive NHL in combination with cyclophosphamide, doxorubicin, vincristine, and prednisone (CHOP) or other anthracycline-based chemotherapy regimens; chronic lymphocytic leukemia (CLL) previously untreated and previously treated CD20-positive CLL in combination with fludarabine and cyclophosphamide (FC). Rituximab is also approved for the treatment of granulomatosis with polyangiitis (GPA), Wegener's granulomatosis, and microscopic polyangiitis (MPA) in combination with glucocorticoids. Rituximab is administered by intravenous (IV) infusion and should not be administered concomitantly with cisplatin. Dosages and frequency vary based on disease treated. See full prescribing information for complete administration instructions.

Q5124

Q5124 Injection, ranibizumab-nuna, biosimilar, (Byooviz), 0.1 mg

Ranibizumab-nuna is a monoclonal antibody produced by recombinant DNA technology using a strain of *E. coli* bacteria. The drug binds to receptor sites of human vascular endothelial growth factor A (VEGF-A) and inhibits its activity. VEGF-A has been shown to cause new vascularization and leakage of blood vessels in the eye and contributes to the progression of age-related macular degeneration. Ranibizumab is indicated as a treatment for neovascular or wet, age-related macular degeneration (AMD); macular edema following retinal vein occlusion (RVO); and myopic choroidal neovascularization (mCNV). It is supplied in a single use vial of 0.05 ml (10 mg/ml). The drug is administered by intravitreal injection only. Recommended dosage is 0.5 mg once monthly. Length of treatment depends on the condition treated. See full prescribing information for complete administration and dosage instructions. This code reports the biosimilar formulation of ranibizumab.

Q5125

Q5125 Injection, filgrastim-ayow, biosimilar, (Releuko), 1 mcg

Filgrastim-ayow is a leukocyte growth factor indicated as a treatment of adult and pediatric patients for febrile neutropenia, who are receiving myelosuppressive therapy for nonmyeloid malignancies; to reduce time to neutrophil recovery and fever duration following chemotherapy treatment for acute myeloid leukemia (AML); reduce duration of neutropenia and neutropenia-related sequelae from chemotherapy for nonmyeloid malignancies followed by bone marrow transplantations (BMT); and to reduce incidence and duration of sequelae of severe neutropenia in patients with congenital, cyclic, or idiopathic neutropenia. It is supplied in single dose vials of 300 mcg/ml or 480 mcg/1.3 ml administered via short intravenous (IV) infusions over 15 to 30 minutes, and in prefilled syringes of 300 mcg/0.5 ml and 480 mcg/0.8 ml administered via subcutaneous (SC) injection. The recommended dosage and route of administration varies based on the condition treated. SC administration of less than 0.3 ml (180 mcg) by prefilled syringes is not recommended due to potential of dosing errors. See full prescribing information for complete administration instructions.

Q5126

Q5126 Injection, bevacizumab-maly, biosimilar, (Alymsys), 10 mg

Bevacizumab-maly is a vascular endothelial growth factor inhibitor, indicated for the treatment of metastatic colorectal cancer in combination with 1) intravenous fluorouracil-based chemotherapy for first- or second-line treatment, or 2) fluoropyrimidine-irinotecan- or fluoropyrimidine-oxaliplatin-based chemotherapy for second-line treatment in patients who have progressed on a first-line bevacizumab product-containing regimen. Other indications include first-line non-squamous non-small cell lung cancer; recurrent glioblastoma; metastatic renal cell carcinoma; persistent, recurrent, or metastatic cervical cancer; and epithelial ovarian, fallopian tube, or primary peritoneal cancer. It is supplied in a single dose vial of 100 mg/4 ml (25 mg/ml) or 400 mg/15 ml (25 mg/ml) requiring dilution in 100 ml of 0.9% sodium chloride. It should not be administered or diluted with dextrose solution. Administered as an intravenous infusion, recommended dosage and frequency is dependent upon the condition treated. See full prescribing information for complete administration instructions.

Q9001-Q9003

Q9001 Assessment by chaplain services

Q9002 Counseling, individual, by chaplain services

Q9003 Counseling, group, by chaplain services

These codes report services of clinically trained Chaplains in their provision of medical service to veterans. Chaplains provide a range of pastoral and spiritual care and counseling services. These services include in-depth assessment, evaluation, and treatment (consultation, counselling, support) as part of a comprehensive bio-psycho-social-spiritual approach to include assessment of intrinsic/extrinsic spirituality, determining spiritual preference and practice, as well as determining the patient's coping mechanisms, well-being, and spiritual care development goals that are unique to patient, family, and/or caregiver needs. Report Q9001 for assessment; Q9002 for individual counseling; and Q9003 for group counseling services.

Q9004

Q9004 Department of Veterans Affairs Whole Health Partner Services

This code reports services of the Department of Veterans Affairs' Whole Health Partners to assist veterans in navigating the health care system and find resources to meet their individual goals. Whole Health Partners provides a safe environment for veterans to share their experiences, reach out into veteran communities, and improve access to health education and information.

Q9950

Q9950 Injection, sulfur hexafluoride lipid microspheres, per ml

Sulfur hexafluoride lipid-type A microsphere is an ultrasound contrast agent. It is indicated for patients who have had suboptimal echocardiograms, for better visualization of the left ventricular chamber and to better delineate the left ventricular border. It is administered intravenously with a 2 ml bolus injection during an echocardiography procedure. An additional 2 ml injection can be given during the procedure to enhance imaging.

Q9951

Q9951 Low osmolar contrast material, 400 or greater mg/ml iodine concentration, per ml

Low osmolar contrast material (LOCM) is a type of iodinated radiology contrast media that has a substantially lower concentration of particles contained in solution than high osmolar contrast material at the same iodine concentration. LOCM is supplied in radiological diagnostic procedures when the patient is known to have sensitivity to standard high osmolar contrast material or when other sensitivities or medical conditions exist that can increase the chances of a reaction in the patient. Contrast material is the dye that physicians use in diagnostic procedures to enable them to visualize the best picture possible and hence help to diagnose a patient's illness/disease, locate the point of the abnormality, or to assist in determining the extent of disease. LOCM is reported per ml based on the iodine concentration.

Q9953

Q9953 Injection, iron-based magnetic resonance contrast agent, per ml

Magnetic resonance imaging (MRI) is a radiation-free, noninvasive technique to produce high-quality sectional images of the inside of the body in multiple planes. MRI uses the natural magnetic properties of the hydrogen atoms in our bodies that emit radiofrequency signals when exposed to radio waves within a strong electromagnetic field. These signals are then processed and converted by the computer into high-resolution, three-dimensional, tomographic images. Iron is a common metal with strong magnetic properties. Various forms of the metal are used to enhance an MRI. The iron is administered intravenously and is taken up by reticuloendothelial cells, allowing greater detail to be captured by the MRI. The iron-based solution congregates in the spleen and liver allowing for the detection and evaluation of lesions. Dosage depends on patient body weight with a recommended dose of 0.05 ml per kg.

Q9954

Q9954 Oral magnetic resonance contrast agent, per 100 ml

Magnetic resonance imaging (MRI) is a radiation-free, noninvasive technique to produce high-quality sectional images of the inside of the body in multiple planes. MRI uses the natural magnetic properties of the hydrogen atoms in our bodies that emit radiofrequency signals when exposed to radio waves within a strong electromagnetic field. These signals are then processed and converted by the computer into high-resolution, three-dimensional, tomographic images. Oral MRI contrast may be composed of several paramagnetic metals including magnetite, gadolinium, or iron. The contrast is administered orally and is distributed through the gastrointestinal system enhancing its delineation from other adjacent organs and tissues. Recommended dose is 600 ml.

Q9955-Q9957

Q9955 Injection, perflexane lipid microspheres, per ml

Q9956 Injection, octafluoropropane microspheres, per ml

Q9957 Injection, perflutren lipid microspheres, per ml

Octafluoropropane and perflutren are two names for the same substance with the chemical name of octafluoropropane. Perflutren lipid microspheres are octafluoropropane gas encapsulated in lipid shells. Perflexane lipid microspheres is a similar product that encapsulates perfluorohexane in lipid spheres. When exposed to ultrasound waves, the spheres resonate or echo back strong signals that enhance echocardiogram imaging. They are indicated for use in suboptimal echocardiograms to opacify the left ventricular chamber and enhance delineation of the left ventricular endocardial border.

Q9958-Q9964

Q9958 High osmolar contrast material, up to 149 mg/ml iodine concentration, per ml

Q9959 High osmolar contrast material, 150-199 mg/ml iodine concentration, per ml

Q9960 High osmolar contrast material, 200-249 mg/ml iodine concentration, per ml

Q9961 High osmolar contrast material, 250-299 mg/ml iodine concentration, per ml

Q9962 High osmolar contrast material, 300-349 mg/ml iodine concentration, per ml

Q9963 High osmolar contrast material, 350-399 mg/ml iodine concentration, per ml

Q9964 High osmolar contrast material, 400 or greater mg/ml iodine concentration, per ml

High osmolar contrast material (HOCM) refers to a water-soluble, iodinated, monomeric, ionic radiology contrast material. Contrast material is the dye physicians use in diagnostic procedures to enable them to visualize abnormalities as clearly as possible so that they can diagnose a patient's illness/disease, locate the point of the abnormality, or determine the extent of disease. HOCM is a type of iodinated radiology contrast media that has a higher concentration of particles contained in solution than low osmolar contrast material at the same iodine concentration. HOCM is supplied in radiological diagnostic procedures when the patient does not have sensitivity to standard high osmolar contrast material or other medical conditions that would preclude the use of the higher particle concentration. HOCM is reported per ml based on the iodine concentration. High osmolar contrast is administered via intravenous push.

Q9965-Q9967

Q9965 Low osmolar contrast material, 100-199 mg/ml iodine concentration, per ml

Q9966 Low osmolar contrast material, 200-299 mg/ml iodine concentration, per ml

Q9967 Low osmolar contrast material, 300-399 mg/ml iodine concentration, per ml

Low osmolar contrast material (LOCM) is a type of iodinated radiology contrast media that has a substantially lower concentration of particles contained in solution than high osmolar contrast material at the same iodine concentration. LOCM is supplied in radiological diagnostic procedures when the patient is known to have sensitivity to standard high osmolar contrast material or when other sensitivities or medical conditions exist that can increase the chances of a reaction in the patient. Contrast material is the dye that physicians use in diagnostic procedures to enable them to visualize the best picture possible and hence help to diagnose a patient's illness/disease, locate the point of the abnormality, or to assist in determining the extent of disease. LOCM is reported per ml based on the iodine concentration.

Q9968

Q9968 Injection, nonradioactive, noncontrast, visualization adjunct (e.g., methylene blue, isosulfan blue), 1 mg

This code represents nonradioactive, noncontrast, visualization enhancing substances that are not represented by other specific HCPCS Level II codes. For example, methylene blue and isosulfan blue are both water-soluble chemicals to stain or mark internal structures. Both may be injected to delineate lymph nodes or to identify the sentinel node in breast cancer.

Q9969

Q9969 Tc-99m from nonhighly enriched uranium source, full cost recovery add-on, per study dose

Modern medical imaging frequently employs the use of radioisotopes, which are widely used in cardiac imaging predominantly for the elderly (Medicare) population. The radioisotope used in the majority of such diagnostic imaging services is Technetium-99 (Tc-99m). This radioisotope is currently produced in legacy reactors outside of the U.S. using highly enriched uranium (HEU). Molybdenum-99 (Mo-99) may be used to manufacture technetium-99m generators. Report Molybdenum-99 for Tc-99m from non-highly enriched uranium source, full cost recovery add-on, per study dose. Any dose of Tc-99m that can be traced to a Mo-99 supply containing no more than 5 percent HEU sourced Mo-99 shall be considered to be completely derived from non-HEU sources for the purposes of payment, and any compliance practices that support it. To put it another way, a product identified as non-HEU sourced must be at least 95 percent derived from non-HEU sources.

Q9982-Q9983

Q9982 Flutemetamol F18, diagnostic, per study dose, up to 5 mCi

Q9983 Florbetaben F18, diagnostic, per study dose, up to 8.1 mCi

Flutemetamol F18 and Florbetaben F18 are diagnostic radiopharmaceuticals used with PET scans of the brain that bind with $\hat{I}^2$-amyloid aggregates. These radiopharmaceuticals use fluorine (F-18) that decays by positron ($\hat{I}^2$+) emission and has a half-life of 109.77 minutes. The uptake of the radiopharmaceuticals can be used to estimate $\hat{I}^2$-amyloid neuritic plaques in adult patients with cognitive impairment. These radiopharmaceuticals are used to confirm the presence of amyloid, but cannot establish a diagnosis of Alzheimer's disease or other cognitive disorders or predict development of dementia or other neurologic conditions. The recommended dosage for Flutemetamol F18 is 185 MBq (5 mCi in a maximum 10 ML volume) given in a single intravenous injection within 40 seconds. The recommended dosage for Florbetaben F18 is 300 MBq (8.1 mCi in a maximum 10 ML volume), given in a single, slow intravenous push.

Q9991-Q9992

Q9991 Injection, buprenorphine extended-release (Sublocade), less than or equal to 100 mg

Q9992 Injection, buprenorphine extended-release (Sublocade), greater than 100 mg

Buprenorphine extended release is a partial opioid antagonist for the treatment of adult patients with moderate to severe opioid dependence. It is a Schedule III narcotic under the Controlled Substances Act. Because of the Drug Abuse Treatment Act, it can only be prescribed and administered by providers meeting qualifying requirements who have notified the Secretary of Health and Human Services (HHS) of their intent to prescribe it for opioid dependence treatment. Those providers must have a unique identification number to be included on every prescription. Buprenorphine extended release should be used in conjunction with a complete treatment program that includes patient counseling and psychosocial support. The patient must have first begun treatment with induction and dose adjustment of a transmucosal (sublingual tablet or buccal film) buprenorphine-containing product. After a minimum of seven days, the patient may then be transitioned to monthly injections of buprenorphine extended release. The drug is administered monthly by subcutaneous injection, by a health care provider, to the abdominal area. The recommended dosage is two monthly doses of 300 mg each, followed by 100 mg monthly maintenance doses, with a minimum of 26 days between doses. It is supplied in a prefilled syringe with a 19 gauge 5/8-inch needle. Caution should be used in patients who are also taking CYP3A4 inhibitors and inducers or serotonergic drugs.

R

R0070-R0076

R0070 Transportation of portable x-ray equipment and personnel to home or nursing home, per trip to facility or location, one patient seen

R0075 Transportation of portable x-ray equipment and personnel to home or nursing home, per trip to facility or location, more than one patient seen

R0076 Transportation of portable EKG to facility or location, per patient

These HCPCS Level II codes represent the charge for transporting portable equipment and personnel to a site to provide diagnostic imaging services or record an electrocardiogram. Payers will sometimes reimburse these additional charges. These codes should be reported conjunction with the CPT radiology codes (70000 series) and only when the x-ray equipment used was actually transported to the location where the image was taken. These codes would not apply to x-ray equipment or an electrocardiograph stored in the location where the service was performed.

S

S0012

S0012 Butorphanol tartrate, nasal spray, 25 mg

Butorphanol tartrate nasal spray is a schedule IV controlled substance. It is a synthetic opioid analgesic used for the management of moderate to severe pain. The most common indication is in the management of migraines. Although the action of the drug is not known, it binds with opiate receptors in the central nervous system and alters not only the perception of pain, but the emotional response as well.

S0013

S0013 Esketamine, nasal spray, 1 mg

Esketamine nasal spray is an N-methyl D-aspartate (NMDA) receptor antagonist. It is indicated for use in conjunction with an oral antidepressant for treatment-resistant depression (TRD) in adults. TRD is defined as a major depressive disorder (MDD) in adults who have not responded adequately to at least two different antidepressants of adequate dose and duration in the current depressive episode. This code reports 1 mg.

S0014

S0014 Tacrine HCl, 10 mg

Tacrine hydrochloride is a reversible cholinesterase inhibitor. Cholinesterase is an enzyme that catalyzes the breakdown of acetylcholine, a neurotransmitter. Early changes in the brain of Alzheimer's patients result in a deficiency of acetylcholine. This deficiency is thought to account for some of the mild to moderate dementia characteristic of Alzheimer's disease. Tacrine hydrochloride inhibits the breakdown of and increases the concentration of acetylcholine in the cerebral cortex. The drug is indicated as a treatment for mild to moderate dementia of Alzheimer's disease. Tacrine hydrochloride is self-administered orally in dosages ranging from 10 to 40 mg four times a day.

S0017

S0017 Injection, aminocaproic acid, 5 g

Aminocaproic acid is an amino acid that inhibits fibrinolysis. After long-term use, this medication distributes throughout extravascular and intravascular compartments of the body, penetrating red blood cells and other tissue cells. It is used to treat fibrinolytic bleeding that may frequently be associated with surgical complications following heart surgery and portacaval shunt, hematological disorders such as aplastic anemia, abruptio placentae, hepatic cirrhosis, and neoplastic diseases such as carcinoma of the prostate, lung, stomach, and cervix. It may also be used to treat urinary fibrinolysis associated with complications following severe trauma, anoxia, shock, complications following prostatectomy, nephrectomy, or nonsurgical hematuria accompanying polycystic or neoplastic diseases of the genitourinary system. Aminocaproic acid can be administered via intravenous infusion or orally.

S0020

S0020 Injection, bupivicaine HCl, 30 ml

Bupivacaine hydrochloride (HCl) is a local anesthetic that blocks the feeling of pain by inhibiting the conduction of nerve impulses. The order of loss of nerve function is pain, temperature, touch, proprioception, and skeletal muscle tone. It is often used for dental procedures and during labor and delivery. Bupivacaine can be administered by infiltration, caudal injection, lumbar epidural injection, peripheral nerve block, retrobulbar block, or sympathetic block. Bupivacaine is not recommended for intravenous or regional anesthesia (Bier Block).

S0021

S0021 Injection, cefoperazone sodium, 1 g

Cefoperazone sodium is a broad spectrum antibiotic. It is used to treat respiratory tract infections, skin infections, and urinary tract infections. Susceptible bacteria include *S. pneumoniae, H. influenzae, S. aureus, S. pyogenes, P. aeruginosa, Klebsiella pneumoniae, E. coli, Proteus mirabilis, Enterobacter* species; anaerobic gram-negative bacilli, *Pseudomonas aeruginosa, Klebsiella, Clostridium*; anaerobic gram-positive cocci, *N. gonorrhoeae* , and *S. epidermidis*. The usual dose is two to four grams per day administered at 12-hour intervals in equally divided doses. Cefoperazone is administered via intramuscular injection or intravenous infusion.

S0023

S0023 Injection, cimetidine HCl, 300 mg

Cimetidine is a histamine H2 receptor antagonist that inhibits the action of histamine at the histamine H2 receptors of the parietal cells. It inhibits gastric acid secretions. It is used in treatment and maintenance therapy for duodenal ulcers, short-term treatment of gastric ulcers, gastroesophageal reflux disease (GERD), prevention of upper gastrointestinal bleeding in critically ill patients, and for the treatment of pathological hypersecretory conditions (i.e., Zollinger-Ellison syndrome, systemic mastocytosis, multiple endocrine adenomas).

S0028

S0028 Injection, famotidine, 20 mg

Famotidine is a histamine H2 receptor antagonist that inhibits the action of histamine at the histamine H2 receptors of the parietal cells. It inhibits gastric acid secretions. It is used for treatment and maintenance therapy for duodenal ulcers, short-term treatment of gastric ulcers, gastroesophageal reflux disease (GERD), prevention of upper gastrointestinal bleeding in critically ill patients, and for the treatment of pathological hypersecretory conditions (i.e., Zollinger-Ellison syndrome, systemic mastocytosis, multiple endocrine adenomas). Famotidine can be administered orally and via intravenous infusion.

S0030

S0030 Injection, metronidazole, 500 mg

Metronidazole is an antibacterial and antiprotozoal. It is thought to work in an anaerobic environment by entering the organism and being reduced by intracellular electron transport proteins. Because of this alteration to the metronidazole molecule, a concentration gradient is maintained that promotes the drug's intracellular transport. Presumably, free radicals are formed that, in turn, react with cellular components, resulting in the death of the microorganism. Metronidazole is effective against the following bacteria and protozoa: *Clostridium* species, *Eubacterium* species, *Peptococcus niger*, *Peptostreptococcus* species, *Bacteroides fragilis* group (*B. fragilis*, *B. distasonis*, *B. ovatus*, B. *thetaiotaomicron*, *B. vulgatus*), *Fusobacterium* species, *Entamoeba histolytica*, and *Trichomonas vaginalis*. Metronidazole is used to treat symptomatic trichomoniasis; asymptomatic trichomoniasis, when the organism is associated with endocervicitis, cervicitis, or cervical erosion; asymptomatic consorts; *T. vaginalis* infection; acute intestinal amebiasis (amebic dysentery) and amebic liver abscess; serious infections caused by susceptible anaerobic bacteria, peritonitis, intra-abdominal abscess, and liver abscess; skin infections; inflammatory lesions of rosacea; endometritis; endomyometritis; tubo-ovarian abscess and postsurgical vaginal cuff infection; bacterial septicemia; bone and joint infections; meningitis and brain abscess; pneumonia; empyema; lung abscess; and endocarditis. Metronidazole can be administered topically, orally, or via intravenous infusion. The loading dose is 15 mg/kg of body weight or about 1 gram infused over one hour. Following that, 500 mg is infused over one hour and administered every six hours.

S0032

S0032 Injection, nafcillin sodium, 2 g

Nafcillin sodium is a semisynthetic antibiotic substance derived from 6-amino-penicillanic acid. This is a penicillinase-resistant penicillin and is used to treat infections caused by penicillinase-producing staphylococci that have shown to be susceptible to the drug. The drug can be administered orally or via intramuscular injection, intravenous push, or intravenous infusion.

S0034

S0034 Injection, ofloxacin, 400 mg

Ofloxacin is a broad spectrum antibiotic of the quinolone class. It inhibits the DNA enzymes in bacteria that are required for the DNA to replicate. This drug is chemically different from aminoglycosides, macrolides, and beta-lactam antibiotics, including penicillins, and therefore may be used to treat bacteria resistant to these antibacterials. Ofloxacin is effective against the following bacteria: *Staphylococcus aureus* (methicillin-susceptible strains), *Staphylococcus epidermidis, Enterobacter cloacae, Streptococcus pneumoniae* (penicillin-susceptible strains), *Streptococcus pyogenes, Citrobacter (diversus) koseri, Enterobacter aerogenes, Propionibacterium acnes, Escherichia coli, Haemophilus influenzae, Serratia marcescens, Proteus mirabilis, Klebsiella pneumoniae, Neisseria gonorrhoeae, Proteus mirabilis, Chlamydia trachomatis, Gardnerella vaginalis, Legionella pneumophila, Mycoplasma hominis, Mycoplasma pneumonia, Ureaplasma urealyticum*, and *Pseudomonas aeruginosa*. Some strains of *Pseudomonas aeruginosa* may quickly develop a resistance to ofloxacin during treatment. It is used to treat acute bacterial exacerbations of chronic bronchitis, community-acquired pneumonia, uncomplicated skin infections, conjunctivitis, corneal ulcers, acute uncomplicated urethral and cervical gonorrhea, nongonococcal urethritis and cervicitis, mixed infections of the urethra and cervix, acute pelvic inflammatory disease, uncomplicated cystitis, complicated urinary tract infections, and prostatitis. Ofloxacin can be administered orally, by ophthalmic drops, and via slow intravenous infusion over 60 minutes. It should not be administered via intramuscular injection, subcutaneous injection, or intravenous push.

S0039

S0039 Injection, sulfamethoxazole and trimethoprim, 10 ml

Sulfamethoxazole and trimethoprim is an antibiotic that blocks two necessary steps in the biosynthesis of nucleic acids and proteins that are critical to many

S

bacteria. It is effective against the following bacteria: *Streptococcus pneumoniae, Haemophilus influenzae, Shigella flexneri, Shigella sonnei, Escherichia coli, Klebsiella* species, *Enterobacter* species, *Morganella morganii, Proteus mirabilis*, and *Proteus vulgaris*. Sulfamethoxazole and trimethoprim is indicated in the treatment of *Pneumocystis carinii* pneumonia, enteritis, urinary tract infections, acute otitis media, acute exacerbations of chronic bronchitis, traveler's diarrhea, and for prophylaxis against *Pneumocystis jirovecii* pneumonia in individuals who are immunosuppressed and considered to be at an increased risk of developing *Pneumocystis carinii* pneumonia. Sulfamethoxazole and trimethoprim is administered orally or via intravenous infusion over 60 to 90 minutes. This drug should not be given via rapid intravenous infusion or by intramuscular injection.

S0040

S0040 Injection, ticarcillin disodium and clavulanate potassium, 3.1 g

Ticarcillin disodium and clavulanate is a combination drug consisting of a semisynthetic form of penicillin and clavulanate. Penicillins block the actions of transpeptidase, an enzyme needed to create the cell wall. This weakens the bacterial cell wall causing cellular death. Many bacteria have developed a resistance to penicillin. Resistant bacteria produce an enzyme, penicillinase or beta-lactamase, that protects it from the effects of penicillin. Clavulanic acid or clavulanate binds to the penicillinase and inhibits it from blocking the actions of penicillin. Ticarcillin disodium is indicated for the treatment of infections with susceptible anaerobic, gram-negative, and positive bacteria. Specific conditions and susceptible bacteria include septicemia/bacteremia caused by *Staphylococcus aureus, Escherichia coli, Pseudomonas aeruginosa*, and other *Pseudomonas* species; lower respiratory infections caused by *Staphylococcus aureus, haemophilus influenza, Klebsiella* species; bone and joint infections caused by *Staphylococcus aureus;* skin and skin-structure infections caused by *Staphylococcus aureus, Escherichia coli, Klebsiella* species; urinary tract infections caused by *Escherichia coli, Klebsiella* species, *Pseudomonas aeruginosa* and other *Pseudomonas* species, *Citrobacter* species, *Enterobacter cloacae, Staphylococcus aureus, Serratia marcescens*; gynecological infections caused by *Prevotella melaninogenicus, Enterobacter* species, *Escherichia coli, Klebsiella pneumoniae, Staphylococcus aureus, Staphylococcus epidermidis*; and intra-abdominal infections caused by *Escherichia coli, Klebsiella pneumoniae*, and *Bacteroides fragilis*. The drug is administered via an intravenous infusion.

S0073

S0073 Injection, aztreonam, 500 mg

Aztreonam is a synthetic bactericidal antibiotic originally isolated from chromobacterium violaceum. Aztreonam is effective against gram-negative organisms. Susceptibility studies should be performed prior to the administration of this drug. Susceptible organisms include *Escherichia coli, Klebsiella pneumoniae, Klebsiella oxytoca, Proteus mirabilis, Pseudomonas aeruginosa, Enterobacter* species including *E. cloacae, Citrobacter* species, including *C. freundii, Serratia* species including *S. marcescens*, and *Haemophilus influenzae*.

S0074

S0074 Injection, cefotetan disodium, 500 mg

Cefotetan disodium is an antibiotic that inhibits the cell wall synthesis in bacteria. It is effective against the following bacteria: *Escherichia coli, Haemophilus influenzae, Klebsiella* species, *Morganella morganii, Neisseria gonorrhoeae, Proteus mirabilis, Proteus vulgaris, Providencia rettgeri, Serratia marcescens, Staphylococcus aureus, Staphylococcus epidermidis, Streptococcus agalactiae, Streptococcus pneumoniae, Streptococcus pyogenes, Prevotella bivia, Prevotella disiens, Bacteroides fragilis, Prevotella melaninogenica, Bacteroides vulgatus, Fusobacterium* species, Gram-positive bacilli, *Peptococcus niger*, and *Peptostreptococcus* species. Cefotetan is indicated in the treatment of urinary tract infections, lower respiratory infections, skin infections, gynecological infections, intra-abdominal infections, bone and joint infections, and may be used as a preventive treatment prior to surgery. This drug can be administered via intramuscular injection, intravenous push, or intravenous infusion, usually less than one hour.

S0077

S0077 Injection, clindamycin phosphate, 300 mg

Clindamycin phosphate is an antibiotic used to treat serious, susceptible strains of streptococci, pneumococci, and staphylococci infections. It is used for patients who are allergic to penicillin or for whom penicillin treatment is inappropriate. It is effective against the following bacteria: *Staphylococcus aureus, Staphylococcus epidermidis, Streptococci* (except *Enterococcus faecalis*), *Pneumococci, Bacteroides* species (including *Bacteroides fragilis* group and *Bacteroides melaninogenicus* group), *Fusobacterium* species, *Propionibacterium, Eubacterium, Actinomyces* species, *Peptococcus* species, *Peptostreptococcus* species, *Microaerophilic streptococci*, and *Clostridium perfringens*. The injectable form is administered by intramuscular or intravenous injection followed by an intravenous infusion over 30 minutes. The usual dose is 600 to 1,200 mg per day in two, three, or four equal doses or for more severe infections 1,200 to 2,700 mg per day in two, three, or four equal doses.

S0078

S0078 Injection, fosphenytoin sodium, 750 mg

Fosphenytoin is a prodrug that is converted within the body to the anticonvulsant phenytoin. It is indicated for short-term (five days or less) treatment of status epilepticus, the prevention or control of seizures during neurosurgery, and for short-term parenteral administration when other means of phenytoin administration are unavailable, inappropriate, or less advantageous. It is thought to alter the sodium channels and block the calcium flow across the neuronal membranes, modulate the voltage-dependent calcium channels of neurons, and enhance the sodium-potassium ATPase activity of neurons and glial cells. Fosphenytoin may be administered by intravenous or intramuscular injection or intravenous infusion.

S0080

S0080 Injection, pentamidine isethionate, 300 mg

Pentamidine isethionate is an aromatic diamidine that is an antimicrobial. Its mechanism of action is not completely known. It is thought that the drug interferes with the synthesis of DNA, RNA, and protein causing cell death. Pentamidine isethionate is indicated as a treatment for *Pneumocystis jirovecii* (previously classified as *P. carinii*), trypanosomiasis, and leishmaniasis. The drug may be administered by intramuscular injection, inhalation, or intravenous infusion over one hour. Dosage is usually 300 mg.

S0081

S0081 Injection, piperacillin sodium, 500 mg

Piperacillin is a broad-spectrum antibiotic that works by inhibiting septum and cell wall synthesis in bacteria. It is effective against the following bacteria: Enterococci, including *Enterococcus faecalis, Streptococcus pneumoniae, Streptococcus pyogenes, Acinetobacter* species, *Enterobacter* species, *Escherichia coli, Haemophilus influenzae* (non-lactamase-producing strains), *Klebsiella* species, *Morganella morganii, Neisseria gonorrhoeae, Proteus mirabilis, Proteus vulgaris, Providencia rettgeri, Pseudomonas aeruginosa, Serratia* species, *Anaerobic cocci, Clostridium* species, *Bacteroides* species including *Bacteroides fragilis, Streptococcus agalactiae, Streptococcus bovis, Viridans* group streptococci, *Burkholderia cepacia, Citrobacter diversus, Citrobacter freundii, Pseudomonas fluorescens, Stenotrophomonas maltophilia, Yersinia enterocolitica, Actinomyces species, Eubacterium species, Fusobacterium necrophorum, Fusobacterium nucleatum, Porphyromonas asaccharolytica, Prevotella melaninogenica, and Veillonella* species. Piperacillin is indicated in the treatment of intraabdominal infections including hepatobiliary and surgical infections, urinary tract infections, endometritis, pelvic inflammatory disease, pelvic cellulitis, septicemia, lower respiratory tract infections, skin infections, bone and joint infections, uncomplicated gonococcal urethritis, and may be used as a preventive treatment prior to surgery. It is also effective for treatment of mixed infections and is used to treat infections prior to identification. Piperacillin can be administered via intramuscular injection, intravenous push, or intravenous infusion over 30 minutes. The maximum intramuscular dose is two grams per injection site.

S0088

S0088 Imatinib, 100 mg

Imatinib is an antineoplastic drug that inhibits the bcr-abl tyrosine kinase, the constitutive abnormal tyrosine kinase created by the Philadelphia chromosome abnormality in chronic myeloid leukemia (CML). It inhibits production and induces apoptosis in bcr-abl positive cell lines, as well as fresh leukemic cells from Philadelphia chromosome positive CML. It is also an inhibitor of the receptor tyrosine kinases for platelet-derived growth factor (PDGF) and stem cell factor (SCF), c-kit, and inhibits PDGF- and SCF-mediated cellular events. It is used to treat adults with newly diagnosed Philadelphia chromosome positive chronic myeloid leukemia in chronic phase. It is also indicated for the treatment of patients with Philadelphia chromosome (CML) in blast crisis, accelerated phase, or in chronic phase after failure of interferon-alpha therapy and patients with Kit (CD117) positive unresectable and/or metastatic malignant gastrointestinal stromal tumors (GIST). Imatinib can be used for children with pH + chronic phase CML whose disease has recurred after stem cell transplant or who are resistant to interferon-alpha therapy. The adult dose is 400 to 800 mg per day.

S0090

S0090 Sildenafil citrate, 25 mg

Sildenafil citrate is a selective inhibitor of an enzyme that controls cyclic guanosine monophosphate. The drug is used to treat erectile dysfunction. Penile erection is a hemodynamic process that involves the release of nitric acid by the corpus cavernosum during sexual stimulation. The nitric acid activates the enzyme cyclic guanosine monophosphate, which produces smooth muscle relaxation in the corpus cavernosum and allows the inflow of blood. Another enzyme, phosphodiesterase type 5, controls the tissue concentration of the cyclic guanosine monophosphate. Sildenafil citrate inhibits the neutralizing effect of the phosphodiesterase type 5. Since the local release of nitric acid is initiated by sexual stimulation and the erectile process is catalyzed by nitric acid, this drug has no effect in the absence of sexual stimulation. The drug is self-administered orally in dosages ranging from 25 to 100 mg. The drug may be taken at anywhere from one-half hour to four hours prior to sexual activity.

S0091

S0091 Granisetron HCl, 1 mg (for circumstances falling under the Medicare statute, use Q0166)

Granisetron hydrochloride is a chemical compound that is a selective blocker of serotonin 5-HT3 receptors. It is an antiemetic drug available in oral and injectable forms. Serotonin 5-HT3 receptors are present on the vagal nerve and at sensory nerve endings. Cytotoxic chemotherapy appears to trigger the release of serotonin in the small intestine, which may trigger the 5-HT3 receptors and initiate the vomiting reflex.

S0092

S0092 Injection, hydromorphone HCl, 250 mg (loading dose for infusion pump)

Hydromorphone is a narcotic and opioid analgesic classified as a schedule II controlled substance. This drug binds to opiate nerve center receptors and alters the human pain response, as well as suppressing the cough reflex. It is available in oral and injectable forms. The injectable form can be administered by intramuscular, subcutaneous, and intravenous injection, or by intravenous infusion. Hydromorphone hydrochloride is indicated for the relief of moderate to severe pain.

S0093

S0093 Injection, morphine sulfate, 500 mg (loading dose for infusion pump)

Morphine is an opioid. It acts upon specific receptors in the brain and spinal cord to decrease the feeling of pain and to reduce the emotional response to pain. An implantable infusion pump is considered medically necessary when used to administer opioid drugs (e.g., morphine) and/or clonidine intrathecally or epidurally for treating severe chronic intractable pain in persons who have proven unresponsive to less invasive medical therapy as determined by the following criteria: a) previous medical history that patient has not responded adequately to noninvasive methods of pain control, such as systemic opioids (including attempts to eliminate physical and behavioral abnormalities that may cause an exaggerated reaction to pain); and b) a preliminary trial of intraspinal opioid drug administration undertaken with a temporary intrathecal/epidural catheter to substantiate adequately acceptable pain relief, the degree of side-effects (including effects on the activities of daily living), and acceptance.

S0104

S0104 Zidovudine, oral, 100 mg

Zidovudine (formerly called azidothymidine or AZT) is a synthetic nucleoside analogue used as an antiviral for the treatment of human immunodeficiency virus (HIV) infection and to prevent maternal-fetal transmission of HIV. Zidovudine incorporates itself into the DNA chain preventing elongation and stopping DNA growth. Zidovudine can be administered via intravenous infusion over one hour or orally.

S0106

S0106 Bupropion HCl sustained release tablet, 150 mg, per bottle of 60 tablets

Bupropion hydrochloride is a chemical that is used to treat major depressive disorders and as an aid to smoking cessation. The drug is a weak inhibitor of neuronal uptake of norepinephrine and dopamine. It does not inhibit monoamine oxidase or the reuptake of serotonin. The exact course of action is unknown. Bupropion hydrochloride is tablet form only.

S0108

S0108 Mercaptopurine, oral, 50 mg

Mercaptopurine is a potent chemotherapeutic drug belonging to a class of drugs known as antimetabolites. Antimetabolites resemble nutrients required for cancer cell growth. The cancer cells take up mercaptopurine, which interfere with cancer cell nucleic acid biosynthesis. Specifically, mercaptopurine inhibits the first enzyme unique to the de novo pathway for purine ribonucleotide synthesis. It is not known exactly which of the biochemical effects of mercaptopurine is responsible for cell death. Mercaptopurine is used to treat acute lymphatic and acute myelogenous leukemia. It has also been shown to be effective in the treatment of some chronic myelogenous leukemias and some acute undifferentiated leukemias. Efficacy depends on the particular subclassification of the leukemia. Mercaptopurine may be used in combination with other chemotherapy drugs as an initial treatment to induce remission. It may also be used as maintenance therapy for lymphatic (lymphocytic, lymphoblastic) leukemia. The induction dose varies; however, the usual dose for both children and adults is 2.5 mg/kg of body weight. The maintenance dose is 1.5 to 2.5 mg/kg per day once the patient is in remission. This medication is administered orally.

S0109

S0109 Methadone, oral, 5 mg

Methadone is a synthetic opioid analgesic that has effects similar to those of morphine and heroin. It is a schedule II controlled substance. Methadone is indicated for the treatment of severe pain and also as a substitute drug in the detoxification of heroin dependence. It is available in injectable and self-administrable oral forms. Generally speaking, injections and tablets are administered as pain treatment and the oral solution or dissolved tablets administered as part of a detoxification program. Dosages for pain management vary depending upon the severity of the pain and the response.

S0117

S0117 Tretinoin, topical, 5 g

Tretinoin is a retinoid compound that is a metabolite of vitamin A used as an acne treatment. The exact mode of action of tretinoin is not known, but current evidence suggests that topical application decreases the cohesiveness of follicular epithelial cells, which decreases the formation of comedones and stimulates mitotic activity increasing the production of new cells.

S0119

S0119 Ondansetron, oral, 4 mg (for circumstances falling under the Medicare statute, use HCPCS Q code)

Ondansetron hydrochloride is a chemical compound that is a selective blocker of serotonin 5-HT3 receptors. It is an antiemetic drug available in oral and injectable forms. Serotonin 5-HT3 receptors are present on the vagal nerve and at sensory nerve endings. Cytotoxic chemotherapy appears to trigger the release of serotonin in the small intestine, which may trigger the 5-HT3 receptors and initiate the vomiting reflex. Ondansetron hydrochloride is indicated for the prevention of nausea and vomiting associated with surgery and antineoplastic drugs. The oral version is also indicated for the prevention of nausea and vomiting associated with radiation therapy. The drug is available in oral and injectable versions. The recommended dose is 4 mg or 0.1 mg/kg of body weight administered by intravenous or intramuscular injection. Dosages for the oral version vary from 8 to 24 mg depending on the indication and patient.

S0122

S0122 Injection, menotropins, 75 IU

Menotropins is a purified preparation of gonadotropins extracted from the urine of postmenopausal women. It contains follicle-stimulating hormone (FSH) activity and luteinizing hormone (LH) activity. Menotropins is used to treat infertility in women. The medication is administered for seven to 12 days to stimulate follicular growth in women who do not have primary ovarian failure. Menotropins treatment results in follicular growth and maturation. An additional drug has to be given to induce ovulation. Menotropins is administered by subcutaneous or intramuscular injection.

S0126

S0126 Injection, follitropin alfa, 75 IU

Follitropin alfa contains a human follicle stimulating hormone (FSH) preparation of recombinant DNA origin. FSH, the active component of follitropin alfa, is responsible for follicular growth, maturation, and gonadal steroid production. It is found in genetically modified Chinese hamster ovary (CHO) cells cultured in bioreactors. Follitropin alfa contains no luteinizing hormone (LH) activity. Based on available data derived from physicochemical tests and bioassays, follitropin alfa and follitropin beta are indistinguishable. Follitropin is used to treat infertility in women and to induce spermatogenesis in men with hypogonadotropic hypogonadism. Follitropin alfa stimulates ovarian follicular growth in women who do not have primary ovarian failure. In order to continue the final phase of follicle maturation, resumption of meiosis, and rupture of the follicle in the absence of an endogenous LH surge, human chorionic gonadotropin (hCG) must be given following the administration of follitropin when patient monitoring indicates that appropriate follicular development has occurred. Follitropin alfa is administered with hCG to men with hypogonadotropic hypogonadism to stimulate spermatogenesis. FSH is the primary hormone responsible for spermatogenesis. Follitropin alfa can be administered via subcutaneous injection.

S0128

S0128 Injection, follitropin beta, 75 IU

Follitropin beta contains a human follicle stimulating hormone (FSH) preparation of recombinant DNA origin. FSH, the active component of follitropin alfa, is responsible for follicular growth, maturation, and gonadal steroid production. It is found in genetically modified Chinese hamster ovary (CHO) cells cultured in bioreactors. Follitropin beta has a dimeric structure containing two glycoprotein subunits (alpha and beta). Follitropin beta contains no luteinizing hormone (LH) activity. Based on available data derived from physicochemical tests and bioassays, follitropin alfa and follitropin beta are indistinguishable. Follitropin is used to treat infertility in women and to induce spermatogenesis in men with hypogonadotropic hypogonadism. Follitropin alfa stimulates ovarian follicular growth in women who do not have primary ovarian failure. In order to continue the final phase of follicle maturation, resumption of meiosis, and rupture of the follicle in the absence of an endogenous LH surge, human chorionic gonadotropin (hCG) must be given following the administration of follitropin when patient monitoring indicates that appropriate follicular development has occurred. Follitropin alfa is administered with hCG to men with hypogonadotropic hypogonadism to stimulate spermatogenesis. FSH is the primary hormone responsible for spermatogenesis. Follitropin beta can be administered via subcutaneous or intramuscular injection for women and only by subcutaneous injection for men.

S0132

S0132 Injection, ganirelix acetate, 250 mcg

Ganirelix acetate is a synthetic decapeptide with high antagonistic activity against naturally occurring gonadotropin-releasing hormone (GnRH). The pulsatile release of GnRH stimulates the synthesis and secretion of luteinizing hormone (LH) and follicle-stimulating hormone (FSH). The large increase of GnRH at mid-cycle results in an LH surge. This results in ovulation, resumption of meiosis in the oocyte, and luteinization. Ganirelix is given to women undergoing fertility treatment to prevent the eggs from being released prematurely. The usual dose is 250 micrograms once a day. It is administered via subcutaneous injection during the mid to late portion of the follicular phase.

S0136

S0136 Clozapine, 25 mg

Clozapine is an atypical antipsychotic medication used to treat severely ill schizophrenic patients who do not respond effectively to standard drug treatment. It is considered an atypical antipsychotic medication because its profile of binding to dopamine receptors and its effects on various dopamine-mediated behaviors differ from those exhibited by more typical antipsychotic drug products. Specifically, although it does interfere with the binding of dopamine at D1,

D2, D3, and D5 receptors and has a high affinity for the D4 receptor, it does not induce catalepsy nor inhibit apomorphine-induced stereotypy. It is a tricyclic dibenzodiazepine derivative. Doses can vary from 600 to 900 mg a day. Patients are started on small doses and the amount is gradually increased to obtain a therapeutic dose. Clozapine is administered orally.

S0137

S0137 Didanosine (ddI), 25 mg

Didanosine (ddI) is an antiviral used in combination with other drugs to treat human immunodeficiency virus (HIV). It is a synthetic nucleoside analogue of the naturally occurring nucleoside deoxyadenosine in which the 3-hydroxyl group is replaced by hydrogen. In the cell, didanosine is converted by cellular enzymes to, the active metabolite, dideoxyadenosine 5'- triphosphate, which inhibits the activity of HIV-1 reverse transcriptase both by competing with the natural substrate, deoxyadenosine 5'-triphosphate, and by its incorporation into viral DNA. This causes failure of viral DNA chain elongation. The usual dose is 400 mg for patients weighing > 60 kg and 250 mg for patients weighing < 60 kg. Didanosine is administered orally and should be taken on an empty stomach.

S0138

S0138 Finasteride, 5 mg

Finasteride is a synthetic compound that is a specific inhibitor of an intracellular steroidal enzyme that converts androgen testosterone into dihydrotestosterone (DHT). Development and enlargement of the prostate gland is dependent upon DHT. Finasteride is indicated as a treatment for symptomatic benign prostatic hypertrophy and androgenic alopecia or male pattern baldness. The drug is available in oral form only with a usual dose of 5 mg for treatment of benign prostatic hypertrophy with 1 mg doses used for treatment of hair loss.

S0139

S0139 Minoxidil, 10 mg

Minoxidil is a peripheral vasodilator used to treat hypertension by decreasing peripheral vascular resistance. It is usually used on patients who do not respond adequately to maximum doses of other hypertensive medications and diuretics. It is usually given in conjunction with beta-blockers and diuretics. The recommended dose for adults older than age 12 is 5 mg a day but can be increased to a maximum of 100 mg a day. The recommended dose for children age 12 and younger is 0.2 mg per kg with a maximum dose of 50 mg per day. Minoxidil used in the treatment of hypertension is administered orally. Minoxidil is also available in topical form. The topical form is used as a hair restorer for men and women with certain types of hair loss.

S0140

S0140 Saquinavir, 200 mg

Saquinavir is a chemical complex that is an HIV protease inhibitor. HIV protease is an enzyme required for replication of the HIV virus. Saquinavir binds to the protease active site and inhibits the activity of the enzyme, which prevents cleavage of the virus polypeptides and results in the formation of immature noninfectious virus particles. Saquinavir in combination with ritonavir and other antiretroviral agents is indicated for the treatment of HIV infection. Saquinavir is administered orally and is available in 200 and 500 mg capsules. The recommended dose of saquinavir is 1,000 mg per day to be used in combination with ritonavir and other antiretroviral agents.

S0142

S0142 Colistimethate sodium, inhalation solution administered through DME, concentrated form, per mg

Colistimethate sodium is an antibiotic produced by certain strains of *Bacillus polymyxa*. Colistimethate sodium is anionic and is readily hydrolyzed to a variety of methanesulfonate derivatives. Colistimethate sodium is indicated as a treatment for *Pseudomonas aeruginosa* infections in cystic fibrosis patients, and it has come into recent use for treating multidrug-resistant *Acinetobacter* infection, but resistant forms have been reported. Colistimethate sodium powder for inhalation is administered twice daily for as long as a physician thinks beneficial. Extemporaneously prepared solutions for nebulization should be used promptly after being prepared.

S0145

S0145 Injection, PEGylated interferon alfa-2A, 180 mcg per ml

Interferon alfa-2a pegylated is a covalent conjugate of interferon alfa-2a recombinant. It is a drug that uses a genetically engineered *Escherichia coli* bacterium containing DNA that codes for the human protein. In the pegylated form, a special strand (commonly called a PEG) is attached to the interferon molecule that helps to protect the interferon from being destroyed by the immune system. Interferon alfa-2a pegylated is used to treat chronic hepatitis C with compensated liver disease and HBeAg positive and HBeAg negative chronic hepatitis B with evidence of viral replication and liver inflammation. The recommended dose is 180 micrograms once a week. Interferon alfa-2a is administered via subcutaneous injection.

S0148

S0148 Injection, PEGylated interferon alfa-2B, 10 mcg

Interferon alfa-2b pegylated is a covalent conjugate of interferon alfa-2b recombinant. It is a drug that uses a genetically engineered *Escherichia coli* bacterium containing DNA that codes for the human protein. In the pegylated form, a special strand (commonly called a PEG) is attached to the interferon molecule that helps protect the interferon from being destroyed by the immune system. Interferon alfa-2b is used to treat chronic hepatitis C with compensated liver disease. The recommended dose is 1 microgram per kg on the same day each week for one year. Interferon alfa-2b is administered via subcutaneous injection.

S0155

S0155 Sterile dilutant for epoprostenol, 50 ml

Epoprostenol is a prostaglandin that acts as a direct vasodilator of pulmonary and systemic arteries and an inhibitor of platelet aggregation. It is usually administered parenterally through a permanent indwelling central venous catheter as a long-term medication to treat primary pulmonary hypertension and pulmonary hypertension secondary to scleroderma in NYHA Class III and IV patients. Initial administration may be through a peripheral intravenous infusion until a central venous catheter is established. It is manufactured as a powder that must be reconstituted with sterile diluent specific to the epoprostenol. Dosages vary dependent upon body weight and response. Once a regimen of epoprostenol has been established, it should never be stopped suddenly.

S0156

S0156 Exemestane, 25 mg

Exemestane is an irreversible, steroidal aromatase inactivator. It acts as a false substrate to the aromatase enzyme and binds to the active site of this enzyme in postmenopausal women to cause its inactivation. Exemestane lowers the circulating concentration in postmenopausal women. Many breast cancers have estrogen receptors, and growth of these tumors can be stimulated by estrogen. It is used in adjuvant treatment of postmenopausal women with estrogen receptor positive early breast cancer who have received two to three years of tamoxifen and are switched to exemestane to finish a total of five consecutive years of adjuvant hormonal therapy. Exemestane has proven effective for the treatment of advanced breast cancer in postmenopausal women whose disease has progressed following tamoxifen therapy. The recommended dose is 25 mg once per day after a meal. Exemestane is administered orally.

S0157

S0157 Becaplermin gel 0.01%, 0.5 gm

Becaplermin gel is a human platelet-derived growth factor (PDGF), a substance naturally produced by the body, that helps to promote wound healing. Becaplermin is available as a gel that is applied to the skin, usually once per day. The amount of gel applied depends on the size of the ulcer and may be changed every one to two weeks as the ulcer heals. It is supplied in a 15 gram tube. Becaplermin gel is used to treat ulcers of the foot, ankle, or leg in patients with diabetes. When used in combination with standard ulcer care that includes cleaning, pressure relief, and infection control, it works by bringing the cells that the body uses to repair wounds to the site of the ulcer. The gel may cause localized skin rash.

S0160

S0160 Dextroamphetamine sulfate, 5 mg

Dextroamphetamine sulfate is an amphetamine. Amphetamines are noncatecholamine, sympathomimetic amines with central nervous system (CNS) stimulant activity. They elevate blood pressure, stimulate respirations, and are highly addictive. Dextroamphetamine is used to treat narcolepsy and as part of a treatment regimen in attention deficit disorder with hyperactivity in children ages 3 to 6. The recommended dose is 5 to 60 mg per day depending on the patient. Dextroamphetamine is administered orally.

S0164

S0164 Injection, pantoprazole sodium, 40 mg

Pantoprazole sodium is a compound that inhibits gastric secretions. Pantoprazole is a proton pump inhibitor (PPI) that suppresses the final step in gastric acid production by forming a covalent bond to two sites of the ATPase enzyme system at the secretory surface of the gastric parietal cell. This effect is dose-related and leads to inhibition of both basal and stimulated gastric acid secretion irrespective of the stimulus. This binding results in a period of antisecretory effect that persists longer than 24 hours for all doses tested. This drug is indicated for short-term treatment (seven to 10 days) for patients with gastroesophageal reflux disease (GERD) and a history of erosive esophagitis, and the hypersecretory conditions that may be associated with Zollinger-Ellison syndrome or other neoplastic conditions.

S0166

S0166 Injection, olanzapine, 2.5 mg

Olanzapine is a psychotropic agent that belongs to the thienobenzodiazepine class. It is used to treat schizophrenia, acute mixed or manic episodes associated with bipolar disorder, agitation associated with schizophrenia, and bipolar disorder.

S0169

S0169 Calcitrol, 0.25 mcg

Calcitrol is a form of cholecalciferol that is a parathyroid-like hormone. It increases the ability of the body to absorb vitamin D and to distribute calcium throughout the body. It is indicated for the treatment of hypocalcemia, hypophosphatemia, rickets, osteodystrophy associated with long-term dialysis, and such disorders as hypoparathyroidism and pseudo-hypoparathyroidism. It is available in oral and injectable forms. The injectable form is administered by intravenous injection. Dosages vary from 0.25 to 3 mcg depending upon the form and indication.

S0170

S0170 Anastrozole, oral, 1 mg

Anastrozole is a nonsteroidal aromatase inhibitor. Anastrozole is converted to estrone in adipose tissue of the breast. The estrone is further converted to estradiol, which is the primary source of estrogen in postmenopausal women. Many breast cancers have estrogen receptors and growth of these tumors can be stimulated by estrogen. Anastrozole is used to treat postmenopausal women with hormone receptor positive early breast cancer and for the first-line treatment of postmenopausal women with hormone receptor positive or hormone receptor unknown locally advanced or metastatic breast cancer. Recommended dose is 1 mg per day. Anastrozole is administered orally.

S0171

S0171 Injection, bumetanide, 0.5 mg

Bumetanide is a potent diuretic that is in the class of loop diuretics. It blocks fluid and sodium reabsorption from the kidney's tubules. This medication is used to treat mild to moderate hypertension, edema associated with heart failure, renal disease, and cirrhosis of the liver.

S0172

S0172 Chlorambucil, oral, 2 mg

Chlorambucil is a nitrogen mustard type of antineoplastic drug. It is used as palliative treatment for chronic lymphatic (lymphocytic) leukemia and malignant lymphomas, including lymphosarcoma, giant follicular lymphoma, and Hodgkin's disease. The usual oral dosage is 0.1 to 0.2 mg per kg body weight daily for three to six weeks. Chlorambucil is administered orally.

S0174

S0174 Dolasetron mesylate, oral 50 mg (for circumstances falling under the Medicare statute, use Q0180)

Dolasetron mesylate is a chemical compound that is a selective blocker of serotonin 5-HT3 receptors. It is an antiemetic drug available in oral and injectable forms. Serotonin 5-HT3 receptors are present on the vagal nerve and at sensory nerve endings. Cytotoxic chemotherapy appears to trigger the release of serotonin in the small intestine, which may trigger the 5-HT3 receptors and initiate the vomiting reflex. This code represents 50 mg of oral dolasetron mesylate.

S0175

S0175 Flutamide, oral, 125 mg

Flutamide is a nonsteroidal compound that actively inhibits the uptake of androgen and inhibits the nuclear binding of androgen to target cells. Prostate cancer is known to be androgen sensitive and responds to treatment that counteracts androgenic effects or removal of the androgen source. Flutamide is available only in oral form. It is indicated for use in conjunction with luteinizing hormone-releasing hormone (LHRH) agonists as a treatment for locally confined and metastatic carcinoma of the prostate.

S0176

S0176 Hydroxyurea, oral, 500 mg

Hydroxyurea is an antineoplastic drug used to treat melanoma, resistant chronic myelocytic leukemia, and recurrent, metastatic, or inoperable carcinoma of the ovary, and in conjunction with radiation therapy for primary squamous cell (epidermoid) carcinomas of the head and neck, excluding the lip. Hydroxyurea is administered orally.

S0177

S0177 Levamisole HCl, oral, 50 mg

Levamisole is an antineoplastic drug used as an adjuvant therapy in conjunction with 5-fluorouracil after surgical resection to treat patients with Dukes' Stage C colon cancer. The initial dose is 50 mg every eight hours beginning seven to 30 days after surgery for three days. The maintenance dose is 50 mg every eight hours for three days every two weeks. Levamisole is administered orally.

S0178

S0178 Lomustine, oral, 10 mg

Lomustine is used to treat primary and metastatic brain tumors in patients who have already undergone surgical or radiation therapy, and as secondary therapy in Hodgkin's disease for patients who relapse while being treated with other medications or do not respond to primary therapy. Lomustine is administered orally.

S0179

S0179 Megestrol acetate, oral, 20 mg

Megestrol acetate is an antineoplastic medication used as palliative treatment for advanced carcinoma of the breast or endometrium. Megestrol acetate has a direct cytotoxic effect on tumors in the breast. In metastatic cancer, hormone receptors may be present in some tissues but not others. The receptor mechanism is a cyclic process whereby estrogen produced by the ovaries enters the target cell, forms a complex with cytoplasmic receptor, and is transported into the cell nucleus. Inside the cell nucleus it alters the normal cell function. This medication decreases the number of hormone-dependent human breast cancer cells and can change or eliminate the way estrogen acts upon these cells. It is not known how megestrol acetate acts on endometrial cancer. Recommended dose for breast cancer is 40 mg four times a day. Recommended dose for endometrial cancer is 40 to 320 mg per day in divided doses. The usual treatment lasts two months. Megestrol acetate is administered orally.

S0182

S0182 Procarbazine HCl, oral, 50 mg

Procarbazine hydrochloride is used to treat stage III and stage IV Hodgkin's disease. It is used in combination with other antineoplastic drugs. The recommended dose is 50 mg per m^2 of body surface per day for the first week. After that 100 mg per m^2 of body surface per day should be given until the maximum response is obtained or until thrombocytopenia or leukopenia occurs. When the maximum response is attained, the dose may be maintained at 50 mg per m^2 of body surface per day. Procarbazine is administered orally.

S0183

S0183 Prochlorperazine maleate, oral, 5 mg (for circumstances falling under the Medicare statute, use Q0164)

Prochlorperazine/prochlorperazine maleate is an antiemetic used for severe nausea and vomiting, such as that associated with the administration of chemotherapy and prior to induction of anesthesia to control nausea and vomiting during and after surgery. The drug inhibits nausea and vomiting by acting on the chemoreceptor trigger zone and partially depresses the vomiting center. Prochlorperazine is also indicated for treating adult psychiatric illnesses, including schizophrenia, nonpsychotic anxiety, and mild psychotic disorders. Prochlorperazine is available in injection form for intramuscular (IM) and intravenous (IV) use, in tablets, extended release capsules and syrup for oral administration, and in suppository form. The dosage, route of administration, and frequency of administration depends on the patient's diagnosis, the severity of symptoms, and, in the injectable form, by the patient's weight.

S0187

S0187 Tamoxifen citrate, oral, 10 mg

Tamoxifen citrate is a nonsteroidal antiestrogen used to treat metastatic breast cancer in men and women, ductal carcinoma in situ, and women at high risk to develop breast cancer. High risk is defined as women at least 35 years of age with a five-year predicted risk of breast cancer > 1.67%, as calculated by the Gail Model. In premenopausal women with metastatic breast cancer, tamoxifen citrate is an alternative to oophorectomy or ovarian irradiation. It is believed that patients whose tumors are estrogen receptor positive are more likely to benefit from tamoxifen citrate therapy. It is recommended for postmenopausal women with node positive breast cancer who have undergone mastectomy, axillary dissection, and radiation therapy. Recommended dose is 20 to 40 mg per day. Tamoxifen citrate is administered orally.

S0189

S0189 Testosterone pellet, 75 mg

Testosterone is an anabolic steroid used primarily to treat male hypogonadism. It stimulates targeted tissues to develop normally in androgen-deficient men. Testosterone may also have some anti-estrogen properties, making it useful in treating certain estrogen-dependent breast cancers. This drug is used to treat male hypogonadism, unusually late sexual maturity, myotonia congenita, inflammation and rotation of the testes, undescended testicle, absence of testicles, Klinefelter syndrome, anemia, and in the prevention of breast pain and engorgement in postpartum women.

S0190

S0190 Mifepristone, oral, 200 mg

Mifepristone, also known as RU486, is a synthetic steroid with anti-progestational effects. The drug is used for the medical termination of an intrauterine pregnancy through the 49th day. Mifepristone binds to progesterone receptor sites blocking the effects of progesterone.

S0191

S0191 Misoprostol, oral, 200 mcg

Misoprostol is a synthetic prostaglandin E1 analog. It is used to reduce the risk of gastric ulcers in patients undergoing NSAID treatment who may be at high risk for complications of ulcers, including elderly patients, those with a history of gastric ulcers, and patients with a concomitant debilitating disease. Misoprostol inhibits gastric acid secretion and may have mucosal protective properties. NSAIDs reduce prostaglandin synthesis, and a lack of prostaglandins within the gastric mucosa may lead to diminishing bicarbonate and mucus secretion and may contribute to the mucosal damage caused by these agents. As a synthetic prostaglandin, misoprostol can also induce labor and dilate the cervix. Misoprostol may be used as a sole drug or in combination with mifepristone to induce a medical termination of pregnancy. The recommended dose for treatment of gastric ulcers is 200 mcg four times a day. Misoprostol is administered orally. It is sometimes administered vaginally for the induction of labor or termination of pregnancy.

S0194

S0194 Dialysis/stress vitamin supplement, oral, 100 capsules

Vitamins and minerals are organic compounds that are necessary for the metabolic functioning of the body. Multivitamins are combined forms of vitamins and may include minerals. Multivitamins are usually oral tablets. Pregnant patients, patients on dialysis, patients with malabsorption diseases, and those with deficient diets may need exogenous sources of multiple vitamins. Liquid forms may be added to TPN solutions. Multivitamins are sold over-the-counter and are self-administered orally.

S0197

S0197 Prenatal vitamins, 30-day supply

Vitamins and minerals are organic compounds that are necessary for the metabolic functioning of the body. Multivitamins are combined forms of vitamins and may include minerals. Multivitamins are usually oral tablets. Pregnant patients, patients on dialysis, patients with malabsorption diseases, and those with deficient diets may need exogenous sources of multiple vitamins. Liquid forms may be added to TPN solutions. Multivitamins are sold over-the-counter and are self-administered orally.

S0199

S0199 Medically induced abortion by oral ingestion of medication including all associated services and supplies (e.g., patient counseling, office visits, confirmation of pregnancy by HCG, ultrasound to confirm duration of pregnancy, ultrasound to confirm completion of abortion) except drugs

An induced abortion can be performed in several ways, including surgically or medically. In a medical abortion, certain drugs are taken to cause the abortion. It only can be done early in pregnancy. A medical abortion does not require surgery or anesthesia, but multiple visits to the doctor are needed. There are four types of medical abortion, including mifepristone and misoprostol pills, mifepristone pills and vaginal misoprostol, methotrexate and vaginal misoprostol, and vaginal misoprostol alone. This code reports a medically induced abortion by oral ingestion of medication, including all associated services and supplies (e.g., patient counseling, office visits, confirmation of pregnancy by hCG, ultrasound to confirm duration of pregnancy, ultrasound to confirm completion of abortion) except drugs.

S0201

S0201 Partial hospitalization services, less than 24 hours, per diem

Partial hospitalization is a nonresidential treatment modality that includes psychiatric, psychological, social, and vocational elements under medical supervision. It is designed for patients with moderate to severe mental or emotional disorders. Partial hospitalization patients require less than 24-hour care, but more intensive and comprehensive services than are offered in outpatient treatment programs. Partial hospital (PH) programs are highly intensive, time-limited medical services intended to provide a transition from inpatient psychiatric hospitalization to community-based care or substitute for an inpatient admission.

S0207-S0208

S0207 Paramedic intercept, nonhospital-based ALS service (nonvoluntary), nontransport

S0208 Paramedic intercept, hospital-based ALS service (nonvoluntary), nontransport

Paramedic intercept services are advanced life support (ALS) services provided by an entity that does not provide the ambulance transport. The ambulance transport crew requests the ALS services from an independent, outside source. This additional paramedic meets the ambulance and provides needed services, such as CPR, EKG monitoring, or IV skills.

S0209

S0209 Wheelchair van, mileage, per mile

Wheelchair vans are equipped to transport patients in wheelchairs. These vans are equipped with wide enough door openings to accommodate a wheelchair, as well as wheelchair lifts or ramps to enable to wheelchair to enter and exit the van. The wheelchair must be secured to the van while the van is in motion.

S0215

S0215 Nonemergency transportation; mileage, per mile

Nonemergency transportation is transportation provided to patients who are not in an emergent situation. This code represents the distance traveled in miles.

S0220-S0221

S0220 Medical conference by a physician with interdisciplinary team of health professionals or representatives of community agencies to coordinate activities of patient care (patient is present); approximately 30 minutes

S0221 Medical conference by a physician with interdisciplinary team of health professionals or representatives of community agencies to coordinate activities of patient care (patient is present); approximately 60 minutes

A medical conference is a meeting for review, discussion, and/or care planning related to a medical illness or condition. This meeting includes the patient, the physician, and an interdisciplinary team of health professionals, and may include representatives of community agencies. The purpose of the meeting is to plan and coordinate activities of patient care.

S0250

S0250 Comprehensive geriatric assessment and treatment planning performed by assessment team

A comprehensive geriatric assessment involves evaluation and treatment planning designed to optimize an elderly person's ability to maintain good health, improve quality of life, reduce the need for hospital and long-term care services, and enable independent living. Because of the comprehensive scope of this exam, it must be performed by a multi-disciplinary team of experts that may include physicians, geriatric nurse practitioners, ancillary personnel, social workers, psychologists, physical/occupational therapists, dieticians, and pharmacists. The assessment begins with an examination of the elderly person's current status including physical, mental, and psycho-social health status. The ability to function independently and perform basic activities of daily living are assessed including dressing, bathing, meal preparation, and medication management. The individual's living arrangement, social network, and access to support services is evaluated. Next, current problems related to the status assessment are identified and evaluated as to their potential to cause future problems. Based on these findings a comprehensive care plan is developed that addresses all current and potential problems. Specific interventions are proposed, including recommendations regarding necessary resources and support services. Management of resources is initiated with the elderly person and family to assure that the necessary services will be provided. A plan for ongoing monitoring is provided so modifications to the care plan can be initiated as required.

S0255

S0255 Hospice referral visit (advising patient and family of care options) performed by nurse, social worker, or other designated staff

Hospice is a licensed program that offers an integrated set of services and supplies designed to provide comfort measures and supportive care to terminally ill patients and their families. It may include legal, financial, emotional, or spiritual counseling, in addition to meeting the patient's immediate physical needs.

S0257

S0257 Counseling and discussion regarding advance directives or end of life care planning and decisions, with patient and/or surrogate (list separately in addition to code for appropriate evaluation and management service)

The advance care directive provides a clear statement of the patient's wishes about when to prolong life or withdraw care. This code reports the discussion and the counseling that is done to explain these options to the patient.

S0260

S0260 History and physical (outpatient or office) related to surgical procedure (list separately in addition to code for appropriate evaluation and management service)

Use this code to report the history and physical that is performed outpatient or in the physician's office that resulted in the decision for surgery.

S0265

S0265 Genetic counseling, under physician supervision, each 15 minutes

Individuals who have a family history of certain genetic diseases or disorders, such as cystic fibrosis, sickle cell anemia, Tay-Sachs disease, or other diseases may be referred for genetic counseling. Genetic counseling is a service that includes evaluating family history and medical records, ordering genetic tests, evaluating the test results, and helping the individuals understand the test results and reach decisions based on the results of the testing. Before meeting with a genetic counselor, information about family history, including relatives with genetic disorders, multiple miscarriages, or early or unexplained deaths, should be gathered. A personal history and medical record information related to ultrasounds, prenatal test results, past pregnancies, and medications should also be provided. The counselor reviews the family and personal history information, determines if additional tests are necessary, assists the individuals in obtaining the necessary tests, and conducts a follow-up when the results of testing are available. During the follow-up, the genetic counselor helps the patient understand options and makes any necessary referrals to other health care professionals.

S0270-S0272

S0270 Physician management of patient home care, standard monthly case rate (per 30 days)

S0271 Physician management of patient home care, hospice monthly case rate (per 30 days)

S0272 Physician management of patient home care, episodic care monthly case rate (per 30 days)

Use these codes to report the physician's management of standard, hospice, or episodic care in the home setting. These services are to be reported on a monthly basis and are paid as a case rate.

S

S0273-S0274

S0273 Physician visit at member's home, outside of a capitation arrangement

S0274 Nurse practitioner visit at member's home, outside of a capitation arrangement

Use these codes to report physician or nurse practitioner home care visits that are outside of the capitated case rate.

S0280-S0281

S0281 Medical home program, comprehensive care coordination and planning, initial plan

S0282 Medical home program, comprehensive care coordination and planning, maintenance of plan

The Multi-payer Advanced Primary Care Practice (MAPCP) Demonstration, also referred to as the patient-centered medical home, is a three-year demonstration whose purpose is to promote advanced primary care (APC) principles. Eight states are participating in this initiative. CMS has joined with Medicaid and commercial insurance payers to participate in each of these eight states' existing multi payer medical home initiatives. CMS pays a monthly care management fee for patients who are receiving primary care from APC practices. In certain circumstances, CMS may pay an additional amount to the organization that works with the APC practice by providing community-based care coordination support. CMS also pays an additional amount to the state for administering and evaluating the program. The payment is a per beneficiary monthly amount that is based on the patients under the practice's care. Use these codes to report the MAPCP services.

S0285

S0285 Colonoscopy consultation performed prior to a screening colonoscopy procedure

This code represents a consultation performed prior to a screening colonoscopy procedure. This consultation may include a detailed history and physical, an explanation of the prep required, the risks involved, and any expected recovery time.

S0302

S0302 Completed early periodic screening diagnosis and treatment (EPSDT) service (list in addition to code for appropriate evaluation and management service)

Early periodic screening diagnosis and treatment (EPSDT) is a free service provided to children ages birth through 21 who are eligible for Medicaid. EPSDT enables children to get medical exams, check-ups, follow-up care, and any special care needed to ensure optimum health. EPSDT legislation requires states to provide Medicaid-eligible children with periodic screening, vision, dental, and hearing services. States are required to assess a child's health needs through initial and periodic examinations and evaluations to assure that health problems are diagnosed and treated early, before they become more complex. States must perform the required evaluations according to a standardized schedule, called a periodicity schedule. At a minimum, these screenings must include comprehensive health and developmental history, including assessment of both physical and mental health development; comprehensive unclothed physical exam; appropriate immunizations according to age and health history; laboratory tests, including a lead toxicity screening; health education, including anticipatory guidance; vision and hearing screens; and dental screens. In addition, EPSDT legislation requires states provide any medically necessary inter-periodic health screens and care, even if the service is not available under the state's Medicaid plan to adults. Report this code in addition to the appropriate evaluation and management service.

S0310

S0310 Hospitalist services (list separately in addition to code for appropriate evaluation and management service)

A hospitalist is a board-certified physician specializing in the care of hospitalized patients. The hospitalist is a single point person who oversees each patient's care throughout the hospital stay. The hospitalist makes daily rounds, checks on each patient as needed throughout the day, monitors the patient's in-hospital care, tracks nursing care, and works to coordinate care between the patient's primary care physician and other physician specialists. In addition, the hospitalist coordinates scheduling of tests and procedures that may be required and follows up to make sure test results are reported and reviewed by the appropriate person. Report this code in addition to the code for the appropriate evaluation and management service.

S0311

S0311 Comprehensive management and care coordination for advanced illness, per calendar month

This code represents the comprehensive management and care coordination required in a calendar month for a patient with an advanced illness. This usually includes a multidisciplinary care team to provide more consistent care for high-risk and rising-risk patients. The team members gain a 360-degree longitudinal view of the patient to enable timely and appropriate interventions and reduce unnecessary utilization.

S0315-S0320

S0315 Disease management program; initial assessment and initiation of the program

S0316 Disease management program, follow-up/reassessment

S0317 Disease management program; per diem

S0320 Telephone calls by a registered nurse to a disease management program member for monitoring purposes; per month

Disease management is a system of coordinated health services for patients with specific disease processes, usually chronic conditions. An evolution from managed care and capitated care, disease management seeks to keep costs down and improve patient health through integrative treatments that range from patient education to life style changes and nutrition to inpatient hospitalizations. Most disease management programs are specific to one condition, such as diabetes, asthma, or heart failure.

S0340-S0342

S0340 Lifestyle modification program for management of coronary artery disease, including all supportive services; first quarter/stage

S0341 Lifestyle modification program for management of coronary artery disease, including all supportive services; second or third quarter/stage

S0342 Lifestyle modification program for management of coronary artery disease, including all supportive services; fourth quarter/stage

Lifestyle modification programs for coronary artery disease (CAD) are designed to prevent and possibly even reverse coronary artery disease. These programs may include diet modification, exercise, non-smoking, group support, stress management, and exercise. They target spiritual, psychological, and emotional healing and encourage patients to participate in their own care. The lifestyle modification program is completed over the course of a year and is conducted by a team of professionals, which may include registered dieticians, exercise physiologists, specialists in behavioral health, and nurse case managers. Use these codes to report CAD lifestyle modification program services based on the time frame the services were rendered.

S

S0353-S0354

S0353 Treatment planning and care coordination management for cancer initial treatment

S0354 Treatment planning and care coordination management for cancer established patient with a change of regimen

A treatment plan is a detailed outline of care composed of a list of problems including details on the cancer, goals, methods to achieve the goals, and estimated time necessary to achieve the goals. It may include treatment side effects and the names and addresses of individual providers. The care coordination involves the organization and monitoring of the different types of treatment or services outlined in the treatment plan.

S0390

S0390 Routine foot care; removal and/or trimming of corns, calluses and/or nails and preventive maintenance in specific medical conditions (e.g., diabetes), per visit

Peripheral neuropathy can be caused by many different disease or agents, such as diabetes mellitus or chemotherapeutic drugs. Decreased sensations in the feet can lead to injuries and open wounds. Periodic foot care performed on a routine basis may help to eliminate an issue before it becomes a medical problem. Routine footcare includes removal or trimming of corns, calluses, and toenails.

S0395

S0395 Impression casting of a foot performed by a practitioner other than the manufacturer of the orthotic

Impression casting of a foot is a cast of a foot that is to be used by a podiatrist or orthotist to create a specialized application that can help correct painful conditions and provide assistance in ambulation. Casting materials can be plaster, wax, or a composite material. Impression casting is generally considered a part of the measurements needed to create an orthotic and is not reported separately.

S0400

S0400 Global fee for extracorporeal shock wave lithotripsy treatment of kidney stone(s)

The physician pulverizes a kidney stone (renal calculus) by directing shock waves through a liquid medium. Two different methods are currently available to accomplish this procedure. The physician first uses radiological guidance to determine the location and size of the renal calculus. In the first method, the patient is then immersed in a liquid medium (degassed, deionized water) with shock waves directed through the liquid to the kidney stone. In the second method, the one most often used, the patient is placed on a specially designed treatment table. A series of shock waves is directed through a water-cushion or bellow placed against the patient's body at the location of the kidney stone. Each shock wave is directed to the stone for only a fraction of a second, and the entire procedure generally takes from 30 to 50 minutes. The treatment table is equipped with video x-ray so the physician can view the pulverization process. Over several days or weeks, the tiny stone fragments pass harmlessly through the patient's urinary system and are discharged during urination.

S0500

S0500 Disposable contact lens, per lens

A contact lens is a corrective, therapeutic, or sometimes cosmetic lens placed on the cornea of the eye. Corrective and therapeutic lenses are intended to correct vision problems in place of glasses, or treat ophthalmological conditions such as corneal ulcers. Contact lenses may be made of hard or soft material, may be made to be worn only when awake, or can be made for continuous overnight wear. Disposable lens are intended to be worn for a specified period of time before being discarded, such a daily, two-week, or four-week disposable lens.

S0504

S0504 Single vision prescription lens (safety, athletic, or sunglass), per lens

A single vision lens provides one viewing surface in the lens that is concave on the back surface. This concave shape follows the shape of the eye and allows the back of the lens to stay at the same distance when the eye moves. It is used to treat refractive errors that cause the patient to have trouble seeing near or far distances. Report this code for single vision specialty prescription safety, athletic, or sunglasses, per lens.

S0506

S0506 Bifocal vision prescription lens (safety, athletic, or sunglass), per lens

Bifocal vision eyeglass lenses address the correction of two focal powers for distance and work, such as reading that requires a close up focus. Lenses are made from glass or plastic to the specific level of correction required to improve vision. The lens provides two viewing surfaces in the lens that is concave on the back surface. This concave shape follows the shape of the eye and allows the back of the lens to stay at the same distance when the eye moves. Use this code to report bifocal specialty prescription safety, athletic, or sunglasses, per lens.

S0508

S0508 Trifocal vision prescription lens (safety, athletic, or sunglass), per lens

Trifocal lenses have three visibly identifiable zones of vision divided by two segment lines of variable widths. Trifocal lenses offer three fixed fields of focus (near/intermediate/distant) for patients with higher levels of presbyopia. The lens provides a three viewing surface that is concave on the back surface. This concave shape follows the shape of the eye and allows the back of the lens to stay at the same distance when the eye moves. It is used to treat refractive errors that cause the patient to have trouble seeing near or far distances. Use this code to report trifocal specialty prescription safety, athletic, or sunglasses, per lens.

S0510

S0510 Nonprescription lens (safety, athletic, or sunglass), per lens

Nonprescription lenses do not correct vision but can serve as a protective covering to the eyes for work, sports participation, and as a barrier against UV rays from the sun.

S0512

S0512 Daily wear specialty contact lens, per lens

Daily wear specialty lenses are designed to be worn daily and removed nightly by patients after certain types of surgery and when other types of lenses are unsuitable. These may include astigmatism, patients who have undergone refractive surgery but need additional correction, and patients with penetrating keratoplasty, eye disfigurement, corneal trauma, or corneal degeneration. Report this code per specialty daily wear contact lens.

S0514

S0514 Color contact lens, per lens

Color contact lenses are worn directly on the cornea and may correct vision or be worn for cosmetic purposes. There are four types of colored contact lens: Light-filtering tinted lenses are intended for athletes and sports fans. These lenses enhance certain colors and mute others. For instance, contact lenses for tennis players enhance the color yellow so the tennis balls are easier to see. Visibility tinted lenses contain a mild tint to make the lenses easier to find if they are dropped. Color tinted lenses are opaque and change the color of the eyes. Enhancement tinted lenses are designed to enhance the natural color of the eyes but do not change the color. Report this code for each lens.

S0515

S0515 Scleral lens, liquid bandage device, per lens

Sclera lenses are a specialized type of contact lens that are larger than the regular soft contact lens and are custom made for each eye. They are designed to rest on the sclera of the eye and to vault over the cornea. The vaulted section is filled with a fluid reservoir that serves as a liquid bandage to help patients with diseased or extremely dry corneas. The fluid reservoir helps improve the patient's vision by masking irregularities of the cornea. Report this code per lens.

S0516-S0518

S0516 Safety eyeglass frames

S0518 Sunglasses frames

Frames are rigid or semi-rigid devices that bear lenses that are held in front of the eyes for vision correction or eye protection. Frames are made from many different materials in many different colors and shapes. Use these codes to report frames used with safety glasses or sunglasses.

S0580

S0580 Polycarbonate lens (list this code in addition to the basic code for the lens)

Polycarbonate lenses are developed from small pellets that are heated until melted and then rapidly injected into lens molds after which they are compressed under high pressure and cooled. These lenses are impact-resistant and often used by people participating in sports and for children and others who are apt to drop and scratch the lenses. The lenses are thin and lightweight.

S0581

S0581 Nonstandard lens (list this code in addition to the basic code for the lens)

A nonstandard lens is any lens that deviates from the average in curvature, size, or both. Report this code in addition to the code for the basic lens.

S0590

S0590 Integral lens service, miscellaneous services reported separately

Use this code to report an integral lens service that is not covered by a current HCPCS Level II code.

S0592

S0592 Comprehensive contact lens evaluation

The comprehensive contact lens evaluation includes the general eye examination in addition to measuring the eye's surface and curvature, possibly measuring the size of the pupils in different lighting conditions, measurement of the cornea diameter, tear film evaluation using Schirmer's test or fluorescein staining, and examining the eye's surface to determine the type of contact lens that will best meet the patient's needs.

S0595

S0595 Dispensing new spectacle lenses for patient supplied frame

This code reports the dispensing of new spectacle lenses for patients that supply their own frames. Dispensing services include following prescriptions written by ophthalmologists or optometrists and fitting the completed glasses on the patient.

S0596

S0596 Phakic intraocular lens for correction of refractive error

This lens is designed for people with extreme nearsightedness, from -10 to -20 diopters of myopia (nearsightedness). People with severe vision impairment may not be suitable candidates for cornea-based refractive surgery like LASIK and PRK. These lenses are not used for patients who have a cataract and have their lens replaced. This lens is a small lens implant inserted into the eye through a small incision at the edge of the cornea. The lens is placed behind the iris and in front of the natural crystalline lens without removing the natural lens. It is then adhered to the front of the iris, or colored portion of the eye, to hold it securely.

S0601

S0601 Screening proctoscopy

A screening proctoscopy allows visualization of the inner lining of the anus and rectum that is done through a proctoscope, a straight, rigid, hollow metal or plastic tube with a small light at the end. It is done to screen for polyps, inflammation, bleeding, and cancer and requires an enema or laxative prior to the procedure.

S0610-S0613

S0610 Annual gynecological examination, new patient

S0612 Annual gynecological examination, established patient

S0613 Annual gynecological examination; clinical breast examination without pelvic evaluation

The annual gynecologic (GYN) exam consists of a breast exam, a pelvic exam, and a Pap test. It is done to evaluate risk factors, monitor changes in health over time, evaluate and prescribe use of birth control methods, provide guidance in wellness, and to detect current health problems. Use these codes to report the annual GYN exam, based on whether the patient is new or established or if the GYN exam is a breast exam only.

S0618

S0618 Audiometry for hearing aid evaluation to determine the level and degree of hearing loss

Audiometry is a hearing test to determine the type and degree of hearing loss and to determine if the patient is a candidate for hearing aids. This exam determines if there is a need for further medical assessment or medical clearance for hearing aids.

S0620-S0621

S0620 Routine ophthalmological examination including refraction; new patient

S0621 Routine ophthalmological examination including refraction; established patient

The ophthalmologist or optometrist performs a routine eye (ophthalmological) examination including refraction. A complete eye examination involves a series of tests to evaluate vision and check for eye diseases. A visual exam is performed on the external eye to check the pupils' response to light, the clarity and shininess of the cornea and iris, and the position and movement of the eyes, eyelids, and eyelashes. The provider checks the eye muscles to ensure they are functioning properly. Tests on the eye muscles involve following movement of an object up and down and side to side to detect any eye muscle weakness or uncontrolled movement. A visual acuity test is performed using an eye chart. Following the visual acuity test, a refraction assessment is performed on individuals who need corrective lenses to determine the prescription required. The provider may use a computerized refractor to estimate the prescription, or alternatively a retinoscopy may be performed. A retinoscopy involves shining a light into the eye and measuring the refractive error by evaluating the movement of the light that is reflected by the retina. These results are verified and fine-tuned using a Phoropter, which consists of a series of lenses through which the patient views an eye chart and indicates which lens provides the clearest vision. The provider checks peripheral vision by means of a visual field (perimetry) test. A slit lamp exam is performed. A slit lamp uses an intense line of light to examine the cornea, iris, lens, and anterior eye chamber. The provider performs a glaucoma test, which checks intraocular pressure. The pupils are dilated, and the retina is examined.

S0622

S0622 Physical exam for college, new or established patient (list separately in addition to appropriate evaluation and management code)

A physical exam is required for college admission and, depending on the college, may be an annual requirement. This code describes the college physical exam and is to be reported in addition to the evaluation and management code.

S0630

S0630 Removal of sutures; by a physician other than the physician who originally closed the wound

The physician removes sutures that have been placed by another physician. When a laceration or an incision for a surgical procedure has required suturing, any non-absorbable stitches must be removed. The area is cleansed with an antiseptic cleanser to remove any dried blood and loosen any scar tissue. Sterile forceps are used to lift the suture at the knot. The suture material is then clipped as close to the skin as possible using sterile forceps and removed. When all the sutures are removed, the area is cleaned again with antiseptic. Adhesive strips and a dry dressing may be applied as needed.

S0800

S0800 Laser in situ keratomileusis (LASIK)

Laser in situ keratomileusis (LASIK) is a type of refractive surgery used to correct myopia, hyperopia, and astigmatism. The cornea directs or refracts light to the retina. The shape of the corneal lens can create blurry or multiple images on the retina. An ultraviolet excimer laser, which does not heat surrounding tissue, is used to ablate corneal tissue, reshaping the curvature of the lens. A flap in the cornea is created and pulled back and the laser is used to ablate the underlying corneal tissue in a pattern designed for the patient and the patient's vision problems. LASIK is intended to improve the patient's vision by improving the refraction of light and decreasing the need for glasses or contact lens.

S0810

S0810 Photorefractive keratectomy (PRK)

Photorefractive keratectomy (PRK) is a type of refractive surgery used to correct myopia, hyperopia, and astigmatism. The cornea directs or refracts light to the retina. The shape of the corneal lens can create blurry or multiple images on the retina. An ultraviolet excimer laser, which does not heat surrounding tissue, is used to ablate corneal tissue, reshaping the curvature of the lens. PRK reshapes the surface of the cornea rather than the underlying tissue (as in LASIK). The laser is used to ablate the corneal tissue in a pattern designed for the patient and the patient's vision problems. Photorefractive keratectomy is intended to improve the patient's vision by improving the refraction of light and decreasing the need for glasses or contact lens.

S0812

S0812 Phototherapeutic keratectomy (PTK)

Phototherapeutic keratectomy (PTK) is a type of eye surgery used to treat anterior corneal diseases and scars. PTK is indicated as a treatment for epithelial basement membrane dystrophy, irregular corneal surfaces, shallow corneal scars, corneal opacities, and superficial corneal dystrophies, including granular, lattice, and Reis-Buckler's. An ultraviolet excimer laser, which does not heat surrounding tissue, is used to ablate corneal tissue to produce a smoother, clearer lens. PTK is a therapeutic procedure and is not intended to decrease the need for glasses or contact lenses.

S1001-S1002

S1001 Deluxe item, patient aware (list in addition to code for basic item)

S1002 Customized item (list in addition to code for basic item)

These codes can be used to report the difference between the base model of an item and the deluxe (or customized) model. For example, report the HCPCS Level II code and charge for a base model of hearing aid and on another line of the claim, list these HCPCS Level II codes to represent the deluxe (or customized) hearing aid model along with the difference in charge between the base hearing aid model and the deluxe (or customized) model.

S1015

S1015 IV tubing extension set

An IV tubing extension set is designed to provide longer IV tubing between the access site and the IV fluid source. This may be done to prevent the needle from dislodging and to allow greater mobility for the patient.

S1016

S1016 Non-PVC (polyvinyl chloride) intravenous administration set, for use with drugs that are not stable in PVC, e.g., Paclitaxel

Some drugs and biologicals are unstable in a PVC environment and must be administered using IV tubing that contains no PVC. Use this code to report an IV administration that is PVC free.

S1030-S1031

S1030 Continuous noninvasive glucose monitoring device, purchase (for physician interpretation of data, use CPT code)

S1031 Continuous noninvasive glucose monitoring device, rental, including sensor, sensor replacement, and download to monitor (for physician interpretation of data, use CPT code)

The continuous noninvasive glucose monitoring devise is worn like a watch and has a special sensor. Without breaking the skin, this sensor measures the patient's blood sugar levels. The patient's blood sugar patterns are recorded and analyzed by the physician, who makes any necessary changes in the patient's treatment. This device is considered experimental by most payers. Use these codes to report the purchase or rental of the continuous glucose monitoring device.

S1034

S1034 Artificial pancreas device system (e.g., low glucose suspend [LGS] feature) including continuous glucose monitor, blood glucose device, insulin pump and computer algorithm that communicates with all of the devices

An artificial pancreas device system (APDS) links a group of devices used to detect and react to rising blood glucose levels by combining a glucose sensor, a control algorithm and an insulin infusion device. The APDS parts communicate with each other to automate the process of maintaining blood glucose concentrations at or near a specific target/range. The glucose sensor continuously detects the patient's glucose levels. The sensor then outputs the glucose level to a control system, which then computes the patient's required insulin dosage and directs the insulin pump to deliver the prescribed dosage. The system may also direct the pump to withhold delivery of insulin.

S

S1035-S1036

S1035 Sensor; invasive (e.g., subcutaneous), disposable, for use with artificial pancreas device system

S1036 Transmitter; external, for use with artificial pancreas device system

A tiny electrode called a glucose sensor is inserted under the skin to measure glucose levels in tissue fluid. The glucose sensor has a small adhesive (sticky) patch to hold it in place for a few days and then it must be replaced with a new sensor. The glucose sensor is inserted with a needle, which is removed after the glucose sensor is in place, generally in the abdominal area. The glucose sensor is easily inserted under the skin using an insertion device. The continuous glucose monitoring transmitter is a small, lightweight device that attaches to the glucose sensor, gathers glucose data, and sends it wirelessly to the glucose monitoring unit.

S1037

S1037 Receiver (monitor); external, for use with artificial pancreas device system

The artificial pancreas external receiver (monitor) can be a stand-alone device or built into an insulin pump. The receiver is small and can be attached to a belt, placed in a pocket, or hidden under clothing. The receiver displays the current glucose levels as well as historical trends. Notifications are issued before the patient reaches predetermined low or high glucose limits. When built into an insulin pump, the device automatically holds or delivers insulin.

S1040

S1040 Cranial remolding orthotic, pediatric, rigid, with soft interface material, custom fabricated, includes fitting and adjustment(s)

This code reports the supply of a special cranial remolding orthosis used to treat plagiocephaly. Plagiocephaly refers to misshapen or flattened skull bones and a variety of causes are noted, including premature closure of cranial sutures, birth trauma, torticollis, or repetitive sleeping positions. This type of cranial remolding orthosis consists of a custom-fabricated, helmet-like device structured to address the specific cranial malformation of the infant. The orthosis has a soft interface material for comfort, as many are worn up to 23 hours per day. Some models consist of broad bands with mild elastic properties, while others are fabricated by molding to the patient's skull. The cranial remolding orthosis is designed to address plagiocephaly and manipulate skull development toward a more normal shape, or to maintain skull structure. This code reports the supply, fitting, and any required adjustments of the custom-fabricated, rigid, pediatric, cranial orthosis.

S1091

S1091 Stent, noncoronary, temporary, with delivery system (Propel)

The Propel sinus implant is a self-dissolving device that delivers a sustained, localized, controlled release of the corticosteroid mometasone furoate over a 30-day period. It is indicated as a treatment for chronic sinusitis in adult patients, 18 years and older, having ethmoid sinus surgery. The device is implanted during sinus surgery where it expands to prop open the sinus, support the bony structures inside the nose, and help prevent scar formation. It is absorbed by the body within six weeks after the surgical implant.

S2053-S2054

S2053 Transplantation of small intestine and liver allografts

S2054 Transplantation of multivisceral organs

The transplantation of organs is the removal of a healthy organ or organs from one body, usually a cadaver, and the insertion or attachment of that organ or organs into another body. Transplant types include allografts, which are transplants from the same species; autografts, which are transplants from the same patient as with skin grafts from one part of the body to another; or xenografts, which are transplants from one species to another species.

S2055

S2055 Harvesting of donor multivisceral organs, with preparation and maintenance of allografts; from cadaver donor

Harvesting is the process of removing living, viable organs from a cadaver for transplantation into another party. The organs of the cadaver are kept functioning with medications and machines. In a multivisceral harvest, multiple organs, such as a liver, small intestine, pancreas, and/or stomach, are removed for transplant from the cadaver. A team of physicians, nurses, and technicians remove the multiple organs that are to be transplanted. The blood supply and ducts are dissected free and isolated leaving organs that are to be transplanted together attached when possible. The organs are then perfused with a cold preservation solution and removed from the operative field. The organs remain under refrigeration, specially packed in a sealable container with some preserving solution, and kept on ice in a suitable carrier.

S2060

S2060 Lobar lung transplantation

The human lung is a paired organ composed of a right and left lung. The right lung represents more than one half of the total lung volume and has three lobes: superior, middle, and inferior. The left lung has a smaller volume and is composed of two lobes. In a lobar lung transplant, one of the lobes of one lung, usually a lower or inferior lobe, is transplanted into a recipient to replace the functions of the recipient's diseased lungs. Lobar lung transplants are typically from living donors. They usually replace both diseased lungs with a right lobe and a left lobe from different donors.

S2061

S2061 Donor lobectomy (lung) for transplantation, living donor

There are two human lungs, a right and a left lung. The right lung represents more than one half of the total lung volume and has three lobes: superior, middle, and inferior. The left lung has a smaller volume and is composed of two lobes. In a lobar lung transplant, one of the lobes of one lung, usually a lower or inferior lobe, is transplanted into a recipient to replace the functions of the recipient's diseased lungs. Report this code for the surgery performed to remove a lobe of the lung from a living donor for transplantation into another person.

S2065

S2065 Simultaneous pancreas kidney transplantation

Simultaneous pancreas kidney transplantation is the replacement, during the same operative session, of both a diseased or nonfunctional pancreas and kidney. This dual transplantation has become accepted therapy for patients with insulin-dependent diabetes mellitus who also have diabetic nephropathy. Both organs are removed from the same cadaver.

S2066

S2066 Breast reconstruction with gluteal artery perforator (GAP) flap, including harvesting of the flap, microvascular transfer, closure of donor site and shaping the flap into a breast, unilateral

Gluteal artery perforator (GAP) is breast reconstruction using the gluteal artery perforator flap, which includes harvesting the flap, the microvascular transfer, closure of the donor site, and shaping the flap into a breast. HCPCS Level II code S2066 is a unilateral procedure.

S2067

S2067 Breast reconstruction of a single breast with "stacked" deep inferior epigastric perforator (DIEP) flap(s) and/or gluteal artery perforator (GAP) flap(s), including harvesting of the flap(s), microvascular transfer, closure of donor site(s) and shaping the flap into a breast, unilateral

Deep inferior epigastric perforator/gluteal artery perforator (DIEP/GAP) is breast reconstruction of a single breast with a stacked deep inferior epigastric perforator or superficial inferior epigastric artery (SIEA) flap. This procedure includes harvesting of the flap, microvascular transfer, closure of the donor site, and shaping the new flap into a breast.

S2068

S2068 Breast reconstruction with deep inferior epigastric perforator (DIEP) flap or superficial inferior epigastric artery (SIEA) flap, including harvesting of the flap, microvascular transfer, closure of donor site and shaping the flap into a breast, unilateral

The deep inferior epigastric (DIEP) flap procedure uses tissues harvested from the patient's lower abdomen. The blood vessel that supplies blood to the abdominal muscle is the deep inferior epigastric artery. This artery also has side branches, which travel around or through the muscle to the overlying fat. These side branches or "perforators" are used as the blood supply for the DIEP procedure. As a result, the large abdominal muscle is not cut during the procedure, but the thick fascia (thick overlying tissue found over the muscle) is cut so that the perforators have enough diameter and length to supply blood to the reconstructed area. The superficial inferior epigastric artery (SIEA) flap procedure uses the same tissues as the DIEP flap. However, the blood supply for the DIEP is through the superficial inferior epigastric artery. In the SIEA procedure, neither the abdominal muscle nor its overlying fascia is touched.

S2070

S2070 Cystourethroscopy, with ureteroscopy and/or pyeloscopy; with endoscopic laser treatment of ureteral calculi (includes ureteral catheterization)

Cystourethroscopy is the insertion of a thin tube through the urethra to the bladder for diagnostic examination or to perform therapeutic procedures. A ureteroscopy and/or pyeloscopy is the extension of this tube through the ureter and sometimes into the kidney. A laser is passed through the tube to destroy any calcium deposits or calculi within the ureter. This code includes all components and a ureteral catheterization when performed.

S2079

S2079 Laparoscopic esophagomyotomy (Heller type)

A Heller type esophagomyotomy is the surgical division of the muscles surrounding the esophagus at the point where the esophagus joins the stomach, the sphincter of the esophagogastric junction. The release of the muscles allows swallowed food to pass more easily into the stomach. The procedure is most commonly performed to treat achalasia.

S2080

S2080 Laser-assisted uvulopalatoplasty (LAUP)

Laser-assisted uvulopalatoplasty (LAUP) is an office procedure used to treat snoring and associated obstructive sleep apnea. The uvula is the conic projection from the middle of the roof of the mouth. It is composed of connective tissue, a few glands, and muscle. The uvula contributes to the articulation of the sound of the human voice. The vibrations created by the uvula also contribute to snoring and sleep apnea. After the administration of a local anesthetic, a laser is used to vaporize the uvula and a portion of the palate. LAUP may require up to five treatments spaced four to eight weeks apart.

S2083

S2083 Adjustment of gastric band diameter via subcutaneous port by injection or aspiration of saline

One form of bariatric surgery uses an inflatable silicone device called a gastric band. This band is placed around the patient's stomach to reduce its size. The adjustment of the gastric band, post bariatric surgery, is accomplished by inserting a needle into the port of the band and adding or removing saline. This is done to change the width of the stomach opening.

S2095

S2095 Transcatheter occlusion or embolization for tumor destruction, percutaneous, any method, using yttrium-90 microspheres

Yttrium-90 microspheres are glass or plastic beads containing the radioactive element yttrium-90. These microspheres are released into the common, right, or left hepatic artery to block blood flow to a tumor and provide internal radiation. This procedure is used to treat tumors in the liver. It is a type of selective internal radiation therapy (SIRT). This code represents a percutaneous installation of yttrium-90 microspheres using a catheter.

S2102

S2102 Islet cell tissue transplant from pancreas; allogeneic

An islet cell tissue transplant from the pancreas is an experimental treatment for Type 1 diabetes mellitus. The pancreas is an organ that makes insulin and digestive enzymes that assist the body in the breakdown and use of food. Within the pancreas are clusters of cells called islets of Langerhans. These islets contain different types of cells, including beta cells, that make insulin. A highly purified mixture of enzymes is used to isolate islet cells from the pancreas of a deceased organ donor. The purified islet cells are then injected, under imaging guidance, into the portal vein of the liver. The islet cells attach themselves to blood vessels and begin releasing insulin. The human body treats islet cells just as it would any foreign body and immunosuppressive drugs must be taken.

S2103

S2103 Adrenal tissue transplant to brain

Parkinson's disease is a progressive neurodegenerative disorder caused by impaired dopamine neurons in the area of the brain that controls balance and muscle movement. Dopamine is a neurotransmitter that relays information between neurons and muscles. An adrenal tissue transplant to the brain removes adrenal gland medullary tissue from the patient (autograft) or from another person (allograft) and places the tissue into the corpus striatum of the brain. This is an experimental procedure intended to restore dopamine activity in patients with Parkinson's disease.

S2107

S2107 Adoptive immunotherapy i.e. development of specific antitumor reactivity (e.g., tumor-infiltrating lymphocyte therapy) per course of treatment

Adoptive immunotherapy is a form of immunotherapy that is used for cancer treatment. It consists of removing a patient's own lymphocytes and growing them with a naturally produced growth factor (lymphokine interleukin 2 [IL-2]). These cells are then injected into the tumor site to increase local immune response.

S2112

S2112 Arthroscopy, knee, surgical for harvesting of cartilage (chondrocyte cells)

Normal cartilage is harvested during a knee arthroscopy with biopsy. The cells of the harvested tissue are separated from the cartilage and cultured in a medium. Over the next six weeks, these cells multiply and are stored in the frozen state. After being thawed and going through a final culture process, they are sent to the OR on the day of the implantation surgery. Under general anesthesia, an arthrotomy is done and the chondral lesion is excised and the cultured chondrocytes are injected beneath the periosteal flap.

S2115

S2115 Osteotomy, periacetabular, with internal fixation

A periacetabular osteotomy is performed to correct hip dysplasia. The surgeon makes an incision on the patient's hip area and divides the pelvis bone to separate the hip socket from the rest of the pelvis. The hip socket is rotated until it covers the head of the femur and is internally attached to the bone with the use of screws. Typically, no cast or other support is required by the patient after the surgery.

S2117

S2117 Arthroereisis, subtalar

Arthroereisis is a surgical procedure that limits the movement of a joint. The term subtalar refers to the point in the foot where the talus meets the calcaneus at the ankle. Subtalar implants are placed in the sinus tarsi to act as a spacer and prevent full flexion of the tendons. This procedure is considered an investigational treatment for flat feet and similar foot deformities.

S2118

S2118 Metal-on-metal total hip resurfacing, including acetabular and femoral components

Total hip resurfacing is a surgical alternative to a total hip replacement. A metal cap, which is a hollow mushroom-shape, is placed over the head of the femur. A matching metal cup is used to replace the articulating surfaces of the acetabulum or pelvic socket. Synovial fluid flows between the two components as lubrication when the patient's hip moves. Total hip resurfacing is a less invasive procedure that preserves bone and provides a reduced chance of hip dislocation. This code represents the procedure, as well as the two metal components.

S2120

S2120 Low density lipoprotein (LDL) apheresis using heparin-induced extracorporeal LDL precipitation

Extracorporeal apheresis is a treatment that drains blood from the body, separates out and removes one particular blood component, and returns the blood to the body. Low density lipoprotein (LDL) is one of the five major types of lipoproteins, lipids bound with protein, that transport lipids within the bloodstream. The current theory categorizes LDL as "bad cholesterol" that contributes to cardiovascular disease and other health problems. This code represents LDL apheresis using heparin-induced LDL precipitation. The heparin binds to the LDL molecule, causing it to be removed more easily from the blood. The procedure is usually reserved for cases of severe hyperlipidemia.

S2140-S2142

S2140 Cord blood harvesting for transplantation, allogeneic

S2142 Cord blood-derived stem-cell transplantation, allogeneic

Cord blood harvesting is the process of collecting blood from the umbilical cord after the baby is born and the cord has been clamped. The umbilical cord contains a large amount of stem cells. After harvesting, the blood is usually screened for infectious and hereditary diseases. If there is a substantial amount of clean blood, it is cryogenically stored for future transplantation.

S

S2150-S2152

S2150 Bone marrow or blood-derived stem cells (peripheral or umbilical), allogeneic or autologous, harvesting, transplantation, and related complications; including: pheresis and cell preparation/storage; marrow ablative therapy; drugs, supplies, hospitalization with outpatient follow-up; medical/surgical, diagnostic, emergency, and rehabilitative services; and the number of days of pre- and posttransplant care in the global definition

S2152 Solid organ(s), complete or segmental, single organ or combination of organs; deceased or living donor(s), procurement, transplantation, and related complications; including: drugs; supplies; hospitalization with outpatient follow-up; medical/surgical, diagnostic, emergency, and rehabilitative services, and the number of days of pre- and posttransplant care in the global definition

Transplants are performed to replace destroyed or damaged bone marrow or solid organs with a healthy organ or stem cells. Allogenic transplants use tissues from cadavers or living persons. Autologous transplants use the patient's own tissue. Use these codes to report all transplant-related services in the global period for stem cell and solid organ transplants.

S2202

S2202 Echosclerotherapy

Echosclerotherapy is the use of ultrasound guidance to inject a sclerosing agent into varicose veins. This office procedure is usually performed on large veins that are not visible through the skin.

S2205-S2209

S2205 Minimally invasive direct coronary artery bypass surgery involving mini-thoracotomy or mini-sternotomy surgery, performed under direct vision; using arterial graft(s), single coronary arterial graft

S2206 Minimally invasive direct coronary artery bypass surgery involving mini-thoracotomy or mini-sternotomy surgery, performed under direct vision; using arterial graft(s), two coronary arterial grafts

S2207 Minimally invasive direct coronary artery bypass surgery involving mini-thoracotomy or mini-sternotomy surgery, performed under direct vision; using venous graft only, single coronary venous graft

S2208 Minimally invasive direct coronary artery bypass surgery involving mini-thoracotomy or mini-sternotomy surgery, performed under direct vision; using single arterial and venous graft(s), single venous graft

S2209 Minimally invasive direct coronary artery bypass surgery involving mini-thoracotomy or mini-sternotomy surgery, performed under direct vision; using two arterial grafts and single venous graft

Unlike traditional coronary artery bypass graft (CABG) where the breast bone is divided and the patient is placed on a cardiopulmonary bypass machine to pump blood through the body, minimally invasive direct coronary artery bypass (MIDCAB) surgery is performed through a small, 2 to 5 inch incision between the ribs and does not require use of the bypass machine. A graft is connected to a diseased coronary vessel on a beating heart. MIDCAB surgery results in quicker recovery time, shorter length of stay, less infection rate, smaller incision scar, and less bleeding and blood trauma.

S2225

S2225 Myringotomy, laser-assisted

A laser-assisted myringotomy is performed. A myringotomy is a surgical procedure in which an incision is made in the eardrum to relieve pressure or drain fluid. A laser-assisted procedure uses a laser to create the opening in the eardrum rather than a surgical incision. The laser is less invasive and requires only topical anesthesia.

S2230

S2230 Implantation of magnetic component of semi-implantable hearing device on ossicles in middle ear

Semi-implantable hearing aids have been developed as another option to the external acoustic hearing aids. The semi-implantable hearing device consists of a magnetic component that is implanted in the ossicles of the middle ear, a receiver, and a sound processor. The sound vibrations are received and amplified by the sound processor. These sound pressures are transformed into electrical signals, which are received by the receiver unit. The receiver unit then converts the electrical signals into electromagnetic energy, creating an electromagnetic field with the magnetic component that is implanted on the ossicles. The electromagnetic field causes vibration of the middle ear bones, which is similar to normal vibrations. Use this code to report the implantation of the magnetic component.

S2235

S2235 Implantation of auditory brain stem implant

An auditory brain implant (ABI) is used for patients who have neurofibromatosis type 2, a rare disease in which cranial nerve tumors must be surgically excised. The excision of these auditory cranial nerves requires severing of the nerves and results in complete loss of hearing. In order to restore some sound, an ABI is done. This system includes a receiver/stimulator, a speech processor (pocket sized) that is worn on the body, and a microphone/headset. The receiver/stimulator is implanted behind the ear during surgery. A series of electrodes are implanted into the brainstem. A wire leads from the implanted receiver/stimulator to the implanted electrodes. The speech processor and microphone/headset pick up the sound, which is then changed to electrical impulses and sent to the receiver/stimulator. These impulses travel down the wire to the electrodes and the area that normally receives the electrical signal from the ear is stimulated.

S2260-S2267

S2260 Induced abortion, 17 to 24 weeks

S2265 Induced abortion, 25 to 28 weeks

S2266 Induced abortion, 29 to 31 weeks

S2267 Induced abortion, 32 weeks or greater

An induced abortion is the intentional termination of a pregnancy before the fetus is viable. The abortion may be done for therapeutic reasons or as an elective procedure, and is accomplished with the use of medication or instrumentation. The type of abortion performed can vary depending upon the age of the fetus.

S2300

S2300 Arthroscopy, shoulder, surgical; with thermally-induced capsulorrhaphy

Thermal capsulorrhaphy (TC), also known as thermal capsular shrinkage, is a technique developed to treat shoulder instability. Heat is used to shrink and tighten the connective tissue around the shoulder joint (shoulder capsule). TC was developed to achieve a less invasive treatment for shoulders that are frequently dislocated. TC was originally accomplished with the use of laser. Now, however, the use of radiofrequency is more commonly used in the procedure. This procedure is considered investigational and not covered by most insurance companies.

S2325

S2325 Hip core decompression

The physician performs a hip core decompression of the femoral head. Hip core decompression is used in the treatment of osteonecrosis in patients with small-sized to medium-sized precollapse lesions of the femoral head. Hip core decompression relieves pressure within the rigid structure of the femoral head, thereby relieving joint pain. An incision is made over the femoral head. The soft tissues are divided. Next, one of two techniques may be used to perform the hip core decompression, which involves drilling a small hole or holes in the diseased bone. Using the more traditional technique, a hole is drilled in line with the axis of the femoral neck at the point where the lateral cortex begins to thicken. An 8 to 10 mm wide reamer is used to over-ream the drill hole. A second, newer technique utilizes a 3 mm Steinman pin to create multiple small drill holes in the diseased bone of the femoral head. Surgical instruments are then removed. The surgical area is flushed with normal saline and the incision is closed.

S2340-S2341

S2340 Chemodenervation of abductor muscle(s) of vocal cord

S2341 Chemodenervation of adductor muscle(s) of vocal cord

Chemodenervation is performed of the abductor muscle (S2340) of the vocal cord or the adductor muscle (S2341) of the vocal cord. Chemodenervation is the injection of a pharmacological compound into a nerve to paralyze a muscle or group of muscles. Abductor muscles open and adductor muscles close the vocal folds in the larynx. Chemodenervation of the vocal cord muscles is used to treat spasmodic dysphonia, a condition producing a variety of unusual vocal sounds. There are two main types of spasmodic dysphonia: adductor and abductor. The most common is the adductor type and it results in a strained-strangled sound, producing multiple voice breaks or pitch. Abductor spasmodic dysphonia is a "mirror image" of the adductor type. The vocal folds spasm open and create an involuntary moment of no voice, as well as a weak, breathy voice. The injection of botulinum toxin type A is used to treat both types.

S2342

S2342 Nasal endoscopy for postoperative debridement following functional endoscopic sinus surgery, nasal and/or sinus cavity(s), unilateral or bilateral

Postoperative debridement may be reported for the limited removal of debris, crust, or secretions from the nasal and/or sinus cavity using straight forceps, irrigation, or suction requiring topical anesthesia.

S2348

S2348 Decompression procedure, percutaneous, of nucleus pulposus of intervertebral disc, using radiofrequency energy, single or multiple levels, lumbar

In a typical herniated disc, the annulus fibrosis opens and the nucleus pulposus protrudes and compresses the nerves. Radiofrequency decompression is minimally invasive and was developed as a treatment for patients with low back pain due to herniated disc disease. Under fluoroscopic guidance, a small needle is inserted into the nucleus pulposus of the herniated disc. Radiofrequency is then applied to ablate the tissue and reduce the nucleus pulposus. This procedure is considered experimental and may not be reimbursed by many insurance companies.

S2350-S2351

S2350 Diskectomy, anterior, with decompression of spinal cord and/or nerve root(s), including osteophytectomy; lumbar, single interspace

S2351 Diskectomy, anterior, with decompression of spinal cord and/or nerve root(s), including osteophytectomy; lumbar, each additional interspace (list separately in addition to code for primary procedure)

The physician performs a lumbar discectomy to remove all or part of a herniated intervertebral disc. The patient is placed supine position. The physician makes a transverse incision in the abdominal wall overlying the intervertebral disc. Dissection and careful retraction of the abdominal contents is carried out to the disc. The physician excises the anterior anulus of the disc and uses pituitary forceps to remove as much disc material as possible. A spreader and microscope are used to enhance the evacuation. A drill is used to remove the transverse bar above and below. Graft material is obtained from the ilium and fashioned to fit into the space. The graft is placed into the disc space and traction is released. The muscles fall back into place and the incision is closed with layered sutures.

S2400

S2400 Repair, congenital diaphragmatic hernia in the fetus using temporary tracheal occlusion, procedure performed in utero

A congenital diaphragmatic hernia (CDH) is a birth defect or hole in the diaphragm that permits abdominal contents to pass into the chest cavity. Lung tissue on the affected side usually cannot develop completely. Temporary tracheal occlusion is a blocking of the trachea with the insertion of operative clips or balloons through a fetoscope. This prevents the normal outflow of fluid from the fetus' lungs, which can result in a buildup of secretions. Since this buildup of secretions increases the lung size, the abdominal viscera is gradually forced out of the lung cavity and back into the abdominal cavity. During delivery, the occlusive devices are removed from the trachea. Repair of the diaphragmatic hernia is completed after birth.

S2401

S2401 Repair, urinary tract obstruction in the fetus, procedure performed in utero

Bilateral urinary tract obstruction can lead to distention of the bladder and is often associated with pulmonary hyperplasia. The treatment goal is to assure adequate amniotic fluid volume for the development of the lungs, and to protect the kidneys from increased pressure. A stent or shunt is placed percutaneously to achieve decompression. This procedure allows the urine from the fetus to flow into the amniotic space and bypass the urinary tract. Coverage is based on the type of obstruction among other criteria.

S2402-S2403

S2402 Repair, congenital cystic adenomatoid malformation in the fetus, procedure performed in utero

S2403 Repair, extralobar pulmonary sequestration in the fetus, procedure performed in utero

Congenital cystic adenomatoid malformation (CCAM) is the most common of the congenital pulmonary anomalies. The CCAM cystic lesions, which are identified as overgrowth of the terminal respiratory bronchioles, are normally found in only one part of the lung. Extralobar pulmonary sequestration (EPS) is commonly identified as masses of lung tissue that is not functioning. The extra lobar sections of lung tissue are not connected to the main tracheobronchial system, are drained by the pulmonary venous system, and are mainly supplied by anomalous artery arising from the aorta. Repair of both of these conditions is usually performed by an open in utero resection of the malformed tissue or placement of a shunt (thoracic to amniotic) in cases of large cystic lesions. Coverage of in utero repair is questionable for both conditions.

S2404

S2404 Repair, myelomeningocele in the fetus, procedure performed in utero

The physician repairs a myelomeningocele in a fetus. Myelomeningocele (MMC) is a developmental disorder caused by incomplete closing of the neural tube. It is the most significant, common cause of spina bifida. The spinal cord develops abnormally and is left open, resulting in the protrusion of a spinal cord sac, which is filled with cerebrospinal fluid. MMC results in disorders to the cerebrospinal fluid circulation, brain malformation, impairment to bowel and legs and bladder function, and cognitive impairment. In utero surgery to cover or repair the exposed spinal cord sac is thought to improve neurologic function but is considered experimental. Coverage is dependent on the insurance payer.

S2405

S2405 Repair of sacrococcygeal teratoma in the fetus, procedure performed in utero

The physician repairs a sacrococcygeal teratoma in the fetus. Sacrococcygeal teratoma (SCT) is an encapsulated neoplasm composed of germ cells that is located at the base of the coccyx. It is usually not malignant and is the most common newborn tumor. If the tumor is accompanied by fetal edema, the condition is rapidly progressive and commonly fatal.

S2409

S2409 Repair, congenital malformation of fetus, procedure performed in utero, not otherwise classified

The physician repairs a congenital malformation of the fetus. Most fetal malformations are handled after birth. However, there are some conditions that are considered prudent and safe to perform in utero. Report code for conditions not identified by another code.

S2411

S2411 Fetoscopic laser therapy for treatment of twin-to-twin transfusion syndrome

The physician performs fetoscopic laser therapy for treatment of twin-to-twin transfusion syndrome. Twin-to-twin transfusion syndrome (TTTS) is only found in identical twins that share the same placenta. Usually, the connections are balanced and the blood flows in both directions equally. However, if the connections are not balanced and one fetus (donor) is losing or donating blood to the other fetus (recipient), the donor receives insufficient nutrients and becomes dehydrated. Conversely, the recipient becomes overly large and the amniotic sac fills with excessive fluid and the recipient can develop heart failure when the extra blood volume becomes too excessive. Treatment for TTTS consists of in utero serial reductions of amniotic fluid and/or the use of fetoscopic laser photocoagulation. The laser photocoagulation is done in the OR under local, spinal, or general anesthesia. The fetoscope is placed into the uterus through a tiny incision and the laser is used to seal the blood vessels on the surface of the placenta. This restores the balance of blood and nutrients flowing to the fetuses.

S2900

S2900 Surgical techniques requiring use of robotic surgical system (list separately in addition to code for primary procedure)

A robotic surgical system is used, which utilizes 3-D cameras and miniature instruments to enable the surgeon to make smaller incisions and work more accurately. The surgeon is always in control but has the use of robotic tools to magnify and optimize the view, as well as guiding the surgeon's hands to achieve accurate results. The FDA has cleared two robotic systems for use in certain circumstances and for certain purposes. When using the da Vinci Surgical System, the surgeon sits at a console located several feet from the operating table. The robot has hands attached to a free standing cart. One of the hands holds the camera that has been inserted into the patient. The ZEUS Robotic Surgical System has three arms that are mounted on the operating table. Two of the arms are the extension of the surgeon's right and left arms, and the other holds the endoscope and is voice activated and responds to the surgeon's commands. The surgeon sits at a console and wears special 3-D glasses.

S3000

S3000 Diabetic indicator; retinal eye exam, dilated, bilateral

A dilated retinal eye exam performed on a patient with undiagnosed diabetes may reveal bleeding of the small blood vessels of the eye. Since these vessels are highly sensitive to the toxicity of hyperglycemia, this is frequently an indicator of the presence of the diabetes. Use this code to report a bilateral exam.

S3005

S3005 Performance measurement, evaluation of patient self assessment, depression

A patient depression self assessment is a list of questions or symptoms to which a patient responds. The patient rates his feelings or thoughts on specific issues, including thoughts of suicide, concentration, eating, and irritability. Patient responses are evaluated by a mental health professional to determine the patient's state of mind.

S3600-S3601

S3600 STAT laboratory request (situations other than S3601)

S3601 Emergency STAT laboratory charge for patient who is homebound or residing in a nursing facility

A stat laboratory request indicates that all possible speed and prioritization should be used to procure, analyze, and report the results of the specimen. The results of the stat requests are necessary for an immediate critical or therapeutic decision.

S3620

S3620 Newborn metabolic screening panel, includes test kit, postage and the laboratory tests specified by the state for inclusion in this panel (e.g., galactose; hemoglobin, electrophoresis; hydroxyprogesterone, 17-d; phenylalanine (PKU); and thyroxine, total)

Newborn screening is done on all newborns for certain metabolic, genetic, and endocrine disorders. It can identify infants who may possibly be at risk for one of the disorders that are within the screening panel. The tests included in the panel are based on state requirements. These tests are considered screening tests only. Additional testing is required to determine if an infant truly has one of the conditions identified in the screening.

S3630

S3630 Eosinophil count, blood, direct

Eosinophil granulocytes are white blood cells that are part of the immune system that battle parasites and infections and regulate inflammation. The granules within their cytoplasm contain many chemical mediators that are released while the eosinophil is activated. These chemical mediators are toxic to the parasite and to the host. Eosinophil granulocytes are generally found in the GI tract, ovary, uterus, spleen, and lymph nodes. When present in the lungs, skin, or esophagus, they may signal disease.

S3645

S3645 HIV-1 antibody testing of oral mucosal transudate

The HIV antibody testing of oral mucosal transudate is an alternative to a standard blood test. A specially treated pad is placed in the mouth and rubbed between the lower cheek and the individual's gum. The pad collects oral mucosal transudate, which contains HIV antibodies in a person infected with HIV. It does not test for HIV in the saliva.

S3650

S3650 Saliva test, hormone level; during menopause

Salivary hormone test measures the biologically active component of female hormones in the bloodstream. There are some that use this test to determine the female hormone levels in women prior to initiation of hormone replacement therapy. The test was developed as a means to monitor the titration of an individual's hormone dosage.

S3652

S3652 Saliva test, hormone level; to assess preterm labor risk

Preterm labor is birth of an infant at less than 37 weeks gestation. One of the tests to predict preterm labor is the salivary estriol test. Estriol levels have been known to increase significantly two to four weeks prior to the onset of labor. The test is usually done with a 24-hour urine or serial blood collection. Salivary estriol has been used as a predictor of late preterm birth. Since late preterm birth has low neonatal morbidity rates, the test is rarely used and considered investigational.

S3655

S3655 Antisperm antibodies test (immunobead)

The presence of antibodies in the sperm may be a cause or contributing factor to infertility. Although sperm antibodies may be measured by a variety of techniques, the direct immunobead test (dIBT) is the method of choice. The test is based on the rosette formation between the viable sperm and the plastic beads coated with antiserum to human immunoglobulins. This enables the analysis of class-specific antibodies (IgM, IgA, or IgG) and their site of attachment (e.g., tail, head).

S3708

S3708 Gastrointestinal fat absorption study

A gastrointestinal fat absorption study is a diagnostic test for fat malabsorption. Fat is a valuable nutrient digested by enzymes in the small intestine. The simplest test involves the staining and examination under a microscope of a random fecal specimen.

S3722

S3722 Dose optimization by area under the curve (AUC) analysis, for infusional 5-fluorouracil

This code describes a laboratory test to determine 5-FU plasma levels for patients with colorectal cancer who are being treated with the drug. It allows more precise and accurate dosing than the body surface area methodology used to calculate doses. The information from the test allows the physician to avoid toxic levels and administered optimal levels of 5-FU to the patient to reach the target range. The assay is competitive homogenous two-reagent nanoparticle agglutination immunoassay. It is a unique service that quickly delivers quantitative 5-FU AUC results to the oncologist. This allows the physician to adjust the dose for each treatment cycle to make sure it is in the correct therapeutic range.

S3800

S3800 Genetic testing for amyotrophic lateral sclerosis (ALS)

A genetic disorder is a disease caused in whole or in part by a mutation of a gene. Genetic tests attempt to identify abnormalities in an individual's genes, which include the presence or absence of key proteins whose production is directed by specific genes. Amyotrophic lateral sclerosis (ALS) is a progressive neurodegenerative disease that affects nerve cells in the brain and spinal column. Motor neurons extend from the brain to the spinal column and from the spinal column to muscles. The progressive degeneration of these motor neurons eventually leads to their death and the loss of muscle control. It is estimated that only a very small percentage of ALS, less than 10 percent, is inherited.

S3840

S3840 DNA analysis for germline mutations of the RET proto-oncogene for susceptibility to multiple endocrine neoplasia type 2

DNA analysis is the study of genes or DNA and is used to detect a genetic alteration that is associated with a specific disorder. A germline mutation is a detectable and heritable variation in germ cells that can create mutations in every cell of the offspring. This code describes the DNA analysis of the RET proto-oncogene for the susceptibility of the patient to multiple endocrine neoplasia type 2 (MEN2). MEN2 is a group of medical disorders that include pheochromocytoma, medullary thyroid carcinoma, parathyroid hyperplasia, and mucocutaneous neuroma.

S3841-S3842

S3841 Genetic testing for retinoblastoma

S3842 Genetic testing for Von Hippel-Lindau disease

A genetic disorder is a disease caused in whole or in part by a mutation of a gene. Genetic tests attempt to identify abnormalities in an individual's genes, which include the presence or absence of key proteins whose production is directed by specific genes. Retinoblastoma is a rare type of eye cancer that develops in the retina, usually before the age of 5. Von Hippel-Lindau disease is a rare genetic disorder that arises from a mutation in the von Hippel-Lindau tumor suppressor gene. In this disorder, tumors form in different areas of the brain and body. The tumors may be benign or malignant.

S3844

S3844 DNA analysis of the connexin 26 gene (GJB2) for susceptibility to congenital, profound deafness

DNA analysis and the study of genes is used to detect a genetic alteration associated with a specific disorder. Connexins are gap junction proteins. Gap junctions are specialized intracellular connections between the cytoplasm of two cells that are essential for many physiologic functions. Connexin 26 is a mutation in gene GJB2 that leads to Vohwinkel syndrome as well as keratitis-ichthyosis-deafness syndrome. Vohwinkel syndrome is a mutilating keratoderma disorder with some mild to moderate hearing loss. Keratitis-ichthyosis-deafness syndrome is a disorder characterized by corneal opacification, mild generalized hyperkeratosis or erythematous plaques, and neurosensory deafness.

S3845-S3846

S3845 Genetic testing for alpha-thalassemia

S3846 Genetic testing for hemoglobin E beta-thalassemia

Genetic testing is used to determine mutations or variances in genes that may be responsible for certain conditions or diseases. Genetic testing for thalassemia is usually done by taking a blood sample and looking for mutations in the gene cluster causing the condition. Thalassemia is an inherited disorder that impacts the production of hemoglobin and includes a number of different types of anemia. The number of genes that are affected determines the severity and type of anemia. All types of thalassemia have three components: heme, alpha globin, and beta globin. Thalassemia results in no synthesis or a reduced rate of synthesis of one of the globin chains that make up thalassemia, which can cause abnormal hemoglobin molecules to form. Anemia is usually the only symptom of thalassemia. Alpha thalassemia includes disorders of the alpha hemoglobin chain. Beta thalassemia affects the beta hemoglobin chain.

S3849

S3849 Genetic testing for Niemann-Pick disease

Genetic testing for Niemann-Pick disease is performed. Genetic testing is used to determine mutations or variances in genes that may be responsible for certain conditions or diseases. Niemann-Pick disease is a group of diseases characterized by a buildup of lipids in the brain, liver, and spleen. There are four main types of this disease: A, B, C, and D. Each type can cause different symptoms and affect different organs. Types A and B are diagnosed through a blood test or bone marrow sample to measure the amount of acid sphingomyelin (found in every cell of the body) in the white blood cells. Types B and C are usually tested with a skin biopsy, which is used to study how the cells move and store cholesterol. A sphingomyelinase assay may also be done.

S3850

S3850 Genetic testing for sickle cell anemia

Genetic testing for sickle cell anemia is performed. Genetic testing is used to determine mutations or variances in genes that may be responsible for certain conditions or diseases. Sickle cell anemia is caused by mutations of the HBB gene. Hemoglobin is made up of four units of protein: 2 subunits called alpha-globin and 2 subunits called beta-globin. The HBB gene is responsible for providing direction for making beta-globin. Different versions of beta-globin result from different mutations of the HBB gene. At least one of the beta-globin hemoglobin subunits is replaced with hemoglobin S in sickle cell anemia. In sickle cell anemia, the normally round red blood cells are shaped like a sickle, or crescent moon. These sickle-shaped cells get stuck in the capillaries, can't carry oxygen as well and can damage muscles, bones, and organs. These sickle-shaped cells are destroyed by the body at a more rapid rate than normal blood cells, resulting in anemia. Testing is done through a blood test. It may also be performed through amniocentesis.

S3852

S3852 DNA analysis for APOE epsilon 4 allele for susceptibility to Alzheimer's disease

A DNA analysis for APOE epsilon 4 allele for susceptibility to Alzheimer's disease is performed. Genetic testing is used to determine mutations or variances in genes that may be responsible for certain conditions or diseases. The APOE lipoprotein is a carrier of the cholesterol that is produced in the brain cells and liver. The APOE gene has three alleles (Epsilon 2, 3, and 4). An individual carries two of the APOE alleles. When at least one of epsilons four allele is present, the risk of developing Alzheimer's disease (AD) is 1.2 to 3 times greater depending on the ethnic group. Genetic testing as a diagnostic technique for patients with AD symptoms is considered investigational and not covered by most insurance companies.

S3853

S3853 Genetic testing for myotonic muscular dystrophy

Genetic testing for myotonic muscular dystrophy is performed. Genetic testing is used to determine mutations or variances in genes that may be responsible for certain conditions or diseases and is the definitive test for myotonic dystrophy. Myotonic dystrophy type 1 is caused by DMPK gene mutations. Myotonic dystrophy type 2 is caused from mutations in the CNBP gene. Mutations in each of these genes involve a small segment of DNA that is abnormally repeated many times. This abnormality forms an unstable area of the gene. The resulting changes keep cells in the muscles and other tissues from normal function. Screening for the type 1 locates the specific area on chromosome 19 and measures the size of the DNA expansion. The genetic test for type 2 was developed to measure and isolate the size of the DNA expansion on chromosome 3.

S3854

S3854 Gene expression profiling panel for use in the management of breast cancer treatment

Genetic testing is used to determine mutations or variances in genes that may be responsible for certain conditions or diseases. As a tool to predict the baseline risk of the recurrence of breast cancer after hormonal therapy, surgery, and radiation therapy, several panels of gene expression markers, known as "signatures," have been developed. These are used to aid in the determination of recurrence risk and can help in the decision-making process for patients who prefer to avoid chemotherapy.

S3861

S3861 Genetic testing, sodium channel, voltage-gated, type V, alpha subunit (SCN5A) and variants for suspected Brugada Syndrome

Brugada syndrome is an inherited arrhythmia disorder that causes ventricular fibrillation and increases the risk of sudden cardiac death. Episodes of ventricular tachycardia exist showing a pattern of right bundle branch block and ST segment elevation. Fainting or black-outs can accompany the ventricular fibrillation. A cardiodefibrillator can be implanted to shock the heart back into rhythm. The disease primarily affects males. Several mutations in the gene SCN5A, which encodes for the cardiac sodium channel, have been linked to this syndrome.

S3865-S3866

S3865 Comprehensive gene sequence analysis for hypertrophic cardiomyopathy

S3866 Genetic analysis for a specific gene mutation for hypertrophic cardiomyopathy (HCM) in an individual with a known HCM mutation in the family

A genetic disorder is a disease caused in whole or in part by a mutation of a gene. Genetic disorders can be passed on to family members who inherit the genetic abnormality. Genetic testing can be predictive, used to confirm a diagnosis, or used to determine if a person is a carrier for the disease. Hypertrophic cardiomyopathy (HCM) is a disorder where a portion of the myocardium becomes thickened without any obvious cause. The disorder is a leading cause of sudden cardiac death. In HCM, the sarcomeres or contractile elements replicate causing the muscle cells to increase in size and thicken the heart wall. The normal alignment of the muscle cells is disrupted creating myocardial disarray and the electrical heart functions are disrupted. HCM is most commonly due to a mutation in one of the nine sarcomeric genes resulting in mutated proteins.

S3870

S3870 Comparative genomic hybridization (CGH) microarray testing for developmental delay, autism spectrum disorder and/or intellectual disability

Genetic variations are often seen with developmental delay and other disorders. Standard cytogenetic analysis detects visible chromosomal alterations, such as an extra chromosome band, but smaller defects could not be reliably found. Improvements in molecular cytogenetics have enabled new more accurate and sensitive tests. Array CGH (comparative genome hybridization) is designed to detect cytogenetic imbalances that are smaller than what can be detected through routine chromosome analysis. Probes are used on glass slides as arrays to hybridize a differentially labeled patient and normal DNA. The result is an identification of changes throughout the genome. They are arranged to correspond to genes that are known to affect development. The test will detect loss or duplication of chromosomes on the array.

S3900

S3900 Surface electromyography (EMG)

Surface electromyography is a non-invasive procedure in which surface electrodes, or a scanner containing electrodes, are placed on the skin to determine the overall muscle function and condition. A surface EMG is often considered not as accurate as the needle EMG.

S3902

S3902 Ballistocardiogram

Ballistocardiogram is a graphic recording that determines the blood volume that passes through the heart during a specific time frame, as well as the force of the contraction of the heart. It measures the body's recoil with each heartbeat as the blood is ejected from the ventricle.

S3904

S3904 Masters two step

The Masters 2 step is used to test for coronary insufficiency. It is accomplished by the patient climbing up and down two nine inch high steps while an electrocardiogram records the cardiac activity both during the exercise and at specific time intervals after the exercise is completed.

S4005

S4005 Interim labor facility global (labor occurring but not resulting in delivery)

This code is reported by a facility to identify services rendered to a patient in labor who was transferred to another facility for the delivery.

S4011

S4011 In vitro fertilization; including but not limited to identification and incubation of mature oocytes, fertilization with sperm, incubation of embryo(s), and subsequent visualization for determination of development

The in vitro fertilization (IVF) process is the fertilization of the egg by the sperm outside of the woman's body. After the eggs have been retrieved by the physician from the woman's ovary, the retrieved eggs are examined and the most promising ones are placed in an IVF culture medium. The father's sperm is then separated from his semen and the most mobile sperm are added to the eggs and placed in an incubator. The sperm cell penetrates an egg, usually within a very short time, and fertilizes it. The following day, fertilization is confirmed if the physician sees two pronuclei. Approximately two days after fertilization, a 2-4 cell zygote will appear, becoming an embryo when it divides. Most embryos are observed for two to four days to determine if they are developing normally and qualify to be placed in the uterus. Report this code for in vitro fertilization, including but not limited to identification and incubation of mature oocytes, fertilization with sperm, incubation of embryo(s), and subsequent visualization for determination of development.

S4013-S4014

S4013 Complete cycle, gamete intrafallopian transfer (GIFT), case rate

S4014 Complete cycle, zygote intrafallopian transfer (ZIFT), case rate

In gamete intrafallopian transfer (GIFT) (S4013), the physician mixes previously captured eggs with sperm and draws the mixture into a catheter. The catheter is passed through the cervix and uterus and into the tubes or passed through an abdominal incision and directly into the fimbrial end of the fallopian tube. The physician deposits the eggs and sperm in the tubes, permitting fertilization. In a zygote intrafallopian transfer (ZIFT) (S4014), a physician draws an already fertilized egg into a catheter. The catheter is passed through the cervix and uterus and into the tube where the egg is deposited. GIFT is a one-step procedure while ZIFT is a two-step process. In ZIFT, the egg is collected and fertilized and transferred to the fallopian tube at a later time. GIFT and ZIFT can be done laparoscopically or hysteroscopically.

S4015-S4021

S4015 Complete in vitro fertilization cycle, not otherwise specified, case rate

S4016 Frozen in vitro fertilization cycle, case rate

S4017 Incomplete cycle, treatment cancelled prior to stimulation, case rate

S4018 Frozen embryo transfer procedure cancelled before transfer, case rate

S4020 In vitro fertilization procedure cancelled before aspiration, case rate

S4021 In vitro fertilization procedure cancelled after aspiration, case rate

The in vitro fertilization (IVF) process is the fertilization of the egg by the sperm outside of the woman's body. The physician then implants the fertilized egg in the woman's uterus. An IVF cycle usually takes four to six weeks and the process may have to be done more than once to result in a pregnancy. There are five steps to IVF: (1) Ovarian stimulation: Usually done with fertility drugs, ovarian stimulation takes eight to 14 days. This usually involves the fertilization of more than one egg since not all will develop. The physician may take blood tests and use ultrasound to determine which eggs are ready for the next step. (2) Egg retrieval: The physician performs a transvaginal ultrasound aspiration once the eggs are ready for retrieval. With the use of a mild sedative or other form of anesthesia, the physician inserts a needle into the follicles in the ovary, and removes the eggs with suction. The physician may use a laparoscope if the ovaries cannot be accessed. (3) Insemination: The retrieved eggs are examined and the most promising

S

ones are placed in an IVF culture medium. The father's sperm is then separated from his semen and the most mobile sperm are added to the eggs and placed in an incubator. (4) Fertilization and embryo culture: The sperm cell penetrates an egg, usually within a very short time, and fertilizes it. The following day, fertilization is confirmed if the physician sees two pronuclei. Approximately two days after fertilization, a two to four cell zygote appears, becoming an embryo when it divides. Most embryos are observed for two to four days to determine if they are developing normally and then placed in the uterus. (5) Embryo transfer: Approximately two to three days after fertilization, the embryo is transferred to the uterus. To do this, the physician suspends them in a drop of fluid and draws it into a catheter. The physician then guides the catheter into the uterus. The patient is usually told to rest for one to two hours to prevent any undue stress on her body. A positive pregnancy test results when the embryo attaches to the uterine wall.

S4022

S4022 Assisted oocyte fertilization, case rate

An oocyte is a human female germ cell involved in reproduction (an immature human egg cell). After the eggs have been retrieved by the physician from the woman's ovary, the retrieved eggs are examined and the most promising ones are retrieved. Sperm is then separated from semen and the most mobile sperm are added to the eggs. An assisted fertilization typically involves the injection into the cytoplasm of the egg.

S4023

S4023 Donor egg cycle, incomplete, case rate

The in vitro fertilization (IVF) cycle usually takes four to six weeks. There are five steps to IVF. This code represents two of these steps. 1) Ovarian stimulation: Usually done with fertility drugs, ovarian stimulation takes eight to 14 days. This usually involves the fertilization of more than one egg since not all will develop. The physician may take blood tests and use ultrasound to determine which eggs are ready for the next step. 2) Egg retrieval: The physician performs a transvaginal ultrasound aspiration once the eggs are ready for retrieval. With the use of a mild sedative or other form of anesthesia, the physician inserts a needle into the follicles in the ovary and removes the eggs with suction. The physician may use a laparoscope if the ovaries cannot be accessed.

S4025

S4025 Donor services for in vitro fertilization (sperm or embryo), case rate

The in vitro fertilization (IVF) process is the fertilization of the egg by the sperm outside of the woman's body. The physician then implants the fertilized egg in the woman's uterus. This code represents the management of the services rendered to an egg or sperm donor.

S4026

S4026 Procurement of donor sperm from sperm bank

The in vitro fertilization (IVF) process is the fertilization of the egg by the sperm outside of the woman's body. The physician then implants the fertilized egg in the woman's uterus. This code represents charges for obtaining the sperm from a sperm bank.

S4027

S4027 Storage of previously frozen embryos

Women who undergo fertility treatment often produce numerous eggs that are fertilized but not all implanted. Embryos can be frozen and stored for implant at a later time. The embryos are cryogenically frozen and stored in carefully regulated tanks at a tissue bank until the woman is ready to attempt a pregnancy.

S4028

S4028 Microsurgical epididymal sperm aspiration (MESA)

A microsurgical epididymal sperm aspiration (MESA) is a procedure to retrieve sperm from a man who has a blockage in the reproductive system. A small incision is made in the scrotum and an operating microscope is used to identify the epididymis. The epididymis is a small tube where sperm is concentrated and stored. It is dilated and the fluid is aspirated and examined for the presence of sperm. If sperm is not present, a sample is aspirated from another tubule and examined. If sperm is identified it is processed to use immediately and can be frozen to be used later.

S4030-S4031

S4030 Sperm procurement and cryopreservation services; initial visit

S4031 Sperm procurement and cryopreservation services; subsequent visit

Sperm can be collected and preserved to be used later for artificial insemination. Donors can be someone known to the woman or couple or an anonymous donor. Men who are undergoing treatment that may affect fertility may also freeze sperm for later use. Anonymous sperm donors may sign a contract with a sperm bank to donate a certain number of weeks for a specified length of time. Once the specimen is obtained, it is evaluated and mixed with a substance to protect it during freezing. The sperm are placed in vials and cryopreserved with nitrogen vapor. The frozen vials are placed in liquid nitrogen and stored in cryogenic tanks at a temperature of -196°C (-321°F).

S4035

S4035 Stimulated intrauterine insemination (IUI), case rate

Intrauterine insemination (IUI) is a form of assisted conception. It is the placement of active washed sperm into the uterus at the time that an egg is released. Fertilization occurs within the uterus. Stimulated IUI uses hormones to cause eggs to be released. The sperm is placed in the uterus to coincide with ovulation.

S4037

S4037 Cryopreserved embryo transfer, case rate

This code reports the last stage of a complete in vitro fertilization cycle. During the IVF process, multiple embryos are frozen or cryopreserved for future use. This code represents the transfer of a thawed embryo into a uterus.

S4040

S4040 Monitoring and storage of cryopreserved embryos, per 30 days

Women who undergo fertility treatment often produce numerous eggs that are fertilized but not all implanted. Embryos can be frozen and stored for implant at a later time. The embryos are cryogenically frozen and stored in carefully regulated tanks at a tissue bank until the woman is ready to attempt a pregnancy.

S4042

S4042 Management of ovulation induction (interpretation of diagnostic tests and studies, nonface-to-face medical management of the patient), per cycle

This code reports the first of five in vitro fertilization (IVF) steps. Tests and studies are undertaken to determine if the woman has viable eggs that can be fertilized. Ovarian stimulation, usually done with fertility drugs, takes eight to 14 days. When the mature eggs are ready to be released, either sperm will be placed in the uterus or the eggs will be retrieved for in vitro fertilization.

S4981

S4981 Insertion of levonorgestrel-releasing intrauterine system

Levonorgestrel-releasing intrauterine system is a hormone-releasing system that is used to prevent pregnancy and works for up to five years. It is inserted into the uterus where it delivers a low dose of progesterone directly into the uterus lining. Use this code to report the insertion of the system.

S4989

S4989 Contraceptive intrauterine device (e.g., Progestacert IUD), including implants and supplies

Contraceptive intrauterine devices (IUD) prevent pregnancy by inhibiting fertilization of the egg. Although not entirely known, it is believed that the IUDs affect the way the sperm and egg move and/or affect the lining of the uterus to prevent implantation of the egg. These devices may be a loop, triangle, T-shape, or a coil. The IUD is inserted into the uterus. This code includes the implant and supplies.

S4990-S4991

S4990 Nicotine patches, legend

S4991 Nicotine patches, nonlegend

Nicotine patches are press-on, transdermal patches that release nicotine slowly through the skin. It is a nicotine replacement therapy. The patches help individuals to cope with withdrawal symptoms while they are trying to quit smoking by providing nicotine without the harmful effects from smoke. A legend drug is one that requires a prescription. Non-legend or over-the-counter drugs do not require a prescription.

S4993

S4993 Contraceptive pills for birth control

Birth control pills are oral contraceptives that are taken on a daily basis. Most of these pills contain synthetic estrogen and progestin. The hormones in the pills suppress the pituitary gland to inhibit the development and/or release of the egg, as well as help to prevent sperm from reaching the egg. The mini pill or progestin only pill works by suppressing ovulation and helps to prevent the sperm from reaching the egg.

S4995

S4995 Smoking cessation gum

Nicotine gum is a drug in chewing gum form to aid people in smoking cessation. Small amounts of nicotine are released from the gum, which when absorbed by the body, cuts down on the withdrawal symptoms. It is a nicotine replacement therapy. The individual is cautioned to chew very slowly until a tingling is felt in the mouth and then to hold the gum between the cheek and gum until the tingle is gone. Chew again a few more times until the tingle is felt and then move the gum to another part of the mouth. This should be repeated for 30 minutes. It is estimated that about 3 mg of nicotine is absorbed from a 4 mg piece of gum.

S5000-S5001

S5000 Prescription drug, generic

S5001 Prescription drug, brand name

A generic drug refers to the chemical name of the drug. Although generic drugs are chemically the same as the brand name of the drug, they are usually less expensive. The brand name drug has a trade name. It can only be produced and sold by the company that holds the patent. Brand name drugs may be available over the counter or by prescription only.

S5010

S5010 5% dextrose and 0.45% normal saline, 1000 ml

This code reports a 5% dextrose solution in half amount of normal saline. A 5% dextrose and 0.45% normal saline is a hypotonic fluid replacement that is used to replace fluid when some sodium is required in patients that are not able to maintain adequate oral intake or are restricted from doing so. It hydrates the cells and releases fluid from the vessels. Possible side effects are hypernatremia and circulatory overload.

S5012

S5012 5% dextrose with potassium chloride, 1000 ml

Potassium chloride in 5% dextrose solution is a sterile, nonpyrogenic solution that is used to replace fluid, electrolytes, and calories in patients that are not able to maintain adequate oral intake or are restricted from doing so. Possible side effects include hypervolemia and extravasation.

S5013-S5014

S5013 5% dextrose/0.45% normal saline with potassium chloride and magnesium sulfate, 1000 ml

S5014 5% dextrose/0.45% normal saline with potassium chloride and magnesium sulfate, 1500 ml

These codes report a 5% dextrose solution in half amount of normal saline to which potassium chloride and magnesium sulfate have been added. It is used to replace fluid in patients that are not able to maintain adequate oral intake or are restricted from doing so. Report the code based on the volume of the IV solution.

S5035-S5036

S5035 Home infusion therapy, routine service of infusion device (e.g., pump maintenance)

S5036 Home infusion therapy, repair of infusion device (e.g., pump repair)

Home infusion therapy is intravenous (IV) administration of medication or fluids to patients in their own home. It is done as an alternative to receiving IV therapy in a facility or office setting. Nurses and other specially trained individuals provide the insertion and management services of the IV and IV equipment, such as the IV pump. Use these codes to report routine service and repair of the IV pump and other equipment that is used with the home infusions.

S5100-S5105

S5100 Day care services, adult; per 15 minutes

S5101 Day care services, adult; per half day

S5102 Day care services, adult; per diem

S5105 Day care services, center-based; services not included in program fee, per diem

An adult day care center furnishes professional services to adults in need. These services provide social services, as well as some health care, to adults who require supervision in a safe place during the day that is outside of the home. In a community setting, the attendees are given the services by interdisciplinary professionals that are trained to meet their physical, social, and emotional needs.

S5108-S5116

S5108 Home care training to home care client, per 15 minutes

S5109 Home care training to home care client, per session

S5110 Home care training, family; per 15 minutes

S5111 Home care training, family; per session

S5115 Home care training, nonfamily; per 15 minutes

S5116 Home care training, nonfamily; per session

Training the home care client, family, or non-family is necessary to assure that they understand everything they need to know about the client's care. Examples of possible training topics include when and how to take medication and possible side effects, skin and wound care, monitoring IV sites and tubing, nutritional needs, fall prevention, issues related to a specific disease condition, and when to contact a health care provider.

S5120-S5121

S5120 Chore services; per 15 minutes

S5121 Chore services; per diem

Chore services are homemaking services provided to individuals who want to remain in their homes but are unable to do all of the necessary tasks. Companies are available to provide help with these chores, for example, shopping for groceries and supplies, planning and preparing meals, changing linens, vacuuming, making beds, housecleaning, lawn mowing, snow shoveling, trash removal, and providing transportation.

S5125-S5126

S5125 Attendant care services; per 15 minutes

S5126 Attendant care services; per diem

Attendant care services provide help with the activities of daily living to a patient with a physical disability, for example, help with eating, bathing, dressing, toilet and bathroom needs, and taking medications that are self administered.

S5130-S5131

S5130 Homemaker service, NOS; per 15 minutes

S5131 Homemaker service, NOS; per diem

These codes report any homemaker services that are not explained by another HCPCS Level II code.

S5135-S5136

S5135 Companion care, adult (e.g., IADL/ADL); per 15 minutes

S5136 Companion care, adult (e.g., IADL/ADL); per diem

Adult companion care is the provision of nonmedical services for adults in their home. These services may include homemaking, medication reminders, personal care, and companionship. ADL refers to the activities of daily living, such as bathing, dressing, self-feeding, and walking. IADLs are instrumental activities of daily living that aren't necessary for fundamental functioning, but do assist in independent living in the community. ADLs include housework, grocery shopping, transportation, and managing money.

S5140-S5141

S5140 Foster care, adult; per diem

S5141 Foster care, adult; per month

Adult foster care provides a family setting for adults who are unable to live alone due to developmental, emotional, or physical impairment. These homes provide room and board and general supervision of their needs, which may include help with dressing, eating, and bathing. These codes report adult foster care on a monthly or daily basis.

S5145-S5146

S5145 Foster care, therapeutic, child; per diem

S5146 Foster care, therapeutic, child; per month

Therapeutic foster care services place children with foster families that have received special training in caring for children with specific medical or behavioral needs. Foster parents in these homes require greater training in order to provide more support for these children. These codes report child therapeutic foster care on a monthly or per diem basis.

S5150-S5151

S5150 Unskilled respite care, not hospice; per 15 minutes

S5151 Unskilled respite care, not hospice; per diem

Respite care is intended to help the patient remain living in a home environment by relieving the patient's unpaid caregiver. Typically, the "home environment" includes the home of a friend, foster home, or a licensed group home, but not a nursing home, hospital, or adult day care setting. Respite care does not refer to care provided by the patient's parent, spouse, or unpaid primary care giver. Use these codes to report respite care as a time increment or a per diem.

S5160-S5162

S5160 Emergency response system; installation and testing

S5161 Emergency response system; service fee, per month (excludes installation and testing)

S5162 Emergency response system; purchase only

Individuals who are at high risk of being put in a facility are often able to remain in the home setting with the use of an emergency response system. This system is an electronic device that allows individuals to secure help if an emergency does occur. These individuals who live alone or are alone for a large portion of the day require extensive routine supervision and do not have a regular caregiver. These codes describe the installation and testing of the system (S5160), the monthly service fee (excluding the installation and testing) (S5161), and the purchase of the system (S5162).

S5165

S5165 Home modifications; per service

An individual's physical condition may require physical modifications to the home setting in order to allow him or her to receive care at home and to ensure safety and welfare (e.g., the installation of hand rails).

S5170

S5170 Home delivered meals, including preparation; per meal

Home meal delivery usually includes two meals per day that are delivered to the patient's home or day care center.

S5175

S5175 Laundry service, external, professional; per order

This code reports laundering done by a professional service that usually includes pickup and delivery. It is to be reported on a per order basis.

S5180-S5181

S5180 Home health respiratory therapy, initial evaluation

S5181 Home health respiratory therapy, NOS, per diem

Home health respiratory services provide aid for patients with respiratory problems that may include COPD, emphysema, bronchitis, asthma, and sleep apnea. These services may include nebulizer and aerosol therapy, chest physical therapy, suction and tracheostomy care, monitoring of equipment, oxygen therapy, and patient education. Use these codes to report the initial evaluation and for home health respiratory therapy services that are not described by any other HCPCS Level II code.

S5185

S5185 Medication reminder service, nonface-to-face; per month

At specific times and dates, a medication reminder service automatically contacts the patient by phone, computer, or other personal electronic device and texts, emails, or plays a recorded message reminding the patient to take his or her medications.

S5190

S5190 Wellness assessment, performed by nonphysician

Wellness assessments are analyses of a person's physical and/or mental state performed in the absence of any known disease or symptom. Wellness assessments may also include evaluations of the person's social, emotional, environmental, and spiritual state. Use this code to report wellness assessments performed by a nonphysician practitioner, such as a nurse practitioner, clinical nurse specialist, or physician assistant.

S5199

S5199 Personal care item, NOS, each

Personal care items are used by patients to help meet their personal needs (e.g., razors, dental care products, hygiene products, and skin and hair care products). Report this code when the personal care item is not described by another existing HCPCS Level II code.

S5497-S5502

S5497 Home infusion therapy, catheter care/maintenance, not otherwise classified; includes administrative services, professional pharmacy services, care coordination, and all necessary supplies and equipment (drugs and nursing visits coded separately), per diem

S5498 Home infusion therapy, catheter care/maintenance, simple (single lumen), includes administrative services, professional pharmacy services, care coordination and all necessary supplies and equipment, (drugs and nursing visits coded separately), per diem

S5501 Home infusion therapy, catheter care/maintenance, complex (more than one lumen), includes administrative services, professional pharmacy services, care coordination, and all necessary supplies and equipment (drugs and nursing visits coded separately), per diem

S5502 Home infusion therapy, catheter care/maintenance, implanted access device, includes administrative services, professional pharmacy services, care coordination and all necessary supplies and equipment (drugs and nursing visits coded separately), per diem (use this code for interim maintenance of vascular access not currently in use)

Home infusion therapy is intravenous (IV) administration of medication or fluids to patients in their own home. It is done as an alternative to receiving IV therapy in a hospital setting. Nurses and other specially trained individuals provide the insertion and management services of the IV and IV equipment, such as the IV pump. These codes report the catheter care, including maintaining patency of the catheter and dressing changes, as a per diem charge when it is a stand-alone therapy (not done the same day as an IV administration). Report the code based on whether the catheter care was for a single lumen, more than one lumen, or for an implanted access device that is not currently in use. Report the not otherwise specified code when there is no other HCPCS Level II code that describes the service.

S5517-S5518

S5517 Home infusion therapy, all supplies necessary for restoration of catheter patency or declotting

S5518 Home infusion therapy, all supplies necessary for catheter repair

Home infusion therapy is intravenous (IV) administration of medication or fluids to patients in their own home. It is done as an alternative to receiving IV therapy in a hospital setting. Nurses and other specially trained individuals provide the insertion and management services of the IV and IV equipment, such as the IV pump. These codes report the supplies used to dissolve a blockage from the catheter in order to restore patency or to repair a catheter.

S5520-S5523

S5520 Home infusion therapy, all supplies (including catheter) necessary for a peripherally inserted central venous catheter (PICC) line insertion

S5521 Home infusion therapy, all supplies (including catheter) necessary for a midline catheter insertion

S5522 Home infusion therapy, insertion of peripherally inserted central venous catheter (PICC), nursing services only (no supplies or catheter included)

S5523 Home infusion therapy, insertion of midline venous catheter, nursing services only (no supplies or catheter included)

Home infusion therapy is the intravenous (IV) administration of medication or fluids to patients in their own home. It is done as an alternative to receiving IV therapy in a hospital setting. Nurses and other specially trained individuals provide the insertion and management services of the IV and IV equipment, such as the IV pump. A PICC line is a catheter that is inserted into the arm and threaded through the vein to the superior vena cave, the large blood vessel that leads to the heart. A midline catheter is 6 to 8 inches long and is inserted in the arm near the elbow (basilic, cephalic, or brachial vein) and threaded to the distal axillary vein. Report the appropriate code based on site and whether supplies or catheters are included.

S5550-S5553

S5550 Insulin, rapid onset, 5 units

S5551 Insulin, most rapid onset (Lispro or Aspart); 5 units

S5552 Insulin, intermediate acting (NPH or LENTE); 5 units

S5553 Insulin, long acting; 5 units

Insulin is a hormone secreted by the beta cells of the pancreas that controls the metabolism and cellular uptake of sugars, proteins, and fats. As a drug, it is used principally to control Type I diabetes mellitus. Different forms of insulin may also be used to control blood sugar levels in patients with gestational diabetes to prevent fetal complications caused by maternal hyperglycemia. The use of insulin in Type II diabetes mellitus is typically only for patients who have failed to control blood sugars with diet, exercise, and oral drugs. In the past, insulin for injection was obtained from beef or porcine pancreas. The onset of action, peak effect, and duration of the insulin effects vary with different kinds of insulin. Most insulin now in use is made by recombinant DNA technology and is equivalent to human insulin from an immunological perspective. Dosage varies by the level of control of blood sugar needed. Insulin is administered by subcutaneous injection or by insulin pump.

S5560-S5571

S5560 Insulin delivery device, reusable pen; 1.5 ml size

S5561 Insulin delivery device, reusable pen; 3 ml size

S5565 Insulin cartridge for use in insulin delivery device other than pump; 150 units

S5566 Insulin cartridge for use in insulin delivery device other than pump; 300 units

S5570 Insulin delivery device, disposable pen (including insulin); 1.5 ml size

S5571 Insulin delivery device, disposable pen (including insulin); 3 ml size

An insulin pen is used to inject insulin into a patient. It is comprised of an insulin cartridge and dial. Disposable needles are attached to the pen. The patient is able to use the dial on the device to adjust the dose dispense. There are two types of pens: reusable and disposable. Insulin cartridges are inserted into a reusable pen. The cartridge is replaced when it is empty but the pen is reused. A prefilled pen includes the pen and the insulin cartridge. The whole device is thrown away when it is empty. Insulin is a hormone secreted by the beta cells of the pancreas that controls the metabolism and cellular uptake of sugars, proteins, and fats. As a drug, it is used principally to control Type I diabetes mellitus. Different forms of insulin may also be used to control blood sugar levels in patients with gestational diabetes to prevent fetal complications caused by maternal hyperglycemia. The use of insulin in Type II diabetes mellitus is typically only for patients who have failed to control blood sugars with diet, exercise, and oral drugs. In the past, insulin for injection was obtained from beef or porcine pancreas. Most insulin now in use is made by recombinant DNA technology and is equivalent to human insulin from an immunological perspective. Dosage varies by the level of control of blood sugar needed.

S8030

S8030 Scleral application of tantalum ring(s) for localization of lesions for proton beam therapy

Prior to proton beam radiation therapy of a scleral tumor, the tumor must be localized. A transillumination and/or indirect ophthalmoscopy are performed during the surgery and titanium rings are sutured to the edges of the scleral tumor.

S8035

S8035 Magnetic source imaging

Magnetic source imaging is a combination of two sets of magnetic data. Brain activity is mapped using the magnetic fields generated by the natural electrical currents within the brain. The magnetic activity is gathered using arrays of superconducting quantum interference devices (SQUID). A recording of this mapping is a magnetoencephalogram or MEG. MEG provides maps of neural activity. Magnetic resonance images map blood flow and physical construction. MEG data is then superimposed on an MRI to create a magnetic source image (MSI). MSIs are used to create functional maps of the human cortex during complex cognitive tasks aiding in the targeting of lesions and epileptic foci, and can aid the identification of head trauma and vascular malformations. It has shown some promise in the classification of patients with multiple sclerosis, Alzheimer's disease, and schizophrenia.

S8037

S8037 Magnetic resonance cholangiopancreatography (MRCP)

Magnetic resonance cholangiopancreatography (MRCP) is magnetic resonance imaging that produces detailed images of the hepatobiliary and pancreatic systems. Multiplanar images that are parallel to the biliary tree are obtained. The MR sequence is sensitive to static fluid and does not require contrast agents. Post-processing can create multi-dimensional images of the entire area. MRCP is useful in the diagnosis and level determination of a bile duct obstruction, cystic biliary diseases, primary sclerosing cholangitis, postop complications, cholangiocarcinoma, pancreatic cancer, and chronic pancreatitis.

S8040

S8040 Topographic brain mapping

Topographic brain mapping, also known as brain electrical activity mapping, is an extension of conventional electroencephalography (EEG). It is the computerized analysis of EEG rhythms and evoked potential data. The analysis is used to generate maps of frequency and voltage. It is intended to identify patterns that represent progressive changes in function or deviations from normal brain activity.

S8042

S8042 Magnetic resonance imaging (MRI), low-field

Magnetic resonance imaging (MRI) usually requires a magnetic field of a few Tesla, which is about 10,000 to 100,000 times stronger than earth's magnetic field. Low field MRIs use approximately 30 millitesla fields, which is about 100 times weaker than the earth's magnetic field. Since the strength of the magnet is directly tied to its cost, lower field MRIs are less costly than regular MRIs. Low field MRIs are generally open and there is less danger to patients with pacemakers and metal implants.

S8055

S8055 Ultrasound guidance for multifetal pregnancy reduction(s), technical component (only to be used when the physician doing the reduction procedure does not perform the ultrasound, guidance is included in the CPT code for multifetal pregnancy reduction (59866)

This code reports the technical component of ultrasound guidance for multifetal pregnancy reduction when the physician doing the reduction procedure does not perform the ultrasound. When the physician performing the surgery is also performing the ultrasound guidance, then the guidance is included in the CPT code for multifetal pregnancy reduction. Multifetal pregnancies can result naturally or from the implantation of multiple embryos during an in vitro fertilization cycle. Fetal reductions can be done to reduce twins to a single fetus, triplets to twins, quadruplets to triplets, etc.

S8080

S8080 Scintimammography (radioimmunoscintigraphy of the breast), unilateral, including supply of radiopharmaceutical

A scintimammography is a nuclear medicine scan performed on women who have an abnormal or inconclusive mammogram study. It is used to help determine whether or not a patient needs a biopsy or if multiple biopsies are needed. A radioactive substance is injected into the patient's vein. The substance accumulates in the breast that has abnormal tissue. An imaging device called a gamma camera is used to detect the radioactive material. A computer is used to analyze and measure the abnormal tissue.

S8085

S8085 Fluorine-18 fluorodeoxyglucose (F-18 FDG) imaging using dual-head coincidence detection system (nondedicated PET scan)

A fluorine-18 fluorodeoxyglucose (F-18 FDG) image using dual-head coincidence detection system (nondedicated positron emission tomography or PET scan) is also known as an FDG-single photon emission computed tomography (SPECT), metabolic SPECT, or PET scan using a gamma camera. F-18 FDG is a radiotracer that emits positrons as it decays. These positrons emit paired photons. Dedicated PET scanners consist of multiple detectors that simultaneously detect all high-energy photons emitted at 180 degrees from one another that produce detailed images. SPECT cameras are less expensive than PET scanners and use the photons to provide scintigraphic images reflecting the metabolic activity of the tissues. SPECT cameras can be adapted to read the higher energy photons emitted by F-18 FDG. To screen out lower energy photons, a dual head rotating SPECT camera is operated in coincidence mode, which means that the camera only counts photons that are simultaneously detected at 180 degrees from one another. However, the lower number of detectors in SPECT machines results in a loss of sensitivity and resolution.

S8092

S8092 Electron beam computed tomography (also known as ultrafast CT, cine CT)

Electron beam computed tomography (EBT) is also known as ultrafast CT or cine CT. In a conventional CT scanner, the x-ray source moves along a circle in space around the object to be imaged. In EBT, the x-ray tube does not move. It is large, stationary, and partially surrounds the imaging circle. The x-ray source, or electron-beam focal point, is swept electronically along a tungsten anode in the tube, tracing a large circular arc. This motion can be very fast creating an ultrafast CT. Ultrafast CT scans are needed to image the heart as its rhythm can blur images during conventional CT scans.

S8096

S8096 Portable peak flow meter

Portable peak flow meters are used to monitor the severity of the disease and its response to therapy in patients with asthma, chronic obstructive pulmonary disease, and other respiratory diseases. Home monitoring of peak expiratory flow is recommended by the National Heart, Lung, and Blood Institute for asthma management. The peak flow meter consists of a spring-loaded piston or vane in a drum. A forced expiration through an inlet moves the piston or vane proportional to the maximum flow. Electronic versions measure peak flow and forced expiratory volume in one second and store the measurements.

S8097

S8097 Asthma kit (including but not limited to portable peak expiratory flow meter, instructional video, brochure, and/or spacer)

An asthma kit includes a portable peak expiratory flow meter, instructional video and/or brochure, and/or a spacer. The kit is designed to assist asthmatics in the management of their disease. The physician should provide instructions to the patient on interpreting the peak flow levels, including normal levels, the levels that require the use of an inhaler or nebulizer, and the level requiring immediate emergency care.

S8100-S8101

S8100 Holding chamber or spacer for use with an inhaler or nebulizer; without mask

S8101 Holding chamber or spacer for use with an inhaler or nebulizer; with mask

A holding chamber is a valved container that holds medication that is to be administered. A spacer is a container or tube that slows the delivery of the medication from a pressurized metered dose inhaler. Spacing or controlling the dose allows the medication to more easily and effectively reach the lungs.

S8110

S8110 Peak expiratory flow rate (physician services)

This code reports physician services related to respiratory diseases and the use of peak flow meters. These services may include instructions to the patient on the use of the meter and interpretation of the peak flow levels, including normal levels, the levels that require the use of an inhaler or nebulizer, and the level requiring immediate emergency care.

S8120-S8121

S8120 Oxygen contents, gaseous, 1 unit equals 1 cubic foot

S8121 Oxygen contents, liquid, 1 unit equals 1 pound

Supplemental oxygen is sometimes necessary for people with respiratory illnesses. Oxygen may be contained in stationary or portable canisters or tanks and delivered in a liquid or gaseous state. These codes report the supply of oxygen used to refill the canisters or tanks.

S8130-S8131

S8130 Interferential current stimulator, 2 channel

S8131 Interferential current stimulator, 4 channel

Interferential current stimulator is a device that produces and delivers a high frequency (4000 HZ) carrier wave that has the same signal as a TENS device. The higher frequency penetrates more deeply than a TENS. The current generated stimulates large impulse fibers and can interfere with the transmission of pain signals at the spinal cord level. The stimulation can also be adjusted to stimulate parasympathetic nerve fibers for increased blood flow. The channels carry different frequencies, usually a high and a medium frequency electrical impulse. One channel is usually fixed and the other variable. When combined, the signals produce the desired electrical impulse. In phase electrical waves combine to deliver an amplified electrical impulse. Out of phase waves can cancel all or parts of other electrical waves, thereby decreasing or stopping the signal. Interferential therapy is used for the treatment of deep pain, to promote bone growth in delayed and nonunion fractures, to stimulate muscles to pump blood in venous insufficiency, and to depress the activity of cervical and lumbosacral sympathetic ganglia in patients with arterial constrictor tone. It has also been used to manage acute postsurgical and posttraumatic pain, edema, and inflammation.

S8185

S8185 Flutter device

A flutter device is used to provide positive expiratory pressure therapy for patients with respiratory conditions that produce mucus (e.g., bronchitis, bronchiectasis, asthma, atelectasis, cystic fibrosis, and COPD). The device works by vibrating the airways to loosen the mucus, helping to maintain the patency of the airway by intermittently increasing endobronchial pressure, and facilitates the movement of mucus up through the airways by increasing expiratory airflow. The device resembles a pipe with a mouthpiece at one end and a perforated cover at the opposite end. Inside the device a stainless steel ball rests on a circular cone.

S8186

S8186 Swivel adaptor

A swivel adaptor is used to connect ventilator circuits to endotracheal tubes. They are usually elbow shaped and allow for flexibility and help in maintaining patent airways.

S8189

S8189 Tracheostomy supply, not otherwise classified

Use this code to report supplies used with a tracheostomy that are not described by other HCPCS Level II codes.

S8210

S8210 Mucus trap

A mucus trap is a container used in respiratory section equipment to prevent sputum from going into the suction bottle so it can be sent to the lab for analysis.

S8265

S8265 Haberman feeder for cleft lip/palate

The Haberman feeder is a bottle named after its developer that is used for babies who have impaired ability to suck due to a cleft lip/palate, congenital heart disease, a genetic disorder, or neurological disorders. The bottle has a one-way valve that helps to reduce the air that the baby takes in. It is a soft squeeze bottle that the parent can squeeze to provide an adequate amount of formula to the baby.

S8270

S8270 Enuresis alarm, using auditory buzzer and/or vibration device

An enuresis alarm is a device that sends out a sound or a vibration when moisture reaches the device. It is attached to the child's underwear or pajamas in the area where it would first come in contact with the drop of urine. When the child feels the vibration or hears the alarm, he or she becomes trained to get up and go to the bathroom to empty the bladder. Eventually, the child learns to respond to the sensation of a full bladder by waking up and going to the bathroom prior to the alarm going off.

S8301

S8301 Infection control supplies, not otherwise specified

Infection control supplies include such items as disinfectants, hand sanitizer, latex gloves, sharps containers, etc. This code reports infection control supplies that are not identified by another HCPCS Level II code.

S8415

S8415 Supplies for home delivery of infant

This code reports the supplies used for a home delivery of an infant. Examples include scissors, suction bulb, warm towels and receiving blankets, lubricants, cord care supplies, antiseptic, sterile gauze, OB pads, gloves, waterproof or plastic sheets, and disposable under pads.

S8420-S8429

S8420 Gradient pressure aid (sleeve and glove combination), custom made

S8421 Gradient pressure aid (sleeve and glove combination), ready made

S8422 Gradient pressure aid (sleeve), custom made, medium weight

S8423 Gradient pressure aid (sleeve), custom made, heavy weight

S8424 Gradient pressure aid (sleeve), ready made

S8425 Gradient pressure aid (glove), custom made, medium weight

S8426 Gradient pressure aid (glove), custom made, heavy weight

S8427 Gradient pressure aid (glove), ready made

S8428 Gradient pressure aid (gauntlet), ready made

S8429 Gradient pressure exterior wrap

When the lymphatic fluid accumulates in the interstitial tissue, especially in the subcutaneous tissue, the condition is known as lymphedema. The accumulated fluid causes gradual and progressive enlargement of the affected extremity and is accompanied by increased weight and decreased functional ability among other changes. Lymphedema may be a complication of cancer and the treatments for cancer and is usually progressive. There is no known cure for lymphedema. Gradient pressure aids are pneumatic compression devices that are used to treat lymphedema. Use these codes to report gradient pressure aids, based on the type, if they are custom or ready made, and whether they are medium or heavy weight.

S8430-S8431

S8430 Padding for compression bandage, roll

S8431 Compression bandage, roll

A compression bandage is an elasticized rolled bandage that provides sustained compression for treatment of venous ulcers, lymphedema, and other types of swelling or edema and related conditions. The compression bandage may also be applied as a first aid measure to control bleeding by applying pressure to stop the blood flow from an artery. Compression bandages are often used to reduce the swelling and to stabilize a limb prior to applying a cast or compression garment. Compression bandage padding may be used as an under wrap for a compression dressing or an under cast padding.

S8450-S8452

S8450 Splint, prefabricated, digit (specify digit by use of modifier)

S8451 Splint, prefabricated, wrist or ankle

S8452 Splint, prefabricated, elbow

A splint is a device used to support or immobilize a limb or the spine. It is commonly used right after an injury. A splint may be custom made or prefabricated. These codes represent prefabricated splints, which are usually plastic or metal and attach to the body with Velcro straps. A prefabricated splint requires very little adjustment to fit the limb or digit and does not require any expertise to trim or bend or mold the splint to fit the patient.

S8460

S8460 Camisole, postmastectomy

A camisole is a sleeveless undergarment for women that extends from the chest to the waist. The postmastectomy camisole has pouches and pockets sewn on the inside of the camisole and is worn with or without foam inserts. It may be used for the first six weeks post-breast surgery in place of a bra. The mastectomy camisole can hold four drains: two in the pouch and two in the underarm tabs.

S8490

S8490 Insulin syringes (100 syringes, any size)

A syringe is a simple pump consisting of a plunger in a tube that is used as a drug delivery device. An insulin syringe has a capacity of 1 ml or less and comes attached to a fine gauge needle (27-29 G). The syringe is marked in insulin units. This code reports a package of 100 insulin syringes.

S8930

S8930 Electrical stimulation of auricular acupuncture points; each 15 minutes of personal one-on-one contact with patient

Acupuncture was commonly used in ancient China to treat a wide variety of conditions, symptoms, and behaviors. It involves insertion of very thin needles superficially into various points in the body to produce therapy and healing in other parts of the body. The ear cartilage is thought to contain approximately 200 of these points. In western medicine, pulse electrostimulation of the needles placed in the ear cartilage provide additional stimulation of the acupuncture site.

S8940

S8940 Equestrian/hippotherapy, per session

Equestrian/hippotherapy, also known as therapeutic horseback riding, is the passive use of the movements of a horse to treat patients with cerebral palsy and neuromuscular disabilities. The therapist tries to facilitate normal muscle tone and discourage abnormal posture by using the horse as a treatment modality. The patient is placed in various positions on the horse (e.g., side sitting, prone across the horse, prone lengthwise on the horse, or sitting). The movement of the horse is thought to enhance balance, motor development, and coordination.

S8948

S8948 Application of a modality (requiring constant provider attendance) to one or more areas; low-level laser; each 15 minutes

Low-level laser therapy (LLLT) is a form of phototherapy in which low power photonic energy light is applied to lesions and injuries. It reportedly enhances wound healing, including amputation injuries, infected wounds, burns, and skin grafts. The laser infuses the body's cells with energy. LLLT is noninvasive and works quickly.

S8950

S8950 Complex lymphedema therapy, each 15 minutes

Complex lymphedema therapy (CLT) is a noninvasive treatment for lymphedema. Lymphedema is a result of lymphatic system failure, which causes an accumulation of lymphatic fluid or edema in the soft tissue. CLT is done to restore function of the affected limb by controlling and reducing the amount of swelling. The therapy usually consists of two phases: treatment and maintenance. CLT treatment phase includes light massage, usually for 30 to 60 minutes. The massage stimulates residual lymphatic vessels to transport the excess fluids from the edematous area. The affected limb is then wrapped in compression bandages and is subjected to range of motion movements. The treatments are usually done two to five times a week for two weeks, and then the patient moves on to the maintenance phase where the patient maintains and applies the techniques learned in the treatment phase, including continuing to wear the compressive sleeve during the day and the compression bandage wrap at night.

S8990

S8990 Physical or manipulative therapy performed for maintenance rather than restoration

Maintenance therapy occurs after the goals of the treatment plan have been reached, the therapy is no longer of therapeutic necessity, and it is apparent that no additional functional improvement is occurring or expected to occur. Maintenance therapy is performed to maintain the quality of life, disease prevention, and general health maintenance.

S8999

S8999 Resuscitation bag (for use by patient on artificial respiration during power failure or other catastrophic event)

A resuscitation bag is used to help a person breathe in a medical emergency. It is a hand-held device that consists of an air chamber (that is squeezed to force air into the patient) and a mask that is placed over the nose and mouth of the patient.

S9001

S9001 Home uterine monitor with or without associated nursing services

A home uterine monitor helps to detect preterm labor. The external device is worn in a belt on the abdomen of a pregnant woman twice a day for one to two hours and records contractions that may be too faint for the patient to recognize. The resulting data is transmitted via telephone modem link to nurses who analyze the data and provide assessment and counseling services to the patient on a daily basis. The uterine monitor consists of a guard ring tocodynamometer that is worn as an abdominal belt, a data transmitter, and a data recorder.

S9007

S9007 Ultrafiltration monitor

An ultrafiltration monitor is intended to reduce overfiltration (removal of too much fluid from tissue) and underfiltration (removal of too little fluid) during hemodialysis.

S9024

S9024 Paranasal sinus ultrasound

The paranasal sinuses are mucus lined air filled cavities and include the fontal, maxillary, ethmoid, and sphenoid sinuses. A paranasal ultrasound, which is a noninvasive procedure, may be used to help diagnose sinusitis, focal soft tissue masses, and thickening of the mucosal walls. The ultrasound applicator is placed over the sinuses on the face, including the cheekbones and nose, and high frequency sound waves are used to image the sinuses.

S9025

S9025 Omnicardiogram/cardiointegram

The cardiointegram or omnicardiogram may be used as a substitute for exercise tolerance testing with thallium imaging in patients for whom a resting EKG may be inadequate to identify changes compatible with coronary artery disease. The device is composed of a microcomputer that receives output from a standard 12 lead EKG. A series of integrations is used to transform the voltage versus tine format and produce a graphic representation of the heart's electrophysiologic signals.

S9034

S9034 Extracorporeal shockwave lithotripsy for gall stones (if performed with ERCP, use 43265)

Extracorporeal shock wave lithotripsy is a noninvasive procedure that may be done by dry method (water-filled compressible bags placed over stone area) or wet method (patient is placed in a water bath or submerged). High-intensity shock waves are electrically produced and focused sonographically on the gallstone. The procedure may be done with either epidural or general anesthesia or with the use of IV sedation.

S9055

S9055 Procuren or other growth factor preparation to promote wound healing

Procuren is a human platelet-derived growth factor (PDGF), a substance naturally produced by the body that helps to promote wound healing. An autologous platelet concentrate is prepared from a sample of the patient's blood, processed to separate the platelets, which are treated with a reagent to create a gel that is applied topically to the wound. Autologous platelet-derived products have also been used to treat a variety of acute surgical wounds. Please note that Procuren may no longer be available but that this code is also used to report other growth factor preparations that promote wound healing.

S9056

S9056 Coma stimulation per diem

A coma is a state of unconsciousness that lasts longer than six hours. Coma stimulation is done by a health care professional or a member of the patient's family (who is trained in the stimulation techniques) to increase patient responsiveness. Stimulation is applied to one or more of the patient's five senses, with the intent of facilitating awakening and enhancing the rehabilitative potential of the patient. Various stimuli can be used for each of the senses. These treatments can be given in the hospital, SNF, or patient's home and can range from hourly treatments twice a day to hourly stimulation cycles lasting 15 to 20 minutes 12 to 14 times a day six days a week. Report this code for one daily (per diem) coma stimulation.

S9061

S9061 Home administration of aerosolized drug therapy (e.g., Pentamidine); administrative services, professional pharmacy services, care coordination, all necessary supplies and equipment (drugs and nursing visits coded separately), per diem

An aerosol is a suspension of solid particles or liquid droplets in a gas. Aerosolized drug therapy is used when rapid absorption and localization effects of the drug are required to produce the appropriate response. They are most commonly used in specific lung diseases that cause breathing difficulties; for example, emphysema, asthma, and COPD. In aerosolized drug therapy, drugs are absorbed through the lungs or bronchial airways through tiny droplets. This code reports the administration of aerosolized drug therapy in the home setting and includes the administrative services, professional pharmacy services, care coordination, and all necessary supplies and equipment (e.g. nebulizer) provided on a daily (per diem) basis. The drugs and nursing visits are reported separately.

S9083-S9088

S9083 Global fee urgent care centers

S9088 Services provided in an urgent care center (list in addition to code for service)

Urgent care centers deliver medical care in a facility outside of a hospital emergency room, and typically, the care is unscheduled and on a walk-in basis. The centers are intended to treat patients who are ill or injured and require immediate care but who do not require the services of a hospital emergency department. Unlike hospital emergency departments, urgent care centers are not open 24 hours a day. These codes report urgent care centers as a global service or as an adjunct code (in addition to the code for the specific service).

S9090

S9090 Vertebral axial decompression, per session

Vertebral axial decompression is a therapy for lower back pain due to herniated lumbar discs or degenerative lumbar disc disease. It uses a computer-driven table to control the disc decompression. For the treatment, a pelvic harness is applied to the patient and the patient lies on the special table and is subjected to a series of cycles as the table is slowly extended and a distraction force is applied via the harness. When the desired tension is reached, it is gradually decreased. This repetitive cycle builds up the patient's tolerance to stronger distraction forces. Each session usually includes 15 cycles lasting about 30 minutes, and 10 to 15 daily treatments are generally administered. Use this code to report each session.

S9097

S9097 Home visit for wound care

This code reports a home care visit to care for the patient's wounds, which may include ulcers, burns, pressure sores, open surgical sites, fistulas, tube sites, and tumor erosion sites.

S9098

S9098 Home visit, phototherapy services (e.g., Bili-lite), including equipment rental, nursing services, blood draw, supplies, and other services, per diem

Phototherapy services are prescribed to treat skin disorders, including babies with high bilirubin count. Use this code to report home visits for phototherapy services on a daily (per diem) basis. The code includes all equipment rentals, nursing services, blood draw, supplies and other services.

S9110

S9110 Telemonitoring of patient in their home, including all necessary equipment; computer system, connections, and software; maintenance; patient education and support; per month

Telehealth is the delivery of health-related services via telecommunications equipment, including email, video conferencing, and the transmission of medical images or medical data. The telecommunications most often involve a primary care practitioner with a patient at a remote site and a consulting medical specialist at an urban or referral facility. The originating site is the location of the patient at the time the service is being furnished via a telecommunications system. A fee that is set annually is paid to the originating site. This code represents the telemonitoring of a patient in the home and includes all of the necessary equipment required, including maintenance, patient education and support, and all computer system connections and software. It is billed on a monthly basis.

S9117

S9117 Back school, per visit

Back school may involve one or more instructive sessions where the patient is instructed in anatomy of the spine, the best sleeping positions, and proper body mechanics for standing, lifting, sitting, and doing household chores.

S9122

S9122 Home health aide or certified nurse assistant, providing care in the home; per hour

Home health aides and certified nurse assistants provide routine health care in the patient's home. Their services may include dressing changes, applying topical medications, feeding the patient, monitoring vital signs, and monitoring and reporting changes in health status. They may also provide help with the patient's personal care, including bathing and dressing and help with toileting.

S9123-S9124

S9123 Nursing care, in the home; by registered nurse, per hour (use for general nursing care only, not to be used when CPT codes 99500-99602 can be used)

S9124 Nursing care, in the home; by licensed practical nurse, per hour

These codes report various home care services provided by a registered nurse (RN) or licensed practical nurse (LPN) on an hourly basis. Examples of duties usually performed by skilled nurses include tube feeding, injections, cardiac and respiratory care, and medication management.

S9125

S9125 Respite care, in the home, per diem

Respite care is the provision of short-term temporary care to a person with a chronic illness or disability. The term "respite care" usually refers to relief provided to a primary caregiver. Use this code to report respite care in the home setting on a daily (per diem) basis.

S9126

S9126 Hospice care, in the home, per diem

Hospice care services are designed to address the physical, mental, emotional, and spiritual needs of terminally ill patients and their families. Hospice care is a palliative service that is provided when a cure is not possible. Services focus on keeping the patient comfortable by relieving pain and other symptoms and supporting the family during the terminal phase of the patient's illness. Hospice services also include bereavement counseling following the patient's death. Hospice care is typically delivered by an interdisciplinary health care team of physicians, nurses, social workers, counselors, home health aides, clergy, therapists, and trained volunteers.

S9127-S9131

S9127 Social work visit, in the home, per diem

S9128 Speech therapy, in the home, per diem

S9129 Occupational therapy, in the home, per diem

S9131 Physical therapy; in the home, per diem

These codes report various services provided by different types of qualified professionals in a home health setting on a per diem basis. Home health includes not only traditional private home settings, but also assisted living quarters, group homes, custodial care facilities, or similar type settings that constitute the patient's place of residence.

S9140-S9141

S9140 Diabetic management program, follow-up visit to non-MD provider

S9141 Diabetic management program, follow-up visit to MD provider

A diabetes management program typically includes an overview of diabetes, as well as instruction in stress management, exercise, meal planning, glucose monitoring, medications, and advice about complications. These codes report a diabetes management program follow-up visit to an MD or a non-MD provider.

S9145

S9145 Insulin pump initiation, instruction in initial use of pump (pump not included)

Insulin pumps are used to deliver rapid-acting insulin continuously throughout the day through a catheter that is placed under the skin. The pump replaces the need for periodic injections of insulin. Prior to using the pump, the patient needs to be instructed in correct use, which includes the basal rate (continuous rate that keeps the glucose level in range overnight and between meals), bolus doses (additional insulin that is given to cover the amount of carbohydrates consumed during a meal), and supplemental doses that may be required to treat high blood sugar. The patient also requires instruction on care of the pump while showering, sleeping, and exercising, and what to do if the pump needs to be removed.

S9150

S9150 Evaluation by ocularist

An ocular prosthesis or artificial eye is a prosthetic unit that is designed to maintain the facial shape and to match the remaining eye as closely as possible for patients who have lost an eye as a result of illness or trauma. An ocularist is an individual who is licensed to design, fabricate, and fit the prosthesis. Use this code to report the evaluation done by an ocularist.

S9152

S9152 Speech therapy, re-evaluation

A speech therapy re-evaluation may be done periodically when the clinician notes a significant improvement or decline or a change that was not anticipated when the plan of care was established. Some state and payer guidelines may require re-evaluations at specific times, but the clinician usually determines when a re-evaluation is indicated. A re-evaluation may not be as extensive as the original evaluation since it is focused on the current treatment. A routine, continuous assessment of the patient's progress is inherent in the treatment and should not be considered a re-evaluation. The re-evaluation is focused on the patient's progress toward the established goals and may include the clinician's judgment on continued care, goal modification, and whether to continue or to terminate the treatment. Typically, the documentation should support the need for further measurements and tests by identifying a significant change in the patient's condition, new clinical findings, or a failure to respond to therapy.

S9208-S9209

S9208 Home management of preterm labor, including administrative services, professional pharmacy services, care coordination, and all necessary supplies or equipment (drugs and nursing visits coded separately), per diem (do not use this code with any home infusion per diem code)

S9209 Home management of preterm premature rupture of membranes (PPROM), including administrative services, professional pharmacy services, care coordination, and all necessary supplies or equipment (drugs and nursing visits coded separately), per diem (do not use this code with any home infusion per diem code)

Preterm labor is regular contractions of the uterus that are accompanied by progressive changes in the cervix prior to 37 weeks of gestation. Preterm premature rupture of the membranes (PPROM) is when the membranes rupture before the onset of uterine contractions and prior to 37 weeks gestation. As an alternative to hospital admission, a woman may opt for home management of her preterm labor or PPROM. In addition to bed rest, medications may be given and a uterine monitor may be used. Tocolytic therapy is the use of drugs to inhibit contractions of the uterus. Acute tocolysis is done to reduce or stop contractions of the uterus and to stop or slow down cervical changes during preterm labor. Maintenance tocolysis is done after acute tocolysis to prevent a recurrence of preterm labor after it has been stopped. Antibiotics may be given for PPROM to prevent infection. The home uterine monitor helps to detect preterm labor. The external device is worn in a belt on the abdomen of a pregnant woman twice a day for one to two hours and records contractions that may be too faint for the patient to recognize. The resulting data is transmitted via telephone modem link to nurses who analyze the data and provide assessment and counseling services to the patient on a daily basis. The uterine monitor consists of a guard ring tocodynamometer that is worn as an abdominal belt, a data transmitter, and a data recorder. Use these codes to report all services involved in home management of preterm labor and PPROM on a daily (per diem) basis. Drugs and nursing visits are to be coded separately. Do not use these codes with any home infusion code.

S9211-S9214

S9211 Home management of gestational hypertension, includes administrative services, professional pharmacy services, care coordination and all necessary supplies and equipment (drugs and nursing visits coded separately); per diem (do not use this code with any home infusion per diem code)

S9212 Home management of postpartum hypertension, includes administrative services, professional pharmacy services, care coordination, and all necessary supplies and equipment (drugs and nursing visits coded separately), per diem (do not use this code with any home infusion per diem code)

S9213 Home management of preeclampsia, includes administrative services, professional pharmacy services, care coordination, and all necessary supplies and equipment (drugs and nursing services coded separately); per diem (do not use this code with any home infusion per diem code)

S9214 Home management of gestational diabetes, includes administrative services, professional pharmacy services, care coordination, and all necessary supplies and equipment (drugs and nursing visits coded separately); per diem (do not use this code with any home infusion per diem code)

Gestational hypertension is the development of high blood pressure in the pregnant woman (usually greater than 140/90) after 20 weeks gestation. Postpartum hypertension is the development of high blood pressure after the completion of labor. Postpartum hypertension may occur in the period just after delivery. Preeclampsia is high blood pressure; swelling of the hands, feet, and face; and excess protein in the urine of a pregnant woman after 20 weeks gestation. If untreated, preeclampsia can lead to serious complications for the mother and the baby. Gestational diabetes is glucose intolerance with first recognition or onset during pregnancy. Use these codes to report the home management of any of the conditions listed above on a daily (per diem) basis. Drugs and nursing visits should be coded separately. Do not report these codes with any home infusion per diem code.

S9325-S9328

S9325 Home infusion therapy, pain management infusion; administrative services, professional pharmacy services, care coordination, and all necessary supplies and equipment, (drugs and nursing visits coded separately), per diem (do not use this code with S9326, S9327 or S9328)

S9326 Home infusion therapy, continuous (24 hours or more) pain management infusion; administrative services, professional pharmacy services, care coordination and all necessary supplies and equipment (drugs and nursing visits coded separately), per diem

S9327 Home infusion therapy, intermittent (less than 24 hours) pain management infusion; administrative services, professional pharmacy services, care coordination, and all necessary supplies and equipment (drugs and nursing visits coded separately), per diem

S9328 Home infusion therapy, implanted pump pain management infusion; administrative services, professional pharmacy services, care coordination, and all necessary supplies and equipment (drugs and nursing visits coded separately), per diem

Home infusion therapy is the intravenous (IV) administration of medication or fluids to patients in their own home. It is done as an alternative to receiving IV therapy in a hospital setting. Nurses and other specially trained individuals provide the insertion and management services of the IV and IV equipment, such as the IV pump. These codes report home infusions for the management of pain on a daily (per diem) basis as an infusion, continuous infusion of 24 hours or more, as an intermittent infusion less than 24 hours, or via an implanted pump. Drugs and nursing visits should be coded separately.

S9329-S9331

S9329 Home infusion therapy, chemotherapy infusion; administrative services, professional pharmacy services, care coordination, and all necessary supplies and equipment (drugs and nursing visits coded separately), per diem (do not use this code with S9330 or S9331)

S9330 Home infusion therapy, continuous (24 hours or more) chemotherapy infusion; administrative services, professional pharmacy services, care coordination, and all necessary supplies and equipment (drugs and nursing visits coded separately), per diem

S9331 Home infusion therapy, intermittent (less than 24 hours) chemotherapy infusion; administrative services, professional pharmacy services, care coordination, and all necessary supplies and equipment (drugs and nursing visits coded separately), per diem

Home infusion therapy is the intravenous (IV) administration of medication or fluids to patients in their own home. It is done as an alternative to receiving IV therapy in a hospital setting. Nurses and other specially trained individuals provide the insertion and management services of the IV and IV equipment, such as the IV pump. These codes report home infusions for the administration of chemotherapy on a daily (per diem) basis as an infusion, continuous infusion of 24 hours or more, or as an intermittent infusion less than 24 hours. Drugs and nursing visits should be coded separately.

S9335

S9335 Home therapy, hemodialysis; administrative services, professional pharmacy services, care coordination, and all necessary supplies and equipment (drugs and nursing services coded separately), per diem

Hemodialysis is done to clear waste and extra fluid from the patient's blood by using a special dialyzer. Two needles are placed into the patient's access site: one into an artery and the other into a vein. They are connected to plastic tubing. This tubing carries the blood to the dialysis machine, which cleanses the blood of excess waste and fluids and returns the clean blood back to the body. The dialysis machine pumps the blood through the dialysis system and controls the temperature, pressure, fluid removal, and treatment time. This code reports the administration of hemodialysis. Drugs and nursing visits should be coded separately.

S9336

S9336 Home infusion therapy, continuous anticoagulant infusion therapy (e.g., Heparin), administrative services, professional pharmacy services, care coordination and all necessary supplies and equipment (drugs and nursing visits coded separately), per diem

Heparin is an anticoagulant indicated for the treatment and prevention of blood clots, including pulmonary embolism and deep vein thrombosis. It is also used to ensure patency of indwelling intravenous catheters. Heparin inhibits reactions that lead to the clotting of blood and the formation of fibrin clots. It works by acting as an accelerant in forming antithrombin III-thrombin complex, which deactivates thrombin. This prevents the conversion of fibrinogen to fibrin. Heparin sodium is derived from bovine or porcine pulmonary or intestinal tissue and standardized for anticoagulant activity. This code reports home infusions for the continuous administration of anticoagulant therapy on a daily (per diem) basis. Drugs and nursing visits should be coded separately.

S9338

S9338 Home infusion therapy, immunotherapy, administrative services, professional pharmacy services, care coordination, and all necessary supplies and equipment (drugs and nursing visits coded separately), per diem

Immunotherapy, also known as biological therapy or biotherapy, uses certain characteristics of the immune system to fight diseases, such as cancer, by stimulating the patient's own immune system or by giving the patient immune system components, such as manufactured immune system proteins. This code reports home infusions for the administration of immunotherapy on a daily (per diem) basis. Drugs and nursing visits should be coded separately.

S9339

S9339 Home therapy; peritoneal dialysis, administrative services, professional pharmacy services, care coordination and all necessary supplies and equipment (drugs and nursing visits coded separately), per diem

For end stage renal disease (ESRD) patients, peritoneal dialysis is the most common form of home dialysis treatment. A catheter is placed in the peritoneal cavity of the patient. The catheter remains permanently in the peritoneum. During the treatment, dialysate is drained from the peritoneal cavity and is replaced with fresh dialysate, which is allowed to remain in the peritoneum for several hours. At that time, this solution is drained through the catheter and a new bag of dialysate is put into the peritoneum. The peritoneal dialysis may be continuous (CAPD), which involves two to five daily manual treatments.

Automated peritoneal dialysis is done with the use of a cycler machine. This machine is programmed to perform three to five fluid exchanges while the patient sleeps. This code reports home peritoneal dialysis on a daily (per diem) basis as an infusion, continuous infusion of 24 hours or more, or as an intermittent infusion less than 24 hours. Drugs and nursing visits should be coded separately.

S9340-S9343

S9340 Home therapy; enteral nutrition; administrative services, professional pharmacy services, care coordination, and all necessary supplies and equipment (enteral formula and nursing visits coded separately), per diem

S9341 Home therapy; enteral nutrition via gravity; administrative services, professional pharmacy services, care coordination, and all necessary supplies and equipment (enteral formula and nursing visits coded separately), per diem

S9342 Home therapy; enteral nutrition via pump; administrative services, professional pharmacy services, care coordination, and all necessary supplies and equipment (enteral formula and nursing visits coded separately), per diem

S9343 Home therapy; enteral nutrition via bolus; administrative services, professional pharmacy services, care coordination, and all necessary supplies and equipment (enteral formula and nursing visits coded separately), per diem

Enteral nutrition provides nourishment directly to the digestive tract via a tube for patients whose nutritional needs cannot be met with a regular diet. Feeding tube options include placing a nasogastric or nasoenteric tube through the patient's nose and into the stomach or percutaneous placement of a gastrostomy or jejunostomy tube into the stomach or small intestine. Gravity enteral feedings are poured into the feeding bag and the bag is hung on a pole. The tube from the bag is attached to the feeding tube. Enteral feedings done with a pump are done by connecting the tubes to an electric pump and programming the desired rate. A bolus feeding is achieved by attaching a syringe to the feeding tube and pouring formula into the syringe. It is allowed to flow into the tube by gravity. These codes report home enteral nutrition therapy on a daily (per diem) basis. Drugs and nursing visits should be coded separately.

S9345-S9363

S9345 Home infusion therapy, antihemophilic agent infusion therapy (e.g., Factor VIII); administrative services, professional pharmacy services, care coordination, and all necessary supplies and equipment (drugs and nursing visits coded separately), per diem

S9346 Home infusion therapy, alpha-1-proteinase inhibitor (e.g., Prolastin); administrative services, professional pharmacy services, care coordination, and all necessary supplies and equipment (drugs and nursing visits coded separately), per diem

S9347 Home infusion therapy, uninterrupted, long-term, controlled rate intravenous or subcutaneous infusion therapy (e.g., epoprostenol); administrative services, professional pharmacy services, care coordination, and all necessary supplies and equipment (drugs and nursing visits coded separately), per diem

S9348 Home infusion therapy, sympathomimetic/inotropic agent infusion therapy (e.g., Dobutamine); administrative services, professional pharmacy services, care coordination, all necessary supplies and equipment (drugs and nursing visits coded separately), per diem

S9349 Home infusion therapy, tocolytic infusion therapy; administrative services, professional pharmacy services, care coordination, and all necessary supplies and equipment (drugs and nursing visits coded separately), per diem

S9351 Home infusion therapy, continuous or intermittent antiemetic infusion therapy; administrative services, professional pharmacy services, care coordination, and all necessary supplies and equipment (drugs and visits coded separately), per diem

S9353 Home infusion therapy, continuous insulin infusion therapy; administrative services, professional pharmacy services, care coordination, and all necessary supplies and equipment (drugs and nursing visits coded separately), per diem

S9355 Home infusion therapy, chelation therapy; administrative services, professional pharmacy services, care coordination, and all necessary supplies and equipment (drugs and nursing visits coded separately), per diem

S9357 Home infusion therapy, enzyme replacement intravenous therapy; (e.g., Imiglucerase); administrative services, professional pharmacy services, care coordination, and all necessary supplies and equipment (drugs and nursing visits coded separately), per diem

S9359 Home infusion therapy, antitumor necrosis factor intravenous therapy; (e.g., Infliximab); administrative services, professional pharmacy services, care coordination, and all necessary supplies and equipment (drugs and nursing visits coded separately), per diem

S9361 Home infusion therapy, diuretic intravenous therapy; administrative services, professional pharmacy services, care coordination, and all necessary supplies and equipment (drugs and nursing visits coded separately), per diem

S9363 Home infusion therapy, antispasmotic therapy; administrative services, professional pharmacy services, care coordination, and all necessary supplies and equipment (drugs and nursing visits coded separately), per diem

This group of codes reports daily or intermittent infusion therapy services and supplies, other than drugs and nursing visits. Medication is infused through a vein or the subcutaneous tissue.

S9364-S9368

S9364 Home infusion therapy, total parenteral nutrition (TPN); administrative services, professional pharmacy services, care coordination, and all necessary supplies and equipment including standard TPN formula (lipids, specialty amino acid formulas, drugs other than in standard formula and nursing visits coded separately), per diem (do not use with home infusion codes S9365-S9368 using daily volume scales)

S9365 Home infusion therapy, total parenteral nutrition (TPN); one liter per day, administrative services, professional pharmacy services, care coordination, and all necessary supplies and equipment including standard TPN formula (lipids, specialty amino acid formulas, drugs other than in standard formula and nursing visits coded separately), per diem

S9366 Home infusion therapy, total parenteral nutrition (TPN); more than one liter but no more than two liters per day, administrative services, professional pharmacy services, care coordination, and all necessary supplies and equipment including standard TPN formula (lipids, specialty amino acid formulas, drugs other than in standard formula and nursing visits coded separately), per diem

S9367 Home infusion therapy, total parenteral nutrition (TPN); more than two liters but no more than three liters per day, administrative services, professional pharmacy services, care coordination, and all necessary supplies and equipment including standard TPN formula (lipids, specialty amino acid formulas, drugs other than in standard formula and nursing visits coded separately), per diem

S9368 Home infusion therapy, total parenteral nutrition (TPN); more than three liters per day, administrative services, professional pharmacy services, care coordination, and all necessary supplies and equipment including standard TPN formula (lipids, specialty amino acid formulas, drugs other than in standard formula and nursing visits coded separately), per diem

This group of codes reports daily parenteral services and supplies, other than nursing visits, associated with total parenteral nutrition (TPN). Parenteral nutrition is administered to the patient through a vein. Since the alimentary tract of a patient with severe pathology does not function adequately for ingesting food normally, nutrients to sustain life must be administered by other methods. Parenteral nutrition solutions are based on the composition of ingredients or nutrients in each product. Scalable TPN ingredients are those that may differ based on lab work or that are ordered based on a concentration basis rather than on the total daily TPN volume.

S9370

S9370 Home therapy, intermittent antiemetic injection therapy; administrative services, professional pharmacy services, care coordination, and all necessary supplies and equipment (drugs and nursing visits coded separately), per diem

This code reports intermittent antiemetic injection therapy services and supplies, other than drugs and nursing visits. Medication is infused through a vein or the subcutaneous tissue.

S9372

S9372 Home therapy; intermittent anticoagulant injection therapy (e.g., Heparin); administrative services, professional pharmacy services, care coordination, and all necessary supplies and equipment (drugs and nursing visits coded separately), per diem (do not use this code for flushing of infusion devices with Heparin to maintain patency)

Heparin is an anticoagulant indicated for the treatment and prevention of blood clots, including pulmonary embolism and deep vein thrombosis. It is also used to ensure patency of indwelling intravenous catheters. Heparin inhibits reactions that lead to the clotting of blood and the formation of fibrin clots. It works by acting as an accelerant in forming antithrombin III-thrombin complex, which deactivates thrombin. This prevents the conversion of fibrinogen to fibrin. Heparin sodium is derived from bovine or porcine pulmonary or intestinal tissue and standardized for anticoagulant activity. This code reports home infusions for the intermittent anticoagulant therapy on a daily (per diem) basis. Drugs and nursing visits should be coded separately.

S9373-S9377

S9373 Home infusion therapy, hydration therapy; administrative services, professional pharmacy services, care coordination, and all necessary supplies and equipment (drugs and nursing visits coded separately), per diem (do not use with hydration therapy codes S9374-S9377 using daily volume scales)

S9374 Home infusion therapy, hydration therapy; 1 liter per day, administrative services, professional pharmacy services, care coordination, and all necessary supplies and equipment (drugs and nursing visits coded separately), per diem

S9375 Home infusion therapy, hydration therapy; more than 1 liter but no more than 2 liters per day, administrative services, professional pharmacy services, care coordination, and all necessary supplies and equipment (drugs and nursing visits coded separately), per diem

S9376 Home infusion therapy, hydration therapy; more than 2 liters but no more than 3 liters per day, administrative services, professional pharmacy services, care coordination, and all necessary supplies and equipment (drugs and nursing visits coded separately), per diem

S9377 Home infusion therapy, hydration therapy; more than 3 liters per day, administrative services, professional pharmacy services, care coordination, and all necessary supplies (drugs and nursing visits coded separately), per diem

This group of codes reports daily hydration infusion and supplies, other than drugs and nursing visits. Fluids are administered to the patient through a vein. Hydration is used to treat dehydration and electrolyte imbalance. Scalable hydration ingredients are those that may differ based on lab work or that are ordered based on a concentration basis rather than on the total daily volume.

S9379

S9379 Home infusion therapy, infusion therapy, not otherwise classified; administrative services, professional pharmacy services, care coordination, and all necessary supplies and equipment (drugs and nursing visits coded separately), per diem

Infusion therapy is the administration of fluids through a needle or catheter. The infusion is usually intravenous, but may also refer to intracavity, intramuscular, or epidural routes of administration. Home infusion therapy is the administration of the infusion in the patient's home. This code reports home infusion therapy that is not otherwise described by other more specific HCPCS Level II codes. The code encompasses administrative services, professional pharmacy services, care coordination, and all necessary supplies and equipment except for drugs and nursing visits.

S9381

S9381 Delivery or service to high risk areas requiring escort or extra protection, per visit

This code reports an added charge per visit when an item or service must be delivered in a high crime area. These areas require an escort or extra protection.

S9401

S9401 Anticoagulation clinic, inclusive of all services except laboratory tests, per session

An anticoagulation clinic is an organized outpatient service that monitors and manages the medications used to prevent blood clots. Anticoagulants must be maintained at a level that does not cause too much clotting or too little clotting. There is usually a pharmacist present. The patient's clotting time is determined using an internalized normalized ratio or INR. Medications are then increased or decreased to reach the target INR.

S9430

S9430 Pharmacy compounding and dispensing services

This code reports pharmacy fees for the compounding (or mixing) of drug and drug components and the dispensing of the drug.

S9432-S9435

S9432 Medical foods for noninborn errors of metabolism

S9433 Medical food nutritionally complete, administered orally, providing 100% of nutritional intake

S9434 Modified solid food supplements for inborn errors of metabolism

S9435 Medical foods for inborn errors of metabolism

Medical foods or food supplements are food stuffs designed and formulated to provide appropriate nutrition to patients who have food allergies or specific problems with digestion or absorption. Inborn errors of metabolism are genetic diseases that cause the incomplete breakdown of various substances or the accumulation of toxic substances that interfere with normal cellular function.

S9436-S9437

S9436 Childbirth preparation/Lamaze classes, nonphysician provider, per session

S9437 Childbirth refresher classes, nonphysician provider, per session

Lamaze is a type of childbirth preparation course. Childbirth preparation courses seek to prepare the woman for coping with pain, progressing through labor, and facilitating delivery of the baby. Women are taught techniques to tolerate pain and to assist the body in a natural childbirth. Techniques include movement, massage, breathing, and exercise. Refresher classes are reviews of the childbirth preparation courses for those women who have previously attended a course.

S9438

S9438 Cesarean birth classes, nonphysician provider, per session

Cesarean birth classes are birth preparation classes designed to explain to women the process of labor, reasons for the cesarean section, the procedure itself, and what to expect after the delivery.

S9439

S9439 VBAC (vaginal birth after cesarean) classes, nonphysician provider, per session

Vaginal birth after cesarean (VBAC) classes are birth preparation classes designed to explain to women the process of labor, the procedure itself, what to expect after the delivery, and any complications that may occur due to the prior cesarean section.

S9441

S9441 Asthma education, nonphysician provider, per session

Asthma education may involve one or more instructive sessions where the patient is taught the anatomy of the lungs, lifestyle changes, triggers, attack prevention, and treatment including the use of medication and medication delivery devices. It may also include self-management and self-monitoring tools to help identify the patient's needs and help them maintain quality of life.

S9442

S9442 Birthing classes, nonphysician provider, per session

Birthing classes seek to prepare the woman for all kinds of issues surrounding childbirth, including breathing, coping with pain, progressing through labor, and vaginal or cesarean delivery of the baby. Women are prepared for the changes that pregnancy brings and the care of a newborn.

S9443

S9443 Lactation classes, nonphysician provider, per session

Lactation classes focus on preparation for breastfeeding, cues from the baby, latching on, length of time to feed, nursing bras, breast pumps, and excess breast milk. Trained counselors are usually available to assist mothers who are encountering difficulties.

S9444

S9444 Parenting classes, nonphysician provider, per session

Parenting classes are lessons and training in the art of parenting. Effective parenting skills include communication skills, stress management, empathy, anger and conflict resolution, boundary and limit setting, rewards and discipline, teamwork, and parenting styles. Parenting classes may be taken for personal growth, but are most often undertaken due to court orders.

S9445-S9446

S9445 Patient education, not otherwise classified, nonphysician provider, individual, per session

S9446 Patient education, not otherwise classified, nonphysician provider, group, per session

Patient education represents patient teaching or training that is not described by other HCPCS Level II codes. Group sessions consist of two or more people, while individual sessions are one-on-one.

S9447

S9447 Infant safety (including CPR) classes, nonphysician provider, per session

Infant safety classes train parents and other caregivers on how to provide safe environments for a newborn and infant. Subjects include car seats, cribs and sleep arrangements, poison prevention, and environmental safety. This code includes cardiopulmonary resuscitation.

S9449

S9449 Weight management classes, nonphysician provider, per session

Weight management classes are training and education related to nutrition, physical activity, stress management, and lifestyle and how they relate to health. They are geared to teaching the patient to reach and maintain an ideal weight.

S9451

S9451 Exercise classes, nonphysician provider, per session

Exercise classes are formal programs of bodily activities that maintain physical fitness and overall health. They are usually performed in a group. Instructors may have formal training. There are generally three types of exercise: flexibility, such as stretching; aerobic, such as cycling, tennis, and swimming; and anaerobic, such as weight lifting. Exercise classes can address all three types or only one.

S9452

S9452 Nutrition classes, nonphysician provider, per session

Nutrition is the provision of the appropriate amount of food, water, vitamins, minerals, and related items that allow an organism to function in a safe and healthy manner. Nutrition classes provide organized instruction in the food and foodstuffs necessary for life. Dietitians are health professionals who specialize in nutrition and meal planning and preparation. Classes are usually group activities that discuss generalities. Counseling involves the dietitian and is usually individualized to a single patient.

S9453

S9453 Smoking cessation classes, nonphysician provider, per session

Smoking cessation classes are organized sessions that provide instruction, assistance, and guidance in the discontinuance of smoking. Smoking usually refers to tobacco smoking, but may also apply to other substances. Smoking cessation can be achieved with or without the assistance of health care professionals and with or without the use of medications. Groups of people who are trying to quit smoking can also provide support to each other.

S9454

S9454 Stress management classes, nonphysician provider, per session

Stress management classes are organized education and training on the techniques and methods of controlling levels of stress, particularly chronic stress, to improve life functioning. Medication can be used to decrease feelings of anxiety and stress. Among the other techniques available are yoga, exercise, meditation, deep breathing, progressive relaxation, time management, planning and decision making, and pet therapy.

S9455-S9465

S9455 Diabetic management program, group session

S9460 Diabetic management program, nurse visit

S9465 Diabetic management program, dietitian visit

A diabetes management program is used to teach a patient how to control and monitor blood glucose levels. The program includes techniques to deal with the emotional and physical problems associated with the disease. It also provides education regarding exercise, nutrition, medication, and monitoring.

S9470

S9470 Nutritional counseling, dietitian visit

Nutrition is the provision of the appropriate amount of food, water, vitamins, minerals, and related items that allow an organism to function in a safe and healthy manner. Nutrition classes provide organized instruction in the food and foodstuffs necessary for life. Dietitians are health professionals who specialize in nutrition and meal planning and preparation. Classes are usually group activities that discuss generalities. Counseling involves the dietitian and is usually individualized to a single patient.

S9472

S9472 Cardiac rehabilitation program, nonphysician provider, per diem

A cardiac rehabilitation program is a rehabilitation program for patients who have experienced one or more of the following: an acute myocardial infarction within the preceding 12 months; coronary artery bypass surgery; current stable angina pectoris; heart valve repair or replacement; percutaneous transluminal coronary angioplasty or coronary stenting; heart or heart-lung transplant. Cardiac rehabilitation programs usually include the following components: physician-prescribed exercise each day that items and services are furnished; cardiac risk factor modification; psychosocial assessment; outcomes assessment; an individualized treatment plan detailing how components are used for each patient. This code represents cardiac rehabilitation services provided by a nonphysician provider.

S9473

S9473 Pulmonary rehabilitation program, nonphysician provider, per diem

Pulmonary rehabilitation (PR) is a program to help improve the quality of life for people with chronic breathing problems. PR may include psychological counseling, breathing strategies, exercise training, ways to conserve energy, and education on the patient's lung disease, including how to manage it. This code includes monitoring services and exercise. Pulmonary rehabilitation items and services are usually prescribed for patients who are diagnosed with moderate to severe COPD, when referred by the physician who is treating the chronic respiratory disease. Report this code when pulmonary rehabilitation services are provided by a nonphysician provider.

S9474

S9474 Enterostomal therapy by a registered nurse certified in enterostomal therapy, per diem

Enterostomal therapy is the care of a stoma, which is a surgically created passageway from the internal body cavity to the outside. A registered nurse certified in enterostomal therapy receives specialized training in the ostomy planning and aftercare. The nurse may work with the patient and surgeons to determine the optimal stoma site, provide surgical aftercare, change the appliance, provide stoma and skin care, and instruct the patient or caregiver on these topics. Enterostomal therapy nurses usually also have specialized training in wound care and incontinence care.

S9475

S9475 Ambulatory setting substance abuse treatment or detoxification services, per diem

Ambulatory setting substance abuse treatment or detoxification services are medically supervised mental and behavioral health services provided in an outpatient environment. Patients arrive at points during the day and return home or to another setting at night. This treatment is aimed at patients with substance abuse problems.

S9476

S9476 Vestibular rehabilitation program, nonphysician provider, per diem

A vestibular rehabilitation program is an organized outpatient program that seeks to train patients with chronic or acute vestibular (inner ear) disorders to deal with or alleviate primary and secondary symptoms. The vestibular rehabilitation therapy is usually exercise based, but may include medications that suppress vestibular functions. Exercises may include the coordination of eye and head movements, balance and walking ability, and fitness and endurance with the goals of decreasing dizziness and visual symptoms, improved balance and ambulation, and increased activity levels. An assessment and therapy plan is usually performed by specially trained physical or occupational therapists.

S9480

S9480 Intensive outpatient psychiatric services, per diem

Intensive outpatient psychiatric services are mental and behavioral health treatments provided in an outpatient setting. Generally, they are at least three hours per day for two or more days per week. The services may address substance abuse disorders, mental or behavioral health issues, or both, which are dual diagnosis programs. These programs are usually used as a step down from acute inpatient care, residential care, or a partial hospitalization program. They may also be viewed as a step up from regular outpatient services.

S9482

S9482 Family stabilization services, per 15 minutes

Family stabilization services are programs, activities, and services that provide participants and their families with employment, family dynamics, economic stability, and reduced barriers. The goal is to keep a family together and united as a cohesive, safe, and productive support system and unit. Many programs operate 24 hours a day, seven days a week. Family stabilization services involve as many disciplines as required and coordinate services among all professionals and paraprofessionals.

S9484-S9485

S9484 Crisis intervention mental health services, per hour

S9485 Crisis intervention mental health services, per diem

Crisis intervention mental health services are emergency mental and behavioral health care intended to assist in a crisis situation. Crisis situations may be defined as a person's perception or experience of an event or situation that exceeds the person's current resources or coping mechanisms. Crisis intervention seeks to stabilize the person's mental state and prevent immediate harm to the person or others in contact with that person.

S9490

S9490 Home infusion therapy, corticosteroid infusion; administrative services, professional pharmacy services, care coordination, and all necessary supplies and equipment (drugs and nursing visits coded separately), per diem

This code reports daily infusion therapy services and supplies of corticosteroids, other than drugs and nursing visits. Medication is infused through a vein.

S9494-S9504

S9494 Home infusion therapy, antibiotic, antiviral, or antifungal therapy; administrative services, professional pharmacy services, care coordination, and all necessary supplies and equipment (drugs and nursing visits coded separately), per diem (do not use this code with home infusion codes for hourly dosing schedules S9497-S9504)

S9497 Home infusion therapy, antibiotic, antiviral, or antifungal therapy; once every 3 hours; administrative services, professional pharmacy services, care coordination, and all necessary supplies and equipment (drugs and nursing visits coded separately), per diem

S9500 Home infusion therapy, antibiotic, antiviral, or antifungal therapy; once every 24 hours; administrative services, professional pharmacy services, care coordination, and all necessary supplies and equipment (drugs and nursing visits coded separately), per diem

S9501 Home infusion therapy, antibiotic, antiviral, or antifungal therapy; once every 12 hours; administrative services, professional pharmacy services, care coordination, and all necessary supplies and equipment (drugs and nursing visits coded separately), per diem

S9502 Home infusion therapy, antibiotic, antiviral, or antifungal therapy; once every 8 hours, administrative services, professional pharmacy services, care coordination, and all necessary supplies and equipment (drugs and nursing visits coded separately), per diem

S9503 Home infusion therapy, antibiotic, antiviral, or antifungal; once every 6 hours; administrative services, professional pharmacy services, care coordination, and all necessary supplies and equipment (drugs and nursing visits coded separately), per diem

S9504 Home infusion therapy, antibiotic, antiviral, or antifungal; once every 4 hours; administrative services, professional pharmacy services, care coordination, and all necessary supplies and equipment (drugs and nursing visits coded separately), per diem

This group of codes reports antibiotic, antiviral, or antifungal medication infusion services and supplies, other than drugs and nursing visits. Medication is infused into a vein. The code reported is based on how often the medication is given.

S9529

S9529 Routine venipuncture for collection of specimen(s), single homebound, nursing home, or skilled nursing facility patient

Routine venipuncture needle is the insertion of a needle into a vein to withdraw a specimen of blood for laboratory testing. This code reports this service when performed on a single homebound, nursing home, or skilled nursing facility patient.

S9537

S9537 Home therapy; hematopoietic hormone injection therapy (e.g., erythropoietin, G-CSF, GM-CSF); administrative services, professional pharmacy services, care coordination, and all necessary supplies and equipment (drugs and nursing visits coded separately), per diem

Hematopoietic hormones, such as EPO, G-CSF, or GM-CSF, stimulate the production of various types of blood cells. The blood cells usually need replenishment due to exogenous factors, such as chemotherapy, radiation therapy, or invasive infections. This code includes all services, except for drugs and nursing visits, provided in the patient's home.

S9538

S9538 Home transfusion of blood product(s); administrative services, professional pharmacy services, care coordination and all necessary supplies and equipment (blood products, drugs, and nursing visits coded separately), per diem

A transfusion of blood products is the intravenous infusion of whole blood or blood components into the patient's circulatory system. Blood transfusions are used to replace blood lost during surgery or due to a serious injury, or when the body cannot appropriately create blood due to illness. This code includes all services, except for the blood products, drugs, and nursing visits, provided in the patient's home.

S9542-S9562

S9542 Home injectable therapy, not otherwise classified, including administrative services, professional pharmacy services, care coordination, and all necessary supplies and equipment (drugs and nursing visits coded separately), per diem

S9558 Home injectable therapy; growth hormone, including administrative services, professional pharmacy services, care coordination, and all necessary supplies and equipment (drugs and nursing visits coded separately), per diem

S9559 Home injectable therapy, interferon, including administrative services, professional pharmacy services, care coordination, and all necessary supplies and equipment (drugs and nursing visits coded separately), per diem

S9560 Home injectable therapy; hormonal therapy (e.g., leuprolide, goserelin), including administrative services, professional pharmacy services, care coordination, and all necessary supplies and equipment (drugs and nursing visits coded separately), per diem

S9562 Home injectable therapy, palivizumab, including administrative services, professional pharmacy services, care coordination, and all necessary supplies and equipment (drugs and nursing visits coded separately), per diem

This group of codes reports daily injection therapy services and supplies, other than drugs and nursing visits. Medication is injected intravenously or subcutaneously.

S9590

S9590 Home therapy, irrigation therapy (e.g., sterile irrigation of an organ or anatomical cavity); including administrative services, professional pharmacy services, care coordination, and all necessary supplies and equipment (drugs and nursing visits coded separately), per diem

Irrigation therapy is the steady flow of a solution, usually sterile, across or into a wound, organ, or body cavity. It is intended to wash away cellular debris and surface pathogens and, in doing so, promote healing. This code includes all services, except for drugs and nursing visits, provided in the patient's home.

S9810

S9810 Home therapy; professional pharmacy services for provision of infusion, specialty drug administration, and/or disease state management, not otherwise classified, per hour (do not use this code with any per diem code)

This code represents professional pharmacy services for provision of infusion, specialty drug administration, and/or disease state management in home therapy. This code should only be reported when other HCPCS Level II codes do not adequately describe the type of home therapy.

S9900-S9901

S9900 Services by a Journal-listed Christian Science practitioner for the purpose of healing, per diem

S9901 Services by a Journal-listed Christian Science nurse, per hour

A Christian Science practitioner is an individual who follows the practice of healing through prayer according to the teachings of Christian Science. This is usually a specifically focused prayer affirming the Christian Scientist beliefs. Any Christian Scientist who has taken an intensive two-week course may be called a practitioner. Full-time practitioners usually have been practicing for several years and must be members of the mother church (the global organization headquartered in Boston). To be journal-listed, the practitioner must be a full-time practitioner and must present evidence of three cases of the healing of nonfamily members. Code S9900 is used to report a daily per diem rate and S9901 is used to report an hourly rate.

S9960-S9961

S9960 Ambulance service, conventional air services, nonemergency transport, one way (fixed wing)

S9961 Ambulance service, conventional air service, nonemergency transport, one way (rotary wing)

Fixed wing (FW) ambulance (airplane) conventional air service is the transportation by a fixed wing aircraft that is certified by the Federal Aviation Administration (FAA) as a fixed wing air ambulance along with the provision of a nonemergency transport, one way, medically. Rotary wing (RW) ambulance (helicopter) conventional air service is the transportation by helicopter that is certified by the Federal Aviation Administration (FAA) as a rotary wing ambulance, including the provision of nonemergency transport, one way.

S9970

S9970 Health club membership, annual

Health club membership is an additional preventive medicine benefit offered by various payers. This code represents the annual fees for a health club, also known as a fitness club or gym. The club or gym is a location that houses exercise equipment, may offer exercise classes, and other educational opportunities.

S9975

S9975 Transplant related lodging, meals and transportation, per diem

This code reports the costs of lodging, meals, and transportation for transplant-related companions or care-givers. This code may also report expenses incurred by a living donor.

S9976-S9977

S9976 Lodging, per diem, not otherwise classified

S9977 Meals, per diem, not otherwise specified

These codes report other lodging and meal expenses that are not adequately described by more specific HCPCS Level II codes. These expenses may be reimbursable depending on the circumstances and on payer policy definitions.

S9981-S9982

S9981 Medical records copying fee, administrative

S9982 Medical records copying fee, per page

These codes report charges for reproducing medical or health record pages, electronically or on paper.

S9986

S9986 Not medically necessary service (patient is aware that service not medically necessary)

This code is reported when the provider does not believe the item or treatment is medically necessary, which may result in noncoverage. The reporting of this code also indicates that the patient is aware that the service is not considered medically necessary.

S9988

S9988 Services provided as part of a Phase I clinical trial

Clinical trials are procedures performed in biomedical or health research development that allow different components to be tested in controlled environments in predefined protocols. A phase one trial is a general screening for safety in a small group of people. Phase one trials seek to determine a safe dose range and to identify any side effects. Phase two trials use a larger group of people to establish effectiveness and safety. Phase three is the final phase of a trial and uses a large group of people to confirm effectiveness, monitor side effects, compare the new treatment to commonly used treatments, and to collect further safety issues.

S9989

S9989 Services provided outside of the United States of America (list in addition to code(s) for services(s))

This code indicates that the service identified by another HCPCS Level II code was performed outside of the United States.

S9990-S9991

S9990 Services provided as part of a Phase II clinical trial

S9991 Services provided as part of a Phase III clinical trial

Clinical trials are procedures performed in biomedical or health research development that allow different components to be tested in controlled environments in predefined protocols. A phase one trial is a general screening for safety in a small group of people. Phase one trials seek to determine a safe dose range and to identify any side effects. Phase two trials use a larger group of people to establish effectiveness and safety. Phase three is the final phase of a trial and uses a large group of people to confirm effectiveness, monitor side effects, compare the new treatment to commonly used treatments, and to collect further safety issues.

S9992-S9996

S9992 Transportation costs to and from trial location and local transportation costs (e.g., fares for taxicab or bus) for clinical trial participant and one caregiver/companion

S9994 Lodging costs (e.g., hotel charges) for clinical trial participant and one caregiver/companion

S9996 Meals for clinical trial participant and one caregiver/companion

Transportation, lodging, and meals are not generally reimbursed for participants and caregivers. These codes report these costs when payers do reimburse the expenses.

S9999

S9999 Sales tax

This code reports sales tax charged for medical goods and services in some localities.

T

T1000

T1000 Private duty/independent nursing service(s), licensed, up to 15 minutes

Private-duty or independent nursing services involve individuals who provide nursing care on a one-on-one basis to individual patients. This code applies to services provided by licensed individuals, registered nurse, or licensed vocational/practical nurse.

T1001

T1001 Nursing assessment/evaluation

A nursing assessment or evaluation is the gathering and recording of a patient's physiological, psychological, sociological, and sometimes spiritual status. Data are gathered from a nursing point of view, such as information about the need for assistance in daily activities.

T1002-T1004

T1002 RN services, up to 15 minutes

T1003 LPN/LVN services, up to 15 minutes

T1004 Services of a qualified nursing aide, up to 15 minutes

Services provided by each practitioner are recorded in 15-minute increments.

T1005

T1005 Respite care services, up to 15 minutes

Respite care is the provision of short-term temporary care to a person with a chronic illness or disability. The term "respite care" usually refers to relief provided to a primary caregiver.

T1006

T1006 Alcohol and/or substance abuse services, family/couple counseling

This code represents family or couples counseling in relation to alcohol and/or substance abuse services.

T1007

T1007 Alcohol and/or substance abuse services, treatment plan development and/or modification

This code represents the development of a treatment plan and/or its modification, in relation to alcohol and/or substance abuse services.

T1009

T1009 Child sitting services for children of the individual receiving alcohol and/or substance abuse services

This code represents charges for child-sitting services for children of the individual receiving alcohol and/or substance abuse services.

T1010

T1010 Meals for individuals receiving alcohol and/or substance abuse services (when meals not included in the program)

This code represents charges for meals for individuals receiving alcohol and/or substance abuse services. It is used only when meals are not included in the program.

T1012

T1012 Alcohol and/or substance abuse services, skills development

This code represents skills development, which can be work-related, life skills, coping skills, or similar types of skills that are needed to successfully attain a goal in relation to alcohol and/or substance abuse services.

T1013

T1013 Sign language or oral interpretive services, per 15 minutes

This code represents the use of an interpreter for sign language or oral interpretive communication services.

T1014

T1014 Telehealth transmission, per minute, professional services bill separately

Telehealth is the delivery of health-related services via telecommunications equipment. The term encompasses technology that includes email, video conferencing, and the transmission of medical images or medical data. The telecommunications most often involve a primary care practitioner with a patient at a remote site and a consulting medical specialist at an urban or referral facility. An originating site is the location of the patient at the time the service is being furnished via a telecommunications system. A fee that is set annually is paid to the originating site. This code represents the transmission charge for the originating site. A separate payment is made for the professional fee(s) of the physician or practitioner.

T1015

T1015 Clinic visit/encounter, all-inclusive

An all-inclusive fee for a clinic visit or encounter is a predetermined fee that includes all services related to the visit or encounter in a Federally Qualified Health Center (FQHC) or Rural Health Clinic (RHC). These services include facility charges, physician and professional charges, ancillary services, supplies, and drugs.

T1016-T1017

T1016 Case management, each 15 minutes

T1017 Targeted case management, each 15 minutes

Case management is an effort to improve care and to contain costs by having one party manage or coordinate all care delivered to a patient that usually has certain complex illnesses or injuries, including mental and behavioral health issues. Case management may include, but is not limited to, the evaluation of a condition, the development and implementation of a plan of care, the coordination of medical resources, and the appropriate communication to all parties. Targeted case management is targeted to a specific population subgroup.

T1018

T1018 School-based individualized education program (IEP) services, bundled

A school-based individualized education program (IEP) is mandated by the Individuals with Disabilities Act. An IEP is designed to meet the specific educational needs of a child who may have a disability as defined by federal regulations. The IEP is intended to help the child reach educational goals. The child's needs are identified in an evaluation process. Specific instructions are provided to teachers and related providers so that there is a clear understanding of the disability and its effect on the learning process.

T1019-T1020

T1019 Personal care services, per 15 minutes, not for an inpatient or resident of a hospital, nursing facility, ICF/MR or IMD, part of the individualized plan of treatment (code may not be used to identify services provided by home health aide or certified nurse assistant)

T1020 Personal care services, per diem, not for an inpatient or resident of a hospital, nursing facility, ICF/MR or IMD, part of the individualized plan of treatment (code may not be used to identify services provided by home health aide or certified nurse assistant)

Personal care services are paraprofessional aide services not directly linked to medical or skilled nursing care. Such services may include activities of daily living, such bathing, shopping, and dressing, as part of an individualized plan of treatment. These codes are not reported when a patient has been institutionalized in a hospital, nursing facility, or intermediate care facility or is receiving formal home health services.

T1021

T1021 Home health aide or certified nurse assistant, per visit

This code identifies a per visit charge for the services provided by a home health aide or certified nurse assistant.

T1022

T1022 Contracted home health agency services, all services provided under contract, per day

This code represents the daily rate for all services provided under a contract for home health agency services.

T1023

T1023 Screening to determine the appropriateness of consideration of an individual for participation in a specified program, project or treatment protocol, per encounter

This code represents an encounter for the screening used to determine if an individual should participate in a specified program, project, or treatment protocol.

T1024

T1024 Evaluation and treatment by an integrated, specialty team contracted to provide coordinated care to multiple or severely handicapped children, per encounter

Multiple disabilities encompass a combination of various challenges and special needs that may include speech, learning, visual, hearing, brain injury, mental retardation, and physical mobility. There may also be sensory loss, behavioral problems, or social issues. The characteristics and severity of these disabilities vary. Severe multiple disabilities include cerebral palsy, severe autism, and brain injuries. An integrated specialty team consisting of practitioners from appropriate practices evaluates the individual with the multiple handicaps and determines which services would be necessary to provide care for the individual.

T1025-T1026

T1025 Intensive, extended multidisciplinary services provided in a clinic setting to children with complex medical, physical, mental and psychosocial impairments, per diem

T1026 Intensive, extended multidisciplinary services provided in a clinic setting to children with complex medical, physical, medical and psychosocial impairments, per hour

Multiple disabilities encompass a combination of various challenges and special needs that may include speech, learning, visual, hearing, brain injury, mental retardation, and physical mobility. There may also be sensory loss, behavioral problems, or social issues. The characteristics and severity of these disabilities vary. Severe multiple disabilities include cerebral palsy, severe autism, and brain injuries. A multidisciplinary team provides services in a clinic setting to children with complex medical, physical, medical, and psychosocial impairments.

T1027

T1027 Family training and counseling for child development, per 15 minutes

Family training and counseling for child development is specialized training and education provided to a family to assist with the child's needs and development.

T1028

T1028 Assessment of home, physical and family environment, to determine suitability to meet patient's medical needs

This code represents a visit to and evaluation of an individual's home, physical, and family environment to determine if it is suitable for the patient's medical needs.

T1029

T1029 Comprehensive environmental lead investigation, not including laboratory analysis, per dwelling

This code represents a comprehensive investigation of the lead that may exist in an individual's environment. Lead in the environment may be ingested or inhaled by a child, leading to moderate to severe poisoning that adversely affects the physical and mental health of the individual.

T1030-T1031

T1030 Nursing care, in the home, by registered nurse, per diem

T1031 Nursing care, in the home, by licensed practical nurse, per diem

These codes represent nursing care provided by licensed practitioners in the individual's home.

T1032-T1033

T1032 Services performed by a doula birth worker, per 15 minutes

T1033 Services performed by a doula birth worker, per diem

A doula is a trained professional that provides emotional, informational, and physical support to pregnant clients before, during, and after childbirth. The goal of a doula is to help the patient and family have a healthy, safe, and positive labor and postpartum experience. A doula does not have medical certification like a physician or midwife and does not perform medical procedures. They are there to help with relaxation and breathing techniques, offer advice on labor positions, enhance the support of the patient's co-parent or coach, provide non-medical pain management techniques (i.e., massage, aromatherapy, music, mantras, counter pressure techniques), as well as advocate for the patient's needs with the medical team during labor and the postpartum period. A doula may be present with the patient during a hospital or home delivery. Report T1032 for each 15 minutes of doula services. For T1033 for doula services provided per diem.

T1040-T1041

T1040 Medicaid certified community behavioral health clinic services, per diem

T1041 Medicaid certified community behavioral health clinic services, per month

The Protecting Access to Medicare Act (PAMA) established a demonstration program based on the Excellence in Mental Health Act. Certified community behavioral health clinics (CCBHC) participating in this demonstration project are eligible for enhanced Medicaid payment through a Prospective Payment System (PPS), a methodology used to reimburse providers based on their anticipated costs of serving individuals in their communities. CCBHCs are subject to unique requirements with respect to their partnerships in the health and social service sectors. CCBHCs service delivery is based on the concept of trauma-informed recovery, with services provided outside the traditional four walls of a clinic in settings where providers can better connect with target populations to engage them in care. Report T1040 when reimbursement is on a per diem basis and T1041 when reimbursement is on a monthly basis.

T1502-T1503

T1502 Administration of oral, intramuscular and/or subcutaneous medication by health care agency/professional, per visit

T1503 Administration of medication, other than oral and/or injectable, by a health care agency/professional, per visit

These codes represent the charge for a health care agency or professional to administer oral, intramuscular, subcutaneous, or other forms of medication.

T1505

T1505 Electronic medication compliance management device, includes all components and accessories, not otherwise classified

An electronic medication compliance management device is a computerized medication dispenser that can dispense individual doses of different medications for up to one month. The device is programmed by the patient's health care provider and delivers the prescribed dose at the prescribed time.

T1999

T1999 Miscellaneous therapeutic items and supplies, retail purchases, not otherwise classified; identify product in "remarks"

This code represents the retail purchase of miscellaneous therapeutic items and supplies that are not otherwise classified in HCPCS codes.

T

T2001-T2005

T2001 Nonemergency transportation; patient attendant/escort

T2002 Nonemergency transportation; per diem

T2003 Nonemergency transportation; encounter/trip

T2004 Nonemergency transport; commercial carrier, multipass

T2005 Nonemergency transportation; stretcher van

Nonemergency transportation is the delivery or movement of a person in a nonemergency situation to a medical appointment or destination. It generally denotes the use of an emergency transport vehicle, such as an ambulance.

T2007

T2007 Transportation waiting time, air ambulance and nonemergency vehicle, one-half (1/2) hour increments

This code represents the idle or unloaded waiting time that a transport, air ambulance, or nonemergency vehicle spends waiting for a particular patient.

T2010-T2011

T2010 Preadmission screening and resident review (PASRR) Level I identification screening, per screen

T2011 Preadmission screening and resident review (PASRR) Level II evaluation, per evaluation

Preadmission screening and resident review (PASRR) is a protection for patients with serious mental illness or mental retardation. PASRR is intended to prevent patients from being inappropriately admitted to nursing facilities that cannot provide the specialized care they require. Federal law requires all patients, regardless of payer source, be given a level I identification screening to identify mental illnesses or mental retardation. Level I screens are generally forms completed by hospital discharge planners, community health nurses, or other practitioners defined by state law. Patients who do or may have a mental illness or mental retardation are then referred for a level II evaluation. The level II evaluation is provided to all patients identified in level I and any resident who has experienced a significant change in condition. This level II evaluation is the resident review that is conducted according to federal delineated criteria. Once it is determined that a patient has a mental illness or mental retardation, it must be determined what specialized services are needed and whether the nursing home can provide those services. Types of specialized services and their definition may vary by state.

T2012-T2021

T2012 Habilitation, educational; waiver, per diem

T2013 Habilitation, educational, waiver; per hour

T2014 Habilitation, prevocational, waiver; per diem

T2015 Habilitation, prevocational, waiver; per hour

T2016 Habilitation, residential, waiver; per diem

T2017 Habilitation, residential, waiver; 15 minutes

T2018 Habilitation, supported employment, waiver; per diem

T2019 Habilitation, supported employment, waiver; per 15 minutes

T2020 Day habilitation, waiver; per diem

T2021 Day habilitation, waiver; per 15 minutes

Habilitation is the act of making an individual capable of fitting into and/or functioning in society. The codes indicated here generally refer to people who have disabilities that initially prevent them from functioning independently in society. Habilitation provides the assistance that these people need to attain their goals, wants, and/or needs. Paraprofessionals and professionals usually provide support, training, and any required therapy. Day habilitation may be a full day of directed services or may be an alternate day where recreational activities are the main body of the day.

T2022-T2023

T2022 Case management, per month

T2023 Targeted case management; per month

Case management is an effort to improve care and to contain costs by having one party manage or coordinate all care delivered to patients who have certain complex illnesses or injuries, including mental and behavioral health issues. Case management may include, but is not limited to, the evaluation of a condition, the development and implementation of a plan of care, the coordination of medical resources, and the appropriate communication to all parties. Targeted case management targets a specific population subgroup.

T2024-T2025

T2024 Service assessment/plan of care development, waiver

T2025 Waiver services; not otherwise specified (NOS)

Medicaid may choose to wave certain requirements in conjunction with specialized programs. In these cases, waivers usually refer to permission from the federal government to waive or change certain requirements.

T2026-T2027

T2026 Specialized childcare, waiver; per diem

T2027 Specialized childcare, waiver; per 15 minutes

Specialized childcare usually refers to childcare provided to an individual who has special physical or developmental needs. It may also refer to childcare needed during nonstandard hours, such as overnight, or care for a mildly ill child who cannot attend school or regular daycare. Most states require providers of specialized childcare to be certified, licensed, or otherwise deemed qualified to care for the child. The waiver refers to permission from the federal government to state Medicaid plans to finance services that are not in compliance with federal regulations.

T2028-T2029

T2028 Specialized supply, not otherwise specified, waiver

T2029 Specialized medical equipment, not otherwise specified, waiver

These codes represent specialized supplies or durable medical equipment that is not otherwise identified by other HCPCS Level II codes. The waiver refers to permission from the federal government to state Medicaid plans to finance services that are not in compliance with federal regulations.

T2030-T2031

T2030 Assisted living, waiver; per month

T2031 Assisted living; waiver, per diem

An assisted living facility provides independent living arrangements with varying degrees of medical care and personal and support services. Most are designed to provide assistance with the activities of daily living, such as bathing and dressing. A community dining room or meal service may be available. Minor medical monitoring and assistance may be offered, depending upon state regulations. The waiver refers to permission from the federal government to state Medicaid plans to finance services that are not in compliance with federal regulations.

T2032-T2033

T2032 Residential care, not otherwise specified (NOS), waiver; per month

T2033 Residential care, not otherwise specified (NOS), waiver; per diem

Residential care is long-term care provided in a setting other than the patient's home. These codes report residential care that is not adequately described by other HCPCS Level II codes. Varying degrees of independent living, medical care, and personal and support services may be offered, depending upon state regulations. The waiver refers to permission from the federal government to state Medicaid plans to finance services that are not in compliance with federal regulations.

T2034

T2034 Crisis intervention, waiver; per diem

Crisis intervention is emergency psychological or psychiatric care intended to assist and stabilize individuals who are in an immediate crisis situation. A crisis may refer to any situation where the individual perceives a sudden loss of his/her ability to problem-solve and cope. The waiver refers to permission from the federal government to state Medicaid plans to finance services that are not in compliance with federal regulations.

T2035

T2035 Utility services to support medical equipment and assistive technology/devices, waiver

This code reports charges for utility services, such as water and electricity, needed to support medical equipment and assistive technology devices. The waiver refers to permission from the federal government to state Medicaid plans to finance services that are not in compliance with federal regulations.

T2036-T2037

T2036 Therapeutic camping, overnight, waiver; each session

T2037 Therapeutic camping, day, waiver; each session

Therapeutic camping is used to teach life and coping skills in an outdoor wilderness environment. Therapeutic camping may be directed to individuals with mental health, behavioral health, or medical health needs. The waiver refers to permission from the federal government to state Medicaid plans to finance services that are not in compliance with federal regulations.

T2038

T2038 Community transition, waiver; per service

Community transition is the facilitation of the movement of an individual from an institutional environment to community living. The waiver refers to permission from the federal government to state Medicaid plans to finance services that are not in compliance with federal regulations.

T2039

T2039 Vehicle modifications, waiver; per service

This code reports charges for a vehicle modification necessary for an individual's functioning. The waiver refers to permission from the federal government to state Medicaid plans to finance services that are not in compliance with federal regulations.

T2040-T2041

T2040 Financial management, self-directed, waiver; per 15 minutes

T2041 Supports brokerage, self-directed, waiver; per 15 minutes

Individuals with serious mental health or substance abuse issues that are actively in recovery are expected to prove self-directed care that includes managing finances, paying bills, and similar financial matters. A financial manager or intermediary supervises and supports these functions. A supports broker assists in defining needs, finding the necessary services, and monitoring the service performance. The waiver refers to permission from the federal government to state Medicaid plans to finance services that are not in compliance with federal regulations.

T2042-T2046

T2042 Hospice routine home care; per diem

T2043 Hospice continuous home care; per hour

T2044 Hospice inpatient respite care; per diem

T2045 Hospice general inpatient care; per diem

T2046 Hospice long-term care, room and board only; per diem

Hospice services are provided to patients who are terminally ill with a medical prognosis of less than six months to live. Routine home care includes hospice services provided in the patient's home for a total of eight hours or less. Continuous home care is provided only during a crisis in which the patient requires continuous nursing care to palliate or manage acute medical symptoms. Respite care is short-term inpatient care provided to relieve the family member or other caretaker. General inpatient care is care in an acute care general hospital for pain control and symptom management. Long-term care is hospice care provided to a patient in a long-term care facility.

T2047

T2047 Habilitation, prevocational, waiver; per 15 minutes

Habilitation is the act of making an individual capable of fitting into and/or functioning in society. The codes indicated here generally refer to people who have disabilities that initially prevent them from functioning independently in society. Habilitation provides the assistance that these people need to attain their goals, wants, and/or needs. Paraprofessionals and professionals usually provide support, training, and any required therapy. Day habilitation may be a full day of directed services or may be an alternate day where recreational activities are the main body of the day. Prevocational services teach general work skills and concepts such as attendance, attention span, communication, following directions, motor skills, personal self-care and appearance, problem solving, public transportation use, safety, social skills, and task completion. Report T2047 for prevocational habilitation services in 15-minute increments.

T2048

T2048 Behavioral health; long-term care residential (nonacute care in a residential treatment program where stay is typically longer than 30 days), with room and board, per diem

This code reports a per diem charge for long-term residential behavioral health care. It is to be reported for nonacute care in a residential treatment program where stay is typically longer than 30 days.

T2049

T2049 Nonemergency transportation; stretcher van, mileage; per mile

This code is reported for nonemergency transport of a stretcher patient who is not being medically monitored or treated. Patients most likely transported by stretcher are those individuals who cannot stand or sit independently.

T2050-T2051

T2050 Financial management, self-directed, waiver; per diem

T2051 Supports brokerage, self-directed, waiver; per diem

Individuals with serious mental health or substance abuse issues that are actively in recovery are expected to prove self-directed care that includes managing finances, paying bills, and similar financial matters. A financial manager or intermediary supervises and supports these functions. A supports broker assists in defining needs, finding the necessary services, and monitoring the service performance. The waiver refers to permission from the federal government to state Medicaid plans to finance services that are not in compliance with federal regulations.

T2101

T2101 Human breast milk processing, storage and distribution only

Human breast milk is the liquid produced by the mammary glands for the nourishment of a human infant. Human breast milk is considered the ideal food for newborns. When a mother cannot produce sufficient quantities of breast milk, the physician may prescribe milk donated by nursing mothers who are not biologically related to the child. This milk is maintained in human milk banks. The banks do not charge for the milk itself, but do charge for the collection, processing, and distribution of the milk.

T4521-T4528

T4521 Adult sized disposable incontinence product, brief/diaper, small, each

T4522 Adult sized disposable incontinence product, brief/diaper, medium, each

T4523 Adult sized disposable incontinence product, brief/diaper, large, each

T4524 Adult sized disposable incontinence product, brief/diaper, extra large, each

T4525 Adult sized disposable incontinence product, protective underwear/pull-on, small size, each

T4526 Adult sized disposable incontinence product, protective underwear/pull-on, medium size, each

T4527 Adult sized disposable incontinence product, protective underwear/pull-on, large size, each

T4528 Adult sized disposable incontinence product, protective underwear/pull-on, extra large size, each

Incontinence garments allow the individual to defecate or urinate somewhat discreetly. The garment is intended to absorb and contain the urine and feces. These garments may be disposable or reusable. It may be a flat diaper or a brief. Disposable garments include those commonly found at supermarkets. Flat reusable cloth diapers are generally rectangular with the same thickness throughout. Fit is accomplished by folding. Reusable briefs come in many varieties and may vary from slightly contoured to fully fitted briefs. There are also fully fitted briefs made of patented materials that are designed to be used with internal pads.

Disposable briefs and diapers are intended to be worn once. Adult pull-ons are diapers that can be pulled on like normal undergarments. Protective underwear is intended to further contain any feces or urine and protect outer clothing or bedding.

T4529-T4537

T4529 Pediatric sized disposable incontinence product, brief/diaper, small/medium size, each

T4530 Pediatric sized disposable incontinence product, brief/diaper, large size, each

T4531 Pediatric sized disposable incontinence product, protective underwear/pull-on, small/medium size, each

T4532 Pediatric sized disposable incontinence product, protective underwear/pull-on, large size, each

T4533 Youth sized disposable incontinence product, brief/diaper, each

T4534 Youth sized disposable incontinence product, protective underwear/pull-on, each

T4535 Disposable liner/shield/guard/pad/undergarment, for incontinence, each

T4536 Incontinence product, protective underwear/pull-on, reusable, any size, each

T4537 Incontinence product, protective underpad, reusable, bed size, each

Incontinence garments allow the individual to defecate or urinate somewhat discreetly. The garment is intended to absorb and contain the urine and feces. These garments may be disposable or reusable and may be a flat diaper or a brief. Disposable garments include those commonly found at supermarkets. Flat reusable cloth diapers are generally rectangular with the same thickness throughout. Fit is accomplished by folding. Reusable briefs come in many varieties and may vary from slightly contoured to fully fitted briefs. There are also fully fitted briefs made of patented materials that are designed to be used with internal pads. Some products include an individual disposable liner, shield, guard, pad, or undergarment. Disposable briefs and diapers are intended to be worn once. Underpads and chair pads are intended to provide reusable individual protection.

T4538

T4538 Diaper service, reusable diaper, each diaper

A reusable diaper is a piece of cloth that is intended to absorb and contain the urine and feces. This code represents diapers provided by and maintained by a diaper delivery service.

T4539

T4539 Incontinence product, diaper/brief, reusable, any size, each

This code reports individual disposable pull-on underwear and diapers used for leakage protection and incontinence. These items are used by patients with the inability to voluntarily control bladder or bowel functions or who are unable to use toilet facilities.

T4540-T4545

T4540 Incontinence product, protective underpad, reusable, chair size, each

T4541 Incontinence product, disposable underpad, large, each

T4542 Incontinence product, disposable underpad, small size, each

T4543 Adult sized disposable incontinence product, protective brief/diaper, above extra large, each

T4544 Adult sized disposable incontinence product, protective underwear/pull-on, above extra large, each

T4545 Incontinence product, disposable, penile wrap, each

Incontinence garments, which absorb and contain urine and feces, allow the individual to defecate or urinate somewhat discreetly. These garments may be disposable or reusable and may be flat diapers or briefs. Disposable garments include those commonly found at supermarkets. Flat reusable cloth diapers are generally rectangular with the same thickness throughout. The diapers are fitted by folding. Reusable briefs come in many varieties and may vary from slightly contoured to fully fitted briefs. There are also fully fitted briefs made of patented materials that are designed to be used with internal pads. Some products include an individual disposable liner, shield, guard, pad, or undergarment. Disposable briefs and diapers are intended to be worn once. Underpads and chair pads are intended to provide reusable individual protection. A penile wrap is a disposable pouch that is wrapped around the penis and is designed for light to moderate incontinence.

T5001

T5001 Positioning seat for persons with special orthopedic needs

Adjustable positioning seat cushions provide skin protection and positioning for individuals with paralysis, deformities, scoliosis, poor muscle control, or other conditions. Positioning seat cushions can aid in manipulation or control of objects, can assist in the performance of specific activities, and can provide added balance and support. Adjustable cushions can be adapted to conform to the individual's special orthopedic needs.

T5999

T5999 Supply, not otherwise specified

This code reports supplies that are not otherwise represented by other HCPCS Level II codes.

U

U0001-U0005

U0001 CDC 2019 Novel Coronavirus (2019-nCoV) Real-Time RT-PCR Diagnostic Panel

U0002 2019-nCoV coronavirus, SARS-CoV-2/2019-nCoV (COVID-19), any technique, multiple types or subtypes (includes all targets), non-CDC

U0003 Infectious agent detection by nucleic acid (DNA or RNA); severe acute respiratory syndrome coronavirus 2 (SARS-CoV-2) (coronavirus disease [COVID-19]), amplified probe technique, making use of high throughput technologies as described by CMS-2020-01-R

U0004 2019-nCoV coronavirus, SARS-CoV-2/2019-nCoV (COVID-19), any technique, multiple types or subtypes (includes all targets), non-CDC, making use of high throughput technologies as described by CMS-2020-01-R

U0005 Infectious agent detection by nucleic acid (DNA or RNA); severe acute respiratory syndrome coronavirus 2 (SARS-CoV-2) (coronavirus disease [COVID-19]), amplified probe technique, CDC or non-CDC, making use of high throughput technologies, completed within 2 calendar days from date of specimen collection (list separately in addition to either HCPCS code U0003 or U0004) as described by CMS-2020-01-R2

The 2019-Novel Coronavirus (2019-nCoV or COVID-19) Real-Time RT-PCR Diagnostic Panel is a molecular in vitro diagnostic test intended for presumptive qualitative detection of nucleic acid from COVID-19 in both upper and lower respiratory tract specimens (e.g., naso- or oropharyngeal swabs, sputum, aspirates, etc.) collected from patients that meet Centers for Disease Control and Prevention (CDC) testing criteria. Some patients may have little or no symptoms; others may have severe symptoms, including pneumonia or respiratory distress. Symptoms may appear between two to 14 days following exposure. Healthcare providers base the decision to order the test based on a patient's signs and symptoms compatible with COVID-19, local epidemiology, and if the patient has had close contact with another patient with a suspected or confirmed COVID-19 diagnosis or travel from an area with sustained virus transmission with 14 days of onset of symptoms. The diagnostic panel targets the nucleocapsid gene, including universal detection of SARS-like coronavirus and specific detection of the 2019-nCoV. COVID-19 infection can cause a range of symptoms including fever, cough, and shortness of breath. Report U0001 for testing performed with a CDC test. Report U0002 for testing performed with a non-CDC test. Additional high throughput machines, using a platform that employs automated processing of more than 200 specimens per day (i.e., Roche cobas 6800 System, Abbott m2000 System, etc.), which require more technician training and time intensive quality assurance, have been assigned to additional codes to accurately identify these tests. Report U0003 for high throughput testing for Severe Acute Respiratory Syndrome Coronavirus 2 (SARS-CoV-2) (Coronavirus disease [COVID-19]) by nucleic acid (DNA or RNA), amplified probe technique, or U0004 for high throughput testing for 2019-nCoV Coronavirus, SARS-CoV-2/2019-nCoV (COVID-19), any technique of making use of high throughput technologies as described by CMS-2020-01-R. Code U0003 should be used to identify tests that would otherwise be reported with CPT® code 87635 but are being performed with high throughput technology. Code U0004 should be used to identify tests that would otherwise be reported with U0002 but are being performed with high throughput technology. Report U0005 (in addition to U0003 or U0004) for testing by nucleic acid (DNR or RNA) using amplified probe technique and making use of high throughput technologies that is completed within two calendar days from the date of specimen collection; this applies to testing performed with CDC or non-CDC tests.

V

V2020-V2025

V2020 Frames, purchases

V2025 Deluxe frame

Frames are rigid or semi-rigid devices that bear lenses that are held in front of the eyes for vision correction or eye protection. Frames are made from many different materials in many different colors and shapes. The definition of deluxe is generally left to the manufacturer or the insurer.

V2100-V2102

V2100 Sphere, single vision, plano to plus or minus 4.00, per lens

V2101 Sphere, single vision, plus or minus 4.12 to plus or minus 7.00d, per lens

V2102 Sphere, single vision, plus or minus 7.12 to plus or minus 20.00d, per lens

A single vision lens provides one viewing surface in the lens that is concave on the back surface. This concave shape follows the shape of the eye and allows the back of the lens to stay at the same distance when the eye moves. It is used to treat refractive errors that cause the patient to have trouble seeing near or far distances. The sphere is the strength of the long or short sightedness and its value is in diopters. A plus sign (+) in front of the sphere reading indicates the amount of correction for near sight or reading whereas the minus sign (-) indicates the power of correction for far distance correction. If there is not a correction one way or another, it will be listed as plano, 0.00, or P.

V2103-V2114

V2103 Spherocylinder, single vision, plano to plus or minus 4.00d sphere, 0.12 to 2.00d cylinder, per lens

V2104 Spherocylinder, single vision, plano to plus or minus 4.00d sphere, 2.12 to 4.00d cylinder, per lens

V2105 Spherocylinder, single vision, plano to plus or minus 4.00d sphere, 4.25 to 6.00d cylinder, per lens

V2106 Spherocylinder, single vision, plano to plus or minus 4.00d sphere, over 6.00d cylinder, per lens

V2107 Spherocylinder, single vision, plus or minus 4.25 to plus or minus 7.00 sphere, 0.12 to 2.00d cylinder, per lens

V2108 Spherocylinder, single vision, plus or minus 4.25d to plus or minus 7.00d sphere, 2.12 to 4.00d cylinder, per lens

V2109 Spherocylinder, single vision, plus or minus 4.25 to plus or minus 7.00d sphere, 4.25 to 6.00d cylinder, per lens

V2110 Spherocylinder, single vision, plus or minus 4.25 to 7.00d sphere, over 6.00d cylinder, per lens

V2111 Spherocylinder, single vision, plus or minus 7.25 to plus or minus 12.00d sphere, 0.25 to 2.25d cylinder, per lens

V2112 Spherocylinder, single vision, plus or minus 7.25 to plus or minus 12.00d sphere, 2.25d to 4.00d cylinder, per lens

V2113 Spherocylinder, single vision, plus or minus 7.25 to plus or minus 12.00d sphere, 4.25 to 6.00d cylinder, per lens

V2114 Spherocylinder, single vision, sphere over plus or minus 12.00d, per lens

A single vision lens provides one viewing surface in the lens that is concave on the back surface. This concave shape follows the shape of the eye and allows the back of the lens to stay at the same distance when the eye moves. Spherocylinder single vision eyeglass lenses address the correction of one focal power such as nearsightedness or farsightedness, and astigmatism. The sphere is the strength of the long or short sightedness and its value is in diopters. A plus sign (+) in front of the sphere reading indicates the amount of correction for near sight or reading whereas the minus sign (-) indicates the power of correction for far distance correction. If there is not a correction one way or another, it will be listed as plano, 0.00, or P. The cylinder, also measured in + or -, is the measurement for astigmatism.

V2115

V2115 Lenticular (myodisc), per lens, single vision

Lenticular lenses are designed for very strong prescriptions generally requiring plus or minus 10.00d or higher. The specified prescription power is found in the center of the lens, and the edges are ground down to reduce the weight and thickness of the lens. A myodisc (myopic disk) is a lens with a steep concave curvature that is on the posterior surface of the carrier lens used with low-vision patients that have extreme myopia.

V2118

V2118 Aniseikonic lens, single vision

Aniseikonic lenses are for correction when patients report unequal visual images. This commonly occurs with a cataract, corneal surgical corrections, radial keratotomy, photoreactive keratectomy, laser surgeries, and scleral buckling. The football-shaped lenses have several aspects for correction, including base curve and lens thickness, refractive index, and the difference of magnification between lenses.

V2121

V2121 Lenticular lens, per lens, single

Lenticular lenses are designed for very strong prescriptions generally requiring plus or minus 10.00d or higher. The specified prescription power is found in the center of the lens, and the edges are ground down to reduce the weight and thickness of the lens.

V2199

V2199 Not otherwise classified, single vision lens

A single-vision lens is a piece of glass or plastic shaped to direct light onto the retina so as to produce a clear visual image. Single-vision lenses address either myopia (near-sightedness) or hyperopia (far-sightedness). This code represents a single-vision lens not otherwise classified or described by other HCPCS codes.

V2200-V2202

V2200 Sphere, bifocal, plano to plus or minus 4.00d, per lens

V2201 Sphere, bifocal, plus or minus 4.12 to plus or minus 7.00d, per lens

V2202 Sphere, bifocal, plus or minus 7.12 to plus or minus 20.00d, per lens

Bifocal vision eyeglass lenses address the correction of two focal powers for distance and work such as reading that requires a close-up focus. Lenses are made from glass or plastic to the specific level of correction required to improve vision. The lens provides two viewing surfaces in the lens, which is concave on the back surface. This concave shape follows the shape of the eye and allows the back of the lens to stay at the same distance when the eye moves. The sphere is the strength of the long- or short-sightedness and its value is in diopters. A plus sign (+) in front of the sphere reading indicates the amount of correction for near sight or reading whereas the minus sign (-) indicates the power of correction for far distance correction. No correction one way or another is listed as plano, 0.00, or P.

V2203-V2214

V2203 Spherocylinder, bifocal, plano to plus or minus 4.00d sphere, 0.12 to 2.00d cylinder, per lens

V2204 Spherocylinder, bifocal, plano to plus or minus 4.00d sphere, 2.12 to 4.00d cylinder, per lens

V2205 Spherocylinder, bifocal, plano to plus or minus 4.00d sphere, 4.25 to 6.00d cylinder, per lens

V2206 Spherocylinder, bifocal, plano to plus or minus 4.00d sphere, over 6.00d cylinder, per lens

V2207 Spherocylinder, bifocal, plus or minus 4.25 to plus or minus 7.00d sphere, 0.12 to 2.00d cylinder, per lens

V2208 Spherocylinder, bifocal, plus or minus 4.25 to plus or minus 7.00d sphere, 2.12 to 4.00d cylinder, per lens

V2209 Spherocylinder, bifocal, plus or minus 4.25 to plus or minus 7.00d sphere, 4.25 to 6.00d cylinder, per lens

V2210 Spherocylinder, bifocal, plus or minus 4.25 to plus or minus 7.00d sphere, over 6.00d cylinder, per lens

V2211 Spherocylinder, bifocal, plus or minus 7.25 to plus or minus 12.00d sphere, 0.25 to 2.25d cylinder, per lens

V2212 Spherocylinder, bifocal, plus or minus 7.25 to plus or minus 12.00d sphere, 2.25 to 4.00d cylinder, per lens

V2213 Spherocylinder, bifocal, plus or minus 7.25 to plus or minus 12.00d sphere, 4.25 to 6.00d cylinder, per lens

V2214 Spherocylinder, bifocal, sphere over plus or minus 12.00d, per lens

Bifocal vision eyeglass lenses address the correction of two focal powers for distance and work such as reading that requires a close up focus. Lenses are made from glass or plastic to the specific level of correction required to improve vision. The lens provides two viewing surfaces in the lens that is concave on the back surface. This concave shape follows the shape of the eye and allows the back of the lens to stay at the same distance when the eye moves. The sphere is the strength of the long or short sightedness and its value is in diopters. A plus sign (+) in front of the sphere reading indicates the amount of correction for near sight or reading whereas the minus sign (-) indicates the power of correction for far distance correction. If there is not a correction one way or another, it will be listed as plano, 0.00, or P. The cylinder, also measured in + or -, is the measurement for astigmatism.

V2215

V2215 Lenticular (myodisc), per lens, bifocal

Lenticular lenses are designed for very strong prescriptions generally requiring plus or minus 10.00d or higher. The specified prescription power is found in the center of the lens, and the edges are ground down to reduce the weight and thickness of the lens. A myodisc (myopic disk) is a lens with a steep concave curvature that is on the posterior surface of the carrier lens used with low-vision patients that have extreme myopia.

V2218

V2218 Aniseikonic, per lens, bifocal

Aniseikonic lenses are for correction when patients report unequal visual images. This commonly occurs with a cataract, corneal surgical corrections, radial keratotomy, photoreactive keratectomy, laser surgeries, and scleral buckling. The football-shaped lenses have several aspects for vision correction, including base curve and lens thickness, refractive index, and the difference of magnification between lenses. Bifocal lenses have two visibly identifiable zones of vision divided by a segment line of variable width. Bifocal lenses offer two fixed fields of focus (near/distant) for patients with higher levels of presbyopia.

V2219-V2220

V2219 Bifocal seg width over 28mm

V2220 Bifocal add over 3.25d

Bifocals are corrective lenses with distinct optical regions, each with different corrective features usually treating two different visual problems, e.g., myopia and astigmatism. Most bifocals are created by molding a reading segment into a specific shape, size, and optical power. The most common reading segment is the D-segment that is 28 mm wide.

V2221

V2221 Lenticular lens, per lens, bifocal

Lenticular lenses are designed for very strong prescriptions generally requiring plus or minus 10.00d or higher. The specified prescription power is found in the center of the lens, and the edges are ground down to reduce the weight and thickness of the lens.

V2299

V2299 Specialty bifocal (by report)

Bifocals are corrective lenses with distinct optical regions, each with different corrective features usually treating two different visual problems, e.g., myopia and astigmatism. This code should be reported when the lens is a specialty lens not described by other HCPCS codes. A report usually accompanies the code so as to explain the special qualities or conditions.

V2300-V2302

V2300 Sphere, trifocal, plano to plus or minus 4.00d, per lens

V2301 Sphere, trifocal, plus or minus 4.12 to plus or minus 7.00d per lens

V2302 Sphere, trifocal, plus or minus 7.12 to plus or minus 20.00, per lens

Trifocal lenses have three visibly identifiable zones of vision divided by two segment lines of variable widths. Trifocal lenses offer three fixed fields of focus (near/intermediate/distant) for patients with higher levels of presbyopia. The lens provides three viewing surfaces in the lens, which is concave on the back surface. This concave shape follows the shape of the eye and allows the back of the lens to stay at the same distance when the eye moves. It is used to treat refractive errors that cause the patient to have trouble seeing near or far distances. The sphere is the strength of the long- or short-sightedness, and its value is in diopters. A plus sign (+) in front of the sphere reading indicates the amount of correction for near sight or reading, whereas the minus sign (-) indicates the power of correction for far distance correction. No correction one way or another is listed as plano, 0.00, or P.

V2303-V2314

V2303 Spherocylinder, trifocal, plano to plus or minus 4.00d sphere, 0.12 to 2.00d cylinder, per lens

V2304 Spherocylinder, trifocal, plano to plus or minus 4.00d sphere, 2.25 to 4.00d cylinder, per lens

V2305 Spherocylinder, trifocal, plano to plus or minus 4.00d sphere, 4.25 to 6.00 cylinder, per lens

V2306 Spherocylinder, trifocal, plano to plus or minus 4.00d sphere, over 6.00d cylinder, per lens

V2307 Spherocylinder, trifocal, plus or minus 4.25 to plus or minus 7.00d sphere, 0.12 to 2.00d cylinder, per lens

V2308 Spherocylinder, trifocal, plus or minus 4.25 to plus or minus 7.00d sphere, 2.12 to 4.00d cylinder, per lens

V2309 Spherocylinder, trifocal, plus or minus 4.25 to plus or minus 7.00d sphere, 4.25 to 6.00d cylinder, per lens

V2310 Spherocylinder, trifocal, plus or minus 4.25 to plus or minus 7.00d sphere, over 6.00d cylinder, per lens

V2311 Spherocylinder, trifocal, plus or minus 7.25 to plus or minus 12.00d sphere, 0.25 to 2.25d cylinder, per lens

V2312 Spherocylinder, trifocal, plus or minus 7.25 to plus or minus 12.00d sphere, 2.25 to 4.00d cylinder, per lens

V2313 Spherocylinder, trifocal, plus or minus 7.25 to plus or minus 12.00d sphere, 4.25 to 6.00d cylinder, per lens

V2314 Spherocylinder, trifocal, sphere over plus or minus 12.00d, per lens

Spherocylinder trifocal vision eyeglass lenses address the correction of focal power such as nearsightedness or farsightedness, and/or astigmatism. Trifocal lenses have three visibly identifiable zones of vision divided by two segment lines of variable widths. Trifocal lenses offer three fixed fields of focus (near/intermediate/distant) for patients with higher levels of presbyopia. Lenses are made from glass or plastic to the specific level of correction required to improve vision. The lens provides three viewing surfaces in the lens, which is concave on the back surface. This concave shape follows the shape of the eye and allows the back of the lens to stay at the same distance when the eye moves. The sphere is the strength of the long- or short-sightedness, and its value is in diopters. A plus sign (+) in front of the sphere reading indicates the amount of correction for near sight or reading, whereas the minus sign (-) indicates the power of correction for far distance correction. No correction one way or another is listed as plano, 0.00, or P. The cylinder, also measured in + or -, is the measurement for astigmatism.

V2315

V2315 Lenticular, (myodisc), per lens, trifocal

Lenticular lenses are designed for very strong prescriptions generally requiring plus or minus 10.00d and higher. The specified prescription power is found in the center of the lens, and the edges are ground down to reduce the weight and thickness of the lens. Trifocal lenses have three visibly identifiable zones of vision divided by two segment lines of variable widths. Trifocal lenses offer three fixed fields of focus (near/intermediate/distant) for patients with higher levels of presbyopia.

V2318

V2318 Aniseikonic lens, trifocal

Aniseikonic lenses are for correction when patients report unequal visual images. This commonly occurs with a cataract, corneal surgical corrections, radial keratotomy, photoreactive keratectomy, laser surgeries, and scleral buckling. The football-shaped lenses have several aspects for vision correction, including base curve and lens thickness, refractive index, and the difference of magnification between lenses. Trifocal lenses have three visibly identifiable zones of vision divided by two segment lines of variable widths. Trifocal lenses offer three fixed fields of focus (near/intermediate/distant) for patients with higher levels of presbyopia.

V2319-V2320

V2319 Trifocal seg width over 28 mm

V2320 Trifocal add over 3.25d

Trifocals are corrective lenses with three distinct optical regions, each with different corrective features usually treating two different visual problems, e.g., myopia and astigmatism. Most trifocals are created by molding a reading segment into a specific shape, size, and optical power. The most common reading segment is the D-segment that is 28 mm wide.

V2321

V2321 Lenticular lens, per lens, trifocal

Lenticular lenses are designed for very strong prescriptions generally requiring plus or minus 10.00d or higher. The specified prescription power is found in the center of the lens, and the edges are ground down to reduce the weight and thickness of the lens.

V2399

V2399 Specialty trifocal (by report)

Trifocals are a corrective lens with three distinct optical regions, each with different corrective features usually treating two different visual problems (e.g., myopia and an astigmatism), with the middle region being a neutral or transition piece. Report this code when the lens is a specialty lens not described by other HCPCS Level II codes. A report usually accompanies the code so as to explain the special qualities or conditions.

V2410

V2410 Variable asphericity lens, single vision, full field, glass or plastic, per lens

Aspheric single-vision lenses address the correction of one focal power such as nearsightedness or farsightedness. They are also a higher quality premium lens, used for patients with slight astigmatism and at the early stages of development of presbyopia. Lenses are made from glass or plastic to the specific level of correction required to improve vision. Report this code for a full field, variable asphericity, single-vision lens.

V2430

V2430 Variable asphericity lens, bifocal, full field, glass or plastic, per lens

Aspherical bifocal vision lenses address the correction of two focal powers for distance and work, such as reading, which requires a close-up focus. They are also a higher quality premium lens used for patients with a slight astigmatism and at the early stages or development of presbyopia. Lenses are made from glass or plastic to the specific level of correction required to improve vision. Report this code for a full field, variable asphericity, bifocal lens.

V2499

V2499 Variable sphericity lens, other type

Light passing through a spherical lens is not all directed at a focal point. This imperfection is known as the lens sphericity. It is the degree of deviation from a sphere. The sphericity of a lens is intended to correct the misfocus of the eye. Spherical lenses are usually used for the main vision correction. The lens acts equally in all meridians.

V2500

V2500 Contact lens, PMMA, spherical, per lens

Polymethyl methacrylate (PMMA) spherical contact lenses are rigid lenses worn directly on the cornea to correct vision and have a spherical anterior (convex) surface and spherical posterior optical zone that approximates the curvature of the sclera. Spherical contact lenses have the same corrective power at each part of the lens, which allows the eye to focus and have clear vision. This code is reported per lens.

V2501

V2501 Contact lens, PMMA, toric or prism ballast, per lens

Polymethyl methacrylate (PMMA) toric or prism ballast contact lenses are rigid lenses worn directly on the cornea to correct vision and have a special curvature designed to correct astigmatism. Astigmatism is a visual defect in which the cornea is not perfectly round. Toric lenses are used when conventional soft or rigid lenses do not correct the defect. This code is reported per lens.

V2502

V2502 Contact lens PMMA, bifocal, per lens

Polymethyl methacrylate (PMMA) bifocal contact lenses are rigid lenses worn directly on the cornea to correct vision. Bifocal contact lenses address the correction of two focal powers for distance and work, such as reading, which requires a close up focus. This code is reported per lens.

V2503

V2503 Contact lens, PMMA, color vision deficiency, per lens

Polymethyl methacrylate (PMMA) contact lenses are rigid lenses worn directly on the cornea to correct vision. Color vision deficiency (a.k.a., color blindness) is a defect in the perception of color. This is usually the inability to distinguish between two or more colors such as red and green. This code represents a specially tinted contact lens that helps the person distinguish between the color for which he or she is deficient.

V2510

V2510 Contact lens, gas permeable, spherical, per lens

A spherical gas permeable contact lens is generally a rigid lens worn directly on the cornea to correct vision and has a spherical anterior (convex) surface and spherical posterior optical zone that approximates the curvature of the sclera. Spherical contact lenses have the same corrective power at each part of the lens, which allows the eye to focus and have clear vision. This lens also allows for oxygen exchange. It consists of materials, such as cellulose acetate butyrate, polyacrylate-silicone, or silicone elastomers, that typically do not attract water.

V2511

V2511 Contact lens, gas permeable, toric, prism ballast, per lens

A gas permeable toric contact lens is generally a rigid lens worn directly on the cornea to correct vision and has a special curvature designed to correct for astigmatism (a visual defect in which the cornea is not perfectly round). This lens also allows for oxygen exchange. It consists of materials, such as cellulose acetate butyrate, polyacrylate-silicone, or silicone elastomers, that typically do not attract water and are used when conventional soft or rigid lenses do not correct the defect.

V2512

V2512 Contact lens, gas permeable, bifocal, per lens

A gas permeable bifocal contact lens is generally a rigid lens worn directly on the cornea to correct vision and address the correction of two focal powers for distance and work, such as reading, which requires a close-up focus. This lens also allows for oxygen exchange. It consists of materials, such as cellulose acetate butyrate, polyacrylate-silicone, or silicone elastomers, that typically do not attract water.

V2513

V2513 Contact lens, gas permeable, extended wear, per lens

A gas permeable extended wear contact lens is generally a rigid lens intended to be worn directly on the cornea to correct vision and may be worn for an extended period of time (does not have to be taken out of the eye on a daily basis). This lens also allows for oxygen exchange. It consists of materials, such as cellulose acetate butyrate, polyacrylate-silicone, or silicone elastomers, that typically do not attract water.

V2520

V2520 Contact lens, hydrophilic, spherical, per lens

A spherical hydrophilic (soft) contact lens is worn directly on the cornea to correct vision and has a spherical anterior (convex) surface and spherical posterior optical zone that approximates the curvature of the sclera. Spherical contact lenses have the same corrective power at each part of the lens, which allows the eye to focus and have clear vision. This lens consists of a variety of polymer materials that absorb or attract a certain amount of water and is used when conventional soft or rigid lenses do not correct the defect.

V2521

V2521 Contact lens, hydrophilic, toric, or prism ballast, per lens

A hydrophilic toric contact lens is worn directly on the cornea to correct vision and has a special curvature designed to correct for astigmatism (a visual defect in which the cornea is not perfectly round). This lens consists of a variety of polymer materials that absorb or attract a certain amount of water and is used when conventional soft or rigid lenses do not correct the defect.

V2522

V2522 Contact lens, hydrophilic, bifocal, per lens

A hydrophilic bifocal contact lens is worn directly on the cornea to correct vision and address the correction of two focal powers for distance and work, such as reading, which requires a close up focus. This lens consists of a variety of polymer materials that absorb or attract a certain amount of water, making it more comfortable for the wearer.

V2523

V2523 Contact lens, hydrophilic, extended wear, per lens

A hydrophilic extended wear contact lens is worn directly on the cornea to correct vision and may be worn for an extended period of time (does not have to be taken out of the eye on a daily basis). This lens consists of a variety of polymer materials that absorb or attract a certain amount of water.

V2524

V2524 Contact lens, hydrophilic, spherical, photochromic additive, per lens

A spherical hydrophilic (soft) contact lens is worn directly on the cornea to correct vision and has a spherical anterior (convex) surface and spherical posterior optical zone that approximates the curvature of the sclera. Spherical contact lenses have the same corrective power at each part of the lens, which allows the eye to focus and have clear vision. This lens consists of a variety of polymer materials that absorb or attract a certain amount of water and is used when conventional soft or rigid lenses do not correct the defect. This code represents a contact lens with light-adaptive technology: a combination of benzotriazole UV absorbing monomer and the naphthopyran monomer (photochromic additive) for the attenuation of bright light to protect the cornea and eye from harmful UV radiation transmission.

V2525

V2525 Contact lens, hydrophilic, dual focus, per lens

A hydrophilic dual focus contact lens is worn directly on the cornea to correct vision and treats myopia pathological eye growth. The lens contains multiple rings of correction zones for refraction (vision correction) and the treatment zone provides a defocus signal to slow down the progression of myopia in children, ages 8 to 12 years, at the initiation of treatment. This lens consists of a variety of polymer materials that absorb or attract a certain amount of water, making it more comfortable to wear.

V2530-V2531

V2530 Contact lens, scleral, gas impermeable, per lens (for contact lens modification, see 92325)

V2531 Contact lens, scleral, gas permeable, per lens (for contact lens modification, see 92325)

A scleral contact lens is generally a rigid lens worn directly on the sclera that fits underneath the top and bottom eyelids. These lenses are used for patients who have problems wearing conventional lenses, patients with high refractive errors, or for patients with ocular surface disease. It consists of materials, such as cellulose acetate butyrate, polyacrylate-silicone, or silicone elastomers, that typically do not attract water and allow for oxygen exchange.

V2599

V2599 Contact lens, other type

A contact lens is a device that is worn on the cornea to correct vision problems by helping to refocus light onto the retina. This code represents a contact lens that is not detailed in one of the other HCPCS Level II codes.

V2600

V2600 Hand held low vision aids and other nonspectacle mounted aids

A low vision aid or magnifier is a type of magnifying lens used by patients who have impaired vision. This magnifier is handheld or may be used with another piece of equipment, but is not mounted onto glasses.

V2610

V2610 Single lens spectacle mounted low vision aids

A low vision aid or magnifier is a type of magnifying lens used by patients who have impaired vision. This magnifying aid is used on a single lens and mounted onto glasses.

V2615

V2615 Telescopic and other compound lens system, including distance vision telescopic, near vision telescopes and compound microscopic lens system

Telescopic and other compound lens systems, including distance vision telescopic, near vision telescopes, and compound microscopic lens systems, are devices and systems used to improve the vision of a person with low vision. Low vision is defined as reduced vision that is not corrected by spectacles or contact lens. Low vision can vary from moderate (20/70) to near total blindness (more than 20/1,000). Telescopic lens are usually limited by the diameter of the objective lens and the magnification.

V2623

V2623 Prosthetic eye, plastic, custom

An ocular prosthesis is a device that fits over an orbital implant and under the eyelids that produces the appearance of a normal human eye. It is created for a patient with absence or shrinkage of an eye due to a birth defect, trauma, or surgical removal. Eye prostheses assist in maintaining the internal orbital eye structures by filling in the void created by the missing natural eye. A byproduct of the prosthesis allows for a cosmetic enhancement by allowing the patient to appear to have two eyes. A prosthetic eye may be made out of glass, acrylic, silicone, hydroxyapatite, ceramic, or polyethylene.

V2624-V2626

V2624 Polishing/resurfacing of ocular prosthesis

V2625 Enlargement of ocular prosthesis

V2626 Reduction of ocular prosthesis

An ocular prosthesis is a device that fits over an orbital implant and under the eyelids that produces the appearance of a normal human eye. It is created for a patient with absence or shrinkage of an eye due to a birth defect, trauma, or surgical removal. Eye prostheses assist in maintaining the internal orbital eye structures by filling in the void created by the missing natural eye. A byproduct of the prosthesis allows for a cosmetic enhancement by allowing the patient to appear to have two eyes. A prosthetic eye may be made out of glass, acrylic, silicone, hydroxyapatite, ceramic, or polyethylene. These codes represent work performed on the ocular prosthesis.

V2627

V2627 Scleral cover shell

A scleral cover shell is a device made out of glass or plastic and placed over the cornea and sclera of a damaged eye to give the eye a more natural appearance. It is intended to be worn for a short period of time for cosmetic or reconstructive reasons. It is typically not implanted in the eye.

V2628

V2628 Fabrication and fitting of ocular conformer

An ocular conformer is a temporary eye prosthesis inserted at the completion of the eye surgery and worn for four to eight weeks until a permanent prosthesis is available. This code represents the fabrication and fitting of the ocular conformer.

V2629

V2629 Prosthetic eye, other type

An ocular prosthesis is a device that fits over an orbital implant and under the eyelids that produces the appearance of a normal human eye. It is created for a patient with absence or shrinkage of an eye due to a birth defect, trauma, or surgical removal. Eye prostheses assist in maintaining the internal orbital eye structures by filling in the void created by the missing natural eye. A byproduct of the prosthesis allows for a cosmetic enhancement by allowing the patient to appear to have two eyes. A prosthetic eye may be made out of glass, acrylic, silicone, hydroxyapatite, ceramic, or polyethylene. This code represents a prosthetic eye that is not described by other HCPCS Level II codes.

V2630-V2632

V2630 Anterior chamber intraocular lens

V2631 Iris supported intraocular lens

V2632 Posterior chamber intraocular lens

An intraocular lens (IOL) is an implanted lens used as a replacement for a clouded lens removed in cataract surgery or as a correction for a refraction problem. When inserted to correct refractive errors, the natural lens is usually not removed. Most IOLs are plastic and contain side struts to hold the lens in place. The anterior chamber is the portion of the eye between the cornea and the iris and is filled with aqueous humor. The iris, along with the choroid and ciliary body, is the midportion of the eye. The posterior chamber is the area between the iris and the rear eye walls. The posterior chamber is filled with the vitreous body. Anterior chamber IOLs can negatively impact the endothelial lining creating corneal complications. IOLs supported by the iris are attached by the struts to the midperipheral iris area. It is believed that iris supported IOLs do not impact the corneal endothelium as much as other types. Posterior chamber IOLs are placed in front of, but do not contact, the natural crystalline lens. Posterior chamber IOLs can cause cataract and pigment dispersion.

V2700

V2700 Balance lens, per lens

Corrective lenses of high powers can become very heavy and thick. A balance lens is similar to another corrective lens (single vision or lined bifocal) that is sized and shaped to appear similar to the other corrective lens. Depending on the patient and the lens, balance lenses may also be used to provide a similar weight as the corrective lens.

V2702

V2702 Deluxe lens feature

This code represents a deluxe lens feature that is not adequately described by other HCPCS Level II codes.

V2710

V2710 Slab off prism, glass or plastic, per lens

A slab off prism is a special lens, with the prismatic effect in the lower half of the lens, used to balance a patient's near vision. Patients whose left and right eyes have a significant difference in power could benefit from the use of a slab-off prism. Two lenses with significant power differences produce different prismatic effects as the eyes move from the distance part of the lens to the reading zone. The prism imbalance can be measured when in the reading zone. A compensating prism can then be incorporated into one of the lenses.

V2715

V2715 Prism, per lens

In optometry, a prism is one device used to correct vision problems. Shifting a corrective lens off the axis can make images appear to be displaced in the same way that a prism displaces images. Prisms are used to correct double vision and positive and negative accommodation problems.

V2718

V2718 Press-on lens, Fresnel prism, per lens

A press-on lens, Fresnel prism, is a prism used to correct vision problems and expand the visual field. Shifting a corrective lens off the axis can make images appear to be displaced in the same way that a prism displaces images. Prisms are used to bend the light so that it produces a clear image to the viewer. Fresnel replaced a large heavy prism lens with small segments. His work was originally developed for lighthouses, but it was adapted for optometry. Press-on lenses are thin flexible pieces of vinyl applied to the back of a corrective lens.

V2730

V2730 Special base curve, glass or plastic, per lens

The base curve in optometry is the measure of the general shape of the lens. On a spectacle lens, it is the flatter curvature of the front surface and on a contact lens, it is the curvature of the back surface. The base curve is the radius of the sphere of the back of the lens that the prescription describes. This code represents a lens that has a special base curve.

V2744

V2744 Tint, photochromatic, per lens

Photochromatic tinted lenses are those in which the degree of tint changes in response to changes in ambient light. Report this code for photochromatic tint per lens.

V2745

V2745 Addition to lens; tint, any color, solid, gradient or equal, excludes photochromatic, any lens material, per lens

Tinted lenses are made by putting coatings on the lens material to reduce the amount of light entering the eye. Report this code for the addition of tint to a lens, any color, solid, gradient or equal, excluding photochromatic.

V2750

V2750 Antireflective coating, per lens

Antireflective coating reduces glare on the surface of a lens and also reduces the reflected glare of headlights to improve nighttime driving. Report this code for antireflective coating, per lens.

V2755

V2755 U-V lens, per lens

UV lenses protect eyes from the potentially harmful ultraviolet rays generated from the sun or other light sources by blocking them from penetrating the lens material and reaching the eye. Report this code per lens.

V2756

V2756 Eye glass case

This code reports an eyeglass case. Eyeglass cases hold and protect glasses when they are not being worn.

V2760

V2760 Scratch resistant coating, per lens

Scratch resistant coating is a protective coating applied directly to the lens that reduces the potential for normal scratching or scraping of the lens material, reducing potential lens distortion. Report this code per lens.

V2761

V2761 Mirror coating, any type, solid, gradient or equal, any lens material, per lens

A mirror coating is a highly reflective coating of any color that prevents anyone looking at the lens from seeing anything other than the color of the mirrored lens. Mirror coatings are mainly cosmetic. The person wearing the lens perceives no difference in vision. The coatings are usually applied to sunglasses, but may be applied to any corrective lens. The density of the coating varies with solid mirrors reflecting back more light than other variations. This code represents mirror coating, any gradient or solid, any type, any lens material, per lens.

V2762

V2762 Polarization, any lens material, per lens

Light reflected from a flat surface such as a road or smooth water usually travels in a more horizontal pattern than normal light. Light that travels in one direction more than another is said to be polarized. The polarized light creates a glare that does not allow clear images. Polarized lenses have laminated surfaces that allow only vertically-polarized light to enter, eliminating the glare created by the horizontally-polarized light. The lenses do not prevent glare when the wearer tilts his or her head past 45 degrees. Polarized lenses also reduce the amount of light entering the eye and cannot be used with regular corrective eyeglasses.

V2770

V2770 Occluder lens, per lens

An occluder lens typically is a soft lens that can be worn for up to seven days (extended wear) and is blackened out, blocking vision in the eye wearing it. This type of prosthetic lens in used for treating patients, generally children, with amblyopia, or "lazy eye." The occluder lens forces the development of the amblyopic eye by blocking out all vision in the other eye. This type of lens may also be used in aphakic infants, where patch therapy has failed. This code is reported per lens.

V2780

V2780 Oversize lens, per lens

Oversize lenses are eyeglass lenses that are physically larger than normal lenses. Oversize lenses are sometimes used to create sunglasses that can slip over regular corrective glasses. Most of the time oversize lenses are requested for cosmetic purposes.

V2781

V2781 Progressive lens, per lens

No-line multifocal lenses that provide the needed correction for multiple focal lengths, but do not have a visible seam or line in the lenses are called progressive lenses. Report this code per progressive lens.

V2782-V2783

V2782 Lens, index 1.54 to 1.65 plastic or 1.60 to 1.79 glass, excludes polycarbonate, per lens

V2783 Lens, index greater than or equal to 1.66 plastic or greater than or equal to 1.80 glass, excludes polycarbonate, per lens

The light bending ability of eyeglass lenses is determined by the index of refraction of the lens material. The refractive index is the ratio of the speed of light as it travels through air to the speed of light as it passes through the lenses material. The speed of light is reduced by the amount of its refraction. Lenses that bend light more efficiently have a higher index of refraction than those that bend light less efficiently. Lenses with higher index are thinner and lighter than those lenses of the same power that are made with materials of a lower index. Conventional plastic lenses have a refractive index of approximately 1.50 and glass has an index of 1.52. Any lens material with indexes higher than these are considered high index. High index plastic usually has an index of 1.53 to 1.74. A plastic lens with an index of 1.70 or higher is at least 50 percent thinner than a conventional lens.

V2784

V2784 Lens, polycarbonate or equal, any index, per lens

Polycarbonate is a thin, light material used to create lenses. It has a high impact resistance, which along with its light weight, makes it preferable over other resins. Polycarbonate has a refractive index of 1.59. This lens material blocks both UVA and UVB rays.

V2785

V2785 Processing, preserving and transporting corneal tissue

The cornea is the transparent lens in the front of the eye that covers the iris, the pupil, and the anterior chamber. When the cornea is damaged or diseased it can be replaced, in whole or in part, by a donated cornea from a cadaver. This code reports the cost of processing, preserving, and transporting the corneal tissue.

V2786

V2786 Specialty occupational multifocal lens, per lens

Multifocal lenses are corrective lenses that contain one or more lens powers. Bifocals have two powers, trifocals have three, and progressive lenses have many that gradually change from the top of the lens to the bottom. Occupational multifocal lenses are designed for performing a particular job or hobby and are not intended for general use. For example, there are multifocal lenses designed for car mechanics, as well as golfers. Report this code for specialty occupational multifocal lenses, per lens.

V2787-V2788

V2787 Astigmatism correcting function of intraocular lens

V2788 Presbyopia correcting function of intraocular lens

An intraocular lens (IOL) is an implanted lens used as a replacement for a clouded lens removed in cataract surgery or as a correction for a refraction problem. When inserted to correct refractive errors, the natural lens is usually not removed. Most IOLs are plastic and contain side struts to hold the lens in place. Most traditional IOLs are monofocal, providing vision at only one distance—near, intermediate, or far. Patients will most likely have to have corrective lenses for other distances. Toric lenses are used to correct astigmatisms. Presbyopia is a condition where the eye progressively loses the ability to focus on near objects. It is usually part of the aging process. Both the astigmatism and the presbyopia correcting functions of an intraocular lens are not usually covered by insurance as they are considered premium additions.

V2790

V2790 Amniotic membrane for surgical reconstruction, per procedure

Severe ocular surface diseases, such as Stevens-Johnson syndrome or ocular cicatricial pemphigoid, and injuries damage the corneal epithelial limbus cells. This damage allows the cornea to be enveloped with conjunctival tissue causing scarring and vascularization. A graft is necessary to surgically reconstruct these damaged eyes. An autograft from the patient's undamaged eye may be used or an allograft from the donor's eye may be used. Healthy limbus cells may also be cultivated on an amniotic membrane and transplanted into a severely damaged eye. The membrane provides support and is a carrier for the cultivated cells.

V2797-V2799

V2797 Vision supply, accessory and/or service component of another HCPCS vision code

V2799 Vision item or service, miscellaneous

Report V2797 when the vision supply, accessory, and/or service provided is a component of another HCPCS Level II vision code. This is not to be used to unbundle and report each component separately, but should be used when it is necessary to replace and report only one component of a complex HCPCS Level II code. Report V2799 when the vision service provided is not adequately described by other HCPCS Level II codes.

V5008

V5008 Hearing screening

A hearing screening is a unilateral or bilateral test consisting of the patient's case history, a visual inspection of the ear, pure tone screening within a range of 1000-4000 Hz, speech audiometry, and a self-assessed judgment of hearing difficulty. The screening is conducted by a certified audiologist, speech-language pathologist, or other personnel under the supervision of an audiologist.

V5010-V5020

V5010 Assessment for hearing aid

V5011 Fitting/orientation/checking of hearing aid

V5014 Repair/modification of a hearing aid

V5020 Conformity evaluation

During an assessment for a hearing aid, an audiologist reviews the results of the initial hearing screening with the patient, discusses the type and degree of hearing loss including the configuration of the loss (whether unilateral or bilateral), the options available based on the information gathered, and costs. The audiologist also obtains audiometric measurements and an impression of the ear canal. The hearing aid is fitted during an orientation in which the audiologist explains how to operate the hearing aid. At this fitting, internal controls of the hearing aid are set or programmed. The patient is scheduled for a conformity evaluation to confirm that the hearing aid is meeting the needs of the patient.

V5030-V5040

V5030 Hearing aid, monaural, body worn, air conduction

V5040 Hearing aid, monaural, body worn, bone conduction

A body worn monaural (one ear) air conduction hearing aid is specifically designed with bigger controls for patients who have less dexterity and have a problem with feedback. It consists of a small box that is clipped to clothing or slips inside a pocket. This connects to a lead to an earphone and attaches to the ear-mold. The bone conduction hearing aid is designed for patients who have an abnormality of the ear canal. Due to drainage, a narrow canal, or no canal at all, the patient is precluded from using an air conduction device. The bone conductor is held onto the mastoid bone by an implanted screw or by using a headband. It works by transmitting vibrations through the skull to the inner ear.

V5050-V5060

V5050 Hearing aid, monaural, in the ear

V5060 Hearing aid, monaural, behind the ear

There are two types of in the ear (ITE) monaural hearing aids available. The full shell aid is for mild to severe hearing loss and is the largest and least expensive available. It covers the entire ear opening and is the most versatile of all the hearing aids. The half-shell/conch aid is for mild to moderately severe hearing loss and is the most popular model. Smaller than the full shell, it covers only the bowl portion of the ear. The behind the ear (BTE) model is connected to the ear by an ear-mold and is used mostly by patients with severe hearing loss, although it can be used for any and all forms of hearing loss. This type is more durable and less flexible than the ITE model.

V5070

V5070 Glasses, air conduction

An air conduction hearing system amplifies sound and directs it into the auditory canal with a thin tube. The device is small and discrete and is worn on the eyeglass frame. The use of a thin tube to direct the amplified sound allows natural ambient sound to also reach the ear. The eyeglass frame usually holds corrective lenses.

V5080

V5080 Glasses, bone conduction

A bone conduction hearing system transmits sound through mechanical vibrations to the inner ear. The device is small and discrete and is worn on the eyeglass frame. The eyeglass frame usually holds corrective lenses.

V5090

V5090 Dispensing fee, unspecified hearing aid

This code reports the dispensing fee charged by the supplier for the dispensing of a hearing aid that is unspecified or not described by other HCPCS Level II codes.

V5095

V5095 Semi-implantable middle ear hearing prosthesis

A semi-implantable middle ear hearing prosthesis is an alternative to an external acoustic hearing aid for patients with moderate to severe sensorineural hearing loss. The device consists of three components: a magnetic component, a receiver, and a sound processor. The magnetic component is implanted onto the ossicles of the middle ear. The sound processor receives and amplifies sound vibrations and transforms sound pressure into electrical signals, which are transmitted to the receiver. The receiver changes the electrical signals into electromagnetic energy and creates an alternating electromagnetic field with the magnetic component. In turn this electromagnetic field creates varying forces on the implant that cause the bones of the middle ear to vibrate, similar to normal hearing.

V5100-V5110

V5100 Hearing aid, bilateral, body worn

V5110 Dispensing fee, bilateral

A hearing aid is a device that amplifies, modulates, or conducts sound. There are a number of types and sizes with different components. A body worn hearing aid consists of an ear piece connected by a cord to a case containing a microphone, amplifier, battery, and controls that are worn in a pocket or on a belt. The device is usually the size of a deck of cards.

V5120-V5160

V5120 Binaural, body

V5130 Binaural, in the ear

V5140 Binaural, behind the ear

V5150 Binaural, glasses

V5160 Dispensing fee, binaural

Binaural hearing aids are for both ears and are used concurrently to treat bilateral hearing loss. Advantages of wearing two hearing aids include a better understanding of speech and a better ability to localize speech. Hearing aids worn on the body are usually placed in a pocket or on a belt. Binaural hearing aids may also be worn in the ear, behind the ear, or may be incorporated into eyeglass frames.

V5171-V5221

V5171 Hearing aid, contralateral routing device, monaural, in the ear (ITE)

V5172 Hearing aid, contralateral routing device, monaural, in the canal (ITC)

V5181 Hearing aid, contralateral routing device, monaural, behind the ear (BTE)

V5190 Hearing aid, contralateral routing, monaural, glasses

V5200 Dispensing fee, contralateral, monaural

V5211 Hearing aid, contralateral routing system, binaural, ITE/ITE

V5212 Hearing aid, contralateral routing system, binaural, ITE/ITC

V5213 Hearing aid, contralateral routing system, binaural, ITE/BTE

V5214 Hearing aid, contralateral routing system, binaural, ITC/ITC

V5215 Hearing aid, contralateral routing system, binaural, ITC/BTE

V5221 Hearing aid, contralateral routing system, binaural, BTE/BTE

Contralateral routing of sound (CROS) hearing aids are used for patients with one deaf ear and one ear with normal or near normal hearing. The device placed in the deaf ear is a microphone and transmitter. The microphone picks up sound and transmits to the hearing ear. The transmission can be accomplished through a cord joining both hearing aids or may be wireless. The device placed in the normal ear consists of a receiver and an amplifier. Amplified sound from the deaf ear is directed into the ear canal. Most CROS ear molds are of an open design to allow natural sound into the normal ear.

V5230-V5240

V5230 Hearing aid, contralateral routing system, binaural, glasses

V5240 Dispensing fee, contralateral routing system, binaural

Bilateral routing of sound (BICROS) is similar to a CROS hearing aid, but is used for patients with one deaf ear and one ear that is hard of hearing. The device placed in the deaf ear is a microphone and transmitter. The microphone picks up sound and transmits it to the hearing ear. The transmission can be accomplished through a cord joining both hearing aids or may be wireless. The device placed in the hearing ear consists of a receiver and an amplifier coupled with a regular hearing aid. Signals from both ears are combined and directed into the hearing ear. BICROS ear molds are normally tightly fitted into the ear so as to prevent feedback.

V5241

V5241 Dispensing fee, monaural hearing aid, any type

Monaural hearing aids direct amplified sound to only one ear through a single signal path. Suppliers report this code for the dispensing fee of a monaural hearing aid, any type.

V5242-V5243

V5242 Hearing aid, analog, monaural, CIC (completely in the ear canal)

V5243 Hearing aid, analog, monaural, ITC (in the canal)

Sound is basically a fluctuation of air pressure and a sound wave is a series of continuous variations in time and amplitude on air pressure. When the fluctuations strike the eardrum, the vibrations are transmitted to the inner ear and ultimately the brain and are perceived as sound. When the fluctuations strike a microphone, they induce corresponding fluctuations or vibrations in the voltage or current of the microphone. These fluctuations or vibrations in the voltage or current are analogs of the sound. Analog hearing aids have a volume control that is adjusted by the patient. They are battery operated and work by converting sound waves to an electronic signal. When the volume is adjusted, all of the sounds are uniformly adjusted.

V5244-V5247

V5244 Hearing aid, digitally programmable analog, monaural, CIC

V5245 Hearing aid, digitally programmable, analog, monaural, ITC

V5246 Hearing aid, digitally programmable analog, monaural, ITE (in the ear)

V5247 Hearing aid, digitally programmable analog, monaural, BTE (behind the ear)

Digitally programmable analog hearing aids are battery operated and work by making sound waves larger and breaking them into distinct units. This digital signal is free from distortion and treats soft sounds differently than loud sounds, thus allowing for more clarity of sound, rather than only allowing more volume. The sound waves are converted from an electronic signal and then passed through an A/D converter. These codes all represent digitally programmable analog monaural hearing aids.

V5248-V5249

V5248 Hearing aid, analog, binaural, CIC

V5249 Hearing aid, analog, binaural, ITC

Sound is basically a fluctuation of air pressure and a sound wave is a series of continuous variations in time and amplitude on air pressure. When the fluctuations strike the eardrum, the vibrations are transmitted to the inner ear and ultimately the brain and are perceived as sound. When the fluctuations strike a microphone, they induce corresponding fluctuations or vibrations in the voltage or current of the microphone. These fluctuations or vibrations in the voltage or current are analogs of the sound. Analog hearing aids have a volume control that is adjusted by the patient. They are battery operated and work by converting sound waves to an electronic signal. When the volume is adjusted, all of the sounds are uniformly adjusted.

V5250-V5253

V5250 Hearing aid, digitally programmable analog, binaural, CIC

V5251 Hearing aid, digitally programmable analog, binaural, ITC

V5252 Hearing aid, digitally programmable, binaural, ITE

V5253 Hearing aid, digitally programmable, binaural, BTE

Digitally programmable analog hearing aids are battery operated and work by making sound waves larger and breaking them into distinct units. This digital signal is free from distortion and treats soft sounds differently than loud sounds, thus allowing for more clarity of sound, rather than only allowing more volume. The sound waves are converted from an electronic signal and then passed through an A/D converter. These codes all represent digitally programmable analog monaural hearing aids.

V5254-V5261

V5254 Hearing aid, digital, monaural, CIC

V5255 Hearing aid, digital, monaural, ITC

V5256 Hearing aid, digital, monaural, ITE

V5257 Hearing aid, digital, monaural, BTE

V5258 Hearing aid, digital, binaural, CIC

V5259 Hearing aid, digital, binaural, ITC

V5260 Hearing aid, digital, binaural, ITE

V5261 Hearing aid, digital, binaural, BTE

Sound is basically a fluctuation of air pressure and a sound wave is a series of continuous variations in time and amplitude on air pressure. When the fluctuations strike the eardrum, the vibrations are transmitted to the inner ear and ultimately the brain and are perceived as sound. When the fluctuations strike a microphone, they induce corresponding fluctuations or vibrations in the voltage or current of the microphone. These fluctuations or vibrations in the voltage or current are analogs of the sound. Digital hearing aids convert the analog sound into a sequence of numbers that can be translated back into the analog sound. In its digital state, sound can be augmented to cancel feedback, reduce noise, and enhance speech. Digital hearing aids all contain a digital signal processing unit that translates the analog signals into and out of a digital format.

V5262-V5263

V5262 Hearing aid, disposable, any type, monaural

V5263 Hearing aid, disposable, any type, binaural

Disposable hearing aids are made of a soft material that is intended to last the user approximately 40 days. A disposable hearing aid has a mushroom-shaped tip that fits in the ear canal and can be fitted to most adults.

V5264-V5265

V5264 Ear mold/insert, not disposable, any type

V5265 Ear mold/insert, disposable, any type

An earmold is a device composed of plastic or another soft material that is inserted into the ear for sound conduction, ear protection, or sound reduction. Ear molds are shaped to fit precisely into an individual ear. They can be full, which completely fills the ear canal, providing sound reduction, and protection; or partial, which allows in other sound. Ear molds may contain a BTE hearing aid, components of other types of hearing aids, such as a receiver or processor, or may simply be used to protect the ear by blocking loud noises.

V

V5266

V5266 Battery for use in hearing device

Hearing devices require select batteries to provide power to the listening device. Batteries are available in different brands, sizes, and quantity packs depending on the requirements of the device. This code reports a battery for use in a hearing device.

V5267

V5267 Hearing aid or assistive listening device/supplies/accessories, not otherwise specified

Report this code for hearing aid supplies or accessories that are not adequately described by other HCPCS Level II codes.

V5268

V5268 Assistive listening device, telephone amplifier, any type

Telephone assistive listening devices are used to amplify sound for the hearing impaired. Some of the telephone assistive listening devices available are portable phones, in-line amplifiers, ring signalers, and super phone ringers. This code is reported for any type of telephone amplifier assistive listening device for the telephone.

V5269

V5269 Assistive listening device, alerting, any type

There are two types of alerting assistive listening devices: visual and vibration. The visual alert includes a flashing light, or strobe light, to assist the hearing impaired user in becoming aware of an event such as ringing smoke alarms, doorbells, baby monitors, or alarm clocks. Some patients find that vibrating devices such as pillow shakers or wrist shakers are more effective. This code is reported for an alerting assistive listening device of either type.

V5270-V5271

V5270 Assistive listening device, television amplifier, any type

V5271 Assistive listening device, television caption decoder

An assistive listening device used with a television amplifies the audio signal from the television and is generally transmitted through infrared to a headset. Closed captioning decoders are also available for older models of televisions in which a decoder is not built into the system.

V5272

V5272 Assistive listening device, TDD

A TDD is a telecommunication device for the deaf. These include text telephones and teletype machines. These assistive listening devices allow a person with hearing impairment to use the telephone. The device is connected to a small keyboard that allows the user to type the message to be sent. If both the caller and receiver have TDDs, a printed message is read on a screen. However, if the receiver does not have a TDD, the messages are relayed through an operator.

V5273

V5273 Assistive listening device, for use with cochlear implant

An assistive listening device for use with a cochlear implant is designed to amplify the voice in a setting such as a classroom or boardroom directly to the person with the implant without amplifying background noise. These systems include an infrared system with a jack.

V5274

V5274 Assistive listening device, not otherwise specified

Assistive listening devices improve hearing in a specific situation for people with hearing loss. The device emphasizes the one signal that the person is interested in hearing more clearly. This code represents assistive listening devices that are not adequately described by other HCPCS Level II codes.

V5275

V5275 Ear impression, each

Impressions are made of the ear to obtain a hearing device specifically for the individual. The ear canal is visualized through an otoscope to check for wax buildup, anomalies, and to check the tympanic membrane. A plug made of soft cotton is inserted just beyond the canal to provide a "wall" for the mold and to ease the removal of debris. The impression material is mixed according to the manufacturer's specifications and loaded into a syringe. The tip of the syringe is placed in the canal and then emptied to fill the ear canal, the pinna, concha, and helix. After the material has set for the time indicated, the impression and cotton wall are removed. The audiologist visualizes the canal with the otoscope to be certain all